Lovell and Winter's
Pediatric
Orthopaedics

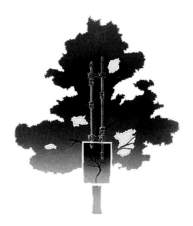

Lovell and Winter's
Pediatric
Orthopaedics

EDITED BY

Raymond T. Morrissy, MD
Medical Director and Chief of Orthopaedics
Scottish Rite Children's Medical Center
Clinical Professor of Orthopaedics
Emory University School of Medicine
Atlanta, Georgia

Stuart L. Weinstein, MD
Ignacio V. Ponseti Professor of Orthopaedic Surgery
University of Iowa College of Medicine
Iowa City, Iowa

With 31 Contributors

Volume **II**
Fourth Edition

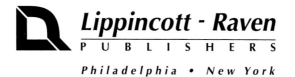

Lippincott - Raven
PUBLISHERS
Philadelphia • New York

Acquisitions Editor: James D. Ryan
Developmental Editor: Delois Patterson
Project Editor: Molly E. Dickmeyer
Production Manager: Caren Erlichman
Production Coordinator: David Yurkovich
Designer: Doug Smock
Compositor: Bi-Comp
Printer: Quebecor/Kingsport

Library of Congress Cataloging-in-Publication Data

Pediatric orthopaedics.
    Lovell and Winter's pediatric orthopaedics / edited by Raymond T.
Morrissy and Stuart L. Weinstein. — 4th ed.
      p.   cm.
    Includes bibliographical references and index.
    ISBN 0-397-51397-6 (set : alk. paper). — ISBN 0-397-51598-7 (vol.
1 : alk. paper). — ISBN 0-397-51599-5 (vol. 2 : alk. paper)
    1. Pediatric orthopedics. I. Lovell, Wood. W. 1915– .
II. Winter, Robert B. 1932–   . III. Morrissy, Raymond T.
IV. Weinstein, Stuart L.V.
    [DNLM: 1. Orthopedics—in infancy & childhood. WS 270 L911 1996]
RD732.3.C48P43 1996
617.3′0083—dc20
DNLM/DLC
for Library of Congress   95-31125
                                            CIP

9   8   7   6   5   4   3   2   1

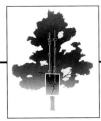

Contributors

Behrooz A. Akbarnia, M.D.
Associate Clinical Professor
Department of Orthopaedic
Surgery
University of California, San Diego,
School of Medicine
San Diego, California;
Adjunct Professor of Orthopaedic
Surgery
St. Louis University School of
Medicine
St. Louis, Missouri

George S. Bassett, M.D.
Associate Professor of
Orthopaedics
University of Southern California
School of Medicine;
Children's Hospital of Los Angeles
Los Angeles, California

Loui G. Bayne, M.D.
Director of Hand Clinic
Scottish Rite Children's Medical
Center;
Clinical Professor of Orthopaedics
Emory University School of
Medicine
Atlanta, Georgia

Michael T. Busch, M.D.
Scottish Rite Children's Medical
Center
Atlanta, Georgia

William G. Cole, M.B.B.S., M.Sc., Ph.D.
Head, Division of Orthopaedic
Surgery
The Hospital for Sick Children;
Professor of Genetics and
Molecular Medicine
University of Toronto
Toronto, Ontario
Canada

Bronier L. Costas, M.D.
Assistant Director of Hand Clinic
Scottish Rite Children's Medical
Center;
Clinical Assistant Professor of
Orthopaedics
Emory University School of
Medicine
Atlanta, Georgia

Donald R. Cummings, C.P.
Director, Prosthetics
Scottish Rite Hospital for Children;
Adjunct Faculty
Prosthetic/Orthotics Program
University of Texas Southwestern
Medical School at Dallas
Dallas, Texas

Jon R. Davids, M.D.
Director, Motion Analysis
Laboratory
Shriners Hospital
Greenville, South Carolina

Dennis P. Devito, M.D.
Scottish Rite Children's Medical
Center
Atlanta, Georgia

James G. Gamble, M.D., Ph.D.
Professor of Orthopaedic Surgery
Stanford University School of
Medicine;
Lucile-Salter Packard Children's
Hospital at Stanford
Stanford, California

Michael J. Goldberg, M.D.
Professor and Chairman
Department of Orthopaedics
Tufts University School of
Medicine and New England
Medical Center
Boston, Massachusetts

Walter B. Greene, M.D.
Professor of Orthopaedic Surgery
and Pediatrics
University of North Carolina
School of Medicine
Chapel Hill, North Carolina

Richard H. Gross, M.D.
Professor of Orthopaedic Surgery
and Pediatrics
Medical University of South
Carolina
Charleston, South Carolina

H. Theodore Harcke, M.D.
Professor of Radiology and
Pediatrics
Jefferson Medical College
Philadelphia, Pennsylvania;
Chairman, Department of Medical
Imaging
Alfred I. duPont Institute
Wilmington, Delaware

John A. Herring, M.D.
Chief of Staff
Scottish Rite Hospital for Children;
Professor of Orthopaedic Surgery
University of Texas Southwestern
Medical Center
Dallas, Texas

Douglas K. Kehl, M.D.
Department of Orthopaedic
Surgery
Scottish Rite Children's Medical
Center;
Associate Clinical Professor of
Orthopaedic Surgery
Emory University School of
Medicine
Atlanta, Georgia

Richard E. Lindseth, M.D.
Professor of Orthopaedic Surgery
Indiana University School of
Medicine
Indianapolis, Indiana

v

Randall T. Loder, M.D.
Assistant Professor of Surgery
Section of Orthopaedics
University of Michigan School of
Medicine
Ann Arbor, Michigan

John E. Lonstein, M.D.
Clinical Associate Professor
Department of Orthopaedic
Surgery
University of Minnesota Medical
School;
Staff, Minnesota Spine Center
Gillette Children's Hospital
St. Paul, Minnesota

Gary M. Lourie, M.D.
Assistant Director of Hand Clinic
Scottish Rite Children's Medical
Center;
Clinical Assistant Professor of
Orthopaedics
Emory University School of
Medicine
Atlanta, Georgia

Raymond T. Morrissy, M.D.
Medical Director and Chief of
Orthopaedics
Scottish Rite Children's Medical
Center;
Clinical Professor of Orthopaedics
Emory University School of
Medicine
Atlanta, Georgia

Vincent S. Mosca, M.D.
Associate Professor of
Orthopaedics
Chief, Pediatric Orthopaedics
University of Washington School of
Medicine;
Director, Department of
Orthopaedics
Children's Hospital and Medical
Center
Seattle, Washington

Colin F. Moseley, M.D.
Clinical Professor of Orthopaedics
University of California, Los
Angeles, UCLA School of
Medicine;
Chief of Staff
Shriners Hospital for Crippled
Children
Los Angeles, California

Thomas S. Renshaw, M.D.
Professor of Orthopaedic Surgery
and Pediatrics
Yale University School of Medicine
New Haven, Connecticut

David D. Sherry, M.D.
Assistant Professor of Pediatrics
University of Washington School of
Medicine
Director of Clinical Pediatric
Rheumatology
Children's Hospital and Medical
Center
Seattle, Washington

Paul D. Sponseller, M.D.
Associate Professor and Head
Division of Pediatric Orthopaedics
Johns Hopkins University School
of Medicine
Baltimore, Maryland

Dempsey S. Springfield, M.D.
Visiting Orthopaedic Surgeon
Massachusetts General Hospital;
Associate Professor of
Orthopaedics
Harvard Medical School
Boston, Massachusetts

J. Andy Sullivan, M.D.
Chairman
Department of Orthopaedic
Surgery and Rehabilitation,
University of Oklahoma Health
Sciences Center College of
Medicine
Oklahoma City, Oklahoma

George H. Thompson, M.D.
Professor of Orthopaedic Surgery
and Pediatrics
Case Western Reserve University
School of Medicine;
Director, Pediatric Orthopaedics
Rainbow Babies and Children's
Hospital
Cleveland, Ohio

Vernon T. Tolo, M.D.
John C. Wilson, Jr, Professor of
Orthopaedics
University of Southern California
School of Medicine;
Head, Division of Orthopaedics
Children's Hospital
Los Angeles, California

William C. Warner Jr, M.D.
Assistant Professor of Orthopaedics
University of Tennessee, Memphis,
College of Medicine
Staff
The Campbell Clinic
Memphis, Tennessee

Stuart L. Weinstein, M.D.
Ignacio V. Ponseti Professor of
Orthopaedic Surgery
University of Iowa College of
Medicine
Iowa City, Iowa

David J. Zaleske, M.D.
Associate Professor of
Orthopaedics
Harvard Medical School;
Chief, Pediatric Orthopaedic Unit
Massachusetts General Hospital
Boston, Massachusetts

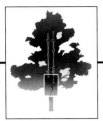

Contents

VOLUME 2

32 The Role of the Orthopaedic Surgeon in Child Abuse 1315

Behrooz A. Akbarnia

Lovell and Winter's
Pediatric
Orthopaedics

Volume **II**

Lovell & Winter's Pediatric Orthopaedics, fourth edition, edited by Raymond T. Morrissy and Stuart L. Weinstein. Lippincott–Raven Publishers, Philadelphia © 1996.

Chapter 17

Scoliosis

John E. Lonstein

Deformities of the spine probably were the most neglected area in orthopaedics during the first half of this century. There has been tremendous progress in this field over the last 35 years, consisting of a better understanding of the possible causes, with new approaches and devices leading to improved nonoperative and operative treatment. Despite all changes, the fundamentals and principles have remained the same.

The classification of spine deformities used in this chapter is that of the Scoliosis Research Society (Appendix 17-1). The classification evolves with new advances regarding the causes of spinal deformities. A glossary of terms has been developed by the Scoliosis Research Society that attempts to standardize definitions and reduce confusion in discussing this branch of orthopaedics (Appendix 17-2). In the past, there has been much confusion about the terms *major*, *primary*, *secondary*, *compensatory*, *structural*, *nonstructural*, *postural*, and *functional*. With the use of this glossary, these terms should be better defined and understood.

PATIENT EVALUATION

History

As in all fields of medicine, the taking of an adequate and complete history is important. Frequently this is ignored in the field of spine deformities, but it is essential in making an accurate diagnosis and treatment decisions.

The history of the detection of the spinal deformity is obtained by inquiring into when and in what manner the deformity was first noted (e.g., school screening, back asymmetry, pain, elevated shoulder, prominent hip). Is the deformity progressive, and has the the progression been documented, either clinically or on radiographs, indicating the need for immediate active treatment? Does a history of pain point to some pathology (e.g., tumor, ruptured disc) as an underlying condition causing the pain and curve? What treatment has been used?

A family history of spine deformity indicates an inherited or familial type of spinal deformity (e.g., idiopathic scoliosis, muscular dystrophy). A history of weakness, numbness, tingling sensation, or awkwardness of gait points to a neurologic basis to the deformity, which can be confirmed by a family history of neurologic disease. Past illnesses, infections, and tumors and the treatment point to the possible cause of the spinal deformity (e.g., postradiation, postlaminectomy). A history of shortness of breath with or without exertion indicates decreased pulmonary function, usually due to a severe thoracic deformity.

It is also important to ask about any previous treatment. Has the patient seen another doctor? What was that doctor's opinion? Was a radiograph taken and treatment prescribed? Was a brace applied? Was surgery performed? What kind of surgery? All the details concerning the surgery, postoperative immobilization, activities, restrictions, and problems are obtained through the history and the collection of prior records and radiographs.

One of the most important aspects of spinal problems is growth, because it is growth that produces the progression of spinal deformities. It is of the utmost importance to determine the status of growth. Is there active growth? If the patient is a girl, have menses begun? Are there signs of puberty, such as the development of pubic hair in both genders and breasts in girls? Boys should be asked about any change of voice and the onset of facial hair growth.[5,148]

Physical Examination

The physical examination of the patient with a spinal deformity involves an assessment of more than the spine. It must be remembered that scoliosis, kyphosis, and lordosis are only the symptoms of an underlying disease process, and every effort must be made to identify this process. It is unfortunate that the most common type of scoliosis is idiopathic, with the cause still unknown. A diagnosis of idiopathic scoliosis is made after all other possible causes of the spinal deformity are excluded, the diagnosis being one of exclusion. It is easy to call all cases of scoliosis in children idiopathic, when in reality the cause can be a spinal cord tumor, syringomyelia, congenital anomaly, or Friedreich ataxia. Failure to obtain a complete history and perform a complete physical examination results in failure to diagnose these conditions.

Spine

Physical examination of the spine involves noting the curve and its effect on the torso; all variations that can be measured are. The spine is first assessed in the standing position (Fig. 17-1A). Is there any obvious spinal deformity as evidenced by scoliosis, kyphosis, or lordosis? Where is the deformity: thoracic, thoracolumbar, or lumbar? Is there asymmetry of the neckline indicating a high thoracic curve? Is there waistline asymmetry? Are the iliac crests level? The amount of decompensation or deviation of a plumb line dropped from the seventh cervical vertebra to the gluteal cleft is measured in centimeters.

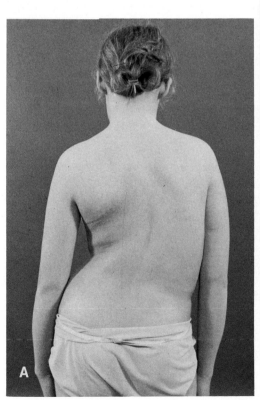
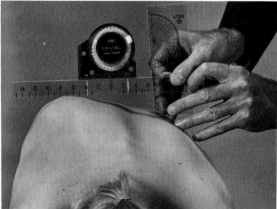
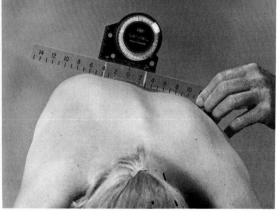

FIGURE 17-1. (A) Back view of patient showing a right thoracic prominence with decompensation of the thorax to the right. (B) Forward-bending view with measurement of the rib rotational prominence in centimeters. (C) Measurement of the rotational prominence in degrees.

The child bends forward toward the examiner, who notes if there is any deviation or spasm on forward bending. When present, this points to cord or cauda equina irritation and is an indication for a bone scan or magnetic resonance image (MRI). The back is inspected, on forward bending with the palms opposed and the arms hanging, for asymmetry or a thoracic or lumbar prominence. The site of any prominence is noted and measured. It must be remembered that the exact etiology of the rotational prominence is unknown, although it is well known that the lateral curvature is accompanied by vertebral rotation with rotation of the attached ribs. Thulborne and Gillespie[154] found no clear relation between the rotational prominence and the vertebral body rotation, the magnitude of the curve, or the rib-vertebral angle difference (RVAD). They postulated that it is due to an asymmetric relation between the pedicles, the laminae, and the transverse processes on the concave versus the concave side of the curve.

To measure the rotational prominence a spirit level is placed at the site of maximal prominence, with the center point over the palpable spinous process. A vertical ruler is placed on the concavity at a point that is an equal distance from the midline because the point of maximal prominence on the convexity is from the midline (Fig. 17-1B). This quantifies the prominence, actually measuring the prominence on the convexity plus the valley on the concavity. In addition, the angle of the prominence can be measured using a spirit level or a Scoliometer, in effect measuring the angle of the prominence on the concavity (Fig. 17-1C).[21]

Anteriorly, any rib prominence of the thoracic cage or rib flaring should be noted. The stage of development of the breasts and pubic hair development are noted and graded using the Tanner system.[148] This is important because it is the most accurate method of determining where the child is in the growth spurt, the range from Tanner 1 to 3 being the most important. Tanner 2 indicates the onset of the adolescent growth spurt, and thus a child with secondary sex characteristics and graded as a Tanner 2 or 3 is in the rapid phase of the growth spurt. The presence of pectus excavatum or carinatum also is noted.

The spine must be appreciated in three dimensions. Is there a pure single-plane deformity (i.e., scoliosis, kyphosis, or lordosis) or is there a combination of these conditions? It must be remembered that the term kyphoscoliosis refers to both scoliosis and true kyphosis and is rarely seen being present in only congenital deformities. The scoliosis and the posterior angulation and the apparent kyphosis in larger degrees of scoliosis are due to the rotation of the spine and actually are kyphosing scolioses.[144] Most patients with idiopathic scoliosis in reality have lordosis in the thoracic spine, not kyphosis.

Neurologic Examination

A neurologic examination is an essential part of every physical examination. It includes an evaluation of the upper and lower extremity reflexes, including the Babinski reflex. The one reflex that usually is not part of a routine examination is the abdominal reflexes; asymmetry or absence of these reflexes can be the first sign of intraspinal pathology. A basic motor and sensory evaluation of all four extremities is important. A Romberg test and finger-to-nose test should be conducted with any present or suspected neurologic disorder.

General Examination

The general examination looks for the presence of any abnormalities that would point to the cause of the spinal deformity. The skin should be examined for the presence of any pigmentation, nevi, lipomas, dermal sinuses, hair patches hemangiomas, café-au-lait pigmentation (a sign of neurofibromatosis), and hyperelasticity (Ehlers-Danlos syndrome).

The head and neck should be examined. The ears should be examined for congenital anomalies, especially preauricular ear tags, a sign of Goldenhar syndrome. A high, arched palate is suggestive of Marfan syndrome, whereas a cleft palate suggests a congenital deformity.

The upper extremities should be examined for any congenital anomalies, joint contractures, joint hyperelasticity, clawing of the fingers, and muscle weakness. The lower extremities are also examined, especially the feet. Foot abnormalities may be the first sign of generalized disorder (e.g., high arch in Charcot-Marie-Tooth syndrome or Friedreich ataxia) or an intraspinal anomaly (e.g., clubfoot and vertical talus can suggest a spinal dysraphism such as diastematomyelia, intraspinal lipoma, or tight filum terminale).

Radiologic Evaluation

Positioning

The nature, site and extent of the spinal deformities are evaluated using radiographs. Upright films form the basis of this evaluation. These are standing views in the coronal and sagittal planes with sitting films obtained in those unable to stand and supine films in infants before they are standing (Fig. 17-2A–C). These are the only views required for the initial evaluation if no treatment is planned. To evaluate the flexibility of a deformity, supine films with bending against the deformity are obtained. These are supine side-bending examination for scoliosis (Fig. 17-2D), hyperextension for kyphosis (Fig. 17-3), and hyperflexion

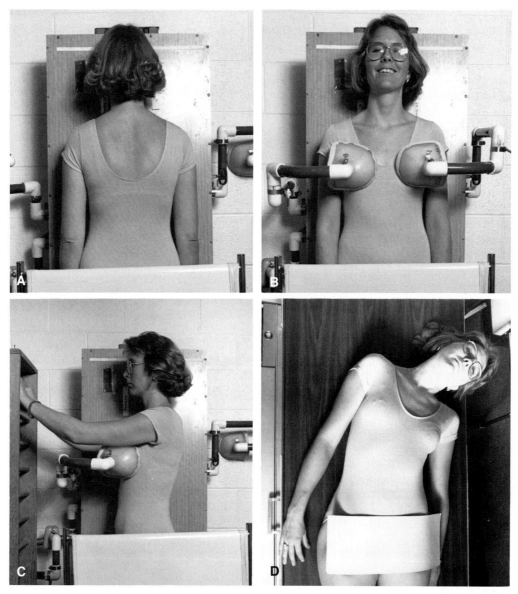

FIGURE 17-2. (**A**) Positioning of the patient for a posteroanterior radiograph. (**B**) Positioning of the patient for an anteroposterior radiograph with appropriate shielding. (**C**) Positioning of the patient for a lateral radiograph with appropriate shielding. The hands grasp a support, and the arms are relaxed and at right angles to the body. (**D**) The position and shielding for taking a maximum voluntary side-bending radiograph.

examination for lordosis. With scoliosis it has been shown that traction is a better corrective force for larger short radius curves, generally over 60 to 70 degrees, with a lateral force being more effective for smaller long radius curves.[158] Thus, for larger curves a film with distraction applied is a more accurate assessment of the curve's flexibility than an active side-bending examination. In children unable to side bend actively, such as young children with neuromuscular deformities, a traction film is obtained to assess flexibility.

In addition to the examinations previously described, additional views are obtained in specific cir-

cumstances. Oblique views are used to assess the integrity and quality of a fusion mass and are used in the lumbosacral area to evaluate the pars interarticularis for integrity in spondylolysis and spondylolysthesis. A Ferguson view of the lumbosacral area (i.e., with the beam angled cranially at 35 degrees) is used to assess the lumbosacral articulation. A Stagnara derotated view of the rotational deformity is used with large deformities to obtain a true coronal plane view of the apex of the deformity and the true magnitude of the scoliosis.[144]

Additional special examinations are obtained in special circumstances, and these include tomography

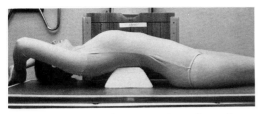

FIGURE 17-3.   To obtain a hyperextension radiograph to evaluate the flexibility of kyphosis the patient is hyperextended over a firm plastic block placed at the apex of the kyphosis, and a cross-table lateral radiograph is taken.

(i.e., laminography), myelography, computed tomography (CT), MRI, and intravenous pyelography (IVP). These techniques are discussed in the following sections.

Radiation Hazards

There is radiation exposure accompanying the taking of radiographs, but it is minimized with the modern techniques, including fast films, rare earth screens, filters for the upright views, and beam collimation, and the position used. One of the concerns is the risk of breast cancer; it has been shown that the risk is less if the posteroanterior position is used instead of the anteroposterior position for standing examinations.[44,120] An alternative is to use the anteroposterior position with the use of breast shields. These should not be hung around the child's neck because the axial loading of the spine actually may increase the curvature present. In addition, after the initial standing film, shielding of the gonads is done using a lead shield attached to an adjustable height pole.

Curve Evaluation

GENERAL.   The radiographs are evaluated generally for any indication of the cause of the spinal deformity. Is the anatomy of the vertebrae, transverse processes, and ribs normal, or are there congenital anomalies or vertebral scalloping and rib spindling indicative of neurofibromatosis? Are the curve patterns typical for idiopathic scoliosis, or they atypical (e.g., a single left thoracic curve)? Is the sagittal profile normal, or is there a change in the normal cervical, thoracic, or lumbar curves? The coronal balance can be measured radiographically as well as clinically with a plumb line dropped from the spinous process of C7. The relation of the thorax to the pelvis is noted, which shows the thoracopelvic balance. In addition, the curves are assessed for pattern, magnitude, and rotation with the spine being evaluated in three dimensions.

PATTERN.   On the coronal view the curves are evaluated, and the pattern is determined. The side of the convexity of the curve determines whether it is a right or left curve. The site of a curve—cervical, cervicothoracic, thoracic, thoracolumbar, lumbar, or lumbosacral—depends on the apical vertebra with the classification following the guidelines laid out in the section on terminology. The curves in idiopathic scoliosis fall into specific patterns. The flexibility of the curve and the cosmetic appearance, especially the size of the rotational prominence, determine the structure of a curve. There may be a single structural thoracic, thoracolumbar, or lumbar curve, or there may be a double pattern with two structural curves. The double patterns are the double thoracic pattern (i.e., upper left thoracic and lower right thoracic), the double thoracic and lumbar pattern, and the double thoracic and thoracolumbar pattern. The least frequent pattern is the multiple curve pattern with three or four short curves. Patterns other than these are atypical and when present point to a cause other than idiopathic because the etiology of the scoliosis, such as long C-curves in neuromuscular deformities and left thoracic curves in intraspinal pathology.

The aim in determining the structural pattern is to decide, when active treatment is necessary, which curve or curves need to be treated. The radiograph may show a right thoracic and left lumbar curve of near equal magnitude. If there is only a significant thoracic prominence on forward bending and the lumbar curve is flexible on supine side-bending evaluation, only the thoracic curve needs treatment. If there are both thoracic and lumbar prominences on forward bending and the two curves are equal structurally on supine side-bending examination, both curves need to be treated.

CURVE MEASUREMENT.   To accurately describe the deformity a method of quantifying the curve is necessary. All current techniques have drawbacks because the spine deformity is three dimensional, and all measurement techniques measure one plane. By combining the coronal and sagittal measurements, the quality and quantity of the deformity can be documented, and the spine can be appreciated in three dimensions. The most widely used and accepted measurement technique is that of Cobb and Lippman.[29]

The first step in this technique is the identification of the end vertebrae of each curve. The upright posteroanterior or lateral radiograph is used for this measurement. The end vertebrae are the vertebrae of the curve that are most tilted from the horizontal. A line is drawn along the upper end plate of the cranial vertebra and the lower end plate of the caudal vertebra, and it is the angle formed by these lines that is measured. This can be done directly with large curves, but is not possible with smaller curves. In these cases perpendicular lines are drawn to these end plate lines on the concavity of the curve, and the angle formed by these perpendiculars is measured (Fig. 17-4A). If the end plate is difficult to see the upper or lower margins of the pedicles can be used for the vertebral margins as long as the pedicle anatomy is normal and the line obtained is parallel to the end plate. In addition, in some curves, two or more vertebrae are parallel at the end of the curve. In these cases the vertebra furthest from the apex of the curve is taken as the end vertebra.

When there is a double curve, both curves are measured. The lower end vertebra of the upper curve is the upper end vertebra of the lower curve; this vertebra is termed the transitional vertebra. Only one line needs to be drawn on this vertebra because the end plates are parallel (Fig. 17-4B). These techniques for identification of the end vertebrae and measurement of the curves apply to scoliosis on the coronal

view and kyphosis and lordosis on the sagittal view (Fig. 17-5).

Once these vertebrae have been identified on the upright film they are used on any additional films to evaluate the curve flexibility. These same end vertebrae are used even though they may not be the maximally tilted vertebrae on these films. This is very important in congenital curves, in which it is essential to use the same vertebrae and the same vertebral lines (end plate, pedicle). Only by being consistent in the measurement technique is it possible to evaluate the flexibility of a curve and follow the curve progression.

ROTATION. An appreciation of the rotation of the curve is important. A small curve without rotation is not a true curve but one that is postural in origin. Rotation assessment also plays a role in the selection of the fusion area, which extends to nonrotated vertebrae cranially and caudally. The rotation is determined by the evaluation of the pedicles and is graded using the

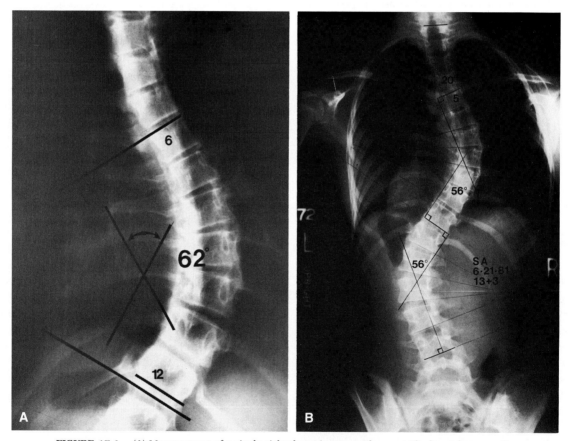

FIGURE 17-4. (A) Measurement of a single right thoracic nerve. The most-tilted vertebrae are the end vertebrae of the curve. A line is drawn along the end plate of each end vertebra, and a line perpendicular to the end plate lines is drawn. The angle of intersection is the curve angle. (B) Measurement of a double curve. A line is drawn along the lower end plate of each vertebra of both curves. The lines converge on the concavity of each curve: on the left for the right thoracic curve and on the right for the left lumbar curve. The most-tilted vertebrae are the end vertebrae of the curves; the end vertebra at the junction of the curves is the transitional vertebra. Lines perpendicular to these end vertebrae are drawn; the angles of intersection are the measurement of the curves.

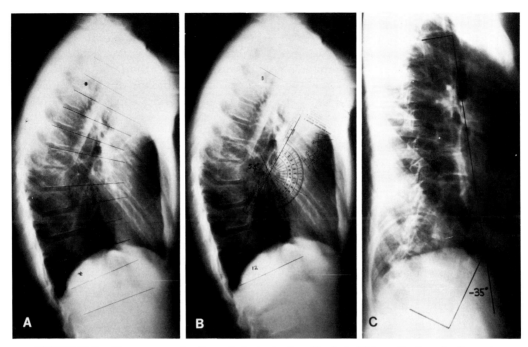

FIGURE 17-5.   Measurement of radiographs for kyphosis and lordosis. (**A**) A standing lateral radiograph with lines drawn along the end plates of all the vertebrae. Note that T3 and T12 are the vertebrae that are most tilted from the horizontal and thus are the end vertebrae. (**B**) Lines perpendicular to the end plates of the end vertebrae are drawn; the angle of intersection is the angle of the kyphosis. (**C**) The same technique is used in thoracic lordosis; the end vertebrae are identified, perpendicular lines are drawn, and the intersection is measured. Because the measurement is less than 0 degrees, the angle of the lordosis is recorded as a negative number (−35 degrees in this example).

system described by Nash and Moe.[121] The pedicle shadows of the vertebra in question, usually the apical or end vertebra of the curve, are used to grade the rotation. In zero rotation the pedicle shadows are equidistant from the sides of the vertebral body. In grade I rotation the pedicle shadow on the convexity has moved from the edge of the vertebra, the symmetry of the pedicle shadows having been lost. In grade III rotation the convex pedicle shadow is close to the center of the vertebral body, with grade II rotation being intermediate between that of grade I and grade III. In grade IV rotation the pedicle shadow is past the center of the vertebral body.

The accurate quantity of the rotation can be measured using the technique described by Pedriolle.[127] This technique also uses the pedicle situated on the convexity of the apical vertebra, measuring the distance from the waist of the vertebra using a torsiometer measuring ruler. This technique is not used on a day-to-day basis but rather in studies.

Maturity

The radiographic evaluation of the maturity of the child is used in conjunction with the clinical assessment (growth, onset of menarche, Tanner staging) to gain an appreciation of the growth potential of the child. The ossification of the iliac crest apophysis for this was originally described by Risser,[136] and his grading system is still used. The ossification usually starts anteriorly at the anterior superior iliac spine and proceeds posteriorly to the posterosuperior iliac spine. The progress of the ossification is divided into quarters and graded as Risser 1 to 4, with a grade 5 being fusion of the ossified apophysis to the ilium. Risser signs of 0 (no ossification) and 1 coincide approximately with a child in the rapidly growing phase of the adolescent growth spurt. A Risser sign of 5 denotes maturity and the cessation of spinal growth.

The vertebral ring apophyses lie at the upper and lower margins of the vertebral body. This secondary ossification center forms a complete ring lying between the cartilage end plate and the annulus. Fusion of the apophysis with the vertebral end plate indicates cessation of all vertebral body (and thus spine) growth potential.

What is of paramount importance is the growth potential of the child, which is related to the skeletal rather than the chronologic age. Using the clinical and radiographic factors mentioned previously, an accurate assessment of the child's growth potential can be estimated. Sometimes all of the factors do not agree, and at these times, an assessment of the bone age is necessary. This is obtained with an anteroposterior radiograph of the right hand and wrist, which is compared with the standards in the Greulich and Pyle atlas.[60] This is used in conjunction with the clinical assessment to obtain an idea of the growth remaining.

Special Studies

LAMINOGRAPHY.   Laminograms are useful for special problems. The most common use is in the better definition of vertebral anatomy, for example in congenital anomalies. It may be difficult to determine the exact nature of a jumbled mass of abnormal bones on a routine film, but the laminogram often can help in appreciating the anomaly. Laminograms in both the anteroposterior and lateral planes allow a three-dimensional appreciation of the abnormal vertebral anatomy. Laminograms also have been useful for the detection of osteoid osteomas and better definition of certain fracture problems, but CT has replaced the laminogram in many cases. Laminography still plays a role in the assessment of congenital spine anomalies because the detail and the anatomy shown are far superior to other methods, such as CT three-dimensional reconstruction.

MYELOGRAPHY.   Myelography is also useful in certain complex problems. An evaluation of the spinal canal is always indicated if there is any suspicion of a spinal cord tumor, spinal dysraphism, or neurologic problems secondary to the curvature. This can be achieved with a myelogram or an MRI scan, the myelogram being easier to interpret in the presence of significant scoliosis. Myelography should always examine the entire spinal canal, never just the lower spine. If there is kyphosis, the patient requires either a high-volume myelogram or supine positioning in order to adequately visualize the cord at the apex of the curve.[56]

Water-soluble myelographic techniques rapidly are replacing the oil-based dyes. For good definition in the lumbar area, especially for dysraphic lesions, water-soluble techniques are virtually mandatory.

COMPUTED TOMOGRAPHY.   This advanced technique is seldom useful in the evaluation of ordinary curvature problems but is highly useful for bone tumors, infections, spinal stenosis, and some fractures. It can be combined with water-soluble myelography, a technique particularly useful for dysraphic problems, tumors, and cystic lesions.

Reformatting of the digital CT information to obtain a coronal, sagittal, or three-dimensional image can be used to better see the spinal anatomy, especially in congenital anomalies. I have found that high-quality supine anteroposterior and lateral radiographs allow a good appreciation of the anatomy, at times with the addition of laminograms for complex deformities. To obtain good three-dimensional CT reconstructions, thin cuts (1–1.5 mm) are necessary; these require a large dose of radiation and are time consuming. In general, the amount of additional information obtained from CT as opposed to routine high-quality radiographs does not justify the large increase in the radiation dose.

MAGNETIC RESONANCE IMAGING.   The MRI is used extensively for evaluation of the spinal canal and its contents. It is used for evaluation or diagnosis of syringomyelia, spinal cord tumors, Arnold-Chiari malformations, and spinal dysraphism. In most cases it has replaced myelography for most of these cases, except for the markedly deformed spine. It is indicated in all cases of congenital spine anomalies with a suspicion of a spinal dysraphism or in which significant operative correction is anticipated in the presence of congenital anomalies. It is also indicated in cases of apparent idiopathic scoliosis to rule out intraspinal pathology, such as with a single left thoracic curve, an atypical curve pattern, or abnormalities on physical examination. In cases that appear to be idiopathic scoliosis, an MRI is indicated. MRI is indicated in all cases of infantile or juvenile idiopathic scoliosis because of the high incidence of intraspinal problems[167] and in cases of adolescent idiopathic scoliosis that show rapid documented progression.

INTRAVENOUS PYELOGRAPHY.   An IVP forms a part of the evaluation of the patient with a spinal deformity in two areas. In congenital spine deformities, because of the high association of renal tract anomalies, an evaluation of the urinary system is essential using renal ultrasonography or an IVP.[95] Usually, ultrasonography is performed first, and if an abnormality is found an IVP should be obtained. In paralytic deformities there is involvement of the bladder and possibly the kidneys, and thus an IVP forms part of evaluation of this patient.

Pulmonary Function Testing

The major reason for treating scoliosis, especially thoracic scoliosis, is preservation of lung capacity. Thus, it can be important to know whether or not pulmonary function has been affected by the curve. In the patient with a significant deformity, it is important to know the extent of the pulmonary effect because this can materially increase the risks of surgery. In addition, patients with thoracic lordosis have decreased pulmonary functions due to the lordosis.[168] These patients have a far greater loss of pulmonary function than would be expected from their posteroanterior radiographs.

Pulmonary function testing evaluates lung volumes and flow rates in the search for restrictive or obstructive disease. The forced vital capacity (FVC) is an easy measure of volume. A decrease in FVC indicates restrictive disease. Forced expiratory volume over 1 second (FEV1) or the ratio of FEV1 to FVC measures obstructive disease. The values on a subject are compared with normal values using patient height, but with spinal deformities this is inaccurate, and the arm span is measured and converted to an estimated height value. The normal range is from 80% to 120% of predicted values, a reduction to 60% of predicted normal values being significant.

In thoracic scoliosis with curves of more than 60 degrees, pulmonary function testing shows a reduction in pulmonary function with mild restrictive disease, and the patient is asymptomatic. The pulmonary function decreases with the increase in the degree of the curve; symptoms of dyspnea on exertion appear with curves of 90 to 100 degrees. Blood gas analysis in patients having this degree of scoliosis shows abnormalities, and respiratory failure and cor pulmonale are risks in patients with long-standing curves of more than 120 degrees. The presence of thoracic lordosis leads to restrictive disease based on the lordosis alone[168]; a thoracic scoliosis of 40 degrees and thoracic lordosis of −25 degrees is associated with marked restrictive disease.

Any patient with pulmonary symptoms should have pulmonary function tests. In addition, these tests should be performed in patients with thoracic curves of more than 90 to 100 degrees and thoracic lordosis of −20 degrees or more.

ADULT SEQUELAE OF UNTREATED SPINAL DEFORMITY

What happens to scoliotic patients who receive no treatment during the growing years? How do they function as adults? Do they have problems related to their spines? These are all very pertinent questions that must be answered before undertaking the active treatment of the growing child. If, indeed, there were no problems in the adult with scoliosis, it would be difficult to justify the stresses, anxieties, and problems encountered in treating the child.

One way to best answer these questions is to document the actual natural history of a group of untreated patients who are now adults. Such documentation is available in several studies. In the study by Nilsonne and Lundgren,[123] 113 patients with idiopathic scoliosis were reviewed an average of 50 years after being seen at a scoliosis clinic from 1913 to 1918. Ninety percent of the patients were located. Forty-five percent were dead; this was twice the expected mortality rate for

the age. Most of the deaths occurred as a result of cardiac or pulmonary disease. There was a noticeable increase in mortality after age 45 years. Of the women, 76% had never married. No patient was engaged in heavy labor, and 47% were on disability pensions, 30% specifically because of their spinal deformities. Ninety percent had symptoms of a bad back. This study shows that severe problems can occur with severe scoliosis, but the original presentation was in the early days of radiography, and no original radiographs were present on review to quantify the magnitude of the scoliosis. In addition, the majority of cases were probably infantile or juvenile idiopathic scoliosis that presented with large initial curves, a situation that is very rare.

In a similar article, Nachemson[117] reviewed 130 patients with various types of scoliosis. Ninety percent of these patients were located for follow-up an average of 35 years later. The mortality rate for the group as a whole was twice that of the population in general. If only thoracic curves were considered, the mortality rate was four times that of the general population. The mortality rate was higher in patients with paralytic and congenital curves. Forty percent of the patients noted backache, and 30% were disabled; the expected rate of disability was 15%. No patient was employed in heavy labor. This is a mixed study with few cases of idiopathic scoliosis, and the comments on Nilsonne's study also apply here.

A third study of the long-term results of untreated idiopathic scoliosis was done by Collis and Ponseti.[32] They attempted to locate the 353 patients reviewed in 1950 by Ponseti and Friedman. This is the only study that used both original and current radiographs. They located and personally examined 105 patients, and an additional 100 patients were reviewed by questionnaire only. The average follow-up was 24 years. Most curves increased after skeletal maturity. Thoracic curves of 60 degrees to 80 degrees progressed the most—an average of 28 degrees. Thoracic curves less than 60 degrees showed an average of only 9 degrees of progression. Lumbar curves of more than 30 degrees progressed an average of 18 degrees, whereas curves of less than 30 degrees did not progress.

The mortality rate was less than that seen in the two Swedish series noted previously, but the length of follow-up was shorter, and there was a much lower percentage of deaths at follow-up. Decreased vital capacity was noted in all thoracic curves over 60 degrees. Dyspnea was noted in 40% of patients, usually in those with thoracic curves of 85 degrees or more. Although 54% of the patients had backache complaints, the authors did not think that this incidence was higher than that of the population as a whole. Only 8 of the 205 patients had been hospitalized for back pain. This study gives a more realistic general expectation of adolescent idiopathic scoliosis and contains data about possible curve increase. It is unfortunate that 148 (42%) of the original patients could not be located, making the follow-up data less accurate. A 50-year follow-up of the same group of patients confirmed the impression of the earlier studies.[157]

The great lesson of these studies is that scolioses are not always static once growth ceases. Some scolioses progress, especially thoracic curves of 60 degrees or more, and these will cause decreased pulmonary function (Fig. 17-6). The question of lumbar curves is less obvious. Undoubtedly, lumbar curves over 50 degrees do tend to progress, but whether there is higher likelihood of back pain is unknown (Fig. 17-7). One condition often quoted as a factor in progression in adult scoliosis is pregnancy. Initial studies suggested that scoliosis progressed during pregnancy, but this was not confirmed. These curves were progressing in adulthood, and the pregnancies were a coincidental occurrence in adulthood. The only true effect of pregnancy on scoliosis was found by Nachemson, in a review of Milwaukee brace–treated patients.[31] The group of patients with multiple pregnancies before age 20 had definite progression after bracing compared with the other patients.

Another way to determine the presence or absence of adult problems in the scoliotic patient is to examine the files of those physicians who might have contact with the scoliosis patient in adult life. If no adults came to these physicians, it could safely be said that adults do not have significant problems. However,

such is not the case. Many patients go to internists and pulmonary physicians because of respiratory failure with or without secondary right heart failure. In many of these there is the pulmonary obstructive component of asthma or smoking, or both, added to the restrictive effect of severe scoliosis. The pathodynamics of "scoliotic heart failure" were well outlined by Bergofsky and colleagues.[13]

Similarly, the orthopaedic surgeon interested in scoliosis sees many adult with scoliosis for a variety of problems. Several series of patients treated in adult life have been reported. The most common complaint is pain especially in lumbar curves. This is the most common problem with which adults with scoliosis present. The previously mentioned studies from Sweden and Iowa give conflicting figures regarding the incidence of back pain. Some of this difference can be attributed to the differences in the populations and social structures. Sweden has a socialized system in which it is easier to be disabled due to scoliosis and back pain and receive a pension, whereas the population in Iowa is mostly rural farmers with a strong work ethic who may not perceive scoliosis as a disability. Additionally, the prevalence of back pain in the general population is as high as 60% in some series.

Some patients come to orthopaedic surgeons because of dyspnea. They are hopeful that the curve can be straightened and their breathing improved. In most cases the dyspnea has other pulmonary or cardiac causes or is due to deconditioning. Some patients are

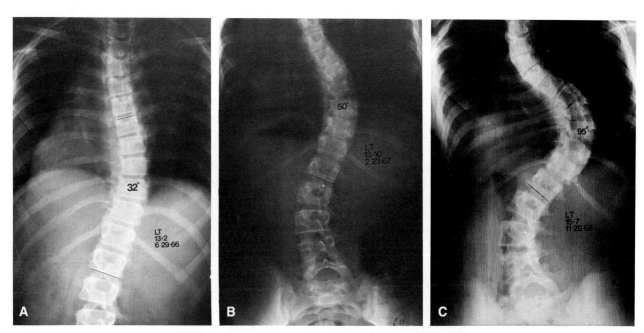

FIGURE 17-6. (**A**) A 13-year-old girl with a 32-degree right thoracic idiopathic scoliosis was placed on observation. (**B**) Only 8 months later, the curve was 50 degrees, well past the chance for bracing. Surgery should have been performed at this point, but the family refused. (**C**) By age 15 years, the curve was 95 degrees. The progression continued so that the curve was 105 degrees at age 17 years and 130 degrees at age 35 years, at which time she presented to the physician with major dyspnea and a marked self-image problem.

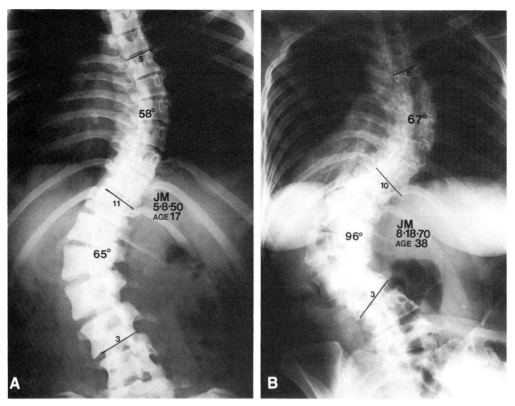

FIGURE 17-7.   (A) A double curve in a 17-year-old girl with a Risser sign of 4+, a right thoracic curve of 58 degrees, and a left lumbar curve of 65 degrees. She was told that she had "nicely balanced curves that should give her no problem in the future." (B) She presented at age 38 years with severe back pain and sciatica in the left leg and progression of her curves to 67 and 96 degrees, respectively.

most concerned about the cosmetic disfigurement of their hump; this can obfuscate their awareness of other symptoms.

Finally, there is a small group of patients who come because of paralysis caused by the spine deformity. They are more likely to be patients with severe kyphosis due to a congenital anomaly or some other cause.[89]

Scoliosis is not necessarily a benign condition. Thoracic curves over 60 degrees, if they are left untreated, lead to reduced pulmonary function, and with severe curves, pulmonary failure and possible early death. Lumbar curves, especially those over 50 degrees, are likely to progress in adult life. These patients have a high likelihood of degenerative disc disease and pain. Therefore, even if cosmetic and emotional factors are not taken into account (and they may be of considerable importance), aggressive treatment of the child with a spinal deformity is justified.

NONSTRUCTURAL SCOLIOSIS

Postural Scoliosis

Although the normal spine is perfectly straight in the frontal plane, there are certain children who do not voluntarily stand perfectly straight. They may slouch and cause one or more curvatures to be present. Usually this is thoracic kyphosis and lumbar lordosis, but there may also be scoliosis of mild degree. It is usually easy to detect the difference between postural and structural scoliosis by a careful physical and x-ray examination. Postural scoliosis is not associated with a prominence on forward bending. It disappears in the prone position and when the child is asked to stand in a straight position. On the radiograph, the curves are different from a structural scoliosis. There is a long curve, usually extending from one end of the spine to the other, without any associated rotation. The supine radiograph is usually perfectly straight and bending films show no areas of structural change. These curves do not progress nor do they become structural.

Leg Length Discrepancy

A difference in the length of the legs will result in a curvature of the spine in the standing position. This is a functional or nonstructural curve in that there is no intrinsic stiffness of the curve in the spine. When the patient is sitting or lying down, the curve disappears (Fig. 17-8). When the leg length difference is corrected, the curve disappears. It is highly doubtful

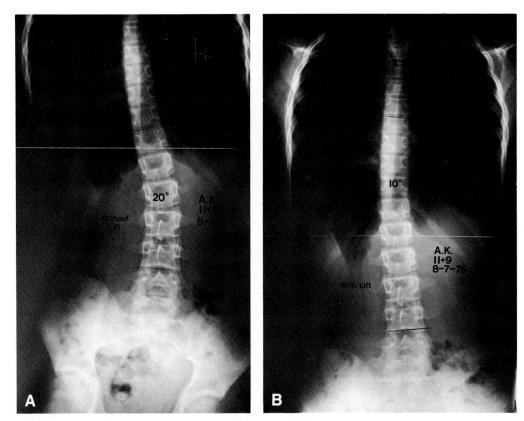

FIGURE 17-8. (A) An 11-year-old girl was seen for a finding of scoliosis, and was found to have a 20-degree right lumbar curve from T11-L3 on the standing radiograph. There is no rotation of the vertebrae in the curve, and a significant leg-length discrepancy is seen. (B) A repeat radiograph was taken of the same patient with a 2.5-cm lift under the right foot. The scoliosis has disappeared.

that the presence of a leg length discrepancy for a long period of time will result in a functional curve becoming structural because humans spend little of their time standing on two feet with balanced weight. When humans walk, they shift weight from one leg to the other. When humans sit, the discrepancy disappears, and humans usually spend a great deal of time lying down. Thus, the inequality of leg length does not act on the spine for more than a small percentage of each day. Neuromuscular conditions that may result in a leg length discrepancy (e.g., poliomyelitis) also can have a structural scoliosis, both conditions being due to the underlying disease.

Hysterical Scoliosis

Hysterical scoliosis has been reported by Blount and Moe.[15] This curve is present in the upright position and may be present in the supine or prone position. It is absent during sleep and also disappears under anesthesia. The curves are long and sweeping, or the patterns are atypical without any rotation radiographically or a rotational prominence on forward bending.[164] In addition, the physical examination may be confusing because it may vary with the examination,

and the examiner may be confused as to whether there is a deformity or not. A supine or prone film may show the absence of a fixed curve, and sometimes the radiograph must be taken under sedation or anesthesia. Before terming the case hysterical, a spinal cord tumor or other neurologic condition must be excluded. Hysterical scoliosis must not be treated by orthopaedic methods, such as exercises, braces, casts, and surgery. This is a psychiatric condition, and it requires consultation with a specialist in this field (Fig. 17-9). Orthopaedic treatment only leads to reinforcement of the underlying condition and fixation of the hysteria.

STRUCTURAL SCOLIOSIS

Idiopathic Scoliosis

Idiopathic scoliosis is the most common form of scoliosis. The child is perfectly healthy and develops a curve sometime during growth. There are three types of idiopathic scoliosis depending on the age of onset: infantile (birth to age 3 years), juvenile (age 3 years to puberty), and adolescent (postpubescent).

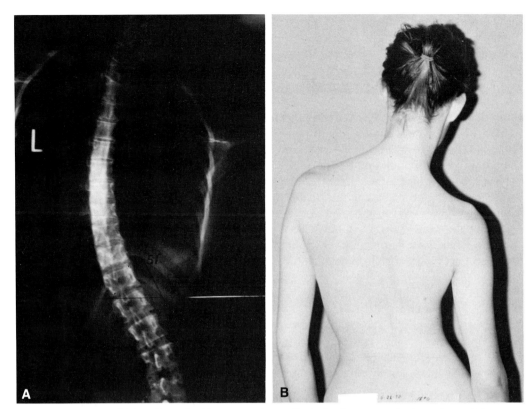

FIGURE 17-9.   (A) A radiograph of long, sweeping scoliosis that has no vertebral rotation and does not resemble an idiopathic scoliosis curve pattern. (B) A photograph of the patient taken at the same visit demonstrates the clinical appearance. This patient had hysterical scoliosis, and the curve eventually disappeared after 3 years of psychiatric treatment.

Prevalence

Two terms are confused in discussing the number of cases of a disease in a population: incidence and prevalence. Incidence refers to the rate of new cases per year of the disease or disorder in the population. Prevalence refers to the number of the population with the disease or disorder. When discussing scoliosis the studies usually give prevalence rates, although they may be called incidence rates.

Early prevalence studies were reviews of a large number of minifilms taken for tuberculosis screening and children referred for scoliosis treatment. These studies were biased to larger curves. The results of school screening programs have shown prevalence rates ranging from 0.3% to 15.3%.[8,19,41,91] This large range reflects differences in detection methods, populations screened, and definitions of scoliosis. In school screening studies when only curves of over 10 degrees are considered, the prevalence is 1.5% to 3.0%.[8,91] The prevalence rate depends on the curve magnitude being 2% to 3% for curves over 10 degrees, 0.3% to 0.5% for curves over 20 degrees, and 0.2 to 0.3% for curves over 30 degrees.[41,160]

There are also differences in the prevalence of the different types of idiopathic scoliosis. Historically, infantile idiopathic scoliosis had been relatively common in Great Britain and rare in North America, but the relative frequencies of the different types of idiopathic scoliosis have been changing in Great Britain. In a study of 157 children with idiopathic scoliosis seen in Edinburgh between 1968 and 1971, 41% had infantile, 7% juvenile and 52% had adolescent curves.[68] The frequencies have changed so that of the 153 children seen at the same clinic 12 years later from 1980 to 1983, 4% had infantile curves, 7% juvenile curves, and 89% had adolescent curves.[102] These changes also were seen in Germany,[98] where the more recent frequencies were similar to those in North America, as shown in a survey of 208 children in Boston, where 0.5% had infantile scoliosis, 10.5% had juvenile scoliosis, and 89% had adolescent idiopathic scoliosis.[135]

Etiology

By definition the cause of idiopathic scoliosis is as yet unknown. Many theories have been proposed, and they are divided into those for the infantile and adolescent types.

INFANTILE IDIOPATHIC SCOLIOSIS.   Infantile idiopathic scoliosis is slightly more common in Europe and occurs more frequently in boys, the left thoracic curve predominating. In a family study conducted in Edinburgh by Wynn-Davies, there was a genetic tendency, but the etiology was thought to be multifactorial.[174,175] Plagiocephaly, a flattening of the posterior occipital prominence on the convexity of the spinal curvature, is commonly associated with infantile idiopathic scoliosis. The plagiocephaly, like the scoliosis, was not present at birth and developed within the first 6 months of life. This suggests a possible postural causation of both the plagiocephaly and the scoliosis. There were associated factors in these children in the family review. These included congenital dislocation of the hip, congenital heart disease, and mental deficiency. In addition, the mothers were older, with a higher incidence of hernias among relatives. Some of these findings have been confirmed in other studies.[27,53,84]

ADOLESCENT IDIOPATHIC SCOLIOSIS. The etiology of adolescent idiopathic is as yet unknown, and studies have focused on the genetic aspects, growth aspects, structural and biochemical changes in the discs and muscle, and central nervous system changes.

Family and population studies point to a hereditary factor to explain the well-known familial pattern.[36,37] The mode of inheritance is uncertain, being regarded as autosomal or gender linked with incomplete penetrance and incomplete expressivity. It has been calculated that if both parents have idiopathic scoliosis, the chance of their children requiring treatment is 50 times that of the normal population.[94] It is important to be aware of this genetic aspect because when one child in a family is detected with idiopathic scoliosis, the physician should examine or suggest evaluation of all the siblings.

Growth has a definite role in idiopathic scoliosis, and a knowledge of normal spinal growth is essential in treating all patients with spinal deformities. This includes total body growth, spinal growth, and the pubertal growth spurt. As demonstrated by Tanner, growth does not proceed uniformly, but there are two periods of rapid growth: from birth to 3 years of age and during the adolescent growth spurt.[148,149] The intervening period from age 3 years to puberty is one of linear growth. Normal growth can be plotted as height attained or as height gain in centimeters per year (i.e., growth velocity); both of these graphs show the pubertal growth spurt.

Total body height is composed of several segments that grow at different rates. The head is relatively large at birth and grows the least, whereas the lower limbs are relatively short at birth and grow the most, the spine being intermediate between the two. The easiest way to measure spine height is to use the sitting height which includes head, pelvis, and spine. The sitting height graph has as similar shape to the total height attained graph, with the same two growth spurts. Pelvic height makes up 18% to 20% of sitting height, and to approximate the spine height the sitting height can be multiplied by .78 in girls and by .85 in boys.[150,151]

DiMeglio and Bonnel investigated spinal growth, concentrating on the thoracic and lumbar spines and measured the growth in three time periods: birth to age 5 years, age 5 to 10 years, and age 10 to 16 years.[42] The thoracic and lumbar spines, T1 to S1, was calculated to be 48% of sitting height, with the thoracic segment accounting for 63% of the T1 to S1 growth and the lumbar spine accounting for the remaining 37% of the growth. Although the thoracic segment grows more than the lumbar segment, the growth per segment in the thoracic spine is 1.1 cm from birth to maturity, compared with 1.6 cm per segment in the lumbar spine.

The relation between the growth spurt and scoliosis increase is well known. This relation between scoliosis and growth was first shown by Duval-Beaupere, who studied 560 girls with scoliosis (500 postpolio and 60 idiopathic) with respect to curve increase and growth, comparing their growth to that of 53 girls without scoliosis.[47,48] The curves increased at a steady rate during growth until a point she called P, when an acceleration of increase occurred until a point she called R, after which the curve increase reached a plateau.

Point P was found to coincide with the onset of the pubertal growth spurt on the growth velocity graph. In girls this coincides with the start of breast and pubic hair development, at Tanner stage 2, which occurs at a chronologic age ranging from 8 to 14 years, generally between 10 and 12 years. In fact, Tanner stage 2 in girls occurs after the onset of the pubertal growth spurt. The total growth spurt lasts approximately 2.5 to 3 years, with the point of maximum growth velocity (peak height velocity) occurring 1 year after the onset of the growth spurt, at a mean age of 12 years. Menarche and the appearance of axillary hair occur 1.5 to 2 years after the onset of the growth spurt at a mean age of 13 years.[24]

In boys the onset of development of pubic hair occurs before the onset of the growth spurt, the latter coinciding with a Tanner stage 2 to 3 (chronologic age, 11–16 years). The growth spurt is longer in boys, lasting 3.5 to 4 years, with peak height velocity occurring at a mean chronologic age of 14 years. Axillary hair appearance and the appearance of facial hair occur after peak height velocity. It must be remembered that all the ages stated are based on a uniform Anglo-Saxon Caucasian population, and cannot be applied to people of African, Asian, Latin American, and

Native American descent. Although the ages do not hold true, the relation between the maturity landmarks (e.g., Tanner stages, menarche) and the growth spurt are constant.

Point R of Duval-Beaupere corresponds to a Risser apophysis ossification sign of 4. Risser 4 corresponds to a cessation of spinal growth, with Risser 5 corresponding to cessation of height increase.[178]

There is a relation between curve increase and growth, and there is a role for growth in the etiology of idiopathic scoliosis. A Swedish study found that girls with adolescent idiopathic scoliosis were significantly taller than their normal peers.[159,161] This was not seen in boys with scoliosis nor in girls at younger ages. These girls started their growth spurts earlier, grew for a longer period, and had a skeletal age more advanced than their unaffected peers, but at the end of growth the height of the girls with scoliosis was equal to that of their unaffected peers.[124]

Some studies on the levels of growth hormone in girls with scoliosis compared with normal girls showed increased levels, whereas others could not confirm this finding.[142,162] Increased levels of growth hormone and somatomedin would explain the early and prolonged growth spurt in adolescent girls with idiopathic scoliosis.

Thoracic idiopathic scoliosis is associated with loss of the normal thoracic kyphosis with hypolordosis in the area of the curve. This has been demonstrated in the work of Dickson and colleagues[39]; whether this is an etiologic factor or part of the pathomechanics is unknown.

Investigators have searched for the etiology in the discs and muscles. Many have reported decreased glucoaminoglycan levels in the apical discs of patients with idiopathic scoliosis, with a concomitant rise in collagen levels.[70,126] Because these changes also were found in nonidiopathic scoliosis,[125] they are secondary to the abnormal stresses on the apical disc in scoliosis.

The paraspinal muscles have been implicated in the cause of idiopathic scoliosis. Electromyographic studies have been inconclusive because increased activity has been found on the convexity of the curve by some investigators,[133,180] whereas others found no difference.[83] Investigators found more type I or slow twitch, red, anaerobic muscle fibers on the convexity of the apical level in idiopathic scoliosis. Abnormalities also were found in muscle spindles, muscle histochemistry, sarcolemma, calcium, phosphorous and zinc concentrations in paravertebral muscles, and platelets because they relate to skeletal muscle. Whether these abnormalities are the cause of the scoliosis or whether they occur secondary to the curve is unknown, but most investigators believe that the latter is the case.

There is a well-known association of scoliosis with neurologic disorders, and therefore an abnormality of the central nervous system is an attractive etiologic theory. Research has concentrated on postural and equilibrium mechanisms by investigating righting reflexes, drift reaction, and optokinetic nystagmus. Postural, equilibrium, and vestibular dysfunction have been found by many authors; however, these findings are not specific for idiopathic scoliosis.[38,176,177] It appears that there may be a postural equilibrium problem in idiopathic scoliosis, and some authors have suggested that the lesion lies in the brain stem.

No single causative factor has been found for idiopathic scoliosis, and it appears that the etiology is probably multifactorial. There may actually be two mechanisms: one for the development of idiopathic scoliosis and another related to curve progression. Genetic, growth, chemical, biomechanical, and neuromuscular factors all seem to be involved. It has been postulated that the mild central nervous system abnormality is genetically determined. With increased growth and the altered viscoelasticity of the discs, the spine biomechanically is less stable, making it susceptible to changes in postural equilibrium. The interrelation of these factors determines whether the curve is progressive or nonprogressive and the extent of the progression.

Presentation

Children who present with idiopathic scoliosis are brought in by their parents because an asymmetry of the back was noted, and a subsequent radiograph showed a curve. In the infantile and juvenile years the parents are most likely to detect this alteration in back contour, whereas in the late juvenile years and adolescence it is more likely detected by routine screening. This is usually performed at school or during a school or sports team physical examination by the pediatrician or family practitioner. Screening is performed using the Adams forward-bending test. This test was first described 130 years ago, and it detects asymmetry of the torso on forward bending.[1] The child bends forward at the waist with feet together, knees straight, and palms opposed. The examiner views the back from the head, comparing the sides of the back for symmetry, viewing the back from the upper thoracic area to the lumbosacral area. The comparison of the sides can be visual alone or with a Bunnell Scoliometer, which measures the difference in degrees, a difference of 5 degrees being positive.[21]

As noted, this screening may occur as part of a routine physical examination by a pediatrician or family physician, or it may be part of a school screening program. Any positive screenings detected by this physician or confirmed from the referred cases are sent for a standing radiograph. Any scoliosis detected is referred for further evaluation and treatment.

There is a lot of controversy regarding routine screening for scoliosis because both British and Canadian task forces have issued statements against routine screening on epidemiologic grounds.[156] They cite lack of evidence of the accuracy of the screening test and lack of a proven method of nonoperative treatment. The controversy has been stimulated lately with the statement of the United States Preventative Services Task Force, which did not endorse routine visits for screening.[156] The policy statement mentioned that screening in the schools may be the only method for all children to be evaluated. There is recent scientific evidence that bracing is effective in altering the natural history of idiopathic scoliosis. In the light of this data it is incumbent on these task forces to reexamine the evidence and issue new recommendations based on these new facts.

Because adolescent idiopathic scoliosis is a treatable condition, early detection is the best approach to ensure early diagnosis and allow optimal treatment results. This early detection was achieved with the establishment of school screening programs using school staff that reduced costs and made the programs cost effective.[8,90,91] There has been a high false-positive referral rate from these screening programs, such as children referred from a screening who on evaluation by a physician are found not to have a rotational prominence. This high false-positive rate of referrals is a problem, and it can be reduced with education and training of the screeners and possibly with the use of the Scoliometer.

One of the side effects of this screening is the increased awareness of scoliosis by families and family physicians. Early detection occurs both at school and during routine evaluations by family physicians. This can be an argument for discontinuing routine school screening, but not all children have routine evaluations with family physicians; therefore, not all cases of scoliosis will be detected without school screening. Routine screening at school should be continued to maintain awareness in the community and to ensure early detection.

The child is evaluated as described previously. After other possible causes of scoliosis are excluded, the diagnosis of idiopathic scoliosis is made. When there is significant pain associated with the scoliosis, further investigation is mandatory to find the cause of the pain. Idiopathic scoliosis is not painful in the pediatric population, and the presence of significant back pain leads to further testing (e.g., additional radiographs, bone scan, MRI, CT).

Infantile Idiopathic Scoliosis

Infantile idiopathic scoliosis classically is described as having an onset before 3 years of age. It is rare in the United States and more common in Europe. It is more common in boys, with the curves usually in a left thoracic or thoracolumbar pattern. The majority of infantile idiopathic curves resolve spontaneously, with the occurrence of the progressive type between 8% and 64%.[68,84] Eighty-five percent of infantile idiopathic scolioses are nonprogressive (Fig. 17-10).

The differentiation of the progressive and nonprogressive varieties has been clarified by the work of Mehta,[106] who used the relation of the head and the neck of the ribs to the vertebral body at the apex of the scoliosis. If the convex rib does not overlap the vertebral body on the anteroposterior radiograph, it is classified as phase I. With progressive deformity the rib overlaps the apical vertebral body, and this is classified as phase II. She also developed a method to measure the difference in the angle at which the rib meets the spine, or the RVAD.

In Mehta's study of 138 cases of infantile idiopathic scoliosis, 86 curves were in phase I. Of these, 46 resolved and 40 progressed.[106] The average RVAD of the resolving group was 11.7 degrees, and 83% had an RVAD of less than 20 degrees. In the remainder of the resolving curves the RVAD decreased in time, despite the Cobb measurement. The average RVAD of the progressive group was 25.5 degrees, and 84% had an RVAD of greater than 20 degrees. If the apical rib head was in phase II, progression was certain, and the RVAD measurement was not necessary. Other studies have confirmed these findings.[27,153] This method has proved helpful but not absolutely reliable in differentiating the prognosis of the cases falling into phase I. These measurements are used to advise the parents regarding the prognosis, and serial radiographic follow-up is necessary every 3 to 4 months.

Mehta also divided progressive infantile idiopathic scoliosis into benign and malignant types. Both demonstrated worsening in the first 5 years of life and gradual progression thereafter with marked deterioration in the adolescent years. The malignant form is more rapidly progressive and difficult to manage.

TREATMENT. No active treatment is necessary for the nonprogressive variety of infantile idiopathic scoliosis, the curves resolving spontaneously without treatment (see Fig. 17-10). These curves are generally less than 35 degrees, and any curve over 35 degrees and any progressive curve need to be treated. The best treatment is the application of a series of well-fitting body casts applied under anesthesia. Serial casts are applied until maximal curve correction has been ob-

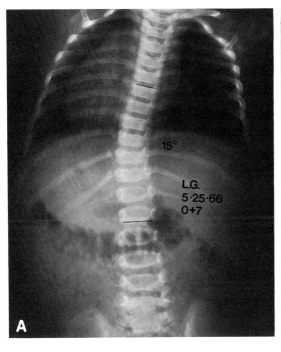

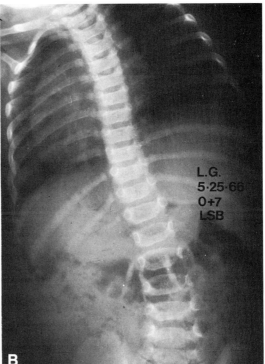

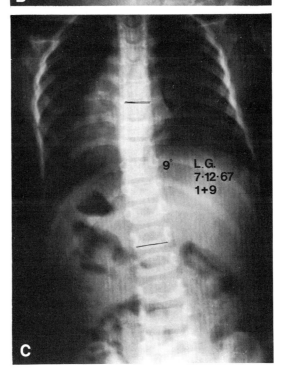

FIGURE 17-10. (**A**) A 7-month-old child presented with a 15-degree left T6-L1 idiopathic scoliosis. (**B**) The supine passive left-side-bending radiograph shows the structural changes in the apex of the curve. This curve was observed and there was no active treatment. (**C**) At the age of 21 months, the curve is resolving spontaneously and was 9 degrees.

tained. At this stage, a Milwaukee brace is fitted and worn on a full-time schedule. This is preferable to a thoracolumbosacral orthosis (TLSO) that, because of its circumferential fit, causes rib pressure with a resultant tubular thorax and reduced pulmonary function.

Some of the progressive curves treated with an aggressive casting program followed by use of the Milwaukee brace have reduction of the RVAD to 0 and straightening of the curve. After a period of bracing allowing the spine to grow in this straightened position with maintenance of this correction, the child is weaned from the brace. If no relapse occurs the brace is discontinued and the child observed to maturity. Mehta and Morel[107] have reported that if the curve is totally corrected prior to the growth spurt there will be no relapse during adolescence.

If curve control cannot be maintained with bracing, usually with the malignant progressive type, surgery is indicated. In the juvenile years this is usually instrumentation without fusion.[97,115] The spine is exposed only at the ends of the curve, and end fusions are performed at the sites of insertion of pediatric hooks. The rod is inserted under the fascia, with external protection in a Milwaukee brace. The rod is lengthened every 6 months and is replaced every 12 to 18 months. Using this technique spinal growth can occur, and the fusion is delayed.

When curve increase occurs, usually at the time of the adolescent growth spurt, a spinal fusion is performed. It has been shown by McMaster and others that curve progression and increased curve rotation occur with a posterior fusion alone.[63,104] With a solid posterior fusion anterior growth continues, which causes the vertebral bodies to increase in height with loss of the disc spaces. This continued anterior growth causes the vertebral bodies to rotate on the solid posterior fusion with increase in the measured curve and increase in the rotational prominence, termed the crankshaft effect.[46] It is more common when there is more growth potential, such as in the juvenile or immature adolescent. In these children fusion should consist of a combined anterior and posterior fusion, the anterior fusion removing the discs and growth plates and eliminating the anterior growth potential. When fusion is necessary, and the child is older, the posterior approach alone is successful. The principles of surgical decision making is the same as in the adolescent.

Juvenile Idiopathic Scoliosis

Idiopathic scoliosis appearing between the ages of 3 years old and puberty, by definition, is classified as juvenile idiopathic scoliosis, and represents 12% to 16% of idiopathic scoliosis. The line between juvenile and progressive infantile idiopathic scolioses and early-onset adolescent idiopathic scoliosis is not well defined. The gender ratio varies; the occurrence of juvenile idiopathic scoliosis is nearly equal between the genders in patients 4 to 6 years of age, but it occurs more often in girls and women later in life.[52,67,155] The incidence of curve patterns also varies from the left thoracic pattern in the young to an an equal incidence of double curves and the right thoracic pattern in older children.[52,67,155]

Mehta classified juvenile idiopathic scoliosis into a number of groups: late-resolving infantile idiopathic scoliosis, benign progressive infantile idiopathic scoliosis, syndromic scoliosis, syringomyelic scoliosis, and early detected adolescent idiopathic scoliosis. Each case of juvenile idiopathic scoliosis must be evaluated to exclude other causes of the scoliosis. The possible presence of intraspinal pathology is important, as in a study of routine MRI scans in a group of juvenile idiopathic scoliosis patients in which 17% showed abnormalities.[167] Routine MRI scans are in order in these children.

In general, one third of the cases of juvenile idiopathic scoliosis are nonprogressive; the other two thirds are progressive at varying rates. The younger the child at presentation with a progressive curve, the larger the ultimate deformity.

TREATMENT.   Smaller curves, those less than 25 degrees, are observed for progression. Follow-up is every 4 to 6 months with repeat standing radiographs. Care must be taken in positioning these children for the radiograph because a change in posture as the image is taken can result in an inaccurate diagnosis of curve increase. Any juvenile presenting with a curve of over 25 degrees should be treated immediately. Curves presenting before 6 years of age are treated in the same manner as the curves of the infantile type as described previously.

Curves first detected in the latter part of the juvenile years that are over 25 degrees or have shown documented progression should be treated nonoperatively. The Milwaukee brace is the orthosis of choice.[75] The brace is worn full time for 18 to 24 months until the curve is controlled. If at this time there is good control with a curve maintained at 20 degrees or less, part-time bracing can be started. A radiograph is taken after the child has been out of the brace for 4 hours. If the curve is still controlled, brace wearing time is reduced to 20 hours per day. Three months later, a radiograph is taken after the patient has been out of the brace for 6 hours; if there is continued curve control, the patient is allowed 6 hours out of the brace at a time. As long as the curve is controlled weaning is continued until the child is using the brace at night only. With continued stability an attempt is made to leave the child out of the brace. If no curve increase occurs, the brace use may be discontinued, even though the child has not reached the growth spurt. Observation continues, watching for curve increase, especially at the time of the adolescent growth spurt. With increase in the curve, bracing is resumed or a spinal fusion is performed.

If, with weaning, the curve increases, bracing remains at full time, this full time wear continues until the growth spurt. If the curve increases at any time, surgery is indicated. Depending on the age of the child at the time of curve increase, the surgery is instrumentation without fusion or a definitive fusion, usually an anterior and posterior approach. In some cases control of the curve continues through the growth spurt till the end of growth, when weaning is instituted (Fig. 17-11).

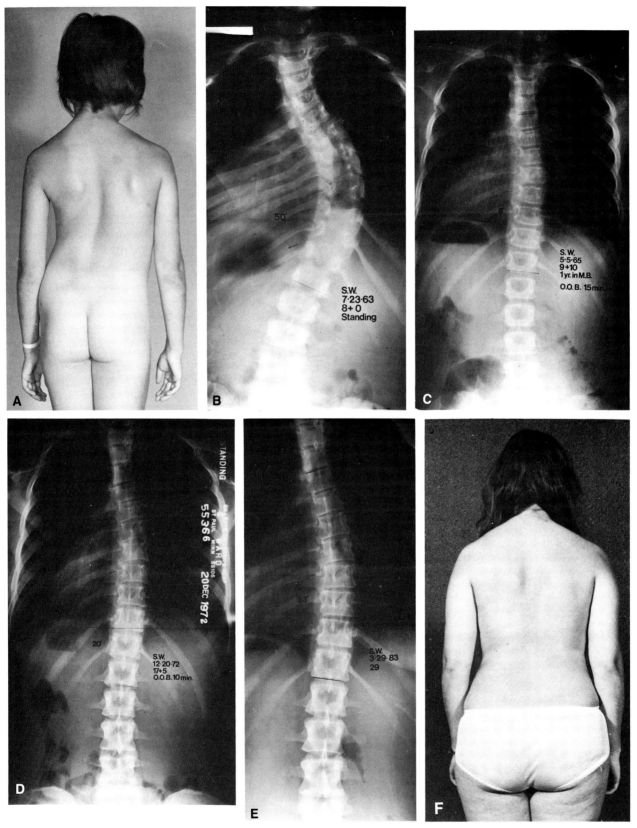

FIGURE 17-11. (A) An 8-year-old girl presented with a right thoracic scoliosis. (B) She had a 50-degree right thoracic T5-L1 curve. (C) After 1 year of Milwaukee brace treatment, her curve measured 8 degrees. Repeated attempts to go from full-time to part-time brace wear failed. (D) After 9 years of full-time orthotic treatment, her curve measured 20 degrees. Weaning from the brace was begun at this time. (E) At age 29 years, after 11 years without the orthosis and three pregnancies, her curve measured 23 degrees. (F) The patient's clinical appearance a few years after brace removal.

The reported success of nonoperative treatment is variable. In a recent large series the surgical rate was 50%, with the most common time of fusion at the onset of the adolescent growth spurt, and good curve control was maintained prior to that.[88] In general, in juvenile idiopathic scoliosis, one third of the children are observed, and two thirds require bracing. Of the latter group, bracing is successful in half of the children, and success is temporary in the rest, who eventually require surgical stabilization.

The surgical decision making regarding selection of the fusion area is the same as in the adolescent as described below. Anterior fusion is used in young and immature adolescents in the same role as in infants to prevent the crankshaft effect.

Adolescent Idiopathic Scoliosis

Most cases of idiopathic scoliosis seen fall into the adolescent category because they are first detected just before or at the time of the adolescent growth spurt. The curves probably begin during the juvenile years and only become apparent when they increase during adolescence. The most common curve patterns are the single right thoracic pattern, followed by the double right thoracic left lumbar and the other patterns described earlier.

PROGRESSION. The progression rates are well documented for adolescent idiopathic scoliosis. Generally, in these studies, progression is defined as a 5-degree increase in the curve from the time of presentation to follow-up with observation. Some studies use a 10-degree increase. It must be remembered that the measurement error in most studies is 3 degrees. These studies are either school screening studies or from a center where children are referred for evaluation and treatment. The progression rates vary tremendously, from 5.2% to 56%[19,22,28,55,85,138] with the lower rates found in school screening studies and the higher rates being reported by a referral center looking at larger curves (Table 17-1).

The factors that are related to curve progression have also been evaluated. These are divided into the factors related to the curve and those related to the child's growth potential. In general, the larger the curve, the greater the incidence of progression. Progression also varied with the curve pattern, a double curve in general being more likely to progress than a single curve. In reviewing all the curve patterns, my colleague and I[85] found that in curves between 5 and 29 degrees the incidence of progression in the different curve patterns was nearly equal except for the single lumbar and single thoracolumbar patterns, in which the incidence of progression was markedly lower.

TABLE 17-1. *Progression of Idiopathic Scoliosis in Adolescence*

	NO. OF PATIENTS	PROGRESSION (%)	CURVE (DEGREES)
Brooks et al[19]	134	5.2	
Rogala et al[138]	603	6.8	
Clarisse[28]	110	35	10–29
Fustier[55]	70	56	<45
Bunnell[22]	326	20	<30
		40	>30
Lonstein and Carlson[85]	727	23	5–29

From Lonstein JE. Idiopathic scoliosis. In: Lonstein JE, Bradford DS, Winter RB, Ogilvie JW. Moe's textbook of scoliosis and other spinal deformities. 3rd ed. Philadelphia; WB Saunders, 1994:221.

When assessing growth potential and curve progression the greater the growth potential available (i.e., the younger the child), the greater the incidence of progression. This can be measured by chronologic or skeletal age, menarchal status, Tanner grading, or Risser sign. The incidence of progression decreases after a girl reaches menarche. With reference to the Risser sign, the incidence of progression is higher in adolescents with a Risser of 0 or 1 compared with those with a Risser of 2 or more[22,85] (Figs. 17-12 and 17-13).

A useful cross-correlation of incidence rates for curves less than 29 degrees was published by me and my colleague.[85] The two factors used were the magnitude of the curve and the maturity of the child determined by the Risser sign. For curves of 20 to 29 degrees in an immature child with a Risser sign of 0 or 1, the incidence of progression was 68%. On the other extreme, for curves less than 19 degrees in a mature adolescent with a Risser sign of 2 or more, the incidence of progression was 1.6%. In the other two groups, one with a smaller curve (<19 degrees) in an immature child (Risser sign of 0 or 1) and the other with a larger curve (20–29 degrees) in a mature child (Risser sign of 2 or more), the incidence of progression is approximately the same: 22% to 23% (Table 17-2). These figures are used for the natural history incidence of progression when evaluating the effectiveness of treatment.

Other clinical factors have been suggested to be related to curve progression. The gender of the child is the most obvious. It is well known that the prevalence of scoliosis detected on school screening has an approximately equal ratio along gender lines, but those requiring treatment are predominantly girls. It would be expected that studies would show different incidences of progression in girls and boys, but this

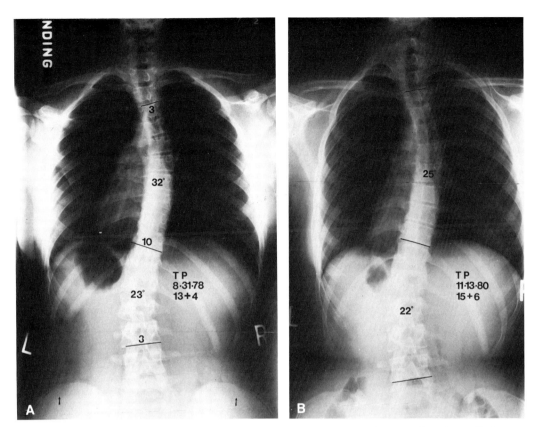

FIGURE 17-12. (A) A 13-year-old girl presented with a 32-degree right thoracic idiopathic scoliosis. She was 9 months postmenarche, and the Risser sign was 2. A Milwaukee brace was recommended, but the patient refused it. (B) After observation for 2 years, the right thoracic curve had not progressed, and it measured 25 degrees. The patient was mature on first presentation and had undergone most of her growth.

is not the case. All large series have too few boys to make any differences found statistically valid.

Other factors thought to be related to curve progression have been evaluated but have not been proven to be of use. These factors include a family history of scoliosis, the rotational prominence, decompensation, and numerous radiographic measurements, such as the RVAD and the vertebral rotation as measured by the Pedriolle method.[85]

TREATMENT. When an adolescent presents with idiopathic scoliosis, a full history and physical examination is performed to exclude other causes of scoliosis. A standing posteroanterior view of the whole spine is obtained, preferably on a 36-inch (90-cm) cassette. With careful positioning of a 14- by 17-inch (35- by 43-cm) cassette, it is possible to assess the spine for the presence of a curve. In juveniles and smaller adolescents this size film can be used. In general, the longer 36-inch cassette is preferred in adolescence because the whole spine is always seen, and a better appreciation of the spinal balance is obtained. An essential part of the examination is a complete neuro-

logic assessment including abdominal reflexes. Absent, decreased, and asymmetric reflexes may be the only sign of intraspinal pathology and indicate the need for an MRI scan. The standing radiograph is assessed with identification of the end vertebrae and measurement of all the curves. There are specific curve patterns in idiopathic scoliosis and if the radio-

TABLE 17-2. *Incidence of Progression of Untreated Adolescent Idiopathic Scoliosis With the Cross-Correlations of Curve Magnitude and Risser Sign*

	CURVE MAGNITUDE	
RISSER SIGN	*<19 degrees*	*20–29 degrees*
0–1	22%	68%
2–4	1.6%	23%

From Lonstein JE, Carlson JM. The prediction of curve progression in untreated idiopathic scoliosis during growth. J Bone Joint Surg [Am] 1984;66:1061.

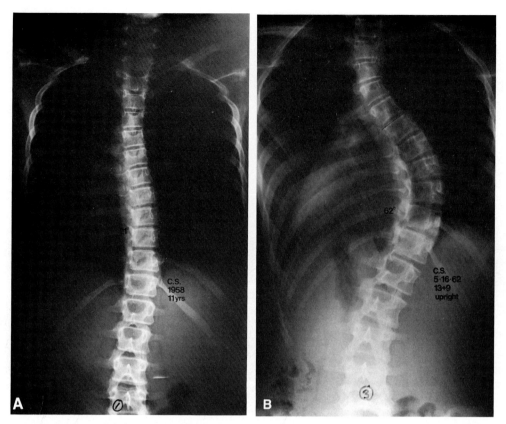

FIGURE 17-13. (A) This 11-year-old girl presented with a 21-degree right thoracic idiopathic scoliosis. She was premenarchal and had a Risser sign of 0. (B) She was followed with periodic evaluations, and 2.5 years later, the curve had progressed to 62 degrees.

graph shows an unusual curve pattern, such as single left thoracic curve, the possibility of nonidiopathic scoliosis must be entertained. Even with a normal neurologic examination and a normal forward-bending evaluation without restriction and deviation an MRI scan is indicated. In cases of a left thoracic curve pattern, studies with routine MRI scans have shown a 20% incidence of intraspinal pathology (Fig. 17-14).[167]

With the history, the physical examination, and the radiographic evaluation the important facts for decision making have been collected. These are the child's growth potential characteristics (i.e., age, Tanner grading, menarchal status in girls, axillary hair development in boys, and Risser grading) and curve characteristics (i.e., curve magnitude and curve pattern). Of importance are Tanner stages 1 and 2; the appearance of Tanner stage 2 indicates the onset of the adolescent growth spurt. The onset of menarche in girls and axillary hair development in both genders occurs after peak height velocity on the adolescent growth curve and indicates that the major portion of the growth spurt is completed and the growth velocity is decreasing. Two other factors that enter into the decision-making process are the cosmetic appearance of the child and any social factors that may have an impact on treatment.

The choices available for treatment are nonoperative and operative. Observation is considered a nonoperative treatment. All curves in the adolescent over 45 to 50 degrees are treated operatively. It must be remembered that the stage of most active growth in the adolescent growth spurt is the stage of increasing growth velocity to the point of peak height velocity and just beyond. Clinically the child is a Tanner stage 2 or 3, which in girls is premenarchal, and has no axillary hair development and a Risser iliac apophysis ossification of 0 or 1. For curves less than 45 degrees, the first question is whether the child is still growing. If the child is at or near the end of growth (i.e., postmenarchal, with axillary hair development and a Risser sign of 3 or more), the curve is followed for progression, with a repeat standing posteroanterior roentgenogram every 4 to 6 months until maturity and the cessation of growth. Larger curves or curves that progress are treated surgically. Some progression can be accepted in smaller curves as the child matures, and as long as the progression is slow the curve remains less than 40 degrees, the cosmetic appearance is satisfactory, and the progression does not continue after the end of growth.

When the child is still growing, the treatment depends on the magnitude of the curve. If the curve is

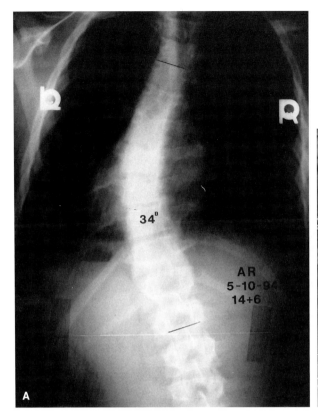
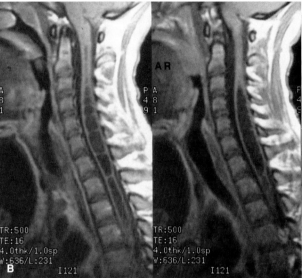

FIGURE 17-14. (**A**) A 14-year, 6-month-old boy presented with a 34-degree left thoracic scoliosis detected during school screening. He was completely asymptomatic, and the physical examination was completely normal except for absence of the left abdominal reflexes. This finding plus the presence of a left thoracic curve—an "abnormal" pattern for idiopathic scoliosis—are indications for further evaluation with a magnetic resonance imaging (MRI) scan. (**B**) The sagittal MRI scan showed a large loculated cervical spinal cord syrinx. The patient was referred to a neurosurgeon for evaluation for decompression through a suboccipital craniectomy.

less than 25 degrees in the growing child and no previous radiographs have been taken, the curve is followed for progression. A repeat roentgenogram is taken after 6 to 8 months for smaller curves (<20 degrees) and after 3 to 4 months for larger curves. A 5-degree increase is progression, and for smaller curves initially less than 19 degrees a 10-degree change is necessary. If the curve progresses, nonoperative treatment is indicated, and with no progression observation continues until maturity and the end of growth. Not all progressive curves need treatment because not all progression is equal. Of importance is the age of the child and the rate of progression. A 12-year-old girl with a Risser sign of 0 who has progression from 20 to 28 degrees over 6 months needs treatment. On the other hand, a 12-year-old girl with a Risser sign of 0 who progresses slowly from 20 to 35 degrees over 3 years to the end of growth does not require active treatment. This applies as long as she is at least 1 or more years postmenarche, has completed growth, is mature with a Risser of 4 or 5, has a good cosmetic appearance, and the curve has stopped progressing. Follow-up should continue into early adulthood to ensure that the progression that had occurred has stopped.

A growing child with a curve of 30 to 40 degrees on the first visit needs immediate treatment, whereas curves between 25 and 29 fall into the gray zone in which many surgeons observe these curves for progression. In the very immature child who is premenarchal with a Risser of 0 or 1 and a curve that is structural, nonoperative treatment should be started immediately.[87] In a more mature child, the curve is closely followed for progression.

NONOPERATIVE TREATMENT. The aim of nonoperative treatment is to control the curve and prevent it from progressing and to obviate the need for surgical stabilization. In addition, the cosmesis of the child should be improved whenever possible. The choices for nonoperative therapy include orthotic treatment, exercises, electrical stimulation, manipulation, and biofeedback. Electrical stimulation of the muscles on the convexity of the curve using implanted or surface electrodes has been used in the past in adolescent idiopathic scoliosis. Early reports showed good results, but these studies included patients still under treatment, with few mature patients and no long-term follow-up.[9,10,16,20,100] Larger studies of a cohort that had completed treatment, with strict definitions of failure and comparisons to natural history, have shown that the results of stimulator treatment are no different than natural history predictions.[3,17,86,147]

Exercises have been used for years in many centers, both during observation and as a form of nonoperative treatment. There is no report documenting the beneficial effect of exercise in controlling or improving progressive curves. Manipulation and biofeedback have been used to treat adolescent idiopathic scoliosis. There are no studies or reports on the results of these treatments and no evidence that they alter the natural history of adolescent idiopathic scoliosis. They should play no role in the treatment of these children.

ORTHOTIC TREATMENT. The indications for orthotic treatment are a growing child who presents with a curve of 30 to 40 degrees or with curves less than 29 degrees who have shown documented progression. Curves of 25 to 29 in the immature (Risser 0, Tanner 1 or 2) child also should be treated immediately. The contraindications for bracing are a child who has completed growth or a growing child who has a curve over 45 degrees or less than 25 degrees without documented progression. True thoracic lordosis, because of the effect of orthoses on the thoracic spine, is also a contraindication to orthotic treatment. Obviously a child with a nonsupportive home situation or a child who refuses to wear a brace is not a candidate for this treatment.

The choices for orthotic treatment are the Milwaukee brace and the TLSO. The first successful orthosis for the treatment of adolescent idiopathic scoliosis was the Milwaukee brace, also known as a cervicothoracolumbosacral orthosis. It consists of a molded pelvic section, which is either custom made[15] or uses a prefabricated module of the Boston system.[51] Attached to the pelvic section are two posterior uprights and one anterior upright connected to a neck ring, and pads are attached to the uprights (Fig. 17-15).

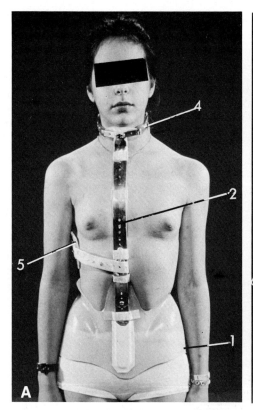 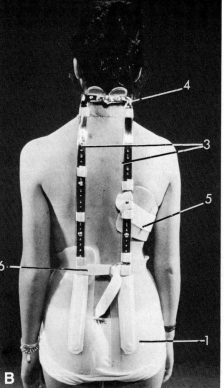

FIGURE 17-15. (**A**) Front and (**B**) back view of a Milwaukee brace. The pelvic girdle is closely contoured to the pelvis, with deep indentations in the waistline, and is cut higher in the front to allow 100 degrees of hip flexion and left low posteriorly to control lumbar lordosis (1). The anterior upright is well centered (2), and the two posterior uprights are parallel (3). The neck ring is attached to these uprights, tilts forward from back to front, and supports the suboccipital pads and throat mold (4); the throat mold does not touch the chin. A thoracic pad for a right thoracic curve is attached by straps to the anterior and posterior uprights (5). A posterior strap connects the pelvic section and is closed snugly (6). On the left side under the pelvic section in the area of the strap is a left lumbar pad.

The TLSO is the generic name for a group of orthoses that are divided into two distinct types: an underarm type and a lower type. Both types of orthoses have a pelvic portion that is like the pelvic section of the Milwaukee brace. The underarm variety extends up to one or both axillae, and the lower type extends only to the lower thoracic area. There are many designs of these orthoses, each being named for the city or center of origin (Fig. 17-16).[12,23,51,99,131]

Historically the Milwaukee brace was used for thoracic and double curves, whereas the TLSO was prescribed for single lumbar and thoracolumbar curves. With widespread use of TLSOs these indications have changed and have become better defined. In general, a TLSO is not used for a thoracic curve with an apex above T8; because of the TLSO's configuration, no corrective force can be applied to a curve apex above this level. For all thoracic curves in which the apex is above T8, a Milwaukee brace is the only effective means of orthotic treatment. For all other curves the choice is between the Milwaukee brace and TLSO. The decision is made by the treating physician based on the patient's age, the cosmetic appearance, the amount of decompensation, and the structure of the curve. Thoracic curve patterns with an apex at or above T8 have to be treated in a Milwaukee brace. These are the double thoracic patterns, which are seen either as the only structural curves or associated with thoracolumbar or lumbar curves.

Once an orthosis is chosen, pads are added that depend on the curve pattern: a trapezius pad for a high thoracic curve, a thoracic pad for a thoracic curve, a combination of an oval and a lumbar pad for a thoracolumbar curve, and a lumbar pad for a lumbar curve. These pads are added to whatever orthosis is prescribed. They are suspended from the uprights in the Milwaukee brace and built into the Milwaukee brace pelvic section or TLSO. Attention must be paid to the sagittal profile of the spine, especially to any hypokyphosis present. In this situation, modifications are made to the brace that prevent an increase of the hypokyphosis and maximize the thoracic pad's corrective force. In the Milwaukee brace, this entails contouring the posterior uprights posteriorly, using a large thoracic pad placed lateral to the posterior upright, and avoiding the use of an anterior outrigger. An anterior gusset is sometimes added. All of these modifications move the corrective vector of the thoracic pad from posterior to posterolateral. The orthopaedic surgeon's understanding of this treatment

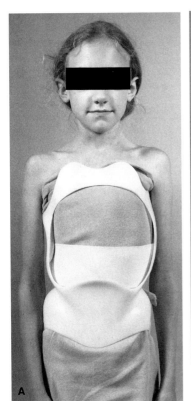
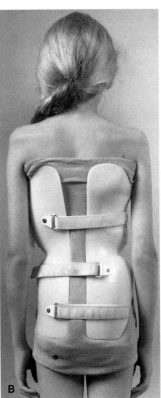
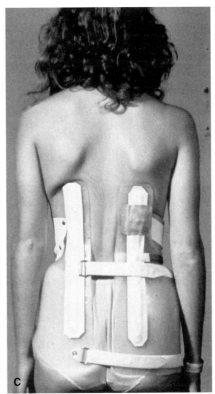

FIGURE 17-16. (**A** and **B**) Underarm thoracolumbarsacral orthosis (TLSO) for treatment of scoliosis. The orthosis extends to the sternum anteriorly with an axillary extension on the left side (**B**). There is pressure over the rotational prominence for a right thoracic curve; opposite this on the left, there is a relief. (**C**) Low-profile TLSO with posterior bars.

leads to better communication with the orthotist when ordering the orthosis, better care of the child (e.g., improved fit of the orthosis), and improved ability to analyze brace problems.

The brace is prescribed for full-time wear with time out for bathing and athletic activity. The child should be encouraged to be active in sports and remain active in these sports in the brace, if possible. Contact sports (e.g., soccer, hockey) are not allowed in the brace, not because the child in the brace will be hurt but to protect the other participants. Should the child play such sports he or she should do so out of the brace. These activities total an average of 2 to 4 hours per day, so that the brace is worn 20 to 22 hours per day. Use of the brace part-time, or only at night, has been advocated by some treating physicians and is widely used in some centers, but there is no literature that proves the effectiveness of this regimen in adolescents. Some small series with short follow-up out of the brace suggest that part-time bracing is effective.[59,131] They do not compare their results to natural history or to full-time use of the brace, and one series states that "the results are not as good as those obtained with full-time wear."[59]

Follow-up should be performed every 4 months with radiographs taken with the child in the brace at every visit. The fit of the brace is checked, and appropriate adjustments are made for growth. Some physicians obtain radiographs of the patient while they are not wearing the brace, but this does not show the effect of the brace on the curve and the child's balance. Weaning from the brace is started at the end of growth, as evidenced by no increase in height, a Risser sign of 4, and 12 to 18 months postmenarche. In boys this weaning begins later because their growth spurt starts later and is longer in duration. The brace is discontinued by slowly decreasing the time the patient spends in the brace or it can be discontinued at once at the end of growth. In many cases, to maintain curve control, gradual weaning is necessary, and there is no way to predict who will be successfully treated by brace discontinuation versus weaning. In addition, it is impossible to reestablish a brace-wearing program in the adolescent once the brace has been discontinued. For these reasons it is better to treat all the children with a gradual weaning program.

A standing posteroanterior radiograph is scheduled 4 hours out of the brace, and this is compared with the most recent radiograph in the brace. If the curve control is maintained, with minimal loss in the curve, the patient is allowed to be out of the brace 4 hours daily. This is repeated every 4 months, with an additional 4 hours out of the brace, on every visit until the child only wears the brace while sleeping. This

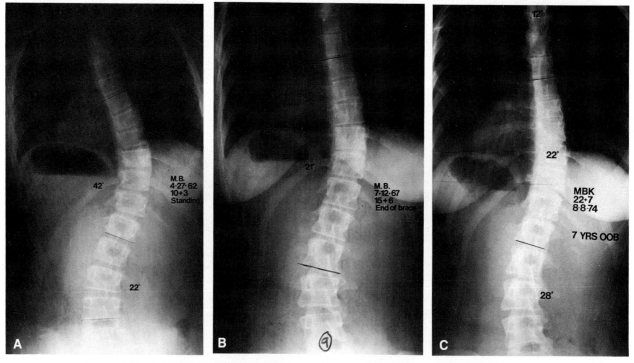

FIGURE 17-17. (**A**) A 10-year-old girl with a 42-degree right thoracic idiopathic scoliosis. She was premenarchal, and the Risser sign was 0. Treatment with a Milwaukee brace was started immediately. (**B**) Five years later, at the completion of orthotic treatment, the curve measured 21 degrees. (**C**) Seven years later, at the age of 22 years, 7 months and after two pregnancies, her curve remained unchanged at 22 degrees.

final stage of wearing the brace is usually during the final 6 to 12 months of treatment. After this a radiograph is obtained 1 week out of the brace, and then bracing is discontinued. This regimen has given the best results of bracing (Figs. 17-17 and 17-18).

RESULTS. Many articles in the literature discuss the results of nonoperative treatment of adolescent idiopathic scoliosis treated with various orthoses, including the Milwaukee brace,[26,50,71,108] the Boston bracing system,[51,78,112,128] the Wilmington brace,[12,130] the Corset Lyonaisse,[109] and the Charleston brace.[131] There are many problems with the reported series. They include juveniles and adolescents as well as different curve magnitudes and different lengths of follow-up. There are no matched, untreated control groups, and the series do not compare the results of bracing with studies of natural history. In addition many studies evaluate the response of curves to the brace rather than the result of curve patterns. For instance, the thoracic curve in the single thoracic pattern is analyzed with the thoracic curves in the double thoracic pattern and the double thoracic and lumbar patterns.

The results in these series are expressed two ways: those who failed bracing and underwent surgical stabilization and those who at follow-up had progressed 5 or more degrees compared with their prebrace curve. The surgical rates vary greatly in the literature, from 3% to 22%, but the series are not comparable because the range of curves varies greatly, with varying follow-up out of the brace. Three series found an increase in the surgical rates with increased curve magnitude.[51,116,146] The indications for surgery are not stated, and they vary from city to city, country to country, and surgeon to surgeon. Some cases of surgery are related to patient factors and not brace failure.

Long-term studies of the Milwaukee brace give similar results, with an initial improvement in the brace and a gradual loss of correction so that at the end of bracing the average curve is 10% to 15% better than the prebrace curve.[26,50,71,108] At follow-up 5 or more years out of the brace the average curve is about the same as the prebrace curve.

Only one study has compared the results with the natural history and concentrated on curve patterns rather than curves. A colleague and I[87] reviewed 1020

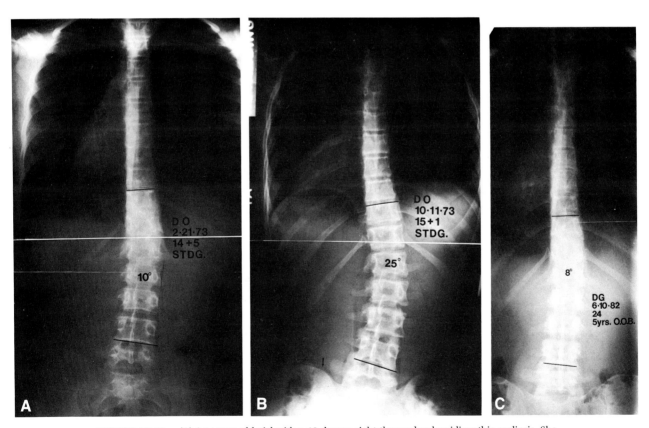

FIGURE 17-18. (**A**) A 14-year-old girl with a 10-degree right thoracolumbar idiopathic scoliosis. She was premenarchal, with a Risser sign of 0. (**B**) After a period of observation, the curve progressed to 25 degrees. At this stage, she was still premenarchal, but the Risser sign was 3+. Because the scoliosis showed definite progression and the patient had growth remaining, she was placed in a thoracolumbarsacral orthosis (TLSO). (**C**) She was treated with full-time wear for 2 years and gradually weaned from the orthosis over an additional 2 years. After being out of the orthosis, at the age of 24 years and after one pregnancy, curve correction was maintained at 8 degrees.

adolescents treated with the Milwaukee brace for an average of 3.8 years, and 54% of the patients had more than 2 years of follow-up out of the brace. Two thirds of the prebrace curves were between 20 and 39 degrees, and the single right thoracic pattern was the most common, constituting one third of the cases. The overall surgical rate was 22%; the most common indications for surgery were an initial response in the brace followed by an increase in the curve with bracing. The surgical rate increased with increased curve magnitude over 30 degrees, and it also increased in immature patients with a Risser sign of 0 or 1 compared with more mature patients with a Risser sign of 2 or more.

The results also were compared with a prediction based on natural history, using the figures from a study from the same center with a similar patient base.[85] Failure of bracing was defined as those patients needing surgery and those who at follow-up had curves that were 5 or more degrees larger than the prebrace curve. The four main curve patterns of 20 to 39 degrees were analyzed. For curves of 20 to 29 degrees and a Risser sign of 0 or 1, the Milwaukee brace results showed a failure rate of 40% compared with a natural history prediction of 68% progression, a statistically significant difference ($P = 0.0001$). With the same curve magnitude and a Risser of 2 or more, the Milwaukee brace had a 10% failure rate compared with a 23% failure rate with natural history. This is also a significant difference ($P = 0.022$). For curves of 30 to 39 degrees, the corresponding figures were 43% versus 57% for a Risser sign of 0 or 1 and 22% versus 43% for a Risser sign of 2 or more. Although the Milwaukee brace results are half those of the natural history predictions, the number of cases in the natural history group is too small to get a statistical validation for this group. These results indicate that the Milwaukee brace alters the natural history of idiopathic scoliosis.

There are only a few series that evaluate the results of the TLSO. Bassett and colleagues[12] reviewed 79 children over the age of 9 years with curves of 20 to 39 degrees treated with the Wilmington TLSO. They found that 30% of the children had progressed 5 or more degrees, the progression rate varying with the curve pattern. The rates were 36% for thoracic curves, 16% for thoracolumbar curves, and 38% for double major curves. This series is a combination of juvenile and adolescent idiopathic scoliosis patients.

Nachemson recently concluded a prospective, multicenter, multinational study of the nonoperative treatment of adolescent idiopathic scoliosis that was funded by the Scoliosis Research Society.[118] All the patients were girls with idiopathic scoliosis and single curves of between 25 and 35 degrees with an apex from T8–L1 and 5 or more vertebrae in the curve. The skeletal age of the girls on presentation was between 10 and 15 years. Each center treated the patients consistent with its views; the patients at each center were observed, treated with electrical stimulation, or treated with a TLSO. Electrical stimulation was found not to be an effective treatment method; the results of stimulation were the same as those of observation. These cases were included with the observation cases to form the natural history group. Using survival analysis, the brace was found to be statistically effective in altering the natural history ($P < 0.0001$). Even if the cases lost to follow-up were regarded as failures, this statistical difference existed ($P = 0.0005$). The failure rate for observation and electrical stimulation was 70% compared with a 40% failure rate of bracing.

These studies show that bracing alters the natural history of adolescent idiopathic scoliosis with statistical significance.

OPERATIVE TREATMENT. Despite the best nonoperative treatment some curves progress. In addition, curves present that are too large or too late for nonoperative treatment. These cases are considered for surgery. The decision to perform surgery is made with a knowledge of natural history. A premenarchal girl with a 40- to 45-degree single right thoracic curve, a Tanner score of 2 to 3, and a Risser sign of 0 either on first presentation or with progression in an orthosis would be considered for surgery. The same curve in a postmenarchal girl with a Tanner score of 4 and a Risser sign of 3 to 4 on first presentation or with progression in an orthosis can be merely observed as long as the cosmetic appearance is acceptable and the curve does not progress.

Thus the indications for operative treatment of idiopathic scoliosis in the adolescent are: 1) A child in the rapid growing phase who presents with a curve of over 40 to 45 degrees, 2) progression to a curve of 40 to 45 degrees while under nonoperative therapy, either in adolescent idiopathic scoliosis or in the juvenile at the onset of the adolescent growth spurt, or 3) curves over 50 to 60 degrees in a mature adolescent.

The decision for surgery must not be based on the Cobb measurement alone. The age and maturity of the child and the growth potential and possibility of progression are important. A 45-degree thoracic curve in an 11-year-old premenarchal girl has a high likelihood of progressing, whereas the same curve in a 17-year-old person who has completed growth is unlikely to progress. The curve pattern is important in deciding whether to operate; a 12-year-old child with a single thoracic curve of 40 degrees is a more likely candidate for surgery than an age-matched patient with a double thoracic and lumbar pattern with

40-degree curves. The cosmetic appearance concerning decompensation, thoracic prominence, and the presence of thoracic lordosis is important.

PREOPERATIVE EVALUATION. The preoperative evaluation includes a full history and physical examination, including a complete neurologic evaluation. Once surgery is recommended, additional radiographs are necessary for the decision-making process. A lateral view is obtained so that the spine can be appreciated in three dimensions, and an evaluation of flexibility of all curves is obtained. Preoperative casting[61,114] or preoperative Cotrel traction were used to possibly correction and reduce the risk of neurologic complications, but it has been shown that traction did not increase correction.[14,40,82] The advent of intraoperative neurologic monitoring has made these techniques obsolete.

When performing a spinal fusion in a patient with adolescent idiopathic scoliosis, decisions have to be made regarding the surgical procedure: the curves needed to be fused, the levels to which they need to be fused, the surgical approach, the instrumentation, and the type of postoperative immobilization. The aim of surgical treatment is correction and stabilization of the deformity with prevention of future progression. This must be performed as safely as possible, with minimal complications and the best clinical and radiologic outcome.

SELECTION OF THE FUSION AREA. In selecting the fusion area the curve pattern is identified, noting the major and compensatory curves. This is achieved by analyzing the clinical appearance and the standing and supine side-bending radiographs. The curve patterns are either a single major pattern (single major thoracic, lumbar, or thoracolumbar) or a double major pattern (double major thoracic, thoracic and lumbar, or thoracic and thoracolumbar). Thoracic idiopathic curves were reviewed by King and colleagues[73] and divided into five curve patterns. King pattern types II and III are the most common; each comprise one third of the series. These five patterns are shown in Table 17-3, in which the classification is based on the clinical appearance and the radiographic evaluation. Two important patterns were identified. A King type II pattern is a structural thoracic curve with a compensatory flexible lumbar curve in which selective fusion of the thoracic curve alone is possible. The unfused lumbar curve spontaneously balances the fused thoracic spine as long as the thoracic curve is not corrected beyond the ability of the lumbar curve to balance. The other important pattern is the double thoracic pattern (King type V), in which fusion of both thoracic curves is necessary.

TABLE 17-3. *Curve Patterns of Thoracic Curves*

Type I
Double thoracic and lumbar curves
Thoracic and lumbar prominences clinically
Both curves cross the midline
Lumbar curve may be larger than the thoracic curve
Both curves are structural with nearly equal flexibility on supine side bending
True double-major curve; both require fusion

Type II
Thoracic and lumbar curves
Minimal lumbar prominence clinically
Both curves across the midline
Lumbar curve is more flexible on supine side-bending examination
False double-major pattern allowing selective fusion of the thoracic curve

Type III
Thoracic curve
Minimal or no decompensation
Lumbar curve does not cross the midline

Type IV
Long thoracic curve
Marked decompensation
Curve reaches the midline at L4, which tilts into the curve

Type V
Double thoracic curve
Positive tilt of T1 with prominent left neckline
High left and right thoracic prominences clinically
Upper left curve structural on side-bending examination

From King HA, Moe JH, Bradford DS, Winter RB. The selection of fusion levels in thoracic idiopathic scoliosis. J Bone Joint Surg [Am] 1983; 65(9):1302.

Once the curve pattern has been identified, all the major curves need to be fused. The most common errors seen are failure to recognize the thoracic curve with a compensatory lumbar curve below (i.e., not differentiating a King type II from a King type I curve pattern) and failure to recognize the double thoracic pattern, usually due to not using a long film cassette.

Determining the level of fusion depends on the identification of the end vertebrae of the curve or curves to be fused and the vertebral rotation.[121] These principles were established years ago by Moe[113,114] and Goldstein[57,58] and confirmed by the review of King.[73] All the vertebrae included in the measured major curve or curves are to be fused. The fusion also must extend from a neutrally rotated (i.e., nonrotated) vertebra cranially to a neutrally rotated vertebra caudally, which is usually the end vertebra of the curve or one vertebra beyond it. In addition, the lower end vertebra of the fusion must be the stable vertebra—that vertebra that lies in the midsacral line (a vertical erected from the spinous process of S1), the vertical line lying within its pedicles. Thus, the caudal end vertebra of the fusion must be neutrally rotated and stable. There are two exceptions to these rules. First, when a single lumbar or thoracolumbar curve is treated with an anterior fusion and instrumentation the extent of the fusion is less than the measured curve. Second, in curves in which the end vertebra is L5, or L5 should be included in the fusion because of rotation, the fusion can be stopped at L4, short of the end vertebra of the planned fusion.

The reliability of these rules was demonstrated by King and colleagues,[73] who reviewed 455 patients with thoracic idiopathic scoliosis treated with spinal fusion and Harrington instrumentation. The average follow-up of this series was 5 years, with a range of 2 to 29 years. The study confirmed the principles of fusion to the neutral and stable vertebra caudally. With fusion short of the stable vertebra the curve became longer, and the unfused caudal vertebrae became part of the curve. Although these rules were established with the Harrington system, they still apply with the new systems as long as overcorrection of the treated curve in relation to the unfused compensatory curve is prevented. The third-generation multiple-hook-and-rod systems can involve rod rotation during correction. This procedure was proposed to derotate the spine and aid correction, but CT scans have shown that this rarely occurs. Just straightening the curve results in some element of derotation with an accompanying reduction in the rotational prominence. This derotation maneuver can result in change in the sagittal contour and decompensation and should not be used routinely.

The principles for hook placement with the multiple-hook-and-rod systems were originally laid out by Cotrel and Dubousset,[35] the selection of the fusion area being similar to that proposed by Moe[73,114] and Goldstein.[57] Although new principles have been proposed for both the selection of the fusion area and for hook patterns, the original principles have never been disproved. Bridwell,[18,81] Shufflebarger,[141] and others[66] have further subclassified the King curve patterns and proposed fusion beyond the stable and neutral vertebra to solve problems encountered with the newer instrumentation systems when the original principles were not followed.

The spine must be appreciated in three dimensions when selecting the area to be fused because the sagittal contour affects the fusion extent. When there is thoracic hyperkyphosis, thoracic hypokyphosis, or thoracic lordosis, the selection of the vertebrae to be fused must consider both the scoliosis and the sagittal deformity. This necessitates extending the fusion cranially to the upper end of the sagittal curve, usually to T2. In the rare case of a thoracolumbar kyphosis, or to adequately treat the abnormal thoracic sagittal curve (true thoracic lordosis), the fusion must extend into the upper lumbar spine.

There is some difficulty in understanding and handling King type II curves because some classify the pattern as a King type II curve and then fuses into part or all of the compensatory lumbar curve. A King type II thoracic pattern is a structural thoracic curve with a more flexible compensatory lumbar curve that allows selective fusion of the thoracic curve alone. It is seen clinically as a balanced torso with a significant thoracic and smaller lumbar rotational prominence on forward bending. Radiographically it is a double-curve pattern in which the apical vertebrae of the two curves lie completely off the midsacral line. The two curves are nearly equal in magnitude, or the thoracic curve is larger. On supine side-bending examination the thoracic curve is more structural, with the lumbar curve being more flexible (i.e., the side-bending magnitude of the lumbar curve is less then the thoracic-bending magnitude, a difference of 7 to 10 degrees or more being the cut off value). This allows selective fusion of the thoracic curve alone, usually to T11, T12, or L1 (Fig. 17-19). With instrumentation, especially the third-generation systems, it is possible to overcorrect the thoracic curve beyond the ability of the compensatory lumbar curve to balance. This should not be done. The orthopaedist should be aware of this possibility with flexible curves and should take an intraoperative radiograph after obtaining correction to ensure that overcorrection of the thoracic curve has not occurred. This is more likely to occur when the rotation maneuver of the third generation systems is used with a flexible spine. In these cases it is prudent to insert the concave rod without rotation and take an intraoperative radiograph.[72]

The thoracic curve patterns that are confused with the King type II pattern are the double major thoracic and lumbar patterns (King type I) and the single thoracic curve pattern (King type III). A patient with a King type I curve is balanced clinically with significant thoracic and lumbar rotational prominences on forward bending. Radiographically, there are thoracic and lumbar curves that are nearly equal or the lumbar curve may be slightly larger; this can look like the King type II pattern. The difference is seen on the supine side-bending evaluation, in which both curves are structurally equal, giving close to equal values on side bending, or the lumbar curve is more structural. In this pattern both curves need to be fused, generally from T4–L4 (Fig. 17-20).

In contrast, the King type III single thoracic pattern is balanced clinically or shows mild decompensa-

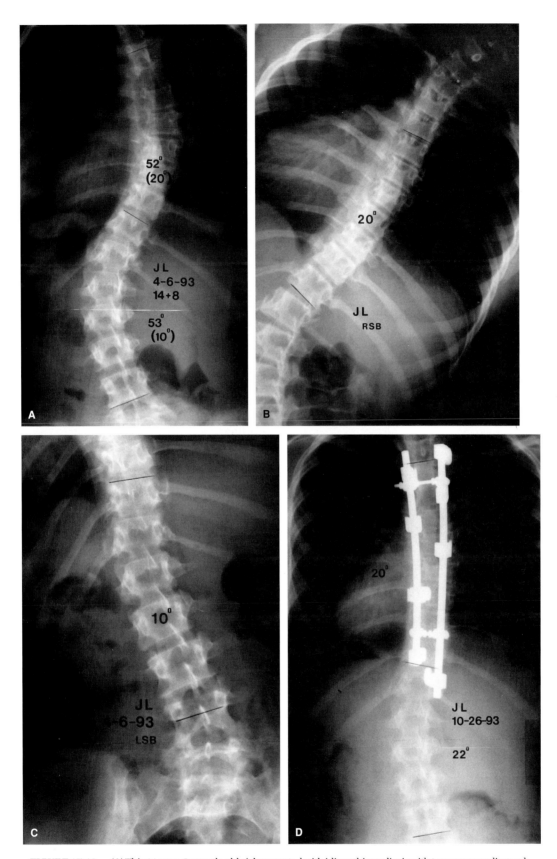

FIGURE 17-19. (A) This 14-year, 8-month-old girl presented with idiopathic scoliosis with two curves radiographically: a right thoracic curve of 52 degrees and a left lumbar curve of 53 degrees. Clinically, she was well balanced with level shoulders and on forward bending had a significant thoracic prominence and a small lumbar prominence. (B) On supine right-side-bending evaluation, the right thoracic curve corrected to 20 degrees. (C) On the supine left-side-bending radiograph, the left lumbar curve corrected to 10 degrees. Selective fusion of the thoracic curve is possible as long as there is not overcorrection of the right thoracic curve. The lower end vertebra of the curve is neutrally rotated and lies on the midsacral line; therefore this vertebra, T11, is the lower end vertebra of the fusion. (D) Fusion was performed from T4-T11, and 8 months postoperatively, the fusion was solid and the thoracic curve was corrected to 20 degrees with the lumbar curve balancing at 22 degrees.

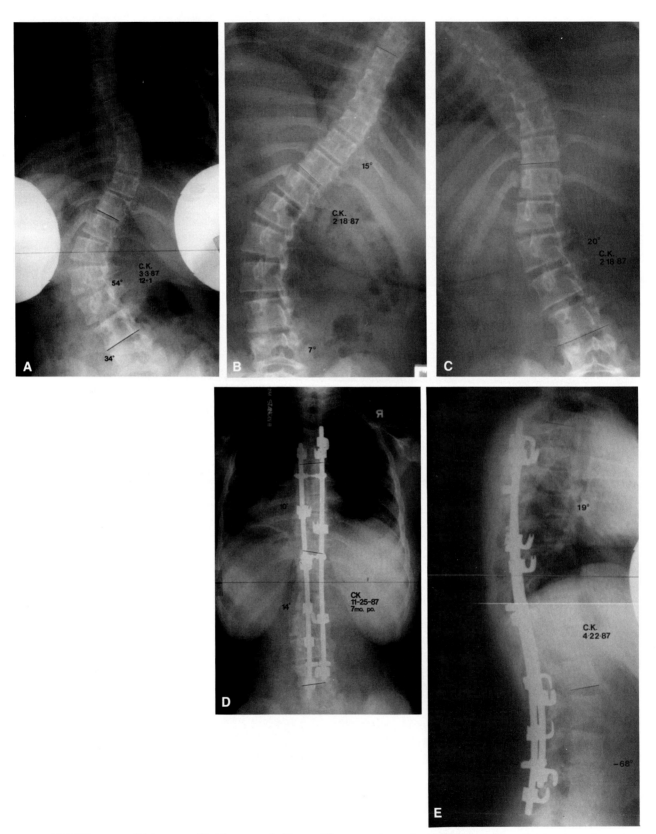

FIGURE 17-20. (A) A 12-year-old girl presented with a rapidly progressing major double idiopathic scoliosis with a right thoracic curve of 43 degrees and a left lumbar curve of 54 degrees. (B) The supine right-side-bending radiograph shows that the right thoracic curve corrected to 15 degrees and the fractional lumbosacral curve to 7 degrees. (C) The lumbar curve corrected to 20 degrees on left-side-bending. (D) Because this is a double curve (King type I), she underwent fusion of both curves from T4-L4. The 7-month postoperative radiograph shows a solid fusion with correction of the thoracic curve to 10 degrees and the lumbar curve to 14 degrees. (E) Lateral radiograph shows maintenance of normal sagittal contours postoperatively. (From Cotrel DF. Dubousset instrumentation and fusion for idiopathic scoliosis. Orthop Clin North Am 1988:19.)

tion to the right and has elevation of the right shoulder. On forward bending there is no lumbar rotational prominence; radiographically there is a larger thoracic curve with a smaller compensatory curve below. The latter curve may be a fractional curve and lie on the midsacral line, or it may be a true curve on which the midsacral line passes through the all the vertebrae of the curve. The apical vertebra does not lie to the left of the midsacral line; this is an essential radiographic feature that differentiates King type II from King type III curves.

The classic double thoracic curve (King type V) is easy to recognize with elevation of the left shoulder and tilt of T1 with elevation of the first rib on the left. Failure to fuse both curves results in further elevation of the first rib and the shoulder with imbalance and a worse cosmetic appearance. A recent article[80] identified another type of double thoracic curve. In this pattern, the radiograph resembles a typical single right thoracic curve, but the shoulders are level rather than an elevated right shoulder, which is typical for a single right thoracic curve. The left hemicurve is not flexible on a left-side-bending evaluation. Failure to recognize this as a double thoracic pattern with fusion to T2 results in elevation of the left shoulder and a worse cosmetic appearance because the shoulders were level preoperatively (Fig. 17-21). The use of these newer systems has resulted in decompensation in some cases, a situation not seen with the earlier systems.

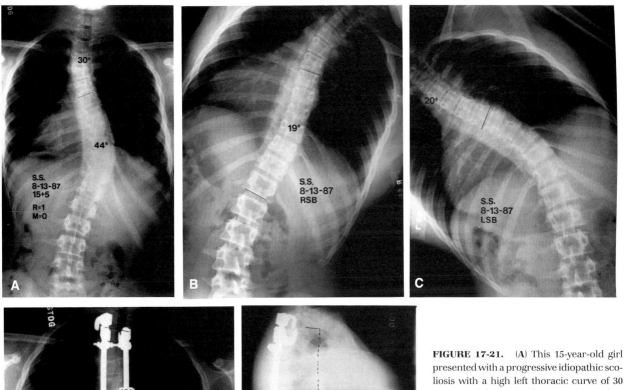

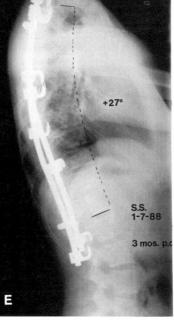

FIGURE 17-21. (**A**) This 15-year-old girl presented with a progressive idiopathic scoliosis with a high left thoracic curve of 30 degrees and a right thoracic curve of 44 degrees. The shoulders are level, but there is elevation of the first rib on the left and a positive tilt of T1. (**B**) The supine right-side-bending radiograph showed correction of the right thoracic curve to 19 degrees. (**C**) The left-side-bending radiograph showed correction of the left thoracic curve to 20 degrees. Both thoracic curves are equally structural and must be included in the fusion, which is a King V curve pattern. (**D**) Three months after posterior fusion with Cotrel-Dubousset instrumentation from T2-L1 the curves measure 19 and 14 degrees, respectively. (**E**) A lateral radiograph at this time shows a normal thoracic kyphosis of 27 degrees. The rod contouring in the thoracolumbar area is to preserve the normal sagittal contour.

In King type II curves in which there is overcorrection of the thoracic curve beyond the ability of the left lumbar curve to correct and balance, results in decompensation to the right. In King type V curves, overcorrection of the right thoracic curve compared with the left thoracic curve, or failure to fuse the left thoracic curve results in elevation of the left shoulder and left neckline. Fusion of a King type II or III pattern beyond the neutral and stable vertebra into the lumbar spine results in decompensation to the left. If a King type III or IV pattern is fused short of the neutral and stable vertebra, there is decompensation to the right (Fig. 17-22).

APPROACH. The possible approaches for the fusion are posterior, anterior, or combined (anterior plus posterior). The posterior approach is the most common used in adolescent idiopathic scoliosis. The surgical technique consists of meticulous subperiosteal exposure, facet excision and packing with autologous bone plugs, and the addition of autologous iliac bone graft. Because of the high fusion rate in children, the surgeon may be tempted to not take an iliac bone graft but rather to use local bone alone or add allograft cancellous bone. This should not be done, and autologous iliac bone should be harvested and used for every posterior fusion. This does not significantly add to the operative time or blood loss, and the use of autograft ensures the best chance of obtaining a solid fusion with sufficient fusion mass.

Instrumentation is added to the fusion procedure to achieve and maintain correction, as discussed below. It must be remembered that the procedure being performed is a spinal fusion, and the instrumentation is an adjunct to the fusion. It is true that the instrumentation portion of the procedure takes the longest and receives the most attention.

An anterior approach is used in the single lumbar and thoracolumbar curve pattern when motion segments can be saved from being included in the fusion area. In these cases the fusion area is only of the central structural area of the curve, which is shorter than the measured curve on the standing radiograph. The fusion area selected includes all the disc spaces that remain wedged open on the convexity of the curve on the supine side-bending evaluation. In addition, the lower end vertebra chosen on the supine side-bending view must at least lie horizontal to the sacrum on the side-bending examination for the the evaluation of the flexibility of the fractional lumbosacral curve (Figs. 17-23 and 17-24). If this correction does not occur on the side-bending examination an anterior procedure alone results in an unbalanced spine. If there is a thoracic curve above the thoracolumbar curve the latter must not be corrected beyond the ability of the thoracic curve to correct on side-bending examination because doing this results in shoulder imbalance.

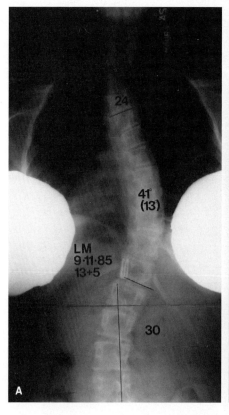 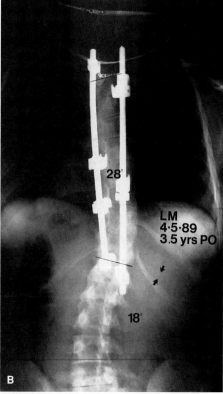

FIGURE 17-22. (A) This 13-year, 5-month-old girl presented with a 41-degree right thoracic idiopathic scoliosis. The curve corrected on side-bending to 13 degrees. This is a single right thoracic curve in the King III pattern. The neutral, stable vertebra is L1; therefore, fusion should extend from T5-L1. (B) Fusion was performed from T5-T12, and this radiograph taken 3.5 years postoperatively shows solid fusion and a right thoracic curve of 28 degrees. Note the mild decompensation to the right and the acute angulation at T12-L1 owing to the fact that she was fused short. She is asymptomatic and continues to be observed.

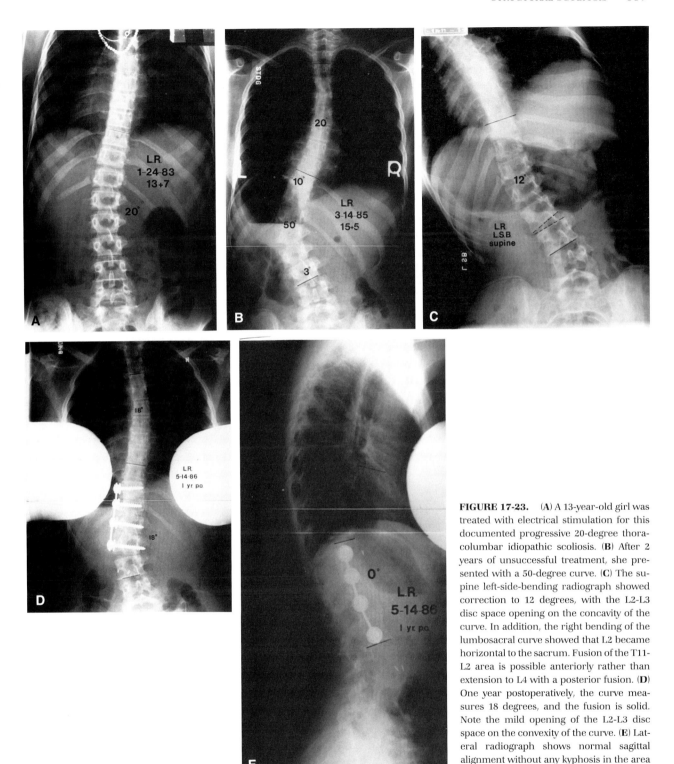

FIGURE 17-23. (**A**) A 13-year-old girl was treated with electrical stimulation for this documented progressive 20-degree thoracolumbar idiopathic scoliosis. (**B**) After 2 years of unsuccessful treatment, she presented with a 50-degree curve. (**C**) The supine left-side-bending radiograph showed correction to 12 degrees, with the L2-L3 disc space opening on the concavity of the curve. In addition, the right bending of the lumbosacral curve showed that L2 became horizontal to the sacrum. Fusion of the T11-L2 area is possible anteriorly rather than extension to L4 with a posterior fusion. (**D**) One year postoperatively, the curve measures 18 degrees, and the fusion is solid. Note the mild opening of the L2-L3 disc space on the convexity of the curve. (**E**) Lateral radiograph shows normal sagittal alignment without any kyphosis in the area of instrumentation and fusion.

The exposure is from the convexity of the curve with radical disc excision, packing of the disc with morselized rib bone, and use of convex compression instrumentation with vertebral body screws.[49,179] Because anterior compression instrumentation tends to produce kyphosis, the presence of preoperative kyphosis in the area of the curve is a contraindication to this approach. This kyphosing effect is lessened with the use of a solid rod with the third generation systems rather than a Dwyer cable or a flexible threaded Zielke rod. The screws are inserted from posterior to anterior to minimize this kyphosing effect, and the anterior annulus is not removed during the discectomy. Some surgeons, to prevent this kyphosing effect of anterior

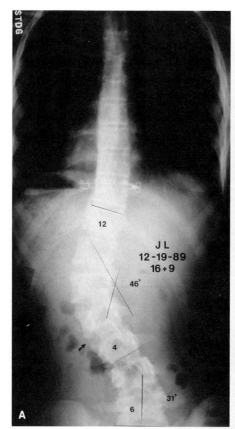

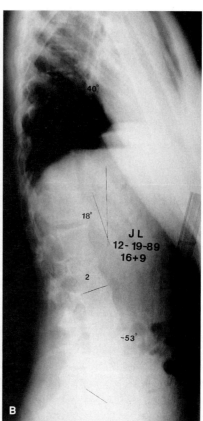

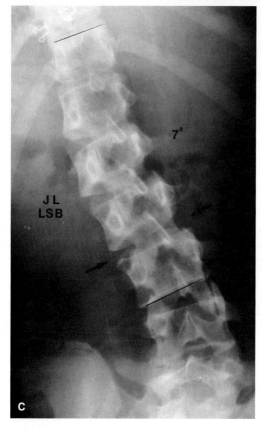

FIGURE 17-24. (**A**) This 16-year, 9-month-old girl presented with a progressive 46-degree left lumbar idiopathic scoliosis. Note that there are six lumbar vertebrae. (**B**) The lateral radiograph shows a 18-degree kyphosis in the area of the curve. (**C**) The left-side-bending radiograph shows correction of the scoliosis to 7 degrees and opening of the L3-L4 disc on the concavity of the curve. (**D**) The right-side-bending radiograph shows that L4 does not correct and become parallel to the sacrum. An anterior fusion and instrumentation is not possible because L3 and L4 do not correct over the sacrum, and there is kyphosis in the area of the curve. A posterior approach is necessary. (**E**) A posterior fusion and Cotrel-Dubousset instrumentation was performed from T11-L4. A radiograph taken 2 years postoperatively shows a solid fusion with a curve of 27 degrees and good balance. Because there were six lumbar vertebrae, three motion segments remain unfused. (**F**) The lateral view postoperatively shows correction of the thoracolumbar kyphosis with a normal sagittal contour. Note the contouring of the rods to maintain this profile.

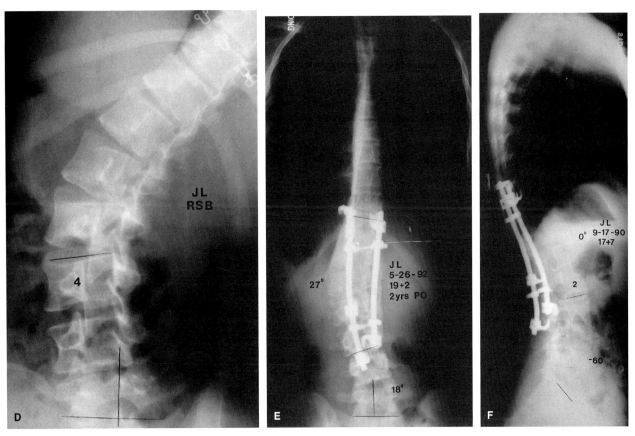

FIGURE 17-24 (*Continued*)

instrumentation, place a piece of rib graft anteriorly in the disc.

The combined approach is used for two indications in the adolescent, for large stiff curves or to prevent the crankshaft effect. The latter is used in the young adolescent before or just at the growth spurt, Risser 0 and Tanner 1. The exact incidence of this possible growth effect is unknown, but it was found in a recent study to be much more common in a child with open acetabular triradiate cartilage.[139] This sign is used as the indicator whether performing an combined or a posterior fusion (Fig. 17-25).

The approach is from the convexity of the curve with excision of the discs and packing of the disc spaces with rib bone. In large curves, if additional correction is desired, a wedge of the end plate is removed using an osteotome so that more shortening on the convexity can occur. This anterior releasing with shortening of the convexity is the principle for large stiff curves. The crankshaft effect is prevented with the disc excision, which removes the growth centers, and anterior growth potential and adds an anterior fusion.

The second-stage posterior fusion and instrumentation is performed 1 week later or under the same anesthetic. Other indications for the combined approach in adolescent idiopathic scoliosis are unusual. These include the presence of a rigid thoracic sagittal deformity (hypokyphosis or hyperkyphosis), which requires an anterior release and fusion for treatment of the sagittal deformity. A rare indication is for a double thoracic and thoracolumbar curve pattern, which can be treated via an anterior fusion and instrumentation for the thoracolumbar curve plus a posterior approach for both curves when it is possible to save a level or two because of the use of the anterior fusion.[76]

INSTRUMENTATION. Instrumentation used with a fusion corrects the deformity and adds stability, allowing ambulation and resulting in a lower pseudarthrosis rate. The original instrumentation was introduced by Harrington[61] and consisted of a distraction rod on the concavity of the curve and a compression rod on the convexity. This system is regarded as the first generation system of spinal instrumentation and consists of a distraction rod alone or distraction and compression rods with or without the the addition of a device for transverse traction (DTT).[7,33] The second-generation systems use segmental fixation with sublaminar (Luque)[92] or spinous process (Drummond) wiring.[43] Modifications of the Harrington system were made with segmental fixation using sublaminar wires or spinous process wires attached to a Harrington rod and a convex Luque rod (Wisconsin system; Fig. 17-26).[45]

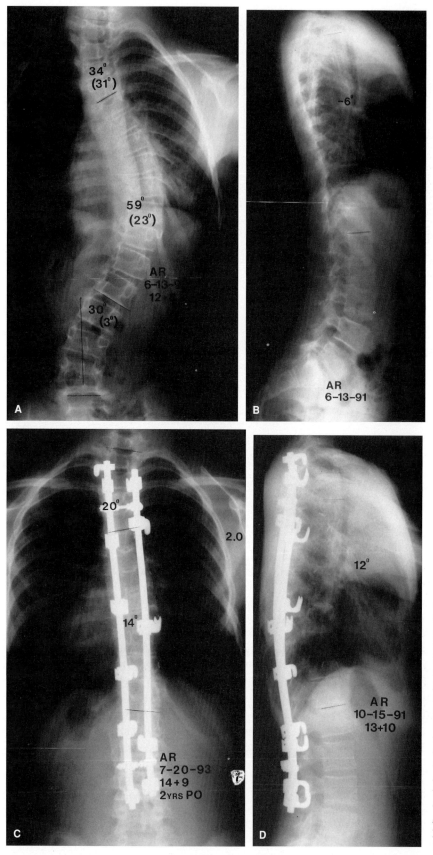

FIGURE 17-25. (**A**) This 12-year, 8-month-old girl presented with a double thoracic idiopathic scoliosis with a high left thoracic curve of 34 degrees and a right thoracic curve of 59 degrees. (**B**) There was an associated thoracic lordosis of −6 degrees, as shown on the lateral radiograph. She was premenarchal with a Risser sign of 0, and open acetabular triradiate cartilages. Because of her age and the curve magnitude, surgery is the treatment of choice. A combined approach is indicated because of her immaturity. (**C**) Two years following a combined anterior and posterior fusion, the fusion is solid, with curves of 20 and 14 degrees, respectively. (**D**) The lateral radiograph shows the rod contouring and improvement of the thoracic sagittal curve to 12 degrees.

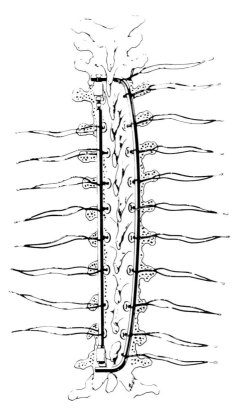

FIGURE 17-26. The Drummond (Wisconsin) system of segmental spinal instrumentation using bilateral spinous process wires with a Harrington distraction rod on the concavity and a Luque rod on the convexity. (Courtesy of Denis Drummond, MD.)

The era of the third-generation systems started in 1984, when Cotrel and Dubousset introduced an instrumentation system consisting of two interlinked rods with multiple hooks on each rod.[34,35] Many similar systems subsequently have been introduced, all consisting of two interlinked rods with multiple hooks (TSRH, ISOLA). The choice of the instrumentation system chosen by the surgeon has not been shown to change the principles of selection of the fusion area.

Anteriorly the Dwyer system was the first system introduced, consisting of vertebral screws introduced on the convexity of the curve with a cable between the screws to give compression.[49] This was modified by Zielke with the use of a threaded rod,[179] which has evolved into a solid rod in the TSRH, synergy, and other systems.

There are many instrumentation options for the scoliosis surgeon, which makes deciding which system to use difficult. In evaluating these options, each of these systems must be considered from many different aspects as discussed by Akbarnia.[2] These include three-dimensional correction, rigidity of fixation, safety, preservation of spinal mobility, technical complexity, training, and cost. There are also the nonscientific factors of prejudice and fads. Factors related to the patient also influence the choice, including curve magnitude and location, sagittal alignment, cosmetic appearance, and the size of the patient.

THREE-DIMENSIONAL CORRECTION. Scoliosis is a three-dimensional deformity, and the effect of the instrumentation on the spine in three dimensions must be considered. The usual manner of assessment of instrumentation is by the effect on the scoliosis using the Cobb measurement. A correction in the initial curve of 40% to 70% is usual. Distraction instrumentation affects the sagittal contour with reduction in the thoracic kyphosis and lumbar lordosis.

The addition of the compression rod increases stability and can reduce thoracic kyphosis. When a square-ended Harrington rod is used with sublaminar wires in the thoracic spine there is an improvement in thoracic hypokyphosis or true thoracic lordosis. The average improvement was 19 degrees in the sagittal contour in one study (Fig. 17-27).[111,165] The use of spinous process wires has been demonstrated to maintain thoracic kyphosis, with an improvement of 4 to 10 degrees.[45,122]

There are few studies that compare different instrumentation systems. Mielke and colleagues[111] compared the treatment of thoracic idiopathic scoliosis with four systems: Harrington distraction rod alone; Harrington distraction rod and compression rods; Harrington distraction rod, compression rods, and a DTT; Harrington distraction rod with sublaminar wires. The average preoperative curves were comparable, and there was no difference in the postoperative correction obtained at surgery and maintained at follow-up. This applied to all the groups described previously, with the exception of the subgroup with sublaminar wires without external support, in which there was a greater loss of correction at follow-up. The degree of correction obtained and maintained with these systems is equal; no system has been shown to offer an advantage in this area.

The other difference found regards the sagittal correction.[111] There was reduced thoracic hyperkyphosis with the use of the Harrington distraction and compression rods and improvement in thoracic lordosis with the use of a Harrington distraction rod with sublaminar wires. All systems, including a technique using segmental fixation with sublaminar wires (Luque or Harrington rod plus sublaminar wires) or spinous process wires (Wisconsin system) and the third-generation systems, are effective in the treatment of thoracic hypokyphosis. When there is true thoracic lordosis, a system with sublaminar wires provides the best correction in the sagittal plane.

The third-generation systems have the capability of three-dimensional correction because of rotation of the concave rod in flexible deformities and rotation of the curve apex transforming the scoliosis into ky-

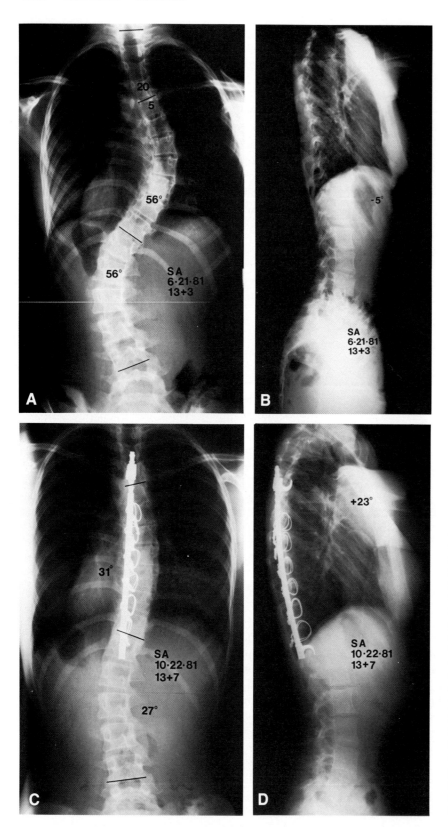

FIGURE 17-27. A 13-year-old girl presented with two 56-degree curves (right thoracic and left lumbar). (**A**) The lumbar curve is more flexible on side-bending (12 degrees for the lumbar curve versus 34 degrees for the thoracic curve). This is classified as a King II pattern, which allows selective fusion of the thoracic curve. (**B**) The lateral view shows thoracic lordosis of −5 degrees. The use of sublaminar wires will improve the correction in the sagittal plane. The patient underwent a posterior fusion from T4-T12 with a kyphotically bent square-ended Harrington rod and sublaminar wires. A thoracolumbarsacral orthosis (TLSO) was used for 4 months postoperatively. (**C**) The thoracic curve was corrected to 31 degrees, with the lumbar curve balancing at 27 degrees. (**D**) A lateral view taken at the same time shows correction of the thoracic lordosis with restoration of thoracic kyphosis to 23 degrees—a 28-degree improvement.

phosis. Because of the potential problems of decompensation reported with King type II curves, King[72] has suggested that not all of these curves should be treated with the rotation maneuver. A thorough assessment and comparison of all these systems is essential with adequate follow-up to compare their effect on the spine in three dimensions and document any advantages one system may possibly have over another.

A distractive force is more effective for curves over 53 degrees, whereas a transverse force is more effective for smaller curves.[158] This and the effect of the instrumentation on the sagittal contour must be considered in the choice of instrumentation.

RIGIDITY OF FIXATION. The quality of the fixation and its rigidity determine the amount of correction obtained at the time of surgery and maintained at follow-up. The larger the number of fixation points the more secure the construct, with a reduced incidence of hook dislodgment and less loss of correction at follow-up. With better quality of fixation less rigid postoperative immobilization is required; some systems require no postoperative immobilization. More rigid fixation also shortens the immobilization time, and it appears to result in faster incorporation of the fusion, although no studies have been performed to prove this.

SAFETY. The safety of the system used, especially the rate of neurologic complications, is important. The use of overdistraction with the Harrington system is a danger.[93] A 0.5% incidence of neurologic complications in idiopathic scoliosis was reported. The use of sublaminar wires in adolescent idiopathic scoliosis resulted in a 17% rate of neurologic complications,[152] although no neurologic complications were reported in another series.[165]

A comparison of the neurologic complications using different instrumentation systems has been reported by the Morbidity Committee of the Scoliosis Research Society.[139a] They reported that the overall incidence of cord problems in idiopathic scoliosis was 0.26%. With the Harrington system, the rate was 0.23%, increasing to 0.60% with the Cotrel-Dubousset system and 0.86% with the use of sublaminar wires. The newer systems report a neurologic rate greater than that of the Harrington distraction rod. These results may reflect early experiences, but these factors must be considered in the choice of instrumentation.

PRESERVATION OF SPINAL MOBILITY. The thoracic spine has little motion, and fusion of the thoracic spine alone does not reduce spinal motion significantly. The lumbar spine, on the other hand, has a lot of mobility, and any fusion will reduce spinal motion. Early studies showed an increase in the incidence of back pain and degenerative changes with fusion to the lower lumbar spine.[30,110] A longer follow-up study was conducted of 172 patients with adolescent idiopathic scoliosis fused with Harrington instrumentation and followed for a minimum of 10 years after spinal fusion (average follow-up, 19 years).[11] This group of patients was compared with an age-, gender-, height-, and weight-matched control group without scoliosis or spine surgery. Patients and control subjects experienced a similar incidence of back pain, and the functional outcome was independent of the caudal extent of the fusion.

The studies to date that evaluate back pain following spinal fusion are relatively short-term follow-up studies because the patients are only in their 30s. Therefore the minimum number of lumbar segments must be fused. This is achieved by following the rules described earlier. The King type II thoracic curve pattern with a compensatory lumbar curve must be recognized, allowing selective fusion of the thoracic curve alone. Whenever possible the single lumbar and thoracolumbar curves should be treated with an anterior fusion and instrumentation, saving one or two lumbar motion segments from the fusion area.

TRAINING. With the introduction of each new instrumentation system the technical complexity increases. Experience is needed with each new system to be able to use the system effectively and assess its role. A surgeon's initial experience with an instrumentation system usually occurs during fellowship. On entering practice this surgeon will most likely choose an instrumentation system based on his or her training and experience rather than the benefits of the system.

COST. The cost of the newer systems is high because the implants cost more and the newer systems are multiple-hook-and-rod systems that require more implants. This increased cost is offset by the fact that no external immobilization usually is required, with no cost for a postoperative brace, and the hospitalization is shorter.

PREJUDICE. Sometimes the choice of instrumentation is based on perceived, nonscientific benefits and advantages. The current fad in new instrumentation may play a role.

Careful monitoring of neurologic function is an essential part of the surgical procedure. This is with the wake-up test of Vauzelle and colleagues[156a] or electronically with spinal cord monitoring using somatosensory evoked potentials (SSEP)[119] or motor evoked potentials (MEP). In SSEP the posterior tibial nerve is stimulated at the ankle, with the stimulus recorded from the cerebral cortex and multiple signals filtered and averaged by a computer. The amplitude of the response as well as the latency between the stimulus and response is measured. Changes are an early warning of possible alteration in the pathway, such as spinal cord damage. In MEP the stimulus is applied to the motor cortex, and the response is read from the muscle. This monitoring is being investigated, and its current clinical role is unclear. The most accurate and cost-effective method of monitoring in adolescent idiopathic scoliosis is the wake-up test. This was first introduced by Vauzelle and colleagues[156a] and consists of reducing the depth of anesthesia after the instrumentation is inserted so that the patient can respond to commands and move the toes and feet. Any electronic technique is an early warning system of possible cord problems, and when this warning occurs a wake-up test is performed. Some sort of monitoring should be used whenever instrumentation is used, but the false-positive and false-negative rate of electronic monitoring is unknown, and a wake-up test should be performed in every case. Electronic monitoring can be performed repeatedly throughout the surgery with the wake-up test performed once the instrumentation is inserted. Any change in neurologic function must be treated with reduction in the distraction or removal of the instrumentation. With the extremely low rate of neurologic complications in surgery for adolescent idiopathic scoliosis, the decreased distractive forces of the third-generation systems, and the cost of monitoring the wake-up test alone is sufficient monitoring in these patients. It must be remembered that it is still possible to have a neurologic problem in the time from the wake-up test to the end of the anesthetic, but this is rare.

POSTOPERATIVE IMMOBILIZATION. With the use of the newer systems with increased internal fixation, it was initially believed that there would be no role for postoperative immobilization. This proved not to be the case with the Luque system and the use of the Harrington rod with sublaminar wiring. Without postoperative immobilization with these systems there is an increased loss of correction and an increased pseudarthrosis rate.[111] The Wisconsin system and the third-generation systems provide excellent maintenance of correction with no apparent increase in the pseudarthrosis rate. It must be remembered that these systems are rigid and for fatigue failure of the instrumentation to occur and a pseudarthrosis to be obvious may take 3 to 4 years. Therefore with the newer systems a minimum follow-up of 5 years is necessary when discussing the pseudarthrosis rate.

Even with these new systems postoperative immobilization is necessary in certain cases. With selective fusion of a thoracic curve, if the lumbar or thoracolumbar curve below it does not balance, the unfused curve needs to be treated nonoperatively. This was never seen with the Harrington system because in these cases postoperative immobilization in a cast was always used, and the lumbar or thoracolumbar curve was always treated. When postoperative immobilization is necessary a postoperative cast or brace is used; a TLSO is the orthosis of choice. The model for the brace is taken standing or supine, the choice depending on the preference of the surgeon. The orthosis, once fitted, is worn full time, with time out for bathing. Brace wearing continues until the end of growth or the unfused curve is controlled.

The postoperative level of activity allowed varies greatly and depends on the surgeon's preference and protocol. I encourage the child to be active postoperatively with a regular walking program, walking up to 1 to 2 miles per day. Running, bicycling, gentle cross-country skiing, horseback riding, swimming (excluding diving), and shooting baskets also are allowed. Bending or twisting are discouraged. The fusion is checked for incorporation after 4 months with supine oblique radiographs, and if satisfactory at this time full activities are allowed. The more active a child is, the better the quality of the fusion mass.

ASSOCIATED PROCEDURES

THORACOPLASTY. In adolescent idiopathic scoliosis, cosmesis is important because it is one of the reasons treatment is sought. Some teenagers openly discuss this aspect of their scoliosis, whereas others require the surgeon to introduce the topic. Surgeons who treat adults know that this is an important aspect of the problem that is generally commented on by the patient postoperatively but rarely preoperatively. The two aspects of the cosmetic effects are the decompensation of the torso in relation to the pelvis with a change in the thoracopelvic relation and the thoracic rotational prominence. With surgical treatment of the scoliosis the spine is rebalanced with restoration of the waistline symmetry and a normal thoracopelvic relation. The effects on the rotational prominence vary, some improving, and some being unchanged. The probable correction of the rotational prominence can be shown clinically preoperatively by actively side bending the thoracic curve while the patient is being examined in the forward-bending position. With curve correction there is often improvement in the prominence, whereas in other cases, usually with a larger and sharper prominence, the correction is less dramatic.

In some cases operative correction of the rotational prominence by thoracoplasty should be considered. This consists of excision of the medial portion of the rib, allowing the lateral rib to rotate and improve the asymmetry. The determining factors in this decision are not only the magnitude of the asymmetry but include the overall contour of the back (sharp or rounded prominence) and the patient's desire for correction. Rib elevations of more than 5 to 6 cm should be considered for correction if desired by the patient, whereas prominences less than 3 cm rarely require correction, Prominences between these numbers fall into the gray zone.

There are two techniques for the thoracoplasty. If an anterior fusion is performed as part of the surgical plan for a large curve, the rib excision can be performed through the thoracotomy, an internal thoracoplasty.[140] The other approach is posterior after correction and instrumentation of the scoliosis.[145] In cases in which the need for a thoracoplasty is questionable, the improvement of the rotational prominence that accompanies the curve correction is evaluated after instrumentation; the decision to perform a thoracoplasty is made at this time.

It must be noted that there is often an increase in the prominence postoperatively, when comparing the follow-up appearance to that immediately postoperatively. In most cases this is an apparent worsening because in the immediate postoperative period there is edema of the paraspinal tissues, especially on the curve concavity, which obscures the cosmetic changes. Once this edema resolves, which may take 6 to 9 months, the true picture is seen. In some cases there is a true increase in the prominence that occurs later with growth. This is unusual and is related to the crackshaft phenomenon.

Congenital Scoliosis

Congenital scoliosis is due to abnormal vertebral development, and the vertebral anomaly is present at birth. Because of this, a curvature is noted much earlier in life in these children than in the typical patient with idiopathic scoliosis.

This early development of the deformity has resulted in a tendency for the young child with congenital scoliosis to receive less than optimum care. Congenital curves tend to be rigid and resistant to correction. The curves are frequently allowed to progress, and because of all the years of growth remaining, large deformities can result. These curves must not be allowed to progress. In many cases early fusion is necessary, which is preferable to allowing severe curves to develop. Early fusion will not stunt the poten-

tial growth because the area of the anomalies and the area that needs to be fused cannot grow in a normal vertical manner because of the undeveloped growth plates.

Classification

The vertebral anomaly is classified into segmentation, formation, and mixed problems that can occur at any part in the vertebral ring (anterior, anterolateral, lateral, posterolateral, or posterior; Fig. 17-28). A hemivertebra is *not* an extra vertebra, but rather the remainder of a vertebra that did not form completely. The anomaly results in a spine deformity because of absent growth potential in the area of the anomaly with the resultant growth in the remainder of the vertebral ring causing the deformity. Depending on where there is loss of growth potential in the ring, the resulting deformity can be pure scoliosis, kyphosis, or lordosis or a combination of scoliosis plus kyphosis or lordosis. The magnitude of the deformity, its behavior, and its rate of progression depend on the type of anomaly and the growth potential of the vertebrae in the area.

Scoliosis

Although it is desirable to be able to associate a certain prognosis with a certain anomaly, this is not always possible. It is best to consider the curve in its general character and see what problem it produces and whether it is progressive, regardless of the specific type of anomaly. Careful documentation of the deformity and the magnitude of the curve by high-quality radiographs and photographs is necessary on the first

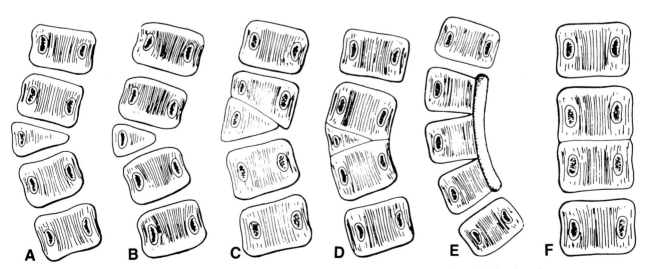

FIGURE 17-28. Anomalies causing scoliosis. (**A**) Wedge vertebra. (**B**) Hemivertebra. (**C**) A hemivertebra nonsegmented on its cranial surface. (**D**) A hemivertebra nonsegmented on both sides. (**E**) A unilateral unsegmented bar. (**F**) A nonsegmented vertebra (bloc vertebra). (From Winter RB. Congenital deformities of the spine. New York: Thieme-Stratton, 1983;12.)

examination. Subsequent serial photography and radiology are important. Children should be followed at 6-month intervals until the end of their growth. Many patients have mild curves that are stable for many years and then suddenly become severe when the adolescent growth spurt begins. Some curves never progress at all and, after being followed for many years, do not result in any significant deformity (Fig. 17-29). These patients, of course, do not require any treatment, and it is foolish to apply an orthosis or perform a fusion for a condition that is neither progressive nor disabling.

Many studies have been performed documenting the natural history of congenital scoliosis. They showed that most curves are progressive, with 10% to 25% being nonprogressive.[77,169] The large study of McMaster and Ohtsuka[105] of 202 patients is the best in this regard. They found that only 11% were nonprogressive, whereas 14% were slightly progressive, and the remaining 75% progressed significantly. The rate of curve increase depended on the area of the spine involved and the type of anomaly. Thoracic curves had the poorest prognosis, with the worst anomaly being a unilateral unsegmented bar (i.e., unilateral failure of segmentation) accompanied by single or multiple convex hemivertebrae (Fig. 17-30). Other anomalies with a poor prognosis are, in order, a unilateral unsegmented bar, double convex hemivertebrae, and a single free convex hemivertebra. The bloc vertebra anomaly (i.e., bilateral failure of segmentation) has the best prognosis.

There are certain anomalies that consistently are associated with progression (e.g., the unilateral unsegmented bar) and are so damaging that the patient with this anomaly should undergo immediate fusion. The unilateral unsegmented bar causes a total lack of growth on the concave side of the curve, and if growth continues on the convex side, a severe deformity results. Once established, this deformity is extremely rigid and virtually impossible to correct except by extraordinary and difficult surgery. Therefore, it is far better to prevent an increase in the deformity than to correct it once it has become severe.

Hemivertebrae may be single or multiple and balanced or unbalanced.[163] They are classified by their relation to the adjacent spine as being incarcerated or nonincarcerated. An incarcerated hemivertebra is "tucked into" the spine and does not change the contour of the spine. The relation of hemivertebrae to the adjacent vertebrae is critical (segmented, semisegmented, or nonsegmented) because it gives an idea of the possible growth potential on the convexity of the curve (see Fig. 17-28). When balanced, contralateral hemivertebrae (i.e., hemimetric segmental displacement or hemimetric shift) often do not progress and do not require treatment. When separated by several segments a double curve is produced, and both curves may progress and require fusion. A single hemiverte-

FIGURE 17-29. (A) A 20-month-old boy with a 33-degree right upper thoracic scoliosis. There are multiple rib synostoses on the left. This is either a unilateral defect of segmentation with a poor prognosis, or a bilateral defect of segmentation with a good prognosis. No active treatment was given, and he was observed for progression. (B) The same patient 28 years later has a 28-degree curve. This indicates a bilateral defect of segmentation with a good prognosis. (From Winter RB. Congenital deformities of the spine. New York: Thieme-Stratton, 1983:61.)

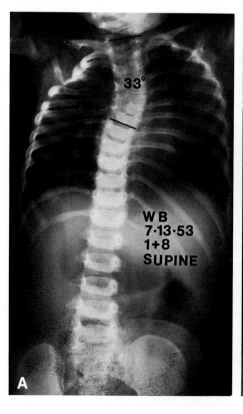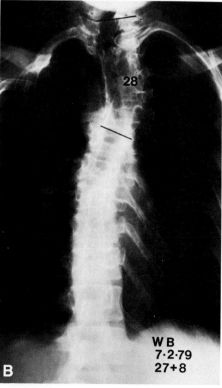

bra, which is the most common anomaly, may or may not cause a progressive deformity, this outcome being difficult to predict.[101] The patient must be carefully followed, and if deformity occurs fusion should be performed. A single hemivertebra at the lumbosacral level produces significant decompensation because there is no room below the hemivertebra for natural compensation to occur. These patients may have a severe list to one side, which is progressive with growth. This list produces a rigid deformity that is extraordinarily difficult to correct.

GENETICS.   The possible genetic origin of congenital spine deformities is intriguing. A study of 337 patients with congenital spinal anomalies found that the majority were sporadic with no risk to subsequent siblings or offspring.[173] Patients with multiple anomalies carried a 5% to 10% risk to subsequent siblings. These findings could not be confirmed at our center in over 1200 congenital deformities, where only about 1% of patients with congenital spinal deformities have a known relative with the problem.[163] Most studies of identical twins show that one twin has the congenital defect and the other does not.[62,129] There are rare reports of both twins with congenital anomalies.[4]

There is only one type of congenital spine anomaly that has a positive family history. This syndrome consists of multiple levels of bilateral failures of segmentation, with multiple fused ribs and often missing segments, and goes by many names: spondylothoracic dysplasia, spondylocostal dysplasia, spondylovertebral dysplasia, and Jarcho-Levin syndrome.[25,69,134] Some of the children die early as a result of respiratory failure. Both recessive and dominant forms of inheritance have been reported.

PATIENT EVALUATION.   Patients with congenital spine anomalies frequently have congenital anomalies involving other organs or systems. It is extremely important that these patients receive a complete evaluation that is not restricted to the spine alone.

The most common associated congenital anomaly is found in the genitourinary tract. Studies of patients with congenital scoliosis revealed a 20% incidence of urinary tract anomalies on routine IVP,[95] whereas Hennsinger's study on cervical anomalies found a higher rate of 33%.[64] This finding is not surprising from an embryologic point of view because the same undifferentiated mesenchyme will differentiate into the vertebra medially and the mesonephros ventrolat-

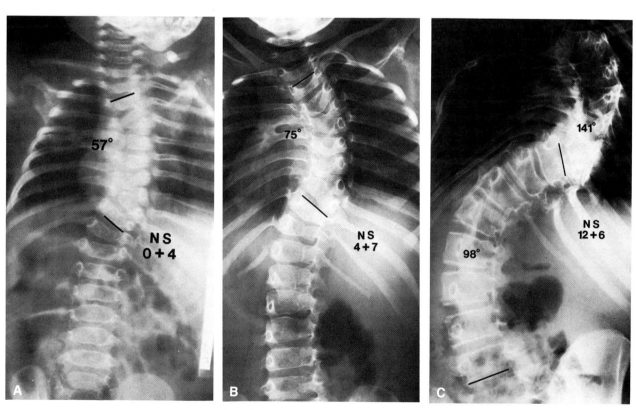

FIGURE 17-30.   (A) A 4-month-old girl with a 57-degree congenital right thoracic scoliosis. There are hemivertebrae on the right and segmentation defects on the left—the most likely of all congenital curves to progress. No treatment was given. (B) At age 4 years, the curve had progressed to 75 degrees. The segmentation defect is more obvious. (C) By age 12 years, her curve had progressed to 141 degrees, and a highly structural 98-degree lumbar curve had appeared. (From Winter RB. Congenital deformities of the spine. New York: Thieme-Stratton, 1983:55.)

erally, the latter forming the kidney and the urinary tract. Many of the anomalies noted do not demand urologic treatment (e.g., unilateral kidney, cross-fused ectopia) because they are anatomic variations with normal renal function. However, 6% of the patients in the study by MacEwen and colleagues[95] were noted to have a life-threatening urologic problem, usually an obstructive uropathy. All patients diagnosed as having a congenital spine anomaly must have a renal tract evaluation (Fig. 17-31). Historically, this evaluation has been performed using an IVP, but renal ultrasonography and MRI have become more common for this function. MRI is used primarily to evaluate the spinal canal in these patients. If an obstructive uropathy is detected during this screening, appropriate urologic procedures should be done before instituting orthopaedic treatment of the scoliosis.

A second area of great concern is the cardiac anomalies. As many as 10% to 15% of patients with congenital scoliosis have been noted to have congenital heart defects.[64,132] These previously may have been undetected. Murmurs should never be attributed to the scoliosis and must be thoroughly evaluated. It is tempting to blame murmurs on distortion of the thorax caused by the scoliosis, but scoliosis does not produce murmurs. Therefore, any murmur must be thoroughly evaluated.

Examination of the back and extremities for evidence of a hidden neurologic disorder is important. There is a high frequency of spinal dysraphism in patients with congenital scoliosis. McMaster reported that about 20% of his patients with congenital scoliosis had some form of dysraphism, such as a tethered spinal cord, fibrous dural bands, diastematomyelia, or intradural lipoma.[103] These neural canal abnormalities frequently are associated with cutaneous changes (e.g., hair patches, dimples, skin pigmentation, hemangiomata) and various abnormalities on the examination of the lower extremities (Figs. 17-32 and 17-33). These include flatfeet, cavus feet, vertical tali, clubfeet, and more subtle changes, such as slight atrophy of one calf, a slightly smaller foot on one side, and asymmetric reflexes. On the other hand, it is possible for a patient to have one of these intraspinal anomalies and have no associated findings. The physician must evaluate the radiographs for any interpediculate widening or midline bony spicules. The use of MRI scans has greatly aided the evaluation of dysraphism. This imaging should be obtained in any patient having neurologic findings, foot deformities, bladder or bowel mal-

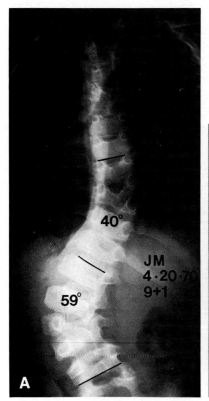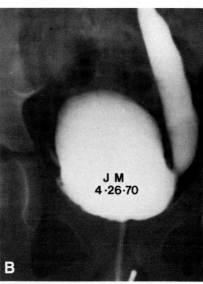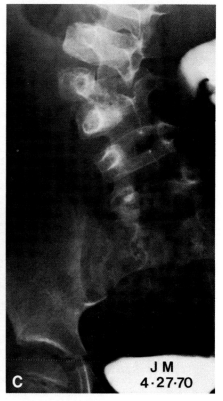

FIGURE 17-31.   (A) A 9-year-old boy with a 59-degree left lumbar congenital scoliosis caused by a hemivertebra. There is a second hemivertebra on the right at T10 with an associated right thoracic scoliosis. (B) An intravenous pyelogram demonstrates uterovesical obstruction with a hydroureter. There were no urinary symptoms. (C) There is associated hydronephrosis of the right kidney.

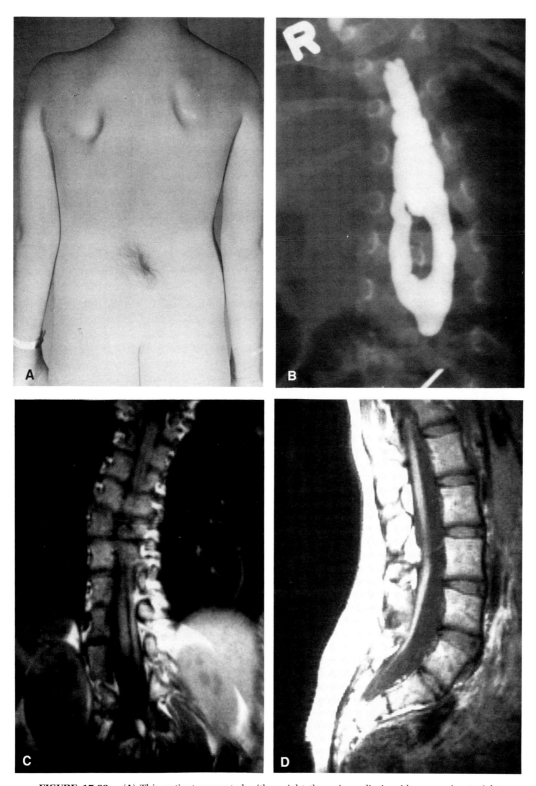

FIGURE 17-32.   (A) This patient presented with a right thoracic scoliosis with a prominent right scapula and a hair patch in the lumbar area. One foot is smaller than the other, and the ankle reflex is absent on the side of the smaller foot. (**B**) A myelogram demonstrates a diastematomyelia. (**C**) A magnetic resonance imaging (MRI) scan shows a diastematomyelia with a split in the spinal cord. This is a fibrous band, not the more common bony spur. (**D**) On the sagittal MRI, the cord extended to the sacral area, with a tight filum terminale for each hemicord.

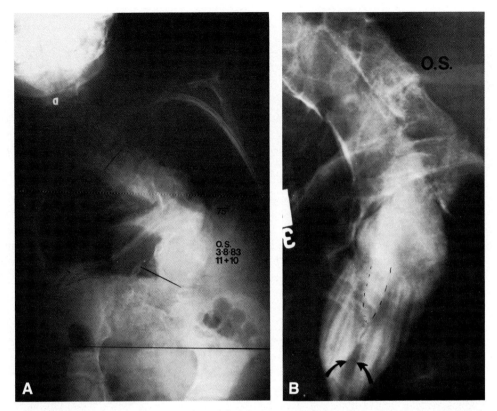

FIGURE 17-33. (A) An 11-year-old boy with a severe congenital scoliosis of 75 degrees also had bilateral talipes equinovarus. (B) A water-soluble myelogram shows a split spinal cord with a low-lying conus and a tight filum terminale.

function, or cutaneous changes overlying the spine or in whom a corrective spinal surgery is planned.[166]

An accurate radiologic evaluation is essential. Supine radiographs should be obtained on all children unable to sit or stand unaided. This view is obtained in older children to accurately see the vertebral anatomy, the upright views showing the deformity. The convex growth is important, and the quality of the bone and disc spaces on the convexity must be clearly seen and inspected. If the disc spaces are present and clearly defined and the convex pedicles clearly formed there is a possibility of convex growth, and the prognosis is poor. On the other hand, if the convex discs are not clearly formed and the convex pedicles are poorly demarcated there is less convex growth potential, and the prognosis is not as bad. It must be remembered that in the first 1 to 2 years of life cartilage forms a significant part of the vertebra, and at this stage prognostication is not as accurate as in the older child.

Routine coronal and sagittal views are obtained initially to appreciate the deformity in both planes; subsequent examinations depend on the deformity that exists. It is important to see the whole spine on both views because multiple anomalies are common, and they may be on opposite ends of the spine, such as one cervical and one lumbosacral anomaly. Accurate vertebral landmarks need to be selected on the end vertebrae of the curves measured, and exactly the same landmarks are used for subsequent radiographs, ensuring the reliability of the evaluation.

ORTHOTIC TREATMENT. Because the primary deformity in congenital scoliosis is in the bones rather than the soft tissues, the curves tend to be rigid; they are not as amenable to orthotic treatment as idiopathic or paralytic curves. Nevertheless, there are definite indications for orthotic treatment of congenital spine deformities. The orthosis of choice is the Milwaukee brace because underarm braces, although they provide effective curve control, do so at the expense of thoracic compression and a reduction of vital capacity, which are undesirable side effects.

A study indicated that certain patients did well in the Milwaukee brace for many years, and a few could even be treated permanently in an orthosis, avoiding surgery.[171] The best results were in patients with mixed anomalies that were flexible and with a progressive secondary curve. The patients who did well had flexible curves with the anomalous vertebrae making up only a part of the curve. The vertebral anomalies were in the cranial, center, or caudal portion of the curve, the curve being much longer than the anomalous area and consisting of normal vertebrae. The brace is effective with a flexible deformity and has no role in a rigid deformity. Orthotic treatment is contraindicated for the treatment of congenital kyphosis. Progressive secondary curves need to be controlled, and the Milwaukee brace is the best method to achieve this.

The other role for orthotic treatment in congenital scoliosis is for the treatment of coronal imbalance, which may be coronal decompensation or head tilt. In coronal decompensation with single or multiple anomalies the Milwaukee brace can be effective in correcting the malalignment, allowing the spine to become balanced with growth. With head tilt in young child with cervicothoracic or upper thoracic anomalies the Milwaukee brace with an occipital pad can correct the head tilt.

The physician must recognize the role of the orthosis when it is used and must monitor this use to ensure that it accomplishes its goal; that is, it must control the curve with acceptable spine alignment. Careful monitoring, both clinically and radiographically, is necessary. If the patient's curve progresses despite the orthosis, fusion must be performed without further delay. The orthosis should only be continued if it successfully controls the curve.

The most common error seen in the treatment of congenital scoliosis with a Milwaukee brace is the attempt to treat a curve that requires surgery. The second most common mistake is the failure to recognize that the orthosis is not doing an adequate job of controlling the curve, allowing curve progression to occur. The current radiograph must always be compared with the radiograph of the last visit as well as with the earliest radiograph available. Because curve progression is slow, averaging 5 to 7 degrees per year, if the current radiograph is compared only with the radiograph of the last visit, any slight difference can be ascribed to measurement error, and progression will be missed.

SURGICAL TREATMENT. Surgery is the most customary treatment of severe or progressive congenital scoliosis. Several types of operative procedures can be applied, and two fundamental questions emerge: What is the best procedure? What is the best age for surgery?

In congenital scoliosis there is no simple answer to these questions. The operative treatment chosen must be tailored to that specific patient. It depends on the age of the patient, the type of deformity (scoliosis, kyphosis, lordosis, or a combination), the area of the deformity, the curve pattern, the natural history of the deformity, and the presence of other congenital anomalies.

Progressive curves should be treated surgically, especially if they do not respond to orthotic treatment. If a 25-degree curve in a 3-year-old child progresses to 35 degrees by age 6 years the curve requires surgical treatment. The tendency is to avoid surgery at this age for fear of stunting the child's growth, but in reality, the child will grow taller if the curve is fused than if a progressive deformity occurs because the area of anomaly is devoid of normal vertical growth potential.

There are four basic procedures for the surgical treatment of congenital scoliosis: posterior fusion, anterior and posterior fusion, convex growth arrest (anterior epiphyseodesis and posterior hemiarthrodesis), and hemivertebra excision. The fusion, posterior or combined, can be in situ or with correction by traction, casting, bracing, or instrumentation. The correction is maintained with casting, bracing, or instrumentation. Because fusion in congenital scoliosis is performed at a much earlier age than in other types of scoliosis, instrumentation becomes an adjunct to the procedure rather than an integral part of the fusion.

POSTERIOR FUSION. The aim of posterior fusion is not curve correction but rather curve stabilization with the prevention of further curve increase.[170] Generally, congenital curves tend to be rigid, and there is little chance of significant correction unless extensive anterior and posterior osteotomies are performed. The fusion must cover the entire measured curve and extend to the central gravity line. Abundant bone graft should be added because a wide, thick fusion mass is necessary to avoid possible bending of the fusion by the intact anterior growth plates. Correction and immobilization are best obtained with a carefully molded Risser cast or with a well-fitting Milwaukee brace (Fig. 17-34).

The use of traction to gain correction is reserved for major curves when it is desired to slowly correct the curve with the patient awake, allowing careful and constant neurologic monitoring rather than more rapid correction with instrumentation. It is used after preliminary removal of a tethering structure, such as a tight filum terminale or a diastematomyelia, or after osteotomy of an unsegmented bar. The traction is obtained either with a halo-gravity device or with the use of a femoral pin on the side of the high pelvis with pelvic obliquity. After the correction has been obtained, it is held with a cast, and the patient is kept nonambulatory for the first 3 to 4 months postoperatively, or the correction is maintained with instrumentation if the child is old enough and the vertebrae are of sufficient size (Fig. 17-35). The use of traction with a posterior fusion alone was the most common method for achieving correction in congenital scoliosis, but in the past 10 years the combined anterior and posterior approach has been used more often.[170]

It must be noted that instrumentation is an adjunct to the posterior fusion, used to obtain or maintain correction. Correction with instrumentation is

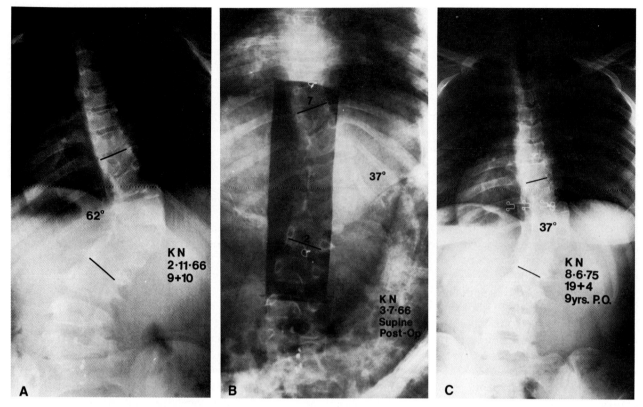

FIGURE 17-34. (A) A 9-year-old girl presented with progressive congenital scoliosis with a 62-degree right thoracolumbar curve owing to two hemivertebrae on the right. Surgical treatment is indicated. (B) Risser localized cast correction gave improvement to 37 degrees. A posterior fusion was performed from T5-L2. (C) At age 19 years, 9 years postoperatively, the fusion is solid and the curve is 37 degrees. Not 1 degree was lost since the time of surgery. (From Winter RB. Congenital deformities of the spine. New York: Thieme-Stratton, 1983:116.)

appropriate for curves in which it is safe to to obtain correction in one procedure with the patient under anesthesia. There must be no evidence of spinal dysraphism, and the curve must be small enough and the child old enough that an anterior approach is not necessary to improve the correction or to ablate the anterior growth plates with the disc excision. Because there are many types of instrumentation available the surgeon should choose the system that best fits the child, the deformity, the safety factors, and the surgeon's experience.

A preoperative MRI is necessary when instrumentation is planned. This rules out any tethering problems as well as any localized spinal stenosis.[167] In addition spinal cord monitoring with the wake-up test is mandatory with the use of instrumentation in congenital spine deformities. Electronic monitoring can be used, but it augments rather than replaces the wake-up test.

COMBINED ANTERIOR AND POSTERIOR FUSION. This has become an increasingly performed procedure for congenital scoliosis. It is used for thoracic, thoracolumbar, or lumbar curves with a poor prognosis, such as good convex growth potential. The multi-

ple discectomies give an anterior growth arrest that reduces or eliminates any bending of the fusion or crankshaft effect, and improved correction usually results because of the multiple disc excisions that are actually multiple convex wedge excisions. Because of the combined approach, the pseudoarthrodesis rate is lower. This approach obviously adds the risks of an anterior procedure, although these are small (Fig. 17-36).

As with a posterior fusion alone, the correction can be obtained externally with traction, a cast, or a brace or internally with instrumentation. The choice depends on the nature, the magnitude, and the flexibility of the deformity; the alignment of the spine (e.g., decompensation, head tilt); and the size and age of the child. In more severe deformities a combination of these methods is applicable, such as multiple discectomies to increase flexibility, traction to safely obtain correction with the patient awake and achieve a balanced spine, and a cast to maintain this correction.

CONVEX GROWTH ARREST. Convex growth arrest is not new; it was first described in 1922.[6,96,137,172] It is achieved by anterior and posterior convex fusion

(*text continues on p. 679*)

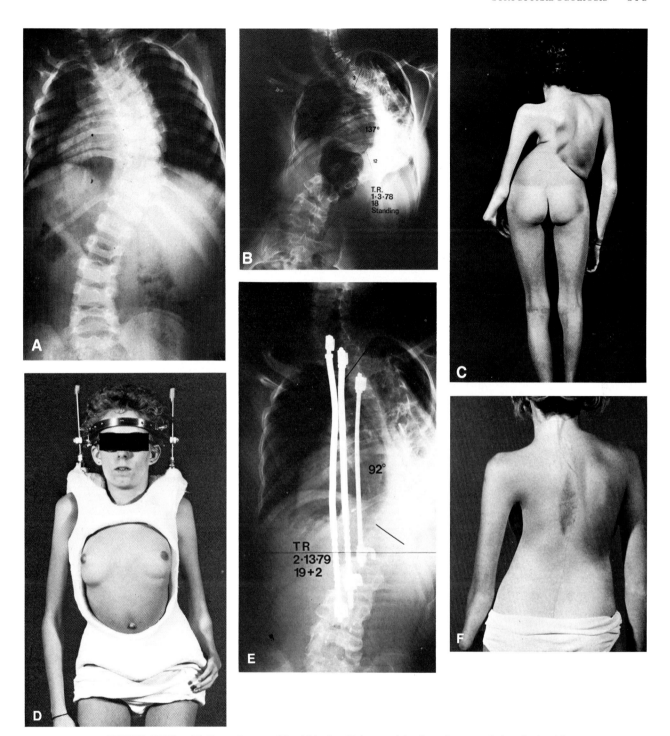

FIGURE 17-35.   (**A**) At age 8 years, this girl had a 60-degree right thoracic congenital scoliosis with two hemivertebrae on the curve convexity. Note the rib gap on the left at T10 and T11. Her spine was not treated, although she was under the care of an orthopaedist for congenital clubfoot and radial clubhand. (**B**) By age 18 years, her scoliosis had increased to 137 degrees. (**C**) Her clinical appearance at age 18 years, at which time she underwent a posterior fusion with three distraction Harrington rods. (**D**) She was immobilized in a halo cast postoperatively. (**E**) A radiograph 1 year after surgery shows a solid fusion with correction to 92 degrees. (**F**) Postoperative photograph. She gained 11 cm in height, and her vital capacity increased by 750 mL. (From Winter RB. Congenital deformities of the spine. New York: Thieme-Stratton, 1983:209.)

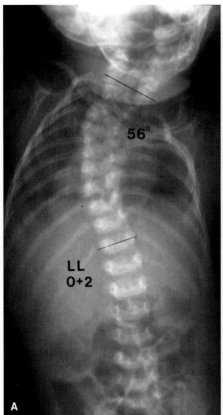

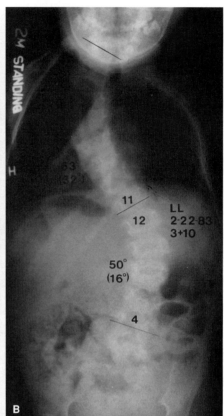

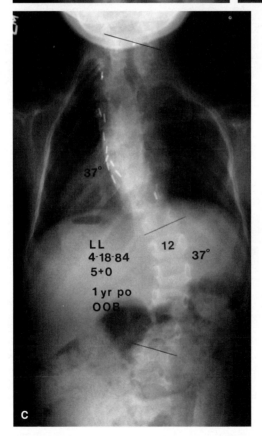

FIGURE 17-36. (A) This girl presented at age 2 months with a left thoracic congenital scoliosis of 56 degrees caused by multiple hemivertebrae on the left. Note the fused ribs on the right and the head tilt to the right. She also had bilateral clubhands. At the age of 9 months, she was placed in a Milwaukee brace to control her head position. (B) At the age of 3 years, 10 months, her curve had progressed to 63 degrees, and she had developed a 50-degree right lumbar secondary curve, which was flexible. She underwent an anterior and posterior thoracic fusion from C7-T10 and was immobilized postoperatively in a cast and kept flat for 4 months. She was then placed back in her brace to control the secondary lumbar curve. (C) A radiograph taken out of the brace 1 year postoperatively shows excellent balance and two curves of 37 degrees. She was kept full time in the brace, all attempts to wean her were unsuccessful because the lumbar curve increased. (D) At the onset of her growth spurt at the age of 14 years, her curves increased to 70 and 77 degrees, respectively, the left thoracic curve increasing because of "adding on" additional vertebrae to the curve. She underwent a right lumbar anterior fusion and a posterior fusion with Cotrel-Dubousset instrumentation. (E) A postoperative radiograph shows correction to 50 and 67 degrees, respectively.

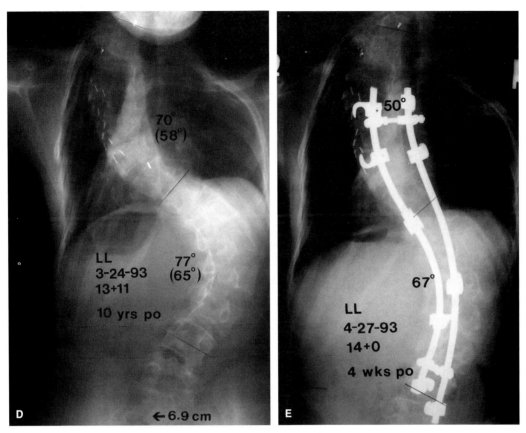

FIGURE 17-36 (*Continued*)

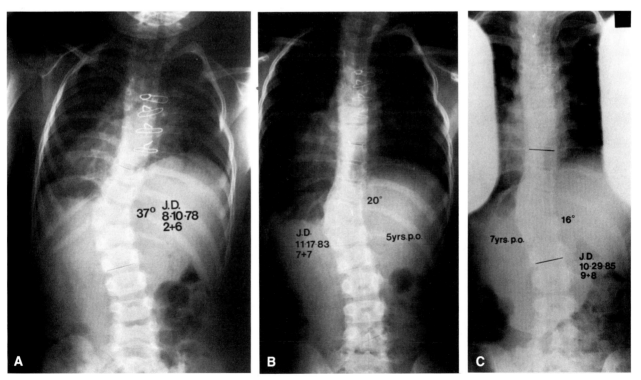

FIGURE 17-37.   (**A**) A 2-year, six-month-old girl presented with progressive congenital thoracolumbar scoliosis caused by a hemivertebra. Treatment options included anterior and posterior fusion, epiphysiodesis, posterior fusion only, and hemivertebra excision. She underwent an anterior and posterior growth arrest, or epiphysiodesis. (**B**) Five years after surgery her curve was 20 degrees. (**C**) Seven years after surgery her curve was 16 degrees. Nine years after surgery, the curve was 10 degrees.

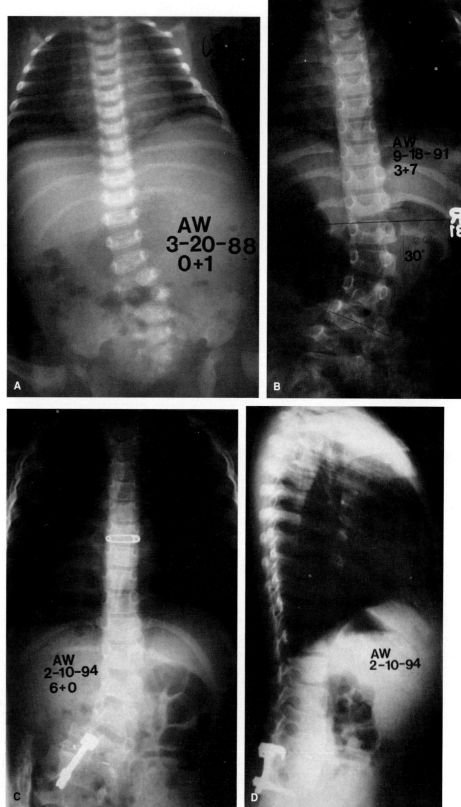

FIGURE 17-38. (A) A 1-month-old girl with an L5 hemivertebra and a small associated curve. (B) At age 3 years, 7 months, the curve had progressed to 30 degrees with a marked shift of her torso to the right because of the lumbosacral hemivertebra. She underwent an anterior and posterior hemivertebra excision with fixation using Cotrel-Dubousset instrumentation consisting of a screw and hook. (C) Two and one half years after surgery, at the age of 6 years, the fusion is solid, and the correction is shown. (D) Lateral radiograph shows the normal sagittal contours.

(i.e., anterior hemiepiphyseodesis and posterior hemi-arthrodesis) and was designed to arrest excessive convex growth and allow the concave growth to occur and correct the deformity. It is indicated in cases with a progressive scoliosis or marked scoliosis on presentation with single or adjacent convex hemivertebrae and a chance for concave growth with normal or near-normal concave growth plates. To be successful the surgery must be performed when there are a sufficient number of years of growth remaining, such as in a child younger than 5 years, and it is contraindicated if there is any kyphosis in the area of the anomaly. Another indication for convex growth arrest is in cases with a marked potential for bending of the fusion, such as a young patient with healthy convex growth. In these cases removal of the convex growth forces is essential to achieve the best result.

The anterior and posterior procedures are performed under the same anesthetic. It is essential to address the whole measured curve, sometimes adding a normal level to the convex fusion to increase the possibility of curve improvement by concave growth. The child is placed in a postoperative body cast with leg extensions because correction usually can be obtained in the segments adjacent to the hemivertebra. The cast is trimmed appropriately so that the chest tube, which is inserted more anteriorly than normal, can be removed from under the cast. The child is kept nonambulatory for 3 to 4 months, the cast is removed, and the child is placed in a well-fitting Milwaukee brace, which is worn full time for 12 to 18 months. The use of an orthosis after fusion in a young child is necessary because at 4 months postoperatively the fusion mass is continuous but immature, and continued support is necessary to achieve a strong mature solid fusion. This protection is actually necessary in all cases of fusion in the young child (Fig. 17-37).

HEMIVERTEBRA EXCISION. Hemivertebra excision is essentially an anterior and posterior wedge osteotomy, which is combined with correction and fusion. It is used for rigid angulated scoliosis in which compensation cannot be achieved with other methods.[79] It is usually applied in the lumbosacral area for a lumbosacral hemivertebra, which causes decompensation because there is no spine below the hemivertebrae to allow compensation.[54,65,74,143] There is no way to achieve a balanced spine other than by a wedge excision, which is best performed before 5 years of age, before the secondary curve has developed structural changes. The hemivertebra and the adjacent discs are excised using a lumbotomy approach, and a corresponding wedge of the hemivertebra and the pedicle are removed posteriorly with a fusion of the adjacent vertebrae. Depending on the age of the child and the size of the vertebrae, the correction is maintained with

a body cast with a leg extension or with the use of internal fixation, usually a compression system on the convexity of the excised segment, with the use of hooks and pedicle screws. Internal fixation is preferable. Postoperatively the child is immobilized in a body cast, usually with a leg extension, and is nonambulatory for 3 to 4 months (Fig. 17-38).

In rare cases there are dystrophic changes at the level of the hemivertebra with insufficient bone stock for compression instrumentation. In such a case, a preliminary convex hemifusion is performed posteriorly, followed by excision of the wedge 9 to 12 months later, after the hemifusion is solid and can support the instrumentation.

References

1. Adams W. Lectures on pathology and treatment of lateral and other forms of curvature of the spine. London: Churchill Livingstone, 1865.
2. Akbarnia B. Selection of methodology in surgical treatment of adolescent idiopathic scoliosis. Orthop Clin North Am 1988;19:319.
3. Akbarnia B, Keppler L. Lateral electrical surface stimulation for the treatment of adolescent idiopathic scoliosis. Analysis based on progression risk. J Pediatr Orthop 1986;6:369.
4. Akbarnia BA, Heydarian K, Ganjavian MS. Concordant congenital spine deformity in monozygotic twins. J Pediatr Orthop 1983;3(4):502.
5. Anderson M, Hwang S, Green W. Growth of the normal trunk in boys and girls during the second decade of life. J Bone Joint Surg [Am] 1965;47:1554.
6. Andrew T, Piggott H. Growth arrest for progressive scoliosis: combined anterior and posterior fusion of the convexity. J Bone Joint Surg [Br] 1985;67:193.
7. Armstrong G, Connock S. A transverse loading system applied to a modified Harrington instrumentation. Clin Orthop 1985;108:70.
8. Asher M, Green P, Orrick J. A six year report: spinal deformity screening in Kansas school children. J Kansas Med Soc 1980;81:968.
9. Axelgaard J, Brown JC. Lateral electrical surface stimulation for the treatment of progressive idiopathic scoliosis. Spine 1983;8(3):242.
10. Axelgaard J, Nordwall A, Brown JC. Correction of spinal curvatures by transcutaneous electrical muscle stimulation. Spine 1983;8(5):463.
11. Bartie B, Lonstein J, Winter R. Long-term follow-up of idiopathic scoliosis patients fused to the lower lumbar spine. Orthop Trans 1993;17:176.
12. Bassett GS, Bunnell WP, MacEwen GD. Treatment of idiopathic scoliosis with the Wilmington brace. Results in patients with a twenty to thirty-nine-degree curve. J Bone Joint Surg [Am] 1986;68(4):602.
13. Bergofsky E, Turino G, Fishman A. Cardiorespiratory failure in kyphoscoliosis. Medicine 1959;38:263.
14. Bjerkreim I, Carlsen B, Korsell E. Preoperative Cotrel traction in idiopathic scoliosis. Acta Orthop Scand 1982;53(6):901.
15. Blount W, Moe J. The Milwaukee brace. Baltimore: Williams & Wilkins, 1973.
16. Bobechko W, Herbert M, Friedman H. Electrospinal instrumentation for scoliosis: current status. Orthop Clin North Am 1979;10:927.
17. Bradford DS, Tanguy A, Vanselow J. Surface electrical stimula-

tion in the treatment of idiopathic scoliosis: preliminary results in 30 patients. Spine 1983;8(7):757.

18. Bridwell KH, McAllister JW, Betz RR, Huss G, Clancy M, Schoenecker PL. Coronal decompensation produced by Cotrel-Dubousset "derotation" maneuver for idiopathic right thoracic scoliosis. Spine 1991;16(7):769.

19. Brooks HL, Azen SP, Gerberg E, Brooks R, Chan L. Scoliosis: a prospective epidemiological study. J Bone Joint Surg [Am] 1975;57(7):968.

20. Brown JC, Axelgaard J, Howson DC. Multicenter trial of a noninvasive stimulation method for idiopathic scoliosis. A summary of early treatment results. Spine 1984;9(4):382.

21. Bunnell W. An objective criterion for scoliosis screening. J Bone Joint Surg [Am] 1984;66:1381.

22. Bunnell W. A study of the natural history of idiopathic scoliosis. Spine 1986;11:773.

23. Bunnell WP, MacEwen GD, Jayakumar S. The use of plastic jackets in the non-operative treatment of idiopathic scoliosis. Preliminary report. J Bone Joint Surg [Am] 1980;62(1):31.

24. Calvo J. Observations on the growth of the female adolescent spine and its relation to scoliosis. Clin Orthop 1957;10:40.

25. Cantu J, Urrusti J, G R. Evidence for autosomal recessive inheritance of costovertebral dysplasia. Clin Gen 1971;2:149.

26. Carr WA, Moe JH, Winter RB, Lonstein JE. Treatment of idiopathic scoliosis in the Milwaukee brace. J Bone Joint Surg [Am] 1980;62(4):599.

27. Ceballos T, Ferrer-Torrelles M, Castillo F, Fernandez-Paredes E. Prognosis in infantile idiopathic scoliosis. J Bone Joint Surg [Am] 1980;62:863.

28. Clarisse P. Prognostic evolutif des scolioses idiopathiques mineures de 10 degrees to 29 degrees en periode de croissance. Doctoral thesis. Lyon: Univ Claude Bernard, 1974.

29. Cobb J. Outline for the study of scoliosis. Instr Course Lect 1948;5:261.

30. Cochran T, Irstam L, Nachemson A. Long-term anatomic and functional changes in patients with adolescent idiopathic scoliosis treated by Harrington rod fusion. Spine 1983;8(6):576.

31. Cochran T, Nachemson A. Long-term anatomic and functional changes in patients with adolescent idiopathic scoliosis treated with the Milwaukee brace. Spine 1985;10(2):127.

32. Collis DK, Ponseti IV. Long-term follow-up of patients with idiopathic scoliosis not treated surgically. J Bone Joint Surg [Am] 1969;51(3):425.

33. Cotrel Y, Denis F, Galante H. Bilan actuel des 250 premieres arthrodesis vertebrales pour scoliose per grefon tibial. Harrington et dispositif de traction transversale (DTT). Congress de GES. France: St. Etienne, 1976.

34. Cotrel Y, Dubousset J. New segmental posterior instrumentation of the spine. Orthop Trans 1985;9:118.

35. Cotrel Y, Dubousset J, Guillaumat M. New universal instrumentation in spinal surgery. Clin Orthop 1988;227:10.

36. Cowell H, Hall J, MacEwen G. Familial patterns of idiopathic scoliosis. J Bone Joint Surg [Am] 1969;51:1236.

37. Cowell H, Hall J, MacEwen G. Genetic aspects of idiopathic scoliosis. Clin Orthop 1972;86:121.

38. Crisfield R. Scoliosis with external ophthalmoplegia in four siblings. J Bone Joint Surg [Br] 1974;48:484.

39. Dickson RA, Lawton JO, Archer IA, Butt WP. The pathogenesis of idiopathic scoliosis. Biplanar spinal asymmetry. J Bone Joint Surg [Br] 1984;66(1):8.

40. Dickson RA, Leatherman KD. Cotrel traction, exercises, casting in the treatment of idiopathic scoliosis. A pilot study and prospective randomized controlled clinical trial. Acta Orthop Scand 1978;49(1):46.

41. Dickson RA, Stamper P, Sharp AM, Harker P. School screening for scoliosis: cohort study of clinical course. Br Med J 1980;281(6235):265.

42. DiMeglio A, Bonnel F. La rachis en croissance. Paris: Springer-Verlag, 1990.

43. Drummond D, Guadagni J, Keene JS, et al. Interspinous process segmental spinal instrumentation. J Pediatr Orthop 1984;4(4):397.

44. Drummond D, Ranallo F, Lonstein J, Brooks L, Cameron J. Radiation hazards in scoliosis management. Spine 1983;8:741.

45. Drummond DS. Harrington instrumentation with spinous process wiring for idiopathic scoliosis. Orthop Clin North Am 1988;19(2):281.

46. Dubousset J, Herring J, Shufflebarger H. The crankshaft phenomenon. J Pediatr Orthop 1989;9:541.

47. Duval-Beaupere G. The growth of scoliosis patients. Hypothesis and preliminart study. Acta Orthop Belg 1972;38:365.

48. Duval-Beaupere G. Les reperes de maturation dans la surveillance des scoliosis. Rev Chir Orthop 1970;56:56.

49. Dwyer A, Schager M. Anterior approach to scoliosis; results of treatment in 51 cases. J Bone Joint Surg [Br] 1974;56B:218.

50. Edmonsson AS, Morris JT. Follow-up study of Milwaukee brace treatment in patients with idiopathic scoliosis. Clin Orthop 1977;126:58.

51. Emans JB, Kaelin A, Bancel P, et al. The Boston bracing system for idiopathic scoliosis. Follow-up results in 295 patients. Spine 1986;11(8):792.

52. Figueiredo UM, James JI. Juvenile idiopathic scoliosis. J Bone Joint Surg [Br] 1981;1981:61.

53. Fillio N, Thompson M. Genetic studies in scoliosis. J Bone Joint Surg [Am] 1971;53:199.

54. Freedman L, Leong J, Luk K, Hsu L. One stage combined anterior and posterior excision of hemivertebrae in the lower lumbar spine. J Bone Joint Surg [Br] 1987;69:854.

55. Fustier J. Evolution radiologique spontanee des scolioses idiopathiques de moins 45 degrees en periode de croissance. Thesis. Lyon: Univ Claude Bernard, 1980.

56. Gold L, Leach D, Keiffer S, et al. Large volume myelography. Radiology 1970;97:531.

57. Goldstein L. Surgical management of scoliosis. J Bone Joint Surg [Am] 1966;48:167.

58. Goldstein LA. The surgical treatment of idiopathic scoliosis. Israel J Med Sci 1973;9(6):797.

59. Green NE. Part-time bracing of adolescent idiopathic scoliosis. J Bone Joint Surg [Am] 1986;68(5):738.

60. Greulich W, Pyle S. Radiographic atlas of skeletal development of the hand and wrist. 2nd ed. Stanford, CA: Stanford University Press, 1959.

61. Harrington P. Surgical instrumentation for management of scoliosis. J Bone Joint Surg [Am] 1960;42:1448.

62. Hathaway G. Congenital scoliosis in one of monozygotic twins: a case report. J Bone Joint Surg [Am] 1977;59:837.

63. Hefti FL, McMaster MJ. The effect of the adolescent growth spurt on early posterior spinal fusion in infantile and juvenile idiopathic scoliosis. J Bone Joint Surg [Br] 1983;65(3):247.

64. Hensinger R, Lang J, MacEwen G. Klippel-Feil syndrome: a constellation of associated anomalies. J Bone Joint Surg [Am] 1974;56:1246.

65. Holte D, Winter R, Lonstein J, Denis F. Hemivertebra excision and wedge resection in the surgical treatment of patients with congenital scoliosis. J Bone Joint Surg [Am] 1995;77:159.

66. Ibrahim K, Benson L. Cotrel-Dubousset instrumentation for double major right thoracic left lumbar scoliosis, the relation between frontal balance, hook configuration and fusion levels. Orthop Trans 1991;15:1.

67. James J. Idiopathic scoliosis: prognosis, diagnosis and opera-

tive indications related to curve patterns and age of onset. J Bone Joint Surg [Br] 1954;33:36.

68. James J, Lloyd-Roberts G, Pilcher M. Infantile structural scoliosis. J Bone Joint Surg [Br] 1959;41:719.

69. Jarco S, Levin P. Hereditary malformations of the vertebral bodies. Bull Johns Hopkins Hosp 1938;62:215.

70. Kazmin A, Merkureva R. Role of disturbances of glucosaminoglycan metabolism in the pathogenesis of scoliosis. Ortop Travmatol Protez 1971;32:87.

71. Keiser RP, Shufflebarger HL. The Milwaukee brace in idiopathic scoliosis: evaluation of 123 completed cases. Clin Orthop 1976;118:19.

72. King H. Analysis and treatment of type II idiopathic scoliosis. Orthop Clin North Am 1994;25(2):225.

73. King HA, Moe JH, Bradford DS, Winter RB. The selection of fusion levels in thoracic idiopathic scoliosis. J Bone Joint Surg [Am] 1983;65(9):1302.

74. King JD, Lowery GL. Results of lumbar hemivertebral excision for congenital scoliosis. Spine 1991;16(7):778.

75. Koop S. Infantile and juvenile idiopathic scoliosis. Orthop Clin North Am 1988;19:331.

76. Korovessis P. Combined VDS and Harrington instrumentation for treatment of idiopathic double major curves. Spine 1987;12(3):244.

77. Kuhns J, Hormel R. Management of congenital scoliosis. Arch Surg 1952;65:250.

78. Laurner E, Tupper J, Mullen M. The Boston brace in thoracic scoliosis—a preliminary report. Spine 1983;8:388.

79. Leatherman KD, Dickson RA. Two-stage corrective surgery for congenital deformities of the spine. J Bone Joint Surg [Br] 1979;1979:324.

80. Lee C, Denis F, Winter R, Lonstein J. Analysis of the upper thoracic curve in surgically treated idiopathic scoliosis. A new concept of the upper thoracic curve pattern. Spine 1993; 18:1599.

81. Lenke LG, Bridwell KH, Baldus C, Blanke K. Preventing decompensation in King type II curves treated with Cotrel-Dubousset instrumentation. Strict guidelines for selective thoracic fusion. Spine 1992;17(Suppl 8):S274.

82. Letts R, Palakar G, Bobetcko W. Preoperative skeletal traction on scoliosis. J Bone Joint Surg [Am] 1975;57:616.

83. Lihvar G, Putilova A, Tabin V. Statistical and correlation analysis of electrical muscle activity in congenital scoliosis. Ortop Travmatol Protez 1975;36:9.

84. Lloyd-Roberts G, Pilcher M. Structural idiopathic scoliosis in infancy: a study of the natural history of 100 patients. J Bone Joint Surg [Br] 1965;47:520.

85. Lonstein J, Carlson J. The prediction of curve progression in untreated idiopathic scoliosis during growth. J Bone Joint Surg [Am] 1984;66:1061.

86. Lonstein J, Willson S, Beattie C, et al. Results of stimulator treatment of 332 cases of adolescent idiopathic scoliosis. Orthop Trans 1989;13:92.

87. Lonstein J, Winter R. Milwaukee brace treatment of adolescent idiopathic scoliosis—review of 1020 patients. J Bone Joint Surg [Am] 1994;76:1207.

88. Lonstein J, Winter R. Milwaukee brace treatment of juvenile idiopathic scoliosis. Orthop Trans 1989;13:91.

89. Lonstein J, Winter R, Moe J, et al. Neurological deficits secondary to spinal deformity. Spine 1980;5:331.

90. Lonstein JE. Natural history and school screening for scoliosis (Review). Orthop Clin North Am 1988;19(2):227.

91. Lonstein JE, Bjorklund S, Wanninger MH, Nelson RP. Voluntary school screening for scoliosis in Minnesota. J Bone Joint Surg [Am] 1982;64(4):481.

92. Luque ER. Segmental spinal instrumentation for correction of scoliosis. Clin Orthop 1982;163:192.

93. MacEwen G, Bunnell W, Siram K. Acute neurological complications in the treatment of scoliosis. J Bone Joint Surg [Am] 1975;57:404.

94. MacEwen G, Cowell H. Familial incidence of idiopathic scoliosis. J Bone Joint Surg [Am] 1970;52:405.

95. MacEwen GD, Winter RB, Hardy JH. Evaluation of kidney anomalies in congenital scoliosis. J Bone Joint Surg [Am] 1972;54(7):1451.

96. Maclennan A. Scoliosis. Br Med J 1922;2:864.

97. Marchetti P, Faldini A. End fusions in the treatment of severe scoliosis in childhood and early adolescence. Orthop Trans 1978;2:271.

98. Mau H. The changing concept of infantile scoliosis. Int Orthop 1981;5:131.

99. McCollough N, Schultz M, Javech N, Latta L. Miami TLSO in the management of scoliosis: preliminary results in 100 cases. J Pediatr Orthop 1981;1:141.

100. McCollough N. Electrical stimulation in management of idiopathic scoliosis. Instr Course Lect 1985;34:119.

101. McMaster M, David C. Hemivertebra as a cause of scoliosis: a study of 104 patients. J Bone Joint Surg [Br] 1986;68:588.

102. McMaster MJ. Infantile idiopathic scoliosis: can it be prevented? J Bone Joint Surg [Br] 1983;65(5):612.

103. McMaster MJ. Occult intraspinal anomalies and congenital scoliosis. J Bone Joint Surg [Am] 1984;66(4):588.

104. McMaster MJ, Macnicol MF. The management of progressive infantile idiopathic scoliosis. J Bone Joint Surg [Br] 1979;61(1):36.

105. McMaster MJ, Ohtsuka K. The natural history of congenital scoliosis. A study of two hundred and fifty-one patients. J Bone Joint Surg [Am] 1982;64(8):1128.

106. Mehta M. The rib-vertebral angle in the early diagnosis between resolving and progressive infantile scoliosis. J Bone Joint Surg [Br] 1972;54:230.

107. Mehta M, Morel G. The non-operative treatment of infantile idiopathic scoliosis. In: Zorab P, Siezler D, ed. Scoliosis. London: Academic Press; 1979:71.

108. Mellencamp DD, Blount WP, Anderson AJ. Milwaukee brace treatment of idiopathic scoliosis: late results. Clin Orthop 1977;126:47.

109. Michel C, Caton J, Allegre M. The place of a four-piece spinal support in the conservative treatment of scoliosis: a review of 700 cases over 10 years. Orthop Trans 1983;7:130.

110. Michel CR, Lalain JJ. Late results of Harrington's operation. Long-term evolution of the lumbar spine below the fused segments. Spine 1985;10(5):414.

111. Mielke CH, Lonstein JE, Denis F, et al. Surgical treatment of adolescent idiopathic scoliosis. A comparative analysis. J Bone Joint Surg [Am] 1989;71(8):1170.

112. Miller JA, Nachemson AL, Schultz AB. Effectiveness of braces in mild idiopathic scoliosis. Spine 1984;9(6):632.

113. Moe J. Methods and technique of evaluating idiopathic scoliosis. In: AAOS symposium on the spine. St. Louis: CV Mosby; 1969:194.

114. Moe J. Methods of correction and surgical techniques in scoliosis. Orthop Clin North Am 1972;3:17.

115. Moe J, Kharrat K, Winter R, Cummine J. Harrington instrumentation without fusion plus external orthotic support for the treatment of difficult curvature problems in young children. Clin Orthop 1984;185:35.

116. Moe JH, Kettleson DN. Idiopathic scoliosis. Analysis of curve patterns and the preliminary results of Milwaukee-brace treatment in one hundred sixty-nine patients. J Bone Joint Surg [Am] 1970;52(8):1509.

117. Nachemson A. A long-term follow-up study of non-treated scoliosis. Acta Orthop Scand 1968;39:466.

118. Nachemson A, Peterson L. Effectiveness of brace treatment in moderate adolescent scoliosis. Annual meeting of the Scoliosis Research Society, Dublin, Ireland, 1993.

119. Nash C, Brown R. Current concepts review: spinal cord monitoring. J Bone Joint Surg [Am] 1989;71:627.

120. Nash C, Gregg E, Brown R, Pillia M. Risk of exposure to X-rays in patients undergoing long term treatment for scoliosis. J Bone Joint Surg [Am] 1979;61:371.

121. Nash C, Moe J. A study of vertebral rotation. J Bone Joint Surg [Am] 1969;51:223.

122. Neuwirth MG, Drummond DS, Casden AS. Results of interspinous segmental instrumentation in the sagittal plane. J Spinal Dis 1993;6(1):1.

123. Nilsonne U, Lundgren K. Long-term prognosis in idiopathic scoliosis. Acta Orthop Scand 1968;39:456.

124. Nordwall A, Willner S. A study of skeletal age and height in girls with idiopathic scoliosis. Clin Orthop 1975;110:6.

125. Oegema T, Bradford D, Cooper K, Hunter R. Comparison of the biochemistry of proteoglycans isolated from normal, idiopathic scoliotic and cerebral palsy spines. Spine 1983;8:378.

126. Pedrini VA, Ponseti IV, Dohrman SC. Glycosaminoglycans of intervertebral disc in idiopathic scoliosis. J Lab Clin Med 1973;82(6):938.

127. Perdriolle R, Vidal J. Etude de la courbure scoliotique. Rev Chir Orthop 1981;67:25.

128. Peltonen J, Poussa M, Ylikoski M. Three-year results of bracing in scoliosis. Acta Orthop Scand 1988;59(5):487.

129. Peterson HA, Peterson LF. Hemivertebrae in identical twins with dissimilar spinal columns. J Bone Joint Surg [Am] 1967;49(5):938.

130. Piazza M, Basset G. Curve progression after treatment with the Wilmington brace for idiopathic scoliosis. J Pediatr Orthop 1990;10:39.

131. Price CT, Scott DS, Reed F Jr, Riddick MF. Nighttime bracing for adolescent idiopathic scoliosis with the Charleston bending brace. Preliminary report. Spine 1990;15(12):1294.

132. Reckles L, Peterson H, Bianco A, Weidman W. The association of scoliosis and congenital heart defects. J Bone Joint Surg [Am] 1975;57:449.

133. Riddle H, Roaf R. Muscle balance in the causation of scoliosis. Lancet 1975;1:1245.

134. Rimoin D, Fletcher B, McKusick V. Spondylocostal dysplasia. A dominantly inherited form of short trunked dwarfism. Am J Med 1968;45:948.

135. Riseborough E, Wynne-Davies R. A genetic survey of idiopathic scoliosis in Boston, Massachusetts. J Bone Joint Surg [Am] 1973;55:974.

136. Risser J. The iliac apophysis: an invaluable sign in the management of scoliosis. Clin Orthop 1958;11:111.

137. Roaf R. The treatment of progressive scoliosis by unilateral growth arrest. J Bone Joint Surg [Br] 1963;45:637.

138. Rogala EJ, Drummond DS, Gurr J. Scoliosis: incidence and natural history. A prospective epidemiological study. J Bone Joint Surg [Am] 1978;60(2):173.

139. Sanders J, Herring J, Browne R. Posterior arthrodesis and instrumentation in the immature (Risser grade 0) spine in idiopathic scoliosis. J Bone Joint Surg [Am] 1995;77:39.

139a. Scoliosis Research Society. Report of the Morbidity and Mortality Committee. 1987.

140. Shufflebarger H, Smiley K, Roth H. Internal thoracoplasty: a new procedure. Spine 1994;19:840.

141. Shufflebarger HL, Clark CE. Fusion levels and hook patterns in thoracic scoliosis with Cotrel-Dubousset instrumentation. Spine 1990;15(9):916.

142. Skogland L, Miller J. Growth related hormones in idiopathic scoliosis. Acta Orthop Scand 1980;51:779.

143. Slabaugh PB, Winter RB, Lonstein JE, Moe JH. Lumbosacral hemivertebrae. A review of twenty-four patients, with excision in eight. Spine 1980;5(3):234.

144. Stagnara P. Examen du scoliotique. In: Deviations laterales du rachis: scolioses. Encyclopedie mediochirurgicale. Paris: Appareil Locomoteur, 1974.

145. Steel H. Rib resection and spine fusion in correction of convex deformity in scoliosis. J Bone Joint Surg [Am] 1983;65:920.

146. Styblo K. Conservative treatment of juvenile and adolescent idiopathic scoliosis. Doctoral thesis. Leiden: University of Leiden, 1991.

147. Sullivan JA, Davidson R, Renshaw TS, et al. Further evaluation of the Scolitron treatment of idiopathic adolescent scoliosis. Spine 1986;11(9):903.

148. Tanner J. Growth and endocrinology of the adolescent. In: Gardener L, ed. Endocrine and genetic diseases of childhood. Philadelphia: WB Saunders, 1975:14.

149. Tanner J. Growth at adolescence. 2nd ed. London: Blackwell, 1962.

150. Tanner J, Whitehouse R. Clinical longitudinal standards for height, weight, height velocity, weight velocity and stages of puberty. Arch Dis Child 1976;51:170.

151. Tanner J, Whitehouse R, Takaisni M. Standards from birth to maturity for height, weight, height velocity and weight velocity: British children. Arch Dis Child 1966;41:454.

152. Thompson GH, Wilber RG, Shaffer JW, et al. Segmental spinal instrumentation in idiopathic scoliosis. A preliminary report. Spine 1985;10(7):623.

153. Thompson SK, Bentley G. Prognosis in infantile idiopathic scoliosis. J Bone Joint Surg [Br] 1980;1980:151.

154. Thulbourne T, Gillespie R. The rib hump in idiopathic scoliosis: measurement, analysis and response to treatment. J Bone Joint Surg [Br] 1976;64:64.

155. Tolo VT, Gillespie R. The characteristics of juvenile idiopathic scoliosis and results of its treatment. J Bone Joint Surg [Br] 1978;1978:181.

156. United SPTF. Screening for idiopathic scoliosis. J Am Med Assoc 1993;296:2664.

156a. Vauzelle C, Stagnara P, Jouvinroux P. Functional monitoring of spinal cord activity during spinal surgery. Clin Orthop 1973;93:173.

157. Weinstein S, Zavala D, Ponsetti I. Idiopathic scoliosis: long-term follow-up and prognosis in untreated pateints. J Bone Joint Surg [Am] 1981;63:701.

158. White A, Panjabi M. Clinical biomechanics of the spine. Philadelphia: JB Lippincott, 1978:105.

159. Willner S. The proportion of legs to trunk in girls with idiopathic structural scoliosis. Acta Orthop Scand 1975;46:84.

160. Willner S. Prospective prevalence study of scoliosis in southern Sweden. Acta Orthop Scand 1982;53:233.

161. Willner S. A study of height, weight and menarche in girls with idiopathic structural scoliosis. Acta Orthop Scand 1975;46:71.

162. Willner S, Nilssone K, Kastrup K, Bergstrand C. Growth hormone and somatomedin A in girls with adolescent idiopathic scoliosis. Acta Pediatr Scand 1976;65:547.

163. Winter R. Congenital deformities of the spine. New York: Thieme-Stratton, 1983.

164. Winter R. Hysterical (conversion) scoliosis. In: Bradford D, Lonstein J, Ogilvie J, Winter R, eds. Moe's textbook of scoliosis and other spinal deformities. 2nd ed. Philadelphia: WB Saunders, 1987:511.

165. Winter R, Anderson M. Spinal arthrodesis for spinal deformity using posterior instrumentation and sublaminar wiring: a preliminary report of 100 consecutive cases. Int Orthop 1985;9:239.

166. Winter R, Haven J, Moe J, Lagaard S. Diastematomyelia and congenital spine deformities. J Bone Joint Surg [Am] 1974;56:27.

167. Winter R, Lonstein J, Denis F, Koop S. Presence of spinal canal or cord abnormalities in idiopathic, congenital and neuromuscular scoliosis. Orthop Trans 1992;16:135.

168. Winter R, Lovell L, Moe J. Excessive thoracic lordosis and loss of pulmonary function in patients with idiopathic scoliosis. J Bone Joint Surg [Am] 1975;57:972.

169. Winter R, Moe J, Eilers V. Congenital scoliosis: a study of 234 patients treated and untreated. J Bone Joint Surg [Am] 1968;50:1.

170. Winter R, Moe J, Lonstein J. Posterior spinal arthrodesis for congenital scoliosis. J Bone Joint Surg [Am] 1984;66:1188.

171. Winter R, Moe J, MacEwen G, Peon-Vidales H. The Milwaukee brace in the nonoperative treatment of congenital scoliosis. Spine 1976;1:85.

172. Winter RB. Convex anterior and posterior hemiarthrodesis and hemiepiphyseodesis in young children with progressive congenital scoliosis. J Pediatr Orthop 1981;1(4):361.

173. Wynne-Davies R. Congenital vertebral anomalies: etiology and relationship to spina bifida cystica. J Med Genet 1975;12: 280.

174. Wynne-Davies R. Familial (idiopathic) scoliosis: a family survey. J Bone Joint Surg [Br] 1968;50:24.

175. Wynne-Davies R. Infantile idiopathic scoliosis. Causative factors, particularly in the first six months of life. J Bone Joint Surg [Br] 1975;57(2):138.

176. Yamada K, Yamamoto H, Nakagawa Y, et al. Etiology of idiopathic scoliosis. Clin Orthop 1984;184:50.

177. Yamada K, Yamamoto H, Tamura T. Development of scoliosis under neurological basis, particularly in relation to brainstem abnormalities. J Bone Joint Surg [Am] 1974;56:1764.

178. Zaouss A, James J. The iliac apophysis and the evolution of curves in scoliosis. J Bone Joint Surg [Br] 1958;40:442.

179. Zielke K. Ventral derotation spondylodesis: results of treatment of idiopathic lumbar scoliosis. Author's translation. Z Orthop 1982;120:320.

180. Zuk T. Role of spinal and abdominal muscles in the pathogenesis of scoliosis. J Bone Joint Surg [Br] 1962;44:102.

APPENDIX 17-1. *Classification Systems*

CLASSIFICATION OF SCOLIOSIS

Idiopathic
  Infantile
    Resolving
    Progressive
  Juvenile
  Adolescent
Neuomuscular
  Neuropathic
    Upper motor neuron
      Cerebral palsy
      Spinocerebellar degeneration
        Friedreich disease
        Charcot-Marie-Tooth disease
        Roussy-Levy disease
      Syringomyelia
      Spinal cord tumor
      Spinal cord trauma
      Other
    Lower motor neuron
      Poliomyelitis
      Other viral myelitides
      Traumatic
      Spinal muscular atrophy
        Werdig-Hoffmann disease
        Kugelberg-Welander disease
      Myelomeningocoele (paralytic)
    Dysautonomia (Riley-Day
      syndrome)
    Other
  Myopathic
    Arthrogryposis
    Muscular dystrophy
      Duchenne
        (pseudohypertrophic)

    Limb-girdle
    Facioscapulohumeral
    Fiber-type disproportion
    Congenital hypotonia
    Myotonia dystrophica
    Other
Congenital
  Failure of formation
    Wedge vertebra
    Hemivertebra
  Failure of segmentation
    Unilateral bar
    Bilateral (fusion)
  Mixed
Associated with neural tissue defect
  Myelomeningocele
  Meningocele
  Spinal dysraphism
    Diastematomyelia
    Other
Neurofibromatosis
Mesenchymal
  Marfan syndrome
  Homocystinuria
  Ehlers-Danlos syndrome
  Other
Traumatic
  Fracture or dislocation
    (nonparalytic)
  Postirradiation
  Other
Soft tissue contractures
  Postempyema

  Burns
  Other
Osteochondrodystrophies
  Achondroplasia
  Spondyloepiphyseal dysplasia
  Diastrophic dwarfism
  Mucopolysaccharidoses
  Other
Tumor
  Benign
  Malignant
Rheumatoid disease
Metabolic
  Rickets
  Juvenile osteoporosis
  Osteogenesis imperfecta
Related to lumbosacral area
  Spondylolysis
  Spondylolisthesis
  Other
Thoracogenic
  Postthoracoplasty
  Postthoracotomy
  Other
Hysterical
Functional
  Postural
  Secondary to short leg
  Due to muscle spasm
  Other

(continued)

APPENDIX 17-1 *(Continued)*

CLASSIFICATION OF KYPHOSIS

Postural	Inflammatory	Developmental
Scheuermann disease	Tuberculosis	Achondroplasia
Congenital	Other infections	Mucopolysaccharidoses
Defect of segmentation	Ankylosing spondylitis	Other
Defect of formation	Postsurgical	Tumor
Mixed	Postlaminectomy	Benign
Paralytic	Post–body excision (e.g., tumor)	Malignant
Polio	Postirradiation	Primary
Anterior horn cell	Metabolic	Metastatic
Upper motor neuron	Osteoporosis	
Myelomeningocele	Senile	
Posttraumatic	Juvenile	
Acute	Osteogenesis imperfecta	
Chronic	Other	

CLASSIFICATION OF LORDOSIS

Postural	Paralytic	Contracture of hip flexors
Congenital	Neuropathic	Secondary to shunts
	Myopathic	

From Scoliosis Research Society. Report of the Morbidity and Mortality Committee. 1987.

APPENDIX 17-2   ***Glossary***

Adolescent scoliosis: Spinal curvature developing after the onset of puberty and before maturity.

Adult scoliosis: Spinal curvature existing after skeletal maturity is attained (i.e., after closure of epiphyses).

Apical vertebra: The vertebra most deviated from the vertical axis of the patient.

Cervical curve: Spinal curvature that has its apex between C2 and C6.

Cervicothoracic curve: Spinal curvature that has its apex at C7 and T1.

Compensation: Accurate alignment of the midline of the skull over the midline of the sacrum.

Compensatory curve: A curve, which can be structural, above or below a major curve that tends to maintain normal body alignment.

Congenital scoliosis: Scoliosis due to congenitally anomalous vertebral development.

Double structural curve (scoliosis): Two structural curves in the same spine that balance each other.

Double thoracic curve (scoliosis): Two structural curves that have their apices within the thoracic spine.

End vertebra: The most cephalad vertebra of a curve whose superior surface or the most caudad vertebra of a curve whose inferior surface tilts maximally toward the concavity of the curve.

Fractional curve: A curve that is incomplete because it returns to the erect position. Its only horizontal vertebra is its caudad or cephalad one.

Full curve: A curve in which the only horizontal vertebra is at the apex.

Gibbus: A sharply angular kyphos.

Infantile scoliosis. Spinal curvature developing during the first 3 years of life.

Juvenile scoliosis: Spinal curvature developing between the skeletal ages of 4 years and the onset of puberty.

Kyphos: An abnormal kyphosis.

Kyphoscoliosis: Lateral curvature of the spine associated with either increased posterior or decreased anterior angulation in the sagittal plane in excess of the accepted normal for that area.

Lordoscoliosis: Lateral curvature of the spine associated with an increase in anterior curvature or a decrease in posterior angulation in the sagittal plane in excess of normal for that area.

Lumbar curve: Spinal curvature that has its apex from L2–L4.

Lumbosacral curve: Spinal curvature that has its apex at L5 or below.

Major curve: The most apparent curve and usually the most structural.

Nonstructural scoliosis: Spinal curvature without structural characteristics (*See* Structural curve.)

(continued)

APPENDIX 17-2 (*Continued*)

Pelvic obliquity: Deviation of the pelvis from the horizontal in the frontal plane.

Primary curve: The first or earliest of several curves to appear. Usually the most structural curve.

Structural curve: The segment of spine with a fixed lateral curvature. It is not necessarily the major or primary curve. Radiographically, it is identified in supine lateral side-bending or traction films by the failure to demonstrate normal flexibility.

Thoracic curve (scoliosis): Curve with its apex between T2 and T11.

Thoracolumbar curve: Spinal curvature that has its apex at T12, L1, or the T12–L1 interspace.

Adapted from Scoliosis Research Society. Report of the Morbidity and Mortality Committee. 1987.

Lovell & Winter's Pediatric Orthopaedics, fourth edition,
edited by Raymond T. Morrissy and Stuart L. Weinstein.
Lippincott–Raven Publishers, Philadelphia © 1996.

Chapter

18

Kyphosis

William C. Warner Jr.

Kyphosis is a curvature of the spine in the sagittal plane in which the convexity of the curve is directed posteriorly. Lordosis is a curvature of the spine in the sagittal plane in which the convexity of the curve is directed anteriorly.[204] The thoracic spine and the sacrum normally are kyphotic, and the cervical spine and the lumbar spine normally are lordotic.[133] Although several authors have tried to define normal kyphosis of the thoracic spine and normal lordosis of the lumbar spine, these studies have shown much variability in what is considered normal.[52,123,124,139,164,186,206] The ranges of normal kyphosis and lordosis change with increasing age and vary according to gender and the area of the spine involved.[52,123,124,139] The degree of kyphosis or lordosis that is considered normal or abnormal depends on the location of the curvature and the age of the patient. For example, 30 degrees of kyphosis is normal in the thoracic spine but abnormal in the thoracolumbar junction.

For the purposes of this chapter, the guidelines established by the Scoliosis Research Society for normal thoracic kyphosis and lordosis are used. They define the normal range of thoracic kyphosis as 20 to 40 degrees and that of lumbar lordosis as 30 to 60 degrees.[112] The thoracolumbar junction should have no kyphosis or lordosis.[16] Lumbar lordosis begins at L1–2 and increases gradually until the L3–4 disc space. The apex of normal thoracic kyphosis is the T6–7 disc space.[16,77]

Initially, during fetal and intrauterine development, the entire spine is kyphotic. During the neonatal period, the thoracic, lumbar, and sacral portions of the spine remain in a kyphotic posture. Cervical lordosis begins to develop when a child starts holding his head up. When an upright posture is assumed, the primary and secondary curves begin to develop. The primary curves are thoracic and sacral kyphosis, and the secondary or compensatory curves in the sagittal plane are cervical and lumbar lordosis. These curves balance each other so that the head is centered over the pelvis.[52,104,160]

Cutler[45] and Fon[65] showed that the ranges of normal thoracic kyphosis and lumbar lordosis are dynamic, progressing gradually with growth. During the juvenile and adolescent growth periods, thoracic kyphosis and lumbar lordosis become more pronounced and take on a more adult appearance. Differ-

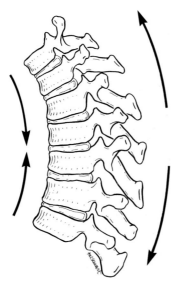

FIGURE 18-1. Forces that contribute to kyphotic deformity of the thoracic spine. The anterior vertebral bodies are in compression, and the posterior vertebral elements are in tension. (Adapted from White AA, Panjabi MM. Practical biomechanics of scoliosis and kyphosis. In: White AA, Panjabi MM, eds. Clinical biomechanics of the spine. Philadelphia: JB Lippincott, 1990:155.)

ences also exist between male and female spines.[164] Normal thoracic kyphosis and spine mobility are different in boys and girls. Mellin[123,124] has shown that during the juvenile and adolescent periods, girls have less thoracic kyphosis and thoracic spinal mobility than do comparable boys. Thoracic kyphosis also tends to progress with age. Fon[65] showed that from 30 to 70 years of age, women have a progressive increase in kyphosis, from a mean of 25 degrees to 40 degrees. Men also show a definite progression with age, but at a lower rate.

Different forces are exerted on the spine depending on the presence of kyphosis or lordosis. In the upright position, the spine is subjected to the forces of gravity, and several structures maintain its stability: the disc complex (nucleus pulposus and annulus), the ligaments (anterior longitudinal ligament, posterior longitudinal ligament, ligamentum flavum, apophyseal joint ligaments, and interspinous ligament), and the muscles (the long spinal muscles, the short intrinsic spinal muscles, and the abdominal muscles). Alteration in function resulting from paralysis, surgery, tu-

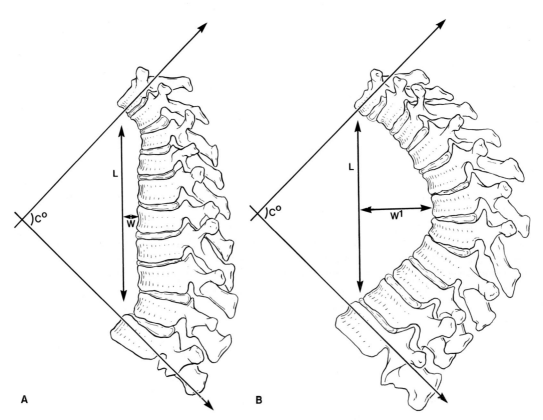

FIGURE 18-2. The two spinal curvatures represented by these drawings are different in magnitude; however, using Cobb's method to measure the deformities, the degrees of curvature are identical. The differences in the curves are more accurately reflected when the length of the curves (L) and their respective widths (W and W¹) are taken into consideration. (Adapted from Voutsinas SA, MacEwen GD. Sagittal profiles of the spine. Clin Orthop 1986;210:235.)

TABLE 18-1 *Disorders Affecting the Spine That Result in Kyphosis*

I. Postural disorders

II. Scheuermann kyphosis

III. Congenital disorders
    a. Defect of formation
    b. Defect of segmentation

IV. Paralytic disorders
    a. Poliomyelitis
    b. Anterior horn cell disease
    c. Upper motor neuron disease
      (e.g., cerebral palsy)

V. Myelomeningocele

VI. Posttraumatic
    a. Acute
    b. Chronic
    c. With or without cord damage

VII. Inflammatory
    a. Tuberculosis
    b. Other infection

VIII. Postsurgical
    a. Postlaminectomy
    b. Post–body (tumor) excision

IX. Inadequate fusion
    a. Too short
    b. Pseudoarthrosis

X. Postirradiation
    a. Neuroblastoma
    b. Wilms tumor

XI. Metabolic
    a. Osteoporosis
      1. Senile
      2. Juvenile
    b. Osteogenesis imperfecta

XII. Developmental
    a. Achondroplasia
    b. Mucopolysaccharidosis
    c. Other

XIII. Collagen disease (e.g., Marie-Strümpell)

XIV. Tumor
    a. Benign
    b. Malignant

XV. Neurofibromatosis

From Winter RB, Hall JE. Kyphosis in childhood and adolescence. Spine 1978;3:285.

mor, or infection, or alteration in growth potentials, can cause a progressive kyphotic deformity in a child.[204]

Both compressive and tensile forces are produced by the action of gravity on an upright spine (Fig. 18-1). With normal thoracic kyphosis, the compressive forces borne by the anterior element are balanced by the tensile forces borne by the posterior element. In a lordotic spine, the compressive forces are posterior and the tensile forces are anterior. These forces of compression and tension on the spinal physes can cause changes in normal growth, and a growth deformity can be added to a biomechanical deformity to cause a pathologic kyphosis.[204]

Voutsinas and MacEwen[201] believe that relative differences in forces applied to the spine are reflected more accurately by the length and width of a kyphotic curve than by just the degree of the curve. For example, curves that are longer and wider (farther from the center of gravity) have more of a pathologic force about the spine and, therefore, are more likely to cause deformity in an immature spine (Fig. 18-2).

Winter and Hall[211] classified disorders that result in kyphosis of the spine. Only the more common causes are presented in this chapter; the other causes are discussed elsewhere in this text (Table 18-1).

POSTURAL KYPHOSIS

Postural kyphosis is a flexible deformity of the spine and is a common complaint of juvenile and adolescent patients. Usually, the parents are more concerned about the postural roundback deformity than the adolescent is, and these parental concerns typically are what bring the patient to the physician's office. The physician's role in this situation is to rule out more serious causes of kyphosis. Postural kyphosis should be differentiated from pathologic types of kyphosis, such as Scheuermann disease or type II congenital kyphosis. When observed from the side, patients with postural roundback have a gentle rounding of the back while bending forward (Fig. 18-3). Patients with Scheuermann disease and congenital kyphosis have a sharp angular kyphosis or gibbus on forward bending when observed from the side. Radiographs are usually necessary to rule out pathologic types of kyphosis. Patients with postural kyphosis do not have radiographic vertebral body changes, and the deformity is completely correctable by changes in position or posture. This deformity is common in patients who are taller than their peers and in young adolescent girls undergoing early breast development, who tend

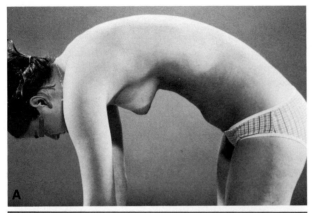

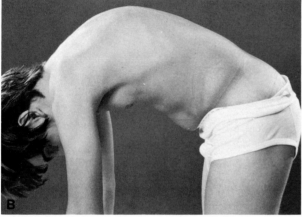

FIGURE 18-3. (A) Lateral view of normal spinal contour on forward bending. (B) Lateral view of a patient with Scheuermann disease on forward bending. Note the break in the normal contour of the spine. (Courtesy of Robert Winter, M.D., Minneapolis.)

to stoop because they are self-conscious about their bodies.[203]

No active medical treatment is necessary. Bracing is not indicated. Exercises have been suggested and may help maintain better posture, but adherence to such a therapy program is difficult for juveniles and young adolescents. This problem is treated best by patient and, more important, parent education and observation.[207]

CONGENITAL KYPHOSIS

Congenital kyphosis occurs because of abnormal development of the vertebrae. This can consist of a failure of developing segments of the spine to form or to separate properly.[208] The spine can be stable or unstable, or it can become unstable with growth.[56] Spinal deformity in congenital kyphosis usually progresses with growth, and the amount of progression is directly proportional to the number of vertebrae involved, the type of involvement, and the amount of remaining normal growth in the affected vertebrae.[56]

Van Schrick[199a] in 1932 and Lombard and Legenissel[106] in 1938 initially described two basic types of congenital kyphosis: a failure of formation of part or all of the vertebral body and a failure of segmentation of part or all of the vertebral body. Winter[208,216] developed the most useful classification of congenital kyphosis; it divides the deformity into three types. Type I is a failure of formation of all or part of the vertebral body (Fig. 18-4A). Type II is a failure of segmentation of one or multiple vertebral levels (Fig. 18-4B). Type III is a mixed form that has elements of both failure of formation and failure of segmentation. Dubousset[55] also classified congenital kyphosis. His classification is similar to that of Winter except for his type III, which includes rotatory dislocation of the spine. Either classification can be subdivided further into deformities with and without neurologic compromise. Both classifications and the presence or absence of neurologic compromise are useful for making treatment decisions, because each type of congenital kyphosis has a distinct natural history and risk of progression. The presence of neurologic compromise also affects the type of treatment recommended.

Most vertebral malformations that cause spinal deformity occur between the 20th and 30th days of fetal development.[56,148,216] Tsou[197,198] concluded that congenital kyphosis and congenital scoliosis occur during different periods of spinal development. He divided the development of the spine into an embryonic period (the first 56 days) and a fetal period (from 57 days to birth). During the embryonic period, hemivertebra formation or aplasia of part of the vertebrae and failure of segmentation causes scoliosis. Tsou believes that the causes of congenital kyphosis occur in the fetal period during the cartilaginous phase of development. Failure of formation occurs in this cartilaginous phase

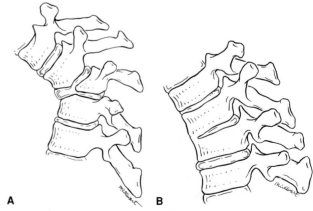

FIGURE 18-4. (A) Congenital kyphosis caused by failure of formation of the vertebral body (type I). (B) Congenital kyphosis caused by failure of segmentation (type II). (Courtesy of Robert Winter, M.D., Minneapolis.)

when half of the centrum of the vertebral body forms a functionally inadequate growth cartilage. Failure of formation varies from complete aplasia that involves the pars and the facet joints and makes the spine unstable, to involvement of only the anterior one third to one half of the vertebral body. This type of failure of formation also can cause scoliosis if one side of the vertebra is involved more than the other side (Fig. 18-5). Failure of segmentation is believed to be an osseous metaplasia of the annulus fibrosus,[128,197,198] which acts as a tether against normal growth and causes spinal deformity. The height of the vertebral bodies is relatively normal, but the depth of the ossification of the annulus fibrosus varies. Ossification also can be delayed, with a period of normal growth followed by spontaneous ossification.

The natural history of congenital kyphosis is well known and based on the type of congenital kyphosis: failure of formation (type I) or failure of segmentation (type II). The natural history of type III congenital kyphosis is less well understood. Both type I and type II deformities tend to be progressive, with the greatest rate of progression occurring during the adolescent growth spurt. Failure of formation (type I deformity) produces a much more malignant kyphosis, with a rate of progression that averages 7 degrees a year.[216] Type I deformities have a much higher incidence of neurologic involvement and paraplegia than do type II deformities.[216] Neurologic problems are increased

in patients with this type of deformity because they tend to have an acute angular kyphosis over a short segment, which places the spinal cord at high risk for compression at the level of acute angulation. Type II deformities generally progress at an average rate of 5 degrees a year and rarely result in neurologic problems because involvement of several segments produces a more gradual kyphosis.[121]

Patients with congenital kyphosis often have other anomalies. Intraspinal abnormalities have been reported to occur in 5% to 18% of patients with congenital kyphosis and congenital scoliosis,[20] but a more recent study by Bradford[26] indicates that the incidence may be greater. He found that six of eight patients with congenital kyphosis had spinal cord abnormalities visible on magnetic resonance imaging (MRI). Even though the proposed time of development of deformity may be different from that of congenital scoliosis, other nonskeletal anomalies, such as cardiac, pulmonary, renal, and auditory disorders or Klippel-Feil syndrome,[73] can be associated with congenital kyphosis.

Dubousset[55] has suggested that certain forms of type II congenital kyphosis (failure of segmentation) may be inherited. These patients have a failure of segmentation with delayed fusion of the anterior vertebral elements, which is not visible on radiographs until 8 or 10 years of age. Dubousset[55] described one family in which three individuals had delayed ossification and congenital kyphosis, and another family in which the grandmother, mother, and two sisters had the deformity. Progression of this kyphosis can be significant during the adolescent growth spurt and should be observed closely.

Patient Presentation

The diagnosis of a congenital spine problem usually is made by a pediatrician before the patient is seen by an orthopaedist. The deformity may be detected before birth on prenatal ultrasonography[31] or noted as a clinical deformity in the newborn nursery. If the deformity is mild, congenital kyphosis can be overlooked until a rapid growth spurt makes the condition more obvious. Some mild deformities are found by chance on radiographs that are obtained for other reasons.

Physical examination usually reveals a kyphotic deformity at the thoracolumbar junction or in the lower thoracic spine. An attempt should be made to determine the rigidity of the deformity by flexion and extension of the spine. A detailed neurologic examination should be performed, looking for any subtle signs of neurologic compromise. Associated musculoskeletal and nonmusculoskeletal anomalies should be sought on physical examination.

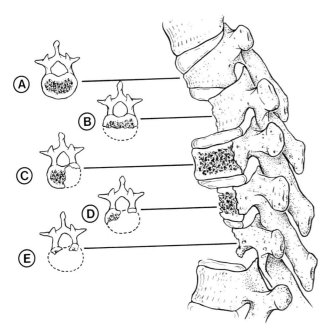

FIGURE 18-5. The five most common patterns of congenital vertebral hypoplasia and aplasia are illustrated in lateral and transverse views. Types B and E tend to produce pure congenital kyphosis. (Adapted from Tsou PM. Embryology of congenital kyphosis. Clin Orthop 1977;128:18.)

High-quality, detailed anteroposterior and lateral radiographs provide the most information in the evaluation of congenital kyphosis (Fig. 18-6). Failure of segmentation and the true extent of failure of formation may be difficult to detect on early films because of incomplete ossification. Flexion and extension lateral radiographs are helpful to determine the rigidity of the kyphosis and possible instability of the spine. Anteroposterior and lateral tomography can be helpful to demonstrate the type of congenital kyphosis and the vertebral anatomy. Computed tomographic (CT) scans with three-dimensional reconstructions also can help identify the amount of vertebral body involvement and determine whether more kyphosis or scoliosis might be expected. CT scans can only identify the nature of the bony deformity and the amount of cartilage anlage. They do not show the amount of growth potential in the cartilage anlage and, therefore, only allow an estimate of possible progression to be made. MRI should be done in most cases because of the significant incidence of intraspinal abnormalities. In addition, the location of the spinal cord and any areas of spinal cord compression due to kyphosis can be seen on MRI. The cartilage anlage also can be seen in patients with failure of formation (Fig. 18-7); however,

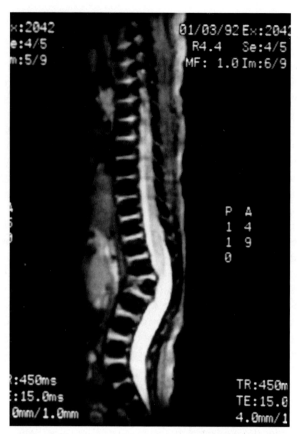

FIGURE 18-7. Magnetic resonance image of type I congenital kyphosis. Failure of formation of the anterior vertebral body is demonstrated, but the growth potential of the involved vertebra cannot be determined. Note the pressure on the dural sac.

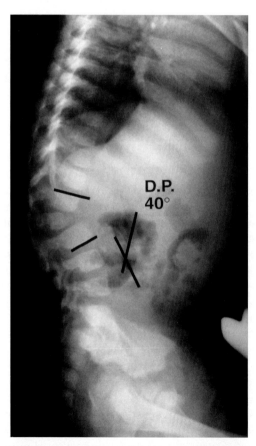

FIGURE 18-6. A 2-year-old child with type I congenital kyphosis measuring 40 degrees. Radiograph demonstrates failure of formation of the anterior portion of the first lumbar vertebra.

as with CT scans and plain radiographs, MRI cannot reveal how much growth potential is present in the cartilage anlage and can only help to estimate the probability of a progressive deformity.

Ultrasonography has been used in the early prenatal (20 weeks of gestation) diagnosis of this condition and is helpful for evaluating the renal system for any occult abnormalities.[31] Myelograms have been used to document spinal cord compression, but have been largely replaced by MRI. If myelography is used, images should be taken in the prone and supine positions. Myelograms obtained in only the prone position may miss information about spinal cord compression because of pooling of dye around the apex of the deformity. Myelography can be used in conjunction with CT scanning after injection to add to the diagnostic information obtained.

Treatment

Because the natural history of this condition is continued progression, surgery usually is the preferred method of treatment.[208] If the deformity is mild, or if the diagnosis is uncertain, close observation may be a treatment option. However, observation of a congenital kyphotic deformity must be used with caution and the physician must not be lulled into a false sense of security if the deformity progresses only 3 to 5 degrees over a 6-month period. If the deformity is observed over 2 to 3 years, it will have progressed 20 to 30 degrees and cannot be easily corrected.

Brace treatment has no role in the treatment of congenital kyphosis unless compensatory curves are being treated above or below the congenital kyphosis.[73,115,208] Bracing a rigid structural deformity such as congenital kyphosis neither corrects the deformity nor stops the progression of kyphosis.

Surgery is the recommended therapy for congenital kyphosis. The type of surgery depends on the type of deformity, the size of the deformity, the age of the patient, and the presence of neurologic deficits. Procedures can include posterior fusion, anterior fusion, both anterior and posterior fusion, and anterior osteotomy and posterior fusion. Fusion can be performed with or without instrumentation.

Treatment of Type I Deformities

Treatment of type I deformities can be divided into three stages: early with mild deformity, late with moderate or severe deformity, and late with severe deformity and with spinal cord compression.

EARLY TREATMENT OF MILD DEFORMITIES. For type I deformities with a known average progression rate of 7 degrees a year, the best treatment is early posterior fusion. If the deformity is less than 50 or 55 degrees and the patient is younger than 5 years of age, posterior arthrodesis alone, extending from one level above the kyphotic deformity to one level below, is recommended.[73,208,213,216] Winter[209,213] found that this predictably controlled the progressive kyphotic deformity, and that the deformity improved with growth in many cases. The improvement seen with growth probably is due to normal growth from the anterior end plates of the vertebrae one level above and below the congenital kyphotic vertebrae that are included in the posterior fusion. Anterior and posterior fusion predictably halts the progression of the kyphotic deformity, but does not allow for the possibility of some correction of the deformity with growth because of ablation of the anterior physes. The ablation of any growth potential of the remaining involved vertebral body anteriorly produces the most reliable results in stopping the progression of a congenital type I kyphotic deformity when this is combined with a posterior fusion.[208,213]

LATE TREATMENT OF MODERATE TO SEVERE DEFORMITIES. In older patients with type I kyphotic deformities, posterior arthrodesis alone may be successful if the kyphosis is less than 50 to 55 degrees.[127,216] If the deformity is more than 55 degrees (which usually is the case in deformities detected late), anterior and posterior arthrodesis produces more reliable results and is recommended.[127,216] Anterior arthrodesis alone will not correct the deformity. Any correction of the deformity requires anterior strut grafting with temporary distraction and posterior fusion, with or without posterior compression instrumentation. The posterior instrumentation should be regarded more as an internal stabilizer than as a correction device.[208] Correction by instrumentation should be avoided in rigid, angular curves because of the high incidence of neurologic complications. If anterior strut grafting is performed, the strut graft should be placed anteriorly under compression. When an associated scoliosis is present, the kyphosis should be approached from the concave side of the scoliosis to place the strut grafts under compression. If no correction is attempted and the goal of surgery is just to stop progression of the kyphosis, a simple anterior interbody fusion combined with a posterior fusion can be performed. The use of skeletal traction (halo-pelvic, halo-femoral, or halo-gravity) to correct the deformity is tempting but is not recommended because of the risk of paraplegia.[215] In a patient with a rigid gibbus deformity, traction pulls the spinal cord against the apex of the rigid kyphosis, causing neurologic compromise (Fig. 18-8).

LATE TREATMENT OF SEVERE DEFORMITIES WITH CORD COMPRESSION. Late treatment of a severe congenital kyphotic deformity with spinal cord compression is difficult. If congenital kyphosis causes spinal cord compression, anterior decompression is indicated. The compression is created by bone or disc material pressing into the front of the spinal cord, and this can be decompressed only by an anterior procedure; laminectomy has no role in the treatment of this condition.[211] For associated scoliosis, the anterior approach should be on the concavity of the scoliosis to allow the spinal cord to move both forward and into the midline after decompression. After adequate decompression has been achieved, the involved vertebrae are fused with an anterior strut graft. This is followed by a posterior fusion, with or without posterior stabilizing instrumentation. Postoperative support with a cast, brace, or halo cast usually is required.

Treatment of Type II Deformities

Treatment of type II deformities can be divided into early treatment of mild deformities and late treatment of severe deformities, as outlined by Mayfield.[121] If a type II kyphosis is mild and is detected early, posterior fusion with compression instrumentation

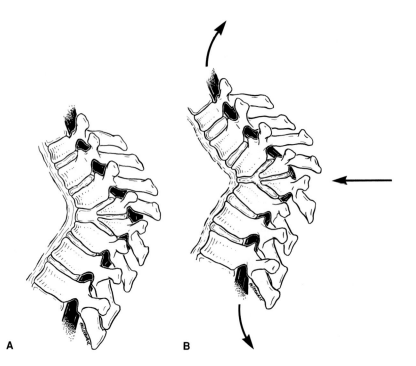

FIGURE 18-8. The effect of traction on a rigid congenital kyphosis. (**A**) The apical area does not change with traction, but the adjacent spine is lengthened. (**B**) The spine and thus the spinal cord lengthen, producing increased tension in the spinal cord and aggravation of any neurologic deficits. (Adapted from Lonstein JE, Winter RB, Moe JH, et al. Neurologic deficit secondary to spinal deformity. Spine 1980;5:331.)

A   B

can be performed. The kyphosis must be less than 50 degrees for a posterior fusion alone to have a good chance of success. The posterior fusion should include all the involved vertebrae, plus one vertebra above and one vertebra below the congenital kyphosis.

Compression instrumentation can be used more safely in type II deformities because the kyphosis is more rounded and over several segments instead of sharply angular as in type I deformities. If the deformity is severe and is detected late, correction can be obtained only by performing anterior osteotomies and fusion, followed by posterior fusion and compression instrumentation.[121]

Complications of Treatment

Some of the more frequent complications of treatment of congenital kyphosis are pseudarthrosis, progression of kyphosis, and paralysis. Pseudarthrosis and progression of the kyphotic deformity can be minimized by performing anterior and posterior fusions for deformities of more than 50 degrees. The posterior fusion should extend from one level above to one level below the involved vertebrae. If scoliosis is present, the anterior approach should be on the concave side of the scoliotic deformity instead of the convex side, so that graft is placed under compression. Paralysis is perhaps the most feared complication of spinal surgery. The risk of this complication can be lessened by not attempting correction or instrumentation of rigid curves. The use of halo traction in rigid congenital kyphotic deformities has been associated with an increased risk of neurologic compromise.[215] Another

long-term problem is low back pain, which occurs in 38% of patients because of an increased compensatory lumbar lordosis.

SCHEUERMANN DISEASE

Scheuermann disease is a common cause of structural kyphosis in the thoracic, thoracolumbar, and lumbar spine. Scheuermann originally described this rigid juvenile kyphosis in 1920; it is characterized by vertebral body wedging that is believed to be caused by a growth disturbance of the vertebral end plates[158,159] (Fig. 18-9).

Scheuermann disease can be divided into two distinct groups: a typical form and an atypical form. These two types are determined by the location and natural history of the kyphosis, including symptoms occurring during adolescence and after growth is completed. Typical Scheuermann disease is a thoracic kyphosis with a well-established natural history during adolescence and after skeletal maturity. In contrast, atypical Scheuermann disease is located in the thoracolumbar junction or in the lumbar spine, and its natural history is less well understood.

Typical Scheuermann disease consists of a rigid thoracic kyphosis in a juvenile or adolescent spine. The apex of kyphosis usually is located between T7 and T9.[6] The reported incidence of typical Scheuermann deformities in the general population ranges from 0.4% to 10%.[23,29,130,174] Reported male-to-female ratios vary in the literature. Scheuermann originally reported a male preponderance of 88%.[158] Most reports in the literature note either a slight male preponder-

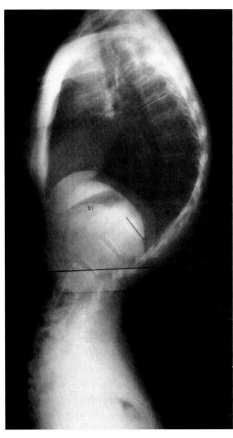

FIGURE 18-9.   Lateral radiograph of a patient with Scheuermann disease and an 81-degree kyphotic deformity. Note the narrowing of the intervertebral disc spaces and the irregularity of the vertebral end plates. There is an associated increase in lumbar lordosis below the kyphotic deformity.

ance or an equal male-to-female ratio.[63,64,126,130,174,196] Bradford[29] has been the only one to show an increased incidence of Scheuermann disease in women.

The onset of Scheuermann disease occurs at about 10 years of age. Usually, radiographic evidence of Scheuermann disease is not detectable in patients younger than 10 years of age because the ring apophysis is not yet ossified. Until the ring apophysis ossifies, vertebral body wedging and irregularity of the end plate are difficult to measure.

Sorensen[174] noted a high familial predilection, and Halal[76] in a study of 5 families and McKenzie[122] in a study of 12 families suggested that the disease may be inherited in an autosomal dominant fashion with a high degree of penetrance. Additional support for a genetic basis for this condition is provided in a report by Carr[37] of Scheuermann disease occurring in identical twins.

Many possible etiologies have been suggested for Scheuermann disease but the true cause remains unknown. Scheuermann believed that the kyphosis was caused by a form of avascular necrosis of the ring apophysis that led to a growth disturbance resulting in

a progressive kyphosis with growth.[158,159] The problem with this theory is that the ring apophysis contributes little to the longitudinal growth of the vertebrae.[17,18] Schmorl[162] described a herniation of disc material through the cartilaginous end plate, known as Schmorl nodes. He believed that the herniation of disc material occurred because of a weakened end plate, resulting in abnormal growth of the anterior end plate, which in turn causes the kyphosis. The problem with this theory is that Schmorl nodes were found outside the area of kyphosis and in patients who did not have a kyphotic deformity. Ferguson[62] suggested that persistence of an anterior vascular groove altered the anterior growth of the vertebral body, but Aufdermaur[7,8] and Ippolito[89] were unable to document growth disturbances around the anterior vascular groove and concluded that persistence of an anterior vascular groove was a sign of immaturity of the spine. Lambrinudi[103a] postulated that Scheuermann disease resulted from upright posture and a tight anterior longitudinal ligament. The fact that no cases of Scheuermann disease have been found in quadruped animals lends support to this theory.[165] This has led to the more popular belief that the anterior end plate changes are caused by mechanical forces, in response to Wolff's law or the Heuter-Volkmann principle. Compression forces in the anterior growth plate cause a decrease in growth in the area of kyphosis. Indirect support for this argument can be found in the changes in the wedging of the involved vertebral bodies and the reversal of these changes when bracing or casting is used in the immature spine. Scoles[165] also supports this theory by demonstrating disorganized endochondral ossification similar to that seen in Blount disease. He concludes that the changes in endochondral ossification are the result of increased pressure on the vertebral growth plate.

Ascani[5,6] found that patients with Scheuermann disease tended to be taller than normal for their chronologic and skeletal ages, and that their bone age tended to be more advanced than their chronologic age. Because he found increased growth hormone levels in these patients, Ascani[5,6] suggested that the increased height and the advanced skeletal age could be caused by the increased growth hormone. The increased height and more rapid growth may make the vertebral end plates more susceptible to increased pressure and result in the changes seen in Scheuermann disease. The increased growth hormone levels noted by Ascani also may lead to a relative osteoporosis of the spine, which may predispose the spine to the development of Scheuermann disease.

Bradford[23,25] Burner,[32] and Lopez[111] reported that Scheuermann kyphosis may be caused by a form of juvenile osteoporosis. Lopez advanced several theories for the associated osteoporosis in patients with

Scheuermann disease: it may be secondary to pain or an inflammatory process that caused a disuse osteoporosis, it may be the underlying cause of Scheuermann disease, it may be a reflection of a lag in mineralization caused by transient accelerated growth in these patients, or it may be only an associated finding with no role in the etiology of Scheuermann kyphosis. Gilsanz,[68] on quantitative CT scans, and Scoles,[165] on single-photon absorptiometric analysis, found no evidence of osteoporosis in patients with Scheuermann kyphosis when compared to normal research subjects. Gilsanz[68] suggested that the differences in his report and reports showing osteoporosis could be related to the technique used to determine osteoporosis.

What is shown by the histologic studies of Ascani,[5] Ippolito,[89] and Scoles[165] is that an alteration in endochondral ossification occurs. Whether this altered endochondral ossification is the cause or the result of kyphosis is not known. Ippolito[89] found a decrease in the number of collagen fibers and an increase in proteoglycan content, and collagen fibers were thinner than normal. Some areas of the altered end plate showed direct bone formation from cartilage instead of the normal growth plate sequences for ossification. These studies help support the belief that Scheuermann kyphosis is an underlying growth problem of the anterior vertebral end plates that results in kyphosis.

Other conditions reported in patients with Scheuermann disease include endocrine abnormalities,[129] hypovitaminosis,[98] inflammatory disorders,[129,189] dural cysts,[5] and spondylolysis.[134] Ogilvie[134] found a 50% incidence of spondylolysis in the 18 patients he reviewed. He believed the reason for the increased incidence of spondylolysis was the increased stress being placed on the pars interarticularis as a result of the associated compensatory hyperlordosis of the lumbar spine in Scheuermann disease.[134,189]

Mild to moderate scoliosis is present in about one third of patients with Scheuermann disease,[114] but the curves usually are small, about 10 to 20 degrees. Scoliosis associated with Scheuermann disease usually has a benign natural history. The scoliotic curve rarely is progressive and usually does not require treatment. Deacon[47,48] divided scoliotic curves found in patients with Scheuermann disease into two types based on the location of the curve and the rotation of the vertebrae into or away from the concavity of the scoliotic curve. In type I curves, the apex of scoliosis and kyphosis are the same and the curve is rotated toward the convexity. This rotation of the scoliotic curve is opposite from what is normally seen in idiopathic scoliosis. Deacon suggested that the difference in direction of rotation is due to the scoliosis occurring in a kyphotic spine instead of the hypokyphotic or lordotic spine that is common in idiopathic scoliosis. In type II curves, the apex of scoliosis is above or below the apex of kyphosis and the scoliotic curve is rotated into the concavity of the scoliosis, more like idiopathic scoliosis.

Clinical signs of Scheuermann disease usually occur around the time of puberty. Scheuermann disease has not been reported in patients younger than 10 years of age. The clinical feature that distinguishes postural kyphosis from Scheuermann kyphosis is rigidity. Often, mild Scheuermann disease is believed to be postural because the kyphosis can be more flexible in the early stages than in later stages. Usually, the patient seeks treatment because of a parent's concern about "poor posture." Sometimes, the poor posture has been present for several months or longer, or the parents may have noticed a recent change during a growth spurt. Attributing kyphotic deformity in a child to poor posture often causes a delay in diagnosis and treatment.

Pain can be the predominant clinical complaint rather than deformity. The pain generally is located over the area of the kyphotic deformity, but also can occur in the lower lumbar spine if compensatory lumbar lordosis is severe. Back pain usually is aggravated by standing, sitting, or physical activity. The distribution and intensity of the pain vary according to the age of the patient, the stage of the disease, the site of the kyphosis, and the severity of the deformity. Pain usually subsides with the cessation of growth, although it continues in the thoracic spine in some cases. More commonly, after growth is completed, patients complain of low back pain caused by the compensatory or exaggerated lumbar lordosis.

Most symptoms related to Scheuermann disease occur during the rapid growth phase. During the growth spurt, pain is reported by 22% of patients, but as the end of the adolescent growth spurt approaches, this figure reaches 60%. Some authors believe that when growth is complete, the pain recedes completely except for well-circumscribed perispinal discomfort.[72,87,88] In adult patients with Scheuermann disease, pain is located in and around the posterior iliac crest. This pain is thought to result from arthritic changes at T11 and T12 because the posterior crest is supplied by this dermatome. Stagnara[184,185] believes that the mobile areas above and below the rigid segment are the source of pain.

Symptoms also depend on the apex of kyphosis. Murray[130] noted that if the apex of kyphosis was in the upper thoracic spine, patients had more pain with everyday activities. The degree of kyphosis also has been correlated with symptoms. It seems logical that the larger the kyphosis, the more likely it is to be symptomatic, but Murray[130] found that curves between 65 and 85 degrees produced the most symptoms, whereas curves of more than 85 degrees and less than 65 degrees produced fewer symptoms. However, in patients with thoracolumbar or lumbar kyphosis (atypical Scheuermann disease), activity decreased as the degree of kyphosis increased.

In a patient with Scheuermann disease, a thorough examination of the back and a complete neurologic evaluation are essential. With the patient standing, the shoulders appear to be rounded and the head protrudes forward. The anterior bowing of the shoulders usually is caused by tight pectoralis muscles. Angular kyphosis is seen best when the patient is viewed from a lateral position and is asked to bend forward. Normally, the back exhibits a gradual rounding with forward bending, but in patients with Scheuermann disease, an acute increase in the kyphosis of the thoracic spine or at the thoracolumbar junction is evident. Stagnara[187] found cutaneous pigmentation to be common at the most protruding spinous process at the apex of the kyphosis, probably the result of friction exerted by the backs of chairs and clothing. He believes that this finding alone should lead to further investigation for vertebral kyphosis. Compensatory lumbar and cervical lordosis, with forward protrusion of the head, further increases the anterior flexion of the trunk. Associated hamstring and hip flexor muscle tightness usually is present.

The kyphotic deformity will have some form of rigidity and will not correct completely with hyperextension. Larger degrees of kyphosis are not necessarily more rigid, and the amount of rigidity will vary with the age of the patient.[130]

The neurologic evaluation usually is normal but must not be overlooked. Spinal cord compression has been reported occasionally in patients with Scheuermann disease.[39,100,105,153,217] Three types of neural compression have been reported: ruptured thoracic disc, intraspinal extradural cyst, and mechanical cord compression at the apex of kyphosis. However, spinal cord compression and neurologic compromise are rare. Bouchez[21] found that only 1% of patients with a paralyzing disc herniation had Scheuermann disease. In patients with spinal cord compression caused by the kyphosis alone, Ryan[153] suggests that the factors influencing the onset of cord compression are the angle of kyphosis, the number of segments involved, and the rate of change of the angle of kyphosis. He also believes that neurologic compromise may be secondary to impairment of the anterior blood supply to the cord.

Natural History

Many early studies suggested a poor natural history for Scheuermann disease and recommended early treatment to prevent severe deformity, pain, impaired social functioning, embarrassment about physical appearance, myelopathy, degeneration of the disc spaces, spondylolisthesis, and cardiopulmonary failure. Despite these reports, few long-term follow-up studies of Scheuermann disease were performed until that of Murray.[130] Findings by Travaglini,[196] Murray,[130] and Lowe[114] suggest that the clinical and functional natural history of the disease tends to be benign.

The kyphotic deformity progresses rapidly during the adolescent growth spurt. Bradford[27] noted that more than half his patients who required brace treatment had progression of their deformities before such treatment. Little is known about progression of the kyphosis after growth is completed and whether it is similar to that in scoliosis. Whether the kyphosis will continue to progress during adulthood after a certain degree of kyphosis has been reached is not known. What is known is that patients with Scheuermann kyphosis have more intense back pain, jobs that require relatively little physical activity, less range of motion of the trunk in extension, and different localization of back pain.[130] Pulmonary function actually increases in these patients until their kyphosis is more than 100 degrees. Compared with normal individuals, patients with Scheuermann kyphosis have no significant differences in self-esteem, social limitations, or level of recreational activities. The number of days they miss from work because of back pain also is similar. The data regarding the natural history of Scheuermann disease suggest that although patients may have some functional limitations, their lives are not seriously restricted and they have few clinical or functional problems.[130]

Radiographic Examination

The most important radiographic views are standing anteroposterior and lateral views of the spine. The amount of kyphosis present is determined by the Cobb method on a lateral radiograph of the spine. This is accomplished by selecting the cranial- and caudal-most tilted vertebrae in the kyphotic deformity. A line is drawn along the superior end plate of the most cranial vertebra and the inferior end plate of the most caudal vertebra. Lines are drawn perpendicular to the lines along the end plates and the angle they form is the degree of kyphosis.[40] Normal kyphosis is between 20 and 40 degrees.[112] The criterion for diagnosis of Scheuermann disease on a lateral radiograph is more than 5 degrees of wedging of at least three adjacent vertebrae.[174] The degree of wedging is determined by drawing one line parallel to the superior end plate and another line parallel to the inferior end plate of the vertebra and measuring the angle formed by their intersection. Bradford believes that three wedged vertebrae are not necessary for the diagnosis, but rather an abnormal, rigid kyphosis is indicative of Scheuermann disease.[22] The vertebral end plates are irregular and the disc spaces are narrowed. The anteroposior diameter of the apical vertebra frequently is increased[35,165] (Fig. 18-10). Associated Schmorl nodes often are seen in the vertebrae in the kyphosis.[35] Flexibility is determined by taking a lateral radiograph with the patient lying over a bolster placed at the apex of the deformity to hyperextend the spine. The bolster should be placed at the apex of the deformity to maximize the amount of correction seen on a hyperextension radiograph. Sometimes it is difficult to distinguish the vertebral end plates, and lateral tomography or xeroradiography is needed,[200] but this increases radiation exposure to the patient. MRI and CT scans are necessary only if the patient has unusual symptoms or positive neurologic findings. An anteroposterior or posteroanterior radiograph of the spine should be obtained to look for associated scoliosis or vertebral body anomalies. The patient's skeletal maturity can be estimated from a radiograph of the left hand and wrist or from the Risser sign on the anteroposterior radiograph of the spine.

Treatment

Treatment options for Scheuermann disease are observation, nonoperative methods, and surgery. Observation is an active form of treatment. If the deformity is mild and nonprogressive, the kyphosis can be observed every 6 months with lateral radiographs. The

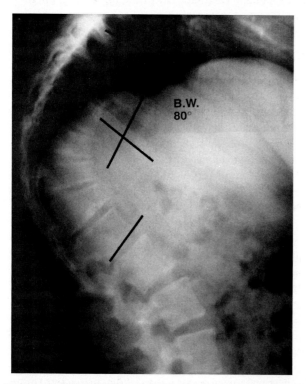

FIGURE 18-10. Lateral radiograph of a patient with Scheuermann disease demonstrates the kyphotic deformity seen in this disorder. Note the irregularity of the vertebral end plates and the anterior vertebral body wedging.

parents and patient must understand the need for regular follow-up visits. If the deformity begins to progress, another form of treatment, such as bracing, casting, or surgery, may be indicated.

Nonoperative methods include exercise, physical therapy, electrical stimulation, bracing, and casting. Exercise and physical therapy alone will not permanently improve kyphosis that is caused by skeletal changes. The improvement seen with these methods is due to improved muscle tone and correction of bad posture. The goals of physical therapy are to increase flexibility of the spine, correct lumbar hyperlordosis, strengthen extensor muscles of the spine, and stretch tight hamstring and pectoralis muscles. The efficacy of this treatment method has not been proven, and although it may improve the postural component of Scheuermann disease, its effect on a rigid kyphosis is questionable.

Electrical stimulation has been reported to improve and prevent the progression of scoliotic and kyphotic deformities.[9] Most of the studies on electrical stimulation have been for scoliotic curves and not kyphotic curves. Because the efficacy of this treatment method in scoliosis is questionable, electrical stimulation is not recommended as therapy for Scheuermann disease.

Other nonoperative treatment methods can be divided into active correction systems (braces) and passive correction systems (casts). For either a brace or a cast to be effective, the kyphotic curve must be flexible enough to allow correction of at least 40%.[6]

The Milwaukee brace is the brace recommended for the treatment of Scheuermann disease (Fig. 18-11). A low-profile brace without a chin ring and with anterior shoulder pads can be used for curves with an apex at the level of T9 or lower. The indications for brace treatment are spine immaturity and increased kyphosis with radiologic evidence of Scheuermann disease. The brace initially is worn full-time for an average of 12 to 18 months. If the curve is stabilized and no progression is noted after this time, a part-time brace program can be started. If no progression is noted with part-time bracing, a nighttime bracing program is used until skeletal maturity is reached. Gutowski[74] has shown that part-time bracing is as effective as full-time bracing and is associated with improved patient compliance. Despite initial improvement, several authors have noted a significant loss of correction after the discontinuation of brace treatment.[61,126,154] Montgomery[126] believes that if permanent correction of kyphosis is possible, a change in vertebral wedging should be seen before bracing is discontinued. Even though some loss of correction can occur after bracing is discontinued, it still is effective in obtaining some correction of the kyphosis and possibly reversing vertebral body wedging, or at least pre-

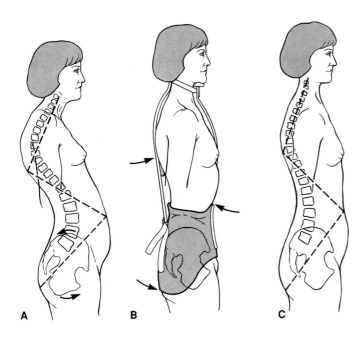

FIGURE 18-11. (A) Patient with Scheuermann kyphosis has thoracic kyphosis, compensatory lumbar lordosis, anterior protrusion of the head, and rotation of the pelvis. (B) Patient with Scheuermann kyphosis in a Milwaukee brace. The placement of the pelvic girdle, posterior thoracic pads, occipital pads, and neck ring encourage correction of the kyphosis. (C) Correction of kyphosis after Milwaukee brace treatment. (Courtesy of Robert Winter, M.D., Minneapolis.)

venting any progression of the kyphotic deformity (Fig. 18-12).

De Mauroy and Stagnara[46] developed a therapeutic regimen for patients with Scheuermann disease that uses serial casts for correction. This method consists of three stages. First, a physical therapy program is started in preparation for the casts. Next, three anti-gravity casts are applied on separate occasions. The casts are changed at 45-day intervals to obtain gradual correction of the deformity at each cast change. The third stage involves the use of a plastic maintenance brace that is worn until skeletal maturity is reached. Although the reported results of this method of treatment have been good,[46] the Milwaukee brace is still the preferred nonoperative treatment method in North America.

Surgical correction of kyphosis usually requires both anterior and posterior surgery[24,78,113,131] (Fig. 18-13). A posterior procedure alone can be considered if the kyphosis can be corrected to and maintained at less than 50 degrees while a posterior fusion occurs.[135,175,190] The spine can be instrumented with Harrington compression rods[28,42] or a posterior Cotrel-Dubousset type of instrumentation system.[168] If Harrington compression rods are used for posterior instrumentation, the ¼-inch rods are used. Even when ¼-inch Harrington compression rods are used, a brace or cast should be applied after surgery to prevent rod breakage until a solid fusion is obtained. When a Cotrel-Dubousset or similar type of instrumentation system is used, postoperative immobilization may not be required. Anterior instrumentation for Scheuermann disease has been reported but is not widely used.[102]

When anterior and posterior surgery is performed for Scheuermann disease, the anterior release and fusion are performed first, followed by the posterior fusion and instrumentation. The posterior fusion and instrumentation can be performed on the same day as the anterior release and fusion, or they can be done as a staged procedure. The posterior instrumentation should include at least three sets of hooks above the apex and at least two sets of hooks below the apex of the kyphosis. The fusion and instrumentation should extend into the normal lordotic segments. If the fusion and instrumentation end in the kyphotic deformity, a junctional kyphosis at the end of the instrumentation is likely to develop. The type of instrumentation used determines whether postoperative immobilization is needed. This immobilization can consist of a brace or a Risser body cast.

POSTLAMINECTOMY KYPHOSIS

Laminectomy is performed most often in children for the diagnosis and treatment of spinal cord tumors, but also may be needed in other conditions, such as neurofibromatosis and syringomyelia.[107] Although deformity after laminectomy is unusual in adults, it is common in children because of the unique, dynamic nature of the growing spine.[38,75,110,191] Postlaminectomy deformities usually are kyphotic but can be scoliotic.

The pathophysiology of postlaminectomy kyphotic deformity can be multifactorial. Deformity of the spine after multiple laminectomies can be caused by skeletal deficiencies (anterior column, facet joint, laminae), ligamentous deficiencies, neuromuscular imbalance,

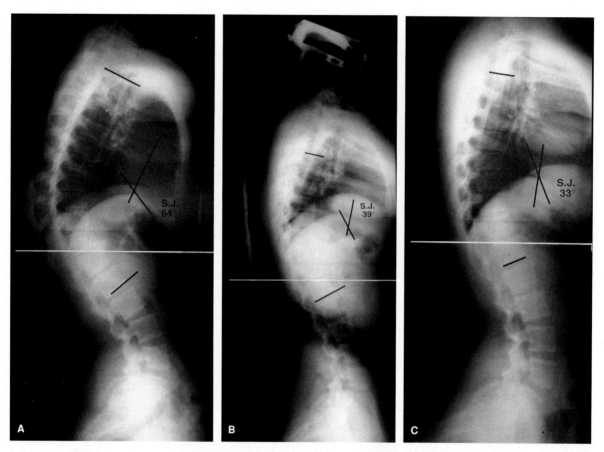

FIGURE 18-12. (**A**) A 15-year-old girl with a 64-degree thoracic kyphosis secondary to Scheuermann disease. (**B**) Lateral radiograph of the patient in a Milwaukee brace with the kyphotic deformity improved to 39 degrees. (**C**) Lateral radiograph obtained after the patient completed brace treatment; the kyphotic deformity has improved to 33 degrees.

effects of gravity, and progressive osseous deformity resulting from growth disturbances.[107] Panjabi[136] and colleagues showed that with loss of the posterior stabilizing structures caused by removal of the interspinous ligaments, spinous processes, and laminae, the normal flexion forces placed on the spine produce a kyphosis. Gravity places a flexion moment on the spine, producing compression on the anterior vertebrae and discs and tension on the remaining posterior structures. This may explain why postlaminectomy deformities occur most often in the cervical and thoracic spine, and rarely in the lumbar spine. Gravity tends to cause a kyphosis in the cervical and thoracic spine, whereas it accentuates the usual lordosis of the lumbar spine.

Skeletal deficiencies also can produce deformity. The most important structure noted to influence the development of postlaminectomy deformity is the facet joint.[33,51,110] If the facet joint is removed or damaged during surgery, deformity is likely. In addition, any secondary involvement of the anterior column by tumor or surgical resection adds to the risk of instability and deformity after laminectomy.

Paralysis of muscles that help stabilize the spine also can add to a postlaminectomy deformity, because these muscles are unable to resist the normal flexion forces placed on the spine by gravity and by the normal flexor muscles of the spine. Yasuoka[218] noted increased wedging of the vertebrae and excessive motion after laminectomy in children but not in adults. The increased wedging is caused by increased pressure on the cartilaginous end plates of the vertebral bodies. With time, the increased pressure decreases growth in the anterior portion of the vertebrae according to the Heuterman-Volkman principle (Fig. 18-14). Excessive spinal motion in children after laminectomy can be attributed to the facet joint anatomy in the cervical spine (more horizontal facets) and the increased ligamentous laxity of growing children.

Kyphosis is the most common deformity, although scoliosis also can occur, either as the primary deformity or in association with kyphosis. The incidence of postlaminectomy kyphotic deformity ranges from 33% to 100%[219] and depends on the age of the patient and the level of the laminectomy. Generally, the deformity is more likely in younger patients and after more ceph-

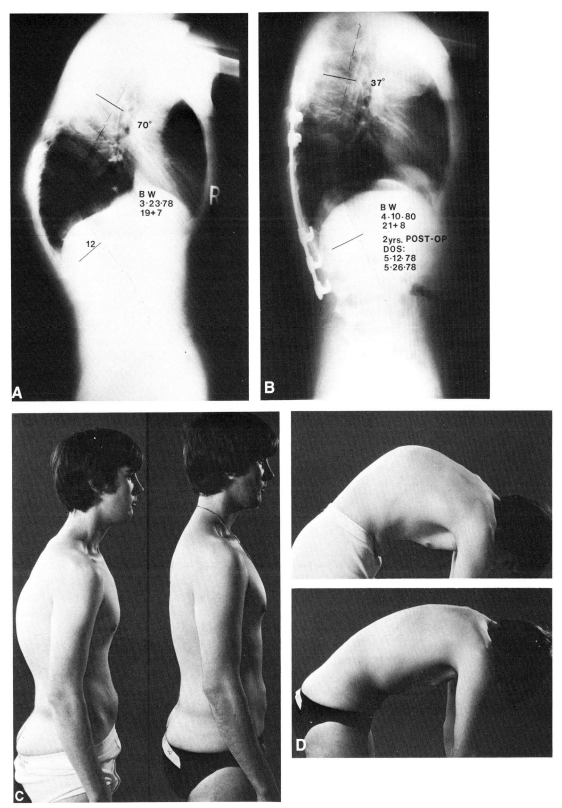

FIGURE 18-13.   (**A**) A 19-year-old man with a 70-degree lower thoracic Scheuermann kyphosis was treated by anterior ligament release and interbody fusion, followed by posterior instrumentation and fusion. (**B**) Two years after surgery, the kyphosis is 37 degrees. (**C**) Standing photographs before and 2 years after surgery. (**D**) Forward-bending photographs before and 2 years after surgery. (Courtesy of Robert Winter, M.D., Minneapolis.)

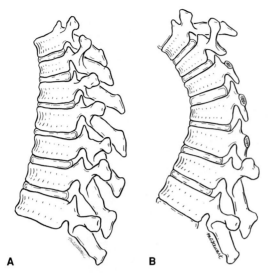

FIGURE 18-14. Drawings of the thoracic spine before and after repeated laminectomy demonstrate the effects on growth of the vertebral bodies. **(A)** Before laminectomy, the anterior vertebral bodies are rectangular in configuration. **(B)** The spine that has had multiple laminectomies will have increased compression anteriorly because of loss of posterior supporting structures. This compression results in less growth in the anterior portion of the vertebral body than in the posterior portion. In time, this will result in wedging of the vertebral bodies, causing a kyphotic deformity. (Adapted from Peterson HA. Iatrogenic spinal deformities. In: Weinstein SL, ed. The pediatric spine: principles and practice. New York: Raven Press, 1994:651.)

alad laminectomy. For example, Yasuoka[218] found that spinal deformity occurred in 46% of patients younger than 15 years of age but in only 6% of patients 15 to 24 years of age. All the patients between 15 and 24 years of age in whom deformity developed were 18 years of age or younger. Yasuoka[219] and Fraser[67] found that higher levels of laminectomy were associated with a greater chance of deformity. Deformity occurred after 100% of cervical spine laminectomies, after 36% of thoracic laminectomies, and after none of the lumbar laminectomies in their study.[219]

Postlaminectomy deformity can occur early in the postoperative period or gradually over time. Kyphotic deformities have been reported to occur as late as 6 years after surgery.[75,219] Progression of postlaminectomy kyphosis also can be sudden or gradual, or the deformity may progress significantly only during the adolescent growth spurt.

The natural history of postlaminectomy spinal deformity is varied and depends on the age of the patient at the time of surgery, the location of the laminectomy, and the integrity of the facet joint. Three types of postlaminectomy kyphosis have been described in children: instability after facetectomy, hypermobility between vertebral bodies associated with gradual rounding of the spine, and wedging of vertebral bodies caused by growth disturbances.[138]

Kyphosis due to instability after facetectomy tends to be sharp and angular. This deformity usually occurs in the immediate or early postoperative period and can cause associated loss of neurologic function (Fig. 18-15). Gradual rounding of the kyphotic deformity is seen more often when the facet joints are preserved. Kyphosis increases gradually over time because of the stress placed on the remaining posterior structures. If the spine is immature when the laminectomy is performed, the resulting kyphosis can inhibit the growth of the anterior growth plates of the involved vertebrae. Unequal growth results in wedging of the vertebrae and a progressive kyphotic deformity that is accelerated during the adolescent growth spurt.

Other associated conditions also can add to or cause kyphotic deformities, including spinal cord tumors, neurologic deficits, intraspinal pathology (hydromyelia), and radiotherapy.

Treatment of postlaminectomy kyphosis is difficult, and it is best to prevent the deformity from occurring. The facet joints should be preserved whenever possible during laminectomy. Localized fusion at the time of facetectomy or laminectomy may help prevent progressive deformity.[36] Because of the loss of bone mass posteriorly, however, localized fusion may not produce a large enough fusion mass to prevent kyphosis. Even so, this approach is advocated because it may produce enough bone mass posteriorly to stabilize what otherwise would be a severe progressive deformity.

After surgery in which the laminae have been removed, bracing has been suggested to prevent deformity,[171,188] although no studies have documented the efficacy of this form of treatment. After the deformity has occurred and started to progress, bracing is ineffective in preventing further progression.[107,110]

For progressive or marked deformity, spinal fusion is recommended, although the patient's long-term prognosis should be considered before making definitive treatment plans. If the prognosis for survival is poor, spinal fusion may not be appropriate. However, given the availability of effective treatment protocols for tumors and the improved survival rates, fusion is almost always indicated for progressive deformity. Combined anterior and posterior spinal fusion is preferred in most patients because of the frequency of pseudarthrosis after either procedure alone.

Lonstein[107] reported pseudarthrosis in 57% of patients after posterior fusion and in 15% of patients after anterior fusion. Anterior and posterior fusion can be performed on the same day or as staged procedures. When the anterior procedure is performed, care must be taken to remove all the physes back to the posterior longitudinal ligament. Leaving some of the physis in the vertebral body can cause an increase in the deformity. When the posterior procedure is performed, in-

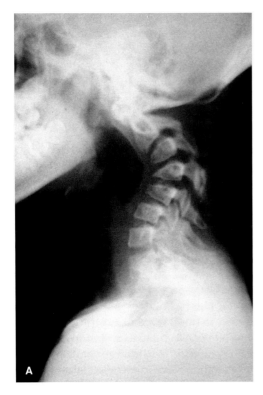

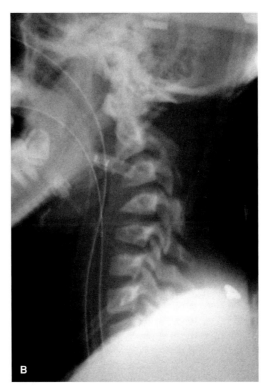

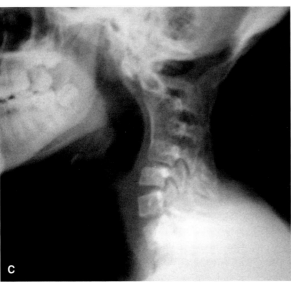

FIGURE 18-15. Radiographs of a 13-year-old girl treated for a low-grade astrocytoma. She underwent resection of the tumor and a portion of the occiput and the laminae of C1–C4, followed by radiotherapy of 5400 cGy. (**A**) A progressive cervical kyphosis developed. Note wedging of the anterior vertebral body. (**B**) Radiograph in halo traction demonstrates partial reduction of the kyphosis. (**C**) Postoperative radiograph after anterior and posterior fusion.

strumentation of the involved spine is desirable but not always possible, because of the absence of posterior elements. The development of pedicle screw fixation has been helpful in allowing the use of posterior instrumentation for postlaminectomy kyphosis. When it can be performed safely, this procedure provides secure fixation while the spinal fusion is maturing. If the deformity is severe or long-standing, anterior release followed by halo traction or a halo cast with an Ilizarov device[70] can be used to obtain gradual correction.[66]

A technique known as laminoplasty may lessen the chance of progressive deformity. This approach involves suturing the laminae back in place after removing them, or removing just one side of the laminae and allowing them to hinge open like a book to expose the spinal cord and then suturing that side of the laminae back in place.[90,140,141] This may provide only a fibrous tether connecting the laminae to the spine, but reported results have been promising. Another promising technique is to hinge the laminae open in a lateral direction after dividing them in the midline. This provides a lateral trough for the placement of bone graft for a lateral fusion.[167] Hopefully, the use of these techniques will decrease the incidence of this deformity.

RADIATION KYPHOSIS

The longitudinal growth of a vertebral body takes place through normal endochondral ossification, similar to the longitudinal growth of the metaphyses of long bones. Bick and Copel[17,18] demonstrated this on histologic sections in fresh autopsy specimens of vertebral bodies taken from research subjects ranging in age from 14 weeks of fetal development to 23 years of age. This endochondral ossification at the physeal growth plate is radiosensitive.[17,18,57,58,80,81,143] Engel[57,58] and Arkin[4] were able to produce spinal deformities in experimental animals using radiation. Arkin[3] was the first to report a case of spinal deformity caused by radiation in humans. Since these reports, it has become clear that exposing an immature spine to radiation can produce spinal deformity, including scoliosis, kyphoscoliosis, lordoscoliosis, and kyphosis.

The three most common solid tumors of childhood in which radiation therapy is part of the treatment regimen and in which the vertebral column is included in the radiation fields are neuroblastoma, Wilms tumor, and medulloblastoma. Early in the history of radiation therapy, survival rates were poor and spinal deformities were not as prevalent. With improved treatment protocols and survival rates, the incidence of spinal deformities has increased. The degree of growth inhibition of the spine is related to the accumulated radiation dose and the age of the child when the spine is irradiated. Progression is directly dependent on the remaining growth potential in the irradiated vertebrae. The younger the child and the greater the accumulated radiation dose, the greater the chance of deformity.[96,97,132,142,146,152,202,205] The most severe growth changes occur in patients who are 2 years of age or younger at the time of irradiation. Initial vertebral changes usually occur 6 months to 2 years after radiation exposure,[54,152] but the deformity may not become apparent until years later after a period of growth.[97,146]

Hinkel,[80,81] Barr,[11] and Reidy[143] found that growth is slowed when a physis is exposed to 600 cGy and completely inhibited when it is exposed to 1200 cGy. Reports of radiation involving the spinal column show that an accumulated dose less than 1000 cGy does not produce a detectable inhibition of vertebral growth,[132,147] whereas a dose of 1000 to 2000 cGy causes a temporary inhibiting effect on growth. Sometimes this is manifested as a transverse growth arrest line in the vertebra that gives the appearance of a bone within a bone. A dose of radiation between 2000 and 3000 cGy causes irregularity or scalloping of vertebral end plates, diminishing axial height, and possibly a flattened, beaked vertebra.[97,132,146,147,152,173,199] A dose of 5000 cGy causes bone necrosis.[151] The effect that radia-

tion has on soft tissue also affects the progression of spinal deformity. The soft tissue anterior to the spine and the abdominal muscle can become fibrotic and act as a tether with growth, adding to the deformity of the spine as the child grows.[116]

The incidence of spinal deformity after irradiation of the spine has been reported to range from 10% to 100%.[12,34,54,97,137,146,147,202] These rates are decreasing because of shielding of growth centers, symmetric field selection, and decreased total accumulated radiation doses. The last of these changes has resulted from an increase in the use and effectiveness of chemotherapeutic regimens that reduce the need for large doses of radiation. Early reports showed an increased incidence of scoliotic deformities with the use of asymmetric fields, but the incidence of kyphotic postirradiation deformities has increased with the use of symmetric radiation fields.[99]

Any child who has received irradiation to the spine should be observed carefully for the development of spinal deformity. Because the development of deformity is related to the amount of disordered growth in the vertebral bodies that were affected by irradiation, it depends to a large extent on the amount of growth left in the spine when irradiation was started and on the amount of damage to the physes caused by irradiation, which correlates directly with the accumulated radiation dose. If the dose of radiation is large enough to cause permanent damage to the physis, the deformity will be progressive. Postirradiation scoliosis and kyphosis both progress more rapidly during the adolescent growth period.[99,146,173,202] Before the adolescent growth spurt, the deformity may remain relatively stable or progress at a steady rate. Severe curves can continue to progress even after skeletal maturity, and these patients may require observation indefinitely.

Radiographic evaluation of a postirradiation deformity should include standard posteroanterior and lateral radiographs of the spine. Occasionally, tomograms or CT scans with sagittal or coronal reconstruction are needed for better delineation of the vertebral body deformities. The spinal cord is evaluated best with MRI. Neuhauser[132] described the roentgenographic changes in irradiated spines. The earliest changes were alterations in the vertebral bodies within the irradiated section of the spine caused by impairment of endochondral growth at the vertebral end plates. Growth arrest lines produced a bone-within-a-bone picture. This occurred in 28% of patients in a study by Riseborough.[146] Other radiographic changes were end plate irregularity, with an altered trabecular pattern and decreased vertebral body height. This pattern was the most common radiographic change reported by Riseborough (83%).[146] Contour abnormalities causing anterior narrowing and beaking of the vertebral bodies, much like those seen in patients with conditions that affect endochondral ossification (e.g., Morquio syndrome, achondroplasia), were the third type of radiographic change noted by Neuhauser.[132]

Treatment

Milwaukee brace treatment has been recommended for progressive curves, but generally has been ineffective for postirradiation kyphosis,[99,146] especially in patients with soft tissue contractures contributing to the deformity. The irradiated skin also may be of poor quality, making long-term brace wear difficult. If progression occurs, spinal fusion with or without instrumentation should be performed, regardless of the age of the patient. Bone quality is poor, and arthrodesis can be difficult to obtain after a single attempt. Anterior and posterior fusion are recommended.[53,99,119,138,146] This fusion mass should extend at least one or two levels above and below the end of the kyphosis. The posterior fusion mass may require reexploration and repeated bone grafting at 6 months, and cast immobilization may need to be prolonged for 6 to 12 months. Posterior instrumentation should be used whenever feasible because it adds increased stability while the fusion mass is maturing and may allow for some limited correction of the kyphotic deformity (Fig. 18-16).

Correction of postirradiation kyphosis is difficult. Typically, these curves are rigid, and soft tissue scarring and contractures often further hamper correction. Healing can be prolonged and pseudarthrosis is common. Infection is a frequent complication in these patients because of poor vascularity of the irradiated tissue.[146] Because viscera also can be damaged by irradiation, bowel obstruction, perforation, and fistula formation can occur after spinal fusion. This can be difficult to differentiate from postoperative cast syndrome, and the treating physician should be aware of this complication.[166]

MISCELLANEOUS CAUSES OF KYPHOTIC DEFORMITIES

Spinal deformity in the sagittal plane occurs in some patients with skeletal dysplasia. The natural history of spinal deformity varies with the type of deformity and the type of dysplasia. Some sagittal plane deformities that appear severe at birth or in infancy improve spontaneously with growth, whereas others continue to progress and eventually can cause paraplegia. A knowledge of the various skeletal dysplasias and the natural history of sagittal plane deformities in each is necessary to prevent overtreatment and undertreatment.

Achondroplasia

Treatment of spinal problems is required most often in patients with achondroplasia. The most common sagittal plane deformity in achondroplastic dwarfs is thoracolumbar kyphosis.[193–195] The kyphosis usually is detected at birth and is accentuated when the child is sitting because of the associated hypotonia in these infants.[195] Ambulation is delayed until about 18 months of age, but after ambulation begins, the thoracolumbar kyphosis tends to improve. According to Lonstein,[108] thoracolumbar kyphosis resolves in 70% of achondroplastic dwarfs and persists in 30%. One third of these patients, or 10% of achondroplastic dwarfs with thoracolumbar kyphosis, have progressive kyphosis[108] (Fig. 18-17).

A lateral radiograph of the thoracolumbar spine during infancy shows anterior wedging of the vertebrae at the apex of the kyphosis.[59] In patients whose thoracolumbar kyphosis resolves, the anterior vertebral body wedging also improves. When the kyphosis is progressive, anterior vertebral body wedging persists.

If no improvement in the thoracolumbar kyphosis is evident by 3 years of age, a thoracolumbarsacral orthosis is recommended to try to prevent progression of the kyphosis.[101,169,170,212] Indications for surgery are documented progression of a kyphotic deformity, kyphosis of more than 40 degrees in a child older than 5 or 6 years of age, or neurologic deficits related to the spinal deformity.[193–195] Distinguishing between neurologic deficits that result from a kyphotic deformity and those associated with lumbar stenosis, which is common in achondroplastic dwarfs, can be difficult. A thorough physical examination and diagnostic studies, such as myelography, CT, and MRI, are necessary to determine appropriate treatment. Most patients with progressive thoracolumbar kyphosis require combined anterior and posterior fusion. Instrumentation is not recommended in these patients because of the small size of the spinal canal and the lack of epidural fat, which make instrumentation hazardous.

Pseudoachondroplasia

Kyphotic deformities also can occur in children with pseudoachondroplasia and are caused by multiple vertebral body wedging in the thoracolumbar and thoracic spine. The kyphotic deformity in patients with pseudoachondroplasia differs from that in patients with achondroplasia. In patients with pseudoachondroplasia, the kyphosis involves multiple levels and is less acutely angular than the deformity in patients with achondroplasia, which involves only one or two levels. Bracing may prevent progression of this deformity, but surgery is indicated if progression occurs. Spinal

(text continues on p. 708)

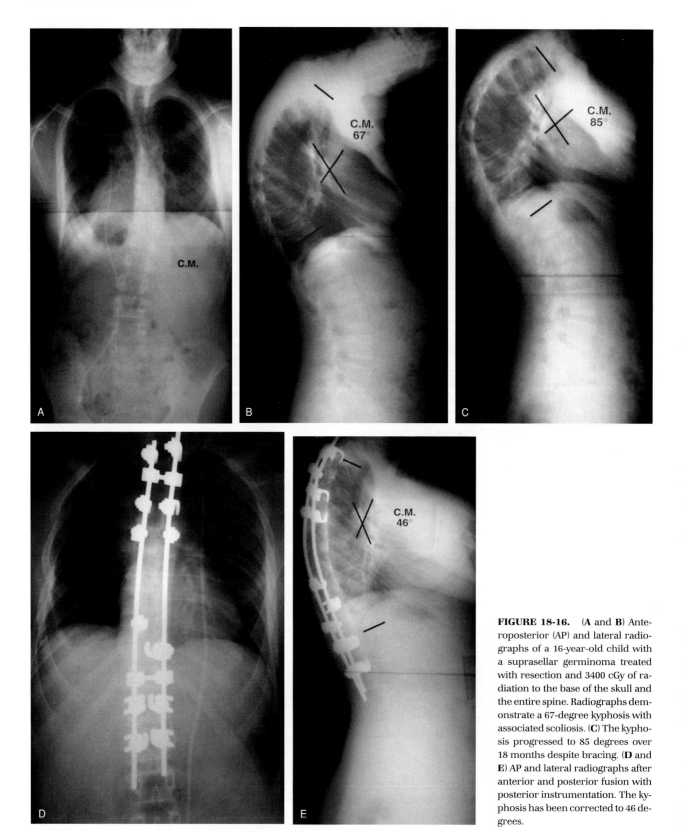

FIGURE 18-16. (**A** and **B**) Anteroposterior (AP) and lateral radiographs of a 16-year-old child with a suprasellar germinoma treated with resection and 3400 cGy of radiation to the base of the skull and the entire spine. Radiographs demonstrate a 67-degree kyphosis with associated scoliosis. (**C**) The kyphosis progressed to 85 degrees over 18 months despite bracing. (**D** and **E**) AP and lateral radiographs after anterior and posterior fusion with posterior instrumentation. The kyphosis has been corrected to 46 degrees.

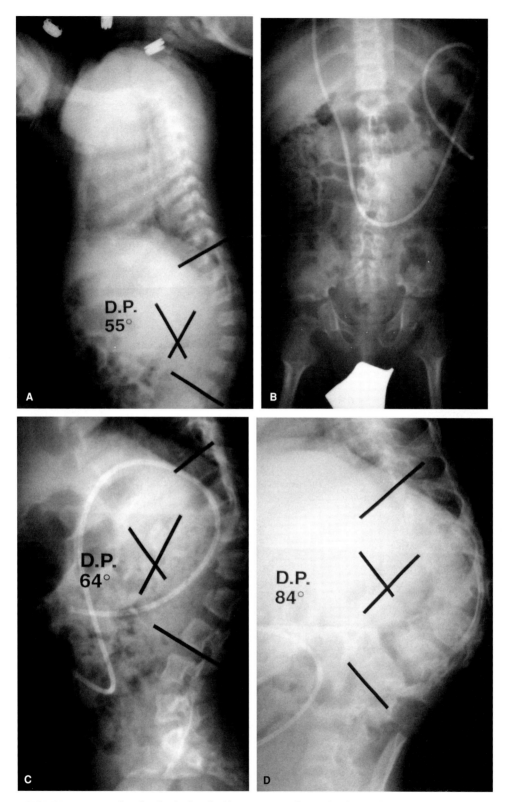

FIGURE 18-17.   Achondroplastic dwarf with progressive thoracolumbar kyphosis. (**A**) Lateral radiograph at 1 year of age shows a 55-degree thoracolumbar kyphosis. (**B**) Anteroposterior radiograph at 5 years of age shows narrowing of the lumbar interpedicular distance characteristic of achondroplasia. (**C**) Lateral radiograph at 5 years of age reveals a 64-degree kyphosis. (**D**) Lateral radiograph at 9 years of age shows an 84-degree thoracolumbar kyphotic deformity.

fusion with instrumentation can be performed safely in patients with pseudoachondroplasia because there is no associated stenosis of the spinal canal as in patients with achondroplasia.[41,93,195]

Spondyloepiphyseal Dysplasia Congenita

Thoracolumbar kyphotic deformities in patients with spondyloepiphyseal dysplasia congenita usually are mild and nonprogressive, and seldom require treatment.[93,195]

Diastrophic Dwarfism

Midcervical kyphosis frequently occurs in patients with diastrophic dwarfism. Progressive cervical kyphosis can be stabilized with a spinal fusion.[79,93,195] There are insufficient data to recommend posterior fusion alone or combined anterior and posterior fusion. If a posterior fusion is performed, the increased incidence of cervical spina bifida in diastrophic dwarfism must be considered during dissection.

Mucopolysaccharidosis

Patients with any of the mucopolysaccharidoses can develop kyphotic spine deformities at the thoracolum-

bar junction. In patients with Hurler syndrome (type I), the vertebral bodies have an anterior beaking at the level of the kyphotic deformity. This kyphosis usually is not progressive and rarely requires treatment because most children with Hurler syndrome die before 10 years of age. Kyphotic deformities in patients with Hunter syndrome (type II) also rarely require treatment because the kyphosis rarely is progressive and patients do not often survive past 20 years of age.[15] Thoracolumbar kyphosis in patients with Morquio syndrome (type IV) is associated with anterior vertebral body defects in the form of anterior beaking of the vertebrae. This kyphosis remains constant with growth and rarely progresses. Patients with Maroteaux-Lamy syndrome (type VI) have a longer life span and can develop progressive kyphosis, which should be treated with bracing. If progression is not halted with bracing, anterior and posterior fusion may be indicated.[93,195]

Marfan Syndrome

Marfan syndrome is a generalized disorder of connective tissue that affects the supporting structures of the body, especially those in the musculoskeletal system. Scoliosis is the most common spinal deformity in pa-

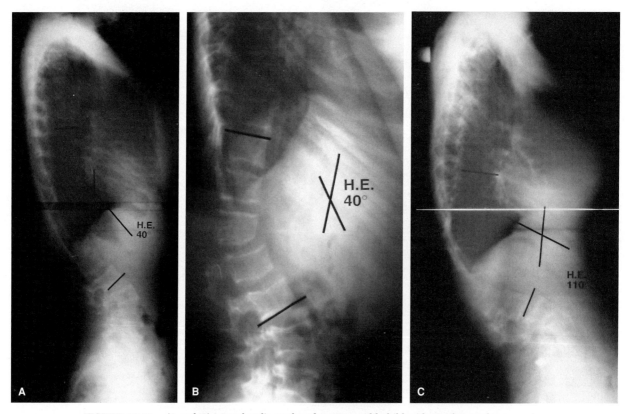

FIGURE 18-18.   (**A** and **B**) Lateral radiographs of a 17-year-old child with Marfan syndrome and a 40-degree progressive thoracolumbar kyphosis. (**C**) Lateral radiograph of the same patient 3 years later shows that the thoracolumbar kyphosis has progressed to 110 degrees.

tients with Marfan syndrome, followed by thoracic lordosis and associated lumbar kyphosis.[2,14,19,95,149,157,192] About two thirds of patients with Marfan syndrome have thoracic lordotic deformities,[69,103] and in some, the thoracic lordosis becomes severe enough to compromise respiration. With the lordotic posture of the thoracic spine, an associated kyphosis or relative kyphosis usually develops in the lumbar spine. The third most common spinal deformity associated with Marfan syndrome is thoracolumbar kyphosis, which affects about 10% of patients (Fig. 18-18). These spinal deformities usually occur during the juvenile growth period before the adolescent growth spurt.[103]

Brace treatment has been recommended to try to halt the progression of spinal deformity, but Birch and Herring[19] found this approach to be ineffective in their patients. Correction of kyphotic deformities requires anterior and posterior spinal fusion with segmental instrumentation.[19] Thoracic lordosis is corrected by posterior segmental instrumentation to correct the lordotic deformity, followed by posterior fusion.[210] Complications are more frequent after surgical correction of spinal deformity in patients with Marfan syndrome than after spinal surgery in other patients.[19]

Posttraumatic Deformities

Kyphosis can occur as a result of trauma to the spinal column or the spinal cord. The deformity can occur at the fracture site or it can result from paralysis after spinal cord injury.[117,120,144,145] Kyphosis at the fracture site is acute and spans a short segment of vertebrae. Paralytic kyphosis is a long, C-shaped deformity that spans many vertebral segments. Kyphosis at a fracture site requires surgical intervention for correction. Brace treatment has been ineffective for progressive paralytic kyphosis,[49,145] and surgery is indicated for paralytic kyphosis of more than 60 degrees. If the kyphosis is flexible and can be reduced to less than 50 degrees, posterior fusion with segmental instrumentation can be performed. If the kyphosis is rigid and cannot be reduced to less than 50 degrees on preoperative bending x-ray films, anterior release and fusion should be followed by posterior fusion and segmental instrumentation.[144,145]

Tuberculosis

Childhood spinal tuberculosis is a disease more malignant in extent and degree of abscess formation but with less associated paraplegia than tuberculosis in adults.[82] The most frequent site of spinal tuberculosis in children is the thoracolumbar junction and its adjacent segments. Tuberculosis infection usually destroys the anterior elements of the spine and results in a significant angular kyphosis at the infected site. With differential growth of the intact posterior elements, the kyphosis increases.[82]

All forms of active spinal tuberculosis are treated with a complete course of chemotherapy. First-line drugs are streptomycin, isoniazid, and rifampicin, and second-line drugs are ethambutol and pyrazinamide.[1] Chemotherapy is combined with surgical debridement in most patients. The only indications for chemotherapy alone are medically high-risk patients and, occasionally, patients who have early disease with little bony destruction.[82] Surgery consists of anterior debridement and placement of strut grafts to prevent further increase in the kyphotic deformity.[10,86,91,176–183] Some correction of the kyphosis may be obtained at the time of surgery. Kyphosis also can be a problem in patients with healed spinal tuberculosis.[84] The infected area of the anterior spine usually fuses, and continued growth posteriorly causes progressive kyphosis that can result in paraplegia. The presence of neurologic symptoms is an indication for anterior decompression and fusion, which can be followed by posterior fusion and instrumentation.

Neurofibromatosis

Kyphoscoliosis is common in patients with neurofibromatosis. The kyphosis is the predominant feature and usually measures more than 50 degrees. The vertebral bodies frequently are deformed and attenuated at the apex of the kyphosis.[43,85] The kyphosis typically is sharp and angular over a relatively small number of vertebral segments. Severely angular kyphosis can cause neurologic compromise.[43,44,125] Lonstein[109] found cord compression due to spinal curvature from neurofibromatosis to be second only to congenital kyphosis as a cause of spinal cord compression.

Treatment of kyphoscoliosis in patients with neurofibromatosis begins with a thorough physical examination for neurologic abnormalities. MRI is performed to demonstrate any intraspinal lesions, such as pseudomeningocele, dural ectasia, or neurofibroma, which may cause impingement on the spinal cord during instrumentation.[163] Any intraspinal lesions should be treated before spinal fusion and instrumentation are undertaken. Because posterior fusion alone has resulted in a high rate of pseudarthrosis (65%),[214] anterior and posterior spinal fusion combined with posterior instrumentation is recommended. Abundant autogenous bone graft and prolonged immobilization may be required to obtain a solid fusion in these patients, and repeated bone grafting 6 months after the initial surgery may be required.[43]

Juvenile Osteoporosis

Idiopathic juvenile osteoporosis is an acquired systemic condition that consists of generalized osteoporosis in otherwise normal prepubertal children. Although idiopathic juvenile osteoporosis is uncommon, associated kyphosis and back pain are common in patients with this condition.

Schippers[161] first described this condition in 1939, and since that time, other authors have described its clinical findings and natural history.[13,50,60,83,92,94,118,155,172] The etiology of idiopathic juvenile osteoporosis is unknown. Laboratory values of serum calcium, phosphorus, alkaline phosphatase, parathyroid hormone, and osteocalcin are normal. The collagen type and ratios from skin biopsy samples also are normal. There have been some reports of a slight decrease in 1,25-dihydroxyvitamin D,[118,150,156] but the significance of this finding is not known. Low serum calcitonin levels also have been reported, but treatment with calcitonin has not proven to be beneficial.[30,92] In contrast, Saggese[155] noted normal serum calcitonin levels in his patients. Green[71] believes that a mild deficiency of 1,25-dihydroxyvitamin D can explain most of the findings in idiopathic juvenile osteoporosis. During rapid growth phases, the deficiency is discovered because growth requirements cannot keep pace, causing a relative osteoporosis. When puberty occurs, the increase in sex hormone overcomes the deficit in 1,25-dihydroxyvitamin D and the relative osteoporosis improves. This theory has yet to be proved.

Clinically, these patients complain of insidious onset of low back pain and lower extremity pain. This occurs during the prepubertal period and is slightly more common in boys than girls. Vertebral collapse or wedging with resulting kyphosis is common. Brenton[30] classified idiopathic juvenile osteoporosis into mild, moderate, and severe types. Patients with the mild type had only back pain and vertebral fractures; those with the moderate type had back and lower extremity pain and fractures, with some limitation of activities but eventual return to normal function; and those with the severe form had back and lower extremity pain and fractures. Both metaphyseal and diaphyseal fractures can occur in the lower extremities. Patients with severe disease improve clinically but do not return to normal activity after puberty.

Plain radiographs show wedging or collapse of the vertebral bodies. A "codfish" appearance of the vertebral bodies can occur, with the superior and inferior borders of the vertebrae becoming biconcave (Fig. 18-19). Because of the osteoporosis, tomograms may be necessary to better delineate the spinal deformity. Other studies that can be useful to follow the progress of this disease are single-photon absorptiometry, dual-photon absorptiometry, and quantitative CT scanning.[92,118,155] The problems with these tests are that normal ranges for adolescents and children are variable and have not been standardized.

Idiopathic juvenile osteoporosis is a diagnosis of exclusion. Other diseases that must be considered include metabolic bone diseases, leukemia, Cushing syndrome, lysinuric protein intolerance, type I homocystinuria, and osteogenesis imperfecta. The natural history of this condition is spontaneous improvement or remission at the onset of puberty. Associated kyphosis tends to improve after the onset of puberty.

Treatment of idiopathic juvenile osteoporosis involves modification of activities, possible calcium supplementation and vitamin D supplementation, and supportive treatment of spinal deformities. A balance must be obtained between restriction of activities to prevent fractures and excessive restriction of activities that will increase osteoporosis. If a significant progressive kyphosis develops, the Milwaukee brace is the treatment of choice.[94] The brace is worn until there is evidence of improvement of the osteoporosis. Operative therapy for this condition has been associated with a high complication rate because the poor bone quality makes instrumentation and fusion difficult.[13]

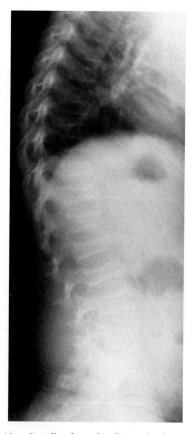

FIGURE 18-19. Standing lateral radiograph of a 10-year-old girl with idiopathic juvenile osteoporosis shows diffuse osteopenia, multiple "codfish" vertebrae in the thoracic and lumbar spine, and "coin" vertebrae in the upper thoracic spine secondary to extreme collapse. (From Green WB. Idiopathic juvenile osteoporosis, ed. 1. New York: Raven Press, 1994:933.)

References

1. Antituberculosis regimens of chemotherapy. Bull Int Union Tuberc Lung Dis 1988;63:60.

2. Amis J, Herring JA. Iatrogenic kyphosis: a complication of Harrington instrumentation in Marfan syndrome. J Bone Joint Surg [Am] 1984;66:460.

3. Arkin AM, Pack GT, Ransohoff NS, Simon N. Radiation-induced scoliosis: a case report. J Bone Joint Surg [Am] 1950;32:401.

4. Arkin AM, Simon N. Radiation scoliosis: an experimental study. J Bone Joint Surg [Am] 1950;32:396.

5. Ascani E, Borelli P, Larosa G, et al. Malattia di Scheuermann. I: studio ormonale. In: Gaggia A, ed. Progressi in patologia vertebrale, vol 5. Bologna: Le Cifosi, 1982:97.

6. Ascani E, LaRossa G. Scheuermann's kyphosis. New York: Raven Press, 1994:557.

7. Aufdermaur M. Juvenile kyphosis (Scheuermann's disease): radiology, histology and pathogenesis. Clin Orthop 1981; 154:166.

8. Aufdermaur M, Spycher M. Pathogenesis of osteochondrosis juvenilis Scheuermann. J Orthop Res 1986;4:452.

9. Axelgaard J, Nordwall A, Brown JC. Correction of spinal curves by transcutaneous electrical muscle stimulation. Spine 1983;8:463.

10. Bailey HL, Gabriel M, Hodgson AR, Shin JA. Tuberculosis of the spine in children: operative findings and results in one hundred consecutive patients treated by removal of the lesion and anterior grafting. J Bone Joint Surg [Am] 1972;54:1633.

11. Barr JS, Lingley JR, Gall EA. The effect of roentgen irradiation on epiphyseal growth. I. Experimental studies upon the albino rat. AJR Am J Roentgenol 1943;49:104.

12. Barrera M, Roy LP, Stevens M. Long-term follow-up after unilateral nephrectomy and radiotherapy for Wilms' tumour. Pediatr Nephrol 1989;3:430.

13. Bartal E, Gage J. Idiopathic juvenile osteoporosis and scoliosis. J Pediatr Orthop 1982;2:295.

14. Beneux J, Rigault P, Poliquen JC. Les deviations rachidiennes de la maladie de Marfan chez l'enfant. Etude de 10 cas. Rev Chir Orthop Reparatrice Appar Mot 1978;64:471.

15. Benson PF, Button LR, Fensom AH, Dean MF. Lumbar kyphosis in Hunter's disease (MPS II). Clin Genet 1979;16:317.

16. Bernhardt M, Bridwell KH. Segmental analysis of the sagittal plane alignment of the normal thoracic and lumbar spines and the thoracolumbar junction. Spine 1989;14:17.

17. Bick EM, Copel JW. The ring apophysis of the human vertebra. Contribution to human osteogeny II. J Bone Joint Surg [Am] 1951;33:783.

18. Bick EM, Copel JW, SS. Longitudinal growth of the human vertebra. A contribution to human osteogeny. J Bone Joint Surg [Am] 1950;32:803.

19. Birch JG, Herring JA. Spinal deformity in Marfan syndrome. J Pediatr Orthop 1987;7:546.

20. Blake NS, Lynch AS, Dowling FE. Spinal cord abnormalities in congenital scoliosis. Ann Radiol (Paris) 1986;29:237.

21. Bouchez B, Arnott G, Combelles G, Pruvo J. Compression medullaire par hernie kiscale dorsale. Rev Neurol (Paris) 1986;142:154.

22. Bradford DS. Juvenile kyphosis. Clin Orthop 1977;128:45.

23. Bradford DS. Vertebral osteochondrosis (Scheuermann's kyphosis). Clin Orthop 1981;158:83.

24. Bradford DS, Ahmed KB, Moe JH, et al. The surgical management of patients with Scheuermann's disease: a review of twenty-four cases managed by combined anterior and posterior spine fusion. J Bone Joint Surg [Am] 1980;62:705.

25. Bradford DS, Brown DM, Moe JH, et al. Scheuermann's kyphosis. A form of osteoporosis? Clin Orthop 1976;118:10.

26. Bradford DS, Heithoff KB, Cohen M. Intraspinal abnormalities and congenital spine deformities: a radiographic and MRI study. J Pediatr Orthop 1991;11:36.

27. Bradford DS, Moe JH, Montalvo FJ, et al. Scheuermann's kyphosis and roundback deformity: results of Milwaukee brace treatment. J Bone Joint Surg [Am] 1974;56:740.

28. Bradford DS, Moe JH, Montalvo FJ, Winter RB. Scheuermann's kyphosis. Results of surgical treatment by posterior spine arthrodesis in twenty-two patients. J Bone Joint Surg [Am] 1975;57:439.

29. Bradford DS, Moe JH, Winter RB. Kyphosis and postural roundback deformity in children and adolescents. Minn Med 1973;56:114.

30. Brenton DP, Dent CE. Idiopathic juvenile osteoporosis. In: Bickel H, Stern J, eds. Inborn errors of calcium and bone metabolism. Baltimore: University Park Press, 1976:222.

31. Broekman BA, Dorr JP. Congenital kyphosis due to absence of two lumbar vertebral bodies. JCU J Clin Ultrasound 1991;19:303.

32. Burner WL, Badger VM, Sherman FC. Osteoporosis and acquired back deformities. J Pediatr Orthop 1982;2:383.

33. Butler JC, Whitecloud TS. Postlaminectomy kyphosis: causes and surgical management. Orthop Clin North Am 1992;23:505.

34. Butler MS, Robertson WW Jr, Rate W, et al. Skeletal sequelae of radiation therapy for malignant childhood tumors. Clin Orthop 1990;251:235.

35. Butler RW. The nature and significance of vertebral osteochondritis. Proceedings of the Royal Society of Medicine 1955;48:895.

36. Callahan RA, Johnson RM, Margolis RN, et al. Cervical facet fusion for control of instability following laminectomy. J Bone Joint Surg [Am] 1977;59:991.

37. Carr AJ. Idiopathic thoracic kyphosis in identical twins. J Bone Joint Surg [Br] 1990;72:144.

38. Cattell HS, Clark GL Jr. Cervical kyphosis and instability following multiple laminectomies in children. J Bone Joint Surg [Am] 1967;49:713.

39. Cloward RB, Bucy PC. Spinal extradural cyst and kyphosis dorsalis juvenilis. AJR Am J Roentgenol 1937;38:681.

40. Cobb J. Outline for the study of scoliosis. Instr Course Lect 1948;5:261.

41. Cooper RR, Ponseti IV, Maynard JA. Pseudoachondroplastic dwarfism. J Bone Joint Surg [Am] 1973;55:475.

42. Coscia MF, Bradford DS, Ogilvie JW. Scheuermann's kyphosis: results in 19 cases treated by spinal arthrodesis and L-rod instrumentation. Orthop Trans 1988;12:255.

43. Crawford AH. Neurofibromatosis. In: Weinstein SL, ed. The pediatric spine: principles and practice. New York: Raven Press, 1994:619.

44. Curtis BH, Fisher RL, Butterfield WL, Saunders FP. Neurofibromatosis with paraplegia: report of 8 cases. J Bone Joint Surg [Am] 1969;51:843.

45. Cutler WB, Friedman E, Genovese-Stone E. Prevalence of kyphosis in a healthy sample of pre and postmenopausal women. Am J Phys Med Rehabil 1993;72:219.

46. De Mauroy JC, Stagnara P. Resultats a long terme du traitement orthopedique. Aix en Provence: 1978:60.

47. Deacon P, Berkin C, Dickson R. Combined idiopathic kyphosis and scoliosis. An analysis of the lateral spinal curvature associated with Scheuermann's disease. J Bone Joint Surg [Br] 1985;67:189.

48. Deacon P, Flood BM, A DR. Idiopathic scoliosis in three dimensions: a radiographic and morphometric analysis. J Bone Joint Surg [Br] 1984;66:509.

49. Dearolf WWI, Betz RR, Vogel LC, et al. Scoliosis in pediatric spinal cord-injured patients. J Pediatr Orthop 1990;10:214.

50. Dent CE, Friedman M. Idiopathic juvenile osteoporosis. Q J Med 1965;134:177.

51. Dietrich U, Schirmer M, Veltrup K, et al. Post laminectomy kyphosis and scoliosis in children with spinal tumors. Neurol Orthop 1989;7:36.

52. DiMeglio A, Bonnel F. Growth of the spine. In: Raimondi AJ, Choux M, Di Rocco C, eds. The pediatric spine I. New York: Springer-Verlag, 1989:39.

53. Donaldson DH. Scoliosis secondary to radiation. In: Bridwell HK, DeWald RL, eds. The textbook of spinal surgery. Philadelphia: JB Lippincott, 1991:485.

54. Donaldson WF, Wissinger HA. Axial skeletal changes following tumor dose radiation therapy. J Bone Joint Surg [Am] 1967;49:1469.

55. Dubousset J. Congenital kyphosis. In: Bradford DS, Hensinger RM, eds. The pediatric spine. New York: Thieme, 1985:196.

56. Dubousset J. Congenital kyphosis and lordosis. In: Weinstein SL, ed. The pediatric spine: principles and practice. New York: Raven Press, 1994:245.

57. Engel D. An experimental study on the action of radium on developing bones. Br J Radiol 1938;11:779.

58. Engel D. Experiments on the production of spinal deformities by radium. AJR Am J Roentgenol 1939;42:217.

59. Eulert J. Scoliosis and kyphosis in dwarfing conditions. Arch Orthop Trauma Surg 1983;102:45.

60. Evans RA, Dunstan CR, Hills E. Bone metabolism in idiopathic juvenile osteoporosis: a case report. Calcif Tissue Int 1983;35:5.

61. Farsetti P, Tudisco C, Caterini R, Ippolito E. Juvenile and idiopathic kyphosis. Long-term follow-up of 20 cases. Arch Orthop Trauma Surg 1991;110:165.

62. Ferguson AB Jr. The etiology of pre-adolescent kyphosis. J Bone Joint Surg [Am] 1956;38:149.

63. Fisk JW, Baigent ML, Hill PD. Incidence of Scheuermann's disease. Preliminary report. Am J Phys Med Rehabil 1982;61:32.

64. Fisk JW, Baigent ML, Hill PD. Scheuermann's disease. Clinical and radiological survey of 17 and 18 year olds. Am J Phys Med Rehabil 1984;63:18.

65. Fon GT, Pitt MJ, Thies AC Jr. Thoracic kyphosis: range in normal subjects. AJR Am J Roentgenol 1980;134:979.

66. Francis WR Jr, Noble DP. Treatment of cervical kyphosis in children. Spine 1988;13:883.

67. Fraser RD, Paterson DC, Simpson DA. Orthopaedic aspects of spinal tumours in children. J Bone Joint Surg [Br] 1977;59:143.

68. Gilsanz V, Gibbens DT, Carlson M, King J. Vertebral bone density in Scheuermann disease. J Bone Joint Surg [Am] 1989;71:894.

69. Goldberg MJ. Marfan and the marfanoid habitus. In: Goldberg MJ, ed. The dysmorphic child: an orthopaedic perspective. New York: Raven Press, 1987:83.

70. Graziano GP, Herzenberg JE, Hensinger RN. The halo-Ilizarov distraction cast for correction of cervical deformity. J Bone Joint Surg [Am] 1993;75:996.

71. Green WB. Idiopathic juvenile osteoporosis. New York: Raven Press, 1994:933.

72. Greene TL, Hensinger RN, Hunter LY. Back pain and vertebral changes simulating Scheuermann's disease. J Pediatr Orthop 1985;5:1.

73. Guille JT, Forlin E, Bowen JR. Congenital kyphosis. Orthop Rev 1993;22:235.

74. Gutowski WT, Renshaw TS. Orthotic results in adolescent kyphosis. Spine 1988;13:485.

75. Haft H, Ransohoff J, Carter S. Spinal cord tumors in children. Pediatrics 1959;23:1152.

76. Halal F, Gledhill RB, Fraser FC. Dominant inheritance of Scheuermann's juvenile kyphosis. Am J Dis Child 1978;132:1105.

77. Hammerberg KW. Kyphosis. In: Bridwell KH, DeWald RL, eds. The textbook of spinal surgery. Philadelphia: JB Lippincott, 1991:857.

78. Herndon WA, Emans JB, Micheli LG, Hall JE. Combined anterior and posterior fusion for Scheuermann's kyphosis. Spine 1981;6:125.

79. Herring JA. The spinal disorders in diastrophic dwarfism. J Bone Joint Surg [Am] 1978;60:177.

80. Hinkel CL. The effect of roentgen rays upon the growing long bones of albino rats. Quantitative studies of the growth limitation following irradiation. AJR Am J Roentgenol 1942;47:439.

81. Hinkel CL. The effect of roentgen rays upon the growing long bones of albino rats II. Histopathological changes involving endochondral growth centers. AJR Am J Roentgenol 1943;49:321.

82. Ho EKW, Leong JCY. Tuberculosis of the spine. In: Weinstein SL, ed. The pediatric spine: principles and practice. New York: Raven Press, 1994:837.

83. Hoekman K, Papapoulos SE, Peters ACB, Bijvoet OLM. Characteristics and bisphosphonate treatment of a patient with juvenile osteoporosis. J Clin Endocrinol Metab 1985;61:952.

84. Hsu LCS, Cheng CL, Leong JCY. Pott's paraplegia of late onset: the cause of compression and results after anterior decompression. J Bone Joint Surg [Br] 1988;70:534.

85. Hsu LCS, Lee PC, Leong JCY. Dystrophic spinal deformities in neurofibromatosis, treated by anterior and posterior fusion. J Bone Joint Surg [Br] 1980;66:495.

86. Hsu LCS, Leong JCY. Tuberculosis of the lower cervical spine (C2–7): a report on forty cases. J Bone Joint Surg [Br] 1984;66:1.

87. Huskisson EC. Measurement of pain. Lancet 1974;:779.

88. Ippolito E, Bellocci M, Montanaro A, et al. Juvenile kyphosis: an ultrastructural study. J Pediatr Orthop 1985;5:315.

89. Ippolito E, Ponseti IV. Juvenile kyphosis: histological and histochemical studies. J Bone Joint Surg [Am] 1981;63:175.

90. Ishida Y, Suzuki K, Ohmori K, et al. Critical analysis of extensive cervical laminectomy. Neurosurgery 1989;24:215.

91. Ito H, Tsuchiya J, Asami G. A new radical operation for Pott's disease. J Bone Joint Surg 1934;16:499.

92. Jackson EC, Strife CF, Tsang RC, Marder HK. Effect of calcitonin replacement therapy in idiopathic juvenile osteoporosis. Am J Dis Child 1988;142:1237.

93. Jones ET, Hensinger RN. Spinal deformity in individuals with short stature. Orthop Clin North Am 1979;10:877.

94. Jones ET, Hensinger RN. Spinal deformity in idiopathic juvenile osteoporosis. Spine 1981;6:1.

95. Joseph KN, Kane HA, Milner RS, et al. Orthopaedic aspects of the Marfan phenotype. Clin Orthop 1992;277:251.

96. Katz LD, Lawson JP. Radiation-induced growth abnormalities. Skeletal Radiol 1990;19:50.

97. Katzman H, Waugh T, Berdon W. Skeletal changes following irradiation of childhood tumors. J Bone Joint Surg [Am] 1969;51:825.

98. Kemp FH, Wilson DC. Some factors in the aetiology of osteochondritis of the spine. Br J Radiol 1947;20:410.

99. King J, Stowe S. Results of spinal fusion for radiation scoliosis. Spine 1982;7:574.

100. Klein DM, Weiss RL, Allen JE. Scheuermann's dorsal kyphosis and spinal cord compression: case report. Neurosurgery 1986;18:628.

101. Kopits SE. Thoracolumbar kyphosis and lumbosacral hyperlordosis in achondroplastic children. In: Nicoletti B, Kopits SE, Ascani E, McKusick VA, eds. Human achondroplasia: a multidisciplinary approach. New York: Plenum Press, 1988: 241.

102. Kostuik JP. Anterior Kostuik-Harrington distraction systems. Orthopedics 1985;11:1379.

103. Kumar SJ, Guille JT. Marfan syndrome. In: Weinstein SL, ed. The pediatric spine: principles and practice. New York: Raven Press, 1994:665.

103a. Lambrinudi L. Adolescent and senile kyphosis. BMJ 1934; 2:800.

104. LeMire RJ. Intrauterine development of the vertebrae and spinal cord. In: Raimondi AJ, Choux M, Di Rocco C, eds. The pediatric spine, vol I. New York: Springer-Verlag, 1989:20.

105. Lesoin F, Leys D, Rousseaux M, et al. Thoracic disk herniation and Scheuermann's disease. Eur Neurol 1987;26:145.

106. Lombard P, Legenissel. Cyphoses congenitales. Rev Orthop 1938;22:532.

107. Lonstein JE. Post-laminectomy kyphosis. Clin Orthop 1977; 128:93.

108. Lonstein JE. Treatment of kyphosis and lumbar stenosis in achondroplasia. Basic Life Sci 1986;48:282.

109. Lonstein JE, Winter RB, Moe JH, et al. Neurologic deficit secondary to spinal deformity. Spine 1980;5:331.

110. Lonstein JE, Winter RB, Moe JH, et al. Post-laminectomy spine deformity. J Bone Joint Surg [Am] 1976;58:727.

111. Lopez RA, Burke SW, Levine DB, Scheider R. Osteoporosis in Scheuermann's disease. Spine 1988;13:1099.

112. Lowe T. Mortality-morbidity committee report. Scoliosis Research Society. Vancouver, British Columbia: 1987:

113. Lowe TG. Double L-rod instrumentation in the treatment of severe kyphosis secondary to Scheuermann's disease. Spine 1987;12:336.

114. Lowe TG. Current concepts review, Scheuermann disease. J Bone Joint Surg [Am] 1990;72:940.

115. Lubicky JP, Shook JE. Congenital spinal deformity. In: Bridwell HK, DeWald RL, eds. The textbook of spinal surgery. Philadelphia: JB Lippincott, 1991:365.

116. Makipernaa A, Heikkila JT, Merikanto J, et al. Spinal deformity induced by radiotherapy for solid tumors in childhood: a long-term follow-up study. Eur J Pediatr 1993;152:197.

117. Malcolm BW. Spinal deformity secondary to spinal injury. Orthop Clin North Am 1979;10:943.

118. Marder HK, Tsang RC, Hug G, Crawford AC. Calcitriol deficiency in idiopathic juvenile osteoporosis. Am J Dis Child 1982;136:914.

119. Mayfield JK. Post-radiation spinal deformity. Orthop Clin North Am 1979;10:829.

120. Mayfield JK, Erkkila JC, Winter RB. Spine deformity subsequent to acquired childhood spinal cord injury. J Bone Joint Surg [Am] 1981;63:1401.

121. Mayfield JK, Winter RB, Bradford DS, et al. Congenital kyphosis due to defects of anterior segmentation. J Bone Joint Surg [Am] 1980;62:1291.

122. McKenzie L, Sillence D. Familial Scheuermann disease: a genetic and linkage study. J Med Genet 1992;29:41.

123. Mellin G, Harkonen H, Poussa M. Spinal mobility and posture and their correlations with growth velocity in structurally normal boys and girls aged 13 to 14. Spine 1988;13:152.

124. Mellin G, Poussa M. Spinal mobility and posture in 8 to 16 year old children. J Orthop Res 1992;10:211.

125. Miller A. Neurofibromatosis with reference to skeletal changes, compression myolytis and malignant degeneration. Arch Surg 1936;32:109.

126. Montgomery SP, Erwin WE. Scheuermann's kyphosis: long-term results of Milwaukee braces treatment. Spine 1981;6:5.

127. Montgomery SP, Hall JE. Congenital kyphosis. Spine 1982;7:360.

128. Morin B, Poitras B, Duhaime M, et al. Congenital kyphosis by segmentation defect: etiologic and pathogenic studies. J Pediatr Orthop 1985;5:309.

129. Muller R. Endokrine Storungen und Morbus Scheuermann. Acta Med Scand 1969;139:99.

130. Murray PM, Weinstein SL, Spratt KF. The natural history and long-term follow-up of Scheuermann kyphosis. J Bone Joint Surg [Am] 1993;75:238.

131. Nerubay J, Katznelson A. Dual approach in the surgical treatment of juvenile kyphosis. Spine 1986;11:101.

132. Neuhauser EBD, Wittenborg MH, Berman CZ, Cohen J. Irradiation effects of roentgen therapy on the growing spine. Radiology 1952;59:637.

133. O'Rahilly R, Benson D. The development of the vertebral column. In: Bradford DS, Hensinger RN, eds. The pediatric spine. New York: Thieme, 1985:3.

134. Ogilvie JW, Sherman J. Spondylolysis in Scheuermann's disease. Spine 1987;12:251.

135. Otsuka NY, Hall JE, Mah JY. Posterior fusion for Scheuermann's kyphosis. Clin Orthop 1990;251:134.

136. Panjabi MN, White AAI, Johnson RM. Cervical spine mechanics as a function of transection of components. J Biomech 1975;8:327.

137. Pastore G, Antonelli R, Fine W, et al. Late effects of treatment of cancer in infancy. Med Pediatr Oncol 1982;10:369.

138. Peterson HA. Iatrogenic spinal deformities. In: Weinstein SL, ed. The pediatric spine: principles and practice. New York: Raven Press, 1994:651.

139. Propst-Proctor SL, Bleck EE. Radiographic determination of lordosis and kyphosis in normal and scoliotic children. J Pediatr Orthop 1983;3:344.

140. Raimondi AJ, Gutierrez FA, Di Rocco C. Laminotomy and total reconstruction of the posterior spinal arch for spinal canal surgery in childhood. J Neurosurg 1976;45:555.

141. Rama B, Markakis E, Kolenda H, Jansen J. Reconstruction instead of resection: laminotomy and laminoplasty. Neurochirurgia (Stuttg) 1990;33(Suppl 1):36.

142. Rate WR, Butler MS, Robertson WWJ, D'Angio GJ. Late orthopaedic effects in children with Wilms' tumor treated with abdominal irradiation. Med Pediatr Oncol 1991;19:265.

143. Reidy JA, Lingley JR, Gall EA, Barr JS. The effect of roentgen irradiation on epiphyseal growth. II. Experimental studies upon the dog. J Bone Joint Surg 1947;29:853.

144. Renshaw TS. Paralysis in the child: orthopaedic management. In: Bradford DS, Hensinger RM, eds. The pediatric spine. New York: Thieme, 1985:118.

145. Renshaw TS. Spinal cord injury and posttraumatic deformities. In: Weinstein SL, ed. The pediatric spine: principles and practice. New York: Raven Press, 1994:767.

146. Riseborough EH, Grabias SL, Burton RI, Jaffe N. Skeletal alterations following irradiation for Wilms' tumor: with particular reference to scoliosis and kyphosis. J Bone Joint Surg [Am] 1976;58:526.

147. Riseborough EJ. Irradiation induced kyphosis. Clin Orthop 1977;128:101.

148. Rivard CH, Narbaitz R, Uhthoff HK. Congenital vertebral malformations: time of induction in human and mouse embryo. Orthop Rev 1979;8:135.

149. Robins PR, Moe JH, Winter RB. Scoliosis in Marfan syndrome: its characteristics and results of treatment in thirty-five patients. J Bone Joint Surg [Am] 1975;57:358.

150. Rosskamp R, Sell G, Emmons D, et al. Idiopathische juvenile osteoporose-Bericht uber zwei Falle. Klin Padiatr 1987; 199:457.

151. Rubin P, Duthie RB, Young LW. The significance of scoliosis in postirradiated Wilms' tumor and neuroblastoma. Radiology 1962;79:539.

152. Rutherford H, Dodd GD. Complications of radiation therapy: growing bone. Semin Roentgenol 1974;9:15.

153. Ryan MD, Taylor TKF. Acute spinal cord compression in Scheuermann's disease. J Bone Joint Surg [Br] 1982;64:409.

154. Sachs B, Bradford D, Winter R, et al. Scheuermann kyphosis: follow-up of Milwaukee brace treatment. J Bone Joint Surg [Am] 1987;69:50.

155. Saggese G, Bartelloni S, Baroncelli GI, et al. Mineral metabolism and calcitriol therapy in idiopathic juvenile osteoporosis. Am J Dis Child 1991;145:457.

156. Samuda GM, Cheng MY, Yeung CY. Back pain and vertebral compression: an uncommon presentation of childhood acute lymphoblastic leukemia. J Pediatr Orthop 1987;7:175.

157. Savini R, Cervellati S, Beroaldo E. Spinal deformities in Marfan syndrome. Ital J Orthop Traumatol 1980;6:19.

158. Scheuermann HW. Kyphosis dorsalis juvenilis. Z Orthop Chir 1921;41:305.

159. Scheuermann HW. Kyphosis dorsalis juvenilis. Ugeskr Laeger 1920;82:385.

160. Schijman E. Comparative anatomy of the spine in the newborn, infant and toddler. In: Raimondi AJ, Choux M, Di Rocco C, eds. The pediatric spine, vol I. New York: Springer-Verlag, 1989:1.

161. Schippers JC. Over een geval van "spontane" algemeene osteoporose bij een klein meisje. Maandschrift voor Kindergeneeskd 1939;8:108.

162. Schmorl G. Die pathogenese der juvenilen kyphose. Fortschr Roentgen 1930;41:359.

163. Schorry EK, Stowens DW, Crawford AH, et al. Summary of patient data from a multidisciplinary neurofibromatosis clinic. Neurofibromatosis 1989;2:129.

164. Schultz AB, Sorensen SE, Andersson GBJ. Measurements of spine morphology in children, ages 10–16. Spine 1984;9:70.

165. Scoles PV, Latimer BM, Diglovanni BF, et al. Vertebral alterations in Scheuermann's kyphosis. Spine 1991;16:509.

166. Shah M, Eng K, Engler GL. Radiation enteritis and radiation scoliosis. N Y State J Med 1980;80:548.

167. Shikata J, Yamamuro T, Shimizu K, Saito T. Combined laminoplasty and posterolateral fusion for spinal canal surgery in children and adolescents. Clin Orthop 1990;259:92.

168. Shufflebarger HL. Cotrel-Dubousset instrumentation for Scheuermann's kyphosis. Orthop Trans 1989;13:90.

169. Siebens AA, Hungerford DS, Kirby NA. Achondroplasia: effectiveness of an orthosis in reducing deformity of the spine. Arch Phys Med Rehabil 1987;68:384.

170. Siebens AA, Kirby N, Hungerford DS. Orthotic correction of sitting abnormality in achondroplastic children. In: Nicoletti B, Kopits SE, Acsani E, McKusich VA, eds. Human achondroplasia: a multidisciplinary approach. New York: Plenum Press, 1988:313.

171. Sim FH, Svien JH, Bickel WH, Janes JM. Swan-neck deformity following extensive cervical laminectomy: a review of twenty-one cases. J Bone Joint Surg [Am] 1974;56:564.

172. Smith R. Idiopathic osteoporosis in the young. J Bone Joint Surg [Br] 1980;62:417.

173. Smith R, Davidson JK, Flatman GE. Skeletal effects of orthovoltage and megavoltage therapy following treatment of nephroblastoma. Clin Radiol 1982;33:601.

174. Sorensen KH. Scheuermann's juvenile kyphosis. Clinical appearances, radiography, aetiology and prognosis. Copenhagen: Munksgaard, 1964.

175. Speck GR, Chopin DC. The surgical treatment of Scheuermann's kyphosis. J Bone Joint Surg [Br] 1986;68:189.

176. Medical Research Council Working Party on Tuberculosis of the Spine. A controlled trial of ambulant outpatient treatment and inpatient rest in bed in the management of tuberculosis of the spine in young Korean patients on standard chemotherapy: a study in Masan, Korea. J Bone Joint Surg [Br] 1973;55:678.

177. Medical Research Council Working Party on Tuberculosis of the Spine. A controlled trial of plaster-of-paris jackets in the management of ambulant outpatient treatment of tuberculosis of the spine in children on standard chemotherapy: a study in Pusan, Korea. Tubercle 1973;54:261.

178. Medical Research Council Working Party on Tuberculosis of the Spine. A controlled trial of anterior spinal fusion and debridement in the surgical management of tuberculosis of the spine in patients on standard chemotherapy: a study in Hong Kong. Br J Surg 1974;61:853.

179. Medical Research Council Working Party on Tuberculosis of the Spine. A controlled trial of debridement and ambulatory treatment in the management of tuberculosis of the spine in patients on standard chemotherapy. J Trop Med Hyg 1974;77:72.

180. Medical Research Council Working Party on Tuberculosis of the Spine. A five-year assessment of controlled trials of inpatient and outpatient treatment and of plaster-of-paris jackets for tuberculosis of the spine in children on standard chemotherapy: studies in Masan and Pusan, Korea. J Bone Joint Surg [Br] 1976;58:399.

181. Medical Research Council Working Party on Tuberculosis of the Spine. Five-year assessments of controlled trials of ambulatory treatment, debridement and anterior spinal fusion in the management of tuberculosis of the spine: studies in Bulaway (Rhodesia) and in Hong Kong. J Bone Joint Surg [Br] 1978;60:163.

182. Medical Research Council Working Party on Tuberculosis of the Spine. A ten-year assessment of a controlled trial comparing debridement and anterior spinal fusion in the management of tuberculosis of the spine in patients on standard chemotherapy in Hong Kong. J Bone Joint Surg [Br] 1982;64:393.

183. Medical Research Council Working Party on Tuberculosis of the Spine. A ten-year assessment of controlled trials of inpatient and outpatient treatment and of plaster-of-paris jackets for tuberculosis of the spine in children on standard chemotherapy: studies in Masan and Pusan, Korea. J Bone Joint Surg [Br] 1985;67:103.

184. Stagnara P, De Mauroy C, Willard B. Traitment des cyphoses regulieres. Ann Med Physique 1975;18:1.

185. Stagnara P. In: Gaggi A, ed. Modern trends in orthopaedics. Cyphoses thoraciques regulieres pathologiques. 1982:268.

186. Stagnara P, DeMauroy JC, Dran G, et al. Reciprocal angulation of vertebral bodies in a sagittal plane: approach to references in the evaluation of kyphosis and lordosis. Spine 1982;7:335.

187. Stagnara P, Fauchet R, Dupeloux J, et al. Maladie de Scheuermann. Pediatrics 1966;21:361.

188. Steinbok P, Boyd M, Cochrane D. Cervical spinal deformity following craniotomy and upper cervical laminectomy for posterior fossa tumors in children. Childs Nerv Syst 1989;5:25.

189. Stoddard A, Osborn JF. Scheuermann's disease or spinal osteochondrosis. Its frequency and relationship with spondylosis. J Bone Joint Surg [Br] 1979;61:56.

190. Sturm PF, Dobson JC, Armstrong GWD. The surgical management of Scheuermann's disease. Spine 1993;18:685.

191. Tachdijian MO, Matson DD. Orthopaedic aspects of intraspinal tumors in infants and children. J Bone Joint Surg [Am] 1965;47:223.

192. Taneja DK, Manning CW. Scoliosis in Marfan syndrome and arachnodactyly. In: Zorab PA, ed. Scoliosis. London: Academic Press, 1977:261.

193. Tolo VT. Surgical treatment of kyphosis in achondroplasia. In: Nicoletti B, Kopits SE, Ascani E, McKusich VA, eds. Human achondroplasia: a multidisciplinary approach. New York: Plenum Press, 1988:257.

194. Tolo VT. Spinal deformity in short-stature syndromes. Instr Course Lect 1990;39:399.

195. Tolo VT. Spinal deformity in skeletal dysplasia. In: Weinstein SL, ed. The pediatric spine: principles and practice. New York: Raven Press, 1994:369.

196. Travaglini F, Conte M. Cifosi 25 anni. Progessi in patolgia vertebrate. In: Goggia A, ed. Le cifosi, vol 5. Bologna, Goggia; 1982;163.

197. Tsou PM. Embryology of congenital kyphosis. Clin Orthop 1977;128:18.

198. Tsou PM, Yau A, Hodgson AR. Embryogenesis and prenatal development of congenital vertebral anomalies and their classification. Clin Orthop 1980;152:211.

199. Vaeth JM, Levitt SH, Jones MD, Holtfreter C. Effects of radiation therapy in survivors of Wilms' tumor. Radiology 1962;79:560.

199a. Van Schrick FG. Dir Angeborene kyphose. Zietr Orthop Chir 1932;56:238.

200. Versfeld GA, Fischer M. Xeroradiography in spinal kyphosis. J Pediatr Orthop 1983;3:482.

201. Voutsinas SA, MacEwen GD. Sagittal profiles of the spine. Clin Orthop 1986;210:235.

202. Wallace WHB, Shalet SM, Morris-Jones PH, et al. Effect of abdominal irradiation on growth in boys treated for a Wilms tumor. Med Pediatr Oncol 1990;18:441.

203. Wenger DR. Roundback. In: Wenger DR, Rang M, eds. The art and practice of children's orthopaedics. New York: Raven Press, 1993:422.

204. White AA, Panjabi MM. Practical biomechanics of scoliosis and kyphosis. In: White AA, Panjabi MM, eds. Clinical biomechanics of the spine. Philadelphia: JB Lippincott, 1990:155.

205. Whitehouse WM, Lampe I. Osseous damage in irradiation of renal tumors in infancy and childhood. AJR Am J Roentgenol 1953;70:721.

206. Willner S, Johnson B. Thoracic kyphosis and lumbar lordosis during the growth period in children. Acta Paediatr Scand 1983;72:873.

207. Winter RB. Spinal problems in pediatric orthopaedics. In: Morrissy RT, ed. Pediatric orthopaedics. Philadelphia: JB Lippincott, 1990:673.

208. Winter R. Congenital kyphosis. Clin Orthop 1977;128:26.

209. Winter RB. Congenital deformities of the spine. New York: Thieme-Stratton, 1983.

210. Winter RB. Thoracic lordoscoliosis in Marfan syndrome: report of two patients with surgical correction using rods and sublaminar wires. Spine 1990;15:233.

211. Winter RB, Hall JE. Kyphosis in childhood and adolescence. Spine 1978;3:285.

212. Winter RB, Herring JA. Kyphosis in an achondroplastic dwarf. J Pediatr Orthop 1983;3:250.

213. Winter RB, Moe JH. The results of spinal arthrodesis for congenital spinal deformity in patients younger than five years old. J Bone Joint Surg [Am] 1982;64:419.

214. Winter RB, Moe JH, Bradford DS, et al. Spine deformities in neurofibromatosis. J Bone Joint Surg [Am] 1979;61:677.

215. Winter RB, Moe JH, Lonstein JE. The surgical treatment of congenital kyphosis: a review of 94 patients age 5 years or older, with 2 years or more follow-up in 77 patients. Spine 1985;10:224.

216. Winter RB, Moe JH, Wang JF. Congenital kyphosis: its natural history and treatment as observed in a study of one hundred and thirty patients. J Bone Joint Surg [Am] 1973;55:223.

217. Yablon JD, Kasdon DL, Levine H. Thoracic cord compression in Scheuermann's disease. Spine 1988;13:896.

218. Yasuoka S, Peterson HA, Laws ER Jr, MacCarty CS. Pathogenesis and prophylaxis of post-laminectomy deformity of the spine after multiple level laminectomy: difference between children and adults. Neurosurgery 1981;9:145.

219. Yasuoka S, Peterson HA, MacCarty CS. Incidence of spinal column deformity after multilevel laminectomy in children and adults. J Neurosurg 1982;57:441.

Lovell & Winter's Pediatric Orthopaedics, fourth edition,
edited by Raymond T. Morrissy and Stuart L. Weinstein.
Lippincott–Raven Publishers, Philadelphia © 1996.

Chapter

19

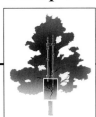

Spondylolysis and Spondylolisthesis

John E. Lonstein

DEFINITIONS

Spondylolysis refers to a defect in the pars interarticularis of the vertebra that is most common at L5 in children and adolescents. The term comes from the Greek *spondylos*, meaning vertebra, and *lysis*, meaning break or defect. *Spondylolisthesis* refers to the slipping forward of one vertebra on the next caudal vertebra and comes from the Greek *spondylos*, meaning vertebra, and *olisthesis*, meaning movement or slipping. Spondylolisthesis was first described by Herbiniaux,[38] a Belgium obstetrician, in 1972. Because the defect is most common at L5, the resultant slip also is most common at this level, with L5 slipping forward on S1.

CLASSIFICATION

The most well known classification is that of Wiltse.[79]

Type I: dysplastic spondylolisthesis, in which a congenital deficiency in the L5–S1 facet joints allows forward slippage of L5 on S1

Type II: isthmic spondylolisthesis, in which a lesion in the pars interarticularis permits the forward slippage and the articular facets are normal.
A. Lytic fracture of the pars
B. Elongated but intact pars
C. Acute pars fracture

Type III: degenerative spondylolisthesis, in which there is degenerative arthritis of the facet joints as well as degeneration of the disc

Type IV: traumatic spondylolisthesis, in which there is an acute fracture in an area of the vertebra other than the pars

Type V: pathologic spondylolisthesis, in which a lesion of the pars or pedicle caused by generalized bone disease allows forward slippage

Only types I and II (Fig. 19-1) occur in children and adolescents, and these are discussed in this chapter (Table 19-1).

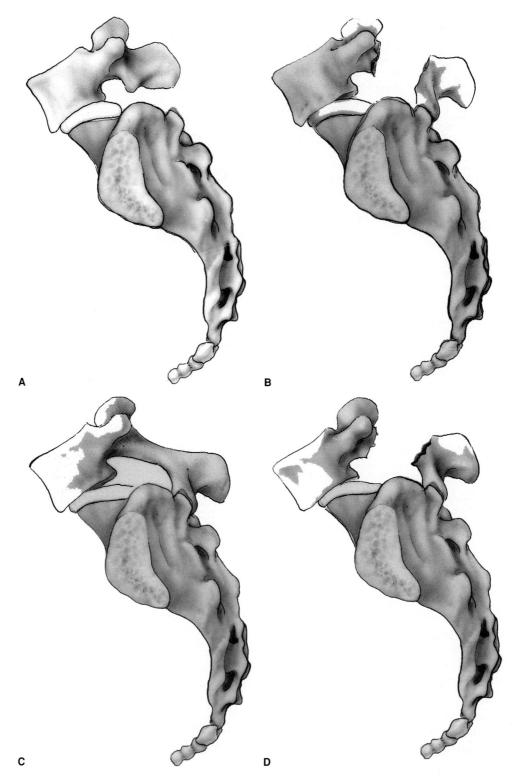

FIGURE 19-1.   In type I or dysplastic spondylolisthesis, there is a congenital deficiency of the L5–S1 facet joints that allows forward slippage of L5 on S1 (**A**). In type II or isthmic spondylolisthesis, there is a lesion of the pars interarticularis that permits the forward slippage. This condition is divided into three groups: (**B**) a lytic lesion of the pars, (**C**) an elongated but intact pars, or (**D**) an acute fracture of the pars.

TABLE 19-1. *Anatomic and Clinical Differences Between Dysplastic and Isthmic Spondylolisthesis*

	DYSPLASTIC	ISTHMIC
L5–S1 facets	Congenitally deficient	Normal
Pars interarticularis	Normal	Defect (lytic or fracture) or elongated
Slip amount	Grade 1 or 2	All grades
Neurologic	Common because of the intact pars	Rare

NATURAL HISTORY

Spondylolysis and spondylolisthesis have never been reported at birth. The incidence of spondylolysis with a pars defect is 4.4% at 6 years of age and rises to the adult rate of 5.5% to 6% by 14 years of age.[3,24] The earliest reported case was in a 3.5-month-old child,[7] and a few other cases have been reported in children younger than 2 years of age. The incidence is higher in boys and lower in persons of African descent.[24,55] The highest incidence is in Alaskan Eskimos (26%), especially those living north of the Yukon River.[69]

The percentage of cases in which spondylolisthesis is associated with spondylolysis has been documented in only one longitudinal study. Fredrickson and colleagues[24] found the rate of associated slippage to be 68% in 5-year-old children, increasing slightly to 74% in adults. In a 20-year follow-up review of 255 patients with spondylolysis and spondylolisthesis, Saraste[57] found an 81% prevalence of spondylolisthesis on initial presentation, but only 23% of the patients were younger than 18 years of age at the time of presentation. These figures suggest that most cases of spondylolysis are associated with spondylolisthesis, although no large population studies have been performed to support this belief.

Two questions are important in discussing the natural history of spondylolysis and spondylolisthesis: How frequently does the slip in spondylolisthesis progress? and How often is pain a problem?

Progression

Progression occurs in a low percentage of cases; it was reported in 4% of Frennered's series[26] and in 5% percent of Saraste's cases.[57] Progression after adolescence was unusual in Fredrickson's series,[24] although some authors have reported progression during adolescence, most likely as a result of disc degeneration.[37,59,70] If progression does occur in adolescence, it tends to happen during the growth spurt, and is more common in girls and in patients with dysplastic spondylolisthesis.[24]

Certain radiographic findings have been identified that are associated with a greater chance of progression. The degree of slippage on presentation has been found to correlate with the likelihood of progression by some authors[3,36,61] but not others.[26,57] The amount of lumbosacral kyphosis, or the slip angle, especially when severe, is associated with progression in growing children. Other changes are found with high-grade slips (e.g., dome-shaped sacrum, trapezoidal L5), but these are secondary to the slip and not predictive of slip progression.[26]

Pain

Pain is the most common presenting symptom of spondylolysis and spondylolisthesis. It probably is caused by the instability resulting from the anatomic lumbosacral lesion that alters the normal biomechanics of the area. In a long-term follow-up study, Saraste[57] found that certain radiographic features correlated with low back symptoms. These were a slip of greater than 25%, L4 spondylolysis or spondylolisthesis, and early disc degeneration at the level of the slip.

ETIOLOGY

The exact etiology of this condition is unknown, but various theories relate it to hereditary factors, a congenital predisposition, trauma, posture, growth, and biomechanical factors.

Hereditary Factors

Family studies have shown a high incidence of spondylolysis and isthmic spondylolisthesis in first-degree relatives of children with these conditions, with the incidence varying from 19% to 69%.[1,27,43,74,83] In a review of the inheritance of spondylolisthesis, Wynne-Davies[83] noted an increased incidence of lesions in affected relatives. Among the 12 patients with dysplastic spondylolisthesis, there were 11 affected first-degree relatives, 10 with isthmic defects and 1 with a dysplastic defect. Among the 35 patients with isthmic spondylolisthesis, there were 17 affected relatives, 14 with isthmic lesions and 3 with dysplastic defects. In addition, there was a higher incidence of spina bifida of S1 in both groups.

Trauma and Biomechanical Factors

Trauma is considered to be a factor in the etiology of spondylolysis and spondylolisthesis. Acute trauma causes the acute traumatic type of spondylolysis. In addition, many cases develop after a traumatic episode. It is unclear whether the trauma is the cause of the lesion or whether it makes an asymptomatic defect symptomatic. Wiltse[80] theorized that spondylolysis is a stress fracture in the pars, and repetitive microtrauma or microstress generally is considered to be a factor in its etiology. Repetitive hyperextension motions, in which the caudal edge of the inferior articular facet makes contact with the pars interarticularis, are believed to be the causative trauma. Circumstantial evidence for this theory is found in the higher incidence of spondylolysis in certain athletes, including female gymnasts,[40] college football linemen,[22,63] and weight lifters,[10] and in patients with Scheuermann disease.[50]

Posture

Spondylolysis has not been reported in adults who have never walked, pointing to the mechanical effects of upright posture in its etiology.[56]

Growth

Proof that growth plays a role in the etiology of spondylolysis is found in the fact that defects do not occur in newborns and that the incidence of the disorder reaches 4% by 6 years of age and rises to adult levels by 14 years of age. Whether this increase in incidence is due to growth alone or to growth combined with adoption of the upright posture is unknown. There also is an increase in the amount of slippage during the adolescent growth spurt.[24]

Thus, the etiology of spondylolysis is multifactorial, in that there is an inherited predisposition that probably manifests as a weakening of the pars interarticularis and the defect occurs with repeated microtrauma. The dysplastic variety with an elongated pars has a strong familial pattern, with congenital abnormalities in the lumbosacral area (i.e., abnormal facet orientation and spina bifida of S1).

PATIENT EVALUATION

History

Spondylolysis and spondylolisthesis usually do not cause symptoms and are detected as incidental findings on pelvic or spinal radiographs obtained for unrelated reasons. Pain is the most common presenting symptom in patients seeking medical attention, who usually are 10 to 15 years of age during the adolescent growth spurt. The pain can be chronic, exacerbated by sports or other physical activities and relieved by rest or restriction of activities. The pain also can follow an acute traumatic episode, often involving hyperextension during sports participation. It manifests as a dull, aching low back discomfort, either localized to the low back or with some radiation into the buttock and posterior thighs. The pain probably is related to the instability resulting from the pars defect. Radicular pain is unusual in adolescents and more common in adults; it occurs at the level of the slip (i.e., L5 root distribution with an L5–S1 spondylolisthesis) and results from nerve compression by the hypertrophic callus at the pars defect or from the foraminal stenosis accompanying the spondylolisthesis.

Parents may bring their children for evaluation of a change in posture or gait, with or without accompanying pain. This is more often the case with spondylolisthesis than with spondylolysis, especially with more marked degrees of slippage. The postural changes noted are a flattening of the buttocks, increased lumbar lordosis, and a waddling gait.

Occasionally, these cases present with scoliosis. This can be typical adolescent idiopathic scoliosis with the spondylolysis or spondylolisthesis detected incidentally during the radiographic evaluation. In a study of 500 consecutive cases of adolescent idiopathic scoliosis, Fisk[23] found the incidence of pars defects to be 6.2%, the same as that in the general population. Patients also can have curve patterns that are atypical for adolescent idiopathic scoliosis and, sometimes, associated lumbosacral pain. The curve can be caused by the spasm associated with the spondylolisthesis and is called spasm scoliosis. The curve can originate at the lumbosacral area, with the maximum rotation at this level. This is due to an asymmetric slip at the lumbosacral area in which one side of L5 has more slip. The scoliosis resulting from this lumbosacral rotation is called an olisthetic curve.

Physical Examination

The physical findings depend on whether pain is one of the presenting symptoms, as well as on the degree of slippage in the spondylolisthesis. The back and gait examination can be completely normal, with no hamstring tightness. With spondylolisthesis, there usually

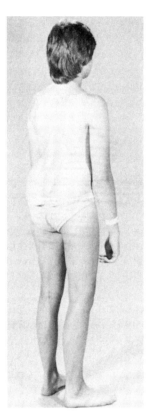

FIGURE 19-2. The typical findings of spondylolisthesis include flattening of the buttocks, lumbosacral kyphosis, a step-off in the lower lumbar area, and the lumbar lordosis.

is some degree of hamstring tightness with restriction of forward bending. Whether this is due to the instability or to nerve root irritation is unknown, but it disappears in the presence of a solid fusion.

With spondylolisthesis and associated pain, there generally is restriction of spine motion in addition to restriction of forward bending. With greater degrees of slippage, there is shortening of the waistline with flattening of the buttocks. A step-off at the lumbosacral area may be visible as well as palpable (Fig. 19-2). A localized area of tenderness to deep palpation also may be elicited in the lumbosacral area. In addition, in these severe slips, the child stands with hips and knees flexed because of the anterior rotation of the pelvis, and the gait is one of short steps because of inability to extend the hips.

Straight leg raising usually is severely restricted by the tight hamstrings. The neurologic examination generally is normal, but can show a diminished or absent ankle deep tendon reflex and weakness of the extensor hallucis longus. Sphincter dysfunction is rare and occurs more commonly with dysplastic spondylolisthesis. Tight hamstrings or pain radiating into the leg alone are *not* indications of a neurologic deficit. There has to be objective evidence of loss, such as a reflex change or muscle weakness.

Scoliosis can be part of the presentation. As mentioned previously, it can be either a typical idiopathic scoliosis or, with more decompensation and spasm, a spasm or olisthetic scoliosis. The pain complaints and neurologic findings can be caused by some pathology other than the spondylolysis or spondylolisthesis, such as a bone, spinal cord, conus, or cauda tumor, disc herniation, or disc space infection. Thus, it is incumbent on the physician to rule out other causes of the back pain with a detailed history, physical examination, radiographs, and adjunctive tests.

Radiologic Evaluation

Routine Views

The initial radiographic evaluation consists of standing posteroanterior and lateral lumbosacral spine films. Full-length views also are taken in the presence of scoliosis, and a full-length lateral film is taken with larger degrees of slippage to evaluate the sagittal spine alignment. The spot lateral film usually shows the defect, especially with bilateral pars defects, and the degree of slippage in spondylolisthesis can be appreciated. The degree of slippage differs in the supine and standing positions: the standing view shows a greater slip and should always be taken.[44] In cases of unilateral defects, there can be sclerosis of the facet, lamina, or pars on the other side. This is due to the increased forces on the intact pars caused by the instability of the area as a result of the unilateral pars defect. The differential diagnosis of the localized sclerosis is an osteoid osteoma, but there is a pars defect and the area of sclerosis is uniform without a central, less sclerotic nidus on tomograms or thin-cut computed tomographic (CT) scans.

To visualize the pars defect better, an oblique view of the lumbosacral area often is necessary. The view is an oblique of the lumbosacral area and not of the lumbosacral spine, so the central x-ray beam must be at the lumbosacral area and not in the midlumbar spine. The pars defect is seen as the well-known "collar" on the "Scotty dog" (Fig. 19-3). In cases in which the defect is strongly suspected but is not seen on the oblique view, a CT scan can be performed. A special technique is used in which 1.5-mm cuts are taken with the scan localized to the vertebra and pars of interest.

Supine flexion and extension views are useful in demonstrating the mobility of the spondylolisthesis, both the amount of slippage and the reduction of the lumbosacral kyphosis. With mobility shown by a change in the amount of slippage or kyphosis on the extension versus the flexion view, instability of articulation is present; a greater change indicates more instability. These views are obtained when surgery is planned, because the information is helpful in as-

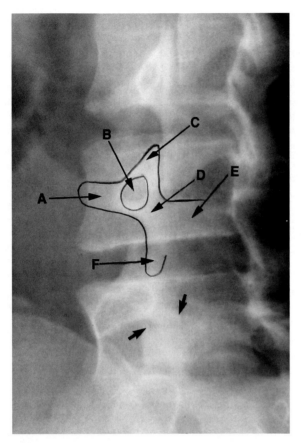

FIGURE 19-3. Oblique lumbosacral radiograph showing the "Scotty dog," which is made up of the following anatomic structures: the nose is the transverse process (A), the eye is the pedicle (B), the ear is the superior articular process (C), the neck is the pars (D), the back is the lamina (E), and the front leg is the inferior articular process (F). At L5, there is a "collar" on the dog (*arrows*), which is the isthmic defect in the pars.

sessing instability and planning postoperative immobilization.

Bone Scan

A bone scan is used in cases involving recent onset of pain or a distinct history of trauma to detect an acute fracture of the pars or to exclude a bony tumor. The examination can be performed using radioactive bone scanning or single-photon emission CT scanning, the latter being more sensitive because it provides better detail.

Computed Tomography or Magnetic Resonance Imaging

Additional imaging is necessary only occasionally. As mentioned previously, a CT scan is used to detect the pars defect in spondylolysis when it is not seen on lateral or oblique radiographs. Imaging of the spinal canal is essential when there is a neurologic deficit.

This can be accomplished using either myelography and CT or magnetic resonance imaging. The area assessed must extend from the lower thoracic region to the sacrum. Cases of spondylolisthesis with a neurologic deficit resulting from a tumor of the conus or cauda equina have occurred. This possibility must be eliminated with imaging studies of the spinal canal.

Measurement[81]

The deformity in spondylolisthesis, usually at the lumbosacral junction, consists of forward slippage of L5 on S1, typically accompanied by rotation of L5 on S1 into lumbosacral kyphosis. The degrees of slippage, kyphosis, and other changes in the lumbosacral anatomy are evaluated on the spot standing lateral radiograph of the lumbosacral area.

SLIP PERCENTAGE. The amount of anterior translation is described most commonly using the Meyerding grading system.[47] This system classifies the slip into five grades: grade I is a slip of 1% to 25%, grade II is a slip of 26% to 50%, grade III is a slip of 51% to 75%, grade IV is a slip of 76% to 100%, and grade V or spondyloptosis is slippage past the anterior border of the sacrum.

The slip can be expressed as a percentage according to the description of Taillard.[71] A line is drawn along the posterior border of the sacrum, and a perpendicular line is drawn at the upper end of the sacrum. The displacement of the posteroinferior corner of L5 from the line along the posterior border of the sacrum is measured. The width of S1 forms the denominator of the calculation, the slip being expressed as a percentage (Fig. 19-4A). In many cases, the upper end of the sacrum is rounded and the measurement of the width of S1 is inaccurate, so the anteroposterior width of L5 is used instead.

SLIP ANGLE. The slip angle measures the amount of lumbosacral kyphosis or sagittal rotation. The kyphosis is measured using the relation of L5 to S1. A line perpendicular to the line at the back of the sacrum described previously forms the sacral measuring line. A line is drawn along the upper end plate of L5, and the angle formed by these two lines is the slip angle, which normally is in lordosis and expressed by a negative sign[81] (Fig. 19-4B). Boxall[9] has used the line along the inferior edge of L5 for measurement, but this edge often is difficult to visualize accurately. In addition, with more marked slips, L5 frequently is trapezoidal in shape, and using the lower edge gives the additive measurement of the kyphosis and the wedging of L5.

The amount of sagittal rotation also can be measured as the angle between the lines drawn along the

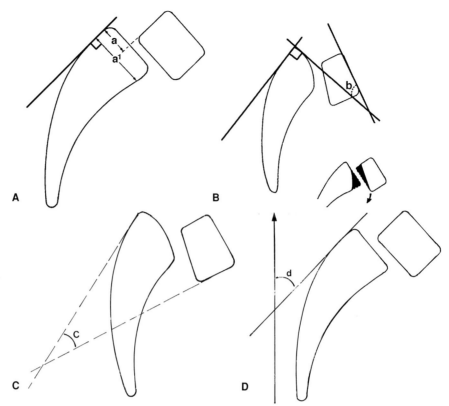

FIGURE 19-4. Measurement of spondylolisthesis. (**A**) Measurement of the amount of forward displacement (a) and of the sagittal diameter of S1 (a^1) allows calculation of the percent slip. (**B**) Measurement of the slip angle (b), which is the kyphosis at the area of the slip (i.e., the L5–S1 kyphosis). As the slip increases, there is a growth inhibition of the anterior lip of S1 and the posterior lip of L5. Because of this, the vertebra becomes trapezoidal, and using the bottom of L5 does not accurately measure the angular deformity. (**C**) Measurement of the sagittal rotation angle (c), which also represents the L5–S1 kyphosis and equals the slip angle. (**D**) Measurement of the sacral inclination (d).

back of the sacrum and along the back of L5. This sagittal rotation angle should equal the slip angle measured previously (Fig. 19-4C).

In larger degrees of slippage (usually >50%), it is seen that L4 shows retrolisthesis on L5, indicating an abnormality of the L4–5 articulation. In these severe slips, the slip angle of L4 in relation to the sacrum also is measured, because this is the effective lumbosacral slip angle after an L4-to-sacrum fusion.

SACRAL INCLINATION. The inclination of the sacrum to the vertical axis is measured by the angle of a line along the posterior edge of the sacrum and the vertical axis (i.e., a line drawn parallel to the edge of the x-ray film; Fig. 19-4D).

ANATOMIC CHANGES. Changes occur in the shape of L5 and S1. The contour of S1 is rounded and dome shaped. The fifth lumbar vertebra becomes trapezoidal in shape, being narrower posteriorly and wider anteriorly.

TREATMENT

Many therapeutic options are available for children with spondylolysis or spondylolisthesis.[82] These include doing nothing, observing, limiting activity, pre-

scribing exercises, bracing, casting, repairing a pars defect, and performing fusion, decompression, and reduction of the slip. The difficulty lies in selecting the best therapy for each child. In making this choice, the following factors should be considered: the presenting complaint; the patient's age and growth potential; the physical findings, especially neurologic signs; and the amount of displacement and slippage (i.e., slip percentage and slip angle). The different treatment approaches in spondylolysis and spondylolisthesis are discussed next, along with the indications for each method.

Spondylolysis

Nonoperative Treatment

OBSERVATION. As noted previously, most cases of spondylolysis are asymptomatic and are detected on radiographs obtained for unrelated reasons. The proper follow-up depends on the child's growth potential. If the child has finished growing, no follow-up is required. If the child is still growing, regular annual visits with spot lateral lumbosacral radiographs are necessary until growth is complete because slippage, when it occurs, can be asymptomatic. The child is allowed to participate in all sports without restriction (Fig. 19-5).

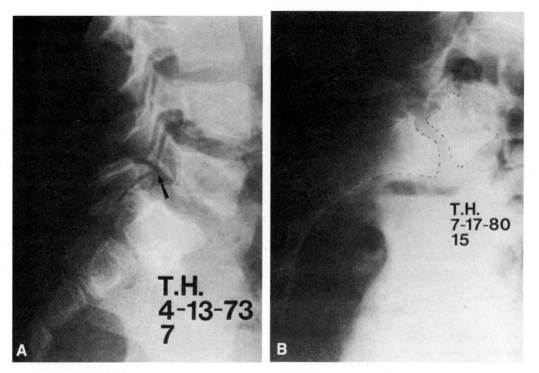

FIGURE 19-5. (A) This 7-year-old boy was seen for lordosis. He was completely asymptomatic, and the radiograph showed a pars defect. He was treated with periodic observation. (B) At 15 years of age, he was still asymptomatic and was an outstanding high-school athlete.

BRACING. If a child has pain, it should be determined whether the symptoms are of recent origin, follow an acute injury, or are of long duration. In cases in which pain follows a definite injury, a technetium single-photon emission CT bone scan is performed to determine whether the pars defect is of recent origin and is an acute fracture. If the scan indicates an acute fracture, immobilization in a cast or brace is used to aid in healing of the pars defect. A brace usually is adequate, but extremely painful cases may require immobilization of this area using a body cast with a leg extension. Healing of the defect has been described, with varying success; healing takes 3 to 4 months and is documented with oblique radiographs or repeated bone scans[54,68,80] (Fig. 19-6).

After healing of the defect, or when the symptoms resolve with immobilization, even with a persistent pars defect, resumption of all activities is allowed. This includes participation in all sporting and athletic activities with no restriction.

REDUCTION OF ACTIVITY. In general, children with symptomatic spondylolysis have long histories of pain with activity. These cases are treated with restriction of activity and abdominal and spinal muscle-strengthening exercises; rest is used only in the rare patients who have severe symptoms. Activity is restricted until symptoms resolve, at which time gradual resumption of activity is initiated. This treatment plan also is used in cases of spondylolysis in which there is a history of a recent injury and the results of a bone scan are negative.

If no relief is obtained with reduction of activity, the use of an orthosis can be suggested to the child and family. Only children with severe symptoms usually agree to this treatment approach. In cases that do not respond to nonoperative treatment, surgery should be offered as an alternative.

Operative Treatment

ARTHRODESIS. A one-level, L5–S1, posterolateral lumbosacral arthrodesis is performed for cases that are not responsive to nonoperative treatment. The procedure is performed through a midline skin incision, with the transverse process and sacral ala approached through a muscle-splitting incision, as described by Wiltse,[78] and the addition of autologous iliac bone graft. Postoperative immobilization can be used, depending on the surgeon's preference and the patient's symptoms. Good results have been reported with no immobilization,[80] immobilization in a corset,[8] and immobilization in a cast.[74] I prefer to immobilize these children using a thoracolumbarsacral orthosis (TLSO) or body cast with a leg extension, using the latter in patients who have more pain or are extremely

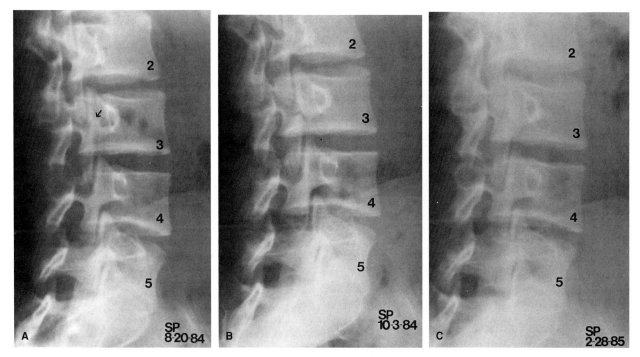

FIGURE 19-6. (**A**) This high-school soccer player was seen for mild, generalized low back pain. Physical examination and radiographs, including this oblique view, were normal. (**B**) Two months later, 10 days after an acute back injury suffered during a soccer game, a pars defect at L3 is clearly visible. (**C**) The patient was placed in an orthosis for 3 months, and 1 month later the lesion had healed, the symptoms had resolved, and the patient had returned to playing sports. (From Winter RB. Spondylolysis and spondylolisthesis in the adolescent: when to do what. Iowa Orthop J 1986;6:36.)

active (Fig. 19-7). Although the rate of success for fusion in spondylolisthesis is superior when a cast with a leg extension is used, no such data exist for fusion in spondylolysis.

REPAIR OF DEFECT. In cases in which the pars defect is at L4 or higher, the preferred approach is direct repair of the defect to maintain normal lumbar motion. This technique was first described by Buck[17] and was popularized by Scott.[42] The pars defect is grafted with spinous process or iliac bone, with wire fixation of the transverse processes to the spinous process (Fig. 19-8). Because the defect is at L4 or above, a TLSO provides adequate postoperative immobilization and is used for 3 to 4 months until fusion has occurred. Healing usually can be seen on oblique radiographs, but if visualization is difficult, tomograms in the oblique plane are used. Good results with healing in all cases have been described by Bradford[16] and others.[31,49,53]

Spondylolisthesis

Nonoperative Treatment

Nonoperative treatment is indicated for slips of less than 30% to 50% in growing children, and for some larger slips in mature adolescents.

OBSERVATION. An asymptomatic slip of less than 50% in an actively growing child should be observed for progression with yearly standing lateral lumbosacral radiographs. This also is the recommended therapy for an asymptomatic slip of less than 50% in a mature adolescent. If there is no change in the slip angle or the amount of slippage, and there are no symptoms, observation should be continued until growth is complete. With an increase in the spondylolisthesis or the appearance of significant pain, surgical stabilization is indicated.

REDUCTION OF ACTIVITIES. Growing children who have low back pain and slips of less than 30% to 50% are advised to limit their exercise and sports participation. After the symptoms subside, these activities can be resumed.

BRACING. If pain does not resolve with restriction of activity, the use of a TLSO may be beneficial.[5,52,68] After the symptoms are relieved, activity is gradually resumed.

Operative Treatment

Surgical stabilization of the spondylolisthesis should be considered for symptomatic children who

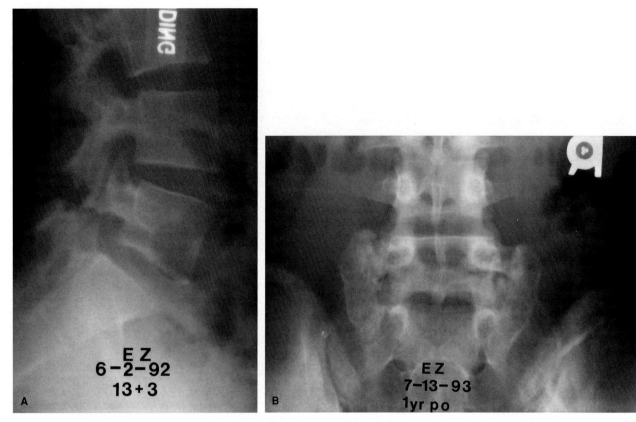

FIGURE 19-7. A patient was seen at the age of 13 years and 3 months with a 1-year history of low back pain. She was a competitive figure skater and, initially, reduction in the amount of time spent skating reduced her symptoms. On this presentation, however, the pain interfered with her daily life. (**A**) The spot lateral lumbosacral radiograph showed an L5 spondylolysis. (**B**) The patient underwent a one-level posterolateral lumbosacral arthrodesis with postoperative immobilization in a one-leg spica cast for 3 months. One year later, she was free of pain and had returned to figure skating, and the radiograph showed a solid posterolateral fusion.

do not respond to nonoperative therapy and in whom pain prevents full participation in normal activities. In addition, growing children with larger slips should undergo fusion because of the degree of slippage. This applies to children or adolescents with slips of over 50%. Mature adolescents with slips of over 50% also should be treated surgically, even in the absence of symptoms.

ARTHRODESIS. The surgical procedure used to treat spondylolisthesis is a posterolateral arthrodesis. The approach is with a midline skin incision, and a midline or paramedian approach to the spine. The midline approach is used when a decompression is performed. When no decompression is necessary, the approach is paraspinal, with an incision through the fascia midway between the posterior iliac crest and the midline. The transverse processes and sacral ala are approached either through or around the paraspinal musculature. Iliac bone graft is placed in this prepared bed on the decorticated transverse processes and adjacent lateral aspect of the superior artic-

ular processes, and on the decorticated sacral ala. In decortication of the sacral ala, it is best to create a cavity in the ala and to place the strips of cancellous graft in this cavity, as described by Hensinger.[35] This places the bone graft more vertically and provides a larger surface area for fusion to the sacrum.

DECISION MAKING. In the surgical treatment of spondylolisthesis, decisions must be made regarding the levels to be fused, the role of decompression, the role of reduction, the need for anterior fusion, the use of instrumentation, and the use of immobilization and bed rest. These decisions depend on the degree of the deformity in terms of slip percentage and kyphosis, the presence of neurologic symptoms and signs, and the mobility of the spondylolisthesis as shown on flexion and extension radiographs.

Levels To Be Fused. The basic procedure is a posterolateral, one-level, L5–S1 fusion. The fusion is extended to L4 with greater degrees of slippage (i.e., >50%) for two reasons. With this degree of slippage,

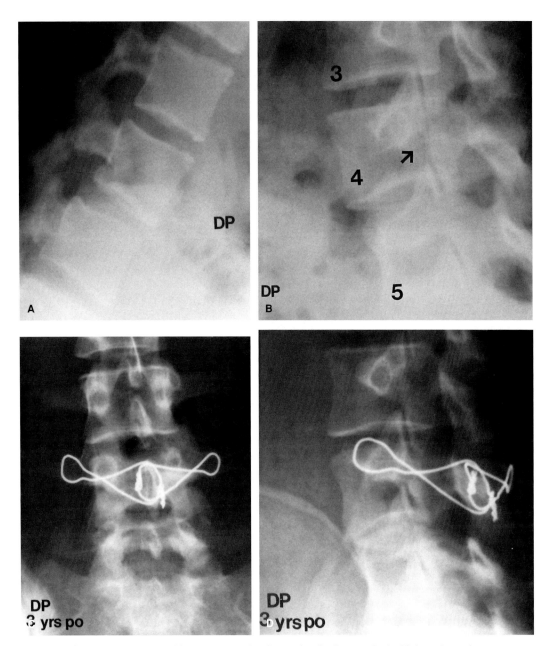

FIGURE 19-8.   A 14-year-old girl was seen for chronic low back pain. She had bilateral pars fractures at L4, as seen on (**A**) lateral and (**B**) oblique radiographs. (*Arrow,* pars defect.) The patient underwent bone grafting with wiring of the defect with a spinous process transverse process wire. (**C**) The wire position is seen on the posteroanterior view and (**D**) the solid fusion is seen on the oblique view. She was rendered free of pain and returned to full activity.

the transverse process of L5 is displaced anterior to the sacral ala, and it is impossible to expose the transverse process of L5 without exposing the transverse process of L4. In addition, bone graft placed from L5 to the ala will be horizontal and under shear forces, whereas graft from the ala to the transverse process of L4 will lie more vertically. A two-level arthrodesis is necessary in a slip of less than 50% in which the transverse process of L5 is small and provides an insufficient bed for the fusion.

DECOMPRESSION. True nerve root compression is evidenced by motor weakness and a sensory deficit, and is confirmed with imaging studies, which also eliminate other possible causes of the neurologic changes (i.e., a spinal cord or cauda tumor). Usually, the L5 root is involved, being compressed at the foraminal level by the proximal part of the pars as it slips forward with the vertebral body, or by the fibrocartilaginous tissue at the pars defect. In rare cases with more marked slips, the nerve root can be trapped

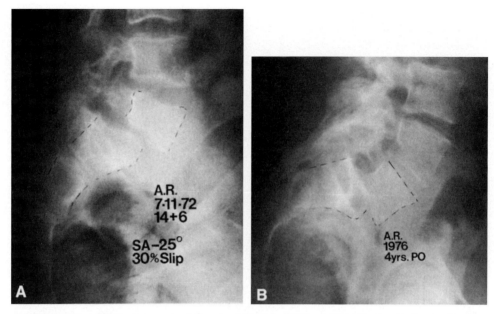

FIGURE 19-9.   A patient was seen at the age of 14 years and 6 months with chronic low back pain. (**A**) The lateral lumbosacral view showed spondylolisthesis with a 30% slip and a −25-degree slip angle. An L4-to-sacrum fusion was performed, followed by postoperative immobilization in a cast. (**B**) Four years after operation, a radiograph shows a solid fusion with no alteration in displacement or slip: a fusion in situ. The patient had complete pain relief.

between the transverse process of L5 and the sacral ala. Cases with true nerve root compression should be treated with nerve root decompression. Tight hamstrings are not a sign of nerve root compression, and no correlation has been found between tight hamstrings and the objective neurologic findings of weakness, sensory deficit, or reflex changes.[9] Cases with tight hamstrings alone require fusion without decompression; after the fusion is solid, the tightness resolves with time.

The basis of decompression is the Gill procedure with removal of the loose lamina.[29] This alone does not decompress the nerve root, and additional dissection and formal nerve root decompression are necessary. Nerve root decompression alone is contraindicated in growing children, and always should be accompanied by spinal fusion.[29,30] Wiltse[78] believes that nerve root decompression rarely is necessary, and that tight hamstrings, abnormal reflexes, and motor weakness recover after posterior fusion alone. I believe that formal decompression of the nerve gives the nerve the best chance of recovery. This must be weighed against the chance of increased slippage that follows decompression and fusion (see following).

REDUCTION.   In treating spondylolisthesis, the question of reduction always comes up. Numerous articles describe different techniques for reduction without documenting improved results after use of the procedure. Fusion in situ, however, has been proven to produce excellent results in high-grade

slips.[33] Many different techniques of reducing spondylolisthesis have been described since the initial description by Jenkins in 1936.[41] These techniques include halo-femoral traction,[34,71,72] cast reduction,[58] instrumentation,[20,32] and the combined anterior and posterior approach.[12,19,51,66]

All this literature makes the topic of reduction controversial and confusing. Distraction instrumentation across the lumbar spine is not recommended because it reduces the lumbar lordosis and has a significant effect on sagittal balance. Of the two deformities in spondylolisthesis—translation and kyphosis—the kyphosis is the more important problem. The degree of instability as shown on flexion and extension radiographs also is important, as is the magnitude of symptoms.

Minor degrees of slippage, usually less than 25%, are treated with fusion in situ unless instability is seen on flexion and extension radiographs (Fig. 19-9). When this is the case, cast reduction is used with immobilization in a single-leg spica cast. In larger degrees of slip translation, or with kyphosis, cast reduction can be used. A single-leg spica cast is applied 5 to 7 days after operation on a Risser frame with the child in traction, a support under the sacrum, and the thigh and pelvis in extension[58] (Fig. 19-10). With larger degrees of slippage (>50%), the fusion extends to L4. In these cases, even with slips of more than 75%, the sagittal relation of L4 to the sacrum in both translation and kyphosis is important. This becomes the effective lumbosacral joint after fusion.[11]

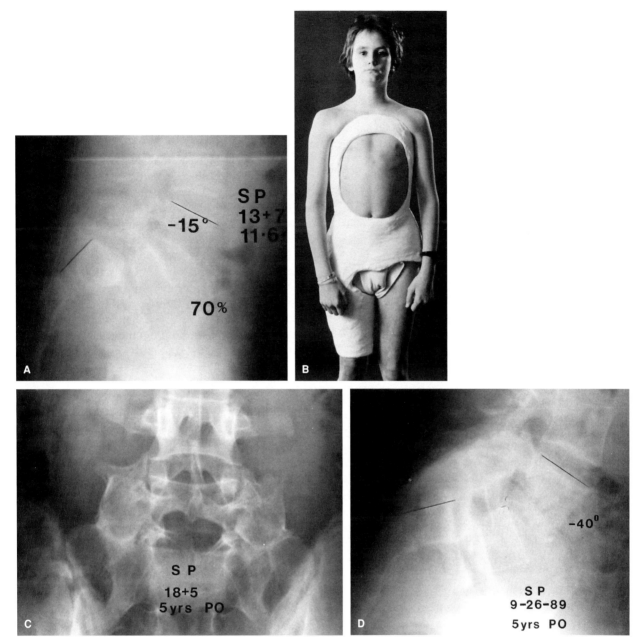

FIGURE 19-10. A patient was seen at the age of 13 years and 7 months with severe low back and leg pain and inability to bend forward. (**A**) The spot lateral lumbosacral view showed a 70% spondylolisthesis with an L5 slip angle of 15 degrees but an L4 slip angle of −15 degrees (**B**). He underwent a posterolateral L4-to-sacrum fusion and, 5 days after operation, had reduction on a Risser frame and was placed in a single-leg spica cast. He wore the leg extension for 4 months and a body cast for an additional 3 months. (From Lonstein JE. Cast techniques. In: Lonstein JE, Bradford DS, Winter RB, Ogelvie JW, eds. Moe's textbook of scoliosis and other spinal deformities. 3rd ed. Philadelphia: WB Saunders, 1994:129.) (**C**) Five years after operation, he was free of pain, his fusion was solid. (**D**) The lateral view showed reduction of the displacement and slip angle with improvement of the L4-to-sacrum slip angle. Note the retrolisthesis of L4 on L5.

With more marked deformities (slips >75%), especially increased lumbosacral kyphosis and spondyloptosis, some degree of reduction may be necessary to realign the lumbar spine over the sacrum in a position that will achieve a solid fusion. Closed reduction with halo-femoral traction or spinous process wiring can result in some reduction. In addition to a posterior fusion, some authors describe the addition of an anterior fusion in such cases.[4,14,15,19,51] An L5 vertebral body resection or vertebrectomy has been described for spondyloptosis. This shortens the lumbar spine and fuses L4 to the sacrum after the vertebrectomy.[28,39] All these more complex reduction techniques are complicated by a significant incidence of radiculopathy, which must be borne in mind during the decision making process.[2,15,45,73]

The role of the combined techniques in the treatment of these severe grades of spondylolisthesis is small, because most cases of spondylolisthesis in children and adolescents are of lesser grades (<50%) and can be treated adequately with posterior fusion and cast reduction alone. More complex reduction techniques rarely are necessary in young patients and may be useful only in reconstructive surgery in this area. The posture in children with severe slips is due in part to the spasm associated with the slip and to pain; when the fusion is solid, the pain disappears and the posture is improved, even with little change in the slip.[33] In my experience, there is little role for these dramatic reduction techniques as long as a solid arthrodesis is achieved. There is no evidence that reduction of slips of over 50% provides better results than can be obtained using fusion without reduction.[33]

ANTERIOR FUSION. The use of anterior fusion in the treatment of spondylolisthesis is reserved for the more severe grades. It can be part of a two-stage procedure in which the anterior fusion is done through a transperitoneal or retroperitoneal approach.[13,25,64,76] In addition, anterior fusion has been described through the posterior approach after a wide decompression, with the interbody fusion performed using a fibular graft inserted through the middle of S1 into the L5 vertebral body.[6,67] This is my preference in cases of spondyloptosis because anterior exposure of this degree of slip is difficult and anterior fusion is beneficial because the posterior fusion is under shear.

INSTRUMENTATION. The initial use of instrumentation in the treatment of spondylolisthesis involved the placement of Harrington distraction rods to reduce the slip. This practice has largely been abandoned because of the effect of distraction on reducing the lumbar lordosis. Transpedicular fixation is commonly used in the lumbar spine in adults for lumbar fusion in various conditions, including spondylolisthesis. It can be used in adolescents for stabilization of the lumbosacral spine, taking the place of the spica cast. Transpedicular fixation can be performed only if the pedicles are large enough to enable placement of the instrumentation. In these cases, internal stabilization with transpedicular fixation is used instead of external immobilization with a spica cast. Some reduction of the spondylolisthesis occurs with positioning on the operating table, with the lumbosacral relation maintained internally by the instrumentation[21] (Fig. 19-11). In many cases, additional fixation caudally is necessary because of the slip angle. Edwards developed a technique of intraoperative reduction of spon-

dylolisthesis using his instrumentation on grade 1 to 4 defects.[2] This approach is time-consuming and associated with a high incidence of radiculopathy, and the need for complete reduction has never been proven.

IMMOBILIZATION AND BED REST. After fusion, a patient may require no immobilization,[77] a corset,[48] a brace, or a unilateral or bilateral spica cast,[35,74] and may be ambulatory or restricted to a period of bed rest. Because fusion is performed to alleviate symptoms, I prefer to use some form of immobilization after surgery, both to slow the patient down and to improve the fusion rate. In a study by Burkus and colleagues[18] of the long-term results of operative treatment of spondylolisthesis, the rate of pseudarthrosis was lower when a cast with a leg extension was used. In addition, all patients who show instability on flexion and extension radiographs should be immobilized after operation. For a routine fusion, cast reduction generally is used, with the patient ambulatory in a single-leg spica cast for about 4 months. Patients who have either significant pain with marked spasm or a larger degree of slippage (>50%–75%) with significant kyphosis seem to do better with a period of bed rest after fusion, which usually is performed posteriorly or using a combined approach. Five to seven days after the fusion, a spica cast is applied with cast reduction and the patient is restricted to bed rest for 3 to 4 months. In this position, the area is at rest and the effect of gravity on the slip is eliminated. After this period, the patient is allowed out of bed in a body cast or brace without a leg extension. After fusion with instrumentation, I prefer to use a TLSO for 3 to 4 months until the fusion is solid. This does not immobilize the lumbosacral area, but rather slows the patient down, preventing vigorous bending or twisting motions.

SCOLIOSIS ASSOCIATED WITH SPONDYLOLISTHESIS. Scoliosis can be associated with spondylolisthesis in two scenarios: spondylolisthesis accompanying adolescent idiopathic scoliosis, or scoliosis caused by spondylolisthesis. The latter can be a spasm curve or result from an asymmetric slip (i.e., olisthetic scoliosis). In this case, the scoliosis and the spondylolysis or spondylolisthesis are assessed separately and treated independently. If the scoliosis requires fusion, it should be treated accordingly, and the same is true for the spondylolisthesis. There is no evidence that a long fusion to L4 results in increased stress on spondylolisthesis with an increase in the slip. Whenever possible, the caudal extent of the fusion should be to L3 to preserve motion segments, even though no concrete scientific evidence exists for possible problems with a fusion to L4. Careful observation of the spondylolisthesis below a fusion is necessary until growth is complete. Scoliosis requiring fusion to L4 and an asymp-

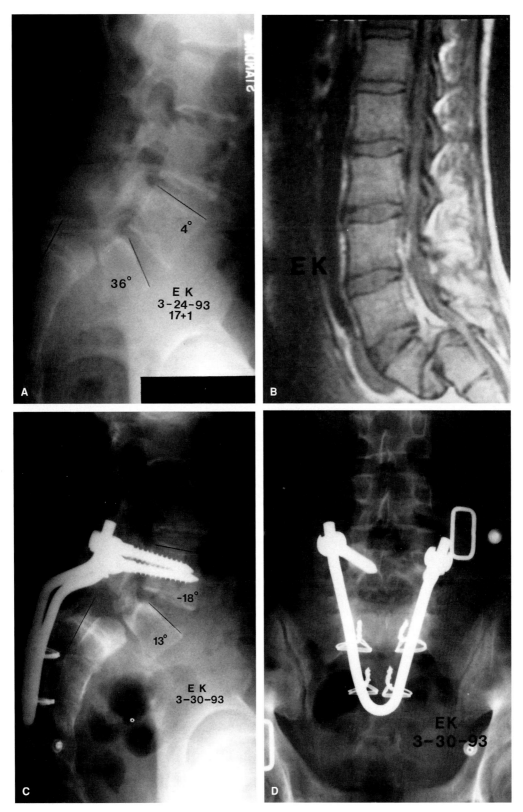

FIGURE 19-11.   A patient was seen at the age of 17 years and 1 month with severe back and right leg pain in an L5 radicular distribution. (**A**) A spot lateral standing lumbosacral radiograph showed a severe spondylolisthesis with a 36-degree L5–S1 slip angle, and a 4-degree L4–S1 slip angle. (**B**) A magnetic resonance imaging scan shows the split lumbosacral disc. The patient underwent a decompression of the L5 nerve roots, an L4–S1 posterolateral fusion with fixation with L4 pedicle screws, and fixation to the back of the sacrum with wiring to S2 and S3 after the technique described by Emans and colleagues.[21] (**C**) The lateral radiograph shows the instrumentation with reduction of the kyphosis and the L4- and L5-to-sacrum slip angles. (**D**) Postoperative posteroanterior radiograph.

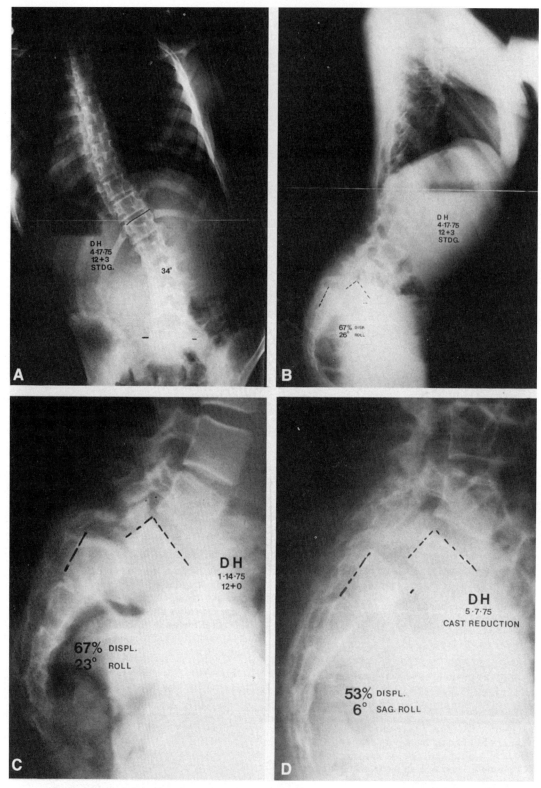

FIGURE 19-12. (A) A patient was seen at the age of 12 years and 3 months with a "spasm" scoliosis, lumbosacral pain, and sciatica. (B) The lateral standing radiograph showed a relatively vertical sacrum, 67% displacement, a 26-degree slip angle, and total lordosis from T1 to L5. Note how the torso is displaced forward in relation to the pelvis. (C) The spot lateral lumbosacral view shows an elongated pars of L5 with a pars defect near the pedicle. (D) The patient was treated by nerve root decompression, L4–S1 transverse process fusion, and partial reduction by double pantaloon cast application in a hyperextended position. The percentage of slip was reduced from 67% to 53%, but more importantly, the slip angle was reduced from 23 to 6 degrees. The patient was nonambulatory for 3 months and then was ambulatory in a body cast for an additional 3 months. (E) At a 2-year follow-up visit, the patient's fusion was solid, she was free of pain, and there was no loss of correction. (F) An anteroposterior view 3 years after surgery shows the solid lumbosacral fusion and total disappearance of the scoliosis

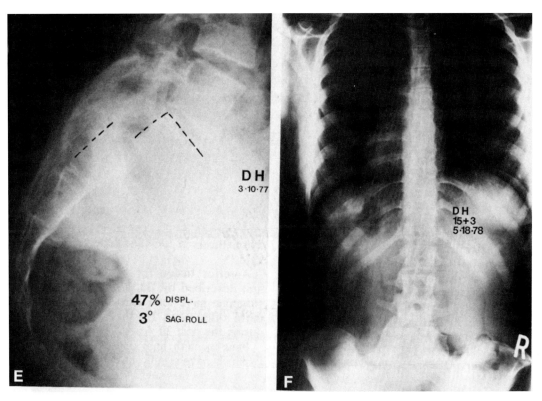

FIGURE 19-12 (*Continued*)

tomatic slip requiring fusion to L4 is rare, and I know of no cases. If this does occur, all attempts must be made to fuse the scoliosis to the upper lumbar spine. This is achieved with an anterior fusion and instrumentation for the lumbar curve and a posterior fusion for both curves. In addition, the spondylolisthesis is treated with a posterior fusion to L4, leaving one or two motion segments between the two fusions.

A spasm scoliosis consists of a long, sweeping curve with a curve pattern that is atypical for adolescent idiopathic scoliosis. It usually is caused by spasm or, rarely, an unequal slip with rotation at the lumbosacral junction. The curve reduces or disappears when the patient is supine. These patients benefit from a period of supine bed rest in a cast after surgery, and the curve disappears with a solid fusion (Fig. 19-12).

COMPLICATIONS

Pseudarthrosis. The pseudarthrosis rate in the literature varies from 0% to 25%.[9,18,35,62,65,75] It is less than 15% in most cases and the higher rate is seen with severe spondylolisthesis.[9] Most of the reported studies are small, and no correlation has been found between the degree of slippage and the rate of pseudarthrosis. The type of postoperative immobilization used is important; in a study by Burkus and colleagues,[18] the rate of pseudarthrosis was lower when a cast with a leg extension was used.

Increased Slippage. Increased slippage, as measured by the amount of displacement or kyphosis, can increase further in the presence of a solid fusion.[9,18,35,62,78] This postoperative increase is more common after posterior dissection, especially with decompression, which tends to remove the midline stabilizing structures, thereby increasing lumbosacral instability. It also is more common with higher degrees of spondylolisthesis that have more displacement or kyphosis (Fig. 19-13). Burkus[18] has shown less slippage with cast reduction after surgery.

Neurologic Complications. Radiculopathy has been described after reduction of spondylolisthesis, and the possibility of this complication must be appreciated if this treatment plan is followed.[2,15,45,73] An L5 lesion is most common and recovery rates vary. If reduction is to be performed, the loose L5 lamina should be removed and the nerve roots visualized so they can be checked repeatedly. When postoperative radiculopathy occurs, it is caused by either nerve compression or neurapraxia. With a mild lesion, the weakness is observed carefully and a methylprednisolone (Medrol) dosepak is used to decrease the nerve root edema. If the pain or weakness does not improve or the lesion becomes more marked in the immediate postoperative period, myelography plus CT is performed to rule out nerve root compression, which would require immediate decompression.

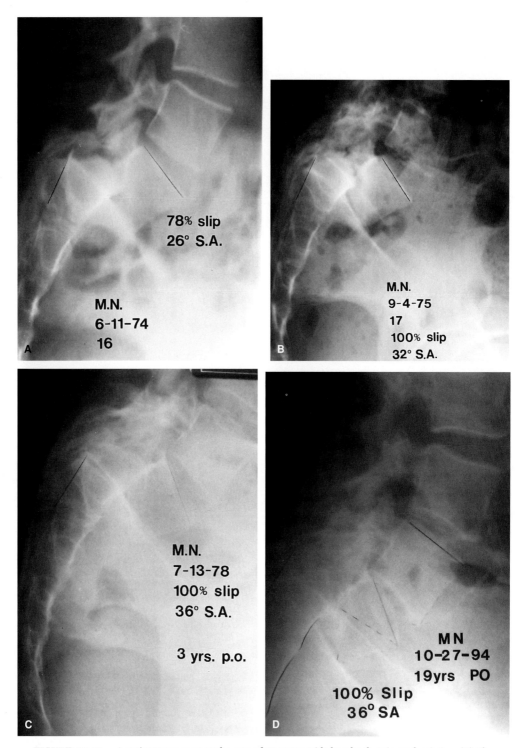

FIGURE 19-13. A patient was seen at the age of 16 years with low back pain and sciatica. (**A**) The spot lateral lumbosacral radiograph showed a 78% displacement and a slip angle (S.A.) of 26 degrees. The patient was treated with 1 decompression and L4-to-S1 posterolateral fusion and after operation was ambulatory in a brace. (**B**) Two months later, a standing radiograph in the brace showed an increase in the displacement to 100% and a slight increase in the slip angle to 32 degrees. (**C**) Three years after operation, the fusion was solid, the patient was free of pain, and the lumbosacral relation was unchanged. (**D**) Nineteen years after operation, the patient remains free of pain without a single degree of change detectable in her radiographs.

Radiculopathy occurring after transpedicular fixation requires immediate evaluation of the screw position in the pedicle with myelography plus CT. Any screw that is not entirely within the pedicle requires urgent exploration with screw replacement or removal. During screw insertion, it is possible to check the medial and inferior pedicle walls by performing a small laminotomy and palpating the pedicle.

Acute postoperative cauda equina syndrome also has been reported after a simple posterolateral fusion without decompression or reduction.[46,60] All but three of the patients in the multicenter report of Schoenecker[60] had severe slips of grade III or IV and preoperative neurologic symptoms or signs implicating the L5 root or cauda. In addition, in these severe slips, magnetic resonance imaging has been shown to demonstrate a split in the lumbosacral disc, with the posterior half indenting the dural sac. Thus, cauda equina syndrome probably is caused by acute neural compression of this disc segment in patients with marked slips and neural elements that already are compressed and, thus, at risk. With the relaxation of muscle tone that accompanies anesthesia, an acute change occurs in the lumbosacral relation, with acute cauda equina compression. This complication can occur in the absence of presenting neurologic signs or symptoms.[46,60]

Even with immediate decompression in these cases, permanent neurologic deficits can remain. Therefore, this complication should be prevented if possible. Any neurologic deficit in a patient with spondylolisthesis should be investigated with additional imaging studies. Any nerve root compression in a patient with severe spondylolisthesis should be decompressed, and this may be an ideal indication for stabilization with pedicle fixation. Careful neurologic follow-up is essential in the immediate postoperative period. If deficits are noted, decompression should immediately follow appropriate imaging studies. Only with knowledge and vigilance can this rare complication be minimized.

References

1. Albanese M, Pizzutillo PD. Family study of spondylolysis and spondylolisthesis. J Pediatr Orthop 1982;2:496.
2. Amundson G, Edwards C, Garfin S. Spondylolisthesis. In: Rothman R, Simeone F, eds. The spine. 3rd ed. Philadelphia: WB Saunders, 1992:913.
3. Baker D, Mc Hollick W. Spondylolysis and spondylolisthesis in children. J Bone Joint Surg [Am] 1956;38:933.
4. Balderston RA, Bradford DS. Technique for achievement and maintenance of reduction for severe spondylolisthesis using spinous process traction wiring and external fixation of the pelvis. Spine 1985;10:376.
5. Bell DF, Ehrlich MG, Zaleske DJ. Brace treatment for symptomatic spondylolisthesis. Clin Orthop 1988;236:192.
6. Bohlman HH, Cook SS. One-stage decompression and posterolateral and interbody fusion for lumbosacral spondyloptosis through a posterior approach. Report of two cases. J Bone Joint Surg [Am] 1982;64:415.
7. Borkow SE, Kleiger B. Spondylolisthesis in the newborn. A case report. Clin Orthop 1971;81:73.
8. Bosworth D, Fielding J, Demarest L, Bonaquist M. Spondylolisthesis: a critical review of a consecutive series of cases treated by arthrodesis. J Bone Joint Surg [Am] 1955;37:767.
9. Boxall D, Bradford DS, Winter RB, Moe JH. Management of severe spondylolisthesis in children and adolescents. J Bone Joint Surg [Am] 1979;61:479.
10. Bradford D. Management of spondylolysis and spondylolisthesis. Instruct Course Lect 1983;32:151.
11. Bradford D. Spondylolysis and spondylolisthesis. In: Lonstein J, Bradford D, Winter R, Ogilvie J, eds. Moe's textbook of scoliosis and other spinal deformities. 3rd ed. Philadelphia: WB Saunders, 1994:415.
12. Bradford DS. Management of spondylolysis and spondylolisthesis. Instr Course Lect 1983;32:151.
13. Bradford DS. Treatment of severe spondylolisthesis. A combined approach for reduction and stabilization. Spine 1979;4:423.
14. Bradford DS, Boachie-Adjei O. Treatment of severe spondylolisthesis by anterior and posterior reduction and stabilization. A long-term follow-up study. J Bone Joint Surg [Am] 1990;72:1060.
15. Bradford DS, Gotfried Y. Staged salvage reconstruction of grade IV and V spondylolisthesis. J Bone Joint Surg [Am] 1987;69:191.
16. Bradford DS, Iza J. Repair of the defect in spondylolysis or minimal degrees of spondylolisthesis by segmental wire fixation and bone grafting. Spine 1985;10:673.
17. Buck JE. Direct repair of the defect in spondylolisthesis. Preliminary report. J Bone Joint Surg [Br] 1970;52:432.
18. Burkus JK, Lonstein JE, Winter RB, Denis F. Long-term evaluation of adolescents treated operatively for spondylolisthesis. A comparison of in situ arthrodesis only with in situ arthrodesis and reduction followed by immobilization in a cast. J Bone Joint Surg [Am] 1992;74:693.
19. DeWald RL, Faut MM, Taddonio RF, Neuwirth MG. Severe lumbosacral spondylolisthesis in adolescents and children. Reduction and staged circumferential fusion. J Bone Joint Surg [Am] 1981;63:619.
20. Edwards C. Reduction of spondylolisthesis: biomechanics and fixation. Orthop Trans 1986;10:543.
21. Emans JB, Waters PM, Hall JE. Technique for maintenance of reduction of severe spondylolisthesis using L4-S4 posterior segmental hyperextension fixation. Orthop Trans 1987;11:113.
22. Ferguson RJ, McMaster JH, Stanitski CL. Low back pain in college football linemen. J Sports Med Phys Fitness 1975;2:63.
23. Fisk JR, Moe JH, Winter RB. Scoliosis, spondylolysis, and spondylolisthesis. Their relationship as reviewed in 539 patients. Spine 1978;3:234.
24. Fredrickson BE, Baker D, McHolick WJ, et al. The natural history of spondylolysis and spondylolisthesis. J Bone Joint Surg [Am] 1984;66:699.
25. Freebody D, Bendall R, Taylor RD. Anterior transperitoneal lumbar fusion. J Bone Joint Surg [Br] 1971;53:617.
26. Frennered AK, Danielson BI, Nachemson AL. Natural history of symptomatic isthmic low-grade spondylolisthesis in children and adolescents: a seven-year follow-up study. J Pediatr Orthop 1991;11:209.
27. Friberg S. Studies on spondylolisthesis. Acta Chir Scand 1939;82(Suppl):56.
28. Gaines RW, Nichols WK. Treatment of spondyloptosis by two stage L5 vertebrectomy and reduction of L4 onto S1. Spine 1985;10:680.

29. Gill G, Manning J, White H. Surgical treatment of spondylolisthesis without spine fusion. J Bone Joint Surg [Am] 1955;37:493.

30. Gill GG. Long-term follow-up evaluation of a few patients with spondylolisthesis treated by excision of the loose lamina with decompression of the nerve roots without spinal fusion. Clin Orthop 1984;182:215.

31. Hambly M, Lee CK, Gutteling E, et al. Tension band wiring-bone grafting for spondylolysis and spondylolisthesis. A clinical and biomechanical study. Spine 1989;14:455.

32. Harrington PR, Dickson JH. Spinal instrumentation in the treatment of severe progressive spondylolisthesis. Clin Orthop 1976;117:157.

33. Harris IE, Weinstein SL. Long-term follow-up of patients with grade III and IV spondylolisthesis. Treatment with and without posterior fusion. J Bone Joint Surg [Am] 1987;69:960.

34. Harris R. Spondylolisthesis. Ann R Coll Surg Engl 1951;8:259.

35. Hensinger R, Lang L, MacEwen G. Surgical management of the spondylolisthesis in children and adolescents. Spine 1976;1:207.

36. Hensinger RN. Spondylolysis and spondylolisthesis in children and adolescents. (Review) J Bone Joint Surg [Am] 1989;71:1098.

37. Henson J, McCall IW, O'Brien JP. Disc damage above a spondylolisthesis. Br J Radiol 1987;60:69.

38. Herbiniaux G. Traite sur divers accouchemens labprieux, et sur polypes de la matrice. Bruxelles: JL DeBoubers, 1782.

39. Huizenga B. Reduction of spondyloptosis with two-stage vertebrectomy. Orthop Trans 1983;7:21.

40. Jackson DW, Wiltse LL, Cirincoine RJ. Spondylolysis in the female gymnast. Clin Orthop 1976;117:68.

41. Jenkins J. Spondylolisthesis. Br J Surg 1936;24:80.

42. Johnson G, Thompson A. The Scott wiring technique for direct repair of lumbar spondylolysis. J Bone Joint Surg [Br] 1992;74:426.

43. Laurent L, Einola S. Spondylolisthesis in children and adolescents. Acta Orthop Scand 1961;31:45.

44. Lowe RW, Hayes TD, Kaye J, et al. Standing roentgenograms in spondylolisthesis. Clin Orthop 1976;117:80.

45. Matthiass HH, Heine J. The surgical reduction of spondylolisthesis. Clin Orthop 1986;203:34.

46. Maurice HD, Morley TR. Cauda equina lesions following fusion in situ and decompressive laminectomy for severe spondylolisthesis. Four case reports. Spine 1989;14:214.

47. Meyerding H. Spondylolisthesis. Surg Gynecol Obstet 1932;54:371.

48. Nachemson A, Wiltse LL. Spondylolisthesis. (Editorial) Clin Orthop 1976;117:2.

49. Nicol RO, Scott JH. Lytic spondylolysis. Repair by wiring. Spine 1986;11:1027.

50. Ogilvie JW, Sherman J. Spondylolysis in Scheuermann's disease. Spine 1987;12:251.

51. Ohki I, Inoue S, Murata T, et al. Reduction and fusion of severe spondylolisthesis using halo-pelvic traction with a wire reduction device. Int Orthop 1980;4:107.

52. Pizzutillo PD, Hummer C. Nonoperative treatment for painful adolescent spondylolysis or spondylolisthesis. J Pediatr Orthop 1989;9:538.

53. Roca J, Moretta D, Fuster S, Roca A. Direct repair of spondylolysis. Clin Orthop 1989;246:86.

54. Roche M. Healing of bilateral fracture of the pars interarticularis of a lumbar neural arch. J Bone Joint Surg [Am] 1950;32:428.

55. Roche M, Rowe C. The incidence of separate neural arch and coincident bone variations. J Bone Joint Surg [Am] 1952;34:491.

56. Rosenberg NJ, Bargar WL, Friedman B. The incidence of spondylolysis and spondylolisthesis in nonambulatory patients. Spine 1981;6:35.

57. Saraste H. Long-term clinical and radiological follow-up of spondylolysis and spondylolisthesis. J Pediatr Orthop 1987;7:631.

58. Scaglietti O, Frontino G, Bartolozzi P, et al. Technique of anatomical reduction of lumbar spondylolisthesis and its surgical stabilization. Clin Orthop 1976;117:165.

59. Schlenzka D, Poussa M, Seitsalo S, Osterman K. Intervertebral disc changes in adolescents with isthmic spondylolisthesis. J Spinal Disord 1991;4:344.

60. Schoenecker PL, Cole HO, Herring JA, et al. Cauda equina syndrome after in situ arthrodesis for severe spondylolisthesis at the lumbosacral junction [see comments]. J Bone Joint Surg [Am] 1990;72:369.

61. Seitsalo S, Osterman K, Hyvarinen H, et al. Progression of spondylolisthesis in children and adolescents. A long-term follow-up of 272 patients. Spine 1991;16:417.

62. Seitsalo S, Osterman K, Poussa M. Scoliosis associated with lumbar spondylolisthesis. A clinical survey of 190 young patients. Spine 1988;13:899.

63. Semon RL, Spengler D. Significance of lumbar spondylolysis in college football players. Spine 1981;6:172.

64. Sevastikoglou JA, Spangfort E, Aaro S. Operative treatment of spondylolisthesis in children and adolescents with tight hamstrings syndrome. Clin Orthop 1980;147:192.

65. Sherman FC, Rosenthal RK, Hall JE. Spine fusion for spondylolysis and spondylolisthesis in children. Spine 1979;4:59.

66. Sijbrandij S. Reduction and stabilisation of severe spondylolisthesis. A report of three cases. J Bone Joint Surg [Br] 1983;65:40.

67. Smith MD, Bohlman HH. Spondylolisthesis treated by a single-stage operation combining decompression with in situ posterolateral and anterior fusion. An analysis of eleven patients who had long-term follow-up. J Bone Joint Surg [Am] 1990;72:415.

68. Steiner ME, Micheli LJ. Treatment of symptomatic spondylolysis and spondylolisthesis with the modified Boston brace. Spine 1985;10:937.

69. Stewart T. The age incidence of neural arch defects in Alaskan natives, considered from the standpoint of etiology. J Bone Joint Surg [Am] 1953;35:937.

70. Szypryt EP, Twining P, Mulholland RC, Worthington BS. The prevalence of disc degeneration associated with neural arch defects of the lumbar spine assessed by magnetic resonance imaging. Spine 1989;14:977.

71. Taillard W. Les spondylisthesis chez l'enfant et l'adolescent. Acta Orthop Scand 1955;24:115.

72. Taillard WF. Etiology of spondylolisthesis. Clin Orthop 1976;117:30.

73. Transfeldt EE, Dendrinos GK, Bradford DS. Paresis of proximal lumbar roots after reduction of L5-S1 spondylolisthesis. Spine 1989;14:884.

74. Turner RH, Bianco A Jr. Spondylolysis and spondylolisthesis in children and teen-agers. J Bone Joint Surg [Am] 1971;53:1298.

75. Velikas EP, Blackburne JS. Surgical treatment of spondylolisthesis in children and adolescents. J Bone Joint Surg [Br] 1981;63:67.

76. Verbiest H. The treatment of lumbar spondyloptosis or impending lumbar spondyloptosis accompanied by neurologic deficit and/or neurogenic intermittent claudication. Spine 1979;4:68.

77. Wiltse L. Spondylolisthesis in children. Clin Orthop 1961;21:156.

78. Wiltse LL, Jackson DW. Treatment of spondylolisthesis and spondylolysis in children. Clin Orthop 1976;117:92.

79. Wiltse LL, Newman PH, Macnab I. Classification of spondylolysis and spondylolisthesis. Clin Orthop 1976;117:23.

80. Wiltse LL, Widell E Jr, Jackson DW. Fatigue fracture: the basic lesion in isthmic spondylolisthesis. J Bone Joint Surg [Am] 1975;57:17.

81. Wiltse LL, Winter RB. Terminology and measurement of spondylolisthesis. J Bone Joint Surg [Am] 1983;65:768.

82. Winter RB. Spondylolysis and spondylolisthesis in the adolescent: when to do what. Iowa Orthop J 1986;6:36.

83. Wynne-Davies R, Scott JH. Inheritance and spondylolisthesis: a radiographic family survey. J Bone Joint Surg [Br] 1979; 61:301.

Lovell & Winter's Pediatric Orthopaedics, fourth edition,
edited by Raymond T. Morrissy and Stuart L. Weinstein.
Lippincott–Raven Publishers, Philadelphia © 1996.

Chapter

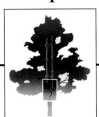

20

The Cervical Spine

Randall T. Loder

Many of the diseases and congenital anomalies affecting the pediatric cervical spine are simply a reflection of aberrant growth and developmental processes. This chapter discusses these diseases and anomalies in this framework. A basic understanding of the normal embryology, growth, and development of the pediatric cervical spine is helpful to understand these conditions. Most of the anomalies and diseases involving the pediatric cervical spine are easily divided into those of the upper (occiput, C1, C2) and lower (C3–C7) segments. This division is a common theme in this chapter.

NORMAL EMBRYOLOGY, GROWTH, AND DEVELOPMENT

Embryology

Occipitoaxioatlas Complex

The occiput is formed from at least four or five somites. All definitive vertebrae develop from the caudal sclerotome half of one segment and the cranial sclerotome half of the next succeeding segment.[173] These areas of primitive mesenchyme separate from each other during fetal growth and then undergo chondrification and subsequent ossification. This chondrification and ossification is a passive process, following the blueprint laid down by the mesenchymal anlage. Because of this sequencing, the cranial half of the first cervical sclerotome remains as a half segment between the occipital and the atlantal rudiments and is known as the proatlas. The primitive centrum of this proatlas becomes the tip of the odontoid process, whereas its arch rudiments assist in the formation of the occipital condyles.[204] The vertebral arch of the atlas separates from its respective centrum, becoming the ring of C1; the separated centrum fuses with the proatlas above and the centrum of C2 below to become the odontoid process and body of C2. The axis forms from the second definitive cervical vertebral mesenchymal segment. The odontoid process is the fusion of the primitive centra of the atlas and the proatlas half segment. The posterior arches of C2 form from only the second definitive cervical segment.

Thus the atlas is made up of three main components: the body and the two neural arches. The axis is made up of four main components: the body, two neural arches, and the odontoid (or five components if the proatlas rudiment is considered).

Vertebrae C3–C7

These vertebrae follow the normal formation schema of all vertebrae.[172] A portion of the mesenchyme from the sclerotomal centrum creates two neural arches that migrate posteriorly and around the neural tube. This eventually forms the pedicles, the laminae, the spinous processes, and a very small portion of the body. The majority of the body is formed by the centrum. An ossification center develops in each of the two neural arches and one in the vertebral center, with a synchondrosis formed by the cartilage between the ossification centers.

Growth and Development

Atlas

Ossification is only present in the two neural arches at birth.[168] These ossification centers extend posteriorly toward the rudimentary spinous process to form the posterior synchondrosis and anteriorly into the articular facet region, forming all the bone present in the facets. Anteromedial to each facet the neurocentral synchondroses form, joining the neural arches and the body; this occurs on each side of the expanding anterior ossification center. The body starts to ossify between 6 months and 2 years, usually in a single center. By 4 to 6 years the posterior synchondrosis fuses, followed by the anterior ones slightly thereafter. The final internal diameter of the pediatric

C1 spinal canal is determined by 6 to 7 years of age. Further growth is obtained only by periosteal appositional growth on the external surface, which leads to thickening and an increased height but without changing the size of the spinal canal.

Axis

The odontoid develops two primary ossification centers that usually coalesce within the first 3 months of life; these centers are separated from the C2 centrum by the dentocentral synchondrosis.[169,171] This synchondrosis is below the level of the C1–C2 facets and contributes to the overall height of the odontoid as well as the body of C2. It is continuous throughout the vertebral body and facets, and it coalesces with the anterior neurocentral synchondroses. These synchondroses progressively close, starting first in the regions of the facets, next at the neurocentral synchondroses, and finally at the dentocentral synchondrosis. This closure occurs between 3 and 6 years of age. The tip of the dens is comprised of a cartilaginous region similar to an epiphysis, the chondrum terminale, which develops an ossification center between 5 and 8 years, becoming the ossiculum terminale. The ossiculum terminale fuses to the remainder of the odontoid between 10 and 13 years of age.

The posterior neural arches are partially ossified at birth, joined by the posterior synchondrosis. By 3 months of age these arches, growing more posteriorly, form the rudimentary spinous process. By 1 year of age ossification fills the spinous process, and by 3 years the posterior synchondrosis has fused. Thus both the posterior and the anterior synchondroses are closed by 6 years of age, and there is again no further increase in spinal canal size after this age.

C3–C7

At birth, all three ossification centers are present.[170] The anterior synchondrosis (i.e., neurocentral synchondrosis) is slightly anterior to the base of the pedicles; it usually closes between 3 and 6 years of age. The posterior synchondrosis is at the junction of the two neural arches; it usually closes by 2 to 4 years of age. In the neonate and young child the articular facets are horizontal but become more vertically oriented as the child ages, reaching the normal adult configuration. They are also more horizontal in the upper cervical spine than in the lower cervical spine. The vertebral bodies enlarge circumferentially by periosteal appositional growth, whereas they grow vertically by endochondral ossification. Secondary ossification centers develop at the tips of the spinous processes and the cartilaginous ring apophyses of the bodies around the time of puberty. These ring apophyses are involved in the vertical growth of the body. These secondary ossification centers fuse with the vertebral body around age 25 years.

Normal Radiographic Parameters

There are certain normal radiographic parameters that indicate pathology of the cervical spine in adults but those in children represent normal developmental processes. These parameters are the atlantooccipital and atlantodens interval (ADI), pseudosubluxation and pseudoinstability, normal cervical spine motion in children, variations in the curvature of the cervical spine that may resemble spasm and ligamentous injury, variations in the presence of skeletal growth and growth centers that may resemble fractures, and anterior soft tissue widening.

Atlantodens Interval and Atlantooccipital Motion

These intervals are determined on lateral flexion and extension views, which should be conducted voluntarily with the patient awake. The ADI is the space between the anterior aspect of the dens and the posterior aspect of the anterior ring of the atlas (Fig. 20-1). An ADI of more than 5 mm on flexion and extension lateral radiographs indicates instability.[129,179] This is more than the 3-mm adult value because of the increased cartilage content of the odontoid and ring of the atlas in children as well as increased ligamentous laxity in children. In extension, overriding of the anterior arch of the atlas on top of the odontoid also can be seen in up to 20% of children.[32]

A mild increase in this interval may indicate a subtle disruption of the transverse atlantal ligament. In adults this ligament ruptures around an interval of 5 mm.[67] In chronic atlantoaxial conditions (e.g., rheumatoid arthritis, Down syndrome, congenital anomalies) the ADI is less useful. In these children, who are frequently hypermobile but do not have a ruptured transverse atlantal ligament, the ADI is increased beyond the 3 to 5 mm range. It is here that the complement of the ADI, or the space available for the cord (SAC), is useful. This space is the distance between the posterior aspect of the dens and the anterior aspect of the posterior ring of the atlas or the foramen magnum. A decrease in the SAC to 13 mm or less may be associated with neurologic problems.[220]

In these patients in which there is an attenuation of the transverse atlantal ligament without rupture, the alar ligament does provide some stability. It acts like a checkrein,[223] first tightening up in rotation and then becoming completely taut as the odontoid process continues to move posteriorly a distance equivalent to its full transverse diameter. This safety zone between the anterior wall of the spinal canal of the atlas, the axis, and the neural structures is an anatomic constant equal to the transverse diameter of the odontoid. This constant defines Steel's rule of thirds: one-third cord, one-third odontoid, and one-third space. The cord can move into this space (safe zone) when the odontoid moves posteriorly because of an attenuated transverse atlantal ligament. It is here where the alar ligament becomes taut, acting as a checkrein and secondary restraint, preventing further movement of the odontoid into the cord. In the chronic situation it is important to recognize when this safe zone has been

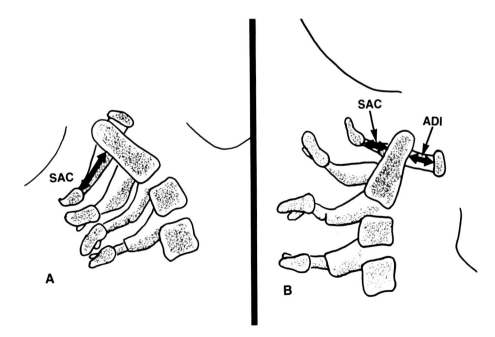

FIGURE 20-1. Lateral view of the atlantoaxial joint. The atlanto dens interval (ADI) is the distance between the anterior aspect of the dens and the posterior aspect of the anterior portion of the ring of the atlas. The space available for the cord (SAC) is the distance between the posterior aspect of the dens and the anterior aspect of the posterior portion of the ring of the atlas. In children, an ADI of 5 mm or larger is abnormal. In teenagers and adults, a SAC of 13 mm or smaller can be associated with canal compromise. In younger children, spinal cord impingement is imminent if the SAC is equal to or less than the transverse diameter of the odontoid. (**A**) The relations in extension. (**B**) The relations in flexion.

exceeded and the child enters the region of impending spinal cord compression. In the case of trauma the alar ligament is insufficient to prevent a fatal cord injury in the event of another neck injury similar to the one that caused the initial interruption of the transverse atlantal ligament.

Normal ranges of motion at the atlantooccipital interval are not well defined. In a series of 40 normal college freshman, the tip of the odontoid remained directly below the basion of the skull in both flexion and extension.[57] Thus the joint should not allow any horizontal translation during flexion and extension. Tredwell and colleagues[237] believe that a posterior subluxation of the atlantooccipital relation in extension of more than 4 mm indicates instability (Fig. 20-2). This can be measured as the distance between the anterior margin of the condyles at the base of the skull and the sharp contour of the anterior aspect of the concave joint of the atlas anteriorly or as the distance between the occipital protuberance and the superior

arch of the atlas posteriorly. Another method to measure this posterior subluxation of the atlantooccipital joint uses the technique of Weisel and Rothman[245] (Fig. 20-3). With this technique, occiput–C1 translation from maximum flexion to maximum extension should be no more than 1 mm in normal adults. These norms in children have not yet been established.

Pseudosubluxation

It is known that the C2–3 and to a lesser extent the C3–4 interspaces in children have a normal physiologic displacement.[12] In a study of 161 children,[32] marked anterior displacement of C2 on C3 was observed in 9% of children between 1 and 7 years old. In some children the anterior physiologic displacement of C2 on C3 is so pronounced that it appears pathologic (pseudosubluxation). To differentiate this from pathologic subluxation, Swischuk[226] has used the posterior cervical line (Fig. 20-4) drawn from the ante-

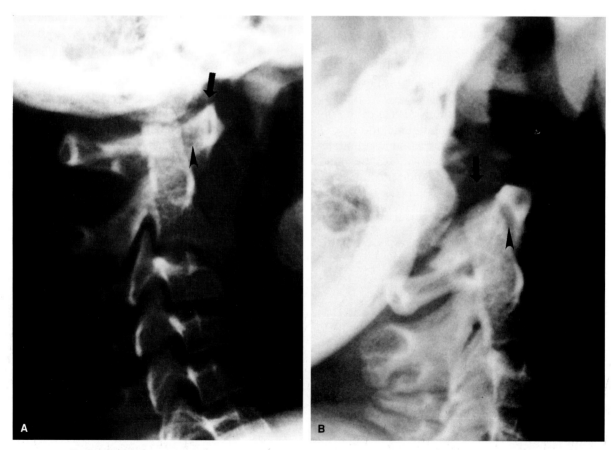

FIGURE 20-2. Lateral (**A**) flexion and (**B**) extension radiographs of an 11-year-old boy with Down syndrome. The child presented with loss of hand control when flexing his neck. Using the method of Tredwell and colleagues,[237] the atlantooccipital distance is measured as the distance between the anterior margin of the condyles at the base of the skull and the sharp contour of the anterior aspect of the concave joint of the atlas. More than 4 mm of posterior translation is abnormal. The atlantooccipital distance (*arrows*) measured 10 mm in extension and 1 mm in flexion. The atlantodens interval (ADI) was 1 mm in extension and 6 mm in flexion, for a total of 5 mm of motion (*arrowheads*). The space available for the cord was 17 mm in flexion and 20 mm in extension. Both occipitoatloid instability (>4 mm posterior translation) and atlantodens hypermobility (5 mm ADI in flexion) were present.

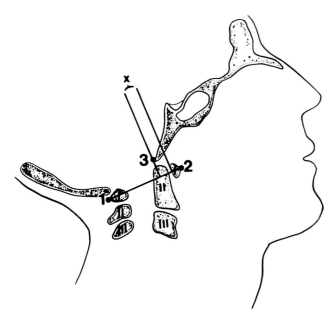

FIGURE 20-3. The method of measuring atlantooccipital instability according to Weisel and Rothman.[245] The atlantal line joins points 1 and 2. A perpendicular line to the atlantal line is made at the posterior margin of the anterior arch of the atlas. The distance (x) from the basion (3) to the perpendicular line is measured in flexion and extension. The difference between flexion and extension represents the anteroposterior translation at the occipitoatlantal joint; in normal adults, this translation should be no more than 1 mm. (From Gabriel KR, Mason DE, Carango P. Occipito-atlantal translation in Down's syndrome. Spine 1990;15:997.)

rior cortex of the posterior arch of C1 to the anterior cortex of the posterior arch of C3. In physiologic displacement of C2 on C3, the posterior cervical line may pass through the cortex of the posterior arch of C2, touch the anterior aspect of the cortex of the posterior arch of C2, or come within 1 mm of the anterior cortex of the posterior arch of C2. In pathologic dislocation of C2 on C3, the posterior cervical line misses the posterior arch of C2 by 2 mm or more.

The planes of the articular facets change with growth. The lower cervical spine facets change from 55 to 70 degrees, whereas the upper facets (i.e., C2–C4) may have initial angles as low as 30 degrees, which gradually change to 60 to 70 degrees. This variation in facet angulation along with normal looseness of the soft tissues, intervertebral discs, and the relative increase in size and weight of the skull compared with the trunk are the major factors responsible for this pseudosubluxation. Because this pseudosubluxation is a normal physiologic condition no treatment is needed.

Normal Lower Cervical Spine Motion

Generally, the interspinous distances increase with increasing age, being the smallest at C4–5 and the largest at C6–7, until 15 years of age, when this distance is largest at C5–6.[10] The anteroposterior displacement from hyperflexion to hyperextension de-

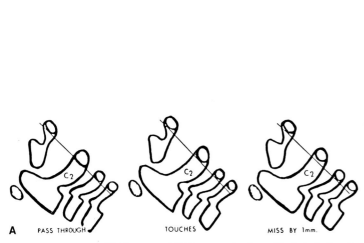

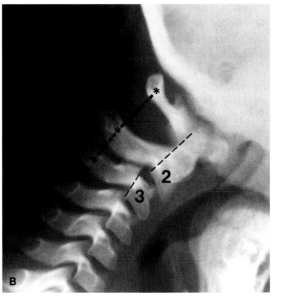

FIGURE 20-4. (A) The posterior line of Swischuk showing the normal limits. Passing through or just behind the anterior cortex of C2 (*left*). Touching the anterior aspect of the cortex of C2 (*center*). Coming within 1 mm of the anterior aspect of the cortex of C2 (*right*). (From Swischuk LE. Anterior displacement of C2 in children: physiologic or pathologic? A helpful differentiating line. Radiology 1977, 122:759. (B) Lateral cervical radiograph of a child with pseudosubluxation at C2–3 shown by a step-off at C2–3 (*dashed line*), but with a normal posterior cervical line (*asterick line*). Also note the anterior wedging of the C3 vertebral body. (From Loder RT, Hensinger RN. Developmental abnormalities of the cervical spine. In Weinstein SL, ed. The pediatric spine: Principals and practice. New York: Raven, 1994:397.)

creases from C2–C3 to C6–C7. The angular displacement is greatest (15 degrees) at C3–4 and C4–5 for children 3 to 8 years of age, the greatest (17 degrees) is at C4–5 for those aged 9 to 11 years of age, and is the greatest (15 degrees) at C5–6 for those aged 12 to 15 years of age.

Variations in the Curvature and Growth of the Cervical Spine That Can Resemble Injury

In the classic study of Catell and Filtzer,[32] 16% of normal children showed a marked angulation at a single interspace, suggestive of injury to the interspinous or posterior longitudinal ligament; 14% showed an absence of the normal lordosis in the neutral position; and 16% showed an absence of the flexion curvature between the second and the seventh cervical vertebrae, which could be erroneously interpreted as splinting secondary to injury.

Spina bifida of the posterior arch or multiple ossification centers of the ring of C1 may mimic fractures. However they are smooth and usually have cortical margins, which can delineate them from fractures. In some children the ring of C1 remains cartilaginous posteriorly, which is usually of no clinical significance.[50] Spina bifida also may occur at other cervical levels, and the overlapping lucent areas on anteroposterior radiographs when crossing a vertebral body may mimic a vertical fracture of the body.

The dentocentral synchondrosis of C2 begins to close between 5 to 7 years of age.[169] However, it can be visible in vestigial forms up to 11 years of age,[32] which can be interpreted erroneously as an undisplaced fracture. Similarly, the apical odontoid epiphysis (i.e., ossiculum terminale) may appear by 5 years of age, although it most typically appears around 8 years of age. This also can be interpreted as a fracture of the odontoid tip.

Wedging of the C3 vertebral body is a normal radiographic finding in 7% of younger children (see Fig. 20-4B).[227] In the face of a traumatic history, a computed tomography (CT) scan documents fracture lines through the body in the case of fracture if it is not known whether the wedging is this normal variation or a true compression fracture. In the lower cervical levels secondary centers of ossification of the spinous processes may resemble avulsion fractures.[32]

CONGENITAL AND DEVELOPMENTAL PROBLEMS

Torticollis

Torticollis is a combined head tilt and rotatory deformity. Torticollis indicates a problem at C1–C2, because 50% of the cervical spine rotation occurs at this joint, whereas a head tilt alone indicates a more generalized problem in the cervical spine. The differential diagnosis of torticollis is large[6] and can be divided into osseous and nonosseous types.

Osseous Types

BASILAR IMPRESSION. Basilar impression is a deformity in which the floor of the skull is indented by the upper cervical spine. The tip of the dens is more cephalad and sometimes protrudes into the opening of the foramen magnum. This may encroach on the brain stem, risking neurologic damage from direct injury, vascular compromise, or cerebrospinal fluid flow alteration.[229]

There are two main types of basilar impression: primary and secondary. Primary basilar impression, the most common type, is a congenital abnormality often associated with other vertebral defects (e.g., Klippel-Feil syndrome, odontoid abnormalities, atlantooccipital fusion, atlas hypoplasia). The incidence of primary basilar impression in the general population is 1%.[27]

Secondary basilar impression is a developmental condition attributed to softening of the osseous structures at the base of the skull. Any disorder of osseous softening can lead to secondary basilar impression.[46] These include metabolic bone diseases (e.g., Paget disease,[58] renal osteodystrophy, rickets, osteomalacia[105]), bone dysplasias and mesenchymal syndromes (e.g., osteogenesis imperfecta,[92] achondroplasia,[252] hypochondroplasia,[251] neurofibromatosis[108]), and rheumatologic disorders[205] (e.g., rheumatoid arthritis, ankylosing spondylitis). The softening allows the odontoid to migrate cephalad and into the foramen magnum.

These patients typically present with a short neck (78% in one series),[46] which is only an apparent deformity because of the basilar impression. They also show asymmetry of the skull and face (68%), painful cervical motion (53%), and torticollis (15%). Neurologic signs and symptoms are often present.[151] Many children will have acute onset of symptoms precipitated by minor trauma.[230] In cases of isolated basilar impression, the neurologic involvement is basically a pyramidal syndrome associated with proprioceptive sensory disturbances (motor weakness, 85%; limb paresthesias, 85%). In cases of basilar impression associated with Arnold-Chiari malformations, the neurologic involvement is usually cerebellar, and symptoms include motor incoordination with ataxia, dizziness, and nystagmus. In both types, the patients may complain of neck pain and headache in the distribution of the greater occipital nerve and cranial nerve involvement, particularly those that emerge from the medulla oblongata (trigeminal [V], glossopharyngeal [IX], vagus [X], and hypoglossal [XII]). Ataxia is a very common finding in children.[230] Hydrocephalus may develop as a result of obstruction of the cerebrospinal fluid flow by obstruction of the foramen magnum from the odontoid.

Basilar impression is difficult to assess radiographically. The most commonly used lines are Chamberlain's,[33] McRae's,[144] and McGregor's[141] in the lateral radiograph (Fig. 20-5). McGregor's line is the best method for screening because the landmarks can be clearly defined at all ages on a routine lateral radiograph. McRae's line is helpful in assessing the clinical significance of basilar impression because it defines the opening of the foramen magnum; in those who are symptomatic the odontoid projects above this line. CT with sagittal plane reconstructions can show the osseous relations at the occipitocervical junction more clearly, and magnetic resonance imaging (MRI) can show the anatomic involvement and impingement of the central nervous system. Occasionally vertebral angiography is needed.[178]

Treatment of basilar impression can be difficult and requires a multidisciplinary approach (orthopaedic, neurosurgical, and neuroradiologic).[149] The symptoms rarely can be helped by custom-made orthoses[104]; the primary treatment is surgical. If the symptoms are due to a hypermobile odontoid then surgical stabilization in extension at the occipitocervical junction is needed. Anterior excision of the odontoid is needed if it cannot be reduced,[150] but it should be preceded by posterior stabilization and fusion. If the symptoms are from posterior impingement, suboccipital decompression and often upper cervical laminectomy are needed. The dura often needs to be opened to look for a tight posterior band.[13,146] Posterior stabilization should also be performed. These are general statements, and each case should be considered individually.

ATLANTOOCCIPITAL ANOMALIES. Occipitocervical synostosis, basilar impression, and odontoid anomalies are the most common developmental malformations of the occipitovertebral junction, with an incidence of 1.4 to 2.5 per 100 children.[133] Both genders are affected equally. These lesions arise from a malformation of the mesenchymal anlages at the occipitovertebral junction.

These children resemble those with the Klippel-Feil syndrome: short, broad necks; restricted neck movements; low hairline; high scapula; and torticollis.[13,146] The skull may be deformed and shaped like a "tower skull." They also may have other associated anomalies, including dwarfism, funnel chest, jaw anomalies, cleft palate, congenital ear deformities, hypospadias, genitourinary tract defects, and syndactyly. Neurologic symptoms can occur during childhood, but more often they present around the age of 40 to 50 years. They progress slowly and relentlessly and can be initiated by traumatic or inflammatory processes. Rarely do they present suddenly or dramatically, although they have been reported as a cause of sudden death. The most common signs and symptoms, in decreasing order of frequency, are neck and occipital pain, vertigo, ataxia, limb paresis, paresthesias, speech disturbances, hoarseness, diplopia, syncope, auditory malfunction, and dysphagia.[83,242]

Standard radiographs are difficult to obtain because of fixed bony deformities; overlapping shadows from the mandible, occiput, and foramen magnum; and the patient's difficulty in cooperating. An x-ray beam directed 90 degrees perpendicular to the skull rather than the cervical spine usually gives a satisfactory view of the occipitocervical junction. The anomaly usually is studied further with tomograms and CT scans. The anterior arch of C1 is commonly assimilated to the occiput, usually in association with a hypoplastic ring posteriorly (Fig. 20-6). The height of C1 also is decreased variably, allowing the odontoid to project upward into the foramen magnum (i.e., the primary basilar impression). The position of the odontoid relative to the opening of the foramen magnum has been described by measuring the distance from the posterior aspect of the odontoid to the posterior ring of C1 or the posterior lip of the foramen magnum, whichever is closer.[145,146] This should be determined

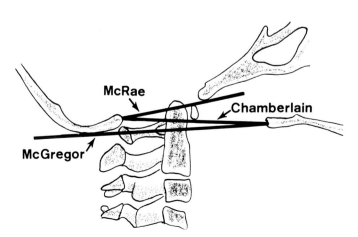

FIGURE 20-5. These landmarks on a lateral radiograph of the skull and upper cervical spine are used to assess basilar impression. McRae's line defines the opening of the foramen magnum. Chamberlain's line is drawn from the posterior lip of the foramen magnum to the dorsal margin of the hard palate. McGregor's line is drawn from the upper surface of the posterior edge of the hard palate to the most caudad point of the occipital curve of the skull. McGregor's line is the best line for screening because of the clarity of the radiographic landmarks in children of all ages.

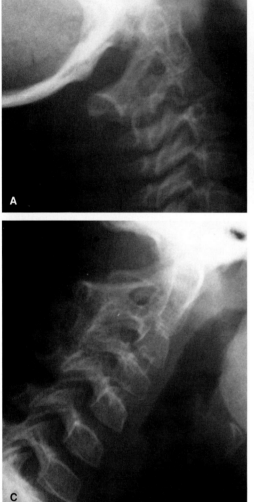

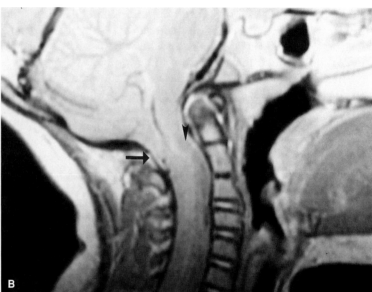

FIGURE 20-6.   This 3-year, 9-month-old girl had a history of vertex headaches for 1 year. One month prior to presentation, she developed a painful, left-sided torticollis. (**A**) Plain lateral radiograph shows fusion of C2–C3 and absence of the ring of C1 with occipitalization. (**B**) The magnetic resonance image shows an Arnold-Chiari malformation, with herniation of the cerebellar tonsils into the foramen magnum (*arrow*). Also note the cordal edema (*arrowhead*). (**C**) The child underwent an occipital decompression and laminectomy to C3, posterior cervical fusion from the occiput to C4, and halo cast immobilization for 4 months. Flexion and extension lateral radiographs 1 year after treatment show solid incorporation of the fusion from C2–C4, with dissolution of the graft from the occiput to C2. However, there is no atlantoccipital instability. The child's symptoms resolved.

in flexion because this position maximizes the reduction in the SAC. If this distance is less than 19 mm, a neurologic deficit is usually present. Lateral flexion and extension views of the upper cervical spine often show up to 12 mm of space between the odontoid and the C1 ring anteriorly[146]; associated C1–C2 instability has been reported to develop eventually in 50% of these patients.[241] The odontoid also may be misshapen or maldirected posteriorly. Up to 70% of these children have a congenital fusion of C2–C3 (see Fig. 20-6). Occipital vertebrac and condylar hypoplasia also can occur.

Myelography in the past, and now MRI, is useful to see the neuropathology. The upper spinal cord or medulla often is encroached on posteriorly by a dural constricting band with resultant neurologic findings. Cerebellar tonsil herniation also can occur.

Compression of the brain stem or upper cervical cord anteriorly occurs from the backward-projecting odontoid. This produces a range of findings and symptoms, depending on the location and degree of compression. Pyramidal tract signs and symptoms (e.g., spasticity, hyperreflexia, muscle weakness, gait disturbances) are most common, although signs of cranial nerve involvement (e.g., diplopia, tinnitus, dysphagia, auditory disturbances) can be seen. Compression from the posterior lip of the foramen magnum or dural constricting band can disturb the posterior columns with a loss of proprioception, vibration, and tactile senses. Nystagmus also occurs frequently as a result of posterior cerebellar compression. Vascular disturbances from vertebral artery involvement can result in brain stem ischemia, manifested by syncope, seizures, vertigo, and unsteady gait. The altered mechanics of the cervical spine may result in a dull, aching pain in the posterior occiput and neck with intermittent stiffness and torticollis. Irritation of the greater occipital nerve may cause tenderness in the posterior scalp.

The natural history of these disorders is not known. The neurologic symptoms may develop so late and progress so slowly because the frequently associated C1–C2 instability progresses with age, and the increased demands placed on the C1–C2 interval produce gradual spinal cord or vertebral artery compromise.

Treatment can be difficult because surgical intervention carries a much higher morbidity and mortality risk than with anomalies of the odontoid.[13,242] For this reason nonoperative methods should be attempted initially. Cervical collars, braces, and traction often help for persistent complaints of head and neck pain, especially following minor trauma or infection. Immobilization may only achieve temporary relief if neurologic deficits are present. Those with evidence of a compromised upper cervical area should take precautions not to expose themselves to undue trauma.

When symptoms and signs of an unstable C1–C2 complex are present, a posterior C1–C2 fusion is indicated. Preliminary traction to attempt reduction is used if necessary. If a reduction is possible and there are no neurologic signs, surgery has an improved prognosis.[13,83,242] Posterior signs and symptoms may be an indication for posterior decompression depending on the evidence of dural or osseous compression. Results vary from complete resolution to increased deficits and death.[13,161] The role of concomitant posterior fusion has not yet been determined, but if decompression, whether anterior or posterior, can destabilize the spine, then concomitant posterior fusion should be strongly considered.

UNILATERAL ABSENCE OF C1. This congenital malformation of the first cervical vertebra arises during fetal life and is in essence a hemiatlas or a congenital scoliosis of C1. Doubousset[52] has described 17 patients with this absence. No definite population incidence is known. The problem often is associated with other anomalies common to children with congenital spine deformities (e.g., tracheoesophageal fistula, other congenital spine deformities).

Two thirds of the children present at birth; the others develop a torticollis and are noticed later. A lateral translation of the head on the trunk with variable degrees of lateral tilt and rotation, best appreciated from the back, is the typical finding. There also may be severe tilting of the eye line. The sternocleidomastoid muscle is not tight, although regional aplasia of the muscles in the nuchal concavity of the tilted side is noted. Neck flexibility is variable and decreases

with age. The condition is not painful. Plagiocephaly can occur and increases as the deformity increases. Neurologic signs (e.g., headache, vertigo, myelopathy) are present in about one fourth of the patients. The natural history is unknown.

Standard anteroposterior and lateral radiographs rarely give the diagnosis, although the open-mouth odontoid view may suggest it. Tomograms and CT scans usually are needed to see the anomaly (Fig. 20-7). The defect can range from a hypoplasia of the lateral mass to a complete hemiatlas with rotational instability and basilar impression. Occasionally the atlas is occipitalized. There are three types of this disorder. Type I is an isolated hemiatlas. Type II is a partial or complete aplasia of one hemiatlas, with other associated anomalies of the cervical spine (e.g., fusion of C3–C4, congenital bars in the lower cervical vertebrae). Type III is a partial or complete atlantooccipital fusion and symmetric or asymmetric hemiatlas aplasia with or without anomalies of the odontoid and the lower cervical vertebrae.

Once diagnosed, entire spinal radiographs should be taken to rule out other congenital vertebral anomalies. Other imaging studies that may be needed are vertebral angiography, myelography, and MRI. Angiography should be performed if operative intervention is

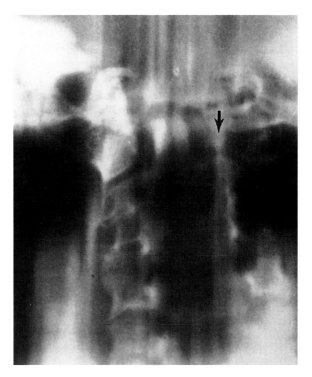

FIGURE 20-7. An anteroposterior tomogram of a 13-year-old girl with a hemihypoplasia of the atlas (*arrow*) and torticollis. Note also the fusion of the second and third cervical vertebrae and basilar invagination. (*From* Dubousset J. Torticollis in children caused by congenital anomalies of the atlas. J Bone Joint Surg [Am] 1986; 68:178.)

undertaken because arterial anomalies (e.g., multiple loops, vessels smaller than normal, abnormal routes between C1 and C2) often are found on the aplastic side. Myelography and MRI also should be done if operative intervention is undertaken because many of these children will have stenosis of the foramen magnum and occasionally an Arnold-Chiari malformation.

The deformity should be observed to document the presence or absence of progression. This observation is primarily clinical (e.g., photographs) because radiographic measurements are difficult if not impossible to obtain. Bracing does not halt progression of the deformity. Surgical intervention is recommended in those patients with severe deformities. Preoperative halo placement is used for gradual correction by using a halo cast over 6 to 8 days until correction has been achieved. An ambulatory method of gradual cervical spine deformity correction has been described using the halo-Ilizarov technique.[82] A posterior fusion from the occiput–C2 or –C3 is then performed, depending on the extent of the anomaly. Decompression of the spinal canal is necessary when the canal size is not ample, either at that time or if projected not to be able to fully accommodate the developed spinal cord. The ideal age for posterior fusion is between the ages of 5 and 8 years, corresponding to the age at which the canal size reaches adult proportions.

FAMILIAL CERVICAL DYSPLASIA. This recently described atlas deformity[197] has an autosomal dominant genetic pattern with complete penetrance and variable expressivity. The epidemiology is not known. Clinical presentation varies from an incidental finding, a passively correctable head tilt, suboccipital pain, or decreased cervical motion to a clunking of the upper cervical spine.

Plain radiographs are difficult to interpret. Various anomalies of C1, most commonly a partial absence of the posterior ring of C1, typically are seen. Various anomalies of C2 also exist, commonly a shallow hypoplastic left facet. Other dysplasias of the lateral masses, facets, and posterior elements and occasionally spondylolisthesis are seen. Occiput–C1 instability is frequently seen; C1–C2 instability rarely is seen. The delineation of this complex anatomy often is seen best with a CT scan and three-dimensional reconstruction (Fig. 20-8). When symptoms of instability are present, an MRI in flexion and extension is recommended to assess the presence and magnitude of neural compression. Neural compression at the occipitocervical junction is created by instability from the malformation.

Nonsurgical treatment is close observation (every 6–12 months) to ensure that no symptoms of instability develop both clinically (e.g., progressive weakness and

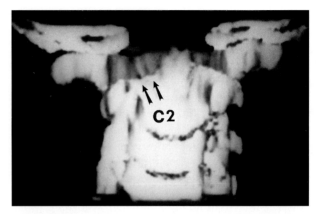

FIGURE 20-8.   A three-dimensional computed tomographic scan of the upper cervical cord in a child with familial cervical dysplasia. The left superior facet of C2 is shallow and hypoplastic (*arrows*). (From Rubin SE, Wagner RS. Ocular torticolis. A review. Surv Ophthalmol 1986;30;366.)

fatigue or objective signs of myelopathy) and radiographically with lateral flexion and extension radiographs. Surgical intervention is recommended for persistent pain, torticollis, and especially neurologic symptoms. A posterior fusion from the occiput to C2 usually is required, with gradual preoperative reduction using an adjustable halo cast.[82]

ATLANTOAXIAL ROTARY DISPLACEMENT. Atlantoaxial rotary displacement is one of the most common causes of childhood torticollis. Rotary displacements are characteristically a pediatric problem, but they may occur in adults. There are several etiologies. Because the resultant radiographic findings and treatment regimens are the same for all pediatric etiologies, I discuss them as a unit and note the individual exceptions where necessary.

The confusing terminology includes rotary dislocation, rotary deformity, rotational subluxation, rotary fixation, and spontaneous hyperemic dislocation.[38,39,68,109,243] The multiple terms used probably indicate a lack of understanding of the pathophysiology and pathoanatomy.

Atlantoaxial rotary subluxation is probably the most accepted term used in describing the common childhood torticollis. *Subluxation* may be misleading because cases of subluxation usually present within the normal range of motion of the atlantoaxial joint. *Rotary displacement* is a more appropriate and descriptive term because this includes the entire range of pathology, from a mild subluxation to a complete dislocation. The majority of these cases recover spontaneously without treatment. Rarely these deformities persist, and the children present with a resistant and unresolving torticollis. This is best termed *atlantoaxial rotary fixation* or *fixed atlantoaxial displacement*. Gradations exist between the very mild, easily correctable rotary displacement and the rigid fixation. Complete atlantoaxial rotary dislocation rarely has been reported in surviving patients.

The radiographic findings of rotary displacement are sometimes difficult to demonstrate. This is because of difficulty in positioning the patient because of associated pain and difficulty in interpreting the radiograph. Malalignment of the head or the x-ray beam, along with congenital anomalies that may occur in this area, make interpretation even more difficult.[66]

With rotary displacement of torticollis, the lateral mass of C1 that has rotated forward appears wider and closer to the midline (medial offset), whereas the opposite lateral mass is narrower and away from the midline (lateral offset). The facet joints may be obscured because of apparent overlapping. The lateral

view shows the wedge-shaped lateral mass of the atlas lying anteriorly where the oval arch of the atlas normally lies, and the posterior arches fail to superimpose because of the head tilt (Fig. 20-9). These findings may suggest occipitalization of C1 because with the neck tilt, the skull may obscure C1. The normal relation between the occiput and C1 is believed to be maintained in children with atlantoaxial rotary displacement. A lateral radiograph of the skull may demonstrate the relative position of C1 and C2 more clearly than a lateral radiograph of the cervical spine. This is because tilting of the head also tilts C1, which creates overlapping shadows and makes interpretation of a lateral spinal radiograph difficult.

The problem with plain radiographs is how to differentiate the position of C1 and C2 in a child with

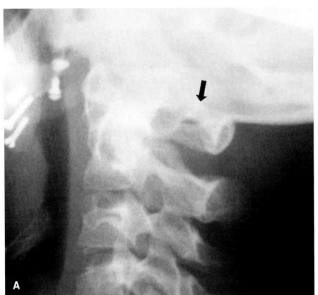

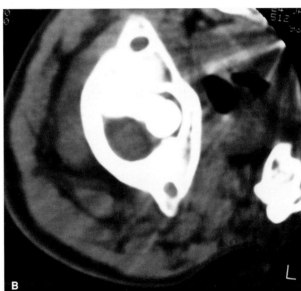

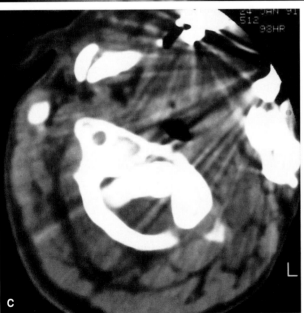

FIGURE 20-9.   Radiographic findings in atlantoaxial rotary subluxation. (**A**) The lateral cervical spinal radiograph. The posterior arches fail to superimpose because of the head tilt (*arrows*). A dynamic computed tomographic scan in a 9-year-old girl with a fixed atlantoaxial rotary displacement with (**B**) the head maximally rotated to the left and (**C**) the head maximally rotated to the right, which in this case does not reach the midline. The ring of C1 is still in the exact relation to the odontoid as in **B**, indicating a fixed displacement.

subluxation from that in a normal child whose head is rotated because both will give the same picture. Open mouth views are difficult to obtain and interpret, and the lack of cooperation and diminished motion on the part of the child often make it impossible to obtain these special views. Cineradiography has been recommended, but the radiation dose is high and patient cooperation may be difficult to maintain because of muscle spasms.[65,66,102] CT scans are helpful in this situation if done properly.[73] A CT scan, when taken with the head in the torticollic position, may be interpreted by the casual observer as showing rotation of C1 on C2. If the rotation of C1 on C2 is within the normal range, as it usually is early on in this condition, then the observer may attribute this rotation to patient positioning. A dynamic rotation CT scan is helpful in this situation. Obtaining views with the head maximally rotated to the right and then to the left side clearly demonstrate atlantoaxial rotary fixation when there is a loss of normal rotation (see Fig. 20-9).

Rotary displacement can be classified into four types (Fig. 20-10)[68]: type I is a simple rotary displacement without an anterior shift, type II is rotary displacement with an anterior shift of 5 mm or less, type III is rotary displacement with an anterior shift greater than 5 mm, and type IV is rotary displacement with a posterior shift. The amount of anterior displacement considered to be pathologic is greater than 3 mm in older children and adults and greater than 4 mm in younger children.[73,85,129] Flexion and extension lateral stress radiographs are suggested to rule out the possibility of anterior displacement.

Type I is by far the type most frequently seen in the pediatric age group. This type is usually benign and frequently resolves on its own. Type II deformity is potentially more dangerous; it must be approached carefully. Types III and IV are very rare, but because of the potential for neurologic involvement and even instant death, management must be approached with great caution.

The multifactorial etiology and pathoanatomy is not known completely.[39,84,99,139,176,243] Several mechanisms are most likely causative. The onset of atlantoaxial rotary displacement may occur spontaneously following minor or major trauma or an upper respiratory infection and after head and neck surgery. The children present with a "cocked-robin" torticollis. The child resists acutely attempts to move the head because of pain. The associated muscle spasm is noted on the side of the long sternocleidomastoid muscle, unlike congenital muscular torticollis because the muscle is attempting to correct the deformity. If the deformity becomes fixed, the pain subsides, but the torticollis may persist, along with a decreased range of motion. In long-standing cases, plagiocephaly and facial flattening may develop on the side of the tilt. Associated fractures rarely may be the cause of the displacement.

Grisel syndrome[84] is a spontaneous atlantoaxial subluxation with inflammation of adjacent neck tissues that is commonly seen in children after upper respiratory infections (Fig. 20-11). Parke and colleagues[176] have shown a direct connection between the pharyngovertebral veins and the periodontal venous plexus and suboccipital epidural sinuses. They believe that this may provide a route for hematogenous transport of peripharyngeal septic exudates to the upper cervical spine and an anatomic explanation for the atlantoaxial hyperemia of Grisel syndrome. Regional lymphadenitis is known to cause spastic contracture of the cervical muscles. This muscular spasm, in the presence of abnormally loose ligaments (hypothetically caused by the hyperemia of the pharyngovertebral vein drainage), could produce locking of the overlapping lateral joint edges of the articular facets. This prevents easy repositioning, resulting in atlantoaxial rotary displacement. Kawabe and colleagues[115] have shown that meniscus-like synovial folds are present in the atlantooccipital and lateral atlantoaxial joints of children but not those of adults, and that the dens-facet angle of the axis is steeper in children than in adults. They postulate that excessive C1–C2 rotation caused by the steeper angle, compounded by ligament

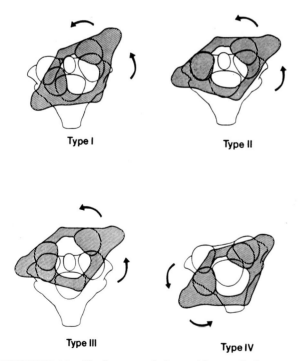

Type I

Type II

Type III

Type IV

FIGURE 20-10. The four types of atlantoaxial rotary displacement. (From Fielding JW, Hawkins RJ. Atlantoaxial rotatory fixation. [Fixed rotatory subluxation of the atlantoaxial joint.] J Bone Joint Surg [Am] 1977;59:37.)

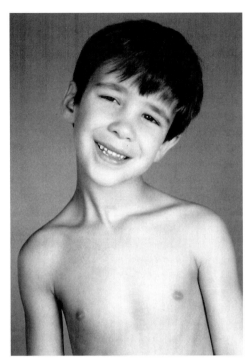

FIGURE 20-11. A 5-year-old boy developed an atlantoaxial rotary subluxation after an upper respiratory viral infection (Grisel syndrome). It rapidly resolved after treatment with a soft collar and mild doses of diazepam.

laxity from an underlying hyperemia, allows the meniscus-like synovial folds to become impinged in the lateral atlantoaxial joint and leads to rotary fixation. The predominance of this syndrome in childhood correlates with the predilection for the adenoids to be maximally hypertrophied and inflamed at this same time and located in the area drained by the pharyngovertebral veins.

A substantial number of the cases have been associated with surgery of the oral pharynx, most frequently tonsillectomy and adenoidectomy and less commonly other head and neck procedures. The hyperemia following the procedure enhances the passage of the inflammatory products into the pharyngovertebral veins.

Most atlantoaxial rotary displacements resolve spontaneously and never come to the attention of the physician. Rarely, however, the deformity becomes fixed. The pain subsides, and the torticollis is persistent. The duration of symptoms and deformity dictates the recommended treatment.[181]

Patients with rotary subluxation of less than 1 week can be treated with immobilization in a soft cervical collar and rest for about 1 week. Close follow-up is mandatory. If spontaneous reduction does not occur with this initial treatment, hospitalization and the use of halter traction, muscle relaxants (e.g., diaze-

pam), and analgesics is recommended next. Patients with rotary subluxation of greater than 1 week but less than 1 month in duration should be hospitalized immediately for cervical traction, relaxants, and analgesics. A halo occasionally is needed to achieve reduction. If after reduction, which is noted clinically and confirmed with a dynamic CT scan, no anterior displacement is noted, then cervical support should be continued only until symptoms have subsided. If their is anterior displacement immobilization should be continued for 6 weeks to allow ligamentous healing to occur. In patients with rotary subluxation for more than 1 month, cervical traction (usually halo skeletal) can be tried for up to 3 weeks, but the prognosis is guarded. These children usually fall into two groups: those whose rotary subluxation can be reduced with halo traction but, despite a prolonged period of immobilization, resubluxate when the immobilization is stopped and those whose subluxation cannot be reduced and is fixed.

When the deformity is fixed, especially when anterior C1 displacement is present, the transverse atlantal ligament is compromised with a potential for catastrophe. In this situation a posterior C1–C2 fusion should be performed. The indications for fusion are neurologic involvement, anterior displacement, failure to achieve and maintain correction, a deformity which has been present for more than 3 months, and recurrence of deformity following an adequate trial of conservative management (at least 6 weeks of immobilization after reduction). Prior to surgical fusion, halo traction over several days is used to obtain as much straightening of the head and neck as possible; a forceful or manipulative reduction should not be performed. Postoperatively the child is simply positioned in a halo cast and vest in the straightened position obtained preoperatively; this can be expected to obtain satisfactory alignment. A Gallie type fusion[79] with sublaminar wiring at the ring of C1 and through and around the spinous process of C2 is preferred rather than a Brooks type fusion,[22] in which the wire is sublaminar at both C1 and C2. This is because of the decreased SAC at C2 with a higher risk of neurologic injury. This wiring does not reduce the displacement but simply provides some internal stability for the arthrodesis. The results for a Gallie fusion overall are very good (Fig. 20-12).[69]

Nonosseous Types

CONGENITAL MUSCULAR TORTICOLLIS. Congenital muscular torticollis, or congenital wry neck, is the most common cause of torticollis in the infant and young child. A disproportionate number of these

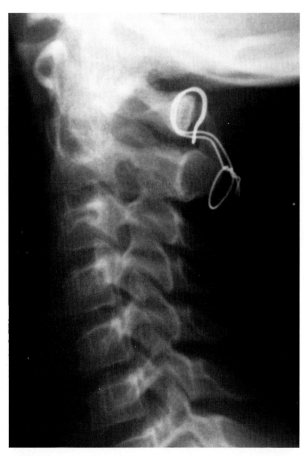

FIGURE 20-12. The child in Figure 20-9 had a fixed deformity that occurred 6 months earlier, immediately after reconstructive maxillofacial surgery for Goldenhar syndrome. It did not respond to traction, including halo traction. She underwent a posterior C1–C2 (Gallie-type) fusion. A solid fusion was present 9 months later; clinically, the patient achieved 80 degrees of rotation to the left and 45 degrees of rotation to the right.

children have a history of a primiparous birth or a breech or difficult delivery. However, this has been reported in children with normal births and even in children born by cesarean section.[126,134] Rarely is there a familial tendency.[231]

Although the exact etiology is not known there are several theories. The most recent is that a compartment syndrome occurs as a result of compression to the soft tissues of the neck at the time of delivery.[44] Histology of resected surgical specimens suggests that the lesion is due to occlusion of the venous outflow of the sternocleidomastoid muscle.[22,247] This blockage may result in a compartment syndrome as manifested by edema, degeneration of muscle fibers, and fibrosis of the muscle body. The muscle fibrosis is variable, ranging from small amounts to the entire muscle. It has been suggested that the clinical deformity is related to the ratio of fibrosis to remaining functional muscle. If ample muscle remains, the sternocleido-

mastoid will probably stretch with growth, and the child will not develop torticollis; if fibrosis predominates, there is little elastic potential, and torticollis will develop. With time the fibrosis of the sternal head may entrap the branch of the spinal accessory nerve to the clavicular head of the muscle, which can then lead to a later progressive deformity.[199] Other authors believe that torticollis is due to in utero crowding because three of four children have the lesion on the right side[127] and 20% have developmental hip dysplasia.[244] The fact that it can occur in children with normal birth histories or in children born by cesarean section challenges the perinatal compartment syndrome theory and supports the in utero crowding theory. The fact that it can occur in families (supporting a genetic predisposition) also questions the compartment syndrome theory. Another theory is primarily neurogenic,[199] supported by histopathologic evidence of denervation and reinnervation. The primary myopathy initially may be due to trauma or ischemia, or both, and involves the two heads of the sternocleidomastoid muscle unequally.

The deformity is due to contracture of the sternocleidomastoid muscle, with the head tilted toward the involved side and the chin rotated toward the opposite shoulder. The clinical features of congenital muscular torticollis depend on the time at which the physician evaluates the child. It is often discovered in the first 6 to 8 weeks of life. If the child is examined during the first 4 weeks of life, a mass or "tumor" may be palpable in the neck.[126] Although the mass may be palpable, it is unrecognized up to 80% of the time.[40] Characteristically it is a nontender, soft enlargement beneath the skin and located within the sternocleidomastoid muscle belly. This tumor reaches its maximum size within the first 4 weeks of life, and then gradually regresses. After 4 to 6 months of life the contracture and the torticollis are the only clinical findings. In some children the deformity is not noticed until after 1 year of age, which questions whether the condition is in fact congenital as well as the perinatal compartment syndrome theory. Because up to 20% of children with congenital muscular torticollis have developmental dysplasia of the hip[244] a very careful examination of the hips should be performed.

If the deformity is progressive, skull and face deformities can develop (plagiocephaly), often within the first year of life. The facial flattening occurs on the side of the contracted muscle and is probably due to the sleeping position of the child.[19] In the United States children usually sleep prone, and in this position it is more comfortable for them to lie with the affected side down. The face therefore remodels to conform to the bed. If the child sleeps supine, reverse modeling of the contralateral skull occurs. In the child who is untreated for many years, the level of the eyes and ears becomes unequal and can result in considerable cosmetic deformity.

Radiographs of the cervical spine always should be obtained to ensure that the deformity is truly a muscular torticollis and is not associated with congenital vertebral lesions of the cervical spine. Plain radiographs of the cervical spine in children with muscular torticollis are always normal, aside from the head tilt and rotation. If any suspicion exists about the status of the hips, appropriate imaging (e.g., ultrasonography, radiographs) should be done, depending on the age of the child and expertise of the ultrasonographer.

The sternocleidomastoid muscle exhibited an abnormal MRI signal in 10 patients with congenital muscular torticollis studied from 4 weeks to 5 years of age. In no case was a discrete mass seen within the sternocleidomastoid muscle.[44] The muscle diameter also increased 2 to 4 times that of the contralateral muscle. In older patients, the signals produced were consistent with atrophy and fibrosis, similar to those encountered in compartment syndromes of the leg and forearm.

Treatment initially consists of conservative measures.[14,29,40,126,134] Good results can be expected with stretching exercises alone, with one series reporting 90% success.[14] These results also may reflect, in some part, a favorable natural history of many of these children. The exercises are performed by the caregivers and guided by the physiotherapist. The ear opposite the contracted muscle should be positioned to the shoulder, and the chin should be positioned to touch the shoulder on the same side as the contracted muscle. When adequate stretching has occurred in the neutral position, the exercises should be graduated up to the extended position, which achieves maximum stretching and prevents residual contractures. Treatment measures to be used along with stretching consist of modifying the child's toys and crib so that the neck is stretched when the infant is reaching for or looking at objects of interest. The exact role of the efficacy of these stretching measures versus a natural history of spontaneous resolution is not known; there are many anecdotal cases of spontaneous resolution.

Surgery is recommended when the deformity persists after 1 year of age. This age has been selected because stretching measures are usually unsuccessful after this age[29,64]; the child's neck and anatomic structures are also larger, making surgery easier. Established facial deformity or a limitation of more than 30 degrees of motion usually precludes a good result, and surgery is required to prevent further facial flattening and further cosmetic deterioration.[29] Asymmetry of the face and skull can improve as long as adequate growth potential remains after the deforming pull of the sternocleidomastoid is removed; good but not perfect results can be obtained as late as 12 years of life.[40] The best time for surgical release is between the ages of 1 and 4 years.[126,239]

Surgical treatments include a unipolar release either at the sternoclavicular or mastoid poles, a bipolar release, and even complete resection. The bipolar release combined with a Z-plasty of the sternal attachment (Fig. 20-13) has yielded 92% satisfactory results in one series, whereas only 15% satisfactory results were obtained with other procedures.[64] The Z-plasty lengthening maintains the V-contour of the neck and cosmesis. Structures that can be injured from surgery are the spinal accessory nerve, the anterior and external jugular veins, the carotid vessels and sheath, and the facial nerve. Skin incisions should never be located directly over the clavicle because of cosmetically unacceptable scar spreading but rather should be made one finger breadth proximal to the medial end of the clavicle and sternal notch and in line with the cervical skin creases. The postoperative protocol can vary from simple stretching exercises to cast immobilization. Some type of a bracing device to maintain alignment

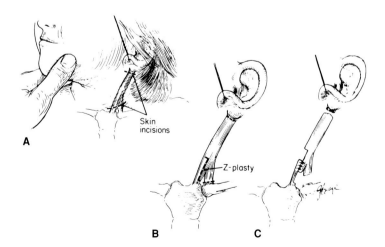

FIGURE 20-13. The Z-plasty procedure for torticollis. (**A**) The location of the skin incisions. (**B**) The clavicular and mastoid attachments of the sternocleidomastoid muscle are cut, and a Z-plasty is performed. Note that the medial aspect of the sternal attachment is preserved. (**C**) The completed procedure after release of the proximal muscle insertion. (From Ferkel RD, Westin GW, Dawson ED, Oppenheim WL. Muscular torticollis. A modified surgical approach. J Bone Joint Surg [Am] 1983;65:894.)

of the head and neck is probably a desirable part of the postoperative protocol.

Neurogenic Types

Although rare, these causes should be considered in the differential diagnosis of any atypical torticollis, especially when the condition is unresponsive or progressive in the face of therapy believed to be appropriate. The major neurogenic etiologies are central nervous system tumors (i.e., of the posterior fossa or spinal cord), syringomyelia with or without cord tumor, Arnold-Chiari malformation, ocular dysfunction, and paroxysmal torticollis of infancy.

Posterior fossa tumors can present with torticollis.[17,228] The ophthalmologic literature[137] has described three children with torticollis, photophobia, and epiphora (tearing). In all three children, the diagnosis was delayed with an initial diagnosis of a local ocular inflammatory condition. The age at presentation ranged from 1 to 23 months. The delay in diagnosis ranged from 5 months to 4 years. The neoplastic diagnosis was not considered initially by the ophthalmologists because the primary signs of posterior fossa tumors are extraocular muscle paresis, nystagmus, and papilledema.

Cervical cord tumors can present with torticollis, often early in their course.[81, 241] Often, these initially are diagnosed as congenital torticollis, obstetric birth palsy, muscular dystrophy, or cerebral palsy.[81] The peculiar, often overlooked signs of the tumor are spinal rigidity, early spinal deformity, and spontaneous or induced vertebral pain. In young children the pain may be expressed as irritability and restlessness.

Radiographic imaging of a child with a potential central nervous system tumor should consist of plain radiographs of the skull and cervical spine followed by CT scan, MRI, and myelography. Vertebral angiography also may be needed, both diagnostically and in neurosurgical planning. A syringomyelia also can be seen with spinal cord tumors.

The Arnold-Chiari malformation (see Fig. 20-6) is a constellation of congenital deformities of the brain stem and cerebellum that is marked by caudal displacement of the hindbrain.[53,248] The deformities may be associated with myelomeningocele (i.e., type II malformation). The Chiari type I malformation is a downward displacement of the medulla oblongata with extrusion of the cerebellar tonsils through the foramen magnum and is encountered in older children. Dure and colleagues[53] described 11 children with Chiari type I malformations in which torticollis was the presenting complaint at 5 years of age in 1 of the 11 children. It also was associated with headaches and paracervical muscle spasm; the torticollis was left sided. As with tumors, the workup of a child with the potential for

a Chiari malformation consists of plain radiographs of the skull and cervical spine followed by central nervous system imaging. MRI is now considered the most reliable and least invasive procedure.[47,53] The treatment is neurosurgical.

Ocular dysfunction also can cause torticollis,[196] usually atypical. The face can be turned about a vertical axis, the head can be tilted to one shoulder with the frontal plane of the face remaining coronal, or the chin can be elevated or depressed. A combination of any of these positions also can occur. Abnormal head position for ocular reasons usually is assumed to optimize visual acuity and maintain binocularity. The orthopaedist can become suspicious that there may be an ocular cause if the head is tilted but not rotated or if the tilt changes when the child is lying versus sitting or standing up. Children with ocular pathology do not have the fibrotic sternocleidomastoid muscle seen in congenital muscular torticollis. Detailed tests conducted by an experienced ophthalmologist are diagnostic (e.g., the Bielschowsky head-tilting test for the vestibuloocular labyrinth pathways and reflex). Treatment of ocular torticollis is usually surgical.

Paroxysmal torticollis of infancy is a rare and unusual episodic torticollis lasting for minutes to days with spontaneous recovery.[177,218] The attacks usually occur in the morning, last from 10 minutes to 14 days, and have a frequency from less than one episode per month to three to four episodes per month. The attacks can be associated with lateral trunk curvature, eye movements or deviations, and alternating sides of torticollis. The children are usually girls (71%), the average age of onset is 3 months (1 week–30 months), and the recovery period is 24 months (6 months–5 years). It has been suggested that paroxysmal torticollis of infancy is equivalent to a migraine headache because of positive family histories for migraines in 29%, or it is a forerunner of benign paroxysmal vertigo of childhood.[218] Whatever the cause, it is usually self-limiting and does not require therapy.

Sandifer Syndrome

This is a syndrome of gastroesophageal reflux, often from a hiatal hernia, and abnormal posturing of the neck and trunk, usually torticollis.[157,189] It commonly is seen either in infancy or in children with cerebral palsy. The torticollis is believed to be an attempt on the part of the child to decrease the esophagitis pain resulting from the gastroesophageal reflux. The majority of patients present in infancy. On occasion the diagnosis may be delayed and not discovered until childhood. The abnormal posturing also may present as opisthotonos or neural tics and often mimics central nervous system disorders. The diagnosis of symptom-causing gastroesophageal reflux frequently is overlooked.[20] The incidence of gastroesophageal reflux is high (up to 40% of infants),[43] with the principal symptoms being vomiting, failure to thrive, recurrent respiratory disease, dysphagia, various neural signs, torticollis, and respiratory arrest. On careful examination of these infants the tight and short sternocleidomastoid muscle or its tumor is not seen, eliminating congenital muscular torticollis. Further workup excludes dysplasias and congenital anomalies of the cervical spine, postinfectious causes, and central nervous system disorders (e.g., extraocular muscle or vestibular apparatus disorders, central nervous system neoplasms). In these situations the physician should consider Sandifer syndrome in the differential diagnosis.

Plain radiographs of the cervical spine should be taken to rule out any congenital anomalies or dysplasias. Contrast studies of the upper gastrointestinal tract usually demonstrate the hiatal hernia and gastroesophageal reflux.[145] Esophageal pH studies may be necessary; many children, both asymptomatic and symptomatic, show evidence of gastroesophageal reflux.[112]

Treatment begins with medical therapy. When this fails fundoplication can be considered. In otherwise normal children this is usually curative.[111]

Klippel-Feil Syndrome

Klippel-Feil syndrome consists of congenital fusions of the cervical vertebrae clinically exhibited by the triad of a low posterior hairline, a short neck, and limited neck motion.[96,117,154,211] There are often other associated anomalies, both in the musculoskeletal and other organ systems. The congenital fusions result from abnormal embryologic formation of the cervical vertebral mesenchymal anlages. This embryologic insult, although as yet unknown, is not limited to the cervical vertebrae and explains the other associated anomalies with the Klippel-Feil syndrome. The incidence of congenital cervical fusion is approximately 0.7%.[23]

These children demonstrate limited neck motion of varying degrees. Approximately one third of the children have an associated Sprengel deformity. The other anomalies associated with the syndrome are scoliosis (both congenital and idiopathic-like),[96] renal anomalies,[147,153] deafness,[143,222] synkinesis (mirror movements),[86] pulmonary dysfunction,[11,18] and congenital heart disease.[163] The radiographs show varying degrees of vertebral fusion, ranging from simple block vertebrae to multiple and bizarre anomalies. There is often an associated scoliosis, which makes interpretation of the radiographs difficult. Flexion and extension lateral radiographs are useful to assess any potential instability. Any segment adjacent to unfused segments may result in hypermobility and neurologic symptoms.[89,123] A common pattern is fusion of C1–C2 and C3–C4, leading to a high risk of instability at the unfused C2–C3 level.[59]

All children with Klippel-Feil syndrome should be further evaluated for other organ system problems. A general pediatric evaluation should be undertaken by a qualified pediatrician to ensure that no congenital cardiac or other neurologic abnormalities exist. Renal imaging should be done in all children; a simple renal ultrasonogram is usually adequate for the initial evaluation.[51] The neural axis is most easily seen with an MRI. An MRI should be obtained whenever any concern for neurologic involvement exists on a clinical basis and prior to any orthopaedic spinal procedure.[194] Simple flexion and extension lateral radiographs should be taken prior to any general anesthetic to rule out any occult instability of the cervical spine. If the flexion and extension radiographs are difficult to interpret, which is common because of the multiple anomalous vertebrae, a flexion and extension CT scan can be useful, especially at the C1–C2 level.

The natural history of children with Klippel-Feil is primarily dependent on the occurrence of severe renal or cardiac problems with subsequent organ system failure and death. Regarding the cervical spine,[182] instability can develop with neurologic involvement, especially in the upper segments or in those with iniencephaly.[182,209] Degenerative joint and disc disease develops in those patients with lower segment instabilities.

Because those children with large fusion areas are at high risk for developing instabilities, strenuous activities should be avoided, especially contact sports. Other nonsurgical methods of treatment are cervical traction, collars, and analgesics when mechanical symptoms appear, which usually occurs in the adolescent or adult patient. Surgical fusion is needed when neurologic symptoms arise from instability. The real dilemma is whether or not prophylactic stabilization should be undertaken for hypermobile segments that are not symptomatic. Unfortunately, no guidelines exist for this problem. The need for decompression at the time of stabilization depends on the exact anatomic circumstance, as will the need for combined anterior and posterior versus simple posterior fusions alone. Surgery for cosmesis alone is usually unwarranted and risky.[18]

Os Odontoideum

Os odontoideum is an anomaly in which the tip of the odontoid process is divided by a wide transverse gap, leaving the apical segment without its basilar support.[70,249] It is rare; the exact incidence is not known. It most likely represents an unrecognized fracture at the base of the odontoid or damage to the epiphyseal plate during the first few years of life. Either of these conditions can compromise the blood supply to the developing odontoid, resulting in the os odontoideum.

The anomaly usually presents with local neck pain and occasionally transitory episodes of paresis, myelopathy, or cerebral brain stem ischemia due to vertebral artery compression from the upper cervical instability. Sudden death rarely occurs.

Radiographically an os odontoideum is seen as an oval or round ossicle with a smooth sclerotic border of variable size and located in the position of the normal odontoid tip. On occasion it can be located near the basioccipital bone in the foramen magnum area. The base of the dens is usually hypoplastic. It is often difficult to differentiate an os odontoideum from nonunion following a fracture. The gap between the os and the hypoplastic dens is wider than in a fracture, usually well above the level of the facets. Tomograms and CT scans are useful to further delineate the bony anatomy and flexion and extension lateral radiographs to assess instability.

The neurologic symptoms are due to cord compression from posterior translation of the os into the cord in extension or the odontoid into the cord in flexion. Increased motion at the C1–C2 level can lead to vertebral artery occlusion and ischemia of the brain stem and posterior fossa structures, resulting in seizures, syncope, vertigo, and visual disturbances. The long-term natural history is unknown.

Those with local pain or transient myelopathies can expect recovery with cervical traction and immobilization. Subsequently, only nonstrenuous activities should be allowed, but the curtailment of activities in the pediatric age group can be difficult. The risk of a small insult leading to catastrophic quadriplegia and death must be weighed.

Surgery is indicated when there is 10 mm or more of ADI, a SAC of 13 mm or less,[220] neurologic involvement, progressive instability, or persistent neck pain. A Gallie fusion is recommended. The surgeon must be careful when tightening the wire so that the os is not pulled back posteriorly into the canal and cord with disastrous consequences. In small children, the wire may be eliminated. In all children, a Minerva or halo cast or vest also is used for at least 6, and often 12, weeks.

Developmental and Acquired Stenoses and Instabilities

Down Syndrome

Because of underlying collagen defects in these children, they can develop cervical instabilities at both the occiput–C1 and C1–C2 levels. The incidence of occiput–C1 instability has been reported to be as high as 60% in children[237] and 69% in adults,[221] and C1–C2

instability has been reported to be as high as 15% to 20%.[237] The instability may occur at more than one level and in more than one plane (e.g., sagittal and rotary planes).

Atlantoaxial instability in children with Down syndrome was first reported by Spitzer and colleagues,[221] in 1961. Subsequently there have been many reports on this instability. Despite these reports, there are none that document the true incidence of atlantoaxial dislocation (in contrast to instability), and there are no long-term studies regarding the natural history of this problem. With the advent of the Special Olympics, there has been much concern regarding the participation of children with Down syndrome and much confusion regarding to the appropriate approach to the problem of cervical instability in these children. Outlined below are the most recent recommendations regarding this problem.

The incidence of atlantoaxial instability in children with Down syndrome has been estimated to be from 9% to 22%,[184,185,237] and it is a gradual, progressive lesion.[26] The incidence of symptomatic atlantoaxial instability is much less and was reported to be 2.6%[184] in a series of 236 Down syndrome patients. Progressive instability and neurologic deficits are more likely to develop in male patients older than 10 years.[26] Children with Down syndrome have a significantly greater incidence of cervical skeletal anomalies, especially persistent synchondrosis and spina bifida occulta of C1, than do normal children.[187] Also, children with both Down syndrome and atlantoaxial instability have an increased frequency of cervical spine anomalies compared with other Down syndrome children without these anomalies.[187] These spinal anomalies may be a contributing factor in the cause of atlantoaxial instability in these children.

The majority of these children are asymptomatic. When symptoms occur, they are usually pyramidal tract symptoms, such as gait abnormalities, hyperreflexia, and quadriparesis. Occasionally local symptoms such as head tilt, torticollis, neck pain, or limited neck mobility exist. Rarely does sudden catastrophic death occur. Neurologic examination is often difficult to perform in these children and difficult to interpret.[237] Because of this difficulty some authors have used somatosensory evoked potentials in assessing these children with equivocal results.[186] There have been a total of 42 documented cases of patients with Down syndrome and symptomatic atlantoaxial subluxation[184] at an average age of 10.5 years. Seven of these 42 patients had a history of injury causing atlantoaxial subluxation with symptoms or augmented preexisting symptoms. There also has been a case report of one asymptomatic patient[184] with long tract signs who became quadriplegic on a trampoline.

Spinal radiographs should be reviewed to determine if there are any associated anomalies, such as persistent synchondrosis of C2, spina bifida occulta of C1, ossiculum terminale, os odontoideum, or other less common anomalies. When the plain radiographs indicate atlantoaxial or atlantooccipital instability of 6 mm or more in an asymptomatic patient, CT and MRI scans in flexion and extension can determine the extent of neural encroachment and cord compression.

The Committee on Sports Medicine of the American Academy of Pediatrics has developed guidelines regarding the overall approach to this problem.[35]

1. All children with Down syndrome who wish to participate in sports that involve possible trauma to the head and neck should have lateral-view roentgenograms of the cervical region in neutral, flexion, and extension positions within the patient's tolerance before beginning training or competition. This recommendation applies to all participants in the high-risk sports who have not previously had normal findings on cervical roentgenograms.

    Some physicians may prefer to screen all patients with Down syndrome routinely at 5 to 6 years of age to rule out atlantoaxial instability.

2. When the distance between odontoid process of the axis and the anterior arch of the atlas exceeds 4.5 mm or the odontoid is abnormal, there should be restrictions on sports that involve trauma to the head and neck, and the patient should be followed up at regular intervals.

3. At the present time, repeated roentgenograms are not indicated for those who have previously had normal findings. Indications for repeat roentgenograms will be defined by research.

4. Persons with atlantoaxial subluxation or dislocation and neurologic signs or symptoms should be restricted in all strenuous activities, and operative stabilization of the cervical spine should be considered.

5. Persons with Down syndrome who have no evidence of atlantoaxial instability may participate in all sports. Follow-up is not required unless musculoskeletal or neurologic signs or symptoms develop.

There is some controversy as to whether the growing child should be screened periodically, even if the initial screening at 5 years of age is normal. I believe that the growing child should be screened every 5 years until mature because of the increase in atlantoaxial motion over time that can develop.[26]

Nonsurgical treatment includes the observation over time, as previously mentioned, and the avoidance of high-risk sports and events, such as gymnastics, diving, the butterfly stroke in swimming, the high jump in track and field, soccer, and any exercises that place pressure on the head and neck muscles. This avoidance should be recommended to all children with an atlantoaxial distance of more than 4.5 mm, as stipulated in guideline 2 listed earlier. This is because an ADI of 5 mm or more indicates that the transverse atlantal ligament is attenuated or disrupted and not competent; the capsular structures and alar ligaments act as secondary restraints. I believe that all children should be stabilized when the interval reaches 10 mm, regardless of the presence or absence of symptoms, because at this point the alar ligaments are the only substantive restraining force.

Atlantooccipital hypermobility recently has been described in Down syndrome children. No guidelines exist regarding the frequency of periodic screening or indications for atlantooccipital fusion except for the symptomatic child. Tredwell and colleagues[237] believe that treatment plans for these children should depend on the amount of room available for the cord rather than absolute values of displacement for both atlantoaxial and atlantooccipital instability. This area requires further investigation.

Posterior cervical fusion at the levels involved is the recommended surgical treatment. The classic technique for posterior C1–C2 fusion uses autogenous iliac crest bone graft with wiring and postoperative halo immobilization. Internal fixation with wiring provides protection against displacement, shortens the time of postoperative immobilization, permits the consideration of using less rigid forms of external immobilization, and is reported to aid in obtaining fusion. However, internal fixation with sublaminar wiring poses added risk. If the instability does not reduce on routine extension films, the patient is at high risk for development of iatrogenic quadriplegia with sublaminar wiring and acute manipulative reduction.[164] For this reason it has been recommended that preoperative traction be used to effect the reduction. If reduction does not occur with traction then only an onlay bone grafting should be performed without sublaminar wiring.[164] I also do not recommend any sublaminar wiring at C2, regardless of the success of reduction because sublaminar wiring at C2 was associated with the only death in a recent series at my institution.[216] If wiring is to be performed, I recommend using pliable, smaller caliber wires.

The Down syndrome patient seems to be at higher risk for postoperative neurologic complications after fusion with instrumentation.[202,215] These complications can range from complete quadriplegia and death to Brown-Séquard syndrome.[216] C2 radiculopathy also has been reported in a patient with Ehlers-Danlos syndrome after a posterior cervical fusion. Another potential cause of neurologic impairment is over-reduction if an unstable os odontoideum is present.[216]

A posterior translation of the ring of C1 and the os fragment into the SAC can occur from this overreduction. In a study of the results of surgical fusion in 35 symptomatic Down syndrome children, 8 made a complete recovery, 14 showed improvement, 7 did not improve, 4 died, and the outcome for 2 is unknown.[184] Patients with long-standing symptoms and marked neural damage showed no or little postoperative improvement, whereas patients with a more recent onset of symptoms usually made an excellent recovery. Other complications that can occur in these children are loss of reduction despite halo immobilization and resorption of the bone graft or nonunion (Fig. 20-14).[202]

The long-term results after cervical fusion are not yet known. Individuals with Down syndrome who undergo short cervical fusions are at risk for developing instability above the level of fusion, such as occiput–C1 after a C1–C2 fusion or C1–C2 after lower level fusions.[156] This later instability occurred in four of five children between 6 months and 7 years after surgery.

Nontraumatic Occipitoatlantal Instability

Nontraumatic occipitoatlantal instability is rare in the absence of any underlying syndrome (e.g., Down syndrome). Georgopoulos and colleagues[80] described

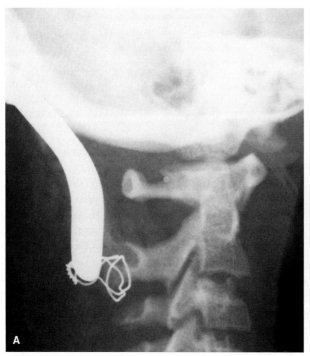

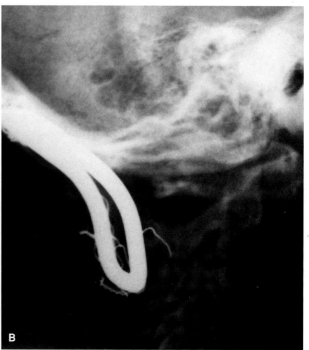

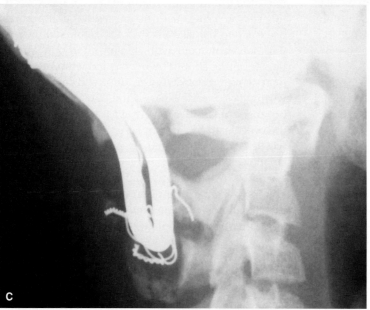

FIGURE 20-14. (A) The child in Figure 20-2 underwent posterior cervical fusion from the occiput to C2 with internal fixation and autogenous iliac crest bone graft. (B and C) Halo-vest immobilization was maintained for 4 months postoperatively and was followed by a Philadelphia collar. Despite this, the boy progressed to a nonunion evidenced by graft resorption, wire breakage, and subsidence of the Luque rectangle, although flexion and extension radiographs 1.5 years postoperatively showed a marked decrease in hypermobility. The atlanto-occipital distance was 4 mm, with only a 1-mm change of the atlantodens interval; the space available for the cord measured 18 mm in flexion and 19 mm in extension. The child's neurologic symptoms also disappeared.

five cases of nontraumatic atlantooccipital instability in children; the etiology was nontraumatic (idiopathic) in two of these children. It was suggested in one study that congenital enlargement of the occipital condyles may have been the etiology by causing an increased motion at this joint. The presenting symptoms were severe vertigo in one 14-year-old boy and nausea with projectile vomiting in one 6-year-old girl. These symptoms are postulated to be a result of vertebrobasilar arterial insufficiency resulting from the hypermobility at the occiput–C1 junction. The diagnosis of instability was suggested by plain radiographs initially and confirmed by cineradiography. Both children were treated with a posterior occiput–C1 fusion with resolution of symptoms.

Cerebral Palsy

Cervical radiculopathy and myelopathy in cerebral palsy[4,54,77,162,192] was first described in the athetoid types and recently has been described in the spastic types. Nishihara and colleagues[162] described nine patients with cervical spondylitic myelopathy complicating athetoid cerebral palsy. All were adults, but two were young adults 19 and 22 years of age. Fuji and colleagues[77] described 10 patients with cervical stenosis secondary to athetoid cerebral palsy, but all of them were adults. Reese and colleagues[192] described three young adults with spastic cerebral palsy and acquired cervical spine impairment in 1991. In all series the symptoms were brachialgia and weakness of the upper extremity with decreased functional use or increased paraparesis or tetraparesis. Some of the patients were not walkers, but in those who were ambulatory there was often a loss of ambulatory ability as a sign of presentation. There was also occasional loss of bowel and bladder control.

Radiographic findings (Fig. 20-15) are narrowing of the spinal canal and premature development of cervical spondylosis; malalignment of the cervical spine with localized kyphosis, increased lordosis, or both; and instability of the cervical spine manifested

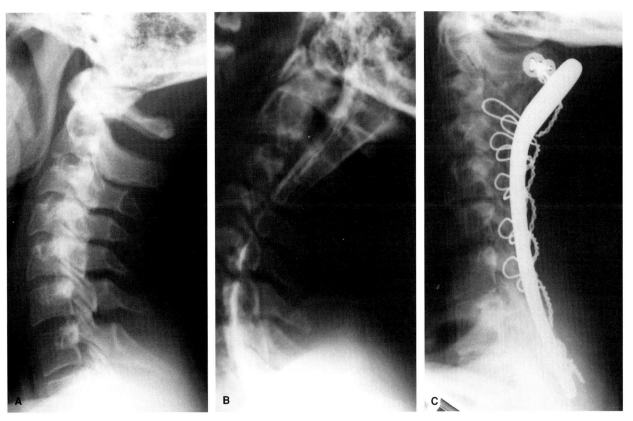

FIGURE 20-15.   A 14-year-old girl with spastic quadriparesis showed progressive loss of upper extremity function with loss of ability to control her wheelchair and feed herself. She also complained of some mild neck pain. (**A**) The lateral radiograph shows marked stenosis from C3–C6, as evidenced by a spinal canal–to–vertebral body ratio (Torg ratio) of <0.8 (**B**) The myelogram shows near complete block of the dye column from C3–C5. This stenosis was treated by posterior laminectomy from C3–C7 and posterior cervical fusion from C2–T1 using Luque rectangle fixation with spinous process and facet wiring. (**C**) Eight months postoperatively, there is stable fixation and solid facet joint fusion. The girl's upper extremity strength is improved, and she is able to feed herself. (*Courtesy of* Dr. Robert Hensinger; from Loder, RT, Hensinger RN. Developmental abnormalities of the cervical spine. In Weinstein SL, ed. The pediatric spine: principles and practice. New York: Raven Press, 1994:397.)

as spondylolisthesis. Flattening of the anterosuperior margins of the vertebral bodies and beak-like projections of the anteroinferior margins are radiographic findings of the spondylosis. Myelography confirms the stenosis and shows disc protrusion, osteophyte projection, and blocks in dye flow. The findings are most commonly at the C3–C4 and C4–C5 levels.

Nerve root and cord compression occurs from the kyphoses, the herniated discs, and the osteophytes. It is believed that these young adults with cerebral palsy develop degenerative cervical stenosis at an earlier age than unaffected people, who develop stenosis in the late fourth and fifth decades of life, because of exaggerated flexion and extension of the neck, causing accelerated cervical degeneration. Exaggerated flexion and extension occurs in patients with athetosis and writhing movements. Difficulty with head control also can cause exaggerated flexion and extension in the spastic cerebral palsy patient.

Treatment is primarily surgical. Anterior discectomy, resection of osteophytes, and interbody fusion have been the most effective methods. Posterior spinal fusion also may be needed. Postoperative immobilization can be a problem, but a halo apparatus seems to be the best treatment and is well tolerated in patients with athetosis.[162] For this reason, some authors recommend a posterior fusion and wiring as well to minimize the amount of time postoperative immobilization is needed.[77] Posterior laminectomy alone[162] is contraindicated in cerebral palsy patients with developmental cervical stenosis because this will increase the instability.

Postlaminectomy Deformity

Cervical kyphosis is common after cervical laminectomy.[7,31,74,214,253] The natural history of postlaminectomy kyphosis is unknown; however the incidence of kyphosis when extensive cervical laminectomies are performed in childhood is nearly 100%. In one study, 12 of 15 children who had undergone a cervical or cervicothoracic laminectomy prior to 15 years of age developed kyphosis.[253] The normal posterior muscular attachments to the spinous processes and laminae, as well as facet capsules, the ligamentum nuchae, and the ligamentum flavum, are violated by the laminectomy. This loss of posterior supporting structures allows for a progressive kyphosis, which eventually can result in neurologic symptoms and deficits. Early radiographic features are a simple kyphosis; later, vertebral body wedging and anterior translations of one vertebral body on another can develop. A late, severe deformity is the swan neck deformity.[214] When these deformities develop, there can be neurologic involvement. These neurologic problems result from cord stretching and compression from the anterior kyphotic vertebral

bodies. MRI is useful to delineate the extent of cord attenuation and compression.

Nonsurgical treatment starts with frequent radiographic follow-up studies after a laminectomy; the role of prophylactic bracing is not yet known. When kyphotic deformities develop, anterior vertebral body fusion with halo cast or vest or a Minerva cast immobilization as soon as the deformity is noted is recommended[74] (Figs. 20-16 and 20-17). The role of a prophylactic posterior fusion at the time of laminectomy is not yet known,[7] nor is the role of osteoplastic laminotomy instead of laminectomy,[101,158] although this approach might not always be amenable to the primary pathology.

Other Syndromes

Fetal Alcohol Syndrome

Fetal alcohol syndrome is a teratogenic syndrome characterized by four major categories: central nervous system dysfunctions, growth deficiencies, facial anomalies, and variable major and minor malformations. The children present with developmental delay, especially in motor milestones, failure to thrive, mild to moderate retardation, mild microcephaly, distinct facies (hypoplasia of the facial bones and circumoral tissues), and congenital cardiovascular anomalies. Abnormal necks are common and are similar to the type found in patients with the Klippel-Feil syndrome. Radiographically congenital fusion of two or more cervical vertebrae occurs in approximately half of the children, resembling the Klippel-Feil syndrome.[132,238] However, the fetal alcohol syndrome is distinctly different than the Klippel-Feil syndrome because the major visceral anomaly in the Klippel-Feil syndrome is the genitourinary system, whereas in the fetal alcohol syndrome it is the cardiovascular system.[238]

The natural history is not known. Radiographic imaging and treatment recommendations regarding the cervical spine are the same as those for the Klippel-Feil syndrome.

Craniofacial Syndromes

Cleft lip and palate is the most common craniofacial anomaly. It can be a solitary finding, or more often it is associated with other syndromes and anomalies. Children with cleft anomalies have a 13% incidence of cervical spinal anomalies compared with the 0.8% incidence of children undergoing orthodontia care for other reasons.[198] This incidence is highest in those with soft palate and submucous clefts (45%). These anomalies, usually spina bifida and vertebral body hypoplasia, are predominantly in the upper cervical spine. The potential for instability is unknown, as is

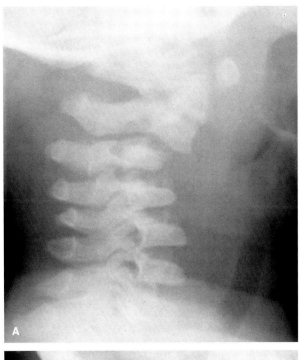

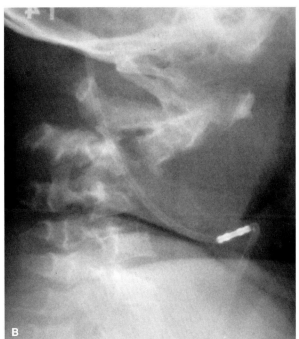

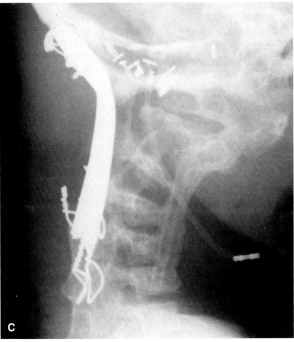

FIGURE 20-16. (A) Lateral cervical spine radiograph of a 9-month-old boy with neurofibromatosis. Note the preexisting cervical kyphosis at C2–3. At the age of 3 years, he underwent a suboccipital craniectomy and cervical laminectomy from C1–C4 for resection of neurofibromata. (B) By the age of 3 years, 10 months, he had developed a 90-degree kyphosis. (C) He underwent combined anterior cervical fusion from C2–C6 with a fibular strut graft and posterior cervical fusion from the occiput to C6 with internal fixation consisting of a Luque U-rod. Three years postoperatively, solid fusion with a residual 70-degree kyphosis is present.

the natural history. No documented information regarding treatment is available; however, the clinician should be aware of this association and make sound clinical judgments as needed.

Craniosynostosis Syndromes

The craniosynostosis syndromes—Crouzon, Pfeiffer, Apert, and Goldenhar—exhibit cervical spine fusions, atlantooccipital fusions, and butterfly vertebrae.[94,131,210] Fusions are more common in Apert syndrome (71%) than in Crouzon syndrome (38%).[94] Upper cervical fusions are most common in Crouzon and Pfeiffer syndromes,[210] whereas in Apert syndrome the fusions are more likely to be complex and involve C5–C6.[94] However, this syndrome variation is not accurate enough for syndromic differentiation. Congenital cervicothoracic scoliosis frequently is seen in Goldenhar syndrome, usually from hemivertebrae.[210]

The cervical fusions are progressive with age; in younger children the vertebrae appear to be separated

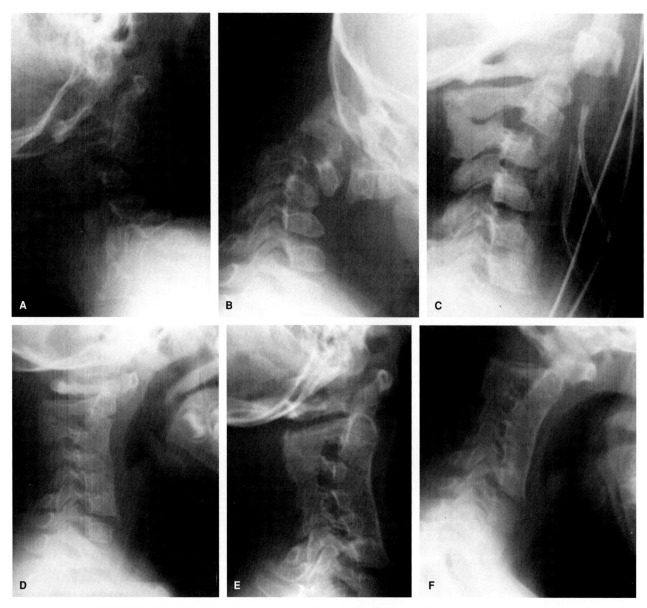

FIGURE 20-17. This girl underwent a cervical laminectomy from C2–C6 for a low-grade astrocytoma of the cervical cord. (**A**) At 1 year 7 months of age, she had a postlaminectomy kyphosis, that was (**A**) 45 degrees in extension and (**B**) 82 degrees in flexion. (**C**) An anterior cervical discectomy and fusion from C2–C6 was performed with autogenous iliac crest strut graft. Immediately postoperative, the kyphosis was corrected to 20 degrees. Halo-vest immobilization was used for 3 months. (**D**) Solid incorporation of the fusion occurred by 6 months postoperatively. At 4 years 7 months of age (**E**) flexion and (**F**) extension lateral radiographs show maintenance of the correction, solid fusion, and no instability at the remaining levels.

by intervertebral discs, but as the children grow older the vertebrae fuse together. There are no specific, standard recommendations for treatment. I recommend following the same principles as in the Klippel-Feil syndrome. The main concern is the potential difficulty with intubation in these children. Odontoid anomalies are rare; however, if any question exists regarding the stability of the cervical spine, lateral flexion and extension radiographs should be obtained.

Skeletal Dysplasias

Skeletal dysplasias are discussed in detail in Chapter 7.

Combined Soft Tissue and Skeletal Dysplasias

NEUROFIBROMATOSIS. Neurofibromatosis is the most common single gene disorder in humans.

The proportion of patients with neurofibromatosis and cervical spine involvement is difficult to assess: 30% of patients in the series of Yong-Hing and colleagues[254] and 44% of those with scoliosis or kyphosis had cervical spine lesions. The children are often asymptomatic.[254] Symptoms, when they do occur, are diminished or painful neck motion, torticollis, dysphagia, deformity, and neurologic signs ranging from mild pain and weakness to paraparesis and quadriparesis.[41,108] Neck masses constituted 20% of presenting symptoms in one study of neurofibromatosis patients.[2]

Radiographic features of neurofibromatosis in the cervical spine are vertebral body deficiencies and dysplasia or scalloping.[42,254] This often is associated with kyphosis and foraminal enlargement. Lateral flexion and extension radiographs are recommended for all neurofibromatosis patients prior to general anesthesia or surgery. MRI is helpful for assessing the involvement of neural structures and dural ectasia. CT scans are useful for evaluating the upper cervical spine complex and bony definition of the neural foramen. The natural history regarding the cervical spine is unknown, but those with severe kyphosis often develop neurologic deterioration.

Surgical indications are cord or nerve root compression, C1–C2 rotary subluxation, pain, and neurofibroma removal.[41,254] Halo cast and vests usually are needed after fusions, with or without internal fixation, which is usually simple interspinous wiring. Kyphosis usually requires anterior and posterior fusions (see Fig. 20-16). If there are no indications for surgical treatment, then the patient should be followed closely. Pseudoarthroses are frequent with isolated posterior fusions.

FIBRODYSPLASIA OSSIFICANS PROGRESSIVA. Fibrodysplasia ossificans progressiva is an inherited, autosomal dominant disorder[114] of connective tissue with progressive soft tissue ossification. The disorder itself is rare; most cases represent new spontaneous mutations. Eventually all patients with this disorder develop cervical spine changes,[88] often starting in childhood. These patients usually present with neck stiffness[36] within the first 5 years of life. No cases of neurologic compromise have been reported. Other general clinical features are big toe malformations, reduction defects of all digits, deafness, baldness, and mental retardation. Early in the course of the disease small vertebral bodies and large pedicles are seen radiographically. Occasionally nuchal musculature ossification also is seen. Later, neural arch fusions are seen. This factor reflects the progressive ossification of the cervical spinal musculature, ligament ossification, and spontaneous fusion of the cervical discs and apophyseal joints. No effective medical treatment is known. Surgical treatment of the cervical spine has not been necessary.

TRAUMA

Injuries to the cervical spine are rare in children and more common in boys than girls. In a recent study, the age- and gender-adjusted incidence was 7.41 per 100,000 population per year[142]; this incidence was much less in children (<11 years of age, 1.19/100,000) compared with adolescents (>11 years of age, 13.24/100,00). The cause of the injury in children is frequently a fall, whereas in adolescents it is frequently due to sports, recreational activities, or motor vehicle accidents. In general, children (<11 years of age) are more likely to sustain ligamentous injuries and injuries to the upper cervical spine, whereas adolescents are more likely to sustain fractures and injuries to the lower cervical spine.[15,142] By the age of 10 years the bony cervical spine has reached adult configurations, and the injuries they sustain are essentially those of the adult. I will therefore concentrate on those injuries sustained in the first decade of life.

Most children with potential cervical spine injuries have sustained polytrauma and frequently arrive immobilized on backboards and cervical collars. If the child is comatose or semiconscious, if there are external signs of head injury, or if the child complains of neck pain then cervical spine radiographs are needed. All children with neck pain involved in a motor vehicle accident with head trauma or who have neurologic signs or symptoms should have cervical spine radiographs.[121,188] The views recommended for this initial screening are the cross-table lateral, the open-mouth odontoid, and anteroposterior views. If the child is too critically ill to be positioned for all views, then the cross-table lateral view is adequate until a complete evaluation can be performed. Cervical spine precautions must be maintained until the a complete evaluation has demonstrated no injury. Once a cervical injury has been identified close scrutiny must be undertaken to ensure that there are no other injuries in the remainder of the axial skeleton.

The child arriving in the emergency suite is often on a standard backboard. Young children have a disproportionately large head, and positioning them on a standard backboard leads to a flexed posture of the neck (Fig. 20-18A).[98] This flexion can lead to further anterior angulation or translation of an unstable cervical spine injury and can also cause pseudosubluxation, which in itself in an injured child can be difficult to interpret. To prevent this undesirable cervical flexion in young children during emergency transport and radiography modifications must be made by either creating a recess for the occiput of the larger head or

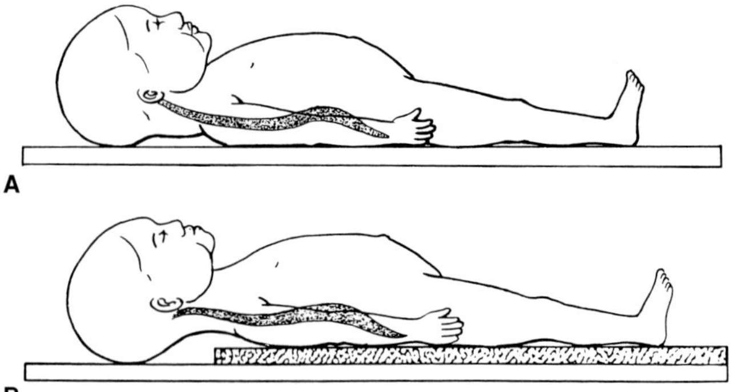

FIGURE 20-18. (A) Positioning a young child on a standard backboard forces the neck into a kyphotic position because of the relatively large head. (B) Positioning a young child on a double mattress, which raises the chest and torso and allows the head to translate posteriorly compensates for the relatively large head. This creates a normal alignment of the cervical spine. (From Herzenberg JE, Hensinger RN, Dedrick DK, Phillips WA. Emergency transport and positioning of young children who have an injury of the cervical spine. The standard backboard may be hazardous. J Bone Joint Surg [Am] 1989;71:15.)

using a double mattress to raise the chest (Fig. 20-18B). A simple clinical guideline is to align the external auditory meatus with the shoulder.

Flexion and extension lateral radiographs may be necessary to determine the stability of the cervical spine; hyperflexion ligamentous injuries may not be seen immediately, and flexion and extension views a few weeks later after the spasm has subsided may document instability. In one series of children with ligamentous injuries of the cervical spine, 8 of 11 children with lower cervical instability were diagnosed between 2 weeks and 4 months after the trauma.[180]

Secondary signs of spinal injury in children often are seen before the actual injury or fracture itself. Malalignment of the spinous processes on the anteroposterior radiograph should be regarded as highly suspicious for a jumped facet. Widening of the posterior interspinous distances should be regarded as highly suspicious for a posterior ligamentous injury. In adults an increase in the retropharyngeal soft tissue space can indicate a hematoma in the setting of trauma and increase the suspicion on the part of the clinician that an upper cervical fracture exists. However, in children the pharyngeal wall is close to the spine in inspiration whereas there may be a large increase in this space with forced expiration, as in a crying child.[5] This should be remembered when considering the significance of prevertebral pharyngeal soft tissue in the cervical spine radiographs of a frightened, crying child.

CT scans are useful to further assess the upper cervical spine, especially the ring of the atlas and occasionally the odontoid. As a rule, CT is not recommended for screening but to further study suspicious areas on plain radiographs or for treatment planning. It should be used to study all fractures of C1. MRI scans are useful to assess the spinal cord and discs.

Fractures and Ligamentous Injuries of the Occipital Complex to the C1–C2 Complex

Atlantooccipital Dislocation

Atlantooccipital dislocation is rare,[25] and most of the children do not survive.[24] With the present rapid response to trauma victims and more aggressive field care, more of these children now survive and present with this problem. These children are usually polytrauma victims with severe head injuries and present with a range of clinical neurologic pictures.[24,25,61] In the past, those who survived had incomplete lesions, often demonstrating cranial nerve dysfunctions and varying degrees of quadriplegia. Many of the children have complete loss of neurologic function below the brain stem and survive only because of outpatient ventilatory support. Other presentations may be a responsive child with hypotension or tachycardia to a complete cardiac arrest. Occasionally, some patients present with normal neurologic examinations.

In severe cases the diagnosis is evident; however, some of the cases do not demonstrate marked radiographic displacement. In the past, a BC/OA ratio greater than 1 (Fig. 20-19A) was used to indicate the presence of atlantooccipital dislocation.[136] This criterion can cause the practitioner to miss isolated distraction injuries, anterior atlantooccipital dislocations that have spontaneously reduced after injury, and posterior atlantooccipital injuries.[25] For this reason, the distance between the tip of the dens and the basion (Fig. 20-19B) has been used, in which a distance of more than 12.5 mm indicates the potential for atlantooccipital dislocation.

The first obstacle in the treatment of this injury is its diagnosis. Once diagnosed, standard respiratory and other supporting measures are given. Early definitive immobilization of the dislocation should be undertaken. The immobilization can be with a halo alone or with supplemental internal fixation and posterior fusion. Traction should be avoided because it can distract the joint and cause further neurologic injury. These children then must be moved rapidly into an upright position to maximize pulmonary care.

Fractures of the Atlas

The Jefferson fracture is rare in children.[136,152] It is caused by an axial load from the head into the lateral masses. Unlike adults, a single fracture through the ring in children may be isolated, hinging on the syn-

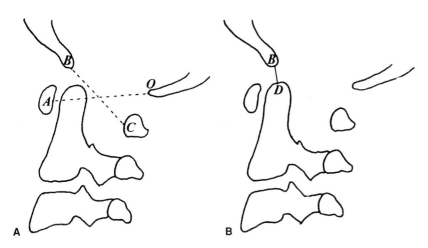

FIGURE 20-19. (A) The BC/OA ratio and (B) the DB distance are used to assess for traumatic atlantooccipital dislocation. (From Bulas DI, Fitz H, Roberts JM, et al. Chronic atlanto-axial instability in Down syndrome. J Bone Joint Surg [Am] 1985; 67:1356.)

chondrosis[152] instead of a double break in the ring. A transverse atlantal ligament rupture may occur as the lateral masses separate, resulting in C1–C2 instability.

CT scans are useful in both the diagnosis of this injury and the assessment of healing. Treatment is usually simple immobilization with a Minerva cast or halo. Rarely is surgery necessary unless rupture of the transverse alar ligament occurs, which renders the spine unstable.

Transverse Atlantoaxial Ligament Ruptures

Transverse atlantoaxial ligament ruptures may occur from either severe or mild trauma.[180] Radiographically the ADI is increased, usually well beyond the normal 5 mm. Adequate ligamentous healing and stability does not occur from simple immobilization. The recommended treatment is reduction in extension, posterior cervical C1–C2 fusion with autogenous bone graft, and immobilization with a halo or Minerva cast. A solid arthrodesis is documented on flexion and extension lateral radiographs after 2 to 3 months of immobilization.

Odontoid Fractures

Odontoid fractures are the most common injuries to the cervical spine in children.[203,206] They are actually physeal fractures of the dentocentral synchondrosis, usually Salter-Hams type I fractures. These may occur after major or minor trauma. Neurologic deficits are rare. These fractures usually displace anteriorly with the dens posteriorly angulated (Fig. 20-20). This fracture usually is seen only on the lateral view. If there is confusion between the mild normal posterior angulation of the dens, which occurs in up to 4% of normal children,[240] dynamic flexion and extension CT scans with sagittal reconstructions can be performed to evaluate for any motion or instability.

Displaced odontoid fractures in children reduce easily with mild extension and posterior translation,

as is typical of all Salter-Hams I type fractures. In most circumstances the simple double mattress technique is all that is needed to obtain a reduction. After a few days of recumbency and early healing the fracture can be immobilized easily by the use of a Minerva cast or halo. As with all physeal fractures, healing is rapid, and immobilization usually can be stopped in 6 to 10 weeks. Flexion and extension lateral radiographs should be taken to confirm union with stability. These fractures, unlike those in adults, do not have a significant nonunion rate requiring subsequent C1–C2 fusion. The intact hinge of anterior periosteum most likely aids in the ease of reduction and accounts for the stability of reduction and rapid healing.

Spondylolisthesis of C2

Spondylolisthesis of C2, also known as a Hangman fracture in adults, is rare in children. It most likely arises from hyperextension. Pizzutillo and colleagues[183] reported on a series of five cases in children. Care must be taken to not confuse this fracture with congenital anomalies that may mimic a Hangman fracture and lead to overtreatment. These fractures readily heal with immobilization in either a Minerva cast or a halo after gentle positioning to obtain a reduction. Traction itself, as with most cervical injuries in children, should be avoided because it usually results in overdistraction with an increased potential for nonunion and more serious neurologic injury. Posterior cervical fusion of C1–C3 is indicated for the rare case of nonunion or instability.

Fractures and Ligamentous Injuries of C3–C7

These injuries are more common in older children and adolescents than in young children.[15,60,142] The typical patterns of fracture usually are compression fractures of the vertebral body or facet fractures and dislocations caused by hyperflexion. These injuries are adult patterns, and standard adult treatment should

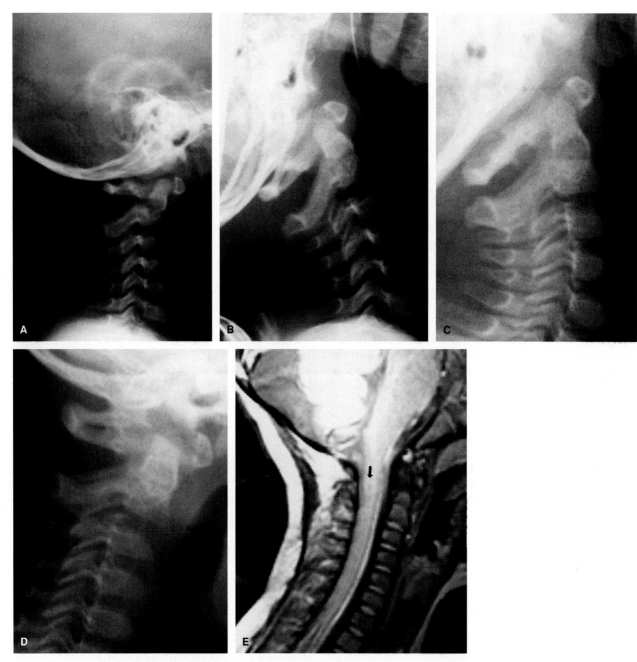

FIGURE 20-20. This 2-year, 9-month-old boy was brought to the emergency department unable to move his upper extremities and withdrew his lower extremities only in response to noxious stimuli. He had a history of falling off couches. On investigation, it became clear that the child had been battered. **(A)** A lateral radiograph demonstrates the odontoid fracture through the dentocentral synchondrosis with anterior angulation and translation. A magnetic resonance image (MRI) scan did not reveal any abnormalities in the cord. **(B)** Simple positioning with a double mattress allowed for reduction of the fracture; the child was maintained on a double mattress for several days to allow for subsidence of cord edema and early healing. He was then placed into a Minverva cast 10 days after the injury. The cast was removed 6 weeks after the injury, followed by immobilization with a soft collar. **(C)** Flexion and **(D)** extension radiographs demonstrated no instability with the healed fracture. **(E)** The child improved remarkably. By 2 months postinjury, he was running and walking without difficulty. There were some subtle upper extremity changes noted by a change in hand dominance from right to left. MRI showed signal changes in the cord (*arrow*), which were interpreted as development of an early posttraumatic syrinx.

be used. Physeal fractures, usually of the inferior end plates, also can occur,[122] which are caused by hyperextension. In older children they are usually ring apophyseal fractures with minimal instability or neurologic damage. In younger children they usually involve the entire end plate. Physeal fractures frequently are not recognized in severely injured children, or they may be noted for the first time at autopsy.[8,122] They have a high incidence of neurologic damage. In these children, simple positioning (e.g., double mattresses; rarely, traction followed by immobilization) is all that is needed for treatment. Because these are physeal injuries healing is rapid.

Traumatic ligamentous instability in children also can occur.[180] The pivot point for younger children is in the upper cervical spine because of their large head size, weak cervical musculature, incompletely ossified wedge-shaped vertebrae, physiologic ligamentous laxity, and horizontal facet joints in this region. The upper cervical spine offers little resistance to traumatic shear forces, which often result in ligamentous instability. The goal is to differentiate this traumatic ligamentous instability from pseudosubluxation using the posterior cervical line. In one study of ligamentous injuries of the cervical spine in children, 7 of 11 injuries occurred at the C2–C3 level. When instability exists, treatment should consist of posterior cervical fusion with Minerva or halo immobilization (Fig. 20-21). Treatment for a mild sprain is immobilization for comfort followed by flexion and extension radiographs several weeks to a few months later to ensure that any late instability does not occur.

Spinal Cord Injury Without Radiographic Abnormality

Spinal cord injury without radiographic abnormality (SCIWORA) occurs in 5% to 55% of all pediatric spinal cord injuries.[174,175] The immature and elastic pediatric spine is more easily deformed than that of an adult. Momentary displacement from external forces may endanger the spinal cord without disrupting bone or ligaments. The four major factors believed to be involved are hyperextension, flexion, distraction, and spinal cord ischemia. Ischemia may arise from direct cord contusion or vascular insufficiency itself.[128]

The neurologic deficit may range from complete cord transection to partial cord deficits. The majority of deficits (78%) are cervical; those people with upper cervical SCIWORA are more likely to have severe neurologic lesions than those with lower cervical SCIWORA. No disruption, malalignment, or other abnormalities are seen on plain radiographs. There is physiologic disruption of the spinal cord that is not necessarily associated with anatomic disruption. The exact pathoanatomy is not known; MRI does not always show cord transection, and myelography often shows only cord edema.

The outcome usually is determined by the presenting neurologic status. Approximately one fourth of the children have a late deterioration in neurologic function. Treatment is controversial. Immobilization in a Guilford brace for 3 months has been recommended by Pang and Pollack, with complete avoidance of all sports. However, in Pang's own series, no instability was noted in any of the children at initial evaluation, and only one child later developed instability on flexion and extension radiographs.[174] Without documented radiographic instability, the biomechanical usefulness of brace immobilization is questionable. Pang however denotes this as treating "incipient instability."[174] Most ligamentous spine injuries, when allowed to heal with simple immobilization, do not return to the stability seen in the preinjury state; fusion usually is needed. It is atypical for SCIWORA to behave differently regarding instability, incipient or otherwise. Regardless of whether the child is braced, close followup of neurologic function is needed. Flexion and extension radiographs after 3 months of bracing should be taken; any late development of instability requires surgical stabilization.

Transient Quadriparesis

Transient quadriparesis is a neuropraxia of the cervical spinal cord with transient quadriplegia that is seen most often in collegiate and professional athletes,[120,232] although there are several cases in younger athletes.[191] The incidence in the National Collegiate Athletic Association is 1.3 per 10,000 athletes per season.[232]

The anteroposterior diameter of the spinal canal is decreased in these athletes. The spinal cord, on forced hyperextension or hyperflexion, is compressed, causing the transient quadriparesis. Sensory changes, such as burning pain, numbness, tingling, and loss of sensation and motor changes ranging from weakness to complete paralysis, are seen. These episodes are transient, and recovery occurs in 10 to 15 minutes; neck pain is not present at the time of injury.

No fractures or dislocations are present. The ratio of the spinal canal to the vertebral body is decreased, with a value of 0.8 used to indicate significant developmental cervical stenosis. Congenital fusions, cervical instability, and intervertebral disc disease also may exist. In children, this spinal canal to vertebral body ratio is not as accurate and is inconsistent in predicting spinal cord concussion.[191] An MRI sometimes is necessary to assess the presence or absence of a herniated nucleus pulposis.

All people with this disorder have resolution of their symptoms. Usually, the only nonsurgical treatments that are needed are collars, analgesics, and

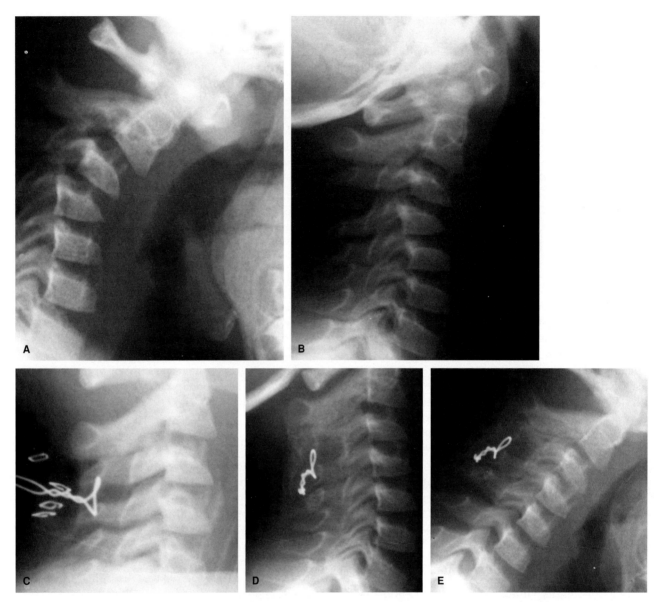

FIGURE 20-21. This 4-year, 9-month old boy was run over by a snowmobile trailer 2 weeks before these radiographs were taken. He had complained of some neck pain and had been treated by chiropractic manipulation during these 2 weeks. (**A**) The flexion and (**B**) extension radiographs demonstrate marked instability at the C3–C4 interspace that does not completely reduce even with extension (*arrow*). (**C**) He was treated by posterior fusion with iliac crest bone graft and interspinous wiring at C3–4, as shown in this intraoperative radiograph. Halo-vest immobilization was used for 3 months. (**D** and **E**). One year postoperatively, there was no instability at the C3–4 level, and there was solid fusion, which had extended to C2 and C5 despite meticulous care not to expose the laminae of C2 and C5 or the interspinous ligaments of C2–3 and C4–5.

antispasmodics. The role of fusions for coexistent instability, discectomy for herniated nucleus pulposus, or decompression for congenital cervical stenosis is not known.

The major concern is whether or not athletic participation should continue, and if so, the risk of a permanent quadriplegia developing with a later episode. This aspect of the natural history is unknown. Torg and colleagues[232] believe that those athletes with

pure developmental spinal stenosis are not predisposed to more severe injuries if they do return to sports and that only those with instability or degenerative changes should be precluded from participation in contact sports. Odor and colleagues[167] found that one third of professional and rookie football players have a spinal canal ratio of less than 0.8 and that it is difficult to make continued play decisions based on this ratio alone. Eisomont and colleagues,[56] however, have shown that smaller cervical canals are correlated with significant neurologic injury in routine trauma. Considering this and the fact that narrowing of the spinal canal correlates even more poorly with spinal cord concussion in children,[191] it is prudent to preclude any child who has had a cervical cord concussion from further contact sports until further epidemiologic data have been established.

Special Injury Mechanisms

Birth Injuries and Battered Children

Birth trauma is one of the most common causes of pediatric spinal cord injury and usually involves the cervical cord.[1,28,124,224,235] Like SCIWORA, the vertebral column is more elastic than the cord, and during delivery with prolonged distraction it is tethered by nerve ends and blood vessels, injuring the cord but not the chondroosseous structures. Damage to the vertebral artery with resultant ischemia of the cord also can occur.[113] In battered children the large head, poorly supported by the cervical musculature, makes the upper cervical spine vulnerable to repeated shaking with either SCIWORA or a fracture.

The diagnosis is difficult, especially with incomplete neurologic injury. Pure transection of the cord itself is rare.[3,212,2332] Temperature regulation dysfunction can cause fevers, reflex movements may be mistaken for voluntary movements, and respiratory distress can occur from paralyzed intercostal muscles. They also may present with a cerebral palsy–like clinical picture later[100,233,234,235] or as sudden infant death syndrome.[235] In one study, the diagnosis was delayed in three of four children, and the delay averaged 4.4 years from birth.[63] Typically, no fractures are seen radiographically; an MRI is often helpful in assessing cord damage.

Some children without complete transection can improve neurologically. Treatment is usually nonsurgical because these are very young infants. Bed rest, respiratory support, and physical therapy to prevent paralytic contractures should be instituted. Older children with bony injuries may need Minerva casts (see Fig. 20-20). Surgical fusion and stabilization rarely is needed.

Car Seat Injuries

Cervical fractures are described with the increased and recent use of infant car seats.[37] When these devices, which clearly make automobile travel safer for children, are not adequately tightened, serious and potentially fatal injuries can occur. The harness must be adjusted periodically to account for

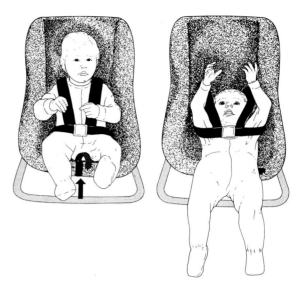

FIGURE 20-22. Placing a child in a car seat without locking the crotch strap (*arrow*) is a dangerous situation and can allow serious injury in a collision. (From Conry BG, Hall CM. Cervical spine fractures and rear car restraints. Arch Dis Child 1987;62:1267.)

normal growth and seasonal changes in clothing thickness. Car seat styles that allow the main lock to be attached to the crotch strap (Fig. 20-22) prevent forward sliding movements, which can apply hyperextension forces to the head, the neck, and the upper chest.

Gunshot Wounds

Spinal injuries from gunshot wounds[119] are increasing and account for one half of the adolescent spinal cord injuries over the last few years.[87] Approximately one third of these injuries involve the cervical spine. Various degrees of neurologic loss are noted, with complete lesions in 75% in one series.[119] Other body areas can be injured as well, which may cause more morbidity than the trauma to the neck itself.

Various degrees of fracture and intracanal bullets are seen radiographically. Other imaging studies, such as arteriograms and esophagograms, often are needed to look for other injuries. Panendoscopy is useful to assess injury to the trachea and esophagus. Spinal decompression is not indicated in either complete or incomplete lesions. Those who undergo decompression have a higher risk of meningitis and spinal instability without any added benefit. For patients with complete injuries, removal of retained bullet fragments from the canal does not improve neurologic outcome. Spinal instability usually does not develop unless laminectomy is performed. Indications for neck exploration are a positive arteriogram, impending airway obstruction, tracheal deviation, widened mediastinum, expanding hematoma, and appropriate pathology on panendoscopy. Routine exploration of the neck and wound is not advised.

INFLAMMATORY AND SEPTIC CONDITIONS

Juvenile Rheumatoid Arthritis

Juvenile rheumatoid arthritis is a chronic synovitis affecting the synovial joints that can affect the joints of the cervical spine as well. The subtypes that usually involve the cervical spine are the polyarticular and systemic onset types; only rarely does the pauciarticular type affect the cervical spine.[95]

Cervical spine involvement usually occurs in the first 1 to 2 years from disease onset and presents with stiffness. Pain and torticollis are rare, and when they occur in a patient with juvenile rheumatoid arthritis other causes should be examined, such as fracture, infection, or tumor. Torticollis was present in only 4 of 92 children in the series of Fried and colleagues[76] and in 1 of 121 children in the series of Hensinger and colleagues.[95] Neurologic findings are also infrequent in these children.

The radiographic features consist of seven types[95]:

1. Anterior erosion of the odontoid process
2. Anteroposterior erosion of the odontoid process (apple-core odontoid; Fig. 20-23)
3. Subluxation of C1 on C2
4. Focal soft tissue calcification appearing adjacent to the ring of C1 anteriorly
5. Ankylosis of the apophyseal joints
6. Growth abnormalities
7. Subluxations between C2 and C7.

The most common radiographic features in children with neck stiffness are the soft tissue calcification at the leading edge of C1, anterior erosion of the odontoid

process, and apophyseal joint ankylosis. Although there may be mild hypermobility at C1–C2 with flexion and extension, few people have true instability or myelopathy. Basilar invagination, which often occurs in adult rheumatoid arthritis, also is rare in juvenile rheumatoid arthritis.[76] The radiographic findings of juvenile rheumatoid arthritis that differ most from those of adult rheumatoid arthritis are late destruction of articular cartilage and bone, growth disturbances, spondylitis with associated vertebral subluxation and apophyseal joint ankylosis, and micrognathia.[138] In five children who had long-standing disease (average age, 19 years), Halla and colleagues[90] described a nonreducible head tilt due to collapse of an atlantoaxial lateral mass.

Other imaging studies are needed in the child with juvenile rheumatoid arthritis and pain. Bone scans and CT scans or tomograms can be useful to pinpoint the exact anatomic location of activity by the bone scan and further study its anatomy with CT. These studies can be helpful to look for occult fractures, infections, and bony tumors.

Odontoid erosion results from the inflammatory synovitis and the pannus of the synovial ring surrounding the odontoid process. The pannus erodes the odontoid anteriorly and posteriorly but leaves the apical and alar ligament attachments free, creating the apple core lesion. This lesion is more susceptible to fracture, both from erosions as well as vascular compromise to the odontoid because the blood supply to the odontoid courses along its side[200] and may be disturbed by the invading pannus. Ankylosis of the apophyseal joints is most common in the systemic onset subtype. In these young children, posterior ankylosis of the immature spine creates a tether, preventing further anterior growth. Decreased disc space height and smaller vertebral bodies, both longitudinally and circumferentially, result.

The treatment is generally nonsurgical in con-

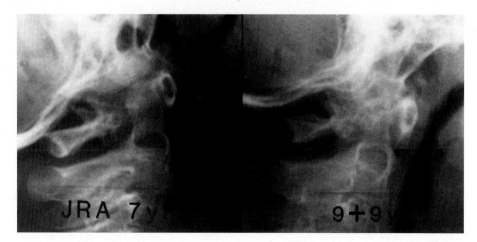

FIGURE 20-23. A boy with polyarticular juvenile rheumatoid arthritis. At 7 years of age, there was only slight erosion of the anterior part of the odontoid, but by 9 years of age, there was an apple-core lesion exhibited by both marked anterior and posterior erosion of the odontoid. (From Hensinger RN, De Vito PD, Ragsdale CG. Changes in the cervical spine in juvenile rheumatoid arthritis. J Bone Joint Surg [Am] 1986;68:189.)

junction with good rheumatologic care. Patients rarely develop flexion deformities; early in the course of the disease a cervical collar may prevent this deformity.[76] A cervical collar also is recommended for those with involvement of the odontoid process or subaxial subluxation whenever they are in an automobile or another mode of travel. If these patients need surgery for any reason, intubation can be difficult because of the micrognathia, flexion deformity, and neck stiffness. Cervical fusion rarely is needed and should be reserved for children with documented instability or progressive neurologic deterioration.

Intervertebral Disc Calcification

The first description of pediatric disc calcification was in 1924, and there are over 100 cases reported in the literature.[219] It is slightly more common in boys (7:5 ratio) than in girls, with an average age at presentation of 8 years (range, 8 days–13 years). It occurs most often in the cervical spine and is especially symptomatic when there. The etiology is unclear. Theories proposed are antecedent trauma (present in 30% of patients) and recent upper respiratory infections (present in 15% of patients, which may only reflect the normally high incidence of upper respiratory infections in children). There is no evidence to suggest metabolic disorders.

The most common clinical presentation is neck pain, which occurs in about half of the children.[219] Torticollis occurs in one fourth of the children. Decreased cervical motion and spinal tenderness also can occur. Radicular signs and symptoms rarely can be seen and never without local symptoms. Myelopathy is rare (3 of 127 cases). The onset of symptoms is abrupt: between 12 and 48 hours. Twenty-three percent of the children are febrile on presentation.

Calcified deposits are seen delineating the nucleus pulposus. The number of calcified discs averages 1.7 per child (Fig. 20-24). No protrusions have been seen in the asymptomatic group; 38% of the symptomatic children have detectable protrusions. Recent reports have also shown vertebral body involvement on MRI.[97]

The pathoanatomy is not known in children. The lesion is known to occur in dogs, in which a chondroid metamorphosis in the nucleus pulposus occurs dur-

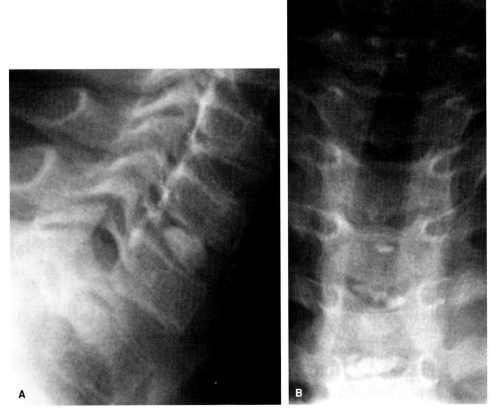

FIGURE 20-24. (A) A 7-year-old boy has symptomatic intervertebral disc calcification at the C6–7 level, as seen on a lateral radiograph. (B) He also has asymptomatic involvement at the T3–4, T4–5, and T5–6 levels, as seen on an anteroposterior radiograph.

ing the first year of life. In children there is no reason to expect an accelerated aging process, as seen in the adult or the dog, whose involvement is found mainly in the lower thoracic spine.[91]

Two thirds of the children are free of symptoms within 3 weeks and 95% by 6 months. The radiographs show regression or disappearance of the calcific deposits in 90%; about half of the radiographic improvement occurs within 6 months. Children who are asymptomatic may not show radiographic regression, even when followed for long periods. Children with multiple lesions show different rates of regression at the different disc levels. In some cases, persistent flattening of the vertebral bodies is noted into adulthood and may result in early degenerative changes.[250]

Because of this natural history, the treatment is symptomatic unless there is spinal cord compression. Analgesics, sedation, and cervical traction can all be used depending on the severity of symptoms. A short trial of a soft cervical collar also may be helpful. Contact sports probably should be avoided. Surgical intervention rarely is needed. One case has been reported in which an anterior discectomy was performed after failure of 6 weeks of conservative management for a severe radiculopathy.[217]

Pyogenic Osteomyelitis and Discitis

Pyogenic osteomyelitis and discitis is a spectrum of disease defined as a symptomatic narrowing of the disc space often associated with fever and infectious-like symptoms and signs. It affects all pediatric age ranges and is more common in boys than girls. The etiology is most likely infectious in nature; in about one third of the children an organism can be isolated, usually *Staphylococcus aureus*.[148,193,246]

Clinically this condition presents with pain, difficulty in walking and standing, fever, and malaise. It usually involves the lumbar spine, with cervical involvement being rare. Early on there is a loss of disc space height; later, end plate irregularities on both sides of the disc appear. Bone scans are very useful to identify the presence of discitis and osteomyelitis in a child with systemic symptoms when the anatomic location cannot be localized on clinical examination. MRIs are consistent with vertebral osteomyelitis.[193] Other helpful diagnostic studies are the erythrocyte sedimentation rate and blood cultures. Disc and bone cultures are necessary if the child does not respond to an initial course of rest and antibiotic treatment.

Many of the children spontaneously improve without treatment. The intervertebral disc space reconstitutes to varying degrees but never to the normal height prior to illness. Sometimes spontaneous vertebral body fusion occurs. Initially nonsurgical treatment is given. This includes rest, immobilization, and intrave-

nous antistaphylococcal antibiotics. Surgery is only necessary when there is no response to nonsurgical management; usually, biopsy and culture to isolate the infectious agent is all that is needed.

Tuberculosis

Mycobacterium tuberculosis infection in the cervical spine is rare, compared with other levels of the spine, but is common in underdeveloped countries. Most likely there will be an increase in North America because of the increasing number of immigrants from Third World countries, the rise of HIV infection, and the emergence of drug-resistant strains. There have been two very thorough reviews of this subject.[62,103] Four of the six patients with upper cervical spine involvement and 24 of 40 with lower cervical spine involvement were children.

In the upper cervical spine the children present with neck pain and stiffness. Torticollis also may be present along with headaches and constitutional symptoms. Neurologic symptoms vary from none to severe quadraparesis. In the lower cervical spine the children present with the same symptoms and also may have dysphagia, asphyxia, inspiratory stridor, and kyphosis. In children younger than 10 years of age more diffuse and extensive involvement is seen with large abscesses but a decreased incidence of paraplegia and quadriplegia. The neurologic symptoms have a gradual onset over a period of 4 to 8 weeks. Sinus formation is not a prominent feature because of the thick cervical prevertebral fascia, which contains the abscess. Cord compression occurs from the abscess and the kyphosis. Cultures and biopsies are not always positive. Because the infection is anterior, most will progress to spinal cord compression and paralysis if left untreated.

Increased width of the retropharyngeal soft tissue space is seen radiographically along with osteolytic erosions. Instability at the C1–C2 level can be seen in some children; rarely is there a fixed C1–C2 rotatory subluxation. A kyphosis is present in one fourth of patients with lower cervical spine involvement. Other useful imaging studies are a chest radiograph and renal studies.

Treatment involves antituberculous chemotherapy in all children. Surgery also is recommended for the cervical spine because it gives rapid resolution of the pain, upper respiratory obstruction, and spinal cord compression. This is in contrast to the thoracic and lumbar spine, in which chemotherapy alone is an established method of treating tuberculosis.[55] Debridement with or without grafting is performed. For children younger that 2 years of age grafting usually is not needed. For children with upper cervical spine involvement consideration should be given to anterior transoral drainage and fusion across the lateral facet joints. Most children need halo traction with reduction prior to drainage, if possible.

HEMATOLOGIC AND ONCOLOGIC CONDITIONS

The primary hematologic condition affecting the cervical spine is hemophilia.[195] The involvement is usually asymptomatic, although patients occasionally may complain of mild neck discomfort. Diminished lateral rotation can be noted on physical examination. Radiographic findings, which begin to occur in adolescence and early adulthood, consist of cystic changes in the vertebral bodies or end plate irregularities. Rarely is C1–C2 instability present. These radiographic changes can occur in patients with all degrees of severity of hemophilia. The pathoanatomy of these changes in the cervical spine is not known.

Although many of these early degenerative changes occur much earlier than in the normal population, the natural history of these premature changes in the hemophiliac populations is not known. At present, other than standard hemophiliac precautions, there are no treatment recommendations.

Benign Tumors

The common benign tumors that can involve the cervical spine in children[16,125] are eosinophilic granuloma, osteoid osteoma and osteoblastoma, osteochondroma, and aneurysmal bone cyst. All can be defined as neoplastic disorders without the propensity to metastasize. Although pathologically and physiologically benign, they can be clinically malignant if their surgical accessibility or risk of recurrence places the neural structures at high risk.

The majority of patients with benign cervical vertebral neoplasms are less than 20 years of age and present with local neck pain.[30,93,125,204] Radicular pain may occur in up to one third of the patients[208]; gross motor or sensory deficits are much less common.[135] Neoplasms can cause torticollis. Probably the most common neoplasm causing childhood torticollis is the osteoid osteoma. In a recent series from my institution, all four children with cervical osteoid osteomas presented with a painful torticollis and decreased neck motion.[190] The incidence in the literature of torticollis ranges from 10% to 100% in children with cervical osteoid osteomas[9,71,110,116,160,266] The pain of an osteoid osteoma classically responds to aspirin or other nonsteroidal antiinflammatory meditations.

With an osteoid osteoma the typical radiographic feature is sclerosis (Fig. 20-25), although it is not always evident. Bone scans are very helpful to locate the lesion; a CT scan is then used to further delineate the anatomy. The osteoid osteoma causes a sclerotic reaction in the surrounding bone but usually does not invade the epidural space. They are usually located in the laminae, followed by the pedicle and the body. An osteoblastoma is usually a mixture of lytic and blastic elements.[201] Bone scans are also positive but usually are not needed to determine the presence or absence of disease because most tumors are seen on plain radiographs. CT scans are very helpful to further assess the anatomy, especially the presence or absence of epidural invasion, which is common in osteoblastomas. They typically are located in the posterior elements. Osteochondromas of the cervical spine[34,72,107,134,165] show the typical radiographic appearances as in any other parts of the body: expansile lesions with intact cortices and normal trabecular patterns, absence of calcification, and absence of soft tissue masses. They can be easily mistaken for osteoblastomas; half of them have multiple osteochondromatosis. The majority arise in the laminae or spinous processes. Aneurysmal bone cysts are typically expansile lytic lesions with a thin rim of cortical bone. CT scans are useful in determining the exact extent and potential involvement and proximity of the vertebral artery and neural elements. Sometimes angiography is needed. Aneurysmal bone cysts usually arise in the posterior elements.[30,93] Eosinophilic granuloma usually exhibits vertebra plana radiographically,[207,215] although not always so.[10] CT scans are useful to determine the potential encroachment on the neural structures. Eosinophilic granuloma usually arises in the vertebral body with varying degrees of involvement and collapse.

The pathoanatomy of these neoplasms is discussed in Chapter 12. In the cervical spine the main concern is for vertebral artery and neural element involvement, which can lead to neurologic dysfunction. The intense inflammatory nature of these lesions, especially that of osteoid osteoma and osteoblastoma, and their proximity to the neural elements causes some nerve root irritation. This root irritation causes pain and muscle spasm, resulting in torticollis. Compressive myelopathy also can occur, especially in those people with epidural compression, such as aneurysmal bone cysts.[30,93,225]

The natural history of these lesions in the cervical spine is unknown because of their rarity. The treatment of eosinophilic granuloma in the cervical spine traditionally has been immobilization (e.g., collars, Minerva casts) and low-dose irradiation. The immobilization is continued until early healing has appeared radiographically. Low-dose irradiation should be reserved only for those lesions with neurologic deficits that are not surgically accessible. Multiple laminectomies should be avoided. Rarely has immobilization

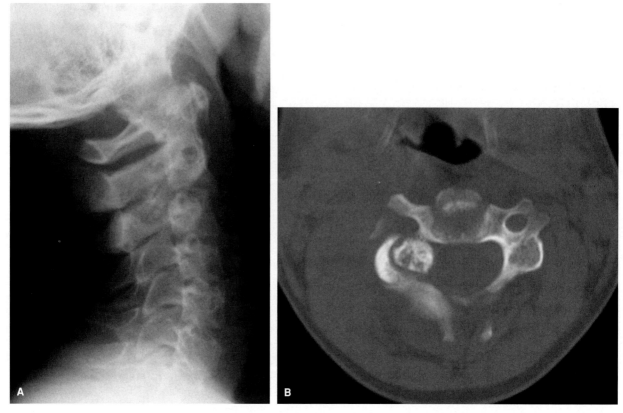

FIGURE 20-25. A 13-year-old boy had a 2-year history of neck pain that did not resolve with long-term chiropractic treatment. (**A**) Plain radiographs show a sclerotic nidus with a surrounding lucency at the level of the C3 pedicle and C2–3 foramen. (**B**) Computed tomography scan confirms the typical appearance of an osteoid osteoma; note the proximity of the lesion to both the foramen and the nerve root as well as the vertebral artery.

alone been used, and one of these children presented with total collapse of the vertebral body.[207] Osteoid osteomas do not undergo malignant transformation. However, continued torticollis and pain may lead to fixed spinal deformities. For this reason I advocate surgical resection. Prophylactic fusion should be performed if the resection renders the spine unstable. The amount of resection necessary to render the spine unstable is not known in children; however, in adults resection of more than 50% of one facet likely leads to segmental instability.[255] Because the development of postlaminectomy cervical instability is even more likely in children than in adults, I recommend an arthrodesis with any degree of facetectomy in children, and strong consideration should be given to an arthrodesis after any degree of laminectomy. Pain relief with complete resection is dramatic. Significant complaints of postoperative pain resembling the preoperative pain either indicates incomplete resection or recurrence. For osteoblastoma and aneurysmal bone cysts, primary treatment is surgical, and nonsurgical treatment is used only as adjunctive therapy. The surgical goal is complete primary excision; however, this is often impossible because of the particular anatomic location of the cysts. In these situations, adjunctive therapy is useful (e.g., radiotherapy for eosinophilic granuloma, embolization for aneurysmal bone cysts if the nondominant vertebral artery is involved).[48,49] Multiple laminectomies should be avoided if at all possible; if necessary, then fusion and stabilization also should be performed. Anterior fusion often is necessary because of insufficient posterior elements after surgical excision; supplemental halo cast or vest or Minerva cast immobilization usually is needed if fusion is required. The overall surgical management is individualized and multidisciplinary (e.g., orthopaedics, neurosurgery, radiotherapy, interventional radiology). Surgical complications include recurrence, pseudarthrosis of the fusion, and neurologic deterioration.

Malignant Tumors

The majority of primary and metastatic malignant tumors involving the cervical spine occur in adults; rarely, the cervical spine in children can be involved by chordoma,[166,213] leukemia, Ewing sarcoma,[75] or metastatic neuroblastoma. These cases are rare.

References

1. Abroms IF, Bresnan MJ, Zuckerman JE, et al. Cervical cord injuries secondary to hyperextension of the head in breech presentations. Obstet Gynecol 1973;41:369.
2. Adkins JC, Ravitch MM. The operative mamagement of von Recklinghausen neurofibromatosis in children, with special reference to lesions of the head and neck. Surgery 1977;82:342.
3. Allen JP, Myers GG, Condon VR. Laceration of the spinal cord related to breech delivery. JAMA 1969;208:1019.
4. Angelini L, Broggi G, Nardocci N, Savoiardo M. Subacute cervical myelopathy in a child with cerebral palsy. Secondary to torsion dystonia? Childs Brain 1982;9:354.
5. Ardran GM, Kemp FH. The mechanism of changes in form of the cervical airway in infancy. Med Radiogr Photogr 1968;44:26.
6. Armstrong D, Pickrell K, Fetter B, Pitts W. Torticollis: an analysis of 271 cases. Plast Reconstr Surg 1965;35:14.
7. Aronson DD, Kahn RH, Canady A, et al. Instability of the cervical spine after decompression in patients who have Arnold-Chiari malformation. J Bone Joint Surg [Am] 1991;73:898.
8. Aufdermaur M. Spinal injuries in juveniles. Necropsy findings in twelve cases. J Bone Joint Surg [Br] 1974;56:513.
9. Azouzi EM, Kozlowski K, Marton D, et al. Osteoid osteoma and osteoblastoma of the spine in children. Report of 22 cases with brief literature review. Pediatr Radiol 1986;16:25.
10. Baber WW, Numaguchi Y, Nadell JM, et al. Eosinophilic granuloma of the cervical spine without vertebrae plana. J Comput Assist Tomogrr 1987;11:346.
11. Baga N, Chusid EL, Miller A. Pulmonary disability in the Klippel-Feil syndrome. A study of two siblings. Clin Orthop 1969;67:105.
12. Bailey DK. The normal cervical spine in infants and children. Radiology 1952;59:712.
13. Bharucha EP, Dastur HM. Craniovertebral anomalies (a report on 40 cases). Brain 1964;87:469.
14. Binder H, Eng GD, Gaiser JF, Koch B. Congenital muscular torticollis: results of conservative management with long-term follow-up in 85 cases. Arch Phys Med Rehabil 1987;68:222.
15. Birney TJ, Hanley Jr EN. Traumatic cervical spine injuries in childhood and adolescence. Spine 1989;14:1277.
16. Bohlman HH, Sachs BL, Carter JR, et al. Primary neoplasms of the cervical spine. Diagnosis and treatment of twenty-three patients. J Bone Joint Surg [Am] 1986;68:483.
17. Boisen E. Torticollis caused by an infratentorial tumour: three cases. Br J Psychiatr 1979;134:306.
18. Bonola A. Surgical treatment of the Klippel-Feil syndrome. J Bone Joint Surg [Br] 1956;38:440.
19. Brackbill Y, Douthitt TC, West H. Psychophysiologic effects in the neonate of prone versus supine placement. J Pediatr 1973;81:82.
20. Bray PF, Herbst JJ, Johnson DG, et al. Childhood gastroesophageal reflux. JAMA 1977;237:1342.
21. Brooks AL, Jenkins EB. Atlanto-axial arthrodesis by the wedge compression method. J Bone Joint Surg [Am] 1978;60:279.
22. Brooks B. Pathologic changes in muscle as a result of disturbances in circulation. Arch Surg 1922;5:188.
23. Brown MW, Templeton AW, Hodges III FJ. The incidence of acquired and congenital fusions in the cervical spine. Am J Roentgenol 1964;92:1255.
24. Bucholz RW, Burkhead WZ. The pathological anatomy of fatal atlanto-occipital dislocations. J Bone Joint Surg [Am] 1979;61:248.
25. Bulas DI, Fitz CR, Johnson DL. Traumatic atlanto-occipital dislocation in children. Radiology 1993;188:155.
26. Burke SW, French HG, Roberts JM, Johnston II CE,

Whitecloud TS, Edmunds Jr. JO. Chronic atlanto-axial instability in Down syndrome. J Bone Joint Surg [Am] 1985;67:1356.
27. Burwood RJ, Watt I. Assimilation of the atlas and basilar impression. A review of 1500 skull and cervical spine radiographs. Clin Radiol 1974;25:327.
28. Byers RK. Spinal-cord injuries during birth. Dev Med Child Neurol 1975;17:103.
29. Canale ST, Griffin DW, Hubbard CN. Congenital muscular torticollis: a long-term follow-up. J Bone Joint Surg [Am] 1982;64:810.
30. Capanna R, Albisinni U, Calderoni P, Campanacci M, Springfield DS. Aneurysmal bone cyst of the spine. J Bone Joint Surg [Am] 1985;67:527.
31. Catell HS, Clark GL Jr. Cervical kyphosis and instability following multiple laminectomies in children. J Bone Joint Surg [Am] 1967;49:713.
32. Catell HS, Filtzer DL. Pseudosubluxation and other normal variations in the cervical spine in children. A study of one hundred and sixty children. J Bone Joint Surg [Am] 1965;47:1295.
33. Chamberlain WE. Baslar impression (platybasia): bizarre developmental anomaly of occipital bone and upper cervical spine with striking and misleading neurologic manifestations. Yale J Biol Med 1939;11:487.
34. Cohn RS, Fielding JW. Osteochondroma of the cervical spine. J Pediatr Surg 1986;21:997.
35. Committee on Sports Medicine, American Academy of Pediatrics. Atlantoaxial instability in Down syndrome. Pediatrics 1984;74:152.
36. Connor JM, Evans DAP. Fibrodysplasia ossificans progressiva. The clinical features and natural history of 34 patients. J Bone Joint Surg [Br] 1982;64:76.
37. Conry BG, Hall CM. Cervical spine fractures and rear car restraints. Arch Dis Child 1987;62:1267.
38. Corner ES. Rotary dislocations of the atlas. Ann Surg 1907;45:9.
39. Coutts MB. Atlantoepistropheal subluxations. Arch Surg 1934;29:297.
40. Coventry MB, Harris LE. Congenital muscular torticollis in infancy. Some observations regarding treatment. J Bone Joint Surg [Am] 1959;41:815.
41. Craig JB, Govender S. Neurofibromatosis of the cervical spine. J Bone Joint Surg [Br] 1992;74:575.
42. Crawford Jr. AH, Bagamery N. Osseous manifestations of neurofibromatosis in childhood. J Pediatr Orthop 1986;6:72.
43. Darling DB, Fisher JH, Gellis SS. Hiatal hernia and gastroesophageal reflux in infants and children: analysis of the incidence in North American children. Pediatrics 1974;54:450.
44. Davids JR, Wenger DR, Mubarak SJ. Congenital muscular torticollis: sequela of intrauterine or perinatal compartment syndrome. J Pediatr Orthop 1993;13:141.
45. Davidson RI, Shilllito Jr. J. Eosinophilic granuloma of the cervical spine in children. Pediatrics 1970;45:746.
46. de Barros MC, Farias W, Ataide L, Lins S. Basilar impression and Arnold-Chiari malformation. A study of 66 cases. J Neurol Neurosurg Psychiatry 1968;31:596.
47. De La Paz RL, Brady TJ, Buonanno FS, et al. Nuclear magnetic resonance (NMR) imaging of Arnold-Chiari type I malformation with hydromyelia. J Comput Assist Tomogr 1983;7:126.
48. Dick HM, Bigliani LU, Michelsen WJ, et al. Adjuvant arterial embolization in the treatement of benign primary bone tumors in children. Clin Orthop 1979;139:133.
49. Disch SP, Grubb Jr. RL, Gado MH, et al. Aneurysmal bone cyst of the cervicothoracic spine: computed tomographic evaluation of the value of preoperative embolization. Case report. Neurosurgery 1986;19:290.
50. Dolan K. Developmental abnormalities of the cervical spine below the axis. Radiol Clin N Am 1977;15:167.

51. Drvaric DM, Ruderman RJ, Conrad RW, et al. Congenital scoliosis and urinary tract abnormalities: are intravenous pyelograms necessary? J Pediatr Orthop 1987;7:441.

52. Dubousset J. Torticollis in children caused by congenital anomalies of the atlas. J Bone Joint Surg [Am] 1986;68:178.

53. Dure LS, Percy AK, Cheek WR, Laurent JP. Chiari type I malformation in children. J Pediatr 1989;115:573.

54. Ebara S, Harada T, Yamazaki Y, et al. Unstable cervical spine in athetoid cerebral palsy. Spine 1989;11:1154.

55. Eighth report of the Medical Research Council Working Party on Tuberculosis of the Spine. A 10 year assessment of a controlled trial comparing debridement and anterior spinal fusion in the management of tuberculosis of the spine in patients on standard chemotherapy in Hong Kong. J Bone Joint Surg [Br] 1982;64:393.

56. Eismont FJ, Clifford S, Goldberg M, Green B. Cervical sagittal spinal canal size. Spine 1984;9:663.

57. El-Khoury GY, Clark CR, Dietz FR, et al. Posterior atlantooccipital subluxation in Down syndrome. Radiology 1986;159:507.

58. Epstein BS, Epstein JA. The association of cerebellar tonsillar herniation with basilar impression incident to Paget's disease. Am J Roentgenol 1969;107:535.

59. Epstein NE, Epstein JA, Zilkha A. Traumatic myelopathy in a seventeen-year-old child with cervical spinal stenosis (without fracture or dislocation) and a C2–3 Klippel-Feil fusion. A case report. Spine 1984;9:344.

60. Evans DL, Bethem D. Cervical spine injuries in children. J Pediatr Orthop 1989;9:563.

61. Evans CM. Traumatic occipito-atlantal dislocation. J Bone Joint Surg [Am] 1970;52:1653.

62. Fang D, Leong JCY, Fang HSY. Tuberculosis of the upper cervical spine. J Bone Joint Surg [Br] 1983;65:47.

63. Farley FA, Hensinger RN, Herzenberg JE. Cervical spinal cord injury in children. J Spin Disord 1992;5:410.

64. Ferkel RD, Westin GW, Dawson ED, Oppenheim WL. Muscular torticollis. A modified surgical approach. J Bone Joint Surg [Am] 1983;65:894.

65. Fielding JW. Cineroentgenography of the normal cervical spine. J Bone Joint Surg [Am] 1957;37:1280.

66. Fielding JW. Normal and selected abnormal motion of the cervical spine from the second cervical vertebra to the seventh cervical vertebra based on cineroentgenography. J Bone Joint Surg [Am] 1964;46:1779.

67. Fielding JW, Cochran GVB, Lawsing III JF, Hohl M. Tears of the transverse ligament of the atlas. A clinical and biomechanical study. J Bone Joint Surg [Am] 1974;56:1683.

68. Fielding JW, Hawkins RJ. Atlanto-axial rotatory fixation. (Fixed rotatory subluxation of the atlanto-axial joint.) J Bone Joint Surg [Am] 1977;59:37.

69. Fielding JW, Hawkins RJ, Ratzan SA. Spine fusion for atlanto-axial instability. J Bone Joint Surg [Am] 1976;58:400.

70. Fielding JW, Hensinger RN, Hawkins RJ. Os odontoideum. J Bone Joint Surg [Am] 1980;62:376.

71. Fielding JW, Keim HA, Hawkins RJ, Gabrielian JZ. Osteoid osteoma of the cervical spine. Clin Orthop 1977;128:163.

72. Fielding JW, Ratzan S. Osteochondroma of the cervical spine. J Bone Joint Surg [Am] 1973;55:640.

73. Fielding JW, Stillwell WT, Chynn KY, Spyropoulos EC. Use of computed tomography for the diagnosis of atlanto-axial rotatory fixation. J Bone Joint Surg [Am] 1978;60:1102.

74. Francis Jr. WR, Noble DP. Treatment of cervical kyphosis in children. Spine 1988;13:883.

75. Freiberg AA, Graziano GP, Loder RT, Hensinger RN. Metastatic vertebral disease in children. J Pediatr Orthop 1993;13:148.

76. Fried JA, Athreya B, Gregg JR, et al. The cervical spine in juvenile rheumatoid arthritis. Clin Orthop 1983;179:102.

77. Fuji T, Yonenobu K, Fujiwara K, et al. Cervical radiculopathy or myelopathy secondary to atheotoid cerebral palsy. J Bone Joint Surg [Am] 1987;69:815.

78. Gabriel KR, Mason DE, Carango P. Occipito-atlantal translation in Down's syndrome. Spine 1990;15:997.

79. Gallie WE. Fractures and dislocations of the cervical spine. Am J Surg 1939;46:495.

80. Georgopoulos G, Pizzutillo PD, Lee MS. Occipito-atlantal instability in children. A report of five cases and review of the literature. J Bone Joint Surg [Am] 1987;69:429.

81. Giuffre R, di Lorenzo N, Fortuna A. Cervical tumors of infancy and childhood. J Neurosurg Sci 1981;25:259.

82. Graziano GP, Herzenberg JE, Hensinger RN. The halo-Ilizarov distraction cast for correction of cervical deformity. J Bone Joint Surg [Am] 1993;75:996.

83. Greenberg AD. Atlantoaxial dislocation. Brain 1968;91:655.

84. Grisel P. Enucleation de l'atlas at tortcollis naso pharyngian. Presse Med 1930;38:50.

85. Grogono BJS. Injuries of the atlas and axis. J Bone Joint Surg [Br] 1954;36:397.

86. Gunderson CH, Solitare GB. Mirror movements in patients with the Klippel-Feil syndrome. Neuropathologic observations. Arch Neurol 1968;18:675.

87. Haffner DL, Hoffer MM, Wiedbusch R. Etiology of children's spinal injuries at Rancho Los Amigos. Spine 1993;18:679.

88. Hall CM, Sutcliffe J. Fibrodysplasia ossificans progressiva. Ann Radiol (Paris) 1979;22:119.

89. Hall JE, Simmons ED, Danylchuk K, Barnes PD. Instability of the cervical spine and neurological involvement in Klippel-Feil syndrome. J Bone Joint Surg [Am] 1990;72:460.

90. Halla JT, Fallahi S, Hardin JG. Nonreducible rotational head tilt and atlantoaxial lateral mass collapse. Clinical and roentgenographic features in patients with juvenile rheumatoid arthritis and ankylosing spondylitis. Arch Intern Med 1983;143:471.

91. Hansen H. A pathological-anatomical study on disc degeneration in dog. Acta Orthop Scand 1952;11(Suppl).

92. Harkey HL, Crockard HA, Stevens JM, et al. The operative management of basilar impression in osteogenesis imperfecta. Neurosurgery 1990;27:782.

93. Hay MC, Paterson D, Taylor TKF. Aneurysmal bone cysts of the spine. J Bone Joint Surg [Br] 1978;60:406.

94. Hemmer KM, McAlister WH, Marsh JL. Cervical spine anomalies in the craniosynostosis syndromes. Cleft Palate J 1987;24:328.

95. Hensinger RN, DeVito PD, Ragsdale CG. Changes in the cervical spine in juvenile rheumatoid arthritis. J Bone Joint Surg [Am] 1986;68:189.

96. Hensinger RN, Lang JE, MacEwen GD. Klippel-Feil syndrome. A constellation of associated anomalies. J Bone Joint Surg [Am] 1974;56:1246.

97. Herring JA, Hensinger RN. Cervical disc calcification. Instructional case. J Pediatr Orthop 1988;8:613.

98. Herzenberg JE, Hensinger RN, Dedrick DK, Phillips WA. Emergency transport and positioning of young children who have an injury of the cervical spine. The standard backboard may be hazardous. J Bone Joint Surg [Am] 1989;71:15.

99. Hess JH, Abelson SM, Bronstein IP. Atlantoaxial dislocation unassociated with trauma and secondary to inflammatory foci of the neck. Am J Dis Child 1935;49:1137.

100. Hillman JW, Sprofkin BE, Parrish TF. Birth injury of the cervical spine producing a "cerebral palsy" syndrome. Am Surg 1954;20:900.

101. Hirabayashi K, Satomi K. Operative procedure and results of expansive open-door laminoplasty. Spine 1988;13:870.

102. Hohl M, Baker HR. The atlanto-axial joint. Roentgenographic and anatomical study of normal and abnormal motion. J Bone Joint Surg [Am] 1964;46:1739.

103. Hsu LCS, Leong JCY. Tuberculosis of the lower cervical spine (C2 to C7). J Bone Joint Surg [Br] 1984;66:1.

104. Hunt TE, Dekaban AS. Modified head-neck support for basilar invagination with brain-stem compression. Can Med Assoc J 1982;126:947.

105. Hurwitz LJ, Shepherd WHT. Basilar impression and disordered metabolism of bone. Brain 1966;89:223.

106. Illingsworth RS. Attacks of unconsciousness in association with fused cervical vertebrae. Arch Dis Child 1956;31:8.

107. Inglis AE, Rubin RM, Lewis RJ, Villacin A. Osteochondroma of the cervical spine. Case report. Clin Orthop 1977;126:127.

108. Isu T, Miyasaka K, Abe H, et al. Atlantoaxial dislocation associated with neurofibromatosis. Report of three cases. J Neurosurg 1983;58:451.

109. Jackson G, Adler DC. Examination of the atlantoaxial joint following injury with particular emphasis on rotational subluxation. Am J Roentgenol 1956;76:1081.

110. Janin Y, Epstein JA, Carras R, Khan A. Osteoid osteomas and osteoblastomas of the spine. J Neurosurg 1981;8:31.

111. Johnson DG, Herbst JJ, Oliveros MA, Stewart DR. Evaluation of gastroesophageal reflux surgery in children. Pediatrics 1977;59:62.

112. Jolley SG, Johnson DG, Herbst JJ, et al. An assessment of gastroesophagela reflux in children by extended pH monitoring of the distal esophagus. Surgery 1978;84:16.

113. Jones EL, Cameron AH, Smith WT. Birth trauma to the cervical spine and vertebral arteries. J Pathol 1970;100:Piv.

114. Kaplan FS, McKluskey W, Hahn G, et al. Genetic transmission of fibrodysplasia ossificans progressive. J Bone Joint Surg [Am] 1993;75:1214.

115. Kawabe N, Hirotani H, Tanaka O. Pathomechanism of atlantoaxial rotatory fixation in children. J Pediatr Orthop 1989;9:569.

116. Kirwan EO, Hutton PAN, Pozo JL, Ransford AO. Osteoid osteoma and benign osteoblastoma of the spine. J Bone Joint Surg [Br] 1984;66:21.

117. Klippel M, Feil A. Un cas d'absence des vertebres cervicales. Nouvelle Icongographie de la Salpétriere 1912;25:223.

118. Kreiger AJ, Rosomoff HL, Kuperman AS, Zingesser LH. Occult respiratory dysfunction in a craniovertebral anomaly. J Neurosurg 1969;31:15.

119. Kupcha PC, An HS, Cotler JM. Gunshot wounds to the cervical spine. Spine 1990;15:1058.

120. Ladd AL, Scranton PE. Congenital cervical stenosis presenting as transient quadriplegia in athletes. J Bone Joint Surg [Am] 1986;68:1371.

121. Lally KP, Senac M, Hardin Jr WD, et al. Utility of the cervical spine radiograph in pediatric trauma. Am J Surg 1989;158:540.

122. Lawson JP, Ogden JA, Bucholz RW, Hughes SA. Physeal injuries of the cervical spine. J Pediatr Orthop 1987;7:428.

123. Lee CK, Weiss AB. Isolated congenital cervical block vertebrae below the axis with neurological symptoms. Spine 1981;6:118.

124. Leventhal HR. Birth injuries of the spinal cord. J Pediatr 1960;56:447.

125. Levine AM, Boriani S, Donati D, Campanacci M. Benign tumors of the cervical spine. Spine 1992;17S:399.

126. Ling CM. The influence of age on the results of open sternomastoid tenotomy in muscular torticollis. Clin Orthop 1976;116:142.

127. Ling CM, Low YS. Sternomastoid tumor and muscular torticollis. Clin Orthop 1972;86:144.

128. Linssen WHJ, Praamstra P, Gabrels FJM, Rotteveel JJ. Vascular insufficiency of the cervical cord due to hyperextension of the spine. Pediatr Neurol 1990;6:123.

129. Locke GR, Gardner JL, Van Epps EF. Atlas-dens interval (ADI) in children. A survey based on 200 normal cervical spines. AJR 1966;97:135.

130. Loder RT, Hensinger RN, Weinstein ed SL. Developmental abnormalities of the cervical spine. The pediatric spine: principles and practice. New York: Raven Press; 1994:397.

131. Louis DS, Argenta LC, Seidman M. The orthopaedic manifestations of Goldenhar's syndrome. Surg Round Orthop 1987:43.

132. Lowry RB. The Klippel-Feil anomalad as part of the fetal alcohol syndrome. Teratology 1977;16:53.

133. Macalister A. Notes on the development and variations of the atlas. J Anat Physiol 1983;27:519.

134. MacDonald D. Sternomastoid tumour and muscular torticollis. J Bone Joint Surg [Br] 1969;51:432.

135. MacGee EE. Osteochondroma of the cervical spine: a cause of transient quadriplegia. Neurosurgery ;4:259.

136. Marlin AE, Williams GR, Lee JF. Jefferson fractures in children. J Neurosurg 1983;58:277.

137. Marmot MA, Beauchamp GR, Maddox SF. Photophobia, epiphora, and torticollis: a masquerade syndrome. J Pediatr Ophthalmol Strabis 1990;27:202.

138. Martel W, Holt JF, Cassidy JT. Roentgenologic manifestations of juvenile rheumatoid arthritis. Am J Roentgenol 1962;88:400.

139. Mathern GW, Batzdorf U. Grisel's syndrome. Cervical spine clinical, pathologic, and neurologic manifestations. Clin Orthop 1989;244:131.

140. McCauley RGK, Darling DB, Leonidas JC, Schwartz AM. Gastroesophageal reflux in infants and children: a useful classification and reliable physiologic technique for its demonstration. Am J Roentgenol 1978;130:47.

141. McGregor M. Significance of certain measurements of skull in diagnosis of basilar impression. Br J Radiol 1948;21:171.

142. McGrory BJ, Klassen RA, Chao EYS, et al. Acute fractures and dislocations of the cervical spine in children and adolescents. J Bone Joint Surg [Am] 1993;75:988.

143. McLay K, Maran AGD. Deafness and the Klippel-Feil syndrome. J Laryng Otol 1969;83:175.

144. McRae DL. Bony abnormalities in the region of the foramen magnum: correlation of the anatomic and neurologic findings. Acta Radiol 1953;40:335.

145. McRae DL. The significance of abnormalities of the cervical spine. Am J Roentgenol 1960;84:3.

146. McRae DL, Barnum AS. Occipitalization of the atlas. Am J Roentgenol 1953;70:23.

147. Mecklenburg RS, Krueger PM. Extensive genitourinary anomalies associated with Klippel-Feil syndrome. Am J Dis Child 1974;128:92.

148. Menelaus MB. Discitis. An inflammation affecting the intervertebral discs in children. J Bone Joint Surg [Br] 1964;46:16.

149. Menezes AH, VanGilder JC, Graf CJ, McDonnell DE. Craniocervical abnormalities: a comprehensive surgical approach. J Neurosurg 1980;53:444.

150. Menezes AHV. Transoral-transpharyngeal approach to the anterior craniocervical junction. J Neurosurg 1988;69:895.

151. Michie I, Clark M. Neurologic syndromes associated with cervical and craniocervical anomalies. Arch Neurol 1968;18:241.

152. Mikawa Y, Watnanbe R, Yamano Y, Ishii K. Fracture through a synchondrosis of the anterior arch of the atlas. J Bone Joint Stag [Br] 1987;69:483.

153. Moore WB, Matthews TJ, Rabinowitz R. Genitourinary anomalies associated with Klippel-Feil syndrome. J Bone Joint Surg [Am] 1975;57:355.

154. Morrison SG, Perry LW, Scott III LP. Congenital brevicollis (Klippel-Feil syndrome). Am J Dis Child 1968;115:614.

155. Mosberg Jr WH. The Klippel-Feil syndrome. Etiology and treatment of neurologic signs. J Nerv Ment Dis 1953;117:479.

156. Msall M, Rogers B, DiGaudio K, et al. Long-term complications

of segmental cervical fusion in Down syndrome. Dev Med Child Neurol 64 1991;33(suppl):5.

157. Murphy Jr WJ, Gellis SS. Torticollis with hiatus hernia in infancy. Sandifer syndrome. Am J Dis Child 1977;131:564.

158. Nakano N, Nakano T, Nakano K. Comparison of the results of laminectomy and open-door laminoplasty for cervical spondylotic myeloradiculopathy and ossification of the posterior longitudinal ligaments. Spine 1988;13:792.

159. Neidengard L, Carter TE, Smith DW. Klippel-Feil malformation complex in fetal alcohol syndrome. Am J Dis Child 1978;132:929.

160. Nemeto O, Moser RP, VanDam BE, et al. Osteoblastoma of the spine. A review of 75 cases. Spine 1990;15:1272.

161. Nicholson JT, Sherk HH. Anomalies of the occipitocervical articulation. J Bone Joint Surg [Am] 1968;50:295.

162. Nishihara N, Tanabe G, Nakahara S, et al. Surgical treatment of cervical spondylotic myelopathy complicating athetoid cerebral palsy. J Bone Joint Surg [Br] 1984;66:504.

163. Nora JJ, Cohen M, Maxwell GM. Klippel-Feil syndrome with congenital heart disease. Am J Dis Child 1961;102:110.

164. Nordt JC, Stauffer ES. Sequelae of atlantoaxial stabilization in two patient with Down's syndrome. Spine 1981;6:437.

165. Novick GS, Pavlov H, Bullough PG. Osteochondroma of the cervical spine: report of two cases in preadolescent males. Skeletal Radiol 1982;8:13.

166. Occhipinti E, Mastrostefano R, Pompili A, et al. Spinal chordomas in infancy. Report of a case and analysis of the literature. Childs Brain 1981;8:198.

167. Odor JM, Watkins RG, Dillin WH, et al. Incidence of cervical spinal stenosis in professional and rookie football players. Am J Sport Meal 1990;18:507.

168. Ogden JA. Radiology of postnatal skeletal development. XI. The first cervical vertebrae. Skeletal Radiol 1984;12:12.

169. Ogden JA. Radiology of postnatal skeletal development. XII. The second cervical vertebra. Skeletal Radiol 1984;12:169.

170. Ogden JA. Skeletal injury in the child. 2nd ed. Philadelphia: WB Saunders; 1990:571.

171. Ogden JA, Murphy MJ, Southwick WO, Ogden DA. Radiology of postnatal skeletal development. XIII. C1–C2 relationships. Skeletal Radiol 1986;15:433.

172. O'Rahilly R, Muller F, Meyer DB. The human vertebral column at the end of the embryonic period proper. 1. The column as a whole. J Anat 1980;131:565.

173. O'Rahilly R, Meyer DB. The timing and sequence of events in the development of the human vertebral column during the embryonic period proper. Anat Embryol 1979;157:167.

174. Pang D, Pollack IF. Spinal cord injury without radiographic abnormality in children—the SCIWORA syndrome. J Trauma 1989;29:654.

175. Pang D, Wilberger Jr JE. Spinal cord injury without radiographic abnormalities in children. J Neurosurg 1982;57:114.

176. Parke WW, Rothman RH, Brown MD. The pharyngovertebral veins: an anatomical rationale for Grisel's syndrome. J Bone Joint Surg [Am] 1984;66:568.

177. Parker W. Migraine and the vestibular system in childhood and adolescence. Am J Otology 1989;10:364.

178. Pásztor E, Vajda J, Piffkó P, Horváth M. Transoral surgery for basilar impression. Surg Neurol 1980;14:473.

179. Pennecot GF, Gouraud D, Hardy JR, Pouliquen JC. Roentgenographical study of the stability of the cervical spine in children. J Pediatr Orthop 1984;4:346.

180. Pennecot GF, Leonard P, Peyrot des Gachons S, et al. Traumatic ligamentous instability of the cervical spine in children. J Pediatr Orthop 1984;4:339.

181. Phillips WA, Hensinger RN. The management of rotatory atlanto-axial subluxation in children. J Bone Joint Surg [Am] 1989;71:664.

182. Pizzutillo PD, Woods MW, Nicholson L. Risk factors in Klippel-Feil syndrome. Orthop Trans 1987;11:473.

183. Pizzutillo PP, Rocha EF, D'Astous J, et al. Bilateral fracture of the pedicle of the cervical vertebra in the young child. J Bone Joint Surg [Am] 1986;68:892.

184. Pueschel SM, Herndon JH, Gelch MM, et al. Symptomatic atlantoaxial subluxation in persons with Down syndrome. J Pediatr Orthop 1984;4:682.

185. Pueschel SM, Scola FH, Perry CD, Pezzullo JC. Atlanto-axial instability in children with Down syndrome. Pediatr Radiol 1981;10:129.

186. Pueschel SM, Findley TW, Furia J, et al. Atlantoaxial instability in Down syndrome: roentgenographic, neurologic, and somatosensory evoked potential studies. J Pediatr 1987;110:515.

187. Pueschel SM, Scola FH, Tupper TB, Pezzullo JC. Skeletal anomalies of the upper cervical spine in children with Down syndrome. J Pediatr Orthop 1990;10:607.

188. Rachesky I, Boyce WT, Duncan B, et al. Clinical prediction of cervical spine injuries in children. Am J Dis Child 1987;141:199.

189. Ramenofsky ML, Buyse M, Goldberg MJ, Leape LL. Gastroesophageal reflux and torticollis. J Bone Joint Surg [Am] 1978;60:1140.

190. Raskas DS, Graziano GP, Herzenberg JE, et al. Osteoid osteoma and osteoblastoma of the spine. J Spin Disord 1992;5:204.

191. Rathbone D, Johnson G, Letts M. Spinal cord concussion in pediatric athletes. J Pediatr Orthop 1992;12:616.

192. Reese ME, Msall ME, Owen S, et al. Acquired cervical spine impairment in young adults with cerebral palsy. Dev Med Child Neurol 1991;33:153.

193. Ring D, Wenger DR, Johnston II C. Pyogenic infectious spondylitis in children: the convergence of discitis and vertebral osteomyelitis. Presented at the annual meeting of the Pediatric Orthopaedic Society of North America, West Sulpher Springs, West Virginia, 1993.

194. Ritterbusch JF, McGinty LD, Spar J, Orrison WW. Magnetic resonance imaging for stenosis and subluxation in Klippel-Feil syndrome. Spine 1991;16:539.

195. Romeyn RL, Herkowitz HN. The cervical spine in hemophilia. Clin Orthop 1986;210:113.

196. Rubin SE, Wagner RS. Ocular torticollis. A review. Survey Opthalmol 1986;30:366.

197. Saltzman CL, Hensinger RN, Blane CE, Phillips WA. Familial cervical dysplasia. J Bone Joint Surg [Am] 1991;73:163.

198. Sandham A. Cervical vertebral anomalies in cleft lip and palate. Cleft Palate J 1986;23:206.

199. Sarnat HB, Morrissy RT. Idiopathic torticollis: sternomastoid myopathy and accessory neuropathy. Muscle Nerve 1981;4:374.

200. Schiff DCM, Parke WW. The arterial supply of the odontoid process. J Bone Joint Surg [Am] 1973;55:1450.

201. Schwartz HS, Pinto M. Osteoblastomas of the cervical spine. J Spin Disord 1990;3:179.

202. Segal LS, Drummond DS, Zanotti RM, et al. Complications of posterior arthrodesis of the cervical spine in patients who have Down syndrome. J Bone Joint Surg [Am] 1991;73:1547.

203. Seimon LP. Fracture of the odontoid process in young children. J Bone Joint Surg [Am] 1977;59:943.

204. Sensenig EC. The development of the occipital and cervical segments and their associated structures in human embryos. Contrib Embryol Carnegie Inst 1957;36:141.

205. Sherk HH, Nicholson JT. Cervico-oculo-acusticus syndrome. Case report of death caused by injury to abnormal cervical spine. J Bone Joint Surg [Am] 1972;54:1776.

206. Sherk HH, Nicholson JT, Chung SMK. Fractures of the odontoid process in young children. J Bone Joint Surg [Am] 1978;60:921.

207. Sherk HH, Nicholson JT, Nixon JE. Vertebra plana and eosinophilic granuloma of the cervical spine in children. Spine 1978;3:116.

208. Sherk HH, Nolan Jr JP, Mooar PA. Treatment of tumors of the cervical spine. Clin Orthop 1988;233:163.

209. Sherk HH, Shjut L, Chung S. Iniencephalic deformity of the cervical spine with Klippel-Feil anomalies and congenital elevation of the scapula. J Bone Joint Surg [Am] 1974;56:1254.

210. Sherk HH, Whitaker LA, Pasquariello PS. Facial malformations and spinal anomalies. A predictable relationship. Spine 1982;7:526.

211. Shoul MI, Ritvo M. Clinical and roentgenological manifestations of the Klippel-Feil syndrome (congenital fusion of the cervical vertebrae, brevicollis). Report of eight additional casea and review of the literature. Am J Roentgenol 1952;68:369.

212. Shulman ST, Madden JD, Esterly JR, Shanklin DR. Transection of spinal cord. A rare obstetrical complication of cephalic delivery. Arch Dis Child 1971;46:291.

213. Sibley RK, Day DL, Dehner LP, Trueworthy RC. Metastasizing chordoma in early childhood: a pathological and immunohistochemical study with review of the literature. Pediatr Pathol 1987;7:287.

214. Sim FH, Svien HJ, Bickel WH, Janes JM. Swan-neck deformity following extensive cervical laminectomy. A review of twenty-one cases. J Bone Joint Surg [Am] 1974;56:564.

215. Smith MD, Phillips WA, Hensinger RN. Complications of fusion to the upper cervical spine. Spine 1991;16:702.

216. Smith MD, Phillips WA, Hensinger RN. Fusion of the upper cervical spine in children and adolescents. An analysis of 17 patients. Spine 1991;16:695.

217. Smith RA, Vohman D, Dimon III JH, et al. Calcified cervical intervertebral discs in children. J Neurosurg 1977;46:233.

218. Snyder CH. Paroxsymal torticollis in infancy. A possible form of labrynthitis. Am J Dis Child 1969;117:458.

219. Sonnabend DH, Taylor TKF, Chapman GK. Intervetebral disc calcification syndromes in children. J Bone Joint Surg [Br] 1982;64:25.

220. Spierings ELH, Braakman R. The management of os odontoideum. J Bone Joint Surg [Br] 1982;64:422.

221. Spitzer R, Rabinowitch JY, Wybor KC. A study of the abnormalities of the skull, teeth, and lenses in mongolism. Can Med Assoc J 1961;84:567.

222. Stark EW, Borton TE. Hearing loss and the Klippel-Feil syndrome. Am J Dis Child 1972;123:233.

223. Steel HH. Anatomical and mechanical considerations of the atlanto-axial articulation. J Bone Joint Surg [Am] 1968;50:1481.

224. Stern WE, Rand RW. Birth injuries to the spinal cord. A report of 2 cases and review of the literature. Am J Obstet Gynecol 1959;78:498.

225. Stillwell WT, Fielding JW. Aneurysmal bone cyst of the cervicodorsal spine. Clin Orthop 1984;187:144.

226. Swischuk LE. Anterior displacement of C2 in children: physiologic or pathologic? A helpful differentiating line. Radiology 1977;122:759.

227. Swischuk LE, Swischuk PN, John SD. Wedging of C-3 in infants and children: usually a normal finding and not a fracture. Radiology 1993;188:523.

228. Taboas-Perez RA, Rivera-Reyes L. Head tilt: a revisit to an old sign of posterior fossa tumors. Bol Asoc Med P R 1984;76:62.

229. Taylor AR, Chakravorty BC. Clinical syndromes associated with basilar impression. Arch Neurol 1964;10:475.

230. Teodori JB, Painter MJ. Basilar impression in children. Pediatrics 1984;74:1097.

231. Thompson T, McManus S, Colville J. Familial congenital muscular torticollis: case report and review of the literature. Clin Orthop 1986;202:193.

232. Torg JS, Pavlov H, Genuario SE, et al. Neurapraxia of the cervical spinal cord with transient quadriplegia. J Bone Joint Surg [Am] 1986;68:1354.

233. Towbin A. Latent spinal cord and brain stem injury in newborn infants. Dev Med Child Neurol 1969;11:54.

234. Towbin A. Central nervous system damage in the human fetus and newborn infant. Am J Dis Child 1970;119:529.

235. Towbin A. Spinal cord and brain stem injury at birth. Arch Pathol 1964;77:620.

236. Towbin A. spinal injury related to the syndrome of sudden death ("crib death") in infants. Am J Clin Pathol 1968;49:562.

237. Tredwell SJ, Newman DE, Lockitch G. Instability of the upper cervical spine in Down syndrome. J Pediatr Orthop 1990;10:602.

238. Tredwell SJ, Smith DF, Macleod PJ, Wood BJ. Cervical spine anomalies in fetal alcohol syndrome. Spine 1982;7:331.

239. Tse P, Cheng J, Chow Y, Leung PC. Surgery for neglected congenital torticollis. Acta Orthop Scand 1987;58:270.

240. Vigoroux RP, Baurand C, Choux M, et al. Les traumatismes du rachis cervical chez l'enfant neurochir. Neurochirurgie 1968;14:689.

241. Visudhiphan P, Chiemchanya S, Somburanasin R, Dheandhanoo D. Torticollis as the presenting sign in cervical spine infection and tumor. Clin Pediatr 1982;21:71.

242. Wadia NH. Myelopathy complicating congenital atlantoaxial dislocation (a study of 28 cases). Brain 1967;90:449.

243. Watson-Jones R. Spontaneous hyperemia dislocation of the atlas. Proc Roy Soc Med 1932;25:586.

244. Weiner DS. Congenital dislocation of the hip associated with congenital muscular torticollis. Clin Orthop 1976;121:163.

245. Weisel SW, Rothman RH. Occipitoatlantal hypermobility. Spine 1979;4:187.

246. Wenger DR, Bobechko WP, Gilday DL. The spectrum of intervertebral disc-space infection in children. J Bone Joint Surg [Am] 1978;60:100.

247. Whyte AM, Lufkin RB, Bredenkamp J, Hoover L. Sternocleidomastoid fibrosis in congenital muscular torticollis: MR appearance. J Comput Assist Tomogrr 1989;13:163.

248. Wilkins RH, Brody IA. The Arnold-Chiari Malformation. Arch Neurol 1971;25:376.

249. Wollin DG. The os odontoideum. Seperate odontoid process. J Bone Joint Surg [Am] 1963;47:1459.

250. Wong CC, Pereira B, Pho RWH. Cervical disc calcification in children. A long term review. Spine 1992;17:139.

251. Wong VCN, Fung CF. Basilar impression in a child with hypochondroplasia. Pediatr Neurol 1991;7:62.

252. Yamada H, Nakamura S, Tajima M, Kageyama N. Neurological manifestations of pediatric achondroplasia. J Neurosurg 1981;54:49.

253. Yasuoka S, Paterson HA, Laws Jr ER, MacCarty CS. Pathogenesis and prophylaxis of postlaminectomy deformity of the spine after multiple level laminectomy: difference between children and adults. Neurosurgery 1981;9:145.

254. Yong-Hing K, Kalamchi A, MacEwen GD. Cervical spine abnormalities in neurofibromatosis. J Bone Joint Surg [Am] 1979;61:695.

255. Zdeblick TA, Zou D, Warden KE, et al. Cervical stability after foraminotomy. J Bone Joint Surg [Am] 1992;74:22.

256. Zwimpfer TJ, Tucker WS, Faulkner JF. Osteoid osteoma of the cervical spine: case reports and literature review. Can J Surg 1982;25:637.

Lovell & Winter's Pediatric Orthopaedics, fourth edition,
edited by Raymond T. Morrissy and Stuart L. Weinstein.
Lippincott–Raven Publishers, Philadelphia © 1996.

Chapter

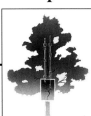

21

The Upper Limb

Loui G. Bayne
Bronier L. Costas
Gary M. Lourie

Malformations of the upper extremity are among the most common congenital abnormalities and the most challenging to treat. Additions and deletions of the anatomic structures pose social and technical challenges for the treating physicians.

In this chapter we outline some general principles for the care of these children. A classification and examples of the individual categories are demonstrated. This chapter provides an overview of the majority of congenital differences of the upper extremity and their possible treatment. The associated problems also are outlined so that the treating physician is sure to treat the entire child rather than just the presenting problem. This chapter is not intended to be a how-to manual. The physician should review many different articles, text books, and other resources so that the global understanding of the problem is achieved before initiating treatment.

GENERAL PRINCIPLES

The emotional impact on the parents of a child with a congenital deformity is overwhelming. Most parents have the initial expectation of a perfect child and often are confronted by many questions and concerns about their newborn child. There may be questions of self-doubt and remorse initially; the surgeon should see the child soon after birth and provide a simple explanation of the problem and outline a program of management for the child. This helps allay the parents' anxiety, because an explanation can be given for the incidence of anomalies, genetic counseling, potential growth and development for the hand, and the role of surgery to improve both cosmetic appearance and functional ability of the hand.

Surgery is seldom an urgent consideration in congenital differences of the upper limb, although the parents and grandparents often want something done early. The size of the hand, anatomic abnormalities, unpredictable growth, and lack of patient cooperation make it extremely difficult to develop and execute a treatment plan. A physician who can sit down and discuss openly and thoroughly with the extended family will go a long way in aiding the treatment of the patient.

The deformities should be divided into those that are amenable to surgery and those in which surgery provides little or no benefit. The objective of reconstructive surgery is to provide the hand with good function and appearance. It is often possible to improve the hand function, but with few exceptions the appearance will not be normal. Therefore the emphasis should be placed on the functional aspect of the problem, but the surgeon also should be attentive to the cosmetic side.

The surgical treatment is to provide the hand with active control for pinch and grasp and a good sensory appreciation for tactile sensation, proprioception, and stereognosis. This implies good sensory skin coverage and appearance as near to normal as possible.

Certain general procedures govern the decision regarding the timing and type of operation. In general, soft tissue procedures are carried out at an early age and bony operations later. This is also true for simple versus complex operations. The use of magnification and increasing literature about congenital differences has allowed us to decrease the age at which we begin to approach these problems.

Because prehension of the hand begins to develop around 1 year of age and is fully developed by 3 years, procedures that affect prehension pattern should be done in the first 2 years. It is usually a mistake to change the prehension pattern that is developed over many years.

Early correction of skeletal development is important. Extra bone, malpositions, and fusions between adjacent bones must be dealt with to allow the child's growth to develop properly. Osteotomy and fusion should be left until a later date. Complicated tendon transfers should be delayed until the child is 3 to 5 years of age, when he or she is better able to cooperate with both the surgeon and the therapist. The primary thrust of the reconstructive surgery should be accomplished by school age to minimize peer reaction and provide the child with the best possible function of the hands to participate in school work.

Most children with congenital differences are mentally normal and have good voluntary control; therefore, the potential for improvement of hand function is significant. The physician must be attentive to the overall condition of the patient who may have associated medical abnormalities. In these cases, or when associated with mentally deficient children, reconstructive procedures may be neither practical nor helpful.

The physician should be attentive to both the patient and the family. As the physician develops a plan for treatment for the patient, care should be directed to the parents so that they have a full understanding regarding their child. Counseling may be advised for parents. The opportunity to talk with other parents whose children have congenital differences is often helpful. Finally, working with a geneticist and understanding the inheritance pattern may help the parents accept the situation and address the possibility of future children having disorders.

There are neither standard abnormalities nor a cookbook treatment for congenital differences of the upper extremity. Many malformations are unusual and require a team approach of the family, the pediatrician, the geneticist, the surgeon, and the therapist. The treatment of congenital abnormalities usually is a long-term project because the child grows until adolescence.

Remember that these children grow and develop with no forgone expectation as to how their hand should look or function. A person's determination may overcome what to some might be considered as a gross functional and cosmetic abnormality. With the whole-team approach, including the support of the extended family, these children can reach their true potential.

INCIDENCE

It is impossible to establish accurately the incidence of congenital differences of the upper extremity because of the definition and reporting data. Congenital abnormalities are defined as those that are present at birth and occur in approximately 6% to 7% of all live births. Multiple anomalies are present in 1% to 2% of live births, but in only 1 in 626 newborns does the abnormality involve the upper extremity.[1] Flatt's Iowa study shows that nearly half of the affected patients had deformities. The most common malformations are polydactyly and syndactyly.[2]

GENETICS AND INHERITANCE

A basic understanding of genetics and inheritance patterns are integral to the care of these children. The guilt of the parents that may be associated with many congenital differences can be lessened when a basic explanation can be provided to the parents and grandparents. The hand surgeon, in conjunction with a geneticist, can help explain to the extended family the problem of developmental sequence, which is defined as a single, localized insult leading to a specific secondary pattern of multiple abnormalities. Three types of sequences have been identified: malformation, deformation, and disruption.

The malformation sequence is a result of poor formation of the fetal tissue. These abnormalities are intrinsic to the developing fetus and are caused by a wide variety of factors. They may be genetic or nongenetic in nature. These defects include failure of formation, segmentation, or differentiation. Duplication and overgrowth are included in this category. The genetic abnormalities may be caused by a mendelian inheritance patterns, recognized chromosomal aberrations, or multifactorial genetic conditions. Other nongenetic factors include teratogens and environmental agents that affect the fetus during the early weeks of development. An example of this type would be radial clubhand, which may occur as an inherited or noninherited disorder.

In the deformation sequence, the fetus is usually normal but environmental factors affect its development. Secondary deformations or distortions are caused by external mechanical forces. One of the most common examples would be the leakage of amniotic fluid and subsequent formation of amniotic bands leading to the occurrence of annular constriction band syndrome of the fingers.

The disruption sequence occurs when tissue breakdown happens in the normal fetus subjective to injury from factors outside the uterus. These may be caused by infection, vascular problems, and mechanical or metabolic factors. The most dramatic of these is the thalidomide changes in the upper extremity producing phocomelia. Cocaine and alcohol abuse also are contributing to the disruption of the newborn child.

An understanding of genetics and inheritance pat-terns are helpful to the hand surgeon in dealing with the family in the early stages of the treatment of the patient. Although the physician may offer a good technical explanation, families may be advised to seek outside support in the form of either counseling or becoming part of a support group, such as Super Kids (60 Clyde Street, Newton, Mass. 02160–2250). This support group will allow parents who have children of similar abnormalities to talk with each other to explore what the future holds for their child. Seeing how other children and parents cope with their specific problem can be helpful to the new parents.

It is important to emphasize to the parents that on the whole their child's development should be normal.[6,11] These children often have normal mental development, and because they are unaware of any difference in their hand because of a lack of previous experience, they will find ways in which to use their hands to accomplish their desired goals. These children should be allowed to find their own ways to use their upper extremities so that they can examine and explore their world.

CLASSIFICATION OF UPPER LIMB MALFORMATIONS

It is difficult to discuss congenital anomalies of the upper extremity without classifying them in the way that is universally acceptable to all medical specialists who treat problems in the upper limb.[3–5] In the past various Greek and Latin names have been used to describe common deficiencies, but these may confuse conditions.[7–9,13] Many terms, such as hemimelia, ectromelia, and eponyms, are no longer being employed.[10,11] A more simplified descriptive terminology that has been adopted by the American Society for Surgery of the Hand, the International Federation of Societies for Surgery of the Hand, and the International Society of Prosthetics and Orthotics now serves as the basic classification.[12] Classification groups similar patterns of deficiency according to the parts that had been affected primarily by the developmental anomaly, whether the insult involves all components of a part (i.e., skeletal and soft tissue) or only the dermal myofascial structures. Malformations are categorized into 7 groups (Table 21-1). A detailed explanation of this classification can be found.[12]

FAILURE OF FORMATION OF PARTS

A group of deformities categorized as failure of formation of parts is distinguished by failure or arrest of the formation of the limb, which may be complete but partial. These deformities seldom are genetically pat-

TABLE 21-1. *Classification of Upper Limb Malformations*

Failure of formation of parts (arrest
  and development)
  Transverse terminal deficiencies
  Longitudinal deficiencies
    Radial ray (radial clubhand)
    Ulnar ray (ulnar clubhand)
    Central ray (cleft hand)
    Intersegmental (phocomelia)
Failure of differentiation
  Soft tissue involvement
    Disseminated
      Arthrogryposis
    Shoulder
    Elbow and forearm
    Wrist and hand
      Cutaneous syndactyly
      Camptodactyly
      Thumb-in-palm deformity
      Deviated or deformed digits
  Skeletal involvement
    Shoulder
    Elbow
      Elbow synostosis
    Forearm
      Proximal radial ulnar synostosis
      Distal radial ulnar synostosis
    Wrist and hand
      Osseous syndactyly
      Synostosis of carpal bones
      Symphalangia
      Clinodactyly
      Delta bone
Congenital tumorous conditions
  Hemangetic
  Lymphatic
  Neurogenic
  Connective tissue
  Skeletal

Duplication
  Whole limb
  Humeral segment
  Radial segment
  Ulnar segment
    Mirror hand
  Digit
    Polydactyly
      Radial (preaxial)
      Central
      Ulna (postaxial)
Overgrowth
  Whole limb
  Partial limb
  Digit
    Macrodactyly
Undergrowth
  Whole limb
  Whole hand
  Metacarpal
  Digit
    Brachysyndactyly
    Brachydactyly
Congenital constriction band syndrome
Generalized skeletal abnormalities
  Chromosomal
    Madelung deformity

terned or inherited. There are two subcategories: transverse and longitudinal (Fig. 21-1).

Transverse Arrest

Transverse arrest is complete absence of the structures distal to a certain point in the upper extremity. They are commonly referred to as *congenital amputations*. The longitudinal arrest is grouped into radial, central, ulnar, and intersegmental deficiencies. These are illustrated in the diagram.

Transverse terminal deficiencies may occur at any level from the shoulder down, but they tend to involve the hand and wrist more frequently. The incidence of these conditions varies; upper arm amputations are reported to be 1 in 270,000 live births, and forearm amputations 1 in 20,000 live births.[3]

The inheritance pattern for transverse deficiencies usually is sporadic. Associated anomalies include those primarily of the musculoskeletal system, such as spina bifida, clubfoot, and radioulnar synostosis. Annular constriction band syndrome also may be seen in association with this condition.

Complete absence of the arm at the level of the proximal humerus is rare. Only during the time of the use of thalidomide or other embryologic toxins has the occurrence of this been common.[11] Bilateral presence of this condition is extremely rare.

Upper third forearm transverse deficiencies are the most common. The clinical appearance and radio-

Transverse   **Longitudinal**

Proximal   Distal   Proximal   Distal

                                                    Radial   Central   Ulnar

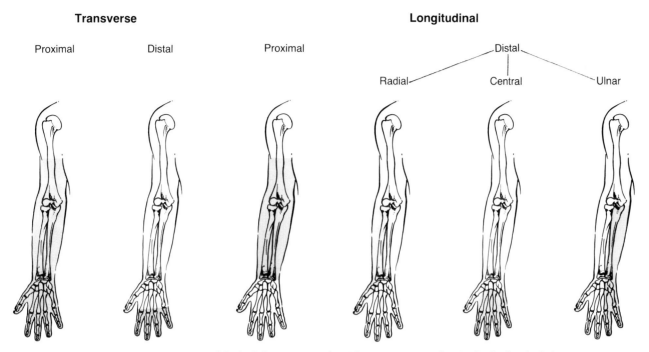

FIGURE 21-1. Congenital limb deficiencies can be either transverse or longitudinal. The shaded portions represent the areas that are either hypoplastic or absent.

graphs characteristically show the upper portion of both forearm bones and a normal elbow (Fig. 21-2).

Treatment in this group of patients is directed toward conservative measures. Prosthesis wear should be introduced at approximately 6 months of age to help facilitate in bimanual tasks. The patients wear the prosthesis part-time because they use the tactile feedback from the normal skin over the end of their transverse amputation. As they become older,

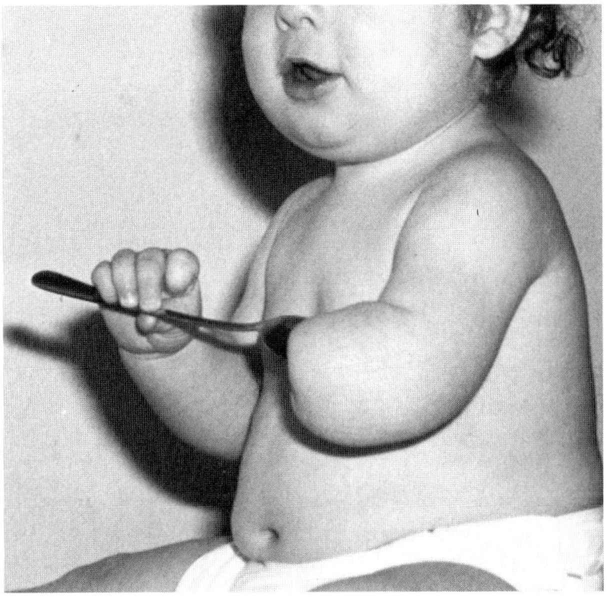

FIGURE 21-2. This child has had a proximal forearm transverse amputation, the most common amputation in the upper extremity.

however, the use of a prosthesis aids them in more complex activity.

Any surgical procedures in this category should be directed toward aiding with prosthetic wear. Techniques such as distraction lengthening and microvascular transfers aid in extending the arm to facilitate prosthetic stability, and although only rarely used when the residual limb is too short to effectively use a prosthesis, it can help the patient in this category.

Radial Deficiencies or Clubhand

Congenital radial deficiency is total or partial absence of parts that occur on the radial (preaxial) border of the upper extremity. The deficiency may range from hypoplasia of the thumb to varying degrees of deficiency of the radius.[17] The most common occurring radial deficiency is complete absence of the radius. The hand has no support except for the ulna and therefore is deviated to the radial side of the forearm, thus giving the appearance of a radial clubhand. The characteristic clinical picture of partial or complete absence of the radius is a forearm slightly bowed to the radial side with a prominent distal ulna. The extremity is two thirds the length of the opposite unaffected extremity, and this disproportion remains throughout growth.[16–21] Typically the hand is deviated radially, the extent being determined by the degree of absence of the radius. The thumb, when present, is defective to some degree.[16] Associated stiffness of the joints of the digits, particularly the index and long

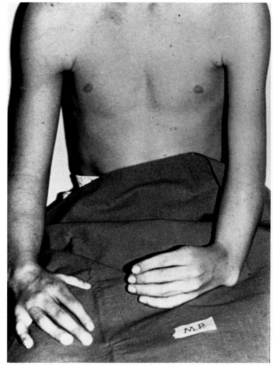
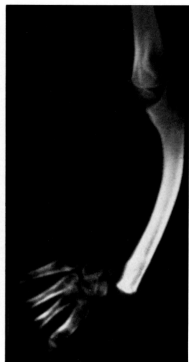

FIGURE 21-3.   The left upper extremity shows a typical radial club-hand deformity. The radiograph shows the complete absence of the radius. The forearm is short, and the hand is not supported because of absence of the radius. The distal ulna forms a prominent knob at the end of the forearm, and the hand is displaced radially.

fingers, is present. The function of the hand is affected by the degree of digital deficiency and loss of wrist support (Fig. 21-3).

As the name radial dysplasia implies, skeletal defects are the hallmark of this clinical entity.[54] The entire involved limb is short. Joint dysfunction, secondary to malformation, may involve the shoulder, the elbow, the carpus, and the small joints of the hand. Any limitation of elbow motion may severely limit hand function by preventing the hands easily reaching the mouth or perineum. Absence of the thumb creates a severe functional handicap because grip is compromised.[54]

Muscle deficiencies vary proportionally with the skeletal defect. Muscles that arise from the medial epicondyle (postaxial) usually are present but not well differentiated distally. The wrist flexors insert variously on the radial side of the wrist and provide a strong radial force. The finger flexors may not be well differentiated and restrict finger function.[21] The muscles that arise from the lateral epicondyle (preaxial) are frequently deficient to some degree and contribute to poor extension of the fingers. The radial wrist extensor insertions on the radial border of the wrist contribute to radial deviation of the hand. When the radius is partially present, a radial anlage may be present and act as a tethering force.[24] The thenar muscles are defective in proportion to the deficiency of the thumb[17] (Fig. 21-4).

Neurovascular deficiencies include absent radial artery and superficial radial nerve. The sensation to the radial side of the hand is supplied by superficial

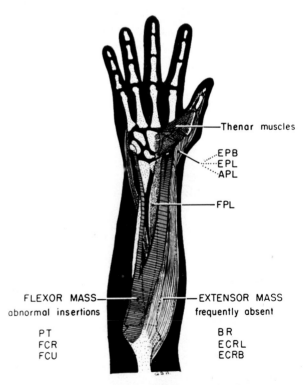

FIGURE 21-4.   Flexor muscles arising from the postaxial border usually are well developed, but their insertion into the preaxial structures are abnormal. When the thumb is absent or hypoplastic, the thenar muscles usually are absent.

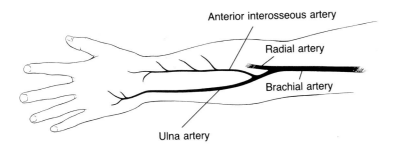

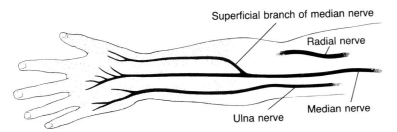

FIGURE 21-5. Arterial anomalies are associated with the radial artery, which usually terminates near the elbow. The anterior interosseous artery takes over the radial artery's distribution to the radial side of the forearm and hand. The radial nerve usually terminates below the elbow, where its sensory distribution is subsumed by the superficial median nerve.

dorsal branch of the median nerve. The normal course of the ulnar and the median nerves and the ulnar artery are unaffected. The ulnar artery is the main source of blood supply to the hand. The anterior interosseous branch of the ulnar artery accompanies the median nerve and supplies the radial side of the extremity (Fig. 21-5). The degree of skeletal deficiency is used to further subclassify the deficiencies into four parts.[17]

TYPE 1: SHORT DISTAL RADIUS. The distal epiphysis of the radius is present but growth of the epiphysis is suppressed, resulting in a shortened radius. The patients have adequate support for the hand with mild radial deviation. The radius is not bowed, the elbow is not affected, the thumb and the radial carpal bones frequently are hypoplastic. Treatment in this group is confined to the thumb deficiency (Fig. 21-6).

TYPE 2: HYPOPLASTIC RADIUS. The radius has a proximal and distal epiphysis, but growth is defective in both areas (Fig. 21-7). The growth of the radius continues but at a slower rate. The forearm is short, and the ulna is thick and bowed to the radial side. The radiographic picture almost resembles a radius in miniature. It would seem appropriate that treatment would be directed toward lengthening of the radius, however, we have not found this to be effective. The distal radial epiphysis does not grow at its usual rate, shortening will recur, and additional lengthening will be necessary to produce adequate support. Repeated lengthenings usually result in progressive contracture of the already hypoplastic musculotendinous units, which usually will further compromise the limited function present in the hand.

TYPE 3: PARTIAL ABSENCE OF THE RADIUS. The radius may be partially absent in the distal, middle, or proximal third. The most frequent occurrence is the absence of the distal and middle third (Fig. 21-8). The presence of the proximal third offers some stability for the elbow. In this type, the hand is not

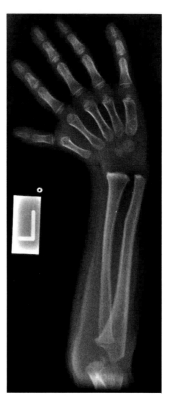

FIGURE 21-6. Type 1, the short distal radius. The distal radial epiphysis is defective. Growth rate is decreased, and a discrepancy between radial and ulnar growth occurs. This condition results in a slightly radially deviated hand.

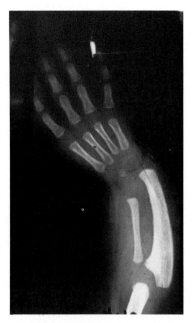

FIGURE 21-7. Type 2, the hypoplastic radius. The radius is present and has a proximal and distal epiphysis, but both are defective, resulting in a small radius that offers no support to the hand.

supported and no stability is provided to maintain good hand and finger function. Treatment is directed to supplying support for the hand.

TYPE 4: TOTAL ABSENCE OF THE RADIUS.

With total absence of the radius (TAR), the hand is completely unsupported and marked radial displacement is present (Fig. 21-9). The soft tissue contracture frequently is severe. Treatment is directed to release of the soft tissue and provide support for the hand.

Using the Bayne classification system,[17] a review of the literature shows that type 4 defects are the most common (Table 21-2). The incidence of thumb absence has been reported to range from 17% to 86%.[31,36,38,46] In their long-term review, Bayne and Klug[17]

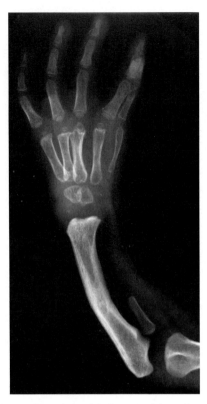

FIGURE 21-8. Type 3, partial absence of the radius. The radius is only partially present, most frequently the proximal one third, as shown here. The hand is unsupported unless it is centralized on the end of the ulna, as shown here. The end of the ulna broadens to accommodate the carpal bones.

reported that thumb absence is most likely to occur when there is complete absence of the radius (Table 21-3). Flatt noted that the TAR syndrome occurs more commonly in type 4 deficiencies when the thumb was normal.[31] In this syndrome the patient presents with thrombocytopenia along with complete absence of the radius. Absence of the thumb also implies associated deficiencies of the scaphoid and trapezium.

TABLE 21-2. *Incidence of Radial Deficiency by Type*

SERIES	*TYPE 1 (%)*	*TYPE 2 (%)*	*TYPE 3 (%)*	*TYPE 4 (%)*
Bayne	23	2	9	67
Lamb		22	3	78
Kato, 1924[35]			15	85
Manske, 1989[257]			10	90
Pardini		30	23	62
Riordan			<50	>50
Schmid			15	85

* Percentage may include lesser-involved types.
† Thirteen percent were unclassified.
Adapted from Urban MA, Ostermann AL. Management of radial dysplasia. Hand Clin 1990;6(4):589.

TABLE 21-3. *Association of Thumb Deficiencies to Radial Deficiencies*

TYPE OF RADIAL DEFICIENCIES	TYPE OF THUMB DEFICIENCIES		
	Normal	Hypoplastic	Absent
Type 1	0	20	3
Type 2	0	1	1
Type 3	0	4	5
Type 4	15	12	40
Total	15	37	49

Occurrence and Etiology

Radial deficiencies occur at a rate varying from 1 in 30,000 to 1 in 100,000 live births.[15,16,19,20] Birch-Jensen's accounts of more than 4 million people gives a more convincing incidence of 1 to 55,000 births.[19]

The etiology of radial deficiencies is still controversial. Familial cases, both with autosomal dominant and recessive inheritance patterns, have been reported.[33] These cases constitute a small number of total cases. Environmental factors, such as viral infections, chemicals, radiation, and drugs have been thought to affect the limb bud in early development. Saunders[44] study in chicks showed that damage to the superior aspect of the apical ectodermal ridge of the embryonic limb bud could produce radial aplasia. Recent studies have shown that interruption of the vascular supply to the limb bud will produce various defects depending on the timing of the vascular deprivation.[33] In humans, the critical period of limb development of the radius is between the fifth and sixth postovulatory weeks.

Associated Anomalies

Radial deficiencies rarely occur as isolated entities; often they are associated with other anomalies and syndromes. An extensive list has ben complied by Goldberg and Bartoshesky[33] (Table 21-4).

Sporadic radial defects that do not demonstrate a recognizable syndrome are not necessarily free of other malformations. Forty percent of the patients with unilateral radial clubhand and 77% of patients with bilateral radial clubhand will have associated malformations.[33] The most frequently associated anomalies and syndromes involve the cardiovascular, gastrointestinal, and genital urinary system. The most common occurrences are the Holt-Oram syndrome, in which the radial longitudinal deficiency is associated with a cardiac septal defect; Fanconi syndrome, which is associated with severe aplastic anemia; the TAR syndrome; trisomy 17; and VATER syndrome, in which a ventricular or vertebral anomaly is associated with an imperforate anus, a tracheoesophageal fistula, and renal anomalies.[25,33]

Treatment

Treatment for the radial clubhand has progressed over the years from no treatment to aggressive surgical correction. The untreated radial clubhand can perform activities of daily living without much difficulty. Surprisingly they can perform many other tasks, but not as fast or with as much precision as other normal hands. The main shortcomings of these patients with radial longitudinal deficiencies are lack of wrist stability, impaired finger function, short forearm, and absent and defective thumb. The wrist and finger motion is decreased because of the mechanical disadvantaged musculotendinous units as they pull across and acutely deviate across the wrist and from distorted intrinsic and extrinsic muscle anatomy. Grip strength is significantly limited,[21–38,46] and these patients have to compensate by using lateral pinch and cylindrical grip,[46] especially notable when missing a thumb (Fig. 21-10).

The adult patient usually has adjusted to the deformity and rarely seeks medical help. If, however, he or she has a child with a similar deformity, the parent will seek medical evaluation. After seeing the results

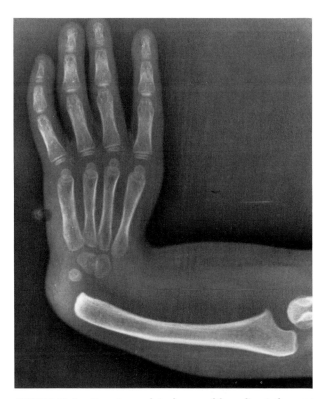

FIGURE 21-9. Type 4, complete absence of the radius, is the most common type of radial dysplasia found in our series. The hand is completely unsupported and rolls around the end of the ulna.

TABLE 21-4. *Differential Diagnosis of Congenital Deficiency of Radius and Radial Ray*

Isolated or sporadic defects	Syndromes with Vertebral Anomalies
Syndromes with blood dyscrasias	VATER association
Fanconi pancytopenia syndrome	1. Complete
Thrombocytopenia–absent radius syndrome	2. Partial-imperforate anus and radial defect
Hypoplastic anemia–triphalangeal thumb syndrome	Cervical rib
Syndromes with congenital heart disease	Klippel-Feil syndrome
Holt-Oram syndrome	Keutel syndrome (costovertebral dysplasia and humero-
Lewis upper limb syndrome	radial synostosis
Syndromes with craniofacial abnormalities	Syndromes with chromosomal abnormalities
Nager acrofacial dystostosis	Trisomy 18
Cleft lip or plate	Deletion and ring chromosomes (D and B)
Radial defect with orofacial malformation	Mental retardation syndromes
Craniosynostosis with radial defects	Seckel syndrome
Duane (eye) radial dysplasia syndrome	Cornelia de Lange syndrome
Laryngeal web and atresia	Teratogenic Syndromes
Hemifacial microsomia	Thalidomide embryopathy
Goldenhar syndrome (oculoauricularvertebral dys-	Aminopterin-induced syndrome
plasia)	Varicella embryopathy
Hanhart micrognathia and limb anomalies	
Juberg-Hayward (orocraniodigital) syndrome	
Levy-Hollister (lacrimoauriculoradiodental) syndrome	

From Goldberg MJ, Bartoshesky LE. Congenital hand anomalies: etiology and associated malformations. Hand Clin 1985;1:405.

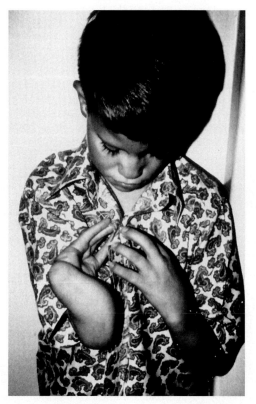

FIGURE 21-10. A young boy with uncorrected bilateral radial longitudinal deficiencies.

that can be obtained, parents usually wish they had chosen surgical management. (Fig. 21-11).

The surgical treatment of the radial clubhand has progressed through the years with its main concern to restore loss of function produced by the deformity. The lack of support of the wrist and hand attracted the attention of most of the early surgeons, starting with Petit in 1733.[41] He felt that by stabilizing the hand, the flexors and the extensors of the fingers could be more effective.

Bone grafts were used by Albee[14] to support the carpus, fixing the proximal end of the bone graft to the ulna in a Y-shaped configuration. Proximal fibular transplants were used by Starr[48] and later by Entin[30] and Riordan[43] to support the carpus. The bone grafts did not grow, and the support to the carpus was soon lost. The fibular physis remained opened for a short time but closed quickly and could not keep up with the growth of the ulna, and the deformity recurred.[40]

Fusion of the wrist is not practical in young children because further shortening of an already shortened forearm is not desirable. Centralization of the carpus over the end of the ulna has become the method of choice because it offers stability of the wrist, which can increase the strength and function of the fingers, allow for growth, and still maintain mobility of the wrist. Centralization has undergone several modifications.

Riordan[43] and others have described placing the carpus over the end of the ulna by releasing the con-

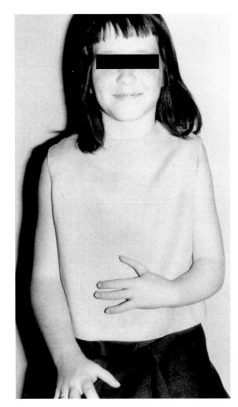

FIGURE 21-11.   This patient's unilateral radial deficiency was centralized at age 3 years. The index finger was pollicized 6 months later. At age 7 years, the appearance and function of the hand are improved.

stricting soft tissue attached to the carpus, then creating a joint by placing the carpus over the flattened end of the ulna, and securing this position with a capsular repair and intermedullary pinning (Fig. 21-12).

This held up well provided splinting was continued to skeletal maturity and soft tissue contracture was not allowed to recur.

Lamb,[38] Lidge,[39] and others[40–45] preferred to notch the carpus by resecting the central carpus and placing the end of the ulna in the notch. This gave good stability to the wrist and helped prevent recurrence of the deformity. The drawback to this method was the decrease in growth of the distal ulna and the limitation of wrist motion. Wrist motion of at least 30 degrees was found to increase overall use of the extremity compared with the patients with stiff wrists. This was observed in our 20-year review of more than 100 extremities.[17]

Lengthening of the radius in patients with hypoplastic type 2 radial deficiencies, where the radius has a proximal and a distal epiphysis but is hypoplastic, has been performed with varied results. The procedure would only be used in type 2 patients who are near skeletal maturity. In young patients, repeated lengthening of the radius would be required to keep up with the ulnar growth. This has not been found effective in improving the function of these patients, and as earlier stated, repeated lengthenings compromises an already hypoplastic musculotendinous unit, which results in further soft tissue contractures. Epiphyseal stapling of the wrist has been advocated in some type 1 and type 2 patients. Results depend on accurate timing of the epiphysiodesis. Stapling has the disadvantage of further shortening the forearm, although this can be effective treatment when there is minimal shortening of the radius.

Kessler[37] has used his skeletal lengthening device to stretch the soft tissues and reduce the hand and carpus over the end of the ulna before percutaneously

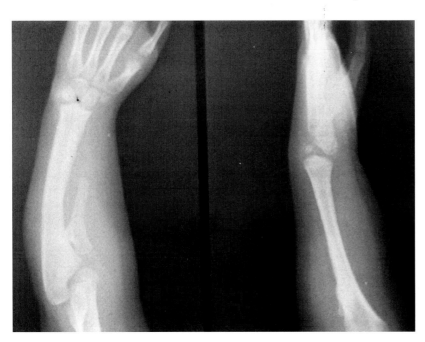

FIGURE 21-12.   This radiograph shows Riordan's method of centralization. The hand is well-placed. The end of the ulna broadens with continued growth, and wrist motion is maintained.

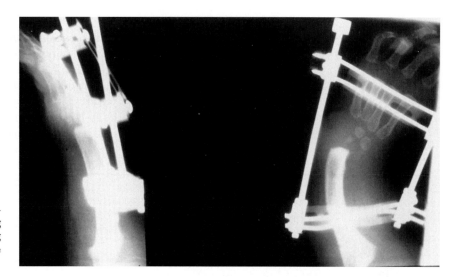

FIGURE 21-13. This radiograph demonstrates Kessler's method of reducing the hand over the end of the ulna by using an external skeletal device to stretch the soft tissues.

pinning the hand and carpus to the ulna with an intramedullary pin. He holds this for a number of months, removes the pin, and provides stability to the hand by continued bracing. This has a disadvantage of not creating a reconstructed capsule joint or providing dynamic balance of the hand over the ulna. The hand position is only maintained by continued splinting. However, preliminary soft tissue stretching with the use of an external fixator has been successful in allowing soft tissue stretching, which then eases the definitive centralization procedure that must be completed at the second operation (Fig. 21-13).

Radialization was devised by Buck-Gramcko.[24] This procedure evolved from the fact that although there were various methods of centralization in current use, recurrences of the deformity were too common. By shifting the hand to the ulnar side of the distal ulna and placing the second metacarpal and scaphoid over the end of the ulna Buck-Gramcko believed that this would create a longer lever arm on the ulnar side. Transferring the extensor carpi radialis and the flexor carpi radialis to the ulnar side of the wrist would balance the hand more effectively (Fig. 21-14). Although his series showed successful results in correcting the deformity, balancing of the muscles can be difficult and zealous tendon transfer may even cause overcorrection toward the ulnar side, which may increase the pressures on the ulnar epiphysis resulting in growth disturbance. Clinically, however, the hand may remain in a better corrected position, improving function.

Problems With Centralization

Recurrent deformity is the most common problem with centralization. Often correction is good initially, but as time passes the deformity recurs. In re-

viewing our cases, we have found several causative factors: inadequate centralization, increased curvature of the distal ulna, inadequate muscle balance, failure to correct initial ulnar bowing greater than 30 degrees, and failure to comply with splinting.[17]

Inadequate centralization is the failure to align the third metacarpal and scaphoid over the center of the ulna. If this is not carried out then the wrist cannot be balanced on the end of the ulna and will be pulled off to the radial side. Figure 21-15 shows the end result of an inadequate centralization of the central carpus over the end of the ulna in which tendon transfer cannot balance the hand resulting in recurrent deformity.

When there is more pressure or tension force on the radial side of the ulna the bone growth follows

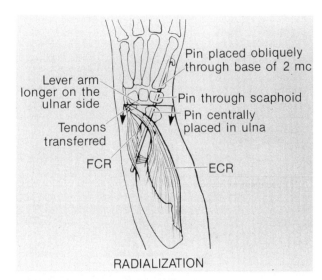

FIGURE 21-14. Buck-Gramcko's method of radialization. The flow carpi radialis (FCR) and exterior carpi radialis (ECR) are transferred to the ulnar side of the wrist to better balance the hand on the end of the ulna.

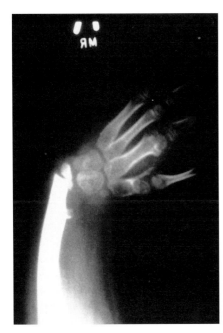

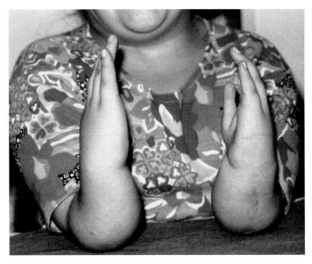

FIGURE 21-17. Patient with bilateral radial defects postcentralization with short forearms.

FIGURE 21-15. Radiograph demonstrating inadequate centralization. The central carpus was not reduced over the end of the ulna. Tendon transfer cannot balance the hand, and the deformity soon will recur.

Wolfe's law and bows to the radial side, causing a recurrence of the deformity. The hand may be well centralized initially, but if the hand is not balanced by adequate tendon transfer on the end of the ulna, the stronger, radially placed muscles will displace the hand. We also found that when initial correction was performed, if the ulna was bowed more than 30 degrees, it was very difficult to balance the hand on the end of the ulna despite tendon transfers.[17] A corrective osteotomy at the time of initial surgery is necessary (Fig. 21-16). When there was poor splint compliance following surgery recurrence of deformity occurred more frequently.[17]

The second problem of centralization was short forearms. In our review, even the patients that had maintained a good correction and were pleased with their results had only one wish: that their forearms could be longer. This presents a real problem with treatment of radial clubhand because ulnar shortening is present even in the untreated patient (Fig. 21-17). Ulnar shortening also can be caused by surgical intervention. Inadequate soft tissue release followed by centralization causes too much pressure on the epiphyseal plate. Interruption of the blood supply to the epiphysis can produce even further shortening of the ulna.

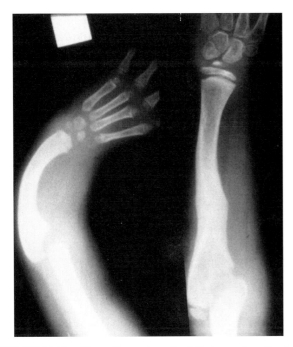

FIGURE 21-16. The radiograph on the left shows ulnar bowing greater than 30 degrees, necessitating an osteotomy to correct the radial angulation. This allows the tendon transfer to help maintain the correction. On the right is the postoperative radiograph 1 year following therapy procedure.

Benefits of Centralization

The advantages of centralization include improved appearance of the hand, an increase in prehensile activities involving the digits, a greater ability to perform more activities, and increased desire to use the hand. Centralization also allows motion of the wrist, which is important to the use of the hand. Centralization of the hand on the end of the ulna allows a pollicization if the index finger to be performed if the patient has a hypoplastic thumb, and this greatly enhances the use of the hand (Fig. 21-18).

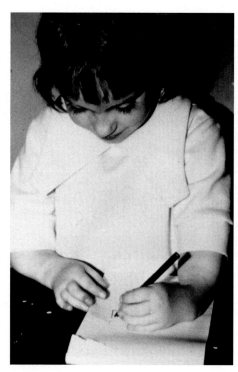

FIGURE 21-18. This patient has had both hands centralized. The cosmetic appearance and the function have been enhanced greatly.

Selection of Patients

Long-term follow-up on patients treated for radial longitudinal deficiencies supports the impression that patients younger than 3 years of age at the time of correction maintain better hand position than patients initially treated at an older age. The primary reason is that in the older patient the soft tissue was more resistant to correction, requiring in some cases an ulnar shortening to reduce the hand over the end of the ulna. The need for more secondary corrective procedures also was present in this subgroup. The patients who had normal fingers and thumb function performed much better than patients with stiff fingers; those patients treated with a pollicization for an absent or unreconstructable hypoplastic thumb showed increased improvement in their prehensile activities.

Patients with severe systemic diseases that are that are not compatible with life, such as Fanconi anemia, are not good candidates for surgery. The same is true for patients with severe digital contractures because they are not improved appreciably because of limited use of the fingers. Patients with elbow extension contractures can be made worse by centralization of the hand because they use the radial deviation of the hand to reach the mouth and take care of their activities of daily living. Those patients with marked webbing of the elbow remain poor candidates for surgery because the shortened neurovascular bundles that usually ac-

company the webbing preclude adequate correction. Recent literature has supported the use of an external fixator for preoperative soft tissue stretching; however, long-term follow-up is needed to recommend its use in the patient with a radial longitudinal deficiency associated with marked webbing of the elbow. The limiting factor is the significantly shortened neurovascular bundles.[37]

Current Treatment

Initial treatment of a patient presenting with a radial longitudinal deficiency at birth begins with serial casting to correct the radial deviation. As already stated, patients with this deformity often have accompanying systemic involvement as a result of the similar embryologic development of other organs. Hematologic and cardiac abnormalities can be seen and must be ruled out. Preoperative evaluation avoids catastrophic intraoperative complications. Once correction of the radial deviation is achieved, usually after 2 to 3 months, an orthoplast splint is fabricated to hold the correction. The definitive surgical centralization usually is performed between 6 months and 1 year of age. Surgical attention to the abnormal radial muscle, the tendons, and the neurovascular structures and thorough understanding of the pathologic anatomy is necessary to avoid inadvertent surgical damage to these anomalous and aberrant structures. Successful surgical centralization is predicated on proper preoperative splinting, stretching, and tendon transfers to help balance the hand on the end of the ulna to maintain the correction. Osteotomy of the ulna is indicated when the bowing is greater than 30 degrees. Thumb reconstruction is helpful in patients with absent or hypoplastic thumbs, and pollicization of the index finger remains the method of choice.

Patients 1 to 3 years of age who first present with the radial longitudinal deficiency usually require an external fixator to stretch the tight radial structures because casting in this age group has been found unsatisfactory. Preoperative stretching greatly enhances the ability to surgically centralize the hand[37] (Fig. 21-19).

Recurrent Deformities

Patients who have undergone centralization and present with early recurrence of their deformity usually require recentralization. The failure often is the result of inadequate release of the tight radial structures or inadequate tendon transfer to maintain the corrected hand on the ulna. In patients who have not reached skeletal maturity and in whom the position of the hand is suboptimal as a result of marked ulnar

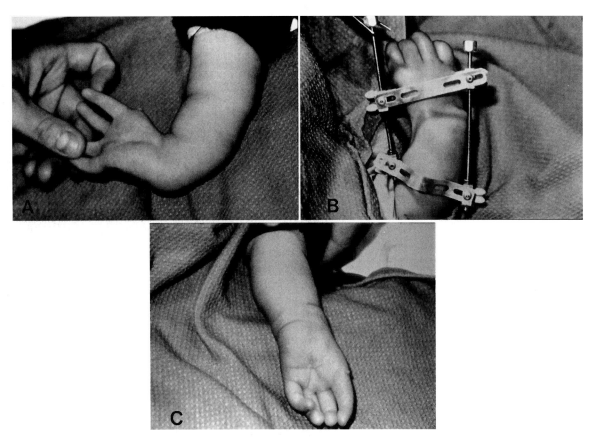

FIGURE 21-19. (A) 1.5-year-old patient had a tight radial contracture. (B) A Kessler-type external skeletal apparatus was used to stretch the soft tissues and reduce the hand over the end of the ulna. (C) Postcentralization, the patient demonstrates good hand position.

bowing, a corrective osteotomy is indicated. Rarely, in patients nearing skeletal maturity, corrective osteotomy may be all that is necessary; however, most of these patients demonstrate severe soft tissue contracture with marked shortening of the ulna and should be treated with gradual skeletal lengthening with simultaneous correction of the angulation (Fig. 21-20).

Skeletal lengthening in the skeletally immature patient does not work well; early recurrence of the deformity is common as a result of soft tissue contracture and the amount of possible progressive bony growth remaining. Therefore, skeletal lengthening in radial longitudinal deficiencies is best indicated in the skeletally mature patient. Problems, however, with progressive digital contractures, associated pin tract problems, and the still relatively high complication rate of injury to closely approximated neurovascular structures still make this form of treatment preliminary in reporting its long-term success.[37] New methods of treating radial dysplasia, either by use of a vascularized fibula epiphyseal transfer or gradual distraction lengthening using an external fixator, still deserve further investigation.[51-56]

Carpal Deformities

After the proximal forearm, the next most common level of terminal transverse absence is at the carpal level. Appearance is characterized by vestigial remnants of the digits that neither grow nor have any functional benefit. Both the remaining bones in the forearm may appear normal, but in general they do not reach the same length as the opposite normal side. Surgical reconstructive procedures at this level are not useful. It is particularly important to remember that valuable sensation is lost when the residual limb is enclosed by a prosthesis.[6] A number of adaptive aids that preserve sensation and increase function may be provided but are rarely used whether the deficiency is unilateral or bilateral.

Metacarpophalangeal Deformities

Deficiencies at the metacarpal phalangeal level range from functioning hypoplastic digits to a vestigial remnant of soft tissue only. These deficiencies occur with similar frequency in all digits. The lack of motion and stability of these digits contributes to the func-

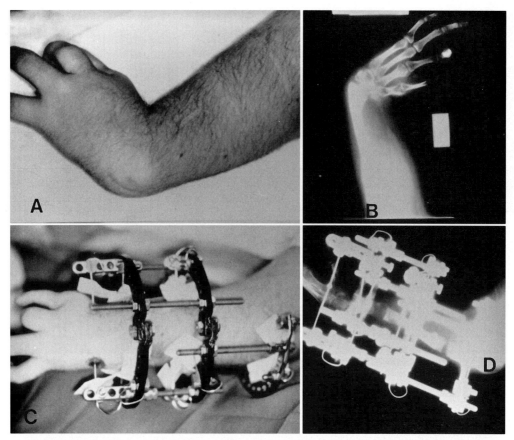

FIGURE 21-20. **(A)** An older patient had recurrent deformity who has reached skeletal maturity. **(B)** Radiograph shows wrist ulna position satisfactory. The end of the ulna is angulated radially. **(C)** Iliazarov skeletal lengthening apparatus is used to stretch the soft tissue and correct the osteotomized distal ulna angulation. **(D)** The ulna was osteotomized proximally, and further lengthening of the ulna was carried out.

tional deficit seen. Treatment is directed toward restoring length to the bony columns and stability to the ligamentous structures to optimize prehensile function. If the digit has the potential to be one third of the normal length then reconstruction is indicated. This can be accomplished in several ways. First, web space deepening may increase the relative length of the present digit. Also, bone grafting, either nonvascular or vascular transfer, such as the toe-to-finger phalanx transfer,[5,8–10] will increase bony length. Gradual distraction-lengthening most recently has proved successful in increasing bony length, and although surgical goals are limited the improvement in length definitely improves pinching, grasping, and other prehensile activities.[5,8–10]

Longitudinal Deficiencies

Intersegmental Deficiencies, or Phocomelia

The intercalary absence of the humerus may be partial or complete. Partial absence of the humerus, although rare, usually occurs in the proximal end and is associated with radial absence distally. A tendency toward weakness of the muscle control of the shoulder is present, but normal elevation is limited and shoulder motion is of little or any functional benefit.

In complete absence of the humerus (i.e., phocomelia), the forearm and hand may project from the shoulder level. The word phocas comes from the word seal, dramatically describing the shortened limb found in this condition. They may appear normal, but the forearm bones frequently are short and deficient in either radial or ulnar components (Fig. 21-21). There also may be associated multiple anomalies of the hand. The deformity was common during the 1950s and 1960s, affecting 60% of infants born to mothers who had taken thalidomide during the first trimester of their pregnancy. Currently, however, these cases tend to occur only sporadically. The incidence of phocomelia is 0.8% of all congenital upper limb abnormalities.

The biggest problem with intersegmental deficiency of the humerus is the functional loss resulting from shortness of the limb, particularly if it is bilateral. At an early age the child's hands, which frequently appear to have some use or function, are able to meet

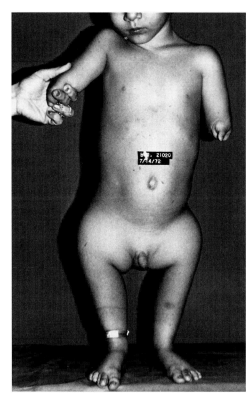

FIGURE 21-21. Bilateral phocomelia. The forearm is absent and the hand, although hypoplastic, is attached to the upper arm.

the mouth and face and may be able to join across the front of the body. As the body size increases the limbs do not grow proportionally. Therefore the ability to reach the face or clasp the other hand in front of the body may be lost.

Phocomelia has been classified into three anatomic types. The first is complete absence of all bones proximal to the hand; the hand is directly attached to the trunk. In the second type, there is absence or extreme hypoplasia of all proximal limb bones so that the hand is attached to a shortened synostosed arm-forearm segment. In the third type the hand attaches directly to the humerus.

Phocomelia can be associated with other congenital defects as well as other syndromes. Clinically they are associated with cleft palate, scoliosis, and Holt-Oram syndrome.[13] Cardiac and musculoskeletal abnormalities are commonly associated because of the development of these structures at the same time in the embryo.

TREATMENT. The goal of treatment is to improve self-care activities that enable the person to be as independent as possible. The shortness of limbs makes activities of daily living increasingly difficult, particularly as the child grows older. Various aids and clothing adjustments can be made by the occupational therapist to help make these children independent,

however, the use of a prosthesis, although theoretically would seem to facilitate the use of a foreshortened limb, in reality is usually rejected by the patient. The adaptive ability of the young child with this deficiency is incredible, and often these individuals become extremely proficient in using both their feet to help with activities of daily living.

There are few indications, therefore, for surgery in phocomelia. In general the management is directed toward correcting any deformity in the arm if that will improve the function of the hand. This may be accomplished by standard web space reconstructions, osteotomies, and tendon transfers to improve digital function. Osteotomy for correction of angulation or distraction lengthening to facilitate bringing one digit into opposition with the other may facilitate activities of daily living. Surgical reconstruction is again directed toward optimization of the deficient hand often present in the phocomelic patient.[2,12]

Central Deficiencies

CLINICAL FEATURES. The terms *central deficiencies, split hand, lobster claw, ectrodactyly,* and *central hypoplasia* all are used to describe cleft hand.[57,59,66,67] The incidence ranges from 0.4 to 0.14 in 10,000 births. The cleft hand usually appears bilaterally, and of those affected, about 60% are boys[79] (Fig. 21-22).

Central deficiencies may be classified into two patterns: typical and atypical.[71] The International Federation of Societies for Surgery of the Hand in 1992 adopted a change to this classification, in which the cleft hand remains *cleft hand*, and the atypical central defect is renamed *symbrachydactyly*. The difference between the two categories was clarified by Buck-

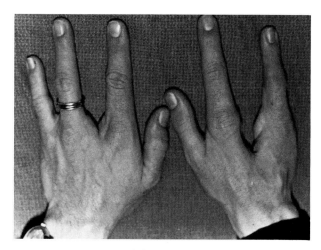

FIGURE 21-22. Central deficiency of the left hand shows absence of the long finger with a minimal cleft. The right hand shows absence of the long and ring fingers with a much deeper cleft.

Gramcko.[60] In true cleft hand there may be malpositioned bones but never rudimentary phalangeal bones or nails.

INHERITANCE.   The cleft hand pattern of central deficiency appears to be more common and is inherited as an autosomal dominant trait.[77] The symbrachydactyly form is sporadic and has no genetic pattern of inheritance.[61] A number of etiologies for the typical cleft hand and symbrachydactyly have been proposed. Although the exact mechanism that produces these defects remains unknown, all seem to share hypoplasia of the apical ectodermal ridge and centripetal suppression of the developing hand plate at approximately 7 weeks of gestation.[71]

ASSOCIATED ANOMALIES.   The most frequently associated anomalies are cleft foot, cleft lip, and cleft palate.[57,70,72,73] The other associations are congenital heart disease, imperforate anus, radial ulnar synostosis, and ectodermal dysplasia.

ANATOMIC PATHOLOGY.   A wide array of anatomic pathologic conditions are present in children with cleft deformities, ranging from central hypoplasia or absence to large central cleft defects with associated syndactyly, carpal coalescence, and multiple metacarpal abnormalities. Syndactyly is closely associated with the cleft hand because of the failure of longitudinal formation of parts.[72,73]

TREATMENT.   In the typical cleft deformity, treatment is directed toward increasing prehension by opposition of the radial and ulnar components. This is achieved by release of the syndactyly in a standard fashion and closing of the cleft in several described methods.[67–69,71,74,75,76,78] It may be necessary to do a ray transfer or rotational angular osteotomy in order to position the digits correctly for function.

If syndactyly is present, it is usually released at the age of 6 months and then closure of the cleft 6 to 12 months later.

In the symbrachydactyly hand, surgery may be of little cosmetic or functional benefit. Often there are so many crossed bones and abnormal soft tissues that the function of the hand is already greatly compromised. Vestigial skin remnants should be removed because they are unstable and may compromise the grasping of the border digits. If the border digits are supple, rotational osteotomies and tendon transfers may be helpful in restoring opposition pinch. In the severe form of a one-digit hand, microvascular or nonvascular toe-to-hand transfers may elongate the bony post and improve opposition for the significantly compromised patient. The existence of even a single bony post, although primitive, will allow the patient to oppose this against the ulnar border of the hand, greatly facilitating pinch and other prehensile activities.

Ulnar Deficiencies

Ulnar clubhand is a convenient label for deficiencies occurring along the ulnar or postaxial border of the upper extremities. The variety of malformations seen in this deficiency are greater than those seen in the radial longitudinal deficiencies. Ulnar deficiencies have a low incidence[83] when compared with other congenital deformities. The ratio of ulnar to radial deficiencies varies from 1 to 4.5 in Flatt's series[88] to the more often quoted ratio of 1 to 10.[71] The male-to-female ratio in deficiency is 3:2 with 25% of the cases being bilateral.[57,59,71]

CLINICAL FEATURES.   The deformity is characterized by ectodactyly, or shortened digits in varying degrees, ulnar deviation of the hand, forearm shortening and bowing, defective elbow motion, and hypoplasia of the humeral segment.[31] Elbow abnormalities are common, including ankylosis of the ulnohumeral joint and dislocation of the radial head. The wrist is abnormal because of the absent ulna, and there is ulnar deviation of the hand of varying degrees, most commonly approximating 30 degrees. Carpal anomalies and fusions are frequently present.[84,96]

In most cases the forearm is shortened, with the radius being shorter than normal and bowed with its concavity toward the ulnar side. Ulnar deviation of the hand is associated with the altered growth of the ulnar side of the distal radial epiphysis. The thumb and index finger may be normal, but the small, ring, and long fingers are frequently abnormal or absent. There may be a wide variation in ectodactyly that is present.[87] Syndactyly is common between the digits that are present as well as stiffness of the digits.

ASSOCIATED ANOMALIES.   Almost half of the patients with ulnar deficiencies insufficiencies have associated defects of the musculoskeletal system.[103] However, unlike radial clubhand, ulnar deficiencies are not related to anomalies of the cardiopulmonary, gastrointestinal, hematopoietic, or genitourinary system. No chromosomal abnormalities have been reported to be associated with ulnar clubhand.[94]

Most reported cases appear to be sporadic and not inherited. There have been no teratogenic factors associated with this abnormality.[86] The existence of the ulnar clubhand with many other syndromes, such as Miller-Pallister, Pillay, Schnizel, Weyars, Reinhardt-Pheiffer, and Langer syndromes and mesomelic dwarfism have been described.[95] One of the most common associated syndromes with ulnar deficiency is the Cornelia de Lange syndrome.[87] This syndrome involves severe mental retardation, a characteristic facies, along with the ulnar longitudinal deficiency.[87] Associated musculoskeletal problems often include clubfoot, spina bifida, mandibular defects, fibular defects, femoral agenesis, and absent patella.[97] The most common associated anomaly is proximal femoral focal deficiency.[103]

CLASSIFICATION. A number of classifications have been proposed.[91,92,95,97] Bayne's[81] classification uses the features that assist in treatment.

Type 1. In hypoplasia of the ulna, both the proximal and the distal ulnar epiphyses are present but growth is suppressed.[37] Because the distal ulnar epiphysis is present there is no fibrous anlage in the ulna. Radial bowing is minimal and generally does not increase with time.

Ulnar deviation of the hand is mild, related only to the minor involvement of the ulnar growth plates. Hand deficiencies do not mirror the involvement of the ulna and may vary from complete absence of digits to only mild hypoplasia of the ulnar digits (Fig. 21-23).

Type 2. Type 2 is the most common form of ulnar deficiency. In this type, an ulnar anlage is present that replaces the distal bony end of the ulna. The radius

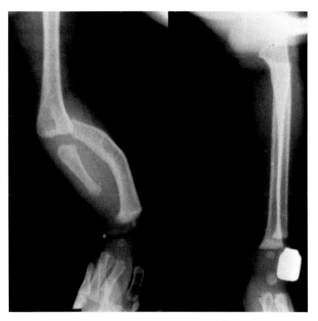

FIGURE 21-24. Type 2, partial absence of the ulna, the most common type in our series.

is bowed, the radial head may be dislocated laterally or posteriorly, and the distal epiphysis is sloped to the ulnar side. The hand is deviated in an ulnar direction with varying degrees of hypoplasia involving the ulnar-sided digits.

The anlage has very poor potential for longitudinal growth, thereby tethering the radius and causing progressive bowing. As the extremity grows, the radial head may become dislocated and interfere with elbow and forearm motion[85] (Fig. 21-24).

Type 3. This type is rare; the ulna is completely absent, and no anlage is present. The radius is usually straight, and the hand is not deviated. Severe deformities in both the carpus and the hand are usually present. The elbow is unstable because of the absence of the ulna, and the head of the radius may be dislocated (Fig. 21-25).

Diagnosis of the type 3 deficiency should be reserved until approximately 1 year of age because the proximal portion of the ulna may not ossify until that time.

Type 4. The proximal radius is fused to the humerus and a small portion of the olecranon also may be fused to the humerus. Although the ulna is completely absent, an anlage usually attaches to the distal radial epiphysis. Severe radial bowing occurs, and ulnar deviation of the hand is present. As with all other types described, there are severe hand anomalies present (Fig. 21-26).

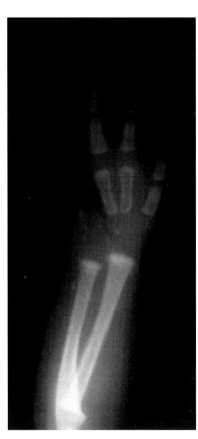

FIGURE 21-23. Type 1, hypoplasia of the ulna with digital deficiencies.

TREATMENT. As always, the fundamental question that should be asked is whether surgery offers an

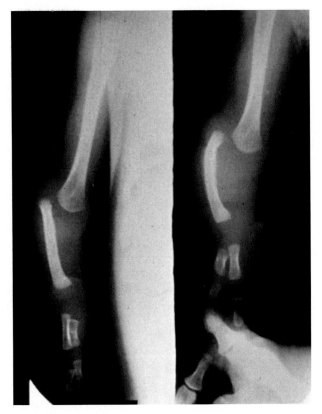

FIGURE 21-25.   Type 3, complete absence of the ulna. This type is rare. The ulnar anlage is absent; the radius is straight but usually displaced proximally.

improvement in the patient's function or merely an improvement in the appearance. The primary goal must always remain improvement in function. Very often a deformed upper extremity will function well and should be left alone. Any attempts to improve the

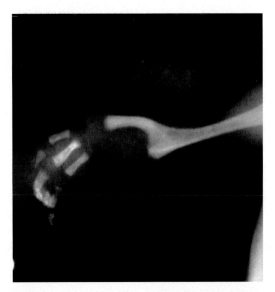

FIGURE 21-26.   Type 4, radiohumeral fusion. The anlage usually is present tethering the hand. The deficiencies in the hand are most prominent.

cosmetic appearance may severely compromise the limited amount of function present. Many authors have concluded that despite a deformed limb, the patient's function with the ulnar longitudinal deficiency is exceedingly good, and minimal surgical intervention is necessary.

If an individual merits surgical intervention based on his or her limitation of function, forearm problems should be dealt with first and the hand anomalies at a later time. When considering the forearm, two problems that surface are the fibrous anlage and the instability of the forearm.[87]

The anlage is present only in type 2 and type 4 ulnar longitudinal deficiencies. The anlage, composed of inelastic fibrocartilage, has poor potential for longitudinal growth.[97] It arises from the ulnar aspect of the humerus or the primary ossification center of the proximal ulnar remnant and inserts on the ulnar side of the carpus, the ulnar side of the distal radial epiphysis, or both. Although not universally accepted, some physicians believe that as growth of the radius proceeds, the unyielding anlage causes progressive bowing of the radius, ulnar tilting of the distal radial epiphysis, proximal migration of the radial head, and ulnar deviation of the hand. Therefore, a logical assumption is to consider excision of the anlage before these secondary deformities occur. Ogden and colleagues,[96] Riordan,[99] Bayne,[81] and others recommend excision of the anlage as early as 6 months of age. Johnson and Omer,[90] Blair and colleagues,[82] Broudy and Smith and colleagues[84] believe that the ulnar anlage does not alone cause the deformities and that excision of it does not significantly affect the development of the deformities. They report that the functional result of nonresection of the anlage is often excellent. A compromise has been proposed by Johnson and Omer[90] that may resolve this controversy. He believes that if ulnar deviation at the wrist is greater than 30 degrees for more than 6 months consideration for resection of the ulnar anlage can be considered. The physician should wait to see both clinical and radiographic evidence that the deformity is occurring before embarking on surgery.

Forearm instability is another problem to be considered in this deficiency. When one of the two bones in the forearm is short or absent there is the potential for instability of the forearm during pronation-supination. Approximately two thirds of these patients have the type 2 deficiency, in which the proximal portion of the ulna will ossify, thereby providing reasonable stability for the elbow and forearm during pronation-supination.

The advantages and disadvantages of fusing the distal radius to the proximal ulna to create a single bone forearm should be carefully weighed in light of the loss of pronation and supination versus the need to gain more stability at the elbow.[93] Evaluation of the opposite extremity as well in association with possible associated anomalies will help in this decision.

Much of the dysfunction in the ulnar clubhand is related to the ectrodactyly, syndactyly, hypoplasia, and malrotation of the hand. This inhibits prehension and dexterity, thereby causing hand weakness. Deformities of the hand and wrist area contribute more to the functional loss of the patient than forearm and elbow deformities. Little controversy exists regarding care of the hand anomalies. Standard techniques for web space deepening, syndactyly release, metacarpal rotational osteotomies, pollicization, and tendon transfers are appropriate measures to improve function of the extremity.

In the infant younger than 6 weeks of age, the decision for treatment is usually easy regardless of the type of deficiency present. The early treatment should be directed toward correction of the ulnar deviation of the hand with serial casting. It is recommended that the cast be applied in pieces, doing the hand and forearm first and then connecting the elbow and upper arm next. These casts need to be changed repeatedly to accommodate growth and skin care. The use of orthoplast splints as the child gets older may facilitate hygiene and allow some time out of the splint to explore their new universe. The down side is the expense of new splints as the arm grows.

When dealing with type 1 or type 3 deficiencies, correction of the hand is easy because of a lack of the ulnar anlage. Soft tissues generally yield to appropriately applied corrective casts. Once the corrected position is obtained, night and nap splints may be applied to preserve the position.

In types 2 and 4, nothing is lost by early casting or splinting, but awareness of the tendency for angulation should be in the surgeons' minds. While maintaining the patient in the splint, the difficult decision of excising the anlage can be weighed depending on how the patient responds to the splinting. If there is increasing resistance to correction, increased bowing of the radius, or dislocation of the radial head the decision may be easier.

If it is apparent that there is tethering along the ulnar side, the decision to excise the anlage may be made as early as 6 months of age. The distal half to two thirds of the anlage should be excised. It is important to ensure that sufficient release along the ulnar side of the carpus is performed in order to allow proper positioning of the hand on the distal radial articular surface. If the radial head is in its proper relation with the humerus no attempt to create a one-bone forearm is made. It is important to ensure that sufficient release along the ulnar side of the carpus is done in order to allow proper positioning of the hand on the distal radial articular surface.

The patient is maintained in an above-elbow plaster cast for 6 weeks followed by an orthoplast brace.

If syndactyly is present between the digits, it is usually corrected at this operation.

When the patient is seen for the first time, between 6 to 18 months of age, types 1 and 3 are treated with splinting if deviation of the wrist warrants this approach. If type 2 or 4 deficiency is present, splinting is still appropriate as an initial step, but experience would suggest that there is a significant resistance to correction of the deformity that is present. If there is already significant deformity present and the indications are met for anlage excision as earlier described, then this can be performed and the surgical technique here is the same as for the younger patient.

If the radial head is already dislocated, radial head excision should be indicated, especially if there is limited active or passive pronation and supination. Because of the instability that may be caused by the radial head excision, creation of a one-bone forearm is easier. However, if there is adequate forearm rotation present, along with the radial head dislocation, then retaining the radial head will give stability to the elbow and even though parents may wish for its excision for cosmetic purposes, this should not be done. Prolonged observation, however, may determine that increased stability gained by a one-bone forearm will be advantageous even at the loss of forearm rotation.

In the few patients with type 4 fusion of the radius to the humerus, excision of the fibrocartilaginous anlage will be necessary. If left, its inelastic nature will impede longitudinal growth and increase ulnar deviation. If the deformity is bilateral this may be severely debilitating because of the inability to reach the mouth. If radiohumeral fusion is combined with rotational deformity of the humerus then surgical correction is necessary. The aim of the operation is to rotate the hand in front of the body, flex the elbow between 60 and 90 degrees, and place the hand midway between pronation and supination. Both of these procedures are done at the point of the ankylosis so that both deformities are corrected at one site. Attention should be given to the neurovascular bundle because rotation and flexion can cause compromise of the vascular structures of the forearm as they pass from posterior to anterior. It often is necessary to consider resection of the bone in order to allow relaxation of the neurovascular bundle.

FAILURE OF DIFFERENTIATION OR SEPARATION OF PARTS

Synostosis

Clinical Features

Synostosis may occur in the upper limb in any place where two bones are adjacent to each other; it may be partial or complete in the transverse or

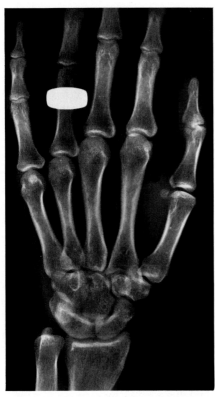

FIGURE 21-27. Example of common carpal synostosis. The lunate and triquetrum are united.

longitudinal plane.[111] Transverse synostosis of the digits is relatively common and known as *complex syndactyly.* Longitudinal synostosis between phalanges is called *symphalangism.*

Transverse synostosis between metacarpals is far less common than longitudinal synostosis. It often involves the ring and little fingers. Approximately 60% to 70% of cases are bilateral.

In the carpal area, a multiplicity of synostoses have been described.[118] The most common fusion is between the lunate and the triquetrum, with the capitate-hamate fusion being the second most common (Fig. 21-27). The incidence of carpal synostosis is 10 times greater in African Americans than in Caucasians.

Synostosis between the radius and ulna occurs in the proximal end of the forearm. Although it is present at birth, it usually is not discovered until early adolescence, when the patient presents with lack of prona-

tion and supination. Initially, it may be more of a synchondrosis, but later the osseous bridge becomes apparent between the radius and the ulna. A large synostosis frequently is accompanied by absence of brachioradialis, pronator teres, pronator quadratus, and supinator muscles. Two types of synostosis are related to the proximal radial and the ulnar junction. Type 1 radioulnar synostosis is complete synostosis, with the radius and ulna fused at their proximal borders for variable distance (Fig. 21-28). Type 2 radioulnar synostosis is a less involved synostosis, which may be only partial; it is just distal to the proximal radial epiphysis and is associated with dislocation of the radial head (Fig. 21-29).

The function of the arm in radioulnar synostosis depends on the severity of the deformity and whether or not it is bilateral. With severe fixed pronation deformity of the forearm, the patient cannot compensate by scapular and glenohumeral motion. In the younger child, activities that would require supination, such as catching a ball, bring this to the parents attention. In the older child, activities requiring supination, such as receiving change, call attention to the problem (Fig. 21-30). The genders are affected equally, and 60% have a bilateral involvement.[113]

At the elbow level, a humeroradioulnar synostosis rarely is seen. Additionally, a synostosis may exist between the humerus and only one of the forearm bones, usually the radius.[111] This can result in considerable shortening of the upper extremity as a result of both the loss of growth attributable to the physes and an inherent congenital shortening.

Inheritance

No specific pattern of inheritance for synostosis of the upper extremity is apparent.[106] As in some cases of phalangeal synostosis, upper extremity synostosis may be autosomal dominant.[119]

Associated Anomalies

Anomalies associated with digital synostosis are numerous and listed in the section under complex syndactyly. Carpal fusions are seen in association with failure of formation in both the upper and lower ex

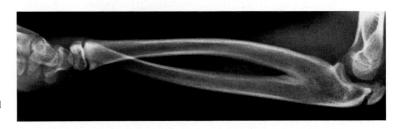

FIGURE 21-28. Type 1 synostosis. The radius and the ulna are fused at their proximal borders.

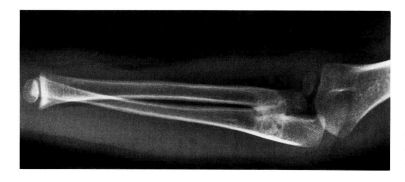

FIGURE 21-29.   Type 2, radioulnar synostosis. The radius and ulna are fused distal to the proximal radial epiphysis.

tremities. These fusions may be manifested as radial, central, and ulnar deficiencies; brachiosyndactyly; and camptodactyly. Many syndromes are associated with carpal fusion. Radioulnar synostosis has been reported primarily in association with general skeletal abnormalities, such as dislocation of the hip, clubfoot, and preaxial dysmelias. It also may be associated with a variety of syndromes, including acrocephalosyndactyly and chromosomal aberrations (XXXY).[109] Humeroradioulnar synostosis seldom is seen without association of other skeletal abnormalities. Although many synostoses occur alone, the presence of any synostosis should alert the examiner to the possibility of other congenital anomalies.

Anatomic Pathology

Because the synostosis may be partial or complete, motion between two adjacent bones may be partial or totally limited. Usually motion is minimal if at all. Radiographically a partial cartilaginous synostosis may exist in the younger patient, but as the patient reaches skeletal maturity the synostosis usually matures to a complete bony union.

In the digits, longitudinal synostosis is seen most often between the proximal and the middle phalanges.

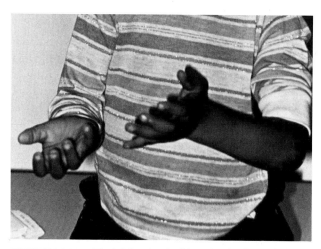

FIGURE 21-30.   The left forearm in this patient has limited supination because of radioulnar synostosis.

The most frequently seen transverse phalangeal synostosis is at the distal phalangeal level.

In the carpus, adjacent synostosis between the lunate and triquetrum is most common but rarely produces a functional disability.

Synostosis in the forearm is almost always proximal and of the two types mentioned previously. The primary defect is that of pronation and supination, and the arm is usually in a pronated or even hyperpronated position.

At the elbow, humeroradioulnar synostosis is the most common synostosis and has a high incidence of associated skeletal abnormalities.

Treatment

Synostosis of the upper extremity should be considered for surgical release if the synostosis interferes with function or growth of the interconnected segments. Complex syndactyly and symphalangism as examples of synostosis are discussed elsewhere. Operations for carpal synostosis are almost never required.

Treatment for radioulnar synostosis is usually not necessary if the patient has mild unilateral deformity or no major functional loss.[106] However, in the presence of bilateral and severe pronation, surgery may be beneficial. Many procedures have been recommended to restore motion, including extensive release of the synostosis, release of the interosseous membrane and radioulnar joints, excision of the distal ulna, interposition of soft tissue, silicone, or a metal swivel.[105,107,109] None of these procedures has produced consistently successful results.

If surgery is required for radioulnar synostosis the only procedure that appears to be useful is that of a rotational osteotomy through the site of the synostosis.[116] The rotational osteotomy has been recommended when pronation is more than 60 degrees either unilaterally or bilaterally.[116] If the deformity is unilateral, the forearm is placed in 20 degrees of pronation. However, if the deformity is bilateral, the dominant side is placed in 30 degrees of pronation and the assistive limb in neutral.[117] In this position, the shoulder rotation permits the child to bring both

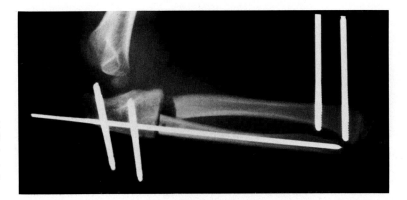

FIGURE 21-31. Rotational osteotomy performed at the level of the synostosis. Up to a 1-cm segment of ulna is resected to allow relaxation of neurovascular structures. The external fixator can provide for gradual correction in the early postoperative period by manipulation of the apparatus.

hands parallel to the tabletop for activities such as writing or using keyboard instruments. Additionally, neutral or mild pronation has a better cosmetic appearance while the patient's arms are at his or her side (Fig. 21-31).

Radioulnar synostosis are not discovered in most patients until early adolescence because of limited dysfunction or adaptation to their limitations. If the osteotomy is contemplated it is recommended early to allow development of normal prehensile patterns. Vascular compromise may limit the degree of rotational osteotomy performed.

Radial Head Dislocation

Clinical Features

Radial head dislocation may occur independently or in association with type 2 radioulnar synostosis. The dislocation may be anterior, posterior, or lateral. Mardam-Bey and Ger[126] report an incidence of 18% anterior, 65% posterior, and 17% lateral.

Both the child and the parent usually do not note the deformity or limited range of motion until the patient is 4 to 5 years of age. The primary physical finding is that of the prominence about the lateral aspect of the elbow (Fig. 21-32).

The radial head dislocation may be either congenital or acquired. To distinguish between congenital and acquired radial head dislocations, a history of bilateral involvement, family history, history of trauma, associated regional abnormalities, dislocation noted at birth, and the radiographic appearance may be helpful in distinguishing the two types. Reports have suggested that the incidence of congenital radial head dislocation is 0.15%.[126,128]

Inheritance

An isolated occurrence of radial head dislocation may be the result of an autosomal dominant trait or occasionally an X-linked recessive trait.[124,130] When associated with multiple exostosis, nail-patella syndrome, and antecubital pterygium syndrome, radial head dislocation is inherited as a dominant genotype. Because of this association with other musculoskeletal defects, a search for other anomalies should be made when radial head dislocation is noted. Approximately 60% of congenital dislocations of the radial head are seen in association with syndromes.

Anatomic Pathology

To distinguish the traumatic from the congenital radial head dislocation, attention is directed to the capitellum. If the capitellum is hypoplastic or absent, the trochlea is partially defective, the ulna is short in relation to the radius, and a dome-shaped radial head is present the dislocation is most likely congenital (Fig. 21-33). Some long-standing posttraumatic dislocations may masquerade as congenital radial head dislocations, illustrating the surprisingly small limitation of function and absence of pain after this injury.

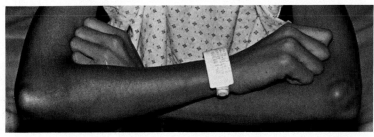

FIGURE 21-32. A 10-year-old girl with posterior dislocations of both elbows first noted 5 years prior to examination because of prominence of the lateral elbow.

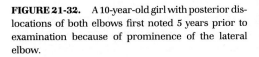

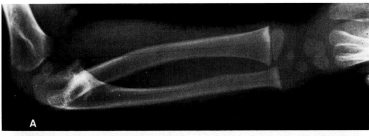

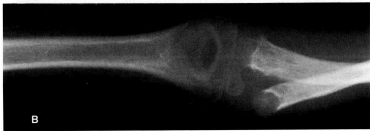

FIGURE 21-33. Congenital radial head dislocation. (**A**) Posterior displacement of the radial head. (**B**) The dome-shaped head and hypoplastic capitellum.

Treatment

The treatment of radial head dislocation should be directed toward alleviating pain, increasing motion, and improving the appearance. In most cases, the deformity has been present for some time with little functional or cosmetic disability. The anterior dislocation represents the most difficulty with motion and the posterior dislocation the least.[126] The motion of rotation is more affected than flexion and extension. There is little change in motion with growth. However, as the child grows, the cosmetic and functional limitations may become apparent.[121,123,125,129]

Treatment of the congenital radial head dislocation or long-standing acquired radial head dislocation is excision of the radial head after skeletal growth is complete. This procedure is indicated only for pain relief and does not improve range of motion of the forearm. The limited motion is probably related to the many surrounding tight soft tissue structures.[126]

Although in theory open reduction of congenital dislocation of the radial head in the infant may have several benefits, there is no evidence that the results justify attempts at the procedure. When only a subluxation of the radial head is noted in the infant distraction lengthening of the ulna has been proposed, which needs further evaluation before it can be recommended.[120,121,129]

Syndactyly

Clinical Features

Syndactyly is a term that means webbed fingers, and the deformity is one of the most common hand anomalies.[132,135] Although it fits into the category of failure of differentiation, it may be seen across a number of different categories of congenital hand problems.

Syndactyly usually is described as complete or incomplete and simple or complex.[134] The complete syndactyly is webbing of the fingers from the commissure to the fingertips. A digit with incomplete syndactyly has webbing extending distally, usually to the middle of the proximal phalanx and not the end of the digit. The syndactyly is simple if the skin alone is joined and complex if the bones of adjacent fingers are fused (Fig. 21-34). Many authors are now proposing an additional

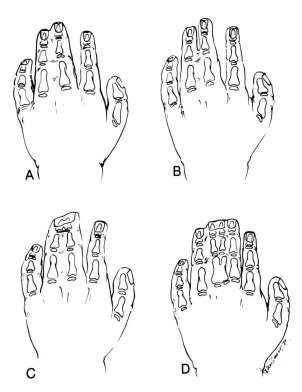

FIGURE 21-34. (**A**) Complete simple syndactyly. (**B**) Incomplete simple syndactyly. (**C**) Complete complex syndactyly manifested by terminal synostosis. (**D**) Variation of complete complex syndactyly with synostosis, duplicate digit, and complete syndactyly.

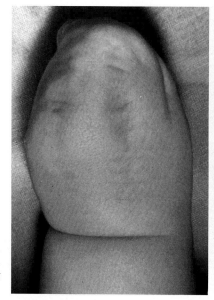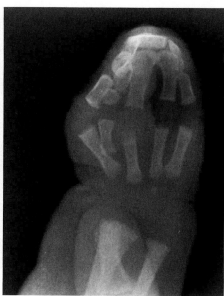

FIGURE 21-35. The Apert hand (acrocephalosyndacyly) is a variation of acrosyndactyly manifested by a severe form of complete complex syndactyly.

category called complicated complex syndactyly. This latter type has features that not only include syndactyly but also clinodactyly, camptodactyly, symphalangism, or associated syndromes, such as Poland, Apert, and amniotic band syndrome.[133,135,140,141] In this category there is more than the simple sharing of a soft tissue envelope with bony connection at the distal portion.

Acrosyndactyly is an adjacent fusion of the digits at their distal ends (Fig. 21-35).[135] There is usually proximal fenestration between the digits distal to the normal web space. *Brachysyndactyly* refers to shortened fingers that are joined on adjacent sides.

The incidence of syndactyly is about 1 in 1650 to 2500 births. Approximately one half of the cases are bilateral and symmetric.[133,134] Syndactyly is twice as common in boys as in girls. The incidence of web involvement is highest between the middle and ring fingers, followed by involvement between the ring and little fingers and between the index and middle fingers. Syndactyly is more prevalent in Caucasians than in African Americans.[134] It is also more common postaxially than preaxially.

Partial syndactyly results in little if any functional impairment. The person usually is able to flex and extend the digits without difficulty, and the inability to adduct the two digits with syndactyly causes no serious handicap. The affected digit continues to grow normally, with minimal deformity or limitation of motion.

Complete simple syndactyly between digits of the same size is likely to result in a small degree of angulation of the digits toward each other. Motion is almost normal, and minimal angular deformity is present. Complete simple syndactyly of the digits of different sizes causes overrotation of the digits toward each other and angulates the larger digit toward the shorter

digit (Fig. 21-36). Angulation, flexion and rotation deformities that exist tend to progress with growth of the digits. Simple complete syndactyly between the thumb and index finger represents the most involved anomaly of this group. Complex syndactyly among fingers of different sizes is more severe than the deformities produced by simple syndactyly.

Inheritance

The literature suggests that 80% of cases of syndactyly are sporadic, however, a familial incidence can be seen as high as 20% to 40%.[132-134]

Associated Anomalies

Syndactyly is seen in association with a variety of syndromes, such as Apert, Poland, and congenital constriction band syndrome. Syndactyly is seen in association with other skeletal problems, visceral problems, and skin dysplasias.

Anatomic Pathology

The most important principle in understanding the anatomy of syndactyly is that there is insufficient skin after release of the two digits. This has been demonstrated by Flatt, who notes the difference between the circumference of two digits held together is less than the sum of the circumference of two separate digits.[134] The underlying soft tissues and bone present more of a varied appearance. Numerous fascial interconnections are present, representing the coalescence of Grayson and Cleland ligaments, which produce a fibrofatty material that is often hypertrophied and contracted.

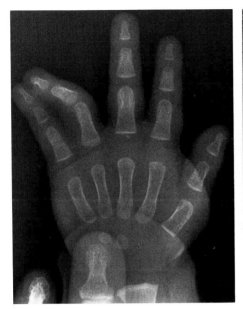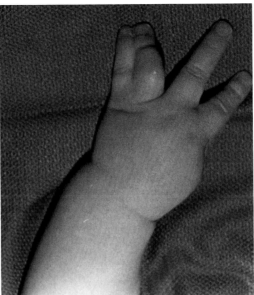

FIGURE 21-36. Syndactyly of adjacent digits of unequal length produces angulation toward the shorter digit.

The next most common problem seen in the anatomy of children with syndactyly is the varied interconnections of muscles and tendons, particularly in those with complex syndactyly. Similar interconnections of nerve and vascular structures also are present, which form an additional problem for surgical separation.

The condition of the joints varies according to the degree of simple or complex involvement. The more simple the syndactyly, the more normal the joints. In the more complex deformities, partial ankylosis, deviations, and instability may be present. The underlying bone abnormalities form a helter-skelter arrangement of interconnections, hypoplasias, and abnormal orientations.

Treatment

Treatment of syndactyly can be a difficult problem that requires good judgment and technical ability. Treatment is not always necessary to maximize function in some forms of incomplete and complete simple syndactyly. However, subtle improvement in function and a greatly enhanced cosmetic appearance are highly valued in our society.

It is important to realize that the sum of the circumference of two adjacent digits is always greater than the singular circumference of two digits in syndactyly. This difference explains why skin grafting is always necessary in the complete syndactyly. However, in incomplete simple syndactyly, especially if the webbing is minimal, there are many ways to approach the release. In the case of the first web space, a four-flap Z-plasty can adequately deepen the cleft between the thumb and the index finger without need for a skin

graft.[142] If incomplete webbing exists between two adjacent fingers, it can be deepened with inverting triangles or a butterfly flap. However, if the webbing extends past the distal third of the proximal phalanx, a more standard type of release should be used, as described by Bauer and colleagues[131] (Fig. 21-37). This type of approach may be used for complete and complex syndactyly. It is essential to remove as much of the fibrofatty material as possible between the two interconnecting digits. Care should be taken around the neurovascular bundle to prevent damage. The arterial supply tends to bifurcate more distally than the digital nerves. The more complex and closer together the syndactyly, the more distal the bifurcation of the neurovascular bundle. It is seldom necessary to ligate the proper digital artery because of the distal bifurcation. If ligation is necessary in a single web involvement, arterial blood supply should be left with the border digit. If three digits are webbed together, the finger requiring web release on both sides is given the benefit of two vascular bundles. In the case of the digital nerve, the fascicles may be dissected apart gently as far proximally as the palm, if necessary. Detailed attention to the fingernails is most important in preventing a deformity of one of the most obvious landmarks of the finger. Defatting of the pulp may facilitate closure of the paronychial fold, although skin grafting is usually necessary. Too tight closure can lead to a deformed nail. Buck-Gramcko has developed a paronychial fold reconstruction technique that produces a superior cosmetic appearance.[132] The use of a paronychial fold graft from the toe also has been used for reconstruction of the nail fold.[133]

If two or more fingers are included in the syndac-

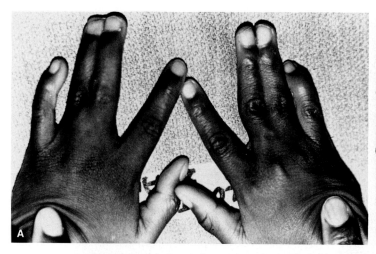 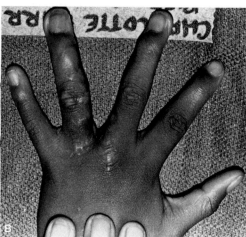

FIGURE 21-37. Surgical treatment of complete simple syndactyly improves functional and cosmetic results. **(A)** Preoperative. **(B)** Postoperative.

tyly, it is not recommended that both sides of the finger be operated on at the same time because this may compromise the vascular supply to the finger. If the index, long, ring, and little fingers are all joined it is best to separate the border digits first. Separation of the central finger usually follows after an interval of 3 months. A similar technique can be used for an approach of complex syndactyly. Because a conjoined distal phalanx and nail are present, it is necessary to sharply transect them longitudinally with a scalpel or osteotome. Complex syndactyly involving the middle and proximal phalanges is rare. In some instances it may be necessary to reconstruct absent collateral ligaments and absent flexor tendon pulleys and even perform reconstructive osteotomies to correct the angulation. This helps promote stability at the joints, prevents bow stringing of the newly separated flexor tendons, and aids in maintaining bony correction. The greater the severity of involvement, the greater the necessity for skin grafting. These severe cases often result in poor joint motion and should be immobilized in some flexion during the healing phase.

Timing of surgery for syndactyly is important. The greater discrepancy between the length of the two digits, the earlier the surgery should be performed. In general, most syndactyly corrections are carried out when the child is between 6 months and 1 year of age.

More detailed descriptions of operative procedures may be found in other texts.[137,139] The important point here is that skin graft is almost always necessary after releasing a complete syndactyly. Postoperative care is designed to immobilize the hand to allow full-thickness skin grafts to adequately heal to the underlying surfaces. This process takes about 2 weeks. It is important to be attentive to the care of the skin grafts because breakdown of the wound or incomplete take of the grafts results in hypertrophic scarring, which

diminishes the desired results and in turn may lead to recurrence of a distally migrating commissure.

Arthrogryposis

Clinical Features

The term *arthrogryposis* derives from the Greek word *gryposis*, meaning "crooking." Arthrogryposis multiplex congenita is not a specific disorder but a symptom complex of congenital joint contractures associated with neurogenic and myopathic disorders. The contractures are always present at birth and usually are not progressive (Fig. 21-38).[152] The clinical picture is characterized by multiple symmetric joint contractures, atrophied extremities, and marked limitation of active and passive motion of the joints involved. The shoulders are adducted and internally rotated and show atrophic shoulder-girdle musculature. The elbows are fixed in extension, and the forearm is pronated. The hands and the wrists are flexed with an ulnar deviation and appear to be cupped. The fingers usually are gathered together, and the thumb is adducted into the palm. The skin appears thin and shiny with some thickening over the joints. The lower extremity involvement tends to mirror that of the upper extremities.

The exact etiology of the syndrome is not known; it is thought to be multifactorial and probably results from a combination of contributing factors. The deformities currently are believed to occur as a component of a large group of heterogenous, neurogenic, and myopathic disorders.

Anatomic Pathology

The pathologic feature that these patients share in common seems to be a defect, whether congenital

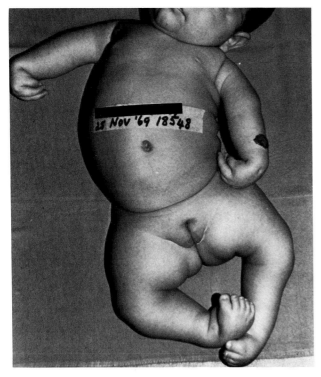

FIGURE 21-38. Arthrogryposis is the symptom complex of joint contracture. The shoulders are narrow and atrophic, the elbows are straight and lack flexion creases, the wrist is flexed, and clubfeet are present.

or acquired, in the motor unit, which is composed of anterior horn cells, roots, peripheral nerves, motor end plates, and muscles.[143,150,153,154] This produces a severe weakness in early fetal development with the immobility leading to hypoplastic joint development and contractures. The neurogenic form is the most common, accounting for approximately 93%, whereas myopathic disorders account for the other 7%.[158] The expression of the degree of involvement in arthrogryposis varies from minimal to severe.

Treatment

In evaluation of the patient for treatment of arthrogryposis multiplex congenita, the physician should consider the patient as a whole.[144] The severity of involvement of the upper and lower extremities determines the feasibility of corrective procedures. These patients almost always have normal intelligence and sensate skin. They have considerable potential for rehabilitation despite the severe limitations from their deformities. The ultimate goal is to provide independent upper extremity function to allow for activities of daily living. Care should be taken not to propose any treatment that will take away any function of the extremities without replacing it with something more productive.[148] These patients demonstrate remarkable adaptability to their limitations, and surgical intervention is often unnecessary.

Treatment of this complex problem begins in the neonatal period. It consists of range of motion exercises and cast stretching of various contractures followed by prolonged splinting.[148,149,151]

If stretching produces sufficient motion functional bracing is instituted to develop normal use patterns. Braces can later be replaced by appropriate tendon transfers to maintain joint motion. Occasionally mobilization of contractures is not possible, and after an adequate trial of 6 months to 1 year with no progress being noted surgical release of contractures may be indicated. This may be done to better optimize planned tendon transfers or to allow for skin care because the contracted skin is prone to breakdown.

The arthrogrypotic patient usually demonstrates very little active abduction of the shoulder; the patient does have limited adductor function. The treatment is designed to mobilize the shoulder through active and passive stretching. If enough range of motion cannot be achieved through therapy to allow approximately 90 degrees of external rotation, which will bring the hand to meet the mouth, then an external rotation osteotomy of the upper third of the humerus may have to be performed. Shoulder fusion is usually not necessary because therapy and compensatory cervical range of motion result in adequate function.

The elbow is fixed in extension with varying, although minimal, degrees of passive motion present. Patients will have more triceps function than biceps function. Dynamic or static splinting is used until 40 to 50 degrees of motion is obtained. When the patient becomes older than 2 years of age, an elastic harness is applied to assist in active flexion (Fig. 21-39). This allows the patient to bring his or her hands to the mouth. In patients whose passive elbow flexion cannot be obtained, posterior capsulotomy and lengthening of the triceps is often necessary to mobilize the elbow.

Active elbow flexion can be provided in several ways depending on the structures that are present.[146,147,159,160,161] If the patient has good wrist and hand flexors, a Steindler flexorplasty can be done.[157] In this procedure the flexor pronator origin is shifted proximal on the humerus, which in its new position will allow for flexion of the elbow. The main drawback to the Steindler flexorplasty is the potential pronation of the forearm and flexion of the elbow it may cause through the advancement of the flexors proximally. Biceps function is more often restored by transfer of the pectoralis major. The pectoral muscles almost always provide good power and may offer some additional mechanical advantage. Other alternatives include the latissimus transfer or a triceps transfer.[146,147,161] The triceps transfer should never be done bilaterally because the patient will require extension at the elbow in at least one arm to help in transfers or using crutches.

The wrist and fingers usually are flexed and devi-

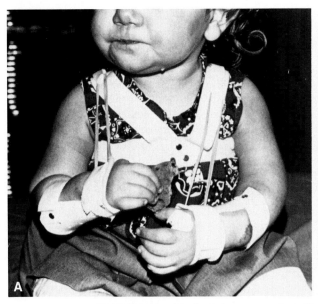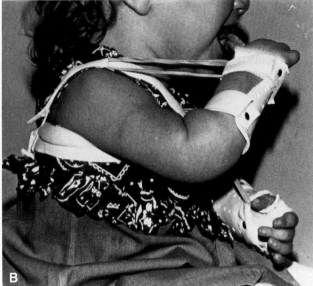

FIGURE 21-39. (A) Elastic harness used to aid flexion of the elbow allows the patient to use the upper extremities in a more natural pattern. (B) Elastic-band tension can be increased or decreased depending on the amount of force needed to allow the hand to reach the mouth.

ated toward the ulna. Persistent wrist flexion contractures may be treated by volar capsulotomy and associated tendon transfer using the flexor carpi ulnaris and radialis to the dorsum of the wrist. In the severely involved wrist that is not passively correctable, Smith[156] recommended performing a proximal row carpectomy, thereby effectively lengthening the contracted structures and placing the wrist in neutral position. This is now augmented by transferring the flexor carpi ulnaris and flexor carpi radialis to the extensor carpi radialis bevis to facilitate extension.[156]

The clutched thumb-in-palm deformities are difficult to correct.[155,156] There is usually a deficient first web space and associated adducted thumb. There also may be a deficiency of the extensor and flexor mechanisms. The skin deficiency is addressed by conventional Z-plasty, rotation, and skin grafts. In severe deformities an abdominal flap may be necessary to make up the severe deficit. Preoperative stretching either with splints or a distraction lengthener may assist in reducing the amount of skin grafting required. The thenar muscles and the adductor pollicis are usually contracted and require a release in the manner described by Matev. The deficiency of tendons is addressed by appropriate tendon transfers when available. If none are available then tenodesis or arthrodesis may be required.

Flexion contractures of the proximal interphalangeal joints usually involve multiple fingers with webbing of the skin. They are extremely difficult to correct.[156] Casting and splinting are the initial treatment modalities followed by active exercises and occupational therapy. These patients develop a remarkable

way of manipulating stiff fingers so they can perform prehensile activities. Surgery seldom improves the function of the fingers.[155] Surgery on these joints may change the arc of motion but generally does not improve the range of motion. For severe contractures that do not allow any functional use of the hand, arthrodesis of the joints in a better position may improve prehensile function by concentrating all motion at the metacarpophylangeal joint.

The primary goal in treating arthrogryposis of the upper extremity is to provide an extremity that may be brought to the mouth for feeding and hygiene and can be used for pushing up to a sitting position or using an ambulatory aid, such as a crutch, if necessary.

Trigger Digits

Clinical Picture

The trigger digit is more likely to present as a fixed, flexed contracture of the interphalangeal joint of the thumb, but clicking and snapping of the digit with motion may be seen.[163,167,179] The metacarpophalangeal joint is often in hyperextension and the interphalangeal joint in flexion (Fig. 21-40). The condition in the child is very similar to that of the adult, except that the thumb is more often involved in the infant.[164] About 25% of cases are noted at birth, with bilateral involvement common. If the contracture is noted at birth, approximately 30% will resolve by 1 year; however, if the problem is noted between the ages of 6 months and 3 years only about 10% to 12% will improve spontaneously.

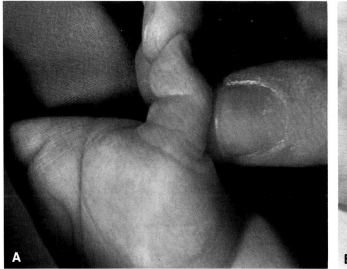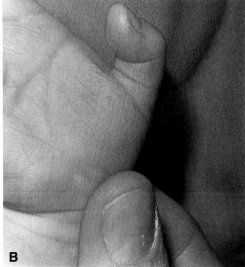

FIGURE 21-40.   Typical trigger finger with the metacarpophalangeal joint in hyperextension and the interphalanged joint in flexion.

There does not appear to be any specific inheritance pattern despite the fact that this may be present at birth.[171,173-176] Ger reported an incidence of 1:2000,[166] whereas Flatt reported the incidence as high as 1:50;[165] the discrepancy may be the result of underreporting and spontaneous resolution of the condition.

Associated Anomalies

Trisomy 13 is the only syndrome to be associated with trigger digits, particularly the thumb.[165] The more important problem with trigger finger is to differentiate it from other thumb abnormalities, particularly clutch thumb anomalies. These include hypoplastic thumb, spastic thumb, and arthrogrypotic thumb.[169,173,174]

Anatomic Pathology

The changes found at the A-1 pulley of the metacarpal phalangeal joint involve the flexor tendon sheath, the tendon, or both. The changes in the pulley are similar to those seen in stenosing tenosynovitis of the adult with narrowing or thickening of the sheath and occasional ganglion formation. The tendon may show a nodule formation at the level of the A-1 pulley.[170] Whether these changes are the result of the trauma of the constriction or there is some other initial deformity to produce the triggering has not been determined.

Treatment

If the diagnosis is made at birth and the trigger is passively extendable, splinting in extension for 6 weeks may overcome the triggering. However, because of poor tolerance of the splint, this usually is not recommended.[162,166-168]

To date both the contracture and the loss of tendon excursion are correctable if the process is treated before the age of 3 years, but the odds of spontaneous resolution are low, and surgical release of this A-1 pulley is recommended after 1 year of age.[166,169]

Surgery in this age group necessitates general anesthesia. Great care must be taken because the digital nerves are close to the midline, especially the radial digital nerve. A small portion of the A-1 pulley is excised and care is taken to preserve the more distal oblique pulley to prevent bowstringing of the flexor pollicis longus. Various approaches have been described, usually made at the level of the metacarpal phalangeal joint. Debulking of the flexor tendon nodule is usually not necessary unless there is a discreet nodule present in the flexor tendon. With the constriction removed the nodule gradually regresses.

The treatment of fingers other than the thumb is similar.

Camptodactyly

Clinical Features

Camptodactyly means bent finger.[177,179] The term is applied to a congenital developmental flexion contracture of the proximal interphalangeal joint of the finger, unrelated to trauma, systemic disease, or neurologic abnormality.[195,197,198] Camptodactyly describes the contracture, which angulates in the anteroposterior plane. This is distinctly different from clino-

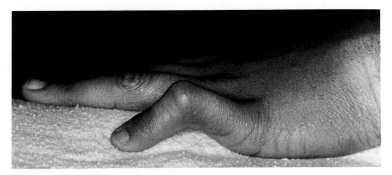

FIGURE 21-41. Camptodactyly. Flexion contracture of the proximal interphalangeal joint most often occurs in the fifth digit but can occur in others.

dactyly, which describes angulation in the radioulnar plane[201,202] (Fig. 21-41).

Three different presentations of camptodactyly have been described: infantile, adolescent, and involvement of other fingers.[186] Much overlap exists and often the adolescent variant may be a progression of the infantile presentation. Engber and Flatt[180] noted that 84% of the patients with this condition developed camptodactyly in the first year of life, whereas only 13% were noted after the onset of age 10.

The overall incidence of camptodactyly in the population is between 1% and 2%, with the little finger being the most frequently involved.[180] About two thirds of cases have bilateral involvement. When only one hand is involved it almost always is the right hand. The typical appearance is that of hyperextension of the metacarpal phalangeal joint to compensate for the flexion contracture at the proximal interphalangeal joint. Pain and swelling are usually absent unless there has been a long-standing deformity.

Although camptodactyly may be present at birth, it is usually not noted until later in childhood. The deformity is usually passively correctable and can be minimized by holding the wrist or metacarpal phalangeal joint in flexion. However, with time, shortening of the skin and tendons occurs until the joint contracture becomes fixed. In more severe involvement, the patients complain of interference with activities, such as typing, playing the piano, or inserting the hand into narrow spaces.

Camptodactyly becomes progressively worse in 80% of cases. The contracture usually increases between the ages of 1 and 4 years and then again between the ages of 10 and 14, which correlates with growth spurts. The deformity usually does not progress past the age of 20 years.

Inheritance

Many cases of camptodactyly are sporadic in origin. There are, however, several cases of autosomal dominant inheritance that have been reported.[181,183,184]

Associated Abnormalities

Camptodactyly is commonly associated with many syndromes, such as trisomy 13, orofaciodigital syndrome, oculodentodigital syndrome, Aarskog syndrome, and cerebrohepatorenal syndrome.[185]

Anatomic Pathology

The basic underlying abnormality is an imbalance between the flexor and the extensor mechanisms. Smith and Kaplan summarize the anatomic pathology by stating "virtually every structure at the base of the finger has been implicated as a deforming factor."[200] The literature suggests that the pathoanatomy of camptodactyly is multifactorial, implicating anomalous flexor tendons, lumbrical muscles, Landsmeer ligaments, dorsal extensor apparatus, volar plate, intrinsic muscles, and circulatory disturbances.[184,185,188,189,191]

Treatment

The operative treatment of camptodactyly remains unpredictable because there is no constant etiology and no single standard method of treatment. If treatment is begun in the early stages, dynamic splinting in the daytime and fixed extension splinting at night may be beneficial. The fixed deformities may be prevented by prolonged diligent splinting; however, tolerance for splinting is usually poor in the child.[182,192]

Surgical treatment, as noted by Engber and Flatt, results in improvement in only 35% of operative cases.[180] Therefore surgical intervention may be less than satisfying. The successful results are obtained only in children operated on under the age of 5 years, as indicated by Miura.[191] Surgical results remain entirely unpredictable.

Numerous operative procedures have been proposed, including lengthening of the flexor digitorum sublimis; the profundus; the release of the palmar fascia, the tendon sheath, the volar plate and collateral ligaments, and the anomalous insertion of lumbrical muscle; and sublimis transfer to the extensor mechanism.[183,186,187,190,194] The splinting provides passive but not active correction of the proximal interphalangeal joint; sublimis transfer to the extensor mechanism is advised by Millesi[190] and Lankford.[187] If an anomalous insertion of the lumbrical muscle is present, resection or transfer may be helpful for improving extension.

It seems reasonable to advise patients with mild deformity to live with their problems. However, if the young child shows progressive deformity and conservative measures of splinting have failed, surgical intervention may be indicated.

In late untreated cases of camptodactyly with severe flexion deformities, treatment is not recommended because of limited improvement that is likely to be achieved. If there are bone or joint problems, reconstructive osteotomy to place the phalangeal head in a better position or arthrodesis of the joint may increase function and relieve pain.[173] Amputation is reserved for only the most extreme problem.

New techniques, such as a hinged proximal interphalangeal distraction lengthening device, may slowly allow for correction of the contracture through stretching of the soft tissues and obviate the need for any reconstructive surgical procedures. More experience and long-term follow-up is needed before this can be recommended.[178]

Clinodactyly

Clinical Features

Clinodactyly describes angular deformity of the finger in the radioulnar plane (Fig. 21-42). The defor-

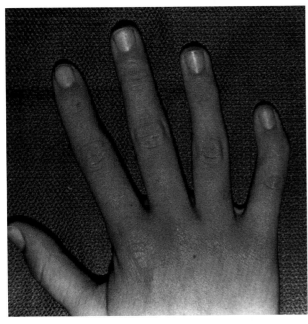

FIGURE 21-42.   Clinodactyly is an ulnar or radial deviation of the digit. Medial deviation is most common, and the fifth digit is involved most often.

mity may occur in any finger, but the little finger is most frequently involved at the distal interphalangeal joint. It more commonly occurs bilaterally and is associated with a middle phalanx that is shorter on the radial than the ulnar side. Function is seldom impaired unless the curvature is severe, and then it may interfere with flexion of the finger.

The clinical importance of clinodactyly is that it may be associated with mental retardation.[219–221,223,224] The incidence of clinodactyly in Down syndrome among this population is reported to be between 35% and 79% as compared with 1% to 19.5% in the Caucasian population.[225] It occurs more often in boys and usually is bilateral.

Inheritance Pattern

Although there are several reported cases of sporadic clinodactyly, it is most often inherited as an autosomal dominant trait.

Associated Anomalies

Clinodactyly is associated with 30 different syndromes. The more important of these syndromes are related to hand and foot abnormalities, such as symphalangism and brachydactyly, chromosomal disorders (e.g., trisomy 21, Klinefelter syndrome, trisomy 18), craniofacial syndromes, Holt-Oram syndrome, Turner syndrome, Cornelia de Lange syndrome, Fanconi anemia, Silver syndrome, and Goltz syndrome.[204–213,215,218–220] Associated anomalies should be looked for when clinodactyly is noted.

Anatomic Pathology

The deformity of clinodactyly results when there is an angulation of the distal interphalangeal joint away from the long axis of the digit. An angulation of more than 10 degrees is regarded as the upper limits of normal. Burke and Flatt[203] believe that there is a greater tendency for the angulation to occur in the middle phalanx because it is the last to ossify.

Care should be taken to distinguish clinodactyly from other forms of bent fingers resulting from a Delta phalanx, triangular ossicle, or triphalangism.

Treatment

Most cases of clinodactyly appear to have problems that are more cosmetic than functional. Splinting is not recommended as an effective method of treatment. Sufficient external forces cannot be applied to affect the growth of the middle phalanx in the small patient. It is preferred to accept the deformity, if minimal. If necessary, surgery is postponed until after the

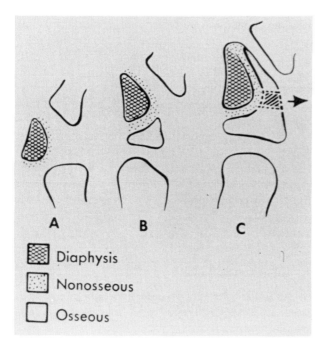

FIGURE 21-43. A trapezoid-shaped bone with a C-shaped epiphysis is shown in developmental stages. This bracketed epiphysis has abnormal longitudinal growth. (Adapted from Green DP, ed. Operative hand surgery. New York: Churchill Livingstone, 1982.)

age of 6 years or until the patient can be more cooperative. Because the deformity is primarily cosmetic, care should be taken with the parents to explain the complications of surgery.

Correction of the angulation is best accomplished by a closing wedge osteotomy of the middle phalanx. Other options include open wedge osteotomy and reversed wedge osteotomy.[203]

Delta Phalanx

Clinical Features

Jones[234] first described the use of the term *delta phalanx* in reporting angular deformities of a finger secondary to an abnormally shaped bone that resembled the Greek letter *delta*. Because similar deformities are found both in the metacarpal and phalangeal bones, it should be referred to delta bone as opposed to delta phalanx. The bone may be triangular, oval, or trapezoidal in shape with an abnormal epiphyseal plate.

The classic delta phalanx is characterized by a triangular or trapezoidal shaped bone with a C-shaped epiphysis (i.e., bracket epiphysis), usually oriented in a semicircular direction. The aberrant epiphysis ossifies from proximal to distal causing unequal longitudinal growth and angulation of the distal portion of the digit (Fig. 21-43). With this longitudinal bracketed diaphysis, progressive angular deformity is inevitable.[227,236] The abnormality is most common in the proximal phalanx of the thumb and the little finger. The deformity most often occurs bilaterally and has a 2:1 ratio of men to women.[244] Involvement of the distal phalanx has never been reported. The border digits commonly deviate toward the rest of the hand[244] (Fig. 21-44). The central digits rarely deviate.

Inheritance Pattern

There is no specific inheritance pattern. Reports support both sporadic occurrence and autosomal dominant inheritance with variable penetrance.[233,244]

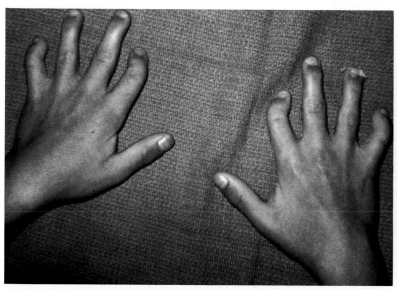
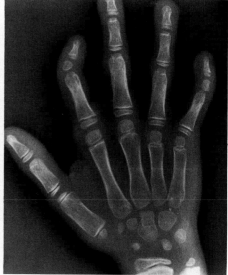

FIGURE 21-44. A delta phalanx is present in the middle phalanx of the index and little fingers. This condition results in clinodactyly.

The inheritance appears to be dependent on the underlying syndrome.

Associated Anomalies

The delta phalanx primarily has been associated with musculoskeletal abnormalities of polydactyly, syndactyly, symphalangism, clinodactyly, diastrophic dwarfism, Holt-Oram syndrome, central hand deficiency, and Poland syndrome.[226,229,231,232,233,237,245]

Anatomic Pathology

Although the etiology of delta bone is unknown, it is clear that there is an abnormal physis and epiphysis surrounding the diaphysis of the phalanx. The different levels of expression have led to a classification by Blevins and Light into three groups:[228]

Group I—longitudinal epiphyseal bracket (LEB): These may take three forms: Complete LEB, incomplete LEB, and complex LEB.

Group II—trapezoidal bone: This bone shows an abnormal distal joint surface with a normal proximal epiphysis. The distal physis may be well developed or a pseudophysis.

Group III—triangular bone: This small triangular-shaped structure does not have a radiographically evident physis during its growth. This type is seen primarily in triphalangeal thumb.

Treatment

The deformity caused by delta phalanx may be unsightly and awkward. If the deformity is of minimal cosmetic and functional disability no treatment should be undertaken.[229,235,238,239,242,243]

Blevins and Light[228] reported a 62% complication rate of their treated delta phalanges, most commonly as a result of premature closure of the physis. This may result in either further angulation or a compromise of longitudinal growth. If surgery is contemplated it should be reserved for older children who have reached skeletal maturity with the angulation remaining unchanged.

Numerous procedures have been described for the correction of this deformity, including open and closed wedge osteotomies.[229,234,240] All procedures are designed to accomplish the recommendation by Smith[240] to realign the abnormal physeal plate perpendicular with the longitudinal axis of the finger.

The most important factors in treating the delta phalanx are to separate the proximal and distal physeal plates from the longitudinal connecting epiphyseal and physeal segment, correct the alignment of the distal and proximal plates by wedge osteotomy, and align the epiphyseal plates perpendicular to the longitudinal axis of the digit.

DUPLICATION

Duplication, or polydactyly, is one of the most common congenital anomalies. Polydactyly can be divided into preaxial, central, and postaxial types. Because of the importance of each they are discussed separately.

Preaxial Polydactyly, or Duplicate Thumbs

Clinical Features

The wide variety of thumb duplications, and even triplications, can be divided into four groups:[248,251,252,255,263,265]

Type I: thumb polydactyly

Type II: polydactyly of an opposable triphalangeal thumb

Type III: a nonopposable triphalangeal thumb, polydactyly of the index finger

Type IV: polysyndactyly

Polydactyly of the thumb is the main type discussed because of its prevalence.

The incidence of preaxial polydactyly is 0.08 in 1000 births in both African-American and Caucasian races.[263,267] There is a slightly higher incidence noted in the Native American and Asian populations. There is a male-to-female ratio of 2.5:1.[254,261] The Wassel-Egawa[251] classification is more commonly used in the literature; however, we prefer the Marks and Bayne[258] classification because it helps in treatment and prognosis (Fig. 21-45). Nearly 50% of the cases will be type 2 in the Marks and Bayne classification or type 4 in the Wassel-Egawa classification.[258,256]

Inheritance

Most reported cases of thumb polydactyly are sporadic. There are, however, some familial cases of inheritance.

Associated Anomalies

In most instances thumb polydactyly is an isolated occurrence. When present with other syndromes it may be associated with musculoskeletal, visceral, hepatic, or nervous systems abnormalities. Holt-Oram

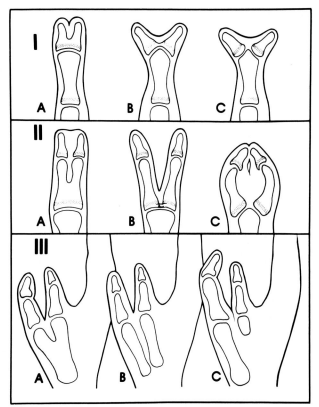

FIGURE 21-45. Classification for thumb duplication. Type 1, duplication of distal phalanx: **(A)** incomplete, **(B)** complete with base joined by cartilage only, **(C)** complete. Type 2, duplication at the proximal phalangeal level: **(A)** incomplete, **(B)** complete with base joined by cartilage, **(C)** complete. Type 3, duplication at the metacarpal level: **(A)** incomplete, **(B)** complete, **(C)** mixed.

and Fanconi syndromes are the best known of these associations.[250]

Anatomic Pathology

Polydactyly of the thumb covers a wide spectrum, from extreme hypoplasia to complete duplication throughout the metacarpal level. The variability of the anatomy is dependent on the amount of duplication. It is similar to the occurrence of a complex syndactyly in which there is a sharing of interconnections of skin, fascial structure, tendons, neurovascular elements, bone, and joints. Although we speak of duplicated thumbs, Ezaki[252] has pointed out that these actually are more of a "split" thumb. The two thumbs that are present are never the size of the normal opposite thumb, indicating that their structures are more shared than duplicated.

Hypoplasia is a central finding in the duplicated digit syndrome. This may produce an accessory thumb of different size, shape, configuration, and stability. It also may be at a different level from the normal thumb (Fig. 21-46). The relations of the accessory thumbs to each other and the rest of the hand is variable.

Treatment

The treatment of polydactyly is designed to improve both the cosmetic and the functional use of the thumb with reconstructive surgery. The surgery should entail not only restoring the proper number of digits but also improving the position, stability, anatomic configuration, and web space.[246,247,249,250,253,257–262,264]

It is commonly advocated that when the duplicate thumb is merely a skin tag that this be tied off in the delivery room and allowed to slough. Frequently this type of treatment results in an unsightly bump at the site of the previous digit, particularly if there is a cartilage anlage remaining. It is usually preferable to excise the supernumerary digit in the newborn nursery. This can be accomplished with the use of local anesthesia and a pacifier. The two vessels may be tied off or cauterized with an ophthalmic cautery. This treatment is not recommended for other types of polydactyly.

Additional surgical treatment of the duplicate thumb is based on the level of duplication and should remove the least functional part with reconstruction of the remaining components (Fig. 21-47). If the function of the two components is equal the appearance of the digits is the deciding factor as to which should be removed. In the case of the thumb it is usually the ulnar thumb that is retained because of the attachment of the collateral ligaments on the ulnar side of the thumb that are necessary for stability in opposition with the other fingers. Most authors follow the 80% principle; that is, if any single portion of the duplication represents 80% of the normal thumb, then that alone is used in the reconstructive process. If it is less than 80%, then tissues from the other duplicated digit are used to augment the larger of the two digits.

It is important to inform the parents that because

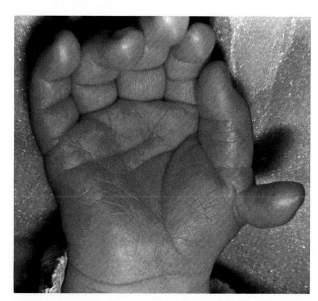

FIGURE 21-46. Incomplete hypoplastic duplication of the thumb.

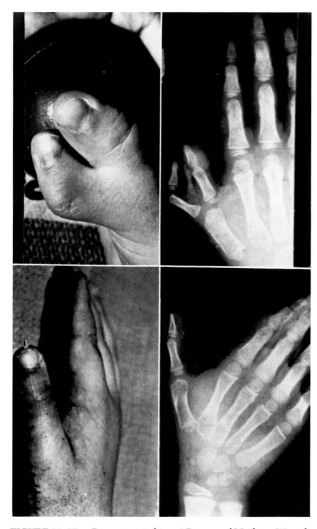

FIGURE 21-47. Reconstructed type 2 Bayne and Marks or Wassel-Egawa type 4 bifid thumb. The hypoplastic radial component is removed; the thumb is realigned by osteotomy, and the radial collateral ligament is reconstructed. The radiographs show the preoperative and postoperative results.

of the shared parts in the duplicated thumb, as well as the necessity to reconstruct many of these anatomic structures and joints, stiffness may result.

Triphalangeal Thumb

Clinical Features

Triphalangeal thumb is characterized by interposition of an extra phalanx between the two phalanges of the thumb (Fig. 21-48). This encompasses a broad spectrum of clinical entities. The extra phalanx varies from a small triangular bone (i.e., delta phalanx) to a normal phalanx in what appears to be a thumbless, five-finger hand. Boys and girls appear to be equally affected, and more than 80% of affected children have bilateral deformities.[274]

The incidence of triphalangeal thumb is 1 in every 25,000 births.[273]

Inheritance

Triphalangeal thumb is inherited as an autosomal dominant trait.[282,286,287] It also has been associated with maternal thalidomide ingestion during pregnancy.[273,283]

Associated Anomalies

Many anomalies are associated with triphalangeal thumb. The most common are polydactyly of the thumb, central deficiencies of the hands and feet, congenital tibial defects, and absence of the pectoral muscles. It also may be part of congenital heart disease, Holt-Oram syndrome, Fanconi aplastic anemia, Blackfan-Diamond syndrome, trisomies 13 through 15, and Junberg-Hayward syndrome.[268,272,275,277,279–281]

Anatomic Pathology

Triphalangeal thumb can be divided into three types:

Type 1: Thumbs with a delta or abnormally shaped phalanx
Type 2: Thumbs with three normal phalanges in excessive length
Type 3: Those hands with five normal fingers and no apparent thumb.

Type 1 triphalangeal thumb includes all abnormally shaped extra phalanges, whether triangular, trapezoid, or rectangular. The distal interphalangeal joint is often incongruous and stiff, especially in the adult. The thumb deviates ulnarward in most cases and only rarely to the radial side. The delta phalanx is located between more normal-appearing distal and proximal phalanges. The more triangular the phalanx, the greater the angulation. The angulation is the result of unequal growth of the delta phalanx.

Type 2 triphalangeal thumb is excessively long but retains its normal proximal location and rotation, which distinguishes it from type III. When the normal thumb is adducted to the index finger its tip normally reaches the middle third of the proximal phalanx. In the type 2 triphalangeal thumb the tip may reach beyond the proximal interphalangeal joint.

Careful observation reveals that the extra long thumb interferes with pinch precision and is cosmetically unappealing. More than one half of these children have contracted first web spaces.[288] This presents a functional deficit by decreasing opposition and limiting grasp between the thumb and the index finger.

Type 3 triphalangeal thumb is really a misnomer: the hand has five normal-appearing fingers and no apparent thumb. More than one half of all triphalangeal thumbs fit into this category.[288] All the fingers

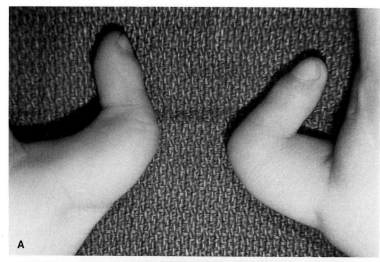

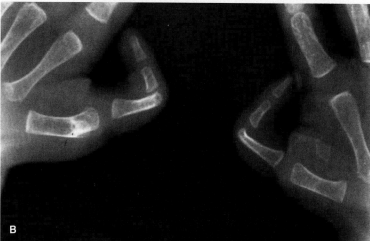

FIGURE 21-48. (A) Clinical photograph and (B) radiograph of a type 2 triphalangeal thumb. There are three normal-shaped phalanges with long, slender appearance, usually with some functional deficit.

are aligned in the same plane. The joints of the most radial digit may be stiff.

Pinch is accomplished between the adducted radial two digits in a clawlike manner. Pinch is weak and many patients develop a widened first web space with rotation of the first finger, such as in pollicization. The palmar grip is usually weak, and the hand serves only as an aid in picking up objects. Most children with this category of triphalangeal thumb have absence of the thenar musculature.[271,273,278,284,288]

Treatment

A conservative approach has no role in the treatment of triphalangeal thumb. The treatment depends on size, stability, and the nature of the angular deformity. It also depends on whether duplication of the adjacent thumb at the site of the triphalangeal digit has occurred.

There are five surgical considerations that are important with triphalangeal thumb:

1. Associated clinical malformations
2. Narrow or contracted thumb-index web space
3. Abnormally shaped extra phalanx
4. Five-fingered hand with all the digits in the same plane
5. Thenar muscle deficiency.

In general, surgery should be performed between 6 months and 2 years of age to allow development of a normal pattern of prehension of the thumb. Surgery is performed only if severe angulation is interfering with normal thumb function. If the child is seen earlier than 1 year of age, Flatt recommends excision of the delta phalanx.[273] He strongly emphasizes the need for adequate collateral ligament reconstruction and Kirschner wire (K wire) fixation for up to 3 months. Early removal of the K-wire may result in an unstable angulated distal phalanx. The earlier the operation is performed, the greater are the chances of good results.

Many surgeons have found this technique disappointing in older adolescents. Several factors are responsible. Joint stiffness and incongruity often prejudice the outcome. Ligament reconstruction frequently fails because of the increased stress involving the everyday use of the digit. This has led to the conclusion that it is better to fuse one or more segments of the triphalangeal thumb.

The goal of surgery in type 2 triphalangeal thumb is reduction of the excessive length. Often the extra phalanx is rectangular, and the appearance is improved by segmental resection of the distal end of the proximal phalanx and the proximal end of the middle phalanx. The neck of the middle phalanx is held in the shaft with K-wires, the extensor mechanism is reefed, and excessive skin is excised later, if necessary. By this procedure, the thumb is shortened and the normal number of joints and phalanges are restored. A simple resection of the extra phalanx is often unsuccessful in restoring normal alignment.

If a web space contracture is present, a four-flap Z-plasty or large dorsal rotation flap is used.[285,289]

In type 3, or five-fingered hand, pollicization of the most radial digital to create a broad web space is needed. This is accomplished by following the procedure described by Barsky,[269] Hertz and Littler,[276] and Buck-Gramcko,[270] in which the digit is shortened, adducted, and pronated to improve function and appearance.[284] Because a large number of five-fingered hands lack appropriate musculature, opponensplasty may be necessary.

Central Polydactyly, or Polysyndactyly

Clinical Features

Central polydactyly involves the index, the long, and the ring fingers and is most often associated with a complex form of syndactyly. The deformity is almost always bilateral, with the ring finger being the most commonly duplicated (Fig. 21-49). It is slightly more common in girls than in boys.[290–293]

Inheritance

Central polydactyly is inherited as an autosomal dominant trait.[292]

Associated Anomalies

Most associated anomalies are of the skeletal system, including syndactyly of the hands and polydactyly of the toes.

Anatomic Pathology

The extra digit in central polydactyly is variable in its presentation. The tendon, bone, and neurovascular supply show great variation, creating a distorted picture. The anomaly often involves complex syndactyly or anomalous phalanges or metacarpals.

Treatment

Surgical approach for central polydactyly should be to release the syndactyly in the first 6 months of life. This early approach is designed to prevent abnormal epiphyseal growth and displacement of normal components that may interfere with growth of the finger.[291,293]

If marked deviation already has occurred, simple removal of the duplicated digit is only part of the solution. More complicated types of surgery, such as osteotomy, reconstruction of soft tissues, and possible arthrodesis, are needed to maintain longitudinal orientation of the digit.

The goal in every patient is to create four normal fingers. If, however, the resultant digits are stiff and unacceptable, Flatt has recommended the creation of a three-fingered hand to maintain the function of the remaining digits.[290]

Postaxial Polydactyly, or Little-Finger Polydactyly

Clinical Features

Little-finger polydactyly is classified into type I, type II, and type III, as outlined by Stelling and Turek.[301] Postaxial polydactyly is seen almost 10 times more

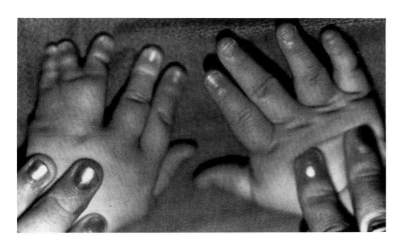

FIGURE 21-49. Central polydactyly. The ring finger is duplicated, and syndactyly is present.

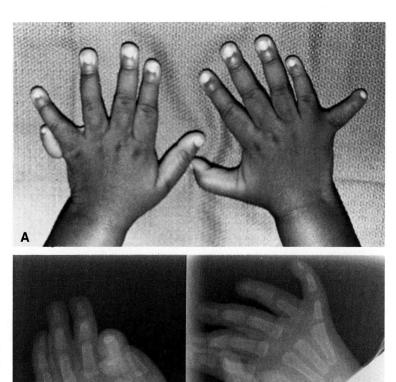

FIGURE 21-50. Polydactyly of the fifth digit. (**A**) The right hand shows a complete duplication of the phalanges of the fifth digit, which is a type II polydactyly. The left hand shows incomplete duplication with no attachment to its adjacent digit, which is a type I polydactyly. (**A1** and **B1**) Radiographs demonstrate the bony characteristics of each.

frequently in African Americans than in Caucasians (1 in 300 to 1 in 3000; Fig. 21-50).[295,304]

Of all the digits that may be duplicated in polydactyly, duplication of the small finger is the most common by a ratio of 8 to 1.[292] The Stelling-Turek type 1 supernumerary digits tend to be bilateral and are almost always on the ulnar side.[301,302]

Inheritance

The well-formed postaxial polydactyly is inherited as an autosomal dominant trait, whereas the skin tag type appears to be a dominant trait with incomplete penetrance.[294]

Associated Anomalies

African-American infants often show postaxial polydactyly as an autosomal dominant trait without associated abnormalities.[297] However, postaxial polydactyly in Caucasian infants has been associated with more than 40 abnormalities.[296,299] The most common local association is syndactyly.[300] Other associations are chromosomal abnormalities (e.g., trisomy 13), eye abnormalities (e.g., Laurence-Moon-Bardet-Biedl syndrome), orofacial abnormalities (e.g., Meckel syndrome), and bone dysplasia (e.g., Ellis-Van Creveld syndrome). Therefore, postaxial occurrence in Caucasian infants requires further evaluation for associated abnormalities.[298]

Anatomic Pathology

As in the case of preaxial polydactyly, postaxial polydactyly represents a variety of anatomic variations. This is characterized by hypoplasia and interconnections of the soft tissue and bones that are often difficult to assess. Radiographic evaluation is essential in classifying the type of duplication for treatment purposes.

Treatment

The treatment of postaxial polydactyly is directed at prevention of further deformity and maintenance of hand function. In type 1 duplications, according to the Stelling and Turek classification, the function of the hand is good, and treatment is directed toward cosmetic appearance by ligation or simple surgical removal at the surgeon's discretion.[301,302] In type 2 duplication, reconstruction is more complicated because the duplicated digit must be deleted and soft tissues from that digit used to reconstruct ligaments and tendons. Osteotomies often are needed to correct deviation. Type 3 duplications represent a complete duplication as a separate ray and can be excised easily.

Surgery should be accomplished when the infant

is 6 to 12 months old to allow development of proper pattern of prehensile function of the hand. The removal of type 1 skin tags obviously may be done much earlier.

General principles of congenital hand reconstruction apply here also. Any excised structure without attention to the adjacent function of the hand or digit is a disservice to the patient. These structures may need to be used for augmentation or stabilization of the adjacent structures. Furthermore, all reconstructive procedures should be finished before school age.

MACRODACTYLY

Clinical Features

Macrodactyly, or gigantism, is a term used to refer to a disproportionately large digit apparent at birth or early childhood. The deformity involves all the structures of the finger, such as the phalanges, the tendon, the nerves, the blood vessels, the fat, the fingernails, and the skin.[306,315] Macrodactyly may be either primary or secondary.

In primary or true macrodactyly all tissue is enlarged such that the finger appears elongated and broadened.[307,309,310,311,316] This type must be distinguished from the secondary type, which results from disorders such as neurofibroma, hemangioma, lymphangioma, arteriovenous fistula, fibrous dysplasia, and lipoma.[305–308,313,318]

Two forms of true macrodactyly have been described.[306] One form is static and consists of a single enlarged digit that is present at birth and subsequently grows proportionally to the other digits. In the second, or progressive, form the digit is not enlarged at birth but begins enlarging in early childhood. The rate of growth is much greater than that of the other digits and frequently results in angular deformity of the digit. The progressive type is more common than the static type.

Macrodactyly is one of the rarest anomalies of the upper extremity. Flatt noted an incidence of 0.9% in the United States.[312] About 95% of cases are unilateral, with the right and the left hands affected equally.[312] The anomaly occurs slightly more often in boys than in girls.[315,316] The index finger is the most frequently involved, with the long finger, the thumb, the ring, and the little fingers following in descending order of frequency. In 70% of cases, multiple finger involvement is present, with the thumb and the index finger the most common, followed by the index and the long fingers.[316] If a single finger is enlarged, it deviates toward the center of the hand. If two digits are involved, they deviate away from each other.

Inheritance

In true macrodactyly there is no familial history of inheritance.[306] Currently its cause remains obscure. Three theories have been postulated: abnormal nerve supply, abnormal blood supply, and abnormal humoral mechanisms.[313] No direct evidence exists that supports either of the latter two.

Associated Anomalies

Macrodactyly is not seen in association with any systemic defects.[316] It does, however, occur in 10% of syndactyly cases.[312,313]

Anatomic Pathology

In macrodactyly all the anatomic structures of the digit become enlarged. Some believe that true macrodactyly is the *forme fruste* of von Recklinghausen neurofibromatosis. Kelikian uses the term *nerve territory oriented macrodactyly* to describe the most common form of macrodactyly.[316] In this occurrence, the most distinctive and consistent change is the aberrations of the digital nerves.[309,310] They become broad, tortuous and covered with a thick epineurium. On the histologic section there is proliferation of fatty infiltration, fibrous endoneurium, and the perineurium, which causes coarseness of the axon cylinders, thereby narrowing the myelin and compressing the axons.[308,320,321]

The bony involvement causes enlargement in the transverse and the longitudinal planes. The bone age for involved fingers appears to be greater than that of normal fingers. Proliferation of the subcutaneous fat with varying amounts of fibrous stoma are present in the fingers of macrodactyly. The skin is usually thickened and the digital arteries also are increased in size. The more distal the involvement, the greater the soft tissue and bony enlargement.

Nerve enlargement may extend proximally into the hand with enlargement of the median nerve producing triggering of the bulbous nerve at the carpal canal level. The close association between peripheral nerve abnormality and macrodactyly has led many to consider the possibility that primary macrodactyly has a neurofibromatosis origin.[307,310,311,313,320]

Treatment

Macrodactyly becomes an obvious enlargement of the digit producing a grotesque deformity that may produce severe psychological changes in a young patient. Because these changes happen early and dramatically out of proportion with the other digits, early intervention is advocated for these young patients. The macrodactylous digit is often cosmetically unsatisfactory as well as stiff. At the cessation of growth, the

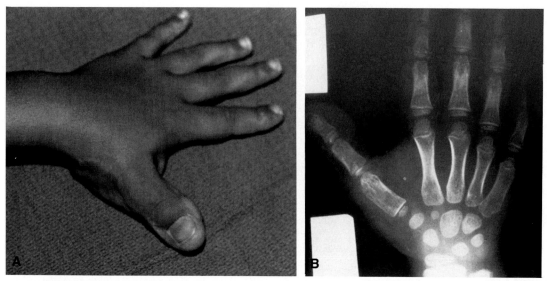

FIGURE 21-51. (A) Patient has persistent soft tissue enlargement following debulking. Bony changes include increased size for length and width. (B) Radiograph demonstrates skeletal change.

involved fingers are 1.5 to 2 times the normal circumference and 1.5 times longer than the other fingers.

Corrective procedures for macrodactyly usually require one or more procedures.[314,322,325] The initial procedure advocated for treatment of macrodactyly includes two stages of soft tissue debulking, size reduction of the soft tissue and bony elements, growth arrest in the form of a epiphysiodesis, arterial ligation, and nerve stripping.[322,325] Even with epiphyseal arrest the longitudinal growth of the finger may be halted, but the finger remains broad and continues to increase in diameter. As soft tissue enlargement proceeds the length of the finger may be normal, but the finger has a bulbous and unattractive appearance. Nerve division has been proposed to eliminate the intrinsic factor; however, it interferes with sensitivity of the finger and has disappointing results in controlling growth of the finger. Although these various procedures of bone shortening and narrowing, defatting of the fingers, and neural stripping may be repeated several times, the resultant digit is often unsatisfactorily stiff and anesthetic. If it inhibits the function of the remainder of the hand ray resection may be considered. However, once ray resection has been carried out, the adjacent digit may begin to adopt a similar behavior, indicating possibly the nerve-mediated origin of this problem.

If epiphysiodesis is recommended it should be carried out at all levels of the digit when the child is 7 or 8 years old. If the child is older the involved finger will be too large for the other fingers to catch up.

If the finger is too large it may be reduced in size by bone shortening at one or more levels, narrowing of the bone structure, defatting of the fingers, and narrowing of the nail and terminal phalanx (Fig. 21-51).[306,319,322] This correction usually is accomplished in

two stages: first by approaching the convex side of the involved digit, then 3 months later by returning to operate on the opposite side. Angular deformity may be corrected by closing-wedge osteotomy. Frequently, soft tissue resection must be performed in two stages to obtain the appropriate results.

When considering reconstruction in the macrodactyly digit, the patient must be aware of the multiple procedures required and the often unsatisfactory results of these procedures. If the resultant digit is unsightly, stiff, and unaesthetic, or if it inhibits the function of the rest of the hand, ray resection may be considered.

CONGENITAL CONSTRICTION BAND SYNDROME

Many names have been ascribed to congenital constriction band syndrome, including Streeter dysplasia, amniotic band syndrome, annular constriction bands, pseudoainhum, and congenital ring constrictions.[326]

Congenital constriction band syndrome may appear anywhere in the body. The most common area is the distal portion of the limbs, particularly the hands.[329,330] The index, the middle, and the ring fingers are affected with almost equal frequency, whereas the little finger and the thumb are rarely involved (Fig. 21-52).[329] Annular constriction bands are twice as common in the upper extremity as in the lower extremity.[326]

Deformities have been grouped into four types by Patterson:

1. Simple ring constrictions
2. Ring constrictions accompanied by fusion of

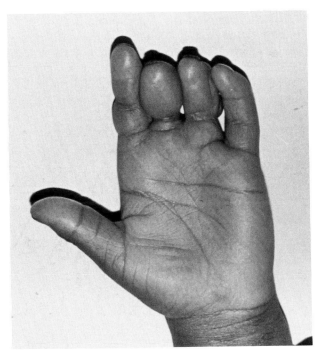

FIGURE 21-52. Congenital constriction band syndrome has many presentations. The thumb and little finger rarely are involved. The index finger shows slight hypoplasia with a partial band. The middle finger shows a severe band proximally, distal ballooning lymphedema, and absence of the distal phalanx. Similar changes are seen in the ring finger.

the distal bony parts, with or without lymphedema

3. Ring constrictions accompanied by fusion of soft tissue parts
4. Intrauterine amputations.[336]

The depth of the constriction band may vary from a small indentation to near strangulation of the distal segment of the digit. Swelling distal to the constriction ring ranges from minimal to severe, which may produce a stiff, functionless digit. The more severe the involvement, the more likely the joints are stiff. The more proximal the involvement, the higher the incidence of neurologic compromise.[326]

Inheritance

Most cases tend to be sporadic although a few familial cases have been reported. The incidence is believed to be between 1 and 5000 to 15,000 births. Boys and girls are affected equally. There is usually the history of some gestational abnormality, and the syndrome is more often seen in association with first pregnancies and premature births.

Causation remains controversial with two major theories predominating: germ plasma defects, as noted by Streeter,[338] and amniotic band constriction, as noted by Kino[331] and Torpin.[340] Temtamy and McKusick

believe that both theories may interplay to produce the ultimate defects.[339] Most patients have a history of abnormal gestational history and appear to have early amnion rupture. Sudden reduction in the fluid volume of the amniotic sac may induce uterine contraction with production of amniotic bands. This gives support to the finding of amniotic bands wrapped around the digits often found in the immediate period after birth.[326]

Associated Anomalies

Annular constriction bands are seen in association with syndactyly, hypoplasia, brachydactyly, symbrachydactyly, symphalangism, and brachydactyly in up to 80% of cases.[329] Other skeletal anomalies include clubfoot, cleft lip, cleft palate, and cranial defects in almost half the patients.[340] Fingernail deformities are common because of acrosyndactyly.[329]

Anatomic Pathology

The annular grooves produced by the constriction band syndrome lie at right angles to the long axis of the bone. The severity of the involvement may vary from a mild depression of the skin to deeper involvement with indentation of the underlying nerves, vessels, and bone. In the acute phase, the distal tissues in the hand are often edematous, and in the chronic stage they are usually thickened and firm. In the acrosyndactyly patient the tips of the digits appear to have fused together with multiple defects in the skin, nail, and underlying bone.

Treatment

Treatment of the congenital constriction band syndrome is directed at two areas: first, the release of the circumferential band to reestablish venous and lymphatic drainage in the distal portions, and second, release of any associated syndactyly.

The treatment of the associated groove should include excision rather than incision. Z-plasties or V-Y-plasties are usually sufficient to release the constriction and reestablish venous-lymphatic flow.[327,328,336] More recently, Upton has emphasized mobilizing the subcutaneous fat as a separate layer in addition to the skin Z-plasty in a better attempt to reduce the significant indentation resulting from the constriction band.[341] Most often surgery is done in two stages, one side of the finger at a time, to prevent vascular compromise from a circumferential operation. Involvement of the soft tissues appears to be more severe on the dorsum than on the volar surface, therefore less dissection is necessary in the areas of the digital vessels and the nerves.[329] In acrosyndactyly, attention is directed first toward separation of the digits if associated constriction rings are not causing compromised circulation.[333] It should be noted that residual limitation of motion of the interphalangeal joints is expected in the patient with acrosyndactyly. If there is circulatory compromise present at birth in the digit these procedures are done expediently. Otherwise they may be delayed until 2 or 3 months of age.

In distal amputations, most children do not require additional surgery. If improvement in prehensile grip is desired, these patients may be helped by web space deepening, phalangeal lengthening, or segmental transposition (Fig. 21-53). Greater attention has been given to microvascular reconstruction in these digits because the proximal portion of these digits have normal anatomic structures. This is in contrast to the

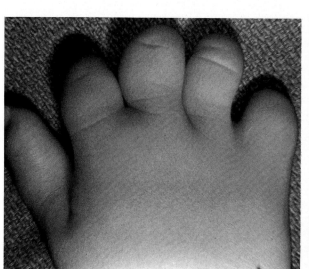
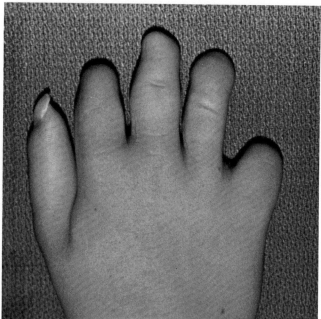
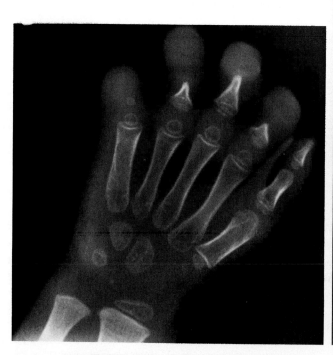
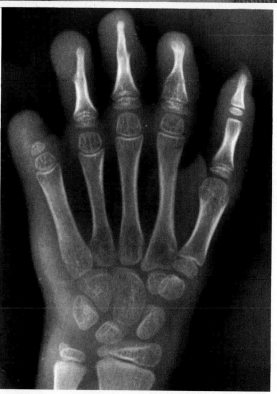

FIGURE 21-53. Terminal absence may be improved with nonvascularized phalangeal toe graft to provide increased length for prehension.

other type of congenital anomalies that are a result of failure formation. Lister[333] and others[334,335] recommend the consideration of toe-to-hand transfer for reconstruction of these more involved patients.

GENERAL SKELETAL ABNORMALITIES

Madelung Deformity

Clinical Features

Madelung deformity is a congenital disorder that does not become clinically obvious until later in childhood, about the age of 8 or 9 years old. It is 4 times more common in girls and is more often bilateral.[354] A classic deformity shows shortening and bowing of the radius with prominence of the ulnar head dorsally, without history of injury or infection. The hand and the wrist appear to be volarly subluxated. Limitation of wrist and forearm motion is usually present, with extension and supination being more affected (Fig. 21-54).

Radiographs show that changes begin at approximately 2 years of age. The ulnar and volar half of the distal radial epiphysis does not grow as rapidly as the radial half. The radius shows a dorsal ulnar curve, decreased longitudinal growth, delayed growth or early fusion of the ulnar half of the distal radial physis, lucency at the ulnar metaphysis of the distal radius, and volar ulnar angulation of the distal radial articular surface.[345] Concomitantly, changes in the ulna show dorsal subluxation and decreased length and enlargement of the ulnar head. The carpus assumes a web-shaped configuration to fit between the radius and the ulna (Fig. 21-55).[345]

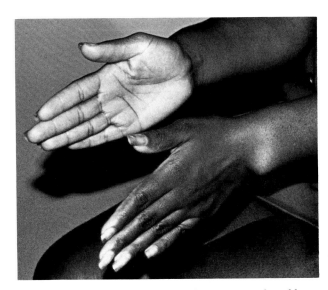

FIGURE 21-54. Madelung deformity demonstrates volar subluxation of the hand, elongated and dorsally prominent ulna, and limited supination.

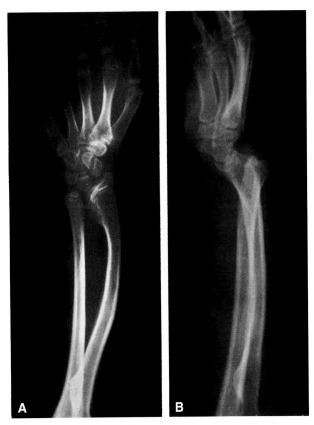

FIGURE 21-55. Radiographic changes in the radius include increased ulnar and volar curve, unequal distal epiphyseal growth, and decreased length. (**A**) Ulnar changes include soral subluxation and relative increased length to radius. (**B**) Carpal bones are wedge-shaped to fit between the radius and the ulna.

Inheritance

Madelung deformity is considered a genetic disorder and is transmitted as an autosomal dominant trait with variable and incomplete penetrance. It is important to distinguish these from other types of deformities that may resemble Madelung deformity but are related to a single traumatic episode, repeated trauma, sickle cell disease, infection, tumors, or other developmental syndromes.

Associated Anomalies

Many other bony abnormalities frequently are associated with Madelung deformity.[350] They include scoliosis, cervical ribs, defects of the humerus, and other bony abnormalities of the lower extremity. The deformity may be seen in syndromes such as Hurler mucopolysaccharidosis, Turner syndrome, and Ollier dyschondroplasia.[354]

Anatomic Pathology

The etiology of Madelung deformity is unknown.[352,356] The ulnar and volar half of the distal radius fails to grow normally. Whether this is a result of musculotendinous anomaly along the volar ulnar surface of the radius that tethers the ulnar half of the radial physis is still debated. Developmentally, the ulnar half of the distal radial physis does appear later and ossifies later than the radial side of the physis. It may represent a primary dyschondroplasia. The end result is the radius curving in the volar ulnar direction while shifting the hand in a volar direction. A gap develops between the distal radius and the ulna, with the carpus wedged into the interosseus space.

Treatment

Deformity of the wrist usually brings the child to seek treatment. It is not essential to treat mild deformities because they are usually painless, and surgical correction does not increase the range of motion of the wrist. Usually, symptomatic treatment is all that is needed. If the pain becomes persistent or the deformity is severe surgical correction may be needed. Surgery should correct the too-long ulna and the radial deformity.

The ulna is shortened by excision of the ulnar head, shortening of the ulna, radioulnar fusion, or epiphysiodesis of the distal ulna.[335-337] There are different methods described to address the deformity of the radius in this condition. Reconstructive osteotomy, usually a biplanar type, has been described to reconstitute the normal radial tilt.[356] This would be better suited for the older, skeletally mature patient. In the younger patient with an open physis, epiphysiodesis, distraction lengthening, and interposition with silicone or collagen has been described.[349-355]

Obstetric Brachial Plexus Injury, or Birth Palsy

Clinical Picture

The occurrence of brachial plexus palsy sustained by the newborn during a difficult delivery has become considerably more infrequent in recent years because of the modern obstetric management.[357]

The incidence of obstetric paralysis has steadily decreased. Hardy noted an incidence of 0.87 in 1000 births in 1981,[368] which is lower than that 1.56 in 1000 from a report by Adler and Patterson[357] in 1938.

Early diagnosis of brachial plexus injury of the newborn is usually not difficult. However, fracture of the clavicle or separation of the proximal humerus can occur at birth and be confused with the obstetric brachial plexus injury. Prompt healing of the fracture, which usually occurs at 7 to 10 days, makes identification of this type injury more clear. In the patient with obstetric brachial plexus injury, the limb usually hangs motionless at the infant's side. Varying degrees of active motion of the upper extremity are usually present while good passive motion is present.

In the child seen at 2 to 3 years of age, the diagnosis may be made by noting the residual deformity secondary to the muscle imbalance despite varying degrees of recovery. The arm may be slightly abducted from the body with notable loss of the humeroscapular motion (Fig. 21-56). Long-standing deformities will be fixed and may be associated with humeral subluxation or dislocation, radial head dislocation, and elbow contractures.

Obstetric brachial plexus injuries may be classified as the following:

Type 1: C4, C5, C6, or Erb palsy (see Fig. 21-56)
Type 2: The entire plexus or Erb-Duchenne-Klumpke palsy
Type 3: C8, T1, or Klumpke palsy

Type I, or Erb palsy, is 4 times more common than the other two types.[357]

Etiology

The cause of nerve injury in obstetric palsy is traction, which usually is the result of fetal malposition; shoulder dystocia; cephalopelvic disproportion; high birthweight associated with maternal diabetes or short, heavy mothers; or the use of forceps. As the newborn is delivered, traction between the head and the shoulder or between the shoulder and the trunk, precipitated by the previously described causes, stretches and injures the child's brachial plexus.

Anatomic Pathology

With involvement of the upper portion of the brachial plexus (type I–Erb palsy of C4, C5, and C6), the appearance is characterized by adduction, internal rotation, and contracture of the shoulder with loss of extension of the elbow. If only mild involvement exists the suprascapular nerve may be the only area of injury with resultant paralysis of the supraspinatus and infraspinatus muscles. When more extensive involvement is seen the deltoid, the external rotators, and the elbow flexors are involved.

In type 1, or whole plexus, obstetric brachial palsy, both motor and sensory deficits usually are present with a virtually flaccid arm.

In type 3, or lower plexus, according to the classification of Klumpke, the muscles of the forearm and the hand, together with the cervical sympathetic system, are paralyzed. This injury involves C8 and T1, and involves limited flexion of the fingers and wrists, poor interosseous function, and Horner syndrome. This third group is rarely seen in its pure form.

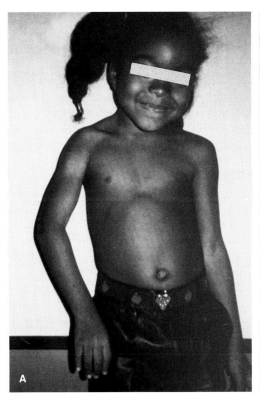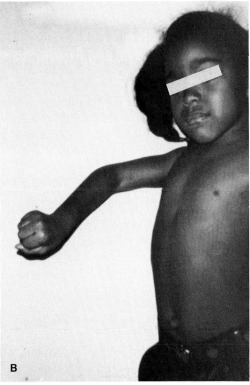

FIGURE 21-56. Patient with Erb palsy shows resting (**A**) and active (**B**) motion. There is residual loss of proximal muscle mass and abduction-external rotation.

Treatment

The natural history of obstetric brachial plexus injury is that about 80% of the children are completely recovered by 12 months of age.[361] Overall treatment should be aimed at preventing contractures in the upper extremity while awaiting neurologic recovery. Most of the children with these types of injuries have excellent recovery of the hand. It is the shoulder function that remains poor. Effort has been directed recently to predict which patients will not improve and to institute earlier treatment to increase the possibility of improvement in function. Several long-term studies now have determined that if the biceps or deltoid is not present by 2 to 3 months of age on physical examination, then its return is usually in doubt.[366,376]

Treatment for the patients who show return of biceps and deltoid function by the second or third month should be observed. In this group intermittent positional splinting may be used, but it is preferable to use range of motion exercises that are carried out at diaper change. Continuous splinting is contraindicated because it may lead to positional contractures, subluxations, and dislocations of the shoulder and elbow. It is important to continue range of motion exercises although the child shows rapid improvement in the early months.

Gilbert and colleagues[366] and Millesi[376] believe that surgical exploration with neurolysis of damaged nerves and grafting of severed nerves is indicated if the infant shows no return of biceps or deltoid function by 2 or 3 months of age. However, Hoffer and colleagues[370] do not share this dismal view; they believe that natural history can improve even in the patient with no biceps function at this age.

If the physician supports the early surgical intervention theory, then at 3 months of age, if there is no biceps function, an electromyogram should be performed. If this shows total absence of electrical activity, then the physician can be confident of avulsion of the corresponding nerve roots. A final evaluation is with cervical myelography, which in skilled hands has a minimal morbidity. The absence of pseudomeningoceles confirms the presence of an extraforaminal lesion. Gilbert and colleagues[366] and Millesi[376] have championed microsurgical techniques for internal neurolysis and interfasicular grafting with demonstrable improvement in these affected children. They showed improvement in deltoid recovery in 80% of cases, biceps recovery in 55% of cases, and improvement in external rotation of the shoulder in 25% of cases. The question that remains unanswered is how many of these children would have improved without surgery.

Often the child does not present until 1 to 2 years of age, at which time contractures about the shoulder may be present. The shoulder usually is adducted and internally rotated. Anterior joint releases may be accomplished by the procedures described by Fairbank[365] and Sever.[380] Active external rotation may be produced by means of tendon transfer of the internal rotators of the shoulder to a more lateral position on the humerus.[361,365,380] L'Episcopo subsequently has added to the above procedures with transfer of the latissimus dorsi and teres major to convert them to external rotators.[374] Further modification has been reported by Hoffer and colleagues,[370] with insertion of the transferred muscles in the posterior aspect of the rotator cuff to facilitate external rotation and glenohumeral abduction.

In our experience, these soft tissue procedures described above have not proven effective. For fixed contractures of 18 months to 3 years, a subscapularis slide may be indicated to permit aid external rotation. A rotational osteotomy is preferable and more predictable than other soft tissue procedures.

Numerous procedures have been described to treat weakness or loss of elbow flexion. The more common procedures for elbow flexion are Clarke pectoral transfer,[363] Steindler flexorplasty,[381] and latissimus or triceps transfer. The pectoral transfer described by Clarke[363] involves a large incision and extensive dissection and can result in significant functional impairment because of loss of pectoralis function. The Steindler flexorplasty involves proximal reattachment of the flexor pronator origin at the elbow to a position on the humerus, which can result in a pronated forearm and inadequate flexion power.[381] The latissimus transfer has the advantage of restoring significant flexion with little residual impairment from its transfer.

Procedures for wrist extension are similar to those for various nerve palsies about the wrist and hand and usually involve transfer of the wrist flexors, either the flexor carpi radialis or the flexor carpi ulnaris to the central extensor carpi radialis brevis.[373] Often a careful physical examination is necessary to identify an appropriate muscle tendon unit for transfer because the wrist flexors may be too weak and, for example, the brachioradialis may be needed for transfer.

Treatment of the patient with the obstetric brachial plexus injury remains an evolving concept as more literature is published supporting early intervention. Still, long-term follow-up is needed to confidentially recommend these newer treatment modalities, and the treating physician must be well-versed in the more established treatment principles in meeting these patients needs.

TRAUMA TO THE PEDIATRIC HAND

This section deals with trauma to the pediatric hand. As the growing child experiences the environment around him or her, the hand is the instrument used in exploration. Unfortunately, it has become the most often injured part of the pediatric patient. Fractures and tendon injuries, along with infections, are common in the pediatric patient, and although knowledge of the pertinent anatomy with principles of treatment usually will effect a satisfactory outcome, the physician must be wary of the old adage that "all children's injuries do well." This section discusses fractures and common tendon injuries along with specific infections involving the pediatric hand.

Skeletal Injuries

There are distinct differences between the skeletal anatomy of the pediatric patient and that of the adult. Unique to the child is an epiphysis, the metabolically active zone responsible for longitudinal growth. Pediatric bones are surrounded by a thick layer of periosteum, which gives protection and allows plasticity to these structures, which can lead to the greenstick fracture unique to the child. The resulting increased osteogenesis allows the child's fracture to heal rapidly and makes the likelihood of nonunion extremely rare (Fig. 21-57).

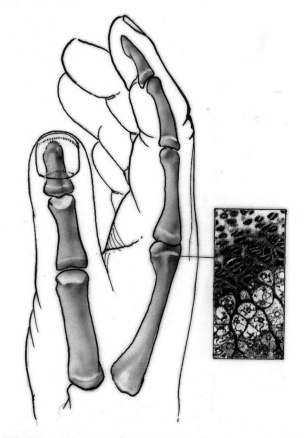

FIGURE 21-57. From the resting zone, the chondrocytes first undergo proliferation, then hypertrophy, and finally provisional calcification, the first step toward bony longitudinal growth. Lack of intercellular collagen in the zone of hypertrophy makes this area prone to injury.

The epiphyseal site in each bone of the child's hand is the most biologically active region, and with the exception of the thumb, each site is found in the proximal aspect of the phalanges and the distal metacarpals, and each site is identical in its anatomic makeup.

With the sound knowledge of this anatomy, most fractures in the pediatric hand can be treated conservatively. In a large series of 276 hand fractures in the patients between the ages of 1 to 11 years of age, Leonard and Dubravcik[396] found that although 41% of these injuries were physeal, only 10% required operative treatment. Hastings and Simmons[394] reported in a review of 354 pediatric hand fractures that in only two patients did a growth disturbance result. Wood[403] has stressed the importance of anatomic reduction, proper confirmation of satisfactory alignment and rotation, and adequate immobilization. Residual displacement of the child's fracture can be accepted if the angulation is close to the biologically active physis, the displacement is within the plane of motion of the joint, and the child has greater than 2 years of growth remaining. Rotational deformity, however, will not remodel. When closed reduction of a metacarpal or a phalangeal fracture is performed it is important to confirm proper clinical rotation of the fingers. With proper rotation all nail beds should be parallel, and finger tips should point to the scaphoid tubercle as the fingers flex toward the palm (Fig. 21-58).

Once closed reduction is performed, immobilization should place the hand in the "safe" position with the metacarpal phalangeal joints in approximately 20 degrees of flexion. This position maintains the collateral ligaments at their full stretch and precludes the development of collateral ligament tightness. Because the pediatric patient has a tremendous ability to destroy a splint or cast in a short time, flexing the elbow 90 degrees and completing the splint or cast above the elbow helps avoid early removal.

It is a mistake, however, to assume that all pediatric fractures do well treated conservatively. If closed reduction cannot obtain or maintain satisfactory alignment, or if the fracture is open, surgical intervention should be performed. The following discussion covers some of the most common and troublesome pediatric fractures involving the hand.

Mallet Finger

A hyperextension injury to the extended digit in the child may result in a mallet finger. The child presents with a flexed or dropped digit at the distal interphalangeal joint and is unable to extend the distal tip of the finger. Although similar in appearance to the adult counterpart, the pathology is different. In a child younger than 3 to 4 years of age, the mallet injury usually results in a Salter-Harris type I or II epiphyseal fracture, with the flexor digitorum profundus flexing the distal metaphysis and the extensor tendon displacing the more proximal physis. In the adolescent patient who is near skeletal maturity the mallet injury usually manifests itself as a Salter-Harris type III injury to the distal phalanx (Fig. 21-59). Treatment involves splinting of the distal interphalangeal joint in full extension for

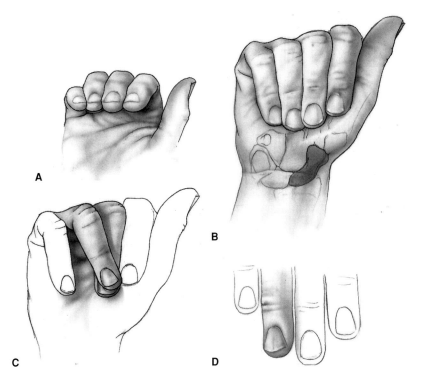

FIGURE 21-58. In the uninjured hand, all nail beds should be parallel, and in flexion all fingertips point to the scaphoid tubercle (**A** and **B**). In malrotation, all fingertips will not point to the scaphoid tubercle, and the nail beds will not be parallel (**C** and **D**).

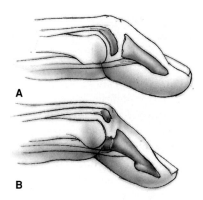

FIGURE 21-59. In the child and the adolescent a mallet finger fracture is very different. (**A**) A Salter type I fracture seen in a child. (**B**) A Salter type III fracture seen in an adult patient nearing skeletal maturity.

approximately 3 to 4 weeks. If anatomic reduction cannot be achieved with the splint in the adolescent variant, open reduction and internal fixation may be necessary[386,388,392,393,399,401] (Fig. 21-60).

Waters and Benson[405] reported two case reports of physeal fracture dislocations of the distal phalanx in a toddler. These cases were originally undiagnosed and only years later did the patient present with a dorsal mass. This represented the dislocated epiphysis from the original injury and only became apparent later when it ossified (Fig. 21-61). Occurring secondary to crush injuries, these two cases report the possibility of dislocation of the epiphysis of the distal phalanx and stress careful physical examination coupled with a high index of suspicion to make the diagnosis and institute early treatment.

Distal Phalanx Fracture and Nail Bed Injury

The most common hand injury in the pediatric patient involves the distal phalanx and accompanying nail bed. This usually results from a crush mechanism with the hand being caught in a door. These fractures are usually an open comminuted fracture with a complex

stellate laceration of the nail bed. It is of utmost importance that all tissue, even of questionable viability, be preserved and loosely sutured because the healing potential in the child is excellent. Because of the preserved soft tissue sleeve, the fracture often receives its stability by simple suture of the laceration.

An injury to the nail bed often accompanies crush fractures to the distal phalanx. Repair of the nail bed, which often is neglected, should receive specific attention because studies have found that up to 50% of patients demonstrated poor results from crush injuries when treated improperly.[403] The nail bed is composed of a germinal and a sterile matrix, with the former being responsible for production of the cells ultimately responsible for the overlying nail plate (Fig. 21-62).

When a subungual hematoma involves more than 25% of the nail it is recommended to remove the nail with a blunt instrument to allow better evaluation of the nail bed.[399] With removal of the nail, laceration through the matrix can be addressed. Using loupe magnification the edges should be trimmed and the nail bed repaired with fine suture. Studies have shown that the new nail plate regenerates only as smoothly as the nail bed below. With completion of the repair, the nail, or if not present, a nonadherent gauze, is placed under the nail bed fold to act as a splint. Not only does this give support to the underlying fracture but also prevents adherence of the overlying nail fold, which may impede growth of the new nail.

Flexor Digitorum Profundus Avulsion and the Reverse Mallet Finger Fracture

An injury that can have significant consequences and that frequently is missed is the flexor digitorum profundus avulsion injury from the distal phalanx, most commonly found in the ring finger. It occurs in the adolescent, usually while playing football, and the patient gives a history of forcible extension of the flexed

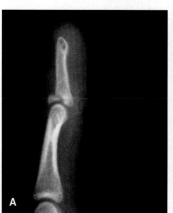

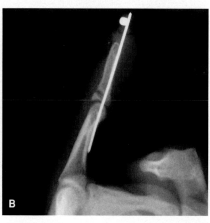

FIGURE 21-60. Radiographs of a Salter type III mallet injury requiring open education and internal fixation.

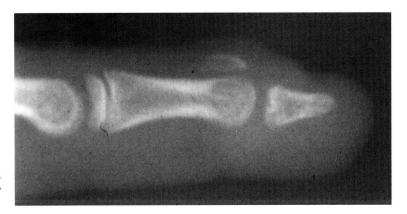

FIGURE 21-61. This dislocated epiphysis was missed at the time of initial presentation. (Courtesy of Waters P, Boston, MA.)

finger while attempting to tackle the opponent. It is also known as the "ring finger jersey injury." The player experiences discomfort in the distal finger and is unable to flex the distal interphalangeal joint actively. This is a pathognomonic sign of the injury that must be sought by the examining physician. Leddy[397] classified this injury into three types, all of which require open surgical repair for return of function (Fig. 21-63). In type 1 injuries, the tendon is avulsed from the bone without being fractured, retracting into the palm and severing all blood supply to the structure. Surgical repair, therefore, must be performed within 7 to 10 days before irreversible changes are initiated. In type 2 injuries, the tendon retracts, often with a small fragment of bone, to the proximal interphalangeal joint, and reinsertion may be successful up to 3 months after injury. In type 3 injuries, a large segment of bone is trapped in the distal interphalangeal joint and surgical repair may be performed up to 3 months after injury. Too often this injury is missed or termed a "jammed finger," and when finally seen, surgical intervention is an impossibility. The importance of recognizing this injury acutely and instituting prompt treatment is of utmost importance.

Phalangeal Neck Fractures, or Supracondylar Fractures

The phalangeal neck fracture involving either the proximal or the middle phalanx is one of the most troublesome pediatric fractures of the hand encountered and carries the worst prognosis if left untreated.[386,388,391–393,399,401–404] These fractures are at the opposite end from where the physis is found and have no potential to remodel. The injury often is caused by a crush mechanism, such as a car door, and on physical examination the only finding may be varying degrees of swelling or ecchymosis. An inadequate radiographic examination is often the source of confusion because the amount of displacement often is not seen. Only a proper anteroposterior and lateral film without overlapping the other fingers shows the classic dorsal dis-

placement that occurs in this type of injury.[391] The lateral radiograph often reveals the distal fragment to be dorsally displaced in relation to the proximal fragment and sometimes rotated up to 100 degrees dorsally. The volar plate and collateral ligaments can become entrapped on the distal fragment, often making the fracture irreducible.

Open reduction and internal fixation are usually

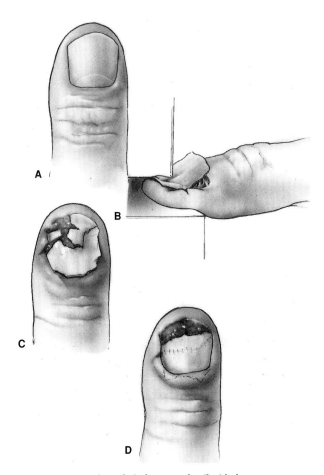

FIGURE 21-62.   (**A** and **B**) The normal nail with the most common mechanism of trauma. (**C**) The resulting stellate laceration of the nail bed often accompanied with distal phalanx fracture. (**D**) The resulting repair of a nail bed with the nail replaced as a stent.

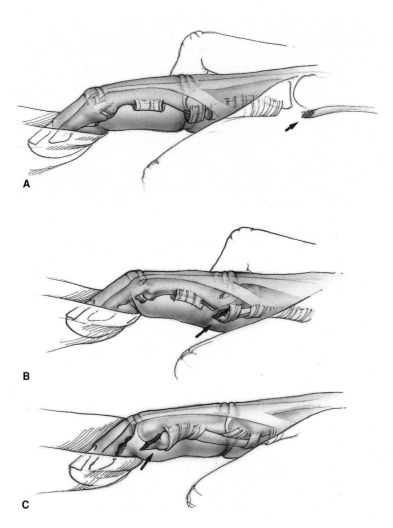

FIGURE 21-63. Leddy classification: (**A**) type 1. (**B**) type 2. (**C**) type 3.

necessary. The fragment is small, sometimes almost entirely composed of cartilage. Through a dorsal extensor tendon splitting incision at the middle phalanx or between the interval of the central slip and lateral band for the proximal phalanx, reduction is obtained and held with two small K-wires. The fracture heals readily, and the pins can be removed between 4 and 6 weeks. Although Dixon and Moon[391] reported successful reduction with percutaneous pinning, most authors advise open reduction (Fig. 21-64).

If this fracture is missed or left untreated, the distal fragment usually heals with significant dorsal displacement resulting in loss of active flexion at the distal interphalangeal joint. Simmons and Peters[400] describe a technique to remove excessive bone in the retrocondylar region to improve motion. Three patients responded with a gain in flexion of 35 to 50 degrees.

Middle Phalanx Fractures

Fractures involving the middle phalanx may be displaced or nondisplaced and usually behave in a spe-

cific manner, depending on the location of the fracture (Fig. 21-65). The flexor digitorum tendon, which inserts on the middle three-fifths of middle phalanx, dictates the direction of the angulation. If the fracture is distal to the insertion of the flexor digitorum superficialis the tendon flexes the proximal fragment and the extensor tendon pulls the distal fragment into extension, resulting in volar angulation (apex volar). Closed reduction is accomplished by traction and flexion of the distal fragment.[403] Conversely, a fracture of the middle phalanx, which is proximal to the insertion of the flexor digitorum superficialis, flexes the distal fragment, whereas the central slip extends the proximal fragment resulting in dorsal angulation (apex dorsal) and requires extension to maintain the position. Overall, in a pediatric hand, fractures of the middle phalanx are relatively rare, tend to be minimally displaced, and heal well with closed reduction and mobilization. However, if there is significant volar or dorsal angulation (>30 degrees) or if there is rotatory malalignment, closed reduction and percutaneous pinning or open reduction and internal fixation may be required.

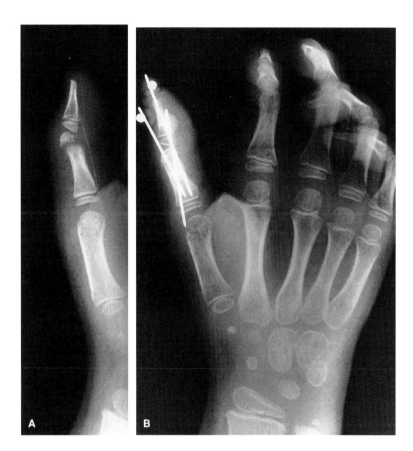

FIGURE 21-64. Displaced supracondylar fractures requiring open reduction and internal fixation with Kirschner wires.

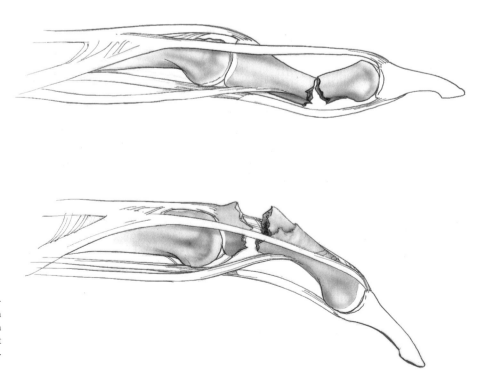

FIGURE 21-65. In treating middle phalanx fractures, the insertion of the flexor superficialis tendon on the middle phalanx is important in determining the position of immobilization.

Intraarticular Fracture of the Proximal Interphalangeal Joint

Fractures at the level of the proximal interphalangeal joint may behave like the adult intercondylar fracture or may be seen as an epiphyseal fracture. The Salter-Harris type III fracture, in which the collateral ligament inserts onto the epiphysis, is involved in this type of injury. This injury, if nondisplaced, will heal well with immobilization; however, if there is displacement greater than 2 mm or involvement of the articular surface of up to 30%, then closed reduction and percutaneous pinning or open reduction and internal fixation is required. If open reduction and internal fixation is required, the fracture is approached in the interval between the lateral band and central slip and fixed with two 0.028-inch K-wires. The K-wires are removed at 4 weeks, and range of motion is started. The intraarticular fracture that involves the head of the proximal phalanx may be intracondylar, either oblique or T-condylar. If the fragments are nondisplaced with no significant step-off at the joint surface simple immobilization in the protective position is all that is required. However, if there is more than 30% joint involvement with greater than 2-mm displacement, surgical intervention is required. It is important to obtain a true lateral of the involved finger because the condylar fragment often is rotated significantly in this plane.

Only with this projection will this be seen. Often, the intercondylar fracture fragment involves only a thin osteochondral slice, and all that may be seen on the radiograph is a flake of bone.

An initially nondisplaced oblique unicondylar fracture frequently slides proximally. If this heals with articular step-off it will lead to traumatic arthritis. Radiographs weekly for the first 2 to 3 weeks are required to avoid missing displacement of the fracture. For the displaced unicondylar or bicondylar fracture, a midlateral approach with incision of one collateral ligament or a dorsal approach between the central slip and lateral band can be performed. In the young child, two small K-wires, 0.028 or 0.035 inch, usually are all that is necessary to hold the fracture, although in the older child (Fig. 21-66) mini screws may be used to hold the reduction and allow for early range of motion.

Fractures of the Shaft of the Proximal Phalanx

Fractures of the shaft of the proximal phalanges are common. They may be transverse, comminuted, or spiral. These fractures should be reduced and held with flexion at the metacarpophalangeal joint. A transverse fracture of the proximal phalanx may heal much

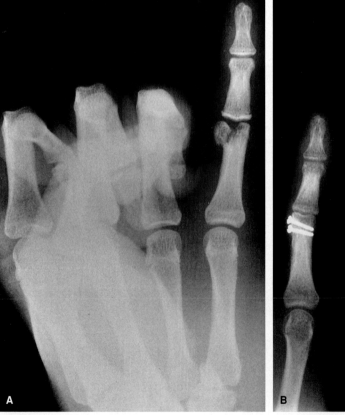
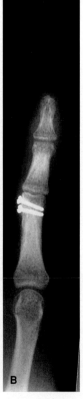

FIGURE 21-66. Radiograph demonstrating (**A**) open reduction and (**B**) internal fixation of a unicondylar fracture.

more slowly than other fractures in the child, requiring up to 6 weeks or more for satisfactory healing. Spiral fractures of the proximal phalanx are often unstable, and if a closed reduction cannot be obtained or maintained, percutaneous pinning or open reduction and internal fixation may be required. Fractures involving the proximal portion of the proximal phalanx have received a significant amount of attention in the literature.

Coonrad and Pohlman[390] reported on the poor results obtained in impacted fractures of the proximal third of the proximal phalanx of the finger in the pediatric patient. This fracture, like its shaft component, usually angulates toward the palm (volar angulation) because of the pull on the intrinsics. If a significant deformity is not corrected limitation of motion results. The intrinsics pull the proximal fragment in a volar direction while the extensors inserting on the base of the midphalanx further shorten the bony column by axial pull. The shortening of the bony column because of the significant volar angulation leaves the extensor tendon in a relatively elongated position and results in inadequate proximal interphalangeal joint extension. Coonrad and Pohlman[390] found that in the younger child, up to 30 degrees of angulation can be accepted, because significant remodeling will occur. However, in the older child, he showed that an uncorrected angulation of 22 degrees or more resulted in significant loss of motion at the metcarpophylangeal joint and poor extension at the proximal interphalangeal joint.[390] Therefore, if satisfactory alignment cannot be maintained, the fracture should be held with cross K-wires for 4 to 6 weeks.

Probably the most common cause of either loss of reduction or failure to obtain a satisfactory reduction is the inability to hold the digit in sufficient flexion in the MP joint to correct the pull of the intrinsics. Any extension permits a loss of reduction, and it is of paramount importance to obtain a true lateral radiograph to confirm proper MP flexion. This is frequently a difficult projection to obtain, but the physician is often amazed at the insufficient flexion seen on the radiograph, even when it appears that the MP joint is in adequate flexion in the cast. If this fracture progresses to a malunion, with the limitation of motion that Coonrad and Pohlman[390] described, the only solution is a dorsal opening wedge osteotomy of the proximal phalanx to correct the deformity.

One of the most common fractures in the pediatric patient is the extraoctave fracture, or the fracture involving the proximal portion of the proximal phalanx, usually in the small finger and presenting with lateral angulation. This injury results from forced ulnar deviation occurring in a fall or when someone grabs the little finger, as can occur when wrestling. The fracture usually is a Salter type II and presents with varying degrees of ulnar deviation. Closed reduction is usually successful in obtaining and maintaining a satisfactory reduction; however, open reduction may be necessary to remove interposed fibrous tissue and entrapped tendons if reduction cannot be maintained. The use of a pencil placed between the fingers to act as a fulcrum has been recommended extensively as a method of closed reduction. Although this technique often works, the epiphysis of the proximal phalanx lies proximal to the web so that the pencil placed between the fingers may be distal to the fracture site and actually block the reduction. The best method to most consistently achieve a closed reduction is to flex the metacarpal phalangeal joint to 90 degrees, which tightens the collateral ligaments thus controlling the proximal fragment. With adduction the distal fragment can be brought into alignment. Immobilization in an ulnar gutter splint for about 3 weeks followed by institution of protective range of motion is usually successful (Fig. 21-67).

With all fractures of the phalanges, the importance of obtaining a proper anteroposterior and true lateral

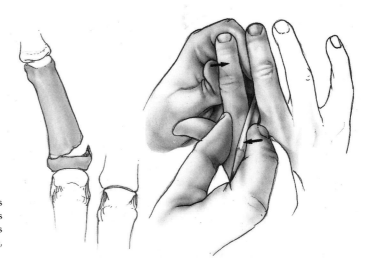

FIGURE 21-67. In the "extra octave" fracture, which is hard to reduce and hold in place, the pencil technique is a way to manipulate this fracture, although some physicians believe that the pencil is distal to the apex of the fracture, which could hinder satisfactory reduction.

radiograph of the involved finger to document not only the extent of angulation but also the adequacy of the closed reduction cannot be underestimated. Campbell[388] has demonstrated a concept to evaluate alignment of phalangeal fractures. Just as a line drawn down the center of the shaft of the radius should always intersect with the center of the capitellum regardless of elbow flexion, a line drawn from the center of the phalangeal neck through the metaphysis should pass through the center of the metacarpal head regardless of flexion. This technique is accurate for anteroposterior, lateral, and oblique films. If the line does not pass through the center of the head, displacement of the involved phalanx as a result of fracture should be suspected.

Metacarpal Fractures

Fractures involving the metacarpal behave differently in the pediatric patient when compared with the adult. The typical "boxer's fracture," involving the distal small finger metacarpal, is usually similar to the adult fracture except for possible physeal involvement. In adults the most common fracture site is the fifth metacarpal, whereas in the child the second and third metacarpal are more frequently involved. Because these metacarpals are less mobile than the ring and small metacarpals less deformity can be accepted.

When displaced, the angulation is usually dorsal (apex dorsal) as a result of the interossei muscles pulling on the distal fragment. Usually the middle and ring metacarpals are less angulated and have less rotatory displacement because of the inherent central stability by the intermetacarpal ligaments. Closed reduction is accomplished with extension of the wrist to relax the extensors, flexion at the MP joint while applying dorsal pressure at the proximal interphalangeal joint, and counterpressure over the metacarpal shaft. Mobilization should be for 3 to 4 weeks followed by range of motion. As much as 60 to 70 degrees of residual dorsal angulation at the ring and small finger can be accepted. However, because of the decreased compensatory motion allowed at the carpometacarpal joint, only 10 to 15 degrees of residual angulation should be accepted at the second and third metacarpal shaft. Again, rotational deformity cannot be accepted, and closed reduction with percutaneous pinning or open reduction and internal fixation may be necessary.

The closed fist injury, or human bite, resulting in an open metacarpal fracture can be a particularly troublesome injury if not seen and cared for early. Any laceration over the metacarpal phalangeal joint, especially in the index finger in the child, must raise suspicion of a human bite. Often the emergency room physician does not consider this, and the child does not give a truthful history. The laceration may be closed and a radiograph not even obtained, and only when the patient presents as early as 12 to 24 hours later with overt infection does the diagnosis become apparent. Radiographs should be obtained to evaluate the fracture and look for air within the soft tissues. Usually, when the hand strikes the mouth, the MP joint is in a flexed position, which allows the tooth to enter and inoculate the joint. The finger is then extended allowing the extensor and capsule to close over the laceration in the joint capsule.

The most common organism seen in this injury is either a Staphylococcus or Streptococcus species, but the organism of notorious repute is a gram negative, facultative anaerobe, Eikinella corrodens. This organism is best grown in a 10% CO_2 medium because of its facultative anaerobic nature. If this injury is suspected, whether or not a fracture is present, the patient should be treated surgically. Skin wound margins should be excised, followed by debridement of the tendon and extension of the arthrotomy into the joint, usually leaving the wound open. Intravenous antibiotics should be given. Usually the E corrodens is sensitive to penicillin, although there has been a 20% resistance documented.[27] Amoxicillin with clavulanate has been recommended to cover not only the Eikinella but the other more common Staphylococcus and Streptococcus species and anaerobes that often are cultured.

Fractures at the base of the thumb metacarpal deserve special attention because they are commonly seen in the pediatric patient. The mechanism of injury, which usually includes an axial, longitudinally directed force against a slightly adducted and flexed metacarpal, causes a Bennett fracture dislocation in the adult; in the child it results in an impacted fracture at the base of the thumb metacarpal. The Bennett fracture dislocation also occurs in the child and is treated the same as in an adult. The impacted fracture at the base of the thumb metacarpal, however, usually presents with radial angulation (Fig. 21-68). In the patient with radial angulation (apex radial), up to 30 degrees of angulation is acceptable because this will remodel. The parents should be warned that a bump will remain for up to 1 year once the cast is taken off. Angulation greater than 30 degrees should be reduced with pressure applied at the base of the thumb and concomitant counter pressure over the head of the metacarpal. Often, in an attempt to provide counterpressure, the metacarpal phalangeal joint is extended, even hyperextended, and this does not correct the deformity.

Ulnar displacement occasionally occurs in this fracture and usually is an unstable injury requiring open reduction with internal fixation. Because the physis is located at the proximal aspect of the thumb metacarpal these injures can involve the physis. Treatment is directed at restoring articular congruity if the

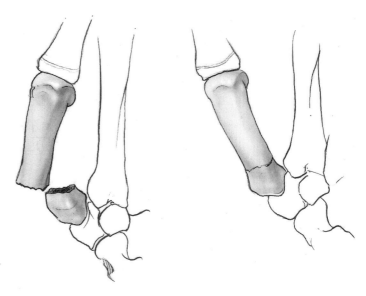

FIGURE 21-68. Closed manipulation and casting of the thumb metacarpal fracture with radial deviation is an easy way to treat this fracture.

physeal fracture is a Salter type III or IV fracture. As seen in the adult Bennett fracture dislocation, the anterior oblique ligament that anchors the first metacarpal to the trapezium is extremely strong, usually holding this fragment while the shaft and base are pulled proximally and radially by the abductor pollicis longus accentuated by the pull of the adductor pollicis. Unlike the adult, the periosteal sleeve is usually intact, which may help in closed reduction. If closed reduction is unsuccessful at maintaining reduction, this fracture dislocation should be treated as in the adult with closed reduction and percutaneous pinning. Occasionally, a complete displacement will buttonhole through the periosteal sleeve precluding a closed reduction and requiring open reduction and internal fixation.

Injury of the Metacarpophalangeal and Proximal Interphalangeal Joints

Joint injuries occur commonly in the pediatric patient. The presentation is different than in the adult because of the physis. The insertion of the collateral ligaments is different for both the proximal interphalangeal and the metacarpophalangeal joints.[387] The collateral ligaments and capsular structures around the joints in the child are much stronger than the epiphyseal plate so that injuries that would cause a dislocation in the adult result in an epiphyseal injury in the child. Bogumill[387] has shown in an anatomic study that the collateral ligament at the level of the proximal interphalangeal joint attaches to the metaphysis, whereas at the metacarpophalangeal joint the attachment is almost exclusively to the epiphysis. This would result in a Salter type III injury at the base of the P1 phalanx, whereas in the middle phalanx a joint injury would more likely result in a Salter type II injury.[387] In the

thumb this is similar to the gamekeeper's injury seen in the adult. If the joint surface involves more than 30% or there is more than 2 mm of displacement, closed reduction with percutaneous pinning or open reduction and internal fixation is required (Fig. 21-69).

Metacarpophalangeal dislocations occur in the pediatric patient and require special attention. The injury occurs with forced hyperextension of the proximal phalanx, most commonly the index finger, usually from a fall on the hand. This injury can be simple or complex and has a special predilection for the pediatric patient. In the simple injury the volar plate tears from the metacarpal head. It usually remains partially intact, allowing a successful closed reduction. In the complex dislocation, the volar plate is completely torn from the metacarpal head and comes to a position dorsal to the metacarpal head, usually precluding a closed reduction. The proximal phalanx is dislocated dorsal to the metacarpal head. It is held in this position because the flexor tendons are displaced toward the ulna, and the lumbrical tendons are displaced in a radial position. The physical examination and the radiographs can help differentiate between the simple and complex dislocation, which is important in instituting proper treatment. In the simple dislocation the proximal phalanx is significantly hyperextended in relation to the metacarpal head, but usually, some bone-to-bone contact remains (Fig. 21-70). Closed reduction is usually successful. Flexion of the wrist, accentuation of the deformity into hyperextension, and then gradual flexion will reduce it. It is important not to apply excessive longitudinal traction to the digit because this may convert a simple to complex injury.

The complex injury always involves a complete tear of the volar plate from the metacarpal head, which is interposed dorsal to the metacarpal head. Clinically there is not the amount of hyperextension seen in the

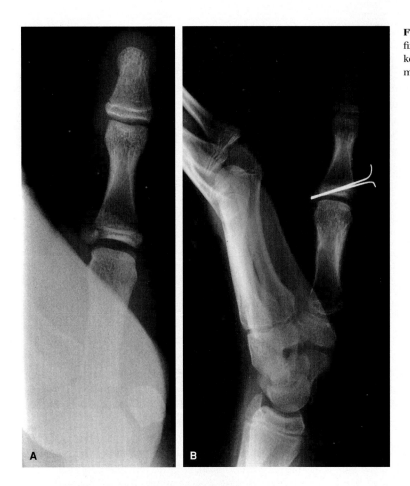

FIGURE 21-69. (A) Open reduction and (B) internal fixation of the displaced Salter type III fracture (gamekeeper's type) in which there were 2 mm of displacement and significant rotation.

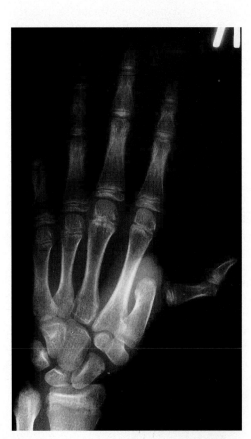

FIGURE 21-70. Radiograph of simple metacarpophalangeal dislocation.

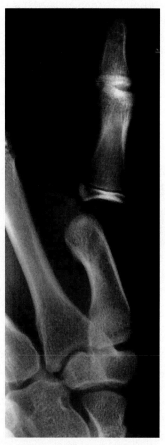

FIGURE 21-71. Radiograph of complex dislocation.

simple variant, and often a dimpling is seen on the volar surface of the palm from the pronounced displacement of the metacarpal head into the palmar fascia. The radiograph demonstrates the metacarpal head and the base of the proximal phalanx to be more parallel. If ossified, a sesamoid may be seen in the joint (Fig. 21-71). Attempts at closed reduction are usually unsuccessful because of the interposed volar plate. One or two attempts at closed reduction may be tried, and often instillation of local anesthetic from a dorsal

approach pushes the displaced volar plate in a volar direction. Open reduction usually is required in this type of injury. There is controversy as to whether a volar or dorsal approach is best. The volar approach, popularized by Kaplan,[395] allows reconstitution of normal anatomy but does place the radial digital nerve at risk because of its altered position. The dorsal approach, popularized by Becton and colleagues,[385] is more forgiving, usually allowing reconstruction of normal anatomy, and if there is a dorsal metacarpal

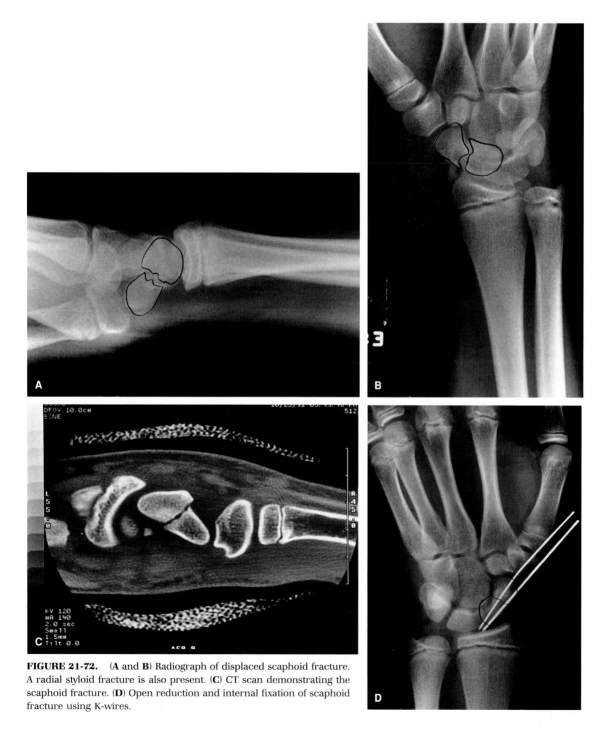

FIGURE 21-72. (A and B) Radiograph of displaced scaphoid fracture. A radial styloid fracture is also present. (C) CT scan demonstrating the scaphoid fracture. (D) Open reduction and internal fixation of scaphoid fracture using K-wires.

fracture present, fixation can be performed at the same time.

Carpal Injuries

Although the distal radius remains the most common site of injury in the pediatric injured physis, the adjacent carpal bones are rarely injured. The significant cartilaginous component in the child's carpus, which ossifies centrifugally, probably protects this area from significant injury. With a hyperdorsiflexion injury to the wrist and forearm area the distal radial epiphysis is usually the site to be injured; however, as this physis closes the scaphoid does become more liable to injury. The scaphoid is the most common bone to be injured in the carpus, and the usual mechanism of injury is a fall onto the outstretched hand. The fracture is usually not displaced and is located in the distal third of the bone.[389] Immobilization in a short-arm thumb spica cast until clinical and radiographic evidence of healing is usually successful; nonunion is rare.

Significantly displaced scaphoid fractures in the pediatric patient, as in an adult, require open reduction and internal fixation (Fig. 21-72).

Recently, fractures of the triquetrum have been described. Letts and Esser[398] reported 15 children with fractures of the triquetrum. The most common mechanism of the injury was a fall onto an outstretched hand, and the most common type was a flake fracture of the triquetrum. All were treated with a short-arm cast with good clinical results. The authors of that study warn that suitable radiographs, including a pronated oblique view, is often necessary to demonstrate this fracture, whose symptoms may be attributed to a sprain of the wrist or Salter type I injury of the distal ulna or radius. Early recognition with expedient treatment usually effects an excellent outcome. However, if the injury is missed it may be a source of chronic wrist pain. Clinical suspicion is important in recognizing this injury, which is localized by pinpoint tenderness dorsally just distal to the ulnar styloid.

References

Upper Limb

1. Conway H, Bowe J. Congenital deformities of the hands. Plast Reconstr Surg 1986;18:2.
2. Flatt AE. The care of congenital hand anomalies. St Louis: CV Mosby, 1977:50.

Classification of Upper Limb Malformations

3. Birch-Jensen A. Congenital deformities of the upper extremities. Odense, Denmark: Endelsbogtrykkeriet and Det Danske Forlag, 1949:15.
4. Blakeslee B, ed. The limb deficient child. Los Angeles: University of California Press, 1963:26.

5. Cowan NJ, Loftus JM. Distraction, augmentation, manoplasty: technique for lengthening digits for the entire hand. Orthop Rev 1978;7(6):45.
6. Lamb DW. General principles of management. In: Lamb DW, Kuczynski K, eds. The practice of hand surgery. London: Blackwell Scientific Publications, 1981;299.
7. MacDonnell JA. Age of fitting upper extremity prosthesis in children. J Bone Joint Surg 1958;40A:655.
8. Matev IB. Thumb reconstruction in children through metacarpal lengthening. Plast Reconstr Surg 1979;64(5):665.
9. May JW, Smith RJ, Peimer CA. Toe to hand free tissue transfer for thumb reconstruction with multiple digit aplasia. Plast Reconstr Surg 1981;67(2):205.
10. O'Brien BMcC, Franklin JD, Morrison WA, MacCleod AM. Microvascular great toe transfer for congenital absence of thumb. Hand 1978;10:113.
11. Rogala EJ, Wynne-Davies R, Littlejohn A, Gormley J. Congenital limb anomalies. Frequency and etiological factors. J Med Genet 1974;11:221.
12. Swanson AB. A classification for congenital limb malformations. J Hand Surg 1976;1:8.
13. Temtamy SA, McKusick VA. Absence deformities as a part of syndromes. Birth Defects 1978;14:73.

Radial Deficiencies (Radial Clubhand)

14. Albee FH. Formation of radius congenitally absent, condition seven years after implantation of bone graft. Ann Surg 1928;87:105–110.
15. Bay K, Levine C. Congenital radial aplasia. Mo Med 1988; 85(2):87.
16. Bayne LG. Radial club hand (radial deficiencies). In: Green DP, ed. Operative hand surgery. 2nd ed. New York: Churchill Livingstone, 1988:261.
17. Bayne LG, Klug MS. Long-term review of the surgical treatment of radial deficiencies. J Hand Surg [Am] 1987;12(2):169.
18. Baync LG, Lovell WW, Marks TW. The radial club hand. In: Proceedings of the American Society for Surgery of the Hand. J Bone Joint Surg [Am] 1970;52(5):1065.
19. Birch-Jensen A. Congenital deformities of the upper extremities. Copenhagen: Ejnar Munksgaard Forlag, 1950.
20. Bora FW Jr, Carniol PJ, Martin E. Congenital anomalies of the upper limb: radial club hand. In: Bora FW Jr, ed. The pediatric upper extremity: diagnosis and management. Philadelphia: WB Saunders, 1986:28.
21. Bora FW Jr, Nicholson JT, Cheema HM. Radial meromelia: the deformity and its treatment. J Bone Joint Surg [Am] 1970;52:966.
22. Bora W Jr, Osterman AL, Kaneda RP, Esterhai J. Radial club hand deformity. J Bone Joint Surg [Am] 1981;63:741.
23. Buck-Gramcko D. Index pollicization. In: Strickland J. The thumb. Churchill Livingstone, 1990.
24. Buck-Gramcko D. Radialization as a new treatment for radial club hand. J Hand Surgery [Am] 1985;10(6):964.
25. Carrol RE, Louis DS. Anomalies associated with radial dysplasia. J Pediatr 1974;84(3):409.
26. Carrol RE. Use of the fibula for reconstruction in congenital absence of the radius. Proceedings of the American Academy of Orthopaedic Surgeons. J Bone Joint Surg [Am] 1966;48:1012.
27. Define D. New surgical treatment of congenital absence of the radius. Proceedings of the Ninth Congress of the Societé Internationale de Chirurgie Orthopaedique et de Traumatologie. Brussels: Imprimerie des Sciences, 1964:653.
28. Dell PC, Sheppard JE. Thrombocytopenia, absent radius syndrome: report of two siblings and a review of the hematologic and genetic features. Clin Orthop 1982;162:129.

29. De Lorme TL. Treatment of congenital absence of the radius by transepiphyseal fixation. J Bone Joint Surg [Am] 1969; 51:117.

30. Entin MA. Reconstruction of congenital aplasia of radial component. Surg Clin North Am 1964;44:1091.

31. Flatt AE. Radial club hand. In: The care of congenital hand anomalies. St Louis: CV Mosby, 1977:286.

32. Frantz CH, O'Rahilly R. Congenital skeletal limb deficiencies. J Bone Joint Surg [Am] 1961;43(8):1202.

33. Goldberg MJ, Bartoshesky LE. Congenital hand anomaly: etiology and associated malformations. Hand Clin 1985;1(3):405.

34. Goldner LJ. Congenital absence of the radius and digital deformities. Inter-Clinic Information Bulletin, 1965.

35. Kato K. Congenital absence of the radius wiht review of the literature and report of three cases. J Bone Joint Surg 1924;22:589.

36. Kelikian H. Radial ray defect. In: Congenital deformities of the hand and forearm. Philadelphia: WB Saunders, 1974:780.

37. Kessler I. Centralization of the radial club hand by gradual distraction. J Hand Surg [Br] 1989;14(1):37.

38. Lamb DW. Radial club hand, a continuing study of sixty-eight patients with one hundred and seventeen club hands. J Bone Joint Surg [Am] 1977;59:7.

39. Lidge RT. Congenital radial deficient club hand. J Bone Joint Surg [Am] 1969;51:1041.

40. Nettelblad H, Randolph MA, Weiland AJ. Free microvascular epiphyseal-plate transplantation. J Bone Joint Surg [Am] 1984; 66(9):1421.

41. Petit JL. Remarques sur un enfant Nouveau-ne, dont les bras e-tainent difformes. Paris: Mem d l'Acad Roy d Sci, 1733:17.

42. Quan L, Smith DW. The VATER Association: Vertebral defects, anal atresia, T.E. Fistula, radial and renal dysplasia: a spectrum of associated defects. J Pediatr 1973;82:104.

43. Riordan CD. Congenital absence of the radius, 15 year follow-up. J Bone Joint Surg [Am] 1955;37:1129.

44. Saunders JW. The proximodistal sequence of origin of the parts of the chick wing and the role of the ectoderm. Exp Zool 1948;108:363.

45. Sayer RH. A contribution to the study of the club hand. Trans Am Orthop Assoc 1893;6:208.

46. Sherik S, Flatt A. The anatomy of congenital radial dysplasia. Clin Orthop 1969;66:125.

47. Smith RJ. The radial club hand. Bull Hosp Jt Dis 1964;25(1):85.

48. Starr DE. Congenital absence of the radius: a method of surgical correction. J Bone Joint Surg [Am] 1945;27(4):572.

49. Swanson AB. A classification for congenital limb malformations. J Hand Surg 1976;1:8.

50. Tachdjian MO. Congenital absence of the radius. In: Pediatric orthopedics. Philadelphia: WB Saunders, 1972:108.

51. Tsai TM. Free epiphyseal transfer. Orthop Trans 1985;9:409.

52. Tsai TM, Ludwig L, Tonkin M. Vascularized fibula epiphyseal transfer: a clinical study. Clin Orthop 1986;228:210.

53. Tsuge K, Watari S. New surgical procedure for correction of club hand. J Hand Surg [Am] 1984;9(9):541.

54. Urban MA, Osterman AL. Management of radial dysplasia. Hand Clin 1990;6(4):589.

55. Watson HK, Beebe RD, Cruz NI. A centralization procedure for radial club hand. J Hand Surg [Am] 1984;9(4):541.

56. Weiland AJ, Kleinert HE, Kutz JE, et al. Free vascularized bone grafts in surgery of the upper extremity. J Hand Surg 1979;4(2):129.

Central Deficiencies

57. Barsky AJ. Cleft hand classification: incidence and treatment. J Bone Joint Surg [Am] 1964;46:1707.

58. Bauer TB, Tondra JM, Trusler HM. Technical modifications and repair of syndactylism. Plast Reconstr Surg 1956;17:385.

59. Birch-Jensen A. Congenital deformities of the upper extremity. Odense Denmark: Enjar Munksgaards Forlag, 1949:46.

60. Buck-Gramcko D. Hanchirurgi, band I, allegmeines wahloperationen. Stuttgart: Thieme, 1981.

61. Flatt AE. The care of congenital hand anomalies. St. Louis: CV Mosby, 1977:265.

62. Graham JB, Bagley CE. Splint hand with unusual complications. Am J Hum Genet 1954;7:44.

63. Kameyama Y. Morphorgenesis of poly- and oliodactylism in the rat fetus due to myleran (busulfan) Teratology 1969;2:262.

64. Kelikian H. Congenital deformities of the hand and forearm. Philadelphia: WB Saunders, 1974:467.

65. Lange M. Grundsatzlicjes uber die Beurteilung der Enstehung und Bewertung atypischer Hand und Fussmissbildungen Verh Dtsch Ortop Des 31 Kongsberg/Pr Z Orthop 1936;31:80.

66. Maisel SDO. Lobster claw deformity of the hands and feet. Br J Plast Surg 1970;23:269.

67. Milford L. The split hand. Presentation at the Symposium on Congenital Hand Deformities sponsored by the American Society for Surgery of the Hand, Atlanta, May 4–6, 1978.

68. Miura T, Komada T. Simple method for reconstruction of the cleft hand with an adducted thumb. Plast Reconstr Surg 1979;64.

69. Muller W. Die angeborenem Fehbildugen der menschlichen Hand. Leipzig: Thieme, 1937.

70. Nutt JN, Flatt AE. Congenital central hand defect. J Hand Surg 1981;6:48.

71. Ogino T. Cleft hand. Hand Clinic 1990;6(4):661.

72. Rogala EJ, Wynne-Davies R, Littlejohn A, Gormly A. Congenital limb anomalies: frequency and etiology factors. J Med Genet 1974;11:221.

73. Rudiger RA, Haase W, Passarge E. Association of extradactyly, extrodermal dysplasia and cleft lip palate. Am J Dis Child 1970;120:160.

74. Saito H, Seki T, Suzuki Y, et al. Operative treatments for various types of cleft hand. Seikeigeha 1978;29:1551.

75. Sandzen SC Jr. Classification and functional management of congenital central defects of the hand. Hand Clin 1985; 1(3):483.

76. Snow JW, Littler JW. Surgical treatment of the cleft hand. Transactions International Society of Plastic and Reconstructive Surgery, Fourth Congress. Rome: Excerpta Medica, 1967;888.

77. Temtamy SA. Genetic factors in hand malformation. Thesis. Baltimore: Johns Hopkins University, 1966.

78. Ube Y. Plastic surgery for the cleft hand. J Hand Surg 1981;6:557.

79. Watari S, Tsuge K. A classification of cleft hands based on clinical findings. Plast Reconstr Surg 1979;64:381.

80. Watari S, Hagiyama Y, Tsuge K. Recent knowledge on cleft hands. Hiroshima J Med Sci 1984;33:81.

Ulnar Deficiencies (Ulnar Club Hand)

81. Bayne LG. Ulnar club hand. In: Green DP, ed. Operative hand surgery. New York: Churchill Livingstone, 1982:261.

82. Blair WF, Shurr DG, Buckwalter JA. Functional status in the ulnar deficiency. J Pediatr Orthop 1983;3:37.

83. Bora FW Jr, Nicholson JT, Cheemah M. Radial meromelia: the deformity and its treatment. J Bone Joint Surg [Am] 1970;52:966.

84. Broudy AS, Smith RJ. Deformities of the hand and wrist with ulnar deficiency. J Hand Surg 1979;4:304.

85. Carroll RE, Bowers WH: Congenital deficiency of the ulna. J Hand Surg 1977;2:169.

86. Downie GR. Limb deficiencies and prosthetic devices. Orthop Clin North Am 1976;7:465.

87. Flatt AE. The care of congenital hand anomalies, 2nd ed. St. Louis: Quality Medical Publishing, 1994:411.

88. Flatt AE. The care of the congenital hand anomalies. St. Louis: CV Mosby, 1977:238.

89. Frantz CH, O'Rahilly R. Congenital skeletal limb deficiency. J Bone Joint Surg [Am] 1961;43:1201.

90. Johnson J, Omer GE Jr. Congenital ulnar deficiency natural history and therapeutic implications. Hand Clin 1985;1:499.

91. Kummel W. Die Mmissbildugen der Extremitaten durch defeckt. Verwachsung und Uberzahl, Atfte 3. Bibliotheca Medica, Kassel, 1895.

92. Laurin CA, Farmer AW. Congenital absence of the ulna. Can J Surg 1959;2:204.

93. Lloyd-Roberts GC. Treatment of defects of the ulna in children by establishing cross union with the radius. J Bone Joint Surg [Br] 1973;55:327.

94. McKusick V. Mendelian inheritance in man. Baltimore: Johns Hopkins Press, 1966:133.

95. O'Rahilly R. Morphological patterns in limb deficiency and duplications. Am J Anat 1951;89:135.

96. Ogden JA, Beall JK, Conlogue GJ, Light TR: Radiology of postnatal skeletal development: 4 distal radius and ulnar skeletal. Radiology 1981;6:255.

97. Ogden JA, Watson HK, Bohne W. Ulnar dysmelia. J Bone Joint Surg [Am] 1976;58:467.

98. Riordan DC. Congenital absence of the ulnar. In: Lovell WW, Winter RB, eds. Pediatric orthopaedics. 2nd ed. Philadelphia: JB Lippincott, 1978:714.

99. Riordan DC. Congenital absence of the radius or ulna. Abstract. J Bone Joint Surg [Br] 1972;54:381.

100. Riordan DC, Mills EH, Aldredge RH. Congenital absence of the ulna. J Bone Joint Surg [Am] 1961;43:614.

101. Roberts AS. A case of deformity of the forearm and hands with an unusual history of hereditary congenital deficiency. Ann of Surg 1886;3:135.

102. Straub LR. Congenital absence of the ulna. Am J Surg 1965;109:300.

103. Swanson AB, Tada K, Yonenobu K. Ulnar ray deficiency: its various manifestations. J Hand Surg [Am] 1984;9:658.

104. Watson HH, Bohne WH. The role of the fibrous band in the ulnar deficient extremities. J Bone Joint Surg [Am] 1971; 53:816.

Synostosis

105. Brady LP, Jewett EL. Treatment for radial ulnar synostosis. South Med J 1960;53:507.

106. Cleary JE, Omer GE. Congenital proximal radial ulnar synostosis natural history and functional assessment. J Bone Joint Surg [Am] 1985;67:539.

107. Dawson HGW. Congenital deformity of the forearm and its operative treatment. Br Med J 1912;2:833.

108. Hansen OH, Anderson NO. Congenital radial ulnar synostosis: report of 37 cases. Acta Orthop Scand 1970;41:225.

109. Kelikian H, Doumanian A. Swivel for proximal radial ulnar synostosis. J Bone Joint Surg [Am] 1957;39:945.

110. Kelikian, H. Congenital deformities of the hand and forearm. Philadelphia: WB Saunders, 1974.

111. McCredie J. Congenital fusion of bones: radiology, embryology and pathogenesis. Clin Radiol 1975;26:47.

112. Minaar AB de V. Congenital fusion between the lunate and the triquetral bones in the South African Bantu. J Bone Joint Surg [Br] 1952;34:45.

113. Mital MA. Congenital radial ulnar synostosis in congenital dislocation of the radial head. Orthop Clin North Am 1976; 7:375.

114. Miura T, Nakamura R, Suzuki M, Kanie J. Congenital radial ulnar synostosis. J Hand Surg [Br] 1984;9:153.

115. Ogino T, Hokino, K. Congenital radial ulnar synostosis: compensatory rotation around the wrist and rotation osteotomy. J Hand Surg [Br] 1987;12:173.

116. Simmons BP, Southmayd WW, Riseborough EJ. Congenital radial ulnar synostosis. J Hand Surg 1983;829.

117. Smith RJ, Lipke RW. Treatment of congenital hand deformities of the hand and forearm. N Engl J Med 1979;300:402.

118. Temtamy SA, McKusick VA. Carpal/tarsal synostosis. Birth Defects 1978;14:502.

119. Temtamy SA, McKusick VA. The genetics of hand malformation. Birth Defects 1978;4:301.

Radial Head Dislocations

120. Almquist EE, Gordon LH, Blue AI. Congenital dislocation of the head of the radius. J Bone Joint Surg [Am] 1966;51:118.

121. Brennan JJ, Krause MEH, Harvey DM. Annular ligament reconstruction for congenital anterior dislocation of the radial heads. Clin Orthop 1963;29:205.

122. Dobyns JH. Congenital abnormalities of the elbow. In: Morrey BF, ed. The elbow and its disorders. Philadelphia: WB Saunders, 1985.

123. Hirayama T, Takeimitsu Y, Yagihara K, Mikita A. Operation for chronic dislocation of the radial head in children: reduction by osteotomy of the ulna. J Bone Joint Surg [Br] 1987;9:639.

124. Kelikian H. Congenital deformities of the hand and forearm. Philadelphia: WB Saunders, 1974:902.

125. Lloyd-Roberts GC, Bucknil TM. Anterior dislocation of the radial head: etiology natural history management. J Bone Joint Surg [Br] 1977;59:402.

126. Mardam-Bey T, Ger G. Congenital radial head dislocation. J Hand Surg 1979;4:316.

127. McKusick VA. Mendelian inheritance in man catalogues of autosomal dominance, autosomal recessive, and X-linked phenotypes. 2nd ed. Baltimore: Johns Hopkins Press, 1968.

128. Mital MA. Congenital radial ulnar synostosis in congenital dislocation of the radial head. Orthop Clin North Am 1976; 7:375.

129. Villa A, Paley D, Katangi MA, et al. Lengthening of the forearm by Ilizarov technique. Clin Orthop 1990;250:125.

130. Wynne-Davis R. Heritable disorders in orthopaedic practice. Oxford: Blackwell Scientific Publications, 1973.

Syndactyly

131. Bauer TB, Tondra JM, Trussler HM. Technical modifications in the repair of syndactylism. Plast Reconstr Surg 1956;17:385.

132. Buck-Gramcko D. Congenital malformations: syndactyly and related deformities. In: Nigst H, Buck-Gramcko D, Millesi H, Lister G, eds. Hand surgery. New York: Thieme, 1988:12.

133. Dobyns JH. Problems and complications in management of upper extremity anomalies. Hand Clin 1986;2:373.

134. Flatt AE. Practical factors in the treatment of syndactylism. In: Littler DW, Cramer LM, Smith JW, eds. Symposium on reconstructive hand surgery. St. Louis: CV Mosby, 1974.

135. Hoover G, Flatt AE, Weiss MW. The hand and Apert's syndrome. J Bone Joint Surg [Am] 1970;52:878.

136. Iowan DCR, Takayama N, Flatt AE. Poland's syndrome: a review of 43 cases. J Bone Joint Surg [Am] 1976;58:52.

137. John EB. Operative Behandlung der Syndaktylie: Zeitpunkt-Technik-Ergebniss E. Theiss: Heinberg 1979.

138. Kelikian H. Congenital deformities of the hand and forearm. Philadelphia: WB Saunders, 1974;939.

139. Norton AT. A new and reliable operation for the cure of webbed fingers. Br Med J 1881;2:931.

140. Temtamy SA. McKusick VA. Syndactyly. Birth Defects 1978;14:301.

141. Wilson MR, Louis DS, Stevenson TR. Poland's syndrome: variable expression in associated anomalies. J Hand Surg [Am] 1988;13:880.

142. Woolf RM, Broadbent TR. The four flap Z-plasty. Plast Reconstr Surg 1972;49:48.

Arthrogryposis

143. Banker BQ. Neuropathologic aspects of arthrogryposis multiplex congenita. Clin Orthop 1985;194:30.

144. Bennett JB, Hansen PE, Grandberry WM, Cain TE. Surgical management of arthrogryposis in the upper extremity. J Pediatr Orthop 1985;5:281.

145. Brown LM, Robson MJ, Sharrad WJW. The pathophysiology of arthrogryposis multiple congenita neurologica. J Bone Joint Surg [Br] 1980;62:291.

146. Bunnell S. Restoring flexion to the paralytic elbow. J Bone Joint Surg [Am] 1951;33:566.

147. Carroll RE, Hill NA. Triceps transfer to restore elbow flexion: the study of fifteen patients with paralytic lesions in arthrogryposis. J Bone Joint Surg [Am] 1970;52:239.

148. Drummond DS, Siller TN, Cruess RL. Management of arthrogryposis multiplex congenita. AAOS Instructional Course Lecture. St. Louis: CV Mosby 1974;23:79.

149. Ferguson AB Jr. Orthopaedic surgery in infancy and childhood. Baltimore: Williams & Wilkins, 1975:438.

150. Fowler M. A case of arthrogryposis multiplex congenita with lesions in the nervous system. Arch Dis Child 1959;34:505.

151. Hansen OM. Surgical anatomy in treatment of patients with arthrogryposis. J Bone Joint Surg [Am] 1961;43:855.

152. Lewin P. Arthrogryposis multiplex congenita. J Bone Joint Surg [Am] 1925;7:630.

153. Lloyd-Roberts GC, Lettn AWF. Arthrogryposis multiplex congenita. J Bone Joint Surg [Am] 1961;43:855.

154. Lloyd-roberts GC, Lettn AWF. Arthrogryposis multiplex congenita. J Bone Joint Surg [Br] 1970;52:494.

155. Mater I. Surgical treatment of spastic thumb and palm deformities. J Bone Joint Surg [Br] 1963;45:703.

156. Smith RJ. The hand deformities of arthrogryposis multiplex congenita. J Bone Joint Surg [Am] 1973;55:883.

157. Stiendler A. Arthrogryposis. Journal of the International College of Surgeons 1949;12:21.

158. Swinyard CA, Black EE. The etiology of arthrogryposis (multiple congenital contracture). Clin Orthop 1985;194:15.

159. Thompson GH, Bilenker RM. Comprehensive management of arthrogryposis multiple congenita. Clin Orthop 1985;194:614.

160. Weeks PM. Surgical correction of upper extremity deformities in arthrogryposis. Plast Reconstr Surg 1965;36:459.

161. Zancolli E, Mitre H. Latissimus dorsi transfer to restore elbow flexion: appraisal of eight cases. J Bone Joint Surg [Am] 1973;55:1265.

Trigger Digits

162. Dinham JM, Meggit DF. Trigger thumbs in children. J Bone Joint Surg [Br] 1974;56:153.

163. Fahey JJ, Bollinger JA. The trigger fingers in adults and children. J Bone Joint Surg [Am] 1954;36:1200.

164. Flatt AE. The care of congenital hand anomalies. 2nd ed. St. Louis: Quality Medical Publishing, 1994:411.

165. Flatt AE. Care of the congenital hand anomalies. St. Louis: CV Mosby, 1977:59.

166. Ger E, Kupcha P, Ger D. The management of trigger thumbs in children. J Hand Surg 1991;16:944.

167. Hudson HW. Snapping thumb in childhood reported eight cases. N Engl J Med 1935;210:854.

168. Jahs SA. Trigger fingers in children. JAMA 1963;107:463.

169. Kelikian H. Congenital deformities in the hand and forearm. Philadelphia: WB Saunders, 1974:902.

170. Sampson SP, Badalament MA, Hurst LC, Seidman J. Pathobiology of the human A1 pulley in trigger finger. J Hand Surg [Am] 1991;16:714.

171. Sprecher EE. Trigger fingers in infants. J Bone Joint Surg [Am] 1949:672.

172. Tsuyuguchi Y, Toda K, Kawaii H. Splint therapy for trigger fingers in children. Arch Phys Med Rehab 1983;64:75.

173. Van Genechten F. Familial trigger thumb in children. Hand 1982;14:56.

174. Weber PC. Trigger thumbs in successive generations of family: a case report. Clin Orthop 1979;143:167.

175. White JW, Jensen WE. Trigger thumbs in infants. Am J Dis Child 1953;85:141.

176. Zadek I. Stenosing tenovaginitis of the thumb in infants. J Bone Joint Surg [Am] 1942;424:326.

Camptodactyly

177. Adams W. On congenital contracture of the fingers and its association with "hammertoe": its pathology and treatment. Lancet 1891;2:165.

178. Cooney WP. Camptodactyly and clinodactyly. In: Carter P, ed. Reconstruction of the child's hand. Philadelphia: Lea & Febiger, 1991.

179. Currariano G, Waldman I. Camptodactyly. AJR 1964;92:1312.

180. Engber WM, Flatt AE. Camptodactyly: an analysis of sixty-six patients in twenty-four operations. J Hand Surg 1977;2:216.

181. Hefner RA. Inheritance of the crooked little figner (streblomicrodactyly). J Hered 1929;20:395.

182. Hori M, Nakamura R, Ninove G, et al. Non-operative treatment of camptodactyly; J Hand Surg [Am] 1987;12:1061.

183. Jones KG, Marmor L, Langford LL. An overview on new procedures in surgery of the hand. Clin Orthop 1974;99:154.

184. Kourtemanche AD, Camptodactyly: etiology and management. Plast Reconstr Surg 1969;44:451.

185. Kilgore ES, Jr, Graham WP III. The hand. Philadelphia: Lea & Febiger, 1977.

186. Koman LA, Toby EB, Poehling GG. Congenital flexion deformities of the proximal phalangeal joint in children; a subgroup of camptodactyly. J Hand Surg [Am] 1990;15:582.

187. Lankford LL. The American Society for Surgery of the Hand Correspondence Club Newsletter, May, 1975.

188. Maeda M, Matsui T. Camptodactyly caused by an abnormal lumbrical muscle. J Hand Surg [Br] 1985;10:95.

189. McFarland RM, Curry GJ, Evans HB. Anomalies of the intrinsic muscles in camptodactyly. J Hand Surg 1983;8:531.

190. Millesi H. Camptodactyly. In: Littler JW, Cramer LM, Smith JW, eds. Symposium on reconstructive surgery. St. Louis: CV Mosby, 1974.

191. Miura T. Non-traumatic flexion deformity of the proximal interphalangeal joint—its pathogenesis and treatment. Hand 1983;15:25.

192. Miura T, Nakamura R, Tamura Y. Longstanding dynamic extended splintage and release of abnormal restraining structures in camptodactyly. J Hand Surg [Br] 1992;17:665.

193. O'Brien JP, Hodgston AR. Congenital abnormality of the flexor digitorum profundus, cause of flexion deformity of the long and ring fingers. Clin Orthop 1974;104:206.

194. Ogino T, Kato T. Operative findings in camptodactyly of the little finger. J Hand Surg [Br] 1992;17:661.

195. Oldfield MC. Camptodactyly Dupuytren's contracture (abridged) proceedings. Roy Soc Med 1954;8:312.

196. Oldfield MC. Camptodactyly flexion contracture of the fingers in young girls. Br J Plast Surg 1956;8:312.

197. Parkes-Weber F. Further rare diseases. London: Staples Press, 1949.

198. Poznanski AK. The hand in radiologic diagnosis. Vol 4. Philadelphia: WB Saunders, 1974:213.

199. Siegert JJ, Cooney WP, Dobyns JH. Management of simple syndactyly; J Hand Surg [Br] 1990;15:181.

200. Smith RJ, Kaplan EB. Camptodactyly in similar atraumatic flexion deformities of the proximal interphalangeal joints of the fingers. J Bone Joint Surg [Am] 1968;50:1187.

201. Stoddard SE. Nomenclature of hereditary crooked fingers. J Hered 1939;30:511.

202. Welch JP, Temtamy SA. Hereditary contracture of the fingers (camptodactyly). J Med Genet 1966;3:104.

Clinodactyly

203. Burke F, Flatt AE. Clinodactyly. A review of a series of cases. Hand 1979;3:269.

204. Doeget C, Thulin HC, Priest JH, et al. Studies of a family with oral facial digital syndrome. N Engl J Med 1968;271 10:73.

205. Dudding BA, Gorlin RJ, Langer LO Jr. Otopalito digital syndrome; a new symptom complex consisting of deafness, dwarfism, cleft palate, characteristic faces and a generalized bone dysplasia. Am J Dis Child 1967;113:214.

206. Gall JC Jr, Stern AM, Cohen MM, et al. Holt-Oram syndrome: clinical and genetic study of a large family. Am J Hum Genet 1966;18:187.

207. Gerald B, Umansky R. Cornelia de Lange syndrome: radiographic findings. Radiology, 1967;88:96.

208. Gorlin RJ, Meskin LH, Peterson WC Jr, Gotz RW. Focal dermal hypoplasia syndrome. Acta Derm Venereol (Stockh) 1963;43:421.

209. Harle TS, Stevenson JR. Hereditary symphalangism associated with carpal and tarsal fusions. Radiology 1967;89:91.

210. Hefke HW. Roentgenologic study of anomalies of hand in 100 cases of mongolism. Am J Dis Child 1940:1319.

211. Hoefnagle D, Gerald PS. Hereditary brachydactyly. Ann Hum Genet 1966;29:377.

212. Holden JD, Akers WA. Golt's syndrome: focal dermal hypoplasia: a combined mesoectodermal dysplasia. Am J Dis Child 1967;114:292.

213. Houston CS. Roentgen findings in XXXY chromosome anomaly. J Can Assoc Radiol 1967;18:258.

214. Langer LO Jr. The roentgenographic features of otopalito digital (OPD) syndrome. Am J Roentgenol 1967:163.

215. Lemili L, Smith DW. The XO syndrome. Study of differentiated phenotype in 25 patients. J Pediatr 1963;63:577.

216. McArthur RG, Edwards JH. Delange syndrome. A report of 20 cases. Can Med Assn J 1967;96:1185.

217. McKusick VA. Heritable disorders of connective tissues. 3rd ed. St. Louis: CV Mosby 1966;122:402.

218. Minagi H, Steinbach HL. Roentgen appearance of anomalies associated with hypoplastic anemias in children. Fanconi's anemia and congenital hypoplastic anemia. AJR 1966;97:100.

219. Mosely JE, Moloshok RE, Freiberger RH. The silver syndrome: congenital asymmetry, short stature and variation of sexual development: roentgen features. AJR 1966;97:74.

220. Ozonoff MB, Steinbach HL, Mamunes P. The trisomy 18 syndrome. AJR 1964;91:618.

221. Poznanski AK. The hand in radiologic diagnosis. Vol. 4. Philadelphia: WB Saunders, 1974:112.

222. Robinson GC, Wood EJ, Miller JR, Baillie J. Hereditary brachy-dactyly and hip disease: unusual radiologic and dermatoglyphic findings in a kindred. J Pediatr 1968;72:539.

223. Rubinowitz JG, Mosley JE, Mitty HA, Hirshorn K. Trisomy 18, esophageal litresia, anomalies of the radius, and congenital hypoplastic thrombocytopenia. Radiology 1989;488.

224. Silver HK. Asymmetry, short stature, variations in sexual development. Am J Dis Child 1964;107:495.

225. Wood V. Clinodactyly. In: Green DP. Operative hand surgery. New York: Churchill Livingstone, 1988:422.

Delta Phalanx

226. Amuso SJ. Diastrophic dwarfism. J Bone Joint Surg [Am] 1968;50:113.

227. Barsky AJ, Congenital anomalies of the hand. J Bone Joint Surg [Am] 1951;33:35.

228. Blevins AD, Light TR. Congenital delta, trapezoidal, and triangular bones in the hand. J Hand Surg (in press).

229. Carstam N, Thenader G. Surgical treatment of clinodactyly caused by longitudinally bracketed diaphysis (delta phalanx). Scand J Plast Reconstr Surg 1975;9:199.

230. Cenani A, Lenz W, Totale Syndaktylie und totale radio-ulnare synostose bei swei bruedern. Z Kinderheilkd 1967;101:181.

231. Flatt AE. The care of congenital hand anomalies. St. Louis: CV Mosby, 1977:157.

232. Hersch AH, DeMarinis F. Stecher RMP. On the inheritance and development of clinodactyly. Am J Hum Genet 1953;5:257.

233. Jaeger M, Refior HJ. The congenital triangular deformity of the tubular bones of the hand and foot. Clin Orthop 1971;81:139.

234. Jones JB. Delta phalanx. J Bone Joint Surg [Br] 1964;46:22.

235. Leclercq C, Moneta MR. The treatment of congenital clinodactyly of the hand. Ital J Orthop Traumatol 1989;15(3):339.

236. Ogden JA, Light TR, Conlogue GJ. Correlative roentgenography and morphology of the longitudinal epiphyseal bracket. Skeletal Radiol 1981;6:109.

237. Poznanski AK, Pratt GB, Manson G, et al. Clinodactyly, camptodactyly, Kirner's deformity and other crooked fingers. Radiology 1969;93:573.

238. Sella EJ. Delta phalanx. Conn Med 1972;36:437.

239. Stover CN, Hayes JT, Holt JF. Diastrophic dwarfism. AJR 1963;89:914.

240. Smith RJ. Osteotomy for delta phalanx: deformity. Clin Orthop 1977;123:91.

241. Taybi H. Diatrophic dwarfism. Radiology 1963;80:1.

242. Theander G, Carstam N, Rausing A. Longitudinally bracketed diaphysis in young children. Acta Radiol Diagn 1982;23:293.

243. Watson HK, Boyes JH. Congenital angular deformity of the digits. Delta phalanx. J Bone Joint Surg [Am] 1967;49:333.

244. Wood VE, Flatt AE. Congenital triangular bones in the hand. J Hand Surg 1977;2:1979.

245. Wood VE. Treatment of central polydactyly. Clin Orthop 1971;74:196.

Duplication

246. Andrew JG, Sykes PA. Duplicate thumbs: a survey results of 20 patients. J Hand Surg [Br] 1988;53:50.

247. Bilhaut M. Guerison d'un puce bifide per un nouveau procede operatoire. Congr Fr Chir 1890;4:576.

248. Buck-Gramcko D. Congenital malformations. Polydactyly. In: Nigst H, Buck-Gramcko D, Millesi H, Lister GD, eds. Hand surgery. Vol 1. New York: Thieme, 1988.

249. Cheng JCY, Chang KM, Ma GFY, Leung PC. Polydactyly of the thumb: a surgical plan based on 95 cases. J Hand Surg 1984;9:155.

250. Dobyns JH, Lipscomb PR, Cooney WP. Management of thumb duplication. Clin Orthop 1985;195:26.

251. Egawa T. Surgical treatment of polydactyly of the thumb. Plast Reconstr Surg 1966;9:97.
252. Ezaki M. Radial polydactyly. Hand Clin 1990;6(4):577.
253. Hartrampf CR. Vasconez LO, Mathes S. Construction of one good thumb from both parts of a congenitally bifid thumb. Plast Reconstr Surg 1974;54:148.
254. Hentz VR, Littler JW. The surgical management of congenital hand anomalies. In: Converse JM, Littler JW, eds. Reconstructive plastic surgery: the hand and upper extremity. Philadelphia: WB Saunders, 1977:3306.
255. Kelikian H. Congenital deformities of the hand and forearm. Philadelphia: WB Saunders, 1974;408.
256. Lister G. Pollex adductus in hypoplasia and duplication of the thumb. J Hand Surg [Am] 1991;16:626.
257. Manske PR. Treatment of the duplicate thumb using ligamentous/periosteal flap. J Hand Surg [Am] 1989;14:733.
258. Marks TW, Bayne LGP. Polydactyly of the thumb: abnormal anatomy and treatment. J Hand Surg 1978;3:107.
259. Mirura T. Duplicated thumb. Plast Reconstr Surg 1982;69:470.
260. Nakamura J, Kanahara K, Endo Y, Hirase Y. Effective use of portions of the supranumerary digit to correct polydactyly of the thumb. Ann Plast Surg 1985;15:7.
261. Palmieri TJ. Polydactyly of the thumb: incidence, etiology, classifications and treatment. Bull Hosp Jt Dis 173;34:200.
262. Tada K, Yonenobu K, Tsuyuguchi Y, et al. Duplication of the thumb: a retrospective review of 237 cases. J Bone Joint Surg [Am] 1983;64:584.
263. Temtamy SA, McKusick VA. Polydactyly. Birth Defects. 1978; 14:364.
264. Tuch BA, Lipp EB, Larsen IJ, Gordon LH. A review of duplicate thumb and its surgical management. Clin Orthop 1977; 125:159.
265. Upton J. Congenital anomalies of the hand and forearm. In: McCarthy J, ed. Plast Surg 1990;8:5213.
266. Wassel HD. The results of surgery for polydactyly of the thumb: a review. Clin Orthop 1969;64:175.
267. Woolf CM, Myrianthopoulos NC. Polydactyly in American Negroes and whites. Am J Hum Genet 1973;25:397.

Triphalangeal Thumb

268. Aase JM, Smith DW. Congenital anemia and triphalangeal thumbs. J Pediatr 1969;74:471.
269. Barsky AJ. Congenital anomalies of the hand and their surgical treatment. Springfield, IL: Charles C. Thomas, 1958.
270. Buck-Gramcko D. Pollicization of the index finger. J Bone Joint Surg [Am] 1971;15:1605.
271. Cotta N, Jaeger M. The familial triphalangia of the thumb and its operative treatment. Arch Orthop Unfallchir 1965;58:282.
272. Diamond LR, Allen DM, Magill FB. Congenital (erythroid) hypoplastic anemia: a 25 year-study. Am J Dis Child 1961;102:403.
273. Flatt AE. The care of congenital hand anomalies. St Louis: CV Mosby, 1977:109.
274. Gates RR. Human genetics. New York: Macmillan, 1946:413.
275. Haas SL. Three-phalangeal thumbs. AJR 1939;42:677.
276. Hertz VR, Littler JW. Adduction, pronation, and recession of the second metacarpal in thumb agenesis. J Hand Surg 1977; 2:113.
277. Jaeger M, Riefor HJ. The congenital triangular deformity of the tubular bones of the hand and foot. Clin Orthop 1971;81:139.
278. Miura T. Triphalangeal thumb and dermatoglyphics. J Hand Surg [Br] 1984;9:151.
279. Phillips RS. Congenital splint foot (lobster claw) and triphalangeal thumbs. J Bone Joint Surg [Br] 1971;53:247.
280. Polinelli U. A case of familial hyperphalangia of the thumbs. Minerva Urol Nefrol 1962;12:373.
281. Poznanski AK, Garn SM, Holt JF. The thumb in the congenital malformation syndromes. Radiology 1971;100:115.
282. Qazi QH, Smithwick EM. Triphalangy of thumbs and great toes. Am J Dis Child 1970;120:255.
283. Rath F. Triphalangie des Daumens als Manifestations from der Thalidomidembryopathie. Wien Klin Wochenschr 1966;78:181.
284. Shiono H, Ogino T. Triphalangeal thumb and dermatoglyphics. J Hand Surg [Br] 1984;9:151.
285. Strauch B, Spinner M. Congenital anomaly of the thumb: absent intrinsics and flexor pollicis longus. J Bone Joint Surg [Am] 1976;58:115.
286. Swanson AB, Brown KS. Hereditary triphalangeal thumb. J Hered 1962;53:259.
287. Temtamy S, McKusick VA. Synopsis of hand malformations with particular emphasis on genetic factors. Birth Defects 1969;3:125.
288. Wood VE. Treatment of the triphalangeal thumb. Clin Orthop 1967;120:188.
289. Woolf RM, Broadbent TR. The four-flap Z-plasty. Plast Reconstr Surg 1972;49:48.

Central Polydactyly

290. Flatt AE. The care of congenital hand anomalies. St Louis: CV Mosby, 1977:233.
291. Tada K, Kurisaki E, Yonenobu K, et al. Central polydactyly—a review of 12 cases and their surgical treatment. J Hand Surg 1982;7:460.
292. Temtamy S, McKusick VA. Synopsis of hand malformations with particular emphasis on genetic factors. Birth Defects 1969;3:125.
293. Wood VE. Treatment of central polydactyly. Clin Orthop 1971;74:196.

Postaxial Polydactyly

294. Barsky AJ. Congenital anomalies of the hand and their surgical treatment. Springfield, IL: Charles C. Thomas, 1958;48.
295. Frazier TM. A note on race-specific congenital malformation rates. Am J Obstet Gynecol 1960;80:184.
296. Kelikian H. Congenital deformities of the hand and forearm. Philadelphia: WB Saunders, 1947;408.
297. McKusick VA. Mendelian inheritance in man. Baltimore: John Hopkins University Press, 1971:237.
298. Nathan PA, Kenniston RC. Crossed polydactyly. J Bone Joint Surg [Am] 1975;57:847.
299. Ruby L, Goldberg MJ. Syndactyly and polydactyly. Orthop Clin North Am 1976;7:361.
300. Simmons BP. Polydactyly. Hand Clin 1985;1:545.
301. Stelling F. The upper extremity. In: Ferguson AB, ed. Orthopaedic surgery infancy and childhood. Baltimore: Williams & Wilkins 1963:304:308.
302. Turek SL. Orthopaedic principles and their applications. Philadelphia: JB Lippincott, 1976:23.
303. Wood VE. Postaxial polydactyly (little finger polydactyly) In: Green DP, ed. Operative hand surgery. 2nd ed. New York: Churchill Livingstone, 1988;479.
304. Woolf CM, Myrianthopoulos NC. Polydactyly in American Negroes and whites. Am J Hum Genet 1973;25:397.

Macrodactyly

305. Amadio PC, Reisman HM, Dobyns JH. Lipofibromatous hematoma of nerve. J Hand Surg [Am] 1988;13:67.

306. Barsky AJ. Congenital anomalies of the hand and their surgical treatment. Springfield, IL: Charles C. Thomas, 158;114.

307. Barsky AJ. Macrodactyly. J Bone Joint Surg [Am] 1967;49:1255.

308. Bell G, Inglis K. Plexiformneuroma. Med J Aust 1925;2:432.

309. Boyes JG. Macrodactylism—a review and proposed management. Hand 1977;9:172.

310. Dell TC. Macrodactyly. Symposium on congenital deformities of the hand. Hand Clinics 1985;1:511.

311. Edgerton MT, Turek DB. Macrodactyly (digital gigantism): its nature and treatment. In: Littler JW, Carmer LM, Smith JW, eds. Symposium on reconstructive hand surgery. Vol. 9. St. Louis: CV Mosby, 1974:157.

312. Flatt AE. The care of congenital hand anomalies. St Louis: CV Mosby. 1977;249.

313. Inglis K. Local gigantism (a manifestation of neurofibromatosis): its relation to geneal gigantism and to acromegaly illustrating the influence of intrinsic factors in disease when development of the body is abnormal. Am J Pathol 1950; 26:1059.

314. Jones KG. Megalodactylism: case report of child treated by epiphyseal resection. J Bone Joint Surg [Am] 1963;45:1704.

315. Kalen V, Burwell DS, Omer GE. Macrodactyly of the hands and feet. Am J Hand Surg 1988;8:311.

316. Kelikian H. Congenital deformities of the hand and forearm. Philadelphia: WB Saunders, 1974:610.

317. Khanna N, Gupta S, Hanna S, Tripathi F. Macrodactyly. Hand 1975;7:212.

318. Klippel M, Trenaunay P. Du Naveus variqueux osteohypertrophique. Arch Med Genet 1990;3:641.

319. Millesi H. Macrodactyly: a case study. In: Littler JW, Cramer LM, Smith JW eds. Symposium on reconstructive hand surgery. Vol. 9. St. Louis: CV Mosby, 1974;173.

320. Moore BH. Macrodactyly and associated peripheral nerve changes. J Bone Joint Surg [Am] 1942;24:617.

321. Temtamy SA, Rogers JG. Macrodactyly, a hemihypertrophy and connective tissue nevi: report of a new syndrome and review of the literature. J Pediatr 1976;89:924.

322. Tsuge K. Treatment of macrodactyly. J Hand Surg [Am] 1985;10:968.

323. Weber FP. Angioma formation in connection with hypertrophy of the limp and hemi-hypertrophy. Br J Dermatol 1907;19:231.

324. Wiedemann HR, Burgio GR, Adlenhoff P, et al. The Proteus syndrome: partial gigantism of the hands and/or feet, nevi, hemi-hypertrophy, subcutaneous tumors, macrocephaly or other skull anomalies and possible accelerated growth and visceral affectations. Eur J Pediatr 1983;140:5.

325. Wood VE. Macrodactyly. In: Green DP, ed. Operative hand surgery. New York: Churchill Livingstone, 1988;491.

Congenital Constriction Band Syndrome

326. Askins G, Ger E. Congenital constriction band syndrome. J Pediatr Orthop 1988;8:461.

327. Baker CJ, Rudolph HA. Congenital ring-contrictions in intrauterine amputations. Am J Dis Child 1971;121:393.

328. Dobyns JH. Segmental digital transposition in congenital hand deformities. Hand Clin 1985;1(3):475.

329. Flatt AE. The care of congenital hand anomalies. St. Louis: CV Mosby 1977;213.

330. Kelikian H. Congenital deformities of the hand and forearm. Philadelphia: WB Saunders, 1974;496.

331. Kino Y. Clinical and experimental studies of the congenital constriction band syndrome with emphasis on its etiology. J Bone Joint Surg [Am] 1975;57:636.

332. Kisler I, Baruch A, Hecht O. Experience with distraction lengthening of digital rays in congenital anomalies. J Hand Surg 1977;2:394.

333. Lister G, Schek ER. The role of microsurgery in reconstruction of congenital hand deformities of the hand. Hand Clin 1985;1:431.

334. Matev I. thumb reconstruction after amputation of the metacarpophalangeal joint by bone lengthening. J Bone Joint Surg [Am] 1970;52:957.

335. May JW, Smith RJ, Peimer CA. Toe to hand tissue transfer for thumb reconstruction with multiple digital aplasia. Plast Reconstr Surg 1981;67:205.

336. Patterson TJS. Congenital ring-constrictions. Br J Plast Surg 1961;14:1.

337. Soiland H. Lengthening a finger with the "on the top" method. Acta Chir Scand 1961;122:184.

338. Streeter GL. Focal deficiencies in fetal tissues and their relation to intrauterine amputation. Contrib Embryol 1930;22:1.

339. Temtamy SA, McKusick VA. Digital and other malformations associated with constriction ring syndrome. Birth Defects 1978;14:547.

340. Torpin R. Fetal malformations caused by amnion rupture during gestation. Springfield, IL: Charles C Thomas, 1968.

341. Upton J, Tam C. Correction of constriction rings. J Hand Surg 1991;16:947.

Madelung Deformity

342. Beals RK, Lovrien EW. Dyschondrosteosis and Madelung's deformity. Report three kindreds and review of the literature. Clin Orthop 1976;116:24.

343. Burrows HJ. An operation for the correction of Madelung's deformity and similar conditions. Proc Roy Soc Med 1937; 30:565.

344. Cronin TD. Syndactylism: the results of zig-zag incision to prevent post-operative contracture. Plast Reconstr Surg 1968; 18:460.

345. Dannenberg M, Anton JI, Speigel MB. Madelung's deformity: consideration of its roentgenological diagnostic criteria. AJR 1939;42:671.

346. Darrach W. Habitual forward dislocation of the head of the ulna. Ann Surg 1913;57:928.

347. Golding JSR, Blackburne JS. Madelung's disease of the wrist and dyschondrosteosis. J Bone Joint Surg [Br] 1976;58:350.

348. Goncalves D. Correction of disorder of the distal radio-ulnar joint by artificial pseudoarthrosis of the ulna. J Bone Joint Surg [Br] 1974;56:462.

349. Karev A, Kess I, Lipsker E. Correction of the Madelung's deformity by means of osteotomy and distraction lengthening. Presented at the Congenital Anomalies of the Upper Extremity Meeting, Lahaina, Maui, Hawaii, June, 1991.

350. Kelikian H. Congenital deformities of the hand and forearm. Philadelphia: WB Saunders, 1974:610.

351. Linscheid RL. Madelung's deformity. American Society for Surgery of the Hand. Correspondence Newsletter 1979;24.

352. Matev I, Karagancheva S. The Madelung deformity. Hand 1975;7:152.

353. Milch H. Cuff resection of the ulna for malunited Colles' fracture. J Bone Joint Surg [Am] 1941;23:311.

354. Neilsen JB. Madelung's deformity: A follow-up study of 26 cases and a review of the literature. Acta Orthop Scand 1977;48:379.

355. Phemister DB. Operative arrestment of longitudinal growth of bones in the treatment of deformities. J Bone Joint Surg [Am] 1933;51:1.

356. Ranawat CS, Defiore J, Straub LR. Madelung's deformity: an end result of surgical treatment. J Bone Joint Surg [Am] 1975;57:772.

Obstetric Brachial Plexus Injury (Birth Palsy)

357. Adler JB, Patterson RL. Erb's palsy: long time results of treatment in eighty-eight cases. J Bone Joint Surg [Am] 1967; 49:1052.

358. Akasaka Y, Hara T, Takahasi M. Restoration of elbow flexion and elbow extension in brachial plexus paralysis by means of free muscle transplantation innervated by intercostal nerve. Ann Hand Surg 1990;9:341.

359. Aziz W, Singer RM, Wolff TW. Transfer of the trapezius for flailed shoulder after brachial plexus injury. J Bone Joint Surg [Br] 1990;72:701.

360. Bonney G, Birch R, Jameson A, Eames R. Experience with vascularized nerve grafts. Clin Plast Surg 1984;11:137.

361. Boome RS, Kaaye JC. Obstetric traction injuries for brachial plexus. Natural history, indication for surgical repair and results. J Bone Joint Surg [Br] 1988;70:571.

362. Bunnell S. Restoring flexion to the paralytic elbow. J Bone Joint Surg [Am] 1951;33:566.

363. Clark JMP. Reconstruction of biceps brachii by pectoral muscle transplantation. Br J Surg 1946;34:180.

364. Dumontier C, Gilbert A. Traumatic brachial plexus injuries in children. Ann Hand Surg 1990;9:351.

365. Fairbank HAT. Birth palsy: subluxation of shoulder joint in infants and young children. Lancet 1913;1:1217.

366. Gilbert A, Tassin JL. Surgical repair of the brachial plexus in obstetric paralysis. Chirurgie 1984;110:70.

368. Hardy AE. Birth injuries of the brachial plexus: incidence and prognosis. In: Rang M. Anthology of orthopaedics. Edinburgh: E & S Livingstone, 1966.

369. Harmon PH. Surgical reconstruction of the paralytic shoulder by multiple muscle transplantation. J Bone Joint Surg [Am] 1950;32:583.

370. Hoffer M, Wickenden R, Roper B. Results of tendon transfer to the rotator cuff. J Bone Joint Surg [Am] 1978;60:691.

371. Kanaya F, Gonzalez M, Park C-M, et al. J Hand Surg [Am] 1990;15:30.

372. Leffert RD. Clinical diagnosis in testing in electromyelographic study in brachial traction injuries. Clin Orthop North Am 1988;237:24.

373. Leffert RD. Brachial plexus injuries. N Engl J Med 1974; 2291:1059.

374. L'Episcopo JB. Tendon transplant in obstetrical paralysis. Am J Surg 1934;25:122.

375. Marshall RW, et al. Operations to restore elbow flexion after brachial plexus injuries. J Bone Joint Surg [Br] 1988;70:577.

376. Millesi H. Surgical management of brachial plexus injuries. J Hand Surg 1977;2:367.

377. Narakas A. Brachial plexus surgery. Clin Orthop North Am 1981;12:303.

378. Schottstaedt ER, Larsen LJ, Bost FC. Complete muscular transposition. J Bone Joint Surg [Am] 1955;27:897.

379. Sedel L. Results of surgical repair in brachial plexus injury. J Bone Joint Surg [Br] 1982;64:54.

380. Sever JW. Obstetrical paralysis: report of eleven hundred cases. JAMA 1925;85:1862.

381. Steindler A. Muscle and tendon transplantation at the elbow. Instr Course Lect 1944;2:276.

382. Wickstrom J. Birth injuries of the brachial plexus; treatment of defects in the shoulder. Clin Orthop 1962;23:187.

383. Zancolli E. Classifications and management of the shoulder in birth palsy. Orthop Clin North Am 1981;12(2):433.

Upper Extremity Trauma Part II

384. Burton NJ. Fractures of the phalanges of the hand in children. Hand 1979;2:134.

385. Becton JL, Christian JD, Goodwin HN, et al. A simplified technique for treating the complex dislocation of the index metacarpal phalangeal joint. J Bone Joint Surg [Am] 1975;57:698.

386. Beatty E, Light TR, Belsole RJ, Ogden JA. Wrist and hand skeletal injuries in children. Hand Clin 1990;4:723.

387. Bogumill GP. A morphologic study of the relationship of collateral ligaments to growth plates in the digits. J Hand Surg 1983;74.

388. Campbell RM. Operative treatment of fractures and dislocations of the hand and wrist region in children. Orthop Clin North Am 1990;21(2):217.

389. Christodoulou AG, Colton CL. Scaphoid fractures in children. J Pediatr Orthop 1986;6:37.

390. Coonrad RW, Pohlman MH. Impacted fractures in the proximal portion of the proximal phalanx. J Bone Joint Surg [Am] 51:1291.

391. Dixon GL, Moon NF. Rotational supracondylar fractures of the proximal phalanx in children. Clin Orthop 1972;83:151.

392. Grad JB. Children's skeletal injuries. Orthop Clin North Am 1986;17:437.

393. Green, DP. Hand injuries in children. Pediatr Clin North Am 1977;24:903.

394. Hastings H II, Simmons BP. Hand fractures in children. Clin Orthop 1984;188:120.

395. Kaplan EB. Dorsal dislocation of the metacarpal phalangeal joint of the index finger. J Bone Joint Surg [Am] 1957;39:1081.

396. Leonard MH, Dubravcik P. Management of fractured fingers in the child. Clin Orthop 1970;73;160.

397. Leddy JP. Avulsions of the flexor digitorum profundus. Hand Clin 1985;1:77.

398. Letts M, Esser D. Fractures of the triquetrum in children. J Pediatr Orthop 1993;13:228.

399. Lourie GM, Bayne LG, Costas BL. Hand injuries in pediatric patient. Hand (newsletter) 1992;2.

400. Simmons BP, Peters TT. Subcondylar fossa reconstruction for malunion of fractures of the proximal phalanx in children. J Hand Surg [Am] 1987;12:1079.

401. Stein F. Skeletal injuries in the hand of children. Clin Plast Surg 1981;8:65.

402. Strickland JW. Bone, nerve, and tendon injures of the hand in children. Pediatr Clin North Am 1975;22:451.

403. Wood VE. Fractures of the hand in children. Orthop Clin North Am 1976;7:527.

404. Wakefield MS. Hand injuries in children. J Bone Joint Surg [Am] 1964;46:1226.

405. Waters PM, Benson LS. Dislocation of the distal phalanx epiphysis in toddlers. J Hand Surg [Am] 1993;18:581.

Lovell & Winter's Pediatric Orthopaedics, fourth edition,
edited by Raymond T. Morrissy and Stuart L. Weinstein.
Lippincott–Raven Publishers, Philadelphia © 1996.

Chapter

22

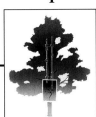

Leg Length Discrepancy and Angular Deformity of the Lower Limbs

Colin F. Moseley

Cases of leg length discrepancy frequently present challenges to the orthopaedic surgeon. The orthopaedic surgeon must understand the mechanisms and concepts of growth, including the relations among age, maturity, and leg length. Because the patient usually presents during the growing years, the orthopaedic surgeon must understand the need to correct the discrepancy as it will exist at maturity and not the discrepancy that is present in the growing child. The surgeon must be conversant with the methods used to analyze

growth and predict future growth and the effects of surgery. The techniques of leg lengthening evolve rapidly, and the orthopaedic surgeon must consider these new techniques in choosing the most appropriate treatment. As surgeons become more confident in their ability to lengthen legs, discrepancies of greater magnitude for correction are accepted, and they must be confident that the improvements in their abilities outweigh the increased risks. The final challenge facing the orthopaedic surgeon is to maintain the perspective of the whole patient and resist the temptation to direct attention solely toward the lengths of the legs, neglecting the other factors that are important in the patient's overall function and cosmesis.

The treatment of leg length discrepancy must be preceded by careful and sometimes difficult education of the patient and parents. In the case of epiphyseodesis, parents frequently find it difficult to understand why a problem in one leg requires an operation on the other normal leg, and they are not pleased at the thought that their child will be shorter. In the case of leg lengthening, the parents and the patients must understand that a fairly high morbidity is associated with this procedure even if things go well because the child must wear an external device for many months and be restricted in recreation and athletics. They also must understand that the risk of complications is high and that these complications can compromise the final result. The orthopaedic surgeon knows that surgery is necessary to correct leg length discrepancy, but parents often are anxious to find some nonsurgical method of stimulating the growth of the short leg. If all other factors were equal, it would be better to correct the leg length discrepancy by lengthening the abnormally short leg than to compensate for the discrepancy by shortening the normal long leg.

EFFECTS

The mechanical and functional effects of leg length discrepancy are immediately apparent. The long-term effects, however, are less understood. Despite a consensus in the orthopaedic and lay communities that leg length discrepancy does have deleterious effects on the spine and the hips, good documentation to support that consensus is lacking.

Mechanisms of Compensation

The child with leg length discrepancy usually compensates better than the adult, probably because of a greater strength-to-weight ratio. The child can compensate for minor degrees of leg length discrepancy by walking on the toes of the short leg with the heel never touching the ground. This can result in a smooth, symmetrical gait that shows no abnormality except for the lack of heel strike on the short side.

The adult, on the other hand, seldom compensates in that fashion but tends to walk with a heel-to-toe gait even on the short side and vault over the long leg. This action produces excessive up and down motion of the pelvis and trunk (Fig. 22-1). Although theoretically it is possible to compensate for the leg length discrepancy by flexing the knee on the long side, this almost never is done by either adults or children, probably because too much physical effort is required to do so.

Gait

Despite evidence to suggest that discrepancies of less than 2.5 cm are not significant,[156] postural sway has been shown to be increased as the result of simulated discrepancies of as little as 1 cm.[130]

Some patients who have had their leg length discrepancies perfectly corrected still show some asymmetry in their gaits by virtue of having knees that are at different levels. Because the segments of the legs act to some extent like pendulums, their natural cadence is controlled by their lengths. Because shorter pendulums swing more quickly, the leg with the low knee and the relatively short tibia tends to swing more quickly during swing phase, which produces asymmetry in the gait or increases the muscular effort of gait in order to control it.

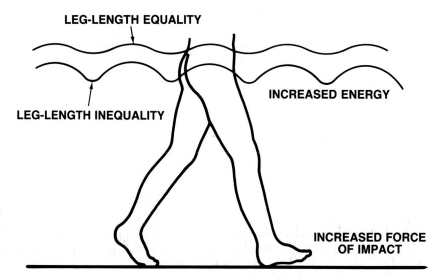

FIGURE 22-1. Motion of pelvis during gait. The amplitude of vertical pelvic motion is increased by leg length discrepancy. The patient vaults over the long leg and descends to plant the heel of the short leg.

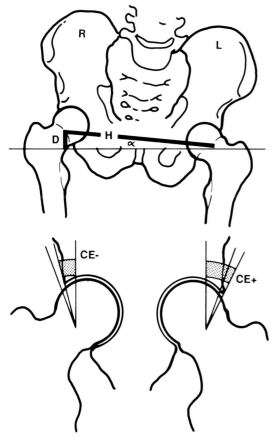

FIGURE 22-2. Decrease in center-edge (CE) angle with pelvic obliquity. The CE angle is decreased on the side of the long leg. Coverage is decreased, and the resulting decrease in the load-bearing area causes an increase in pressure. Such a hip may be susceptible to late degenerative arthritis. (L, left; R, right; adapted from Morscher E. Etiology and pathophysiology of leg length discrepancies. Prog Orthop Surg 1977;1:9.)

Hip

Degenerative arthritis of the hip that is termed idiopathic in the elderly patient may actually be the result of some previously unrecognized minor problem,

such as mild dysplasia, slipping of the capital femoral epiphysis, or possibly leg length discrepancy. In two-legged stance with the legs straight, the patient with leg length discrepancy has a pelvic obliquity with respect to the floor that relatively uncovers the hip of the long leg and increases coverage of the hip of the short leg (Fig. 22-2).

As the leg length discrepancy increases, so does the uncovering on the high side with a decrease in the center-edge angle. This relation is illustrated in Figure 22-3. It is reasonable to suspect that the patient with a leg length discrepancy throughout his or her life may be subject to an increased risk of developing degenerative arthritis in the hip of the long leg.[68] However, there is no documentation to prove this hypothesis. The effect of the leg length discrepancy in decreasing coverage is present only during two-legged stance and perhaps during gait if there is poor compensation. When the patient is in one-legged stance, sitting, or lying down, the effect disappears; most inhabitants of North America spend the majority of their time in one of those positions and not in two-legged stance.

Knee

Although the nature of the relation has not been elucidated, there are reports that leg length discrepancy increases the incidence of knee pain in athletes.[122]

Spine

The effects of leg length discrepancy on the spine also are not clearly established. The parents of young children with leg length discrepancy worry about their children developing degenerative arthritis of the spine, low back pain, and scoliosis. Contradictory evidence exists concerning the possibility that leg length discrepancy causes low back pain in the long term.[67,79,197] In any case, low back pain is rare in the younger child, and parents should be informed of this. Froh and

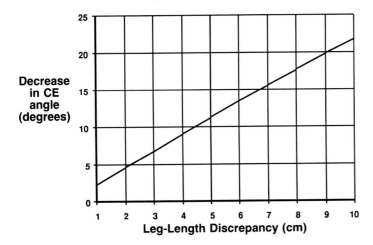

FIGURE 22-3. Relation between leg length discrepancy and center-edge (CE) angle. The CE angle and coverage decrease with increasing leg length discrepancy. For every centimeter of leg length discrepancy, there is a decrease of approximately 2.6 degrees in the CE angle. (Data from Morscher E. Etiology and pathophysiology of leg length discrepancies. Prog Orthop Surg 1977;1:9.)

colleagues looked for an effect of leg length discrepancy on the orientation of the facet joints and found none, whereas Giles and Taylor did find changes in the facet joints of cadavers with leg length discrepancy.[60] Low back pain is a very common complaint in the general population and occurs in patients with leg length discrepancy for the same reasons that it occurs in patients without leg length discrepancy. Radiographs of the spine should be examined carefully to rule out anomalous development of the vertebrae.

Several studies have been performed to determine whether leg length discrepancy leads to scoliosis. Gibson and coworkers assessed 15 patients with leg length discrepancy following femoral fractures and found that after 10 years none had structural scoliosis,[63] but minor structural changes have been reported in such patients.[160] Studies have demonstrated an increased incidence of structural scoliosis in patients with leg length discrepancy when compared with the general population,[186] but it has not been established that the leg length discrepancy has caused the scoliosis. If leg length discrepancy were the cause, the scoliosis is expected to be in the direction that would compensate for the leg length discrepancy, but in up to one third of the cases in these studies, the scoliosis was in the opposite direction[105] (Fig. 22-4). Because the leg length discrepancy affects only the spine during two-legged stance and perhaps during gait, and not at any other

time, some skepticism toward the cause-and-effect hypothesis seems justified. It has been suggested, however, that scoliosis develops more as the result of the dynamic forces of walking and not by the static forces of standing.[202]

If leg length discrepancy has long-term effects on the spine or hips, it is reasonable to suspect that the

TABLE 22-1.   Leg Length as a Function of Skeletal Age

	TOTAL LEG LENGTH (cm)				
Age	+2 SD	+1 SD	Mean	−1 SD	−2 SD
Boys					
1	28.58	27.33	26.08	24.83	23.58
2	36.06	34.37	32.69	31.01	29.32
3	41.81	39.84	37.88	35.92	33.95
4	46.89	44.61	42.32	40.03	37.75
5	51.55	48.97	46.38	43.79	41.21
6	56.06	53.14	50.21	47.45	44.54
7	60.63	57.32	54.01	50.70	47.39
8	64.83	61.25	57.66	54.07	50.49
9	69.14	65.24	61.35	57.45	53.55
10	73.16	68.99	64.82	60.65	56.48
11	77.33	72.80	68.26	63.72	59.19
12	81.83	76.86	71.87	66.88	61.91
13	86.86	81.27	75.66	70.06	64.46
14	90.71	85.03	79.36	73.69	68.01
15	92.32	87.20	82.07	76.95	71.82
16	93.01	88.35	83.70	79.05	74.39
17	93.02	88.66	84.29	79.92	75.56
18	92.95	88.73	84.52	80.31	76.09
Girls					
1	29.02	27.70	26.38	25.06	23.74
2	36.00	34.37	32.74	31.11	29.48
3	42.09	40.09	38.10	36.11	34.11
4	47.75	45.26	42.78	40.30	37.81
5	52.56	49.83	47.09	44.35	41.62
6	57.20	54.04	51.05	47.97	44.90
7	61.75	58.29	54.82	51.35	47.89
8	66.05	62.34	58.61	54.88	51.17
9	70.49	66.38	62.27	58.16	54.05
10	74.99	70.49	66.00	61.51	57.01
11	79.52	74.66	69.81	64.96	60.10
12	85.21	78.28	73.35	68.42	63.49
13	85.75	80.94	76.14	71.34	66.53
14	86.57	82.07	77.57	73.07	68.57
15	86.80	82.43	78.06	73.69	69.32
16	86.90	82.55	78.21	73.87	69.52
17	86.95	82.60	78.25	73.90	69.55
18	86.99	82.63	78.28	73.93	69.57

SD, standard deviation.

Adapted from Anderson M, Messner MB, Green NT. Distribution of lengths of the normal femur and tibia in children from one to eighteen years of age. J Bone Joint Surg [Am] 1964;46:1197.

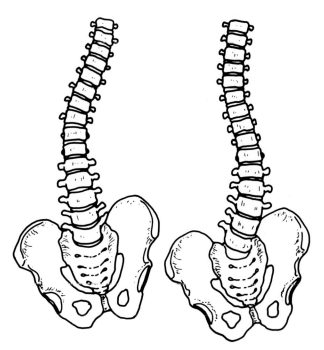

FIGURE 22-4.   Oblique pelvis with scoliosis in compensatory and noncompensatory directions. If leg length discrepancy causes scoliosis, the direction of the spinal curvature is expected to be in the direction that is compensatory for the scoliosis. When scoliosis occurs in the other direction, it must be concluded that the leg length discrepancy is not responsible.

severity of the problem is related to the severity of the discrepancy, the degree to which it remains uncompensated or uncorrected, and the age of the patient at onset.

GROWTH

An understanding of growth is an essential prerequisite to the treatment of patients with leg length discrepancy. The mechanisms of growth are discussed in Chapter 1. In the study of leg length discrepancy we are more concerned with rates and patterns of growth. Growth of the leg is the result of both growth at the four epiphyseal plates at the proximal and distal ends of the tibia and femur and an increase in size of the four adjacent epiphyses. The growth of the epiphyses contributes only 5% to the total growth of the legs, and this usually is ignored in treating patients with leg length discrepancy.

The only good studies relating growth of the legs to age were performed by Anderson and colleagues. Their first study involved populations of girls and boys at various ages from 5 years of age to epiphyseal closure.[10] Their second study was longitudinal in that a group of children was followed until maturity. They published their data in two forms. The first form related the lengths of the femur and the tibia of boys and girls to their ages, from 1 to 18 years.[11] These data can be combined to show the total leg lengths rather than the lengths of the individual bones. The total leg length data are shown here in tabular (Table 22-1) and

graphic forms (Figs. 22-5 and 22-6). The graph showing leg lengths related to age is a useful tool in the analysis of leg length data. They later published their data in the form of a graph showing the growth remaining at the distal femoral and proximal tibial physes of boys and girls related to skeletal age (Fig. 22-7).[9] This graph is also a widely used and valuable tool for decision making in cases of leg length discrepancy.

The four growth plates of the lower limb contribute consistent proportions of growth to their individual bones and to the entire extremity (Fig. 22-8).[71] These percentages are worth remembering because they can be useful in clinical situations. For example, a child with avascular necrosis of the femoral head in infancy can lose a maximum of 15% of future growth of the affected leg, and a child whose distal femoral growth plate was destroyed as a result of infection will loose 38% of the future growth of the leg. Also noteworthy is that the femur is longer than the tibia, consisting of 54% of the total length of the leg compared with 46% for the tibia. In addition, the growth pattern in the lower extremity is the opposite of that in the upper extremity, where most growth is contributed by the plates farthest from the elbow.

The study of growth as it pertains to leg length discrepancy involves the relations among three factors: leg length, maturity, and chronologic age (Fig. 22-9). Although these relations are familiar, some aspects deserve elaboration.

It is evident to all physicians who deal with children that maturation and aging are only loosely related. Some children mature rapidly and go through

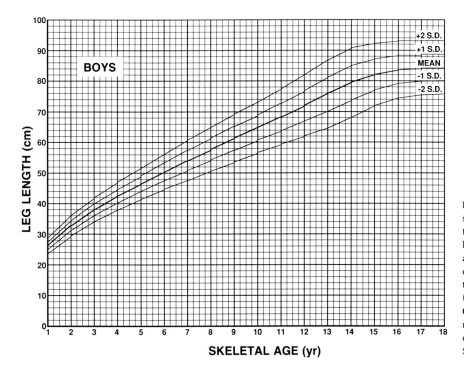

FIGURE 22-5. Total leg length versus skeletal age for boys allows a specific boy to be related to the population by plotting his leg length as a function of his skeletal age. It is useful in the analysis of leg length data because it allows a projection into the future based on the present situation. (Data from Anderson M, Messner MB, Green WT. Distribution of lengths of the normal femur and tibia in children from one to eighteen years of age. J Bone Joint Surg [Am] 1964;46:1197.)

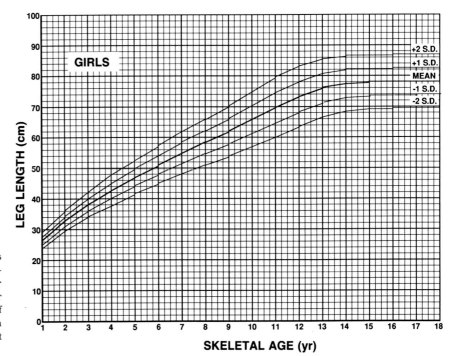

FIGURE 22-6. Total leg length versus skeletal age for girls serves the same purpose for girls as Figure 22-5 serves for boys. (Data from Anderson M, Messner MB, Green WT. Distribution of lengths of the normal femur and tibia in children from 1 to 18 years of age. J Bone Joint Surg [Am] 1964;46:1197.)

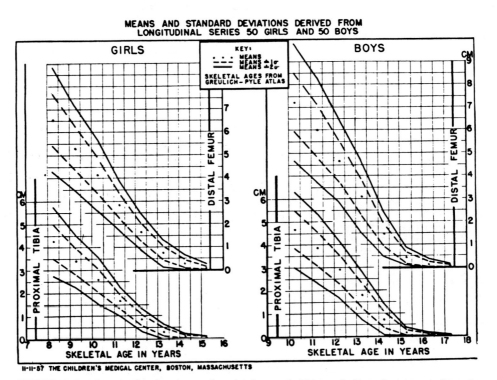

FIGURE 22-7. Green and Anderson growth remaining graph. This graph shows the amount of growth potential remaining in the growth plates of the distal femur and proximal tibia of boys and girls as functions of skeletal age. It is useful in determining the amount of shortening that will result from epiphyseodesis. (From Anderson M, Green WT, Messner MB. Growth and predictions of growth in the lower extremities. J Bone Joint Surg [Am] 1963;45:1.)

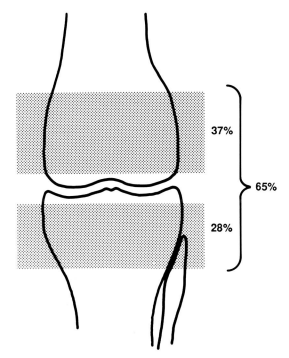

FIGURE 22-8.   The growth plates of the lower limb contribute definite and constant proportions to the growth of the long bones of the leg and the total growth of the limb. These contributions determine the slopes of the reference lines of the straight line graph method and are thus automatically taken into account by it.

their growth spurts early. These children appear tall during the growing years not because they are of a taller growth percentile, but because they are of advanced maturity. Many of these children who are tall for their chronologic ages during early adolescence cease growth early and are shorter than the mean at maturity. Pediatricians, in their studies of stature, and orthopaedic surgeons, in their studies of leg lengths, need a measure of maturity rather than a measure of age. Although leg lengths and chronological age can

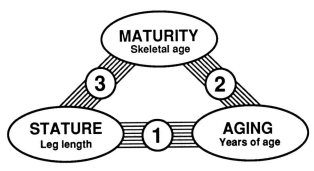

FIGURE 22-9.   Leg length, maturity, and age all change with time, and the way they do so is not identical in every child. The three relations among them can be examined individually, and it is important to do so to understand parents' perceptions and to predict future growth. Relation 2 is maturation, whereas relation 1 and 3 are both growth; but from different perspectives.

be measured accurately and easily, maturity cannot. The best measure of maturity appears to be the development of the bones of the skeleton as seen on radiographs. By comparing the radiographs of a patient with standard radiographs in an atlas, it is possible to derive a number known as the skeletal age. The skeletal age is the age at which the general population reaches the same stage of development as the patient. The skeletal age correlates well with menarche and other signs of maturation, such as the appearance of secondary sexual characteristics, and also correlates more closely with the growth of the legs than does chronologic age. Because skeletal age is determined from an average of the general population, it should be apparent that for any random group of children the mean skeletal age should be equal to the mean chronologic age.

The three relations seen (see Fig. 22-9) among the three aforementioned criteria can be examined individually, and it is instructive to do so. First, consider the relation between growth and chronologic age. This relation is obvious to parents. The parent who is concerned about his or her child being too short or too tall is always comparing the child to classmates and other children of the same age. In this relation, there is steady growth throughout life with a growth spurt in early adolescence and cessation of growth at the age of 16 to 17 in boys and 14 to 15 in girls (Fig. 22-10).[19] Although this relation is the most obvious, it is virtually meaningless without a consideration of maturity, and its variability from child to child presents problems to the treating doctor. A more consistent relation must be used.

The relation between chronologic age and skeletal age is considered next. Although this relation is extremely variable within the population, children tend to pass the various landmarks of maturity in the same orderly and consistent fashion. The child who develops secondary sexual characteristics early also goes through the growth spurt early, reaches menarche early, and has advanced skeletal ages. The implication is that children who mature more quickly or slowly than average do so throughout their growing years, but this is not necessarily so. Some children appear as if they are going through a maturation spurt, during which they mature faster than they age. This maturity spurt tends to coincide with the growth spurt, and the orthopaedic surgeon who is waiting for just the right time to do an epiphyseodesis can be caught unawares. It is as if these children are turning the pages of the skeletal age atlas at a faster rate than normal.

The third relation, that between maturity and growth, correlates more closely than the relation between chronologic age and skeletal age and is of most interest to the orthopaedic surgeon. This is the relation

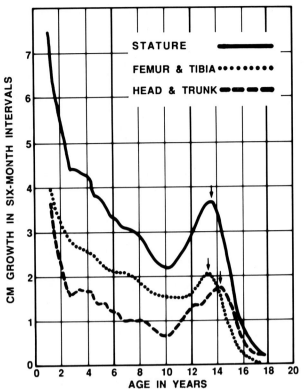

FIGURE 22-10. Green-Anderson growth curve. The examination of growth rate as a function of chronologic age shows a major growth spurt in adolescence. It is of interest to note that no such spurt appears in the growth curve of Figures 22-6 and 22-7. (Adapted from Anderson M, Green WT, Messner B. Skeletal age and the control of bone growth. Instr Course Lect 1960;17:200.)

shown in the data of Green and Anderson (see Figs. 22-5 and 22-6), and it has interesting properties. The first property is that growth is never faster, in either absolute or relative terms, than it is in the newborn. The growth rate continually slows down until it stops completely at maturity. There is no inflection point in the curve, meaning that no growth spurt occurs, as happens when growth is correlated with chronologic age. The disappearance of the growth spurt has two possible explanations. The first is that these curves are derived from averages of a number of patients, and averaging data tend to dampen individual fluctuations that occur at different times. The second, more interesting, explanation is that the growth spurt may be a spurt not only in growth but in maturation as well, with growth maintaining its customary relation to skeletal age.

Although the Green and Anderson study provides good documentation of the relation between skeletal age and leg length for the population studied, there are no corresponding studies of children of other races or of other genetic stocks from within the same race. Therefore it is not certain that the data are reliable in

these cases. On the other hand, the literature contains no reports of consistent errors having been made in the prediction of growth in non-Caucasian children, and therefore it seems reasonable and practical to assume that the same pattern of growth of the legs related to skeletal age is followed by children of all races and that the Green and Anderson data can be used reliably in predicting future growth.

ETIOLOGY

Leg length discrepancy can be classified purely by etiology, but the concepts involved in understanding and treating patients suggest a more logical approach. Leg length discrepancy can result from two types of processes: those that change the length of the leg directly and those that alter its growth. A fracture that heals with overriding is an obvious example of an effect on length with no effect on growth, and injury to the growth plate from osteomyelitis is an example of an alteration in growth rate with no immediate effect on length. These two effects determine whether a discrepancy is static or dynamic and greatly influence the choice of treatment. The causes of leg length discrepancy can be classified according to their effects on length and growth, but the classification system breaks down because certain causes can affect different patients differently, and some affect both length and growth. A fracture, for example, can cause shortening in one patient and overgrowth in another, and a congenitally short femur can be thought of as being both short and retarded in its growth. Such a classification is shown in Table 22-2.

Some patients with asymmetry above or below the legs present as having leg length discrepancy and are treated as such even though their legs may be of equal length. One example is the patient with the neglected, high-riding congenital dislocation of the hip (Fig. 22-11).

Interference With Length

By definition, the only processes that acutely can affect the length of the leg are fractures and dislocations. Whether or not a congenitally short bone has had a direct interference with its length is a moot point because it occurred before birth and it is the inhibition of growth that is the important factor. The terminal hemimelias and proximal focal femoral deficiency and its variants can be thought of as growth inhibition superimposed on a short limb.

Fractures can result in short bones either by overriding or by angular deformity. In the latter case, the shortening often disappears when the angulation is corrected.[82] Sugi and Cole have shown that shortening

TABLE 22-2.   *Classification of Causes of Leg Length Discrepancy*

CLASSIFICATION	BY GROWTH RETARDATION	BY GROWTH STIMULATION
I. Congenital	Congenital hemiatrophy with skeletal anomalies (e.g., fibular aplasia, femoral aplasia, coxa vara), dyschondroplasia (Ollier disease), dysplasia epiphysealis punctata, multiple exostoses, congenital dislocated hip, clubfoot	Partial giantism with vascular abnormalities (Klippel-Trenaunay, Parkes-Weber) Hemarthrosis due to hemophila
II. Infection	Epiphyseal plate destruction due to osteomyelitis (femur, tibia), tuberculosis (hip, knee joint, foot) septic arthritis	Diaphyseal osteomyelitis of femur or tibia, Brodie abscess Metaphyseal tuberculosis of femur or tibia (tumor albus) Septic arthritis Syphilis of femur or tibia Elephantiasis as a result of soft tissue infections Thrombosis of femoral or iliac veins
III. Paralysis	Poliomyelitis, other paralysis (spastic)	
IV. Tumors	Osteochondroma (solitary exostosis) Giant cell tumors Osteitis fibrosa cystica generalisata Neurofibromatosis (Recklinghausen)	Hemangioma, lymphangioma Giant cell tumors Osteitis fibrosa cystica generalisata Neurofibromatosis (Recklinghausen) Fibrous dysplasia (Jaffe-Lichtenstein)
V. Trauma	Damage of the epiphyseal plate (e.g., dislocation, operation) Diaphyseal fractures with marked overriding of fragments Severe burns	Diaphyseal and metaphyseal fractures of femur or tibia (osteosynthesis) Diaphyseal operations (e.g., stripping of periosteum, bone graft removal osteotomy)
VI. Mechanical	Immobilization of long duration by weight-relieving braces	Traumatic arteriovenous aneurysms
VII. Others	Legg-Calve-Perthes disease Slipped upper femoral epiphysis Damage to femoral or tibial epiphyseal plates due to radiation therapy	

From Taillard W, Morscher E. Beinlangenunterschiede. Basel: Kavgev, 1965.

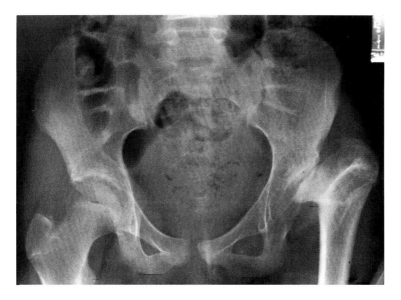

FIGURE 22-11.   High-riding dislocation of hip. This patient has a functional leg length discrepancy that is greater than the actual discrepancy in the lengths of the legs because of the abduction of the short leg.

of up to 10% of the femoral length can be accepted in the treatment of femoral fractures by early spica without causing significant discrepancy.[201] Overgrowth frequently accompanies healing of fractures and can spontaneously correct the shortening.[189] Excessive length can result when excessive force is applied in traction.

Dislocations have a direct effect on length only if they are unreduced.

Inhibition of Growth

The growth of the physis can be slowed by three mechanisms. First, congenital short bones grow more slowly than normal bones as the result of abnormal programming of the genetic mechanism that determines growth rate. Second, the growth plate can be injured in such a way that part or all of it is no longer able to grow and eventually gets converted to solid bone in the form of an epiphyseal bridge or a prematurely closed plate. Any part of the plate that has retained its ability to grow cannot do so effectively because of tethering by the fused part. Third, a change in the environment of the plate can influence its growth rate. Unusual vascular malformations can inhibit growth.[20,56] Children with paralysis usually have shortening of the more severely affected leg presumably because the growth rate of the plate is responsive to the compressive forces across it. The concept that pressure might change the direction of the growth of the plate is commonly known as the Heuter-Volkmann law,[91,214] but the concept was first proposed by Delpech,[13,54] who used casting to cause the distal tibial plate to change its direction of growth to correct an angular deformity of the ankle.

Congenital Shortening

When a patient is born with legs of unequal length that are otherwise normal it is often impossible to know which leg is the abnormal one. Because the more severe cases clearly involve shortening, it is appropriate to think of these cases as hemiatrophy rather than hemihypertrophy, although Beals has stated that the two are separate and distinct clinical syndromes.[21] The dysplasia usually is of the entire limb with some shortening of all components and usually is accompanied by a diminution in girth. Each leg appears to be genetically programmed to be a different size.[163]

Congenitally short bones frequently show qualitative as well as quantitative changes (Fig. 22-12).[161] The congenitally short femur also can show coxa vara, bowing, and hypoplasia of the lateral condyle (Fig. 22-13) and can be associated with anterior cruciate insufficiency,[64,109,111] a short or missing fibula,[62,225] and absence of the lateral rays of the foot. Indeed, the

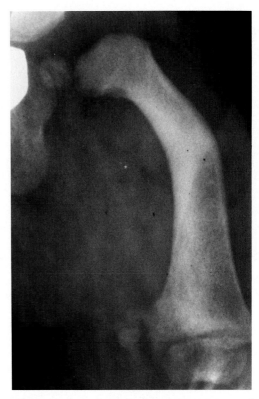

FIGURE 22-12. In proximal focal femoral deficiency, the leg length discrepancy is accompanied by qualitative changes, including coxa vara and bowing.

congenitally short femur commonly is thought of as one variant of proximal focal femoral deficiency.[112] Congenitally bowed tibias frequently are accompanied by leg length discrepancy and hypoplastic feet.[75,92,162] Askins and Ger[15] found that 24% of patients with congenital constriction bands have leg length discrepancy, and Garbarino and colleagues[61] reported short tibias in association with congenital diastasis of the inferior tibiofibular joint.

Trauma

Trauma that injures the epiphyseal plate can slow its rate of growth either by direct injury to the cells responsible for growth or formation of a bony bridge that tethers the epiphysis to the metaphysis. Fractures of the epiphyseal plate have been classified by Salter and Harris, and this classification is useful in anticipating the effect of fractures on future growth.[184] This classification is shown diagrammatically in Figure 22-14. Fractures can wander through all zones of the plate but tend to pass through the part of the plate where its material is weakest and the amount of material is least, the zone of cell hypertrophy. The material in that zone is cartilage that is weaker than bone, and because the cells there are large, the ratio of matrix volume to cell volume is low (Fig. 22-15). It is important

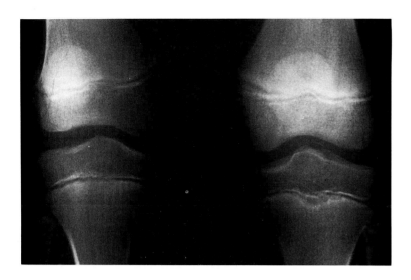

FIGURE 22-13. Hypoplasia of femoral condyle is frequently found in association with congenital shortening of the femur.

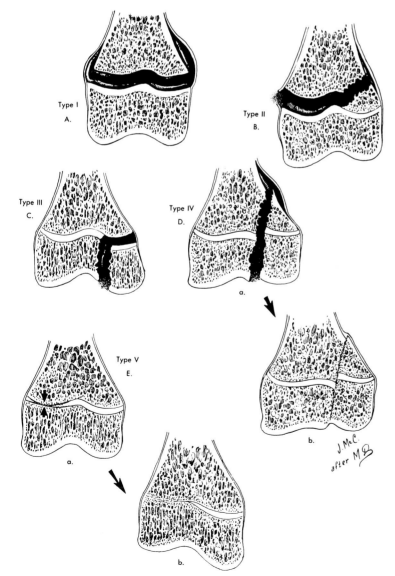

FIGURE 22-14. Salter-Harris classification of epiphyseal fractures. Fractures of types I and II do not cross the part of the growth plate responsible for growth, whereas those of types III and IV do. In the type IV fracture, approximation of epiphyseal bone to metaphyseal bone can result in formation of a bony bridge. (*Adapted from* Salter RB, Harris WR. Injuries involving the epiphyseal plate. J Bone Joint Surg [Am] 1963;45:587.)

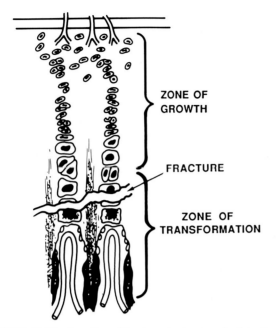

ZONE OF
GROWTH

FRACTURE

ZONE OF
TRANSFORMATION

FIGURE 22-15. Location of fractures in the growth plate. Fractures tend to occur through the part of the growth plate where the matrix is least, although individual fractures may wander from zone to zone.

to note that this part of the plate is involved with the conversion of cartilage to bone and is not primarily responsible for growth that occurs by virtue of cell multiplication and matrix production in the zones nearer the epiphysis.

Because the type I and type II fractures do not pass through the growth zone, they are less likely than other fractures to interfere with growth, although a crush injury, which injures the cells by compression, can accompany any of the other types. This mechanism may account for the higher than expected incidence of growth disturbance in type II fractures of the weight-bearing bones, such as in the distal femur, where growth arrest was found in more than one third of patients.[176] Type III and IV fractures do, however, cross the growth zone and therefore are more likely to result in growth arrest. The type IV fracture in particular can result in a bony bridge when the fracture fragment displaces in the diaphyseal direction (see Fig. 22-14). This is one reason why these fractures must be anatomically reduced. Type V fractures can occur in isolation or can accompany any of the other types. They are insidious because they are not initially recognizable on radiographs and always demonstrate their presence by a disturbance of growth, either shortening or a combination of shortening and angulation, usually in the first year after the fracture. Although the fracture classifications provide guidelines about the likelihood of growth arrest, the orthopaedic surgeon must be wary of giving a definite prognosis

for a given epiphyseal fracture until enough time has elapsed to allow a type V injury to become manifest.

The bony bridge that causes a growth disturbance following physeal fractures usually is discrete and well defined and lends itself to excision if small and peripheral. Bridge resections usually are limited to those that involve less than 50% of the plate in patients who have at least 2 years of growth remaining. Resection of even more extensive bridges can be considered in very young children because, if successful, difficult treatment of severe leg length discrepancy might be avoided. Resection of a bony bridge always should be considered if there is significant growth remaining even if leg length discrepancy is already present. The angular deformity that also can be present because of the bridge can influence treatment of the discrepancy because both deformities can be corrected at once.

Infection

Osteomyelitis adjacent to the plate can result in destruction of physeal cells and disturbance of growth if not treated early.[177] The infection is usually hematogenous osteomyelitis of the metaphysis but can be epiphyseal in infants and follow or precede septic arthritis of the joint. The bony bridge that results from infection is more difficult to treat than that following trauma because it is not so amenable to resection. The bridge tends to be larger, more central, and less discrete than that following trauma and can even consist of multiple small bridges. It is difficult to define by radiograph, is usually more extensive than it appears, and is more difficult to define during resection. There is the danger that minor components of the bridge can be left behind because the usual end point of resection, a continuous line of physis around the resection tunnel, can be achieved despite incomplete resection of all components of the bridge.

Infection tends to produce more serious leg length discrepancy problems than trauma because it occurs so commonly in younger children with so much growth ahead of them. As with trauma, angular deformity and leg length discrepancy can coexist.

Paralysis

Inhibition of growth commonly accompanies weakness or paralysis of the leg, but the mechanism is not clear. It may be true that blood flow to the limb is reduced because of the reduced muscle mass, but this does not necessarily mean that flow to the plate also is reduced. Venous return results partly from muscle activity, and therefore, blood flow to the limb and perhaps to the plate could be reduced as a result of reduced muscle activity and decreased pumping effect. Alternately, abnormal vasomotor control that is part of the basic neurologic abnormality could affect blood flow.

The effect of paralysis and reduced muscle activity can have a more direct effect on the growth rate. The Heuter-Volkmann law suggests that the growth rate of the physis depends on the compression forces across it and frequently is invoked to explain how a spontaneous reorientation of the physis occurs in contributing to the remodeling of angular deformities in the immature child. This mechanism also can explain the decrease in the overall growth rate that occurs in children with muscle weakness.

The parents of children with cerebral palsy frequently are concerned about leg length discrepancy, and minor degrees of discrepancy can be seen in this condition. More often, however, the discrepancy is more apparent than real and results from pelvic obliquity due to hip contractures or asymmetric posturing due to asymmetric spasticity. It is likely that serious discrepancies do not occur more often because even dysfunctional spasticity can be effective, through the Heuter-Volkmann law, in stimulating the physis to grow.

Tumors

Leg length discrepancy can be related to tumors in several ways. The first involves destruction of the plate by direct tumor invasion behaving, in this instance, much like infection.

The second way involves damage to the plate by irradiation used to treat the tumor.[178] Irradiation has a particularly harmful effect because the osteocytes of neighboring bone also are killed, and the bone can take many years to become revascularized and repopulated with healthy osteocytes. The absence of healthy osteoblasts and precursors can complicate the treatment of the ensuing leg length discrepancy by precluding lengthening procedures through the affected bone. Radiation damage to regional soft tissues also can complicate lengthening procedures.[218,221]

The third way that leg length discrepancy can be associated with tumors involves tumors that originate from the cartilage cells of the physis, thereby stealing growth potential from the plate. Examples of this are enchondromatosis and Ollier disease, which can produce growth inhibition of the affected bones,[192] and osteochondromatosis, which frequently results in shortening of the ulna with a Madelung deformity. Although unicameral cysts usually do not result in significant leg length discrepancy, some disturbance of growth can result from aggressive attempts to remove the cyst wall when the cyst is active and immediately adjacent to the plate. Unicameral cysts and fibrous dysplasia cause leg length discrepancy as the result of both growth inhibition and successive fractures with minimal displacement that progressively shorten the leg by small amounts.

Avascular Necrosis

Because the circulation of the physis is derived from the epiphyseal circulation, avascular necrosis of the physis frequently involves the growth plate as well, and these patients can develop leg length discrepancy. This effect may be seen in Legg-Perthes disease and following treatment of developmental dislocation of the hip. Peterson[166] has reported a case in which a discrepancy resulted from a temporary but significant episode of vascular insufficiency during surgery in an infant. This effect, in the case of congenital dislocation of the hip, is maximized by the early age of onset and the years of future growth affected but is moderated by the fact that the growth plate of the proximal femur contributes only about 15% of the growth of the limb. The likelihood of significant discrepancy has been correlated with the pattern of ischemic damage to the head and increases with increasing involvement.[207] That patients with Legg-Perthes disease do not usually develop significant deformity indicates that the vascular damage to the epiphysis does not always significantly affect the physis.[191] Leg length discrepancy also has been reported as a complication of catheterization of the umbilical or femoral artery,[180] presumably due to impairment of the arterial supply to the physis.

Stimulation of Growth

Certain conditions are known to stimulate growth, but although the mechanism is popularly thought to be increased circulation, only circumstantial evidence supports this theory. Attempts to stimulate growth in the treatment of leg length discrepancy have been made by numerous means, including sympathectomy to increase blood flow, insertion of foreign materials next to the physis, stripping and elevation of the periosteum,[108,119,196] surgical establishment of an arteriovenous fistula,[212] short wave diathermy,[55] and electrical stimulation. None of these methods has consistently produced sufficient growth stimulation to be clinically useful,[77,213] but the fact that the arteriovenous fistula does produce stimulation at all supports the hypothesis that increased circulation can be a final common pathway for the conditions that stimulate growth.

Tumor

Vascular malformations, particularly when they involve large portions of the limb, produce growth stimulation that often involves all growth plates of the limb and not just the ones in proximity or those of the involved bone. This stimulation is seen with hemangiomatosis and the Klippel-Trenaunay-Weber syndrome.[165] Stimulation is also seen with certain nonvascular tumors, such as neurofibromatosis, fibrous dysplasia, and Wilms tumor, although an increase in circulation can be the final common pathway in these cases.

Inflammation

Overgrowth of the involved bone is a common feature of chronic osteomyelitis, presumably because of the increased blood flow to the limb as part of the inflammation. Infection therefore can both inhibit and stimulate growth. Overgrowth of the affected limb can be seen in pauciarticular juvenile rheumatoid arthritis,[195] particularly in those cases with onset before the age of 3 years,[215] and also has been reported in a hemophiliac with chronic knee synovitis.[85]

Fracture

Overgrowth usually is seen following fractures of long bones in children and also is believed to result from the increased blood flow to the limb that is part of the healing process.[50] One particularly pernicious example of this effect is the overgrowth of the tibia and valgus deformity that can follow minimally displaced proximal fractures.[107] The mechanism involves overgrowth of the medial side of the tibial growth plate,[88] possibly as the result of tethering by the fibula or by release of the torn medial periosteum.[179,183,204,205]

Overgrowth most commonly occurs following femoral fractures in young children.[5,93] Some studies have reported that the stimulatory effect can last for years, but it is believed to occur principally during the healing and remodeling periods in the first 2 years after the fracture.[164] The stimulation has been reported variously to be greatest in fractures in the proximal third of the femur, the middle third of the femur,[125] and in those fractures with greater degrees of overriding[120] and can be accompanied by overgrowth of the fractured tibia on the same side. Conversely, Meals[137] found that the patient's age and the type and location of the fracture did not influence the extent of overgrowth, although handedness did.

Patterns of Growth

Shapiro has classified the growth patterns of 803 patients with leg length discrepancy into five types.[190] He divided the growth pattern into three phases: the initial phase, when the discrepancy develops; a middle phase, after the acute stage of the disease, when the relative growth rates of the two legs can still be unequal; and a final phase, which leads to the cessation of growth.

This classification can be questioned on the grounds that the study followed the children only to age 13 years and not to maturity, and it evaluated discrepancy related to time, ignoring skeletal age, the shape of the normal growth curve, and the actual growth of the legs. It is possible for children with constant inhibition to have a changing rate of increase in the discrepancy if it parallels the changing rate of growth of the leg. Because normal growth of the legs with respect to time follows "upward slope-deceleration pattern,"[190] it might be suspected that children in this group may in fact have had constant inhibition and not a changing rate.

PATIENT ASSESSMENT

There is a tendency when dealing with patients with leg length discrepancy to concentrate attention on the lengths of the legs and the discrepancy and to ignore other factors that have some importance with respect to the patient's function and the ultimate outcome of treatment. In the choice of treatment goals in this chapter, the importance of a complete and thorough assessment of the patient is emphasized.

History of Discrepancy

A complete history of the patient, the discrepancy, and its previous treatment should be obtained. The cause is important because knowledge of whether length, growth, or both is affected is essential to understanding the growth pattern. Also important is knowledge of the affected plates because this permits an estimation of the future increase in the discrepancy. Parents expect this kind of information on the first visit, and it is important in establishing a good parent-patient-surgeon relationship to be as knowledgeable as possible about the condition and its future. The history of surgery, including surgery to correct angulatory deformity, is needed, because the numeric data concerning leg lengths can be misinterpreted if the examiner is unaware of previous surgery that might have affected the leg lengths.

The history, which delineates the cause, associated deformity, and neuromuscular deficits, is referred to during selection of the treatment goal. That a patient's discrepancy is of congenital origin suggests increased risk and that certain precautionary steps must be taken in conjunction with lengthening. Instability of an adjacent joint can preclude lengthening. Weakness of the leg suggests that the weak leg be left a little short.

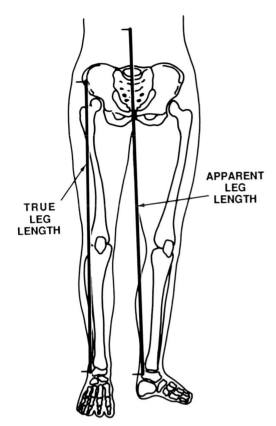

FIGURE 22-16. The measurement of real length is relatively immune from error because of pelvic obliquity. Measurement of apparent length is susceptible to error.

Clinical Assessment

The accuracy and ease of obtaining radiologic measurements of the patient should not blind the physician to the necessity of conducting a careful and complete physical examination. There are two reasons for this. First, the radiographic measurements can be wrong because of artifacts caused by angulatory deformity, positioning, or patient movement. Second, there are important factors not measured by routine radiographs that can be crucial to the outcome of treatment. This latter point is mentioned repeatedly in the section on goal selection. After assessment of the patient is complete, the clinical assessment must be consistent with the radiologic assessment or else an explanation must be sought. Additional radiographs or reexamination can be necessary to discover the reason for the inconsistency.

Leg Length

A tape measure is used to measure the real length of each leg from the anterior superior iliac spine to the tip of the medial malleolus. The apparent length is measured from the umbilicus to the tip of the medial malleolus. The difference between these two measure-

ments is because the apparent length is affected by pelvic obliquity and hip position, the leg on the abducted side appearing shorter, whereas the real length is minimally affected (Fig. 22-16). The patient should be undressed completely for this measurement to avoid tenting of the tape over the clothes. In any case, the tape often tents over or around the knee, impairing the accuracy of the measurement. Although the absolute lengths of the legs measured in this way are not the same as those measured by radiograph because different landmarks are used, the discrepancies should correspond closely.

The medial aspect of the joint line of the knee can be used as a landmark for measuring the segment lengths of the tibia and femur. Although this method is less accurate than the radiologic measurement, it is useful for comparison purposes to avoid errors. The relative heights of the knees can influence treatment decisions.

It is useful to place blocks under the foot on the short side to lengthen the short leg effectively (Fig. 22-17). The block height required to produce a level pelvis should correspond to the measured discrepancy. Blocks also can be used to estimate the amount of correction that feels best to the patient and provides him or her with the best correction. This amount can be different from the measured discrepancy and can

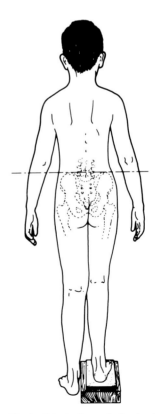

FIGRE 22-17. Placing blocks beneath the heel of the short leg allows assessment of the combined effect of all factors that produce functional leg length discrepancy.

indicate that the goal of treatment should be something other than exact correction of leg length. This assessment is most useful in the mature patient whose discrepancy will not be changing with growth but also can be helpful with immature patients to indicate that exact correction is not the best goal, even though it only measures the present length and does not indicate the desired amount of correction. An even better tool is to provide the patient with a temporary shoe lift and to assess its effect after a period of ambulation. The blocking technique is especially useful for patients with complex deformities because it takes into account the combined effects of asymmetric feet, angulatory deformities, contractures, pelvic obliquity, and spinal balance.

Other Factors

Several factors beside leg length must be assessed, because they affect the measurement of leg length or they will influence the final outcome of the patient's treatment.

The examiner must remain aware that knee and hip flexion contractures tend to shorten the leg, an equinus contracture of the ankle tends to lengthen it, and apparent length also is affected by pelvic obliquity. The term pelvic obliquity has a broader meaning here when used by spinal surgeons, who use it to refer to the relation of the position of the pelvis to that of the spine.[230] In the context of leg length discrepancy, it refers to the relation of the position of the pelvis to that of the legs and is affected both by adduction and abduction contractures of the hips and by spinal deformity. An adduction contracture of the hip causes the leg on that side to appear short and to be functionally short, whereas an abduction contracture has the opposite effects.[106] This situation is common in patients with cerebral palsy and those with the residuals of poliomyelitis. A difference between the measured real and apparent discrepancies indicates that pelvic obliquity is present.

Angular deformity must be assessed because it affects the measurements of leg length and influences the final outcome if it is to be corrected later. Joint stability must be assessed because it pertains particularly to the risks of lengthening. Femoral lengthening is contraindicated in the presence of hip instability. Congenitally short femurs always are associated with laxity of the anterior cruciate ligament and hypoplasia of the lateral femoral condyle (see Fig. 22-13), which predisposes to posterolateral subluxation of the tibial plateau. Lengthening of the tibia can be contraindicated in the presence of an unstable ankle or useless foot, which might be better handled by amputation and prosthetic fitting.

Spinal deformity and balance should be assessed. If there is stiff suprapelvic obliquity such that the axis of the trunk cannot be brought perpendicular to the transverse axis of the pelvis, an equalization of leg lengths will result in imbalance of the trunk, and some modification of that goal will be necessary. Adduction and abduction contractures of the hips produce infrapelvic obliquity with apparent and functional leg length discrepancy.[70]

Weakness and the need for bracing must be assessed because leg length discrepancy in patients with paralysis or weakness is usually best handled by undercorrection, leaving the weak leg short to facilitate swing-through, particularly if the leg is braced with the knee locked in extension. Patients who require bracing of the short leg to walk can have their leg length discrepancy corrected in the brace and may not require surgical correction at all.

Finally, the concerns, compliance, and emotional state of the parents and patient must be taken into account. This aspect is particularly important when lengthening is being considered because this is a long and difficult process requiring understanding and cooperation by all. The challenges of dealing with the length of time for lengthening and for later restriction of activities are always underestimated by parents and patients. If there is a lack of understanding or a suggestion of poor compliance, then another approach may be more appropriate. The surgeon constantly must be aware that patients frequently express concerns about function when they are concerned actually about cosmetic effect, which may be less important when compared with the risks of surgery.

Radiologic Assessment

Leg Lengths

Several methods exist for the radiologic measurement of leg length. These methods universally are more accurate than clinical methods, but each has its advantages and disadvantages. The nonexistent ideal method allows the hip and ankle to be viewed, minimizes radiation, uses only one exposure, uses a film of convenient size, demonstrates angular deformity, has no magnification, gives true readings from a scale on the film, and is inexpensive. The bony landmarks used are the top of the femoral head, the medial condyle, and the ankle. The ankle mortise is slightly saddle shaped, and the midpoint of the saddle can be easily identified. Although these techniques allow the measurement of the femur and tibia individually, these values are not required in analyzing and predicting growth, and the length of the entire leg suffices.

The orthopaedic surgeon must deal with the possibility that films taken over the years have been read by different people using different techniques and landmarks. It is also possible that the scales have been misread or that arithmetic errors have been made in

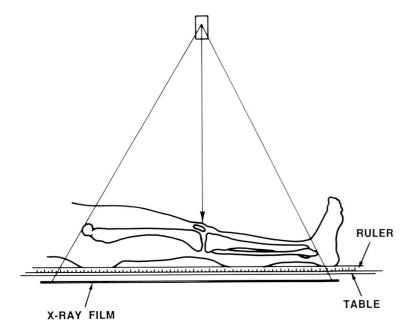

FIGURE 22-18. The diagram of teleoroentgenogram technique reveals angular deformity but is subject to errors of magnification. It is probably the best technique for children who cannot reliably comply with instructions to remain still for multiple exposures.

determining lengths and discrepancies. The surgeon cannot rely on measurements recorded in the patient's record but must review all films before performing surgery to check their accuracy and reliability.

There are four radiologic techniques that measure leg lengths directly and others that provide useful information. The terminology is confusing because names used for these techniques are inconsistent in the literature and use. The term scanogram, for example, was derived from the technique of split scanography, in which the x-ray beam was tightly collimated to a thin transverse slit that exposed the film as the x-ray tube was moved from one end of the leg to the other. Attention should be directed toward the principles involved and not be too concerned with terminology.

The teleoradiograph (Fig. 22-18) is a single exposure of both legs on a long, 35-cm × 90-cm (14-in × 36-in) film. It is taken from a 2-m (6-ft) distance, usually with the patient standing and a radiopaque ruler placed on the cassette. It has the advantage of showing angular deformities and using a single exposure but produces a film that is inconvenient to handle and measurements that are subject to magnification because of parallax of the x-ray beam. There is no significant difference between measurements of the leg taken supine and those taken standing.[45]

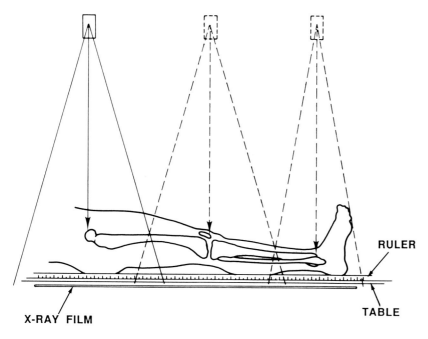

FIGURE 22-19. The orthoroentgenogram technique exposes each joint individually, thereby ensuring that the x-ray beam through each joint is perpendicular to the x-ray film, thereby avoiding errors of magnification.

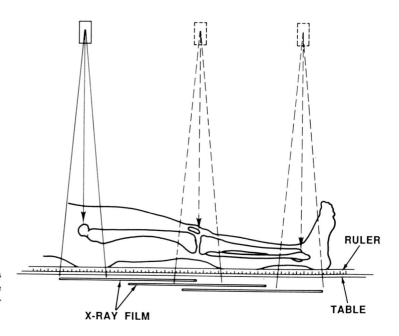

FIGURE 22-20. The scanogram technique avoids magnification error in the same manner as does the orthoroentgenogram and is the preferred technique for children who can remain still for three exposures.

The orthoradiograph (Fig. 22-19) avoids the magnification factor by taking separate exposures of the hip, knee, and ankle so that the central x-ray beam passes through the joints, giving true readings from the scale.[73] The film is still cumbersome, however, and the need for multiple exposures introduces the risk of error because of patient movement.

The scanogram (Figs. 22-20 and 22-21) avoids magnification in the same way but reduces the size of the resulting film by moving the film cassette beneath the patient between exposures.[23] This technique is preferred in children over the age of 5 or 6 years who can be compliant with instructions not to move because it gives true measurements without magnification, but younger children are better assessed using the teleoradiograph.

Positioning for the scanogram must be modified for patients with contractures of the hip or knee. Patients with hip flexion contractures can have accurate measurements made in the reclining position. In those with only knee contractures, the femur can be measured in either the lateral or prone position and the tibia in the lateral position. Assessment of both bones can be performed on one x-ray film in the lateral position if two rulers are used, one parallel to each bone. If a hip contracture is also present the femur must be assessed in the lateral position. The scanogram of both femur and tibia can be done in the lateral position.

Digital radiography appears to be promising in the measurement of leg length.[1,86] Computed tomography can be used to accurately measure the distances between points on the film, and errors from angular deformity are reduced.[66] If the examination is done specifically for this purpose, multiple sections are un-

necessary, the radiation exposure is less, especially with microdose techniques,[6] and the cost is comparable with more traditional techniques.[98,157,206]

Whatever technique is used, it is important to be consistent and, when analyzing data to determine the timing of surgery, not mix true and magnified mea-

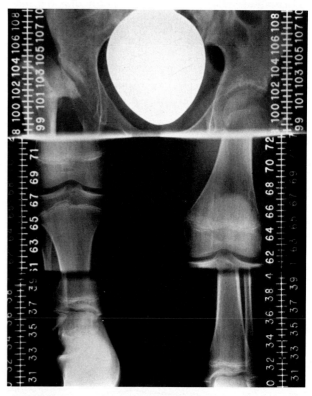

FIGURE 22-21. Scanogram technique allows the images of the three joints to be captured on a film of convenient size by moving the film beneath the patient between exposures.

surements. Because errors are possible with all of these techniques, the resulting measurements should be compared with, and should correspond with, the clinical measurements.

An anteroposterior standing film of the pelvis and hips taken with the legs straight (on blocks if necessary) is occasionally useful in assessing the total combined effects of leg length discrepancy, angular deformity, and asymmetry of the foot and pelvis. The leg length discrepancy is calculated from the heights of the femoral heads from the floor and the height of the blocks. This assessment can supplement the clinical examination done with blocks.

Skeletal Age

All methods of estimating skeletal age involve comparing radiographs of the patient with standards in an atlas. Methods have been described using the bones of the pelvis and hip, the knee, and the hand and wrist.[2,209] The Greulich-Pyle and Tanner-Whitehouse methods are now the only methods commonly used, and both use the hand and wrist. Unfortunately, the estimation of skeletal age is only moderately accurate and is the weak link in the techniques of analysis and prediction of growth.

The Greulich-Pyle atlas[74] consists of reproductions of radiographs of the left hand and wrist of boys and girls that we considered typical for the stated skeletal age. To estimate the skeletal age of the patient a radiograph of the left hand and wrist is taken according to the technique described in the atlas, and this film is then compared with the standard radiographs of the appropriate gender according to qualitative (e.g., the appearance of the hook of the hamate) and quantitative (e.g., the degree of conformity of an epiphysis to its metaphysis) criteria. The standard that most closely matches the patient's radiograph is taken as the skeletal age.

This technique has certain deficiencies. The first is that in some parts of the atlas the standards represent skeletal ages that are far apart, with a gap as great as 14 months. There is a large standard error built into the technique. With practice, it is possible to interpolate between standards, but this practice is difficult and studies have shown significant interobserver and intraobserver errors.[40] A second problem is that some children do not follow the same orderly succession of maturity indicators shown in the atlas, and an arbitrary choice must be made in assigning a skeletal age. Third, some children with leg length discrepancy of congenital origin also have congenital anomalies of the hand and wrist, making it impossible to reliably compare their radiographs with the standards. Finally, one of the features of almost all skeletal age atlases is that the mean skeletal age of a sample of similarly

aged children is equal to their chronologic age so that the skeletal age is, in fact, the best possible predictor of chronologic age. That is, of a random sampling of boys or girls of the stated chronologic age, half would be more developed and half would be less developed than the standard radiograph. Greulich and Pyle however, in selecting standards for their atlas, did not follow this principle exactly, and in some cases, selected radiographs that they believed were more representative. It is important to note that Green and Anderson used the Greulich-Pyle standards in their leg length studies.

The Tanner-Whitehouse method[203] is similar in that it uses radiograph of the hand and wrist but was developed using modern computerized mathematical procedures. It adds a level of refinement and accuracy to the Greulich-Pyle technique by defining and showing examples of successive stages of development of 20 specific bony landmarks (Fig. 22-22). The same standards are used for boys and girls. The patient's radiograph is compared with the standards, and a letter score is assigned to each of the 20 landmarks. The letter score then is converted to a numeric score by consulting a table for the appropriate gender. The sum of these 20 scores represents the level of skeletal maturity attained by the patient and can be converted to years and months with a much smaller standard error than with the Greulich-Pyle technique. Of special interest in dealing with leg length discrepancy is that the bony landmarks can be divided into two groups. Tanner and Whitehouse provide tables for including either the 12 long bone standards of the hand or the eight cuboid bone standards of the wrist in the assessment. When these two approaches give different results, it is reasonable to assume that the long bone standards give a skeletal age that is more pertinent to the growth of the long bones of the leg. The concept that the long bones are more important than the cuboid bones in the context of leg length discrepancy can be useful even with the Greulich-Pyle atlas in allowing the resolution of difficulty in selecting the appropriate standard for a given radiograph.

There are two areas of difficulty with this method. The first is that it is more cumbersome and time consuming than the Greulich-Pyle method, and the second is that it has not been correlated with leg length and cannot be used by orthopaedic surgeons in the analysis of growth. Tanner-Whitehouse skeletal age cannot be used with the Green and Anderson data derived from the Greulich-Pyle method because these two methods give different skeletal ages. This is surprising and probably is related in part to the fact that different populations were used to develop the standards. Whereas Tanner and Whitehouse applied solid mathematical procedures in deriving their scoring system, Greulich and Pyle selected their standards in

Radius

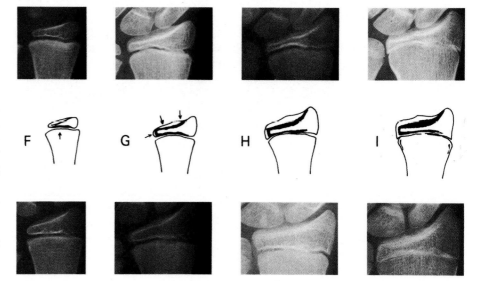

FIGURE 22-22. The Tanner-Whitehouse atlas provides standards like this for twenty different landmarks in the hand and wrist. This technique allows the determination of skeletal age to an accuracy of months but is not consistent with the Greulich-Pyle atlas. (From Tanner JM, Whitehouse RH, Marshall WA, et al. Assessment of skeletal maturity and prediction of adult height ([TW2 method]). London: Academic Press, 1975.)

a somewhat arbitrary fashion for the sake of clarity but in so doing abandoned the basic principle of other skeletal age systems that, for any group of children of the same age, the mean skeletal age should be equal to the chronologic age.

The relation between skeletal age and leg length, although reliable, is not as reliable as we would like it to be, and we must accept the relative inaccuracy of skeletal age estimation. It is still possible to make acceptably accurate predictions.

DATA ANALYSIS

The adult with leg length discrepancy, who has no future growth and no possibility of a changing discrepancy, presents no need to analyze data. The growing child, on the other hand, whose legs may be growing at different rates and whose discrepancy may be changing presents another level of difficulty. The treatment goal must be chosen with respect to maturity; therefore, before performing surgery, the orthopaedic surgeon must be able to predict confidently the situation at maturity. The importance of proper data analysis cannot be overemphasized. Blair and associates[29] reviewed 67 epiphyseodeses and found that correction to within 1 cm had been achieved in only 22 cases, and 35 failures occurred because of incorrect use of the Green and Anderson data.

Three methods are useful in analyzing leg length data: the growth-remaining method, the arithmetic method, and the straight-line graph method. These methods differ significantly in their convenience, com-

plexity, and accuracy, but the analysis moves through the same stages in all three. The first stage is the analysis of past growth, including the determination of the present discrepancy, and depending on the method, the growth percentile and the growth inhibition. The second stage involves the prediction of future growth, including the lengths of the legs and the discrepancy at maturity. The third stage is the prediction of the effects of corrective surgery.

All three methods have their place in the armamentarium of the orthopaedic surgeon. All require a good understanding of the principles of growth and their methodologies to be used properly without error. The three methods are discussed here in general terms, and step-by-step instructions for their use are shown in Figures 22-23, 22-24, and 22-25. Included in those charts are examples of their use in a specific case.

The accuracy of all methods depends to some degree on the nature of available data. The calculation of growth inhibition, for example, is more accurate with data over longer intervals. It is the interval over which data is collected and not the number of visits that is important, and data should be gathered for at least 1 or preferably 2 years. Minor errors in measurement over a short time can lead to major errors in estimating the growth inhibition and major errors in predicting the discrepancy at maturity. An increased number of visits can be useful in recognizing values that are in error because they do not fit the pattern established by other visits. For example, one erroneous radiographic reading can be noticed in a group of other, valid points but can be missed if the patient

Determining Leg Length Discrepancy: The Arithmetic Method

Leg length data

(for examples for all three methods):

Sex: Female

Age (yr)	Skeletal age (yr.)	Right leg length (cm)	Left leg length (cm)
7 + 10	8 + 10	60.0	58.2
8 + 4	9 + 4	64.4	61.9
9 + 3	10 + 3	70.0	66.2

Prerequisite growth information

Distal femoral plate grows 10 mm/yr.
Proximal tibial plate grows 6 mm/yr.

Girls stop growing at 14 years of age.
Boys stop growing at 16 years of age.

A Assessment of past growth

1. Longest time interval for data
= age at last visit - age at first

1. Longest time interval for data
= 9 yr 3 mo - 7 yr 10 mo = 1 yr 5 mo
= 1.42 yr

2. Years of growth remaining
= 14 (16 for boys) - age at last visit

2. Years of growth remaining
= 14 yr - 9 yr 3 mo = 4 yr 9 mo = 4.75 yr

3. Past growth of legs
= present length - first measured length

3. Past growth of:
long leg = 70.0 - 60.0 = 10.0 cm
short leg = 66.2 - 58.2 = 8.0 cm

4. Growth rate of long leg
$= \dfrac{\text{past growth}}{\text{time interval}}$

4. Growth rate of long leg
$= \dfrac{10.0}{1.42} = 7.04$ cm/yr

5. Growth inhibition
$= \dfrac{(\text{growth of long leg - growth of short leg})}{\text{growth of long leg}}$

5. Inhibition
$= \dfrac{(10.0 - 8.0)}{10.0} = 0.2$ cm

B Prediction of future growth

1. Future growth of long leg
= years remaining X growth rate

1. Future growth of long leg
= 4.75 X 7.04 = 33.4 cm

2. Future increase in discrepancy
= future growth of long leg X inhibition

2. Future increase in discrepancy
= 33.4 X 0.2 = 6.7 cm

3. Discrepancy at maturity
= present discrepancy + future increase

3. Discrepancy at maturity
= (70.0 - 66.2) + 6.7 = 10.5 cm

C Prediction of effect of surgery

Effect of epiphysiodesis
= growth rate X years remaining

Effect of epiphysiodesis
Femoral   = 1.0 X 4.75 = 4.75 cm
Tibial   = 0.6 X 4.75 = 2.85 cm
Both   = 1.6 X 4.75 = 7.6 cm

FIGURE 22-23. Step-by-step instructions for use of the arithmetic method. The method presented here is modified from that presented by Menelaus and Westh in that the future increase in discrepancy is calculated from past growth instead of being assumed to be 0.125 inch per year of growth remaining. An example is shown in the panels in the right column.

Determining Leg Length Discrepancy: The Growth-Remaining Method

A Assessment of past growth

1. Growth of both legs
   = present length - first length

2. Present discrepancy
   = length of long leg - length of short leg

3. Growth inhibition
   = (growth of long leg - growth of short leg) / growth of long leg

1. Growth of long leg
   = 70.0 - 60.0 = 10.0 cm

1. Growth of short leg
   = 66.2 - 58.2 = 8.0 cm

2. Present discrepancy
   = 70.0 - 66.2 = 3.8 cm

3. Growth inhibition
   = (10.0 - 8.0) / 10.0 = 0.2 cm

B Prediction of future growth

1. Plot present length of long leg on Green-Anderson leg length graph for appropriate sex

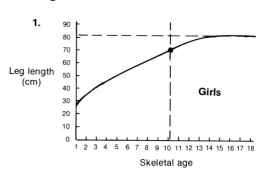

1.

2. Project to right parallel to standard deviation lines until maturity to determine mature length of long leg

3. Future growth of long leg
   = mature length - present length

4. Future increase in discrepancy
   = future growth long X inhibition

5. Predicted discrepancy at maturity
   = present discrepancy + future increase

2. Length of long leg at maturity ‐ 81.1 cm

3. Future growth of long leg
   = 81.1 - 70.0 = 11.1 cm

4. Future increase in discrepancy
   = 11.1 X 0.2 = 2.2 cm

5. Discrepancy at maturity
   = 3.8 + 2.2 = 6.0 cm

C Prediction of effect of surgery

1. The effect of epiphysiodesis of the distal femoral and proximal tibial plates for a given sex and skeletal age can be determined by the Green-Anderson growth = remaining graph.

2. The effect of lengthening is not affected by growth.

1. Correction from proximal tibial arrest
   = 2.7 cm

   Correction from distal femoral arrest
   = 4.1 cm

   Correction from combined arrest
   = 2.7 + 4.1 = 6.8 cm

FIGURE 22-24.   Step-by-step instructions for use of the growth remaining method. An example is shown in the panels in the right column using the same data as in the example in Figure 22-24.

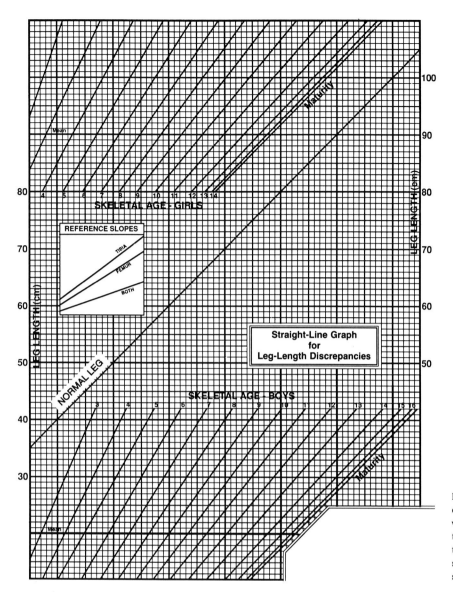

FIGURE 22-25. The straight-line graph comprises three parts: the leg length area with the predefined line for the growth of the long leg, the areas of sloping lines for the plotting of skeletal ages, and reference slopes to predict growth following epiphyseodesis.

makes only one or two visits. The straight-line graph is the only one of the three methods that uses all available skeletal ages, and in that method the accumulation of more skeletal age estimates diminishes the errors in single estimates.

Arithmetic Method

The arithmetic method was first described by White and more recently evaluated by Menelaus and Westh.[139,223] The method is based on the following statements, all of which are first approximations of the true growth pattern described by Green and Anderson.

> Girls stop growing at the age of 14.
> Boys stop growing at the age of 16.
> The distal femoral plate grows 10 mm (3/8 in) per year.

The proximal tibial plate grows 6 mm (1/4 in) per year.
The discrepancy increases by 3 mm (1/8 in) per year.

These approximations are reasonably good during the last years of growth but are inaccurate in young children. The statement that the discrepancy increases by 1/8 in per year is obviously not true in all cases. It is, however, fairly accurate in those children who are in the last few years of growth, whose discrepancies began at birth, whose maturation is not significantly advanced or delayed relative to their chronologic ages, and whose discrepancies are within the clinical range for epiphyseodesis.

Its most significant advantage is its convenience because no special tools are needed for its use. Its disadvantages are that it uses chronologic age rather than skeletal age and is therefore subject to error in children who grow and mature very early or very late. It uses an approximation of the growth curve rather than the growth curve itself and is increasingly inaccurate in young children. If, however, its use is restricted to determining the timing of epiphyseodesis and its application to the patients described earlier, then good results can be anticipated as have been reported by Menelaus.[223] Step-by-step instructions for the use of this method are shown in Figure 22-23.

Fries also has published straight-line approximations to the growth remaining graph, in which the remaining growth in the epiphyses of boys and girls is determined by first-order equations using skeletal age, but this approach lacks the simplicity of the arithmetic method.[59]

Growth Remaining Method

The growth remaining method is based on the data and tables of growth that Green and Anderson published in their two studies.[10,11] These studies are to my knowledge the only good studies published relating leg lengths to chronologic and skeletal age and serve as the foundations of the more accurate methods of analyzing growth. Their graphs describing the lengths of the legs of boys and girls related to age can be used to determine the growth percentile of the child and the future growth of the long leg. Their graph showing the growth remaining in the distal femur and proximal tibia can be used to predict the effects of epiphyseodesis[72] (see Fig. 22-7).

The advantages of this method are that it uses skeletal age, is based on an accurate description of the growth pattern, takes into account the child's growth percentile in predicting future growth, and has been demonstrated to be accurate over decades of use. The disadvantages are that it requires the availability of the two sets of graphs, does not take into account the growth percentile in predicting the effect of epiphyseodesis, and because it uses only the most recent skeletal age estimation, it will be in error to the extent that the skeletal age estimate is in error. An inherent hazard of this method in that the growth remaining graph is so familiar and easy to use that the unwary are tempted to correct the present discrepancy in a growing child, neglecting the steps that involve the prediction of future change. Step-by-step instructions for the use of this method are shown in Figure 22-24.

Straight-Line Graph Method

The straight-line graph method initially was devised as a method of better seeing the relative growth of the legs, and by incorporating the data of Green and

Anderson,[11] the method evolved into a method of recording, analyzing and predicting growth (Fig. 22-26).[153,154] The method is based on two principles: the growth of the legs can be represented graphically by straight lines, and a nomogram can be used to determine the growth percentile from the skeletal age and leg length.

The representation of leg growth by straight lines appears to contradict the Green and Anderson description of growth, in which the growth lines of the legs are clearly curved. It is accomplished by manipulating the scale of the abscissa (X axis) in strict accordance with the Green and Anderson data so that the curve that disappears from the growth lines reappears as an irregularity of that scale. This curve actually appears on the straight-line graph as a variable distance between the skeletal age lines. The important fact is that the straight line is not an approximation of the Green and Anderson data but represents the data just as accurately as did their original graphs. In the absence of active disease or treatment, the relative rates of growth of the two legs stay constant, and the growth line of the short leg also follows a straight line on the graph. This means that the length of the leg is represented on the graph by the vertical position of its growth line and its growth rate by the slope of the growth line. The discrepancy therefore is represented by the vertical distance between the two growth lines and the inhibition by the difference in slope.

The nomogram for skeletal age allows the plotting of points in a way that relates the length of the patient's long leg to the population and, in a sense, depicts the growth percentile. The nomogram is constructed so that all points for the child whose growth pattern follows exactly that described by Green and Anderson lie on a horizontal straight line. In practice, this is rarely the case, partly because of the inaccuracy of estimation of skeletal age, but also in part because of the possibility that children of other races or other genetic stock have different patterns of growth. It is likely that the plotting of every skeletal age point on the nomogram before drawing the horizontal line representing the growth percentile "averages out" the inaccuracies of individual determinations of skeletal age. Similarly, the risk of error due to single estimates of skeletal age is likely to decrease with an increasing number of estimates.

The prediction of the effect of surgery is based on the facts that a change in the length of a leg by lengthening or shortening will be represented on the graph by a vertical shift of its growth line either upward or downward by the appropriate amount without any change in its rate of growth, and conversely, that the effect of an epiphyseodesis will be to decrease the slope of the growth line of the long leg. This is a

Determining Leg Length Discrepancy:
The Straight Line Graph Method

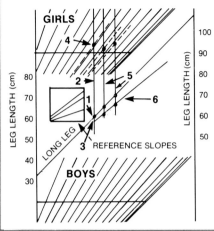

A Assessment of past growth

1. Plot the point for the long leg on the sloping line labeled "LONG LEG" at the appropriate length.

2. Draw a vertical line through that point representing the current assessment.

3. Plot the point for the short leg on the vertical line.

4. Plot the point for skeletal age with reference to the sloping lines in the nomogram.

5. Plot successive visits in the same fashion.

6. Draw a straight line through the short leg points to represent the growth of the short leg.

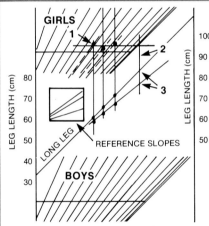

B Prediction of future growth

1. Draw the horizontal straight line that best fits the points previously plotted for skeletal age. The fit to later points is more important than to earlier points. This is the growth percentile line.

2. From the intersection of the growth percentile line with the maturity skeletal age line, draw a vertical line to intersect the growth lines of the two legs. This line represents the end of growth.

3. The points of intersection of the vertical line with the two growth lines indicate the predicted lengths of the legs at maturity.

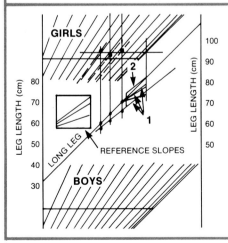

C Prediction of effect of surgery

1. To predict the outcome after epiphysiodesis, draw three lines to the right from the last point for the long leg parallel to the three reference slopes. The intersections of these lines with the vertical line representing the end of growth indicates the predicted lengths of the long leg after the three possible types of epiphysiodesis.

2. To predict the outcome after leg lengthening, draw a line parallel to the growth line of the short leg but elevated above it by the amount of length gained.

FIGURE 22-26. Step-by-step instructions for use of the growth remaining method. The data used are the same as in the example in Figure 22-24.

strict mathematical relation, and because the contributions of the individual growth plates to the overall growth of the leg are known, the future slope of the growth line can be predicted accurately. Reference slopes on the graph depict the slopes to be followed after each of the three possible types of epiphyseodeses: distal femoral, proximal tibial, or both. For example, the slope of the growth line of the leg following a proximal tibial epiphyseodesis will be decreased by the 27% normally contributed by that epiphysis, to 73% of its previous slope. Because the unoperated long leg is defined on the graph as having a slope of 1.0, the slope following that surgery would be 0.73.

The advantages of this method are that it uses skeletal age and the actual growth pattern described by Green and Anderson, takes into account the growth percentile in predicting future growth and the effect of surgery, minimizes errors due to the inaccuracy of skeletal age estimation, facilitates the flagging of erroneous values, and avoids arithmetic with its inherent errors.[169] It is a general tool for analysis, illustration, and prediction in leg length discrepancy and can be used in children with large discrepancies and inhibitions, extreme growth percentiles, and marked delay or advancement of maturation. The disadvantage is that it requires the availability of the straight-line graph and a straight edge. Step-by-step instructions for the use of this method are shown in Figure 22-25.

Patterns of Inhibition

In all three of the preceding methods, the growth inhibition is determined on the basis of past growth and is then used to predict future growth. Evidence supports the assumption that the growth inhibition will remain constant throughout the growing years.[24] Indeed, in my study of patients who went on to have epiphyseodeses, the linear correlation coefficient between the lengths of the two legs was greater than 0.955 in every case.[153,154] This is an extremely close fit and suggests that growth inhibition does indeed remain constant. It should be noted, however, that no children in this group had active disease or were under treatment that could affect growth.

Shapiro also has reported that the growth rate of the femur tends to increase, and that of the tibia to decrease, following a lengthening procedure.[193] This effect is relatively short-lived and is not of sufficient magnitude to affect clinical decisions. Koman and colleagues have demonstrated constant inhibition in unilateral and bilateral proximal focal femoral deficiency,[121] and Hootnick and associates have shown constant inhibition in congenitally short tibias.[95]

The important question for the orthopaedic surgeon concerns the possibility of errors in correction due to changing inhibition. Does changing inhibition cause clinically significant errors in clinical judgment? A partial answer can be derived from my study mentioned earlier, in which the inhibition appeared not to change and the straight-line graph predicted the final outcome within 1 cm in all cases. This suggests that whatever effect changing inhibition has, it is not sufficient to prevent reaching predictions of future growth that are sufficiently accurate for good clinical results.

Inadequate Data

There are certain situations in which patients present late, it is suspected that the time for epiphyseodesis is imminent, and there is insufficient time to accumulate sufficient data for accurate assessment and prediction. In some cases it is still possible to make reliable assumptions about the growth pattern that allow accurate prediction and confident treatment planning.

Consider the situation in which a child presents without any prior data, and the only information available is from that particular visit. The difficulty here is that it is impossible to calculate the growth inhibition and predict the discrepancy at maturity. If, however, the onset of the growth inhibition can be determined, it can be assumed that the legs were of equal length at that time, and using either the Green and Anderson growth graph or the straight-line graph, the length of the long (and therefore the short) leg at that time can be estimated. The growth inhibition can be calculated in the usual way. Likewise, in the case of a congenital discrepancy with inhibition beginning before birth, it can be assumed that the legs were of equal length when there was no length or, in other words, that the growth inhibition is equal to the percentage difference in the length of the legs. This assumption is consistent with the conclusion of Herron and associates.[89]

At times an opinion is sought on the basis of leg length films without skeletal age films when the patient is not immediately available to obtain them. In this case the child's skeletal age can be assumed to be the same as the chronologic age, and this assumption is validated if the development of secondary sexual characteristics and menarche are consistent with the chronologic age.

In certain patients with remote disease that is no longer active, no continuing growth inhibition or accentuation exists. Patients with leg length discrepancy due to stimulation from fracture healing or osteomyelitis or with shortening due to fracture malunion that is more than 2 years old confidently can be assumed to have a static discrepancy. The discrepancy at maturity therefore will be the same as at present, and attention can be directed at correcting the present discrepancy.

Patients with complete destruction of one physis due to trauma or infection can present with an early minimal discrepancy but significant inhibition that, with growth, will certainly lead to a greater discrepancy requiring treatment. In some cases, these children can be treated with an epiphyseodesis of the corresponding plate of the other limb. This plan does not correct the discrepancy but ensures equal inhibition in both legs and an unchanging discrepancy throughout growth.

Sometimes no such assumptions are reasonable, and a reliable decision cannot be made. In these cases, it is best to abandon the possibility of epiphyseodesis and wait until maturity, when the discrepancy can be corrected without error by shortening or lengthening.

DETERMINATION OF TREATMENT GOALS

The choice of the goal of treatment and the choice of the treatment method are two different and independent steps in the treatment of patients with leg length discrepancy and are discussed separately here. The selection of the treatment goal depends heavily on the careful and thorough assessment of the patient, both clinically and radiologically, and the reader is referred back to the earlier sections on patient assessment.

Equal Leg Lengths

Many patients who have leg length discrepancy as an isolated problem, such as those with hemiatrophy, present no difficulty in the choice of treatment goal. Leg length equality at maturity is the appropriate goal.

Unequal Leg Lengths

Many patients do best with less than complete correction. Undercorrection of 1 or 2 cm is best for patients with paralysis of the short leg. The residual discrepancy facilitates clearing of the floor by the weak short leg during the swing phase of gait, and this is even more important in patients who wear braces and have the knee locked in extension in order to ambulate. This situation is a common situation in patients with the residual weakness of poliomyelitis. In patients who cannot walk without braces, the leg length discrepancy usually can be made up in the brace, and corrective surgery may not be indicated.

Level Pelvis

Patients with leg length discrepancy often have asymmetry that extends beyond the legs. Patients with congenital shortening, for example, may have a small foot or hemipelvis, and in these cases perfectly equal leg lengths result in residual pelvic obliquity and tilting of the lumbosacral joint. A similar situation can arise in patients with leg length discrepancy from avascular necrosis of the femoral head following treatment of congenital dislocation of the hip who also have had an innominate osteotomy. These patients should be examined standing with blocks beneath the short leg to relate the desired correction to the leg length discrepancy. The treatment goal can be modified as required.

Vertical Lumbar Spine

Patients with fixed obliquity of the lumbosacral junction cannot achieve a level pelvis and a vertical lumbar spine at the same time. Usually, a vertical lumbar spine and good balance of the spine are more important than a level pelvis, and treatment of the leg length discrepancy should be consistent with the more important goal. It is interesting to consider the possibility that such a patient could benefit from lengthening of the already long leg if the pelvic obliquity were greater than the leg length discrepancy.

Equalization by Prosthetic Fitting

Some discrepancies are too great to be considered for correction. The traditional guideline has been that femurs less than half of the length of the other side and legs that are destined to be more than 15 cm short are candidates for prosthetic fitting. This is often done in conjunction with other procedures, including knee fusion, Syme amputation, and Van Nes rotationplasty. Early reports on the modern techniques being adopted for leg lengthening suggested that we would become more proficient at correcting very large discrepancies with acceptable morbidity.[159] It is my opinion that discrepancies anticipated to be less than 20 cm at maturity can be reasonable candidates for correction by a variety of combined simultaneous or staged shortening and lengthening procedures, but there is no reason for wholesale modification of this guideline.

Correction of Coexisting Problems

The treatment plan must include those intermediate goals that are prerequisites to surgical treatment of the leg length discrepancy itself. These intermediate goals can include stabilization of unstable joints, release of contractures, correction of angular deformity, correction of spinal deformity, completion of partial growth arrests causing angular deformity, and excision of bony bridges in an attempt to restore growth.

TREATMENT

General Principles

In general it is wise to correct coexisting deformities before undertaking correction of the leg length discrepancy. There are two reasons for this. The deformity can adversely affect the outcome of the leg length discrepancy correction or vice versa. The other reason is that the correction of some deformities affects the treatment goal. The correction of angular deformity of the limb usually increases the length of the leg, and the correction of spinal imbalance often changes pelvic obliquity and the desired amount of correction of leg length.

The choice of treatment method is more dependent on the magnitude of the predicted discrepancy at maturity than it is on its etiology. Fairly straightforward guidelines expressed in terms of the magnitude of the predicted discrepancy can be used to choose from among the major treatment categories:

> 0 to 2 cm: No treatment
> 2 to 6 cm: Shoe lift, epiphyseodesis, shortening
> 6 to 20 cm: Lengthening, which may or may not be combined with other procedures
> >20 cm: Prosthetic fitting.

There is some flexibility in these guidelines to account for factors such as environment, motivation, intelligence, compliance, emotional stability, patient and parent wishes, and associated pathology in the limbs.

There are good reasons for the values of these thresholds. It has been shown that discrepancies of less than 2 cm are of no functional or clinical consequence in adults and do not require treatment.[76] Indeed, Rush and Steiner found leg length discrepancy in 71% of new recruits into the United States Armed Forces.[181] Because there is some advantage to being tall,[65,78,134,185] lengthening procedures are preferred by parents and patients, but lengthening is not generally done for discrepancies less than 6 cm because there are other alternatives, and the high morbidity and complication rate of lengthening should be avoided in favor of epiphyseodesis or shortening whenever possible. Because these alternatives are reasonable for corrections of up to 6 cm, they are the procedures of choice. Shortening procedures are usually not appropriate for correction of greater than 6 cm because a disproportionate appearance results that is not pleasing to the patient. It should be noted that epiphyseodesis can be performed to correct a discrepancy of any magnitude in cases in which the long leg is clearly the abnormal leg because it corrects the abnormally long leg and does not result in abnormal proportions in these patients. It is reasonable to consider

patient preference for lengthening over shortening only in the 5 to 6 cm range of correction because there are overriding considerations outside that range.

The site of correction is chosen to leave the patient as symmetrical as possible with knees as level as possible. This involves lengthening the shortest bone or shortening the bone corresponding to the shortest bone on the other side. This principle can be ignored in some cases of correction by epiphyseodesis in which a single plate is arrested to reduce the magnitude of surgery and risk of problems, although a combined femoral and tibial epiphyseodesis might produce the most symmetrical result. It also can be ignored if more time for data gathering allows a more confident prediction of future growth and a more dependable treatment plan. Symmetry of knee height is a secondary consideration to equality of leg length. Knee height is not a factor in function or comfort and is not an important cosmetic factor.

Shoe Lift

A shoe lift is excellent treatment for discrepancies up to 6 cm. It is believed to be less desirable than surgical correction of the discrepancy but is a satisfactory answer for those patients who do not wish or are not appropriate for surgery. The shoe lift is only effective when the patient is walking or is in two-legged stance and is only prescribed for its benefit on gait.

No lift is required for discrepancies less than 2 cm. For larger discrepancies the height of the lift should be less than the discrepancy. For reasons of cosmesis, up to 2 cm of the lift can be put inside the shoe with the remainder, if necessary, on the outside. Lifts higher than 5 cm are poorly tolerated because the muscles controlling the subtalar joint are not strong enough to resist inversion stress, and frequent ankle strains result. If a higher lift is required, an extension up the posterior calf must be added for stability. The optimum height of the lift can be determined by clinical trials in which the lift height is temporarily modified to suit the patient.

Prosthetic Fitting

Prosthetic fitting, often in association with amputation, is a treatment of last resort but is useful for those patients with very large discrepancies and those with deformed and functionally useless feet.[8,132] Discrepancies anticipated to become greater that 15 to 20 cm and those involving a femoral length less than 50% of the other side should be treated in this way.[64] This approach has the significant advantage of involving one hospitalization and one definitive operation. Patients with fibular hemimelia and an unstable ankle do better with this approach than with multiple hospitalizations and surgical procedures in a futile attempt to conserve the foot; the latter situation usually results in late amputation, which is then more difficult to accept.

Children with below-the-knee amputations, such as those amputated for fibular hemimelia, do very well functionally. They have an almost normal walking gait and can participate in recreational and sporting activities. Children who are treated for proximal focal femoral deficiency require above-the-knee prostheses and also function well, although not as well as the former group. Some of the latter can function as below-the-knee prosthesis wearers following a Van Nes rotationplasty, in which the reversed ankle functions as a knee providing active control and motor power to the prosthetic knee.[188]

Although the decision to do an amputation is difficult for the parents of a young child, the children who do best are those who have their surgery and prosthetic fitting early in life. The optimum time for the Syme amputation is toward the end of the first year of life, and for the rotationplasty at about 3 years of age. It is helpful for parents of children who are candidates for these procedures to see older children who have had the same procedure and to talk with their parents.

Epiphyseodesis

Epiphyseodesis has very low morbidity and a very low complication rate and is the treatment of choice for the surgical correction of leg length discrepancy.[71,139,199,226] The operation is effective by slowing the growth rate of the long leg and allowing the short leg to catch up. In planning for this procedure, therefore, it is necessary to take into account the ability of the short leg to catch up by using the growth inhibition to predict the discrepancy at maturity. For all surgical treatments of leg length discrepancy, it is the discrepancy at maturity that should be corrected and not the present discrepancy in a growing child. Epiphyseodesis is a highly acceptable procedure because it is straightforward, does not require postoperative immobilization, and disables the child minimally and for a short time. It is only suitable for those children who have sufficient leg length data to enable a confident prediction of the discrepancy at maturity and who require correction of 2 to 6 cm.[200]

Epiphyseodesis is an all-or-nothing procedure that completely and permanently arrests physeal growth. Thereafter the leg grows at a slower rate, having lost the contribution to growth of the operated physis. The loss is 27% for the proximal tibia plate, 38% for the distal femoral, and 65% for combined epiphyseodesis of both plates. The surgeon thus induces

a known degree of growth inhibition and has before him not a continuous spectrum of shortenings but only three discrete choices. The exact amount of desired shortening can be achieved only by performing the surgery at exactly the correct time. Performing the operation too late results in undercorrection, and performing it too early results in overcorrection. This is in contrast to shortening and lengthening procedures that can be performed at any time.

The prediction of the effect of surgery can be made accurately within 1 cm in almost all cases. Because there is an advantage to being tall,[65,78,134,185] it is better to err on the side of undercorrection than overcorrection, and because slight discrepancies are well tolerated it is best to aim for 0.5 to 1.0 cm of undercorrection by doing the epiphyseodesis slightly later than the time for perfect correction. It should be done in the bone that is opposite the shortest on the other side, although this principle may have to be compromised if future growth is insufficient for such an epiphyseodesis to be effective.

The principle of the surgery is to produce a symmetrical bony bridge that tethers the physis and prevents future growth. The traditional open techniques involve removing a block of bone from the medial and lateral aspects of the plate, extirpating the plate with a curette, and replacing the block of bone in such a fashion as to produce a bony bridge.[168] Phemister described removal of a rectangular block, two thirds on the metaphyseal side and one third on the epiphyseal side of the plate and its replacement in the reversed position (Fig. 22-27). White used a special chisel to remove a square block that later was rotated 90 degrees before replacement, and Blount used a circular trephine to remove a cylindrical block that was rotated in the same way. All of these techniques serve to bridge the physis medially and laterally with solid bone.

Blount produced physeal arrest by placing three staples across the physis both medially and laterally, producing a tethering effect resulting in arrest of growth[7,30,31] (Fig. 22-28). The rationale was that the arrest was temporary and growth would resume following later removal of the staples.[84,136] This concept was attractive because it alleviated the need to make accurate predictions of future growth. Certain patients, however, went on to fuse their physes while the staples were in place, did not resume growth on their removal, and went on to overcorrection of their discrepancies.[35,58] Stapling therefore must be considered to be a permanent form of growth arrest. Staples caused problems by extruding, entering the adjacent joint, or causing overlying bursitis.[37] Growth arrest was occasionally asymmetrical, and a second operation was sometimes necessary to remove the staples. This technique is no longer widely used.

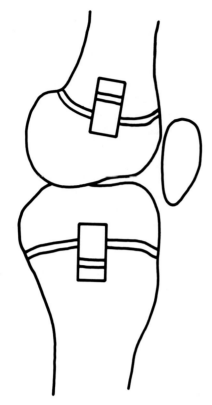

FIGURE 22-27. In epiphyseodesis by the Phemister technique, a rectangular bone block is replaced in reverse position to produce a bar across the growth plate.

Traditional epiphyseodesis requires incisions on both the medial and lateral aspects of the knee, a total of four incisions if both tibial and femoral epiphyseodeses are performed. Canale and others have reported percutaneous techniques developed to avoid unsightly scarring.[39,158] It is done with a drill or burr through small medial and lateral incisions under image intensifier control. This technique has gained wide acceptance and is considered by most to be the technique of choice. Great care must be taken to line up the image intensifier beam perfectly to ensure that the tool is in the plate. The percutaneous technique results in a wider excision of the plate and can be accompanied by excessive bleeding or hematoma formation.

Percutaneous epiphyseodesis can be performed through one incision on the lateral aspect of the plate, or as I prefer, through two incisions, one medial and one lateral. Because the growth plates, particularly the distal femoral, are not perfectly flat, there is a significant technical challenge in making sure that the tip of the tool is in the plate and that it stays there. This challenge increases as the tool gets deeper in the bone and a very large hole is produced in extirpating the medial plate from the lateral aspect. In the distal femur the intercondylar notch intrudes into the posterior aspect of the plate, and it is difficult to reach the posterior part of the medial plate from the lateral aspect without inadvertently entering the notch. Entering the notch can escape the notice of the operator because it not obvious on the anteroposterior view of the image intensifier. This is a serious occurrence because it allows bleeding and perhaps extrusion of bone particles into the knee joint, causing stiffness, and is a reason to avoid postoperative immobilization.

About 50% of the area of the plate should be removed in the pattern shown (Fig. 22-29). This is sufficient to ensure arrest of the physis and maintains enough bone strength through residual plate surrounding periosteum and perichondral ring to make postoperative immobilization unnecessary. Tibial epiphyseodesis should be accompanied by arrest of the proximal fibular physis if the tibial shortening is greater than 2.5 cm.[38]

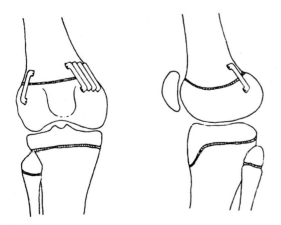

FIGURE 22-28. Epiphyseodesis by stapling. Growth arrest can be accomplished by careful placement of three staples over the medial and lateral aspects of the plate. Growth does not always resume after removal of the staples.

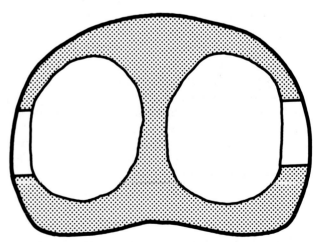

FIGURE 22-29. Area of plate to be removed in epiphyseodesis. Obliteration of medial and lateral circular segments of the plate leaving the central part and the strong periphery successfully stops growth, yet the bone retains sufficient strength to forego immobilization.

Epiphyseodesis has significant advantages over other approaches because of its low morbidity and low complication rate, but there are minor disadvantages.[16,208] It is a compensatory and not a corrective operation in that it makes the normal leg abnormal instead of making the abnormal short leg normal. It results in a decrease in the patient's stature that may be undesirable.

Femoral Shortening

Shortening of the femur has the same indications as epiphyseodesis but is offered to patients who do not meet the prerequisites for epiphyseodesis, either because they are too old or their conditions are such that confident prediction of the discrepancy at maturity cannot be made. It has the advantage over epiphyseodesis that it can be done in the mature patient when the discrepancy is known and unchanging, and the desired degree of correction can be obtained precisely.

Shortening of the tibia also has been performed but is very rarely done except in cases in which the femur does not lend itself to shortening. Although shortening of 7.5 cm in the femur and 5 cm in the tibia have been reported with no loss of function,[117] it is believed that no more than 3 cm of shortening can safely be achieved in the tibia, and it is unusual to perform shortenings of more than 5 cm in the femur. The risk of neurovascular complications is higher in the tibia because of the proximity of neurovascular structures, as is the risk of delayed and nonunion. Fasciotomy is advisable to reduce the risk of compartment syndrome. Internal fixation is more difficult, closed techniques cannot be used because the bone is subcutaneous, and the muscles of the leg are slower to recover strength than those of the thigh.

It is interesting to contemplate the reason for this last factor. The ability of a muscle to adjust to shortening of the underlying bone rests on its ability to remove sarcomeres from the ends of its fibers until the average length of the remaining sarcomeres regains the norm, which is relatively constant throughout the body. The lengths of the hamstring and quadriceps muscles, crossing two joints, are approximately twice as long as the soleus, but more importantly there is an even greater difference in the lengths of the fibers within those muscles. The soleus muscle, requiring high strength and short excursion, has a high number of short fibers oriented obliquely, while the hamstrings, requiring excursion more than strength, have a smaller number of longer fibers oriented longitudinally. The fiber lengths in any muscle are relatively constant, and the fiber length in the hamstrings is much longer than the 4-cm length of fibers in the

soleus muscle.[194] It is not difficult to imagine that a shortening of the tibia of more than 3 cm might completely overwhelm the ability of the fibers of the soleus muscle to accommodate.

The early techniques of shortening involved making step cuts or other complex cuts in the diaphysis of the bone using interfragmentary screws or intramedullary rods for fixation.[141] These techniques are of historical interest only because better techniques with more secure fixation are now available.[116] The two principal techniques in use today are proximal shortening with blade plate fixation and mid-diaphyseal shortening, open or closed, with intramedullary rod fixation. Both approaches provide secure fixation and neither requires postoperative immobilization.

Proximal Shortening

Shortening through the proximal femur at the level of the lesser trochanter with blade plate fixation has the advantage of being proximal to most of the quadriceps origin and therefore does not disadvantage the knee to the same extent as shortening in the midshaft. Patients recover strength and the ability to climb stairs more quickly. This approach leaves a large scar on the lateral thigh and requires a second later operation of moderate magnitude to remove the plate.

Closed Femoral Shortening

Winquist has pioneered a technique that involves the use of a special set of instruments designed to allow the procedure to be performed entirely from within the medullary cavity and without any direct approach to the shaft of the femur.[228,229] The bone is cut by a special eccentric cam saw that is passed down the shaft and cuts through the cortex from within out. The size of the saw required is determined from the outside diameter of the bone, and the femoral shaft is fast reamed to an internal diameter sufficiently large to accept it. The distal cut is made first, and a second cut then is made more proximally at precisely the correct location to give the desired amount of correction. The cuts should be placed so that the cylindrical fragment is removed from the isthmus of the femur where the internal diameter is least, because this provides the best fixation to the rod both proximally and distally. The cylindrical piece of bone can be cut into two sections using a special hook-shaped reverse-cutting osteotome, and the pieces are pushed aside. The gap can then be closed over an intramedullary rod to provide rigid internal fixation. Locking at both ends is desirable to maintain shortening and rotation. A second operation is later required to remove the rod.

The technical complications of this procedure usually result from less than rigid fixation of the fragments, usually due to inadequate reaming without locking. It is apparent, in using an unlocked nail, that if a 5-cm segment of bone is to be removed and 2.5 cm of fixation is desired both proximally and distally, then the bone has to be reamed until 10 cm of the shaft is reamed to the minimum diameter. This in itself can be a problem because the cortex can become very thin at the level of the osteotomies, especially because the reaming is usually eccentric and can lead to fracture of the shaft. Less than rigid fixation can lead to loss of rotational control and opening of the shortening gap, two problems that are difficult to control without locking. Less reaming is necessary for a locked nail, but in that case, the reduced internal diameter of the canal may not allow passage of a cam saw large enough to cut completely through the cortex, and a percutaneous osteotomy may be required to complete the cut. Nevertheless, the benefits of control of position with the locked nail far outweigh this disadvantage, and locking is desirable.

Acute respiratory distress syndrome has been reported during or following closed intramedullary shortening and has been believed to be the result of fat embolization associated with reaming.[57] Possible preventative measures include venting of the distal metaphysis and use of reamers with flutes sufficiently deep to allow the unimpeded egress of reamed material, but the effectiveness of these measures has not been demonstrated. It may be wise not to use this technique until this serious complication can be avoided with certainty.

Although this is an appealing technique, it requires familiarity with the instruments, is technically demanding, and has best results in experienced hands. The major disadvantages are the technical complications and risk of respiratory distress syndrome, as noted above, and the significant quadriceps weakness that results. Patients with greater shortening require 6 to 12 months to regain normal knee control and function.[44] It leaves a small cosmetically acceptable scar, and the later procedure to remove the rod is of lesser magnitude than that required to remove a blade plate.

Growth Stimulation

A technique to stimulate the growth of the short leg so that children discovered early to have growth inhibition could have their growth stimulated to normal, solving the problem, is desired. Many techniques have been used in attempts to accomplish this, but none has been successful enough to be clinically useful. Based on the concept that the periosteum acts as a tether inhibiting growth, circumferential release of the periosteum has been assessed both clinically and experimentally and found to stimulate growth.[127,227] A variety of foreign materials have been implanted next to the growth plate,[32] but the stimulation, if it occurred, was too little and too short-lived to be of use. Sympathectomy[27,83] and surgically constructed arteriovenous fistulae[138,167] temporarily stimulate growth, presumably by altering the circulation to the physis, as does stripping and lifting the periosteum by packing bone beneath it.[108,119,231] However, these techniques have little or no clinical usefulness. Electrical stimulation inconsistently stimulates physeal growth, but even the maximum effect is insufficient to correct clinical discrepancies.[14]

As desirable as this approach might appear, there is no method of growth stimulation available at this time that is useful in the treatment of leg length discrepancy.

Leg Lengthening

Lengthening an abnormally short leg would, at first glance, appear to be the preferable method of dealing with leg length discrepancy because it is a corrective procedure. It involves operating on the abnormal leg to correct its abnormality as opposed to epiphyseodesis and shortening, which make the normal leg abnormal and only compensate for the discrepancy.

Lengthening was first mentioned in the 18th century, in an account of injuries sustained in battle by Ignatius of Loyola. It was next reported by Codivilla at the beginning of this century.[46] A number of advances have been made involving changes in surgical technique or the lengthening apparatus, or both, and each change has been greeted with hopes that it would solve the problems associated with lengthening.[129] The reports in the literature, however, consistently reported difficulties and high complication rates, most reporting more than one complication per patient. Leg lengthening remains a difficult area with unsolved technical and biologic problems. We again find ourselves in an era of enthusiasm with respect to new devices and techniques, but we must learn the lesson of history and temper our enthusiasm until there is solid evidence to support it.

Lengthening is a procedure of last resort and is reserved for those situations in which other methods of correction are inappropriate. Lengthening is inappropriate for patients requiring correction of less than 6 cm because procedures of lesser risk and morbidity can be used. The maximum lengthening possible with traditional methods has been about 8 cm for the femur and 5 cm for the tibia, and therefore patients requiring large corrections may require simultaneous lengthenings of femur and tibia, repeated staged lengthenings of the same bone,[47] or supplementary shortening procedures on the long side. There is a threshold, at about

15 to 20 cm, in which the risks outweigh the benefits and lengthening is abandoned in favor of amputation and prosthetic fitting.

Since Codivilla's report, there have been many techniques described for lengthening the leg. These have included step cuts,[3] periosteal sleeves,[224] onlay cortical grafts,[49] slotted plates,[135] intramedullary rods,[33] and other internal and external devices for gradual controlled lengthening.[69,114,131,172] Transiliac lengthening has been performed and may be indicated in cases of intrapelvic asymmetry and decompensated scoliosis[143] and cases requiring concurrent hip stabilization.[18,123] Techniques of instantaneous lengthening of the femur[42,89,116,149] and tibia[173] have been reported but have not gained widespread support because the amount of length to be gained is limited. Simultaneous shortening of one femur and lengthening of the other with the excised bone segment from the other side has been recommended.[26,235] The Anderson device, using large pins and an external fixator with threaded rods for lengthening, was widely used but confined the patient to bed (Fig. 22-30). Some of the older methods persist in nonindustrialized nations as, for example, double oblique osteotomy followed by elongation by balanced skeletal traction.[232] Many of these methods became obsolete with the introduction of the Wagner device[4] and, later, the Ilizarov and Orthofix devices. Historically, new lengthening technology has been adopted enthusiastically by the orthopaedic community and has been used extensively with great optimism; however, the complication rate has remained high and the patient's course difficult, leading to the realization that the human leg has not made similar advances and that lengthening is still a difficult matter for both surgeon and patient.

I prefer to keep patients in the hospital for 2 weeks after the application of the lengthening device. This allows time for the delay and the patient and parents to understand and become comfortable with the lengthening mechanism, pin site care, an exercise program to maintain mobility and attain ambulation with weight bearing. Not all hospitals can justify such care, and many patients are discharged immediately after the surgical procedure. Patients undergoing lengthening as inpatients should be examined daily with respect to blood pressure, neurologic status, and range of motion. The reading from the scale of the lengthener should be recorded daily and checked to be sure that the lengthening is going according to plan. These assessments also should be made at weekly or biweekly visits after discharge. Roentgenograms are taken at intervals of 2 to 4 weeks to evaluate alignment and the quality of bone in the lengthening gap (i.e., the regenerate). Ultrasonography can be used to measure the lengthening gap[97,128] but is superfluous to the radiograph. The rate of distraction can be modified according to clinical progress or radiologic appearance.

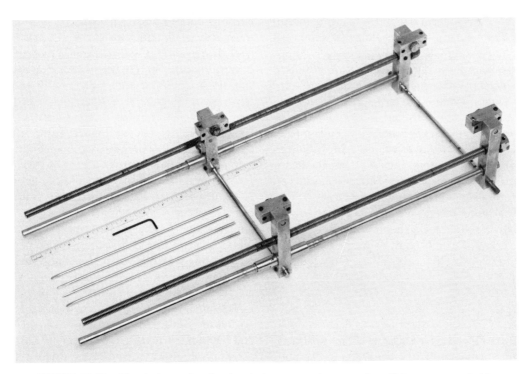

FIGURE 22-30. The Anderson lengthening device was used commonly until it was superseded by the Wagner device. It accomplished stable fixation and gradual lengthening but was not appropriate for application to the femur and confined the patient to bed.

Maintenance of motion is extremely important during the course of lengthening. Patients and parents should be instructed in a home exercise program and range of motion monitored regularly. Stopping the lengthening should be considered if limitation of motion develops that is resistant to a more intensive motion program. Wagner recommended that distraction should not be performed on any given day if the patient cannot achieve 60 degrees of flexion.[219] There is evidence in the literature that all patients regain flexion in the first year after the lengthening,[12] and it appears that maintaining extension is more important. Patients are allowed to ambulate full weight bearing with aids, if necessary. The pin sites are cleaned twice daily and, if necessary, the stab wounds are elongated weekly under local anesthesia to prevent tenting and ischemia of the skin, which could lead to pin tract infection. Cutting pins circumvent the need to release pin sites.

Distraction is discontinued either when the goal has been achieved or an unresolvable complication, usually loss of motion, has supervened. The device is retained until radiographs show consolidation and suggest adequate strength of the regenerate bone. In the consolidation period, dynamization of the device is considered important to subject the bone to cyclic longitudinal loading to stimulate bone formation. If the bone in the lengthening gap is slow to consolidate, the device can be shortened to put the bone under longitudinal compression, either leaving it somewhat shortened or lengthening once again when the regenerate responds. Valid objective guidelines for what constitutes adequate consolidation for removal of the lengthening device has not been established. Findings such as corticalization with three cortices visible on two radiographs and the appearance of a medullary cavity are considered to be signs of adequate strength, but the decision to remove the device is still empiric.

It is possible to protect the tibia externally with a cast or brace after device removal, allowing removal from the tibia earlier than the femur. In addition, the mechanical and anatomic axes of the tibia are colinear, and the bone is subject mainly to compressive forces. This is not the case for the femur, in which the regenerate bone, especially for proximal lengthenings, is eccentric and subject to bending loads. Patients should be restricted from violent body-contact sports for a long time because fractures through the lengthening gap have been reported years later.

Wagner Technique

Wagner developed a lengthening device that was first used in North America in 1973 (Fig. 22-31) and appeared to offer several advantages over older devices, such as the Anderson device (see Fig. 22-30).[216–220] It is unilateral and uses half-pins instead of through-

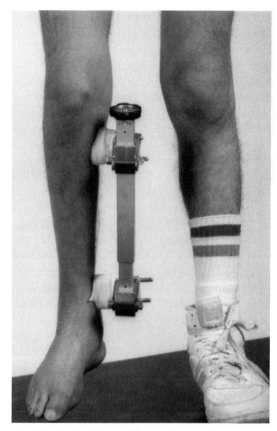

FIGURE 22-31. Patients with the Wagner lengthening device are mobile and can undertake partial weight bearing.

and-through pins that facilitate application to the femur. It is small and light and was the first device to allow the patient to be ambulatory, whereas the older devices required confinement to bed. It is lengthened simply by turning a knob at one end, which can be done by the patient. It is adjustable in two planes—varus-valgus and anteroposterior angulation, but not rotation (Fig. 22-32)—so that minor angulation that occurs during lengthening can be corrected without removing the pins.

The Wagner technique involves at least three surgical procedures. The first involves performing the osteotomy, releasing soft tissues if necessary, and applying the device. At the end of the lengthening phase, a second procedure involves bone grafting the lengthening gap, plating the bone and removal of the lengthener. Months or years later, when the bone has achieved sufficient strength, a third procedure is done to remove the plate (Fig. 22-33). There is a prolonged period of restriction of activities to protect the bone and avoid late fracture.

Although the Wagner device retains its simplicity and utility, the technique largely has been replaced by newer methods that involve neither plating nor grafting and appear to reduce the complication rate.

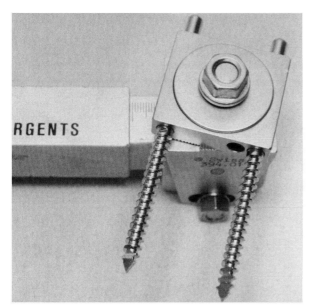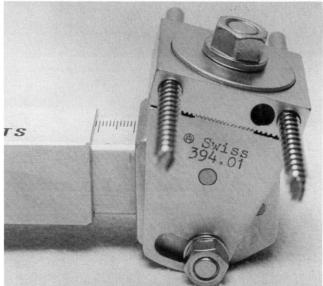

FIGURE 22-32. The Wagner device can be adjusted in two planes but not in rotation. It allows correction of angulation that develops during lengthening but does not allow simultaneous lengthening and gradual correction of angular deformity.

Orthofix Technique

De Bastiani and colleagues have developed a lengthening device, the Orthofix device (Fig. 22-34), which is applied to the bone with two sets of conical screws.[52,53] It is technically similar in operation to the Wagner device but has a more cumbersome method of elongation and is not adjustable once in place. It allows the use of up to three screws in each set, which is an advantage, especially in the proximal femur. Good results have been reported with this method with a complication rate similar to other techniques.[80] The Orthofix external fixator is similar to the lengthener but has ball joints at each end, making it adjustable. Although this device can also be lengthened, the ball joints are not strong enough to withstand the forces of lengthening, even when supported by methyl methacrylate.

Orthofix also produces a second lengthener in which the pin blocks move along a track placed beside the pins (Fig. 22-35). This allows the pin sets to start closer together and provides longer excursion.

Distraction Epiphysiolysis

Distraction epiphysiolysis was pioneered by Ring and more recently reassessed by Monticelli and Spinelli and others.[25,144–147,175,222] It is achieved by applying a distraction force across the physis until it fractures. Lengthening can then be obtained by gradual distraction. This method has the disadvantages that the lysis is sudden, painful, and not well tolerated, and that the physis can be injured, thus compounding the leg

length inequality.[51,81] The complication rate is high[150] and, if it is to be used at all, it should be reserved for children very near the end of growth to minimize the consequences of physeal damage.

Ilizarov Technique

Ring fixators have been developed[100,101,104,147,148,222] (Figs. 22-36 and 22-37) that are more complex and more versatile than the Wagner and Orthofix devices in that they lend themselves to the correction of complex deformities involving more than two segments[99] and can be used to translate segments of bone in the treatment of congenital pseudarthrosis of the tibia.[100] Fixation, at least with the original devices, is accomplished by thin wires passing completely through the bone and the leg attached to complete or partial rings. Modifications to the original techniques have included the capability to use half-pins instead of wires.

Lengthening Over an Intramedullary Rod

In the usual application of any of the external lengthening devices, the device is responsible for both maintaining alignment and achieving distraction. Numerous unsightly scars result because of the multiple percutaneous pins or wires used to achieve sufficient stability and the fact that they must be left in place for a prolonged period, until the bone is strong. It is possible to use an intramedullary rod to maintain alignment during both the distraction and consolidation phases and the external device only to achieve

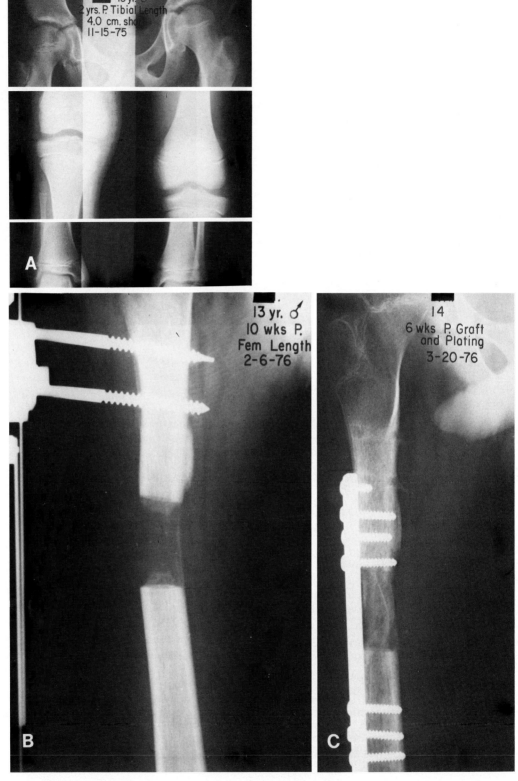

FIGURE 22-33. The technique of Wagner femoral lengthening is demonstrated in a 13-year-old boy with a congenital shortening of the right lower limb who had previously undergone tibial lengthening for a shortening of 8 cm. (**A**) The orthoroentgenogram shows that the lower limb is still 4-cm short. (**B**) Ten weeks after Wagner femoral lengthening, the amount of bone bridging the distraction gap is inadequate; therefore, autogenous bone grafting and plating of the femur were accomplished. (**C**) The results of the plating and grafting procedure.

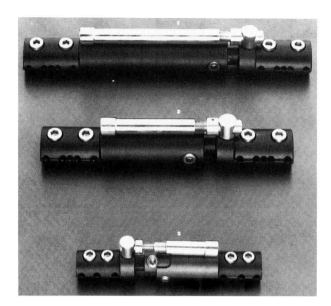

FIGURE 22-34. Standard Orthofix lengthening device. This device is similar in principle to the Wagner device. It does not have ball joints (unlike their external fixator) and is not adjustable once in place. The ability to use three pins in each pin set is an advantage, especially in the proximal femur. (Courtesy of EBI Medical Systems.)

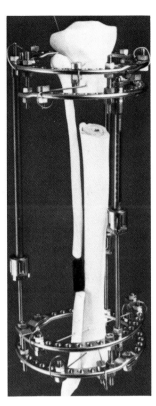

FIGURE 22-36. Ilizarov lengthening device. External fixation is accomplished by tensioned wires fixed to circumferential rings. (From The Ilizarov external fixator, general surgical technique brochure. Memphis, TN: Richards Medical Company, 1988.)

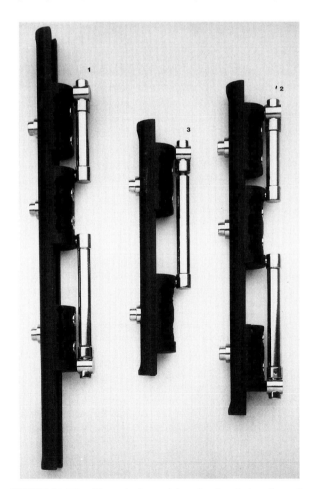

FIGURE 22-35. The orthofix track lengthening device places the lengthening mechanism beside the pins instead of between them, thereby increasing the excursion and obviating device exchange during lengthening. Like the standard device, it is not adjustable once the pins are in place.

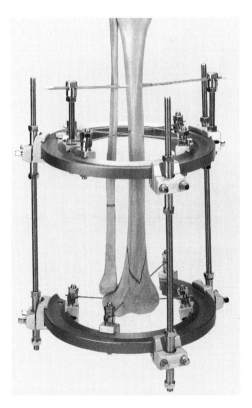

FIGURE 22-37. Monticelli-Spinelli lengthening device, like the Ilizarov device, accomplishes fixation by means of tensioned wires fixed to rings. (Courtesy of Jacquet Orthopedie S.A.)

length.[171] In this way the number of percutaneous tracts can be reduced, and the external device can be removed as soon as the regenerate bone can withstand pure compression loading.

Lengthening over the rod has the disadvantage compared with other lengthening techniques that alignment of the anatomic axis of the femur cannot be changed and that the mechanical axis of the leg cannot be changed. Because the anatomic axes of the femur and tibia are not collinear, elongation in this manner increases valgus of the mechanical axis of the leg. Whether this is a problem depends on the initial configuration of the leg. The correction, if necessary, of preexisting angular deformity or the valgus produced by the lengthening must be performed at another time, when the rod is no longer in place.

There has been reasonable hesitation in using this approach because of the fear of producing a serious intramedullary infection with the intramedullary foreign material in continuity with the exterior through the pin tracts. Although early experience suggests that with care the external device need not contact the rod and that the risk of intramedullary infection is not as great as might be feared, widespread use of this technique should await more definitive reports concerning this and other risks.

The application of this technique is limited to those femurs that are straight enough to accept the rod and, in the case of the femur, children who are old enough not to be at risk for avascular necrosis of the femoral head.

Biologic Factors

Several groups have been working in parallel over the past 3 decades to develop not only improved devices but also improved concepts and methods of lengthening. In particular, Ilizarov, Yakamura, and De Bastiani have contributed new concepts and a new understanding of the biology of lengthening that are more important contributions than the devices themselves.[52,53] Because these techniques overlap in many respects, these biologic concepts are considered in principle; with that foundation, technological issues are considered.

MINIMAL DISTURBANCE OF THE BONE. Corticotomy, a technique in which the cortex is cut but care is taken not to disturb the medullary contents (Fig. 22-38), is important to preserve the intramedullary blood supply of the bone. It is difficult, however, even with careful technique, to avoid disturbance of intramedullary contents, and it has been demonstrated that the intramedullary circulation reconstitutes very quickly, even if interrupted. The current consensus is that it is not necessary to perform a

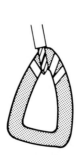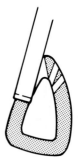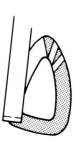

FIGURE 22-38. In the corticotomy technique, care is taken to preserve the contents of the medullary cavity of the bone so that they may make their greatest contribution to osteogenesis during lengthening. Drill holes of controlled depth are made through the anterior cortex; the lateral cortices are cut with a narrow osteotome to avoid entering the medullary cavity; and the posterior cortex is cracked by bending.

corticotomy and care and preservation of the periosteum is more important.

In contrast to the principle of minimal bone disturbance, massive bone production in the lengthening gap following peripheral decortication near the osteotomy has been reported.[124]

LOCATION OF LENGTHENING. Whenever appropriate, the lengthening is done in the metaphysis, where the bone is more active and there are greater numbers of active osteoblasts to participate in the process of regeneration (Fig. 22-39).[34] A second benefit of this location is purely mechanical and is based on the principle that the strength of a structure in bending varies with the fourth power of its diameter. Because the diameter of the metaphysis is so much greater than that of the diaphysis, the bone is stronger for any stage of healing. This allows earlier removal of the fixator with decreased risk of fracture when subjected to bending loads.

It should be noted that the increased strength of the regenerate bone, both from its metaphyseal location and improved quality, is the most important benefit of the newer methods because it allows the avoidance of plating and grafting as in the Wagner technique. No deep wound infections result if there are no deep operations, there are no plate fractures if there are no plates, and there are no bone fractures through screw holes if there have been no screws. In these ways the avoidance of plating avoids some of the serious complications reported in the past.

NUMBER OF LENGTHENING SITES. Devices that lend themselves to fixation of more than two segments of the same bone make it possible to lengthen a single bone both proximally and distally at the same time (Fig. 22-40). Although this theoretically doubles

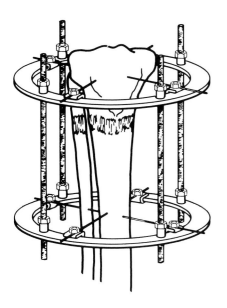
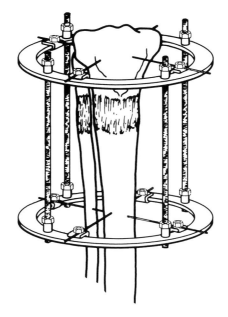

FIGURE 22-39. Metaphyseal lengthening. Elongation through the metaphysis promotes osteogenesis in the lengthening gap because metaphyseal bone is so active, and it promotes strength by the large cross-sectional area.

the rate of bone elongation, the soft tissues do not easily double their elongation rate, and articular cartilage has been shown experimentally in animals to suffer with rapid elongation.[22]

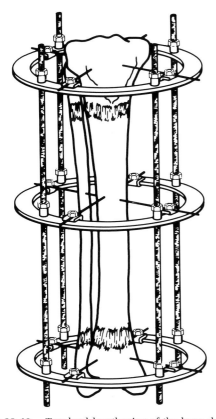

FIGURE 22-40. Two-level lengthening of the bone doubles the rate and reduces the duration of lengthening. It requires fixation of three segments but does not significantly increase the risk or morbidity.

DELAY BEFORE DISTRACTION. It appears beneficial to delay the onset of distraction after the bone sectioning procedure. Guidelines have been established that are as long as possible without risking premature consolidation, which would prevent distraction. Delays of several days for young children, 1 week for adolescents, and 10 days for adults appear appropriate. This delay is to allow the osteogenic process to become established so that osteogenesis can keep up with the elongating gap.

RATE OF DISTRACTION. Ilizarov[100] recommends a distraction rate of 1 mm/day, slower than the 1.5 mm/day used in the Wagner technique. The rationale is that the separation of the bone ends should proceed in advance of the ability of the regenerating bone in the gap to effect union, and too fast a rate will inhibit bone formation. The rate may have to be slowed if radiographs show inadequate regeneration and a widening lucency in the regenerating bone. Faster rates induce ischemia and significant slowing of osteogenesis, but some patients who show excellent regeneration radiologically can have their distraction rate increased. The rate of 1 mm/day also appears to be appropriate for the soft tissues to grow in length in tandem with the bone.[102]

RHYTHM OF DISTRACTION. Increasing the frequency of lengthenings without changing the rate promotes faster consolidation experimentally and reduces the tension stress on the regenerating bone. Lengthening by 0.25 mm four times per day is better than lengthening by 1 mm one time per day, and it appears that gradual continuous elongation, perhaps by a motorized device as suggested by Ilizarov, is ideal.

QUALITY OF REGENERATE BONE. Osteogenesis in the gap begins first in the medulla and expands to fill the gap. Multipotential cells become osteoblasts and form bone without a cartilage foundation in a fashion reminiscent of membranous bone formation. Microscopic examination of the regenerating bone, elongated according to modern concepts, shows that it has a longitudinal orientation, probably because its formation is guided so intimately by the architecture of the osteotomy surface.[103] The architecture of the regenerate resembles haversian bone and is said to be stronger than woven bone and remodel and calcify faster.

THIN WIRES. The ring fixators allow the use of thin (1–2 mm) wires instead of large screws. The wires cause less reaction of surrounding skin and bone, move through the skin more easily, and allow some axial dynamization of the bone fragments. The construct of thin wires with circumferential rings provides rigidity against bending in the sagittal and coronal planes but is not so rigid in the axial direction, allowing slight axial movement in response to applied loads. The cyclic dynamic compression that results is said to promote regeneration of bone in the lengthening gap, and the flexibility of other devices using thick pins can have the same effect.

AMOUNT OF LENGTHENING. It is not known if there is an upper limit to lengthening. Reports on the new techniques suggest that greater lengthening may be possible than was formerly thought. Carroll has shown that permanent changes occur in muscle and joint cartilage with tibial lengthening greater than 11%,[41] and Bell has shown effects on the adjacent joints in animal experiments.[22] These effects may be related more to the rate than the magnitude of lengthening, and the degree to which they occur in human patients is uncertain.

ACTIVITY LEVEL. Patients can be encouraged to be active and full weight bearing from the start and participate in vigorous calisthenics and physical therapy to maintain normal joint motion and muscle strength. Weight bearing takes advantage of the flexibility of the devices to apply dynamic compression to the regenerating bone that is believed to stimulate bone formation.

DYNAMIZATION. The ring fixators have the advantage of allowing dynamic loading of the lengthening gap throughout the period of fixation while they simultaneously control length. The Orthofix device can be dynamized by applying an elastic collar, and when the regenerate bone appears strong enough, the device can be released so that it maintains alignment but not length, thus allowing dynamization, but this cannot be done until the regenerate bone is strong enough to resist shortening. The Wagner device cannot be dynamized but can be put into compression mode when the regenerate bone is strong enough. All of the devices allow some dynamization by virtue of their elasticity and can be made less rigid by the removal of wires or pins in a staged fashion.

LENGTHENING INDEX. This quantity is the number of months of external fixation per centimeter of lengthening. It is generally between 1 and 1.5 months per centimeter and tends to be greater for lesser lengthenings because one component of this time, the interval from the arrest of elongation to the removal, tends to be constant. This number is a guideline to predict the duration of fixation for patients about to undergo lengthening.

Factors Affecting the Choice of Lengthening Hardware

The biologic factors discussed above are, for the most part, device independent. The choice of lengthening device is not, however, completely arbitrary. The devices have certain characteristics that affect their ease of use in specific situations. Because deformity correction often goes hand in hand with lengthening, this discussion includes some aspects of device selection and use in the correction of angular deformity.

GRADUAL VERSUS ACUTE CORRECTION. It is clear that not all deformities need to be corrected gradually. There is a long and successful history of acute correction of deformity by osteotomy with internal or external fixation or no fixation at all. Although there can be advantages in the use of external fixation, in some cases there appears to be no advantage to correcting these deformities gradually, as Ilizarov has proposed.[170]

The question then arises as to the possible advantages or disadvantages of gradual correction if an external fixator is in place in any case to accomplish lengthening. There is good evidence to suggest that, if an external device is already in place for lengthening, either gradual or acute correction of coexisting deformity can achieve good results.[170] Acute correction has the effect of simplifying the lengthening and widens the selection of devices, whereas gradual correction with the Ilizarov or other ring fixator allows the physician to monitor and modify the correction on an ongoing basis.

If the surgeon wishes to perform a gradual deformity correction then the Ilizarov device or another ring fixator is the only choice with the single exception of the Orthofix device with the Garches clamp in the correction of high tibial varus or valgus. Using the Ilizarov apparatus to perform gradual angular correction, with or without lengthening, requires attention to the geometric principles of hinge placement as described by Herzenberg.[90] Careful hinge placement can control both translation and angular correction. Placing hinges so that the axis of rotation is outside the bone can accomplish lengthening and angular correction simultaneously.

THIN WIRES VERSUS HALF-PINS. The Wagner and Orthofix devices require thick half-pins, whereas the Ilizarov device can be used with either thin wires or half-pins. Thin wires appear to pass through the skin more easily but leave twice as many unsightly scars in the skin and tether the muscles in twice as many locations, thereby interfering with knee motion.[34] Loosening of a wire does not result in a loss of position, as with a screw, because the bone is prevented from sliding on the wire by other oblique wires at the same level.

On the other hand, thin wires have a number of disadvantages. They do not lend themselves to fixation of the proximal femur and most prefer half-pins and partial rings at that level. There is a growing trend to the use of half-pins at other levels as well. The wire tension must be adjusted to close to their elastic limit, and it does not take much additional force to stretch the wires plastically, which compromises the rigidity of the frame. Those patients for whom cosmesis is a major motivating force for the lengthening are not pleased with the appearance their leg thereafter.

CONICAL SCREWS. The Orthofix device uses 6-mm pins that taper slightly toward the tip. If they loosen, they can be tightened by advancing them slightly. Conversely, if they are inserted too far, they cannot be retracted without loosening. Screws are also manufactured with cutting edges on one side of the shaft, which, when oriented in the proper direction, facilitate their passage through the skin.

EXCURSION. The standard Orthofix lengthener is limited in its excursion. The short model, for example, has an excursion of only 5 cm, meaning that it will have to be replaced with a longer model if further lengthening is to be attained. The Orthofix track lengthener is available in several lengths and can accommodate any desired excursion. The Wagner device has excursion of more than 15 cm and can accomplish all but the longest lengthenings. The Ilizarov device has the advantage that its external components can be replaced without general anesthesia, and therefore virtually any amount of lengthening or angular correction can be accomplished.

EASE OF REPLACEMENT OF PINS AND WIRES. Because the Ilizarov device allows pins and wires to be placed at almost any level and angle, there is no problem in removing troublesome wires and inserting new ones. The monolateral fixators, on the other hand, are more limited in that the pin clamps have predesignated locations and all pins in one cluster are in the same plane. Replacement of one pin may require replacement of all pins of that cluster.

ABILITY TO PLACE PIN CLUSTERS CLOSE TOGETHER. The Ilizarov apparatus and the Wagner device allow the pin clusters in the proximal and distal segments to be placed as close together as desired. The Orthofix device has the body between the pin clamps so that the pin clusters must be placed far enough apart to accommodate the length of the device. This is a disadvantage in a short bone or if other factors govern pin placement. The Orthofix track lengthener does allow the pin clamps to be placed close to each other.

NUMBER OF PINS IN EACH SEGMENT. The Wagner device permits two pins in each clamp, the Orthofix allows three pins, and the Ilizarov device sets no limits on the number of pins or wires. There can be an advantage to fixation of the proximal femur with more than two pins, especially if the lengthening is through the proximal part of the shaft, and the pins must be placed proximally. In that configuration, the loading is eccentric and three pins provide better fixation with less risk of loosening.

TOTAL NUMBER OF PINS AND WIRES. The Ilizarov apparatus usually requires at least three wires in each segment for a simple lengthening, a total of 12 scars in the skin. The monolateral fixators usually can be applied with only two screws in each segment, producing fewer than half the number of scars and reducing the operative time for the application.

ABILITY TO FIX MORE THAN ONE SEGMENT. The Wagner device only allows fixation of two segments and is incapable of transporting intermediate segments of bone in cases of bone loss. It is also incapable of traversing joints. The Orthofix device and the track lengthener can be assembled to fix more than two segments and, with special clamps and hinges, can traverse joints. The Ilizarov device can be extended to provide fixation of as many segments as required and can be extended across joints with or without hinges.

COMPLEX DEFORMITIES WITH MULTIPLE AXES OF CORRECTION. Only the ring fixators can accomplish gradual correction of deformities in more than one plane. Not only can multiple segments be controlled and multiple hinges incorporated but the system can be modified as correction progresses to met emerging demands.

ABILITY TO ADJUST DEVICE WHILE IN PLACE. The Wagner device can be adjusted in two planes but requires a general anesthetic to do so. Because there is some give in the system with femoral lengthenings with lateral placement of the device tending to go into varus and tibial lengthenings with medial placement tending to go into valgus, it is recommended to begin lengthening with the femur in 10 to 15 degrees of valgus or the tibia in 10 to 15 degrees of varus. The standard Orthofix device is virtually unadjustable, allowing no modification of the orientation of the pins, and once the pins are in place, their track lengthener can be adjusted in only one plane and only if special pin clamps have been used. The Ilizarov method is well suited for continual modification of its configuration by differential lengthening of the individual rods. In addition, its components can be changed and the hinges realigned if required. This can be done without a return to the operating room for anesthesia.

EASE OF ADJUSTING THE LENGTHENING MECHANISM. This is of no concern while patients are hospitalized under the care of trained personnel, but it becomes an issue when they are discharged home. A simple mechanism results in less anxiety and fewer errors. The Wagner mechanism is the simplest with the turn of a single knob. The Orthofix devices require use of a special lengthener that is advanced by turning with a wrench. The Ilizarov device requires elongation of up to three or four rods individually, perhaps by different amounts.

Conclusion

Simple lengthenings can be accomplished by a number of devices, none of which has a clear advantage over another, except that it might be argued that the simplest device capable of solving the problem is advantageous. Gradual correction of complex deformities can present demands that can only be met by a versatile device.

Complications of Lengthening

All studies of leg lengthening, regardless of technique, have reported high complication rates.[28,36,43,48,94,115,133,174,187,198] In our review of 63 Wagner lengthenings in 47 patients, 60% were associated with serious complications that adversely affected the final outcome.[152] Only 40% of patients in this study reached their anticipated lengthening goals with uncompromised function.

Hypertension can be seen during lengthening and can occur suddenly.[17,142,233] The mechanism is not clear, but it resolves dependably with shortening of the lengthening gap and may not recur when lengthening is resumed.

Pin tract inflammation is common and of little consequence in its own right. True pin tract infection usually responds well to local care and systemic antibiotics. It can, however, be elevated to a serious complication by a plating and grafting procedure that is the main reason this technique is no longer commonly used.

Mechanical failure can occur in several modes. Pins can break or loosen and require replacement. Fractures through the lengthening gap or deformation of the bone in the lengthening gap can occur early or late. It can occur soon after removal of the device, indicating that it was removed too soon, or can occur late, while the bone is still remodeling and has not yet regained its normal strength.[126] In my series of Wagner lengthenings, there was one fracture 8 years after the lengthening, which suggests that the bone is extremely slow to remodel and regain full strength and is probably weak even after it looks normal radiologically. Long-term follow-up is important in assessing the results of leg lengthening because complications can occur late.

Subluxation of the knee can occur during femoral lengthening, especially in patients with congenital shortening.[110,152] The subluxation appears to be a posterior subluxation of the lateral tibial plateau and is always preceded by a loss of extension of the knee. Dysplasia or absence of the anterior cruciate ligament and hypoplasia of the lateral femoral condyle are usually found in association with congenitally short femurs[210,211] and contribute to this complication. Routine lengthening of the lateral structures, the biceps tendon and iliotibial band, determined maintenance of knee extension, and avoidance of continued distraction in the face of a knee flexion contracture will avoid knee subluxation.

Dislocation of the hip has been reported, can occur even in the early stages of distraction, and tends to be associated with previous hip surgery and residual instability.[182]

Delayed union is difficult to define in this context, but there is no doubt that certain cases take significantly longer to consolidate than others. True nonunion occurs and is similar in appearance and treatment to posttraumatic nonunion except that it can occur in narrowed and spindle-shaped bone such that it is fragile even when united.

Nerve damage from stretching, entrapment by tense tissues, movement of wires or pins through the tissues, or direct trauma can occur. One study of nerve conduction in six patients undergoing lengthening reported changes in all six.[234]

Karger and colleagues found that femoral lengthenings were more prone to complications than tibial ones, and that the complication rate increased with lengthenings exceeding 25% of the initial bone length.[113] We found that the complication rate is significantly higher in children younger than age 8 years than in older children and this may reflect the inability of younger children to understand instructions and to remain motivated to comply with those of therapists and surgeons.[155] To some extent, the amount of possible lengthening depends on the length of the bone to start with and this is another reason to perform lengthening only in older children whose bones are nearing mature length.

Because of the frequency of concerns, questions, problems, and complications that surround the care of patients undergoing lengthening, it facilitates their management to form a lengthening team in a program with shared responsibilities. A nurse, physical therapist, social worker and a skilled technician are important members of the team and all can assist in the preparation of patients and families for the lengthening and can respond to their ongoing needs and offer support during the lengthening. Families never fully appreciate depth and breadth of the hardship they will face and will require more support than most orthopaedic patients.

Conclusion

Leg length discrepancy and leg lengthening are in a volatile period of changing concepts, ideas and philosophies. Excellent patient care requires comfortable familiarity with the techniques of patient assessment, the methods of prediction of future growth and discrepancy, the factors important in the selection of treatment goals, and the approaches to treatment. Being familiar and up to date with respect to the techniques and philosophies of limb lengthening is challenging but the improvement in our capabilities should be an adequate reward.

ANGULAR DEFORMITY

With the increasing use of external fixators and the increasing favor in which gradual correction of angular deformities is held, the treatment of angular deformities has much in common with the treatment of leg length discrepancy, and therefore the condition is covered here. Although the conditions that caused angular deformity are covered in detail elsewhere in this text, the general principles of the treatment of angular deformities will be dealt with here.

Etiology and Pathogenesis

Angular deformities generally fall into two categories, those that are static and those that are changing. The category of changing discrepancies can also be divided into those that tend to correct spontaneously and those whose natural history is to continue to progress. Static deformities include those that are the result of fractures or surgery and those deformities that have been changing but have ceased to change at or near the end of growth. Deformities that tend to improve include physiologic bowing of childhood and the valgus of the tibia that occurs after high tibial fractures. Those that worsen generally are caused by abnormalities of the growth plate from a number of different causes. They include developmental conditions, such as Blount disease; skeletal dysplasias, such as diastrophic dwarfism; metabolic abnormalities, such as hypophosphatemic rickets; and direct damage to the growth plate as a result of infection, radiation, or trauma.

The principles of treatment of angular deformities in these three groups are different. Deformities that have a tendency to correct spontaneously should be given the chance to do so, and surgical treatment should be considered only after failure to correct spontaneously has been demonstrated. After a deformity is known to be or can be demonstrated to be static, it can be treated at any time. There is usually no reason to defer treatment, regardless of the age of the child. Progressive deformities, on the other hand, deserve a less aggressive approach. Children can tolerate significant angular deformities of the lower limbs without sustaining any damage and, in most cases, without feeling any pain. Even deformities that are severe enough to greatly concern the parents may be well tolerated by the child without harmful effects. Also, the lower the threshold for performing surgical correction, the greater the number of corrections that will be required during the child's growing years. Adoption of a lower threshold result in significantly less morbidity from hospitalizations and postoperative care. For that reason, the deformity should be tolerated for as long as possible to minimize the number of surgical corrections, and the long-term surgical treatment should include the possibility of a last surgical correction at maturity that can be perfect and definitive.

Some progressive deformities in young children can be particularly troublesome. Because the children are growing so fast, the deformity tends to recur quickly after surgical correction, and an unacceptably high number of surgical corrections can be anticipated during the child's growing years. In some of these situations, consideration can be given to completely arresting the growth at the offending epiphysis in order to prevent future progression of the deformity with the view that treatment of the resulting leg length discrepancy entails a lesser morbidity than repeated corrections of the angular deformity.

Radiologic Evaluation

Assessment of angular deformity in the coronal plane is best accomplished by a standing radiograph of both legs with the patellae pointing straight forward. It is important to control the projection in this manner in order to minimize the measurement error due to rotation. Lateral views of the individual bones can be helpful if there is also significant deformity in the sagittal plane. Two types of measurements can be made from these radiographs. The first assesses the angular deformity in the midshaft of the bone and is accomplished by measuring the angle between lines drawn in the proximal and distal diaphyses. The second and perhaps more important type of measurement assesses the mechanical axis of the leg and the tilt of the knee. It is important in this context to measure not only the deviation of the mechanical axis of the leg but also the specific deformities in the distal femur and proximal tibia individually. These measurements are best made by drawing lines to represent the mechanical axis of the individual bones from the center of the hip joint to the center of the knee for the femur and from the center of the knee to the center of the ankle for tibia. A line should then be drawn to represent the transverse access of the knee joint. No convention has been established for this purpose with either or both the femoral condyles or tibial plateau have been used.[96,151] Because the femoral condyles are easier to delineate than the tibial plateau, I prefer to use a transverse line tangent to the two femoral condyles to represent the knee joint for both femur and tibia. Studies have shown that the mechanical axes of the tibia and the femur normally are not perfectly aligned, the mean angle being 1 to 2 degrees of varus. Also, the mean alignment of the distal femur is normally 1 to 1.5 degrees of valgus, and that of the proximal tibia 2 to 3 degrees of varus[151] (Fig. 22-41).

Indications and Goals

For clinical purposes, accepting the errors inherent in measurement and surgical technique, the goal of surgery should be to make the mechanical axes of the femur and tibia colinear and both the knee and the

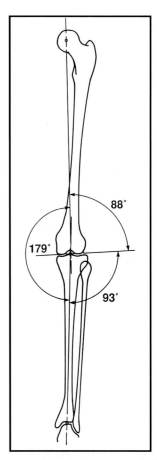

FIGURE 22-41. Normal angular relations in the lower limb. Analysis of lower limb alignment in the general population has shown that the distal femur is in 2 degrees of valgus and the proximal tibia in 3 degrees of varus so that the mechanical axes of the tibia and the femur are 1 degree off colinear. It may be desirable for the surgeon to aim at true colinearity and a perpendicular knee despite these findings.

ankle perpendicular to that line. The actual shapes of the bones are of secondary importance. The shape of the femur is hidden within the musculature of the thigh, but the shape of the tibia, because it is a subcutaneous bone, is more obvious.

There are no long-term prospective studies that have followed children with angular deformities to determine how the development of late osteoarthritis is related to the magnitude of the angular deformity at the end of growth. Several studies, however, have followed angulation due to malunited fractures and have found that angulation predisposes to degenerative arthritis,[118,140] and if uncorrected, both the angulation and the arthritis tend to worsen.[87] The decisions that we make to correct angular deformity are not based on a solid scientific foundation but are based on consideration of cosmesis or an intuitive feeling about the magnitude of deformity that will cause later problems. It is my belief that angular deformities of

15 degrees and greater are generally considered to be candidates for correction at maturity, whereas deformities of lesser magnitude might be tolerated without correction.

Similarly, there are no long-term studies to assist us in determining how much knee tilt can be tolerated in the child without problems in the long term or what the threshold should be for performing osteotomies to achieve ideal alignment of the knee. This is an important consideration in correcting complex deformities in children's lower limbs because the decision on whether to perform osteotomies of one or two bones is based on how much knee tilt is believed to be acceptable.

Patient Assessment

Accurate clinical assessment of angular deformities of the lower limbs can be extremely difficult because the transverse axis of the knee joint can be difficult to control during the examination. It is useful to sit the patient on the edge of the examining table and to attempt to position the limbs so that the transverse axis of the knee joint is exactly parallel to the edge of the table. This can be done visually by rotating the legs so that the patellae are pointing straight forward and observing the knee joint carefully during flexion and extension of the joint. This is much more difficult in practice than it is in principle, and it is very easy to interpret deformity in one plane as a deformity in another. It may be necessary to delay the definitive decision about corrective surgery until the patient is in the operating room and the knee can be examined under fluoroscopy or under direct vision. Fortunately, it is not absolutely necessary to objectively measure the component deformities in each plane in order to perform the corrective surgery.

It is a principle of three-dimensional geometry that significant deviations in two planes actually constitute a deviation in the third plane. The orthopaedic manifestation of this principle is that when there is significant deformity in two planes near the physis of a long bone, then a torsional deformity is also present. Conversely, correction of the angular deformities in both planes can actually constitute a correction of the rotation of the abnormality without any conscious effort to include a derotation component in the osteotomy.

Preoperative Planning

Preoperative planning must include the objectives of a straight mechanical axis and a perpendicular knee and ankle. Note that the concept of "parallel to the floor" is useless in this context because the floor is not available as a valid reference during performance of the surgical procedure. The decisions that must be made concern the number of osteotomies necessary to correct the deformity and the levels at which they should be performed. It is best to perform the osteotomy at the level of the deformity. This can be easy to define in the case of a malunited fracture and difficult to define in the case of the curved bone, as occur in hypophosphatemic rickets. Long curves in the femur can be corrected by a single distal osteotomy because the resulting unusual shape of the bone is well hidden by the musculature of the thigh and has no cosmetic significance. In the subcutaneous tibia, however, more than one osteotomy may be necessary to normalize the shape of the bone although multiple osteotomies are not necessary to satisfy the mechanical demands. The principle of performing the osteotomy at the level of the angulation is difficult to follow in those cases in which the deformity is at the growth plate because the growth plate of the distal femur is partly interarticular and an osteotomy of the tibia at or near the level of the growth plate would violate the part of the growth plate that descends the tibial tubercle. In both of these cases, the osteotomies must be done further from the joint.

If there is deformity in only one bone, then the mechanical goals can be satisfied by a single osteotomy in the deformed bone. If there are deformities in two bones, however, then the situation becomes more difficult, and two or three osteotomies may be required to adequately correct the deformity. In this case the surgeon must decide before performing the first osteotomy how much knee tilt he or she is willing to accept in the final outcome. Any malalignment of the mechanical axis of the leg can be completely corrected by a single osteotomy in the distal femur or proximal tibia. Whereas a single osteotomy can correct the mechanical axis, it cannot ensure that the knee joint will be perpendicular to it and could leave the knee with some tilt. Correction of the mechanical axis and control over the ultimate alignment of the knee may require two osteotomies, one above the knee and one below the knee. This decision can and must be made in advance of surgery. The important principle in this decision is that, if only one osteotomy is performed and the mechanical axis made perfectly straight, then the resulting tilt of the knee will be exactly equal to whatever angular deformity is present on the operated bone. In other words, if there is 15 degrees of varus in the distal femur and 10 degrees of varus in the proximal tibia and the surgeon decides to correct this by performing a distal femoral valgus osteotomy of 25 degrees, then the outcome includes a knee tilt of 10 degrees, the deformity present in the tibia. If the surgeon is able to specify the upper limit of acceptability of knee tilt, then he will be able to decide to perform one osteotomy or two. I have adopted 7 degrees as the upper threshold of acceptable knee tilt, but this is not based on solid scientific evidence. If the angle between the transverse axis of the knee and the mechanical axis of either bone is not within 7 degrees of perpendicular, then that bone requires an osteotomy. Therefore, in the previous example of a femur with 15 degrees varus deformity and tibia with 10 degrees varus deformity, adequate correction of the leg would involve osteotomies of both bones. Conversely, with femoral varus of 15 degrees and tibial varus of only 5 degrees, a single valgus osteotomy of 20 degrees in the distal femur would serve to align the mechanical axis of the two bones and leave the knee tilted only 5 degrees, an acceptable result. A pertinent example is shown in Figure 22-42. A separate decision will have to be made about the need for correction of ankle varus or valgus, but that decision usually does not have a significant bearing on the mechanical axis of the limb because the osteotomy is so close to the point of contact with the floor.

A child with severe deformity in both bones, as is frequently seen in hypophosphatemic rickets, on the other hand, might require osteotomies of the distal femur and proximal tibia, perhaps even the distal tibia, in order to meet the mechanical goals of colinear mechanical axes with the knee and ankle joints both perpendicular to it (Figs. 22-43 and 22-44).

Operative Strategy

The surgeon, having decided preoperatively on the number and locations of corrective osteotomies, must devise an intraoperative strategy to ensure that the operative goals are reached. In the case of the single osteotomy, above or below the knee, the goal is to make the leg straight, to line up the hip joint, the knee joint, and the ankle joint. The operation should be performed with the leg draped free so that it is easy to see. The knee and ankle centers can be determined from anatomic landmarks, and the center of the hip joint can be determined either by an anatomic landmarks or by fluoroscopy. Fluoroscopy adds a reassuring measure of confidence to the procedure. It is an interesting and educational exercise, particularly for those with little experience in these procedures, to make paper cutouts representing the operation preoperatively. This is not necessary, however, and can make the procedure more difficult, leading to error. A more

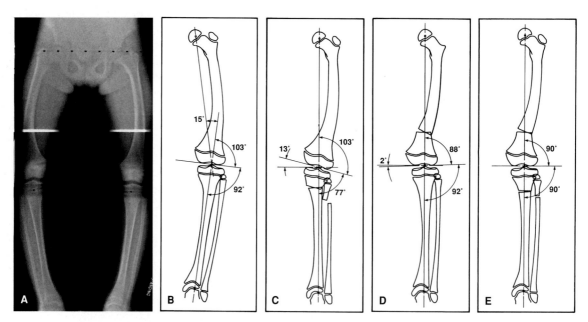

FIGURE 22-42.   Moderate deformity as a result of hypophosphatemic rickets. (**A**) Standing anteroposterior radiograph of a child with hypophosphatemic rickets. (**B**) Measurement of the radiograph shows a total deviation of the mechanical axis of 15 degrees due to varus of the proximal tibia of 2 degrees and varus of the distal femur of 13 degrees. (**C**) Prediction of the result of perfect correction of the mechanical axis by tibial osteotomy only. The knee is left in 13 degrees of lateral downward tilt, which is the deformity present in the unoperated femur. This is not acceptable. (**D**) Prediction of the result of perfect correction of the mechanical axis by femoral osteotomy only. The knee is left in 2 degrees of medial downward tilt, which is the deformity present in the unoperated tibia. This is acceptable. (**E**) Prediction of the result of perfect correction of the mechanical axis by combined distal femoral and proximal tibial osteotomies. The knee is perfectly perpendicular to the mechanical axis. The addition of a tibial osteotomy to avoid 2 degrees of knee tilt would not be worthwhile.

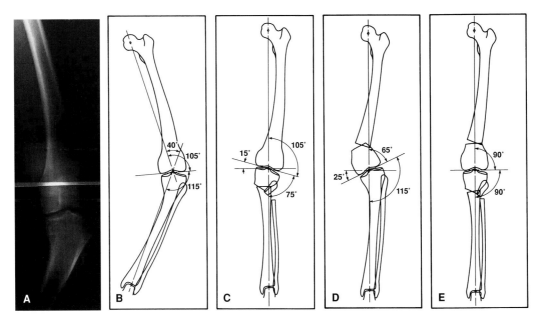

FIGURE 22-43. Severe deformity as a result of Blount disease. (**A**) Standing anteroposterior radiograph of a child with Blount disease. (**B**) Measurement of the film shows a total deviation of the mechanical axis of 40 degrees, varus of the proximal tibia of 25 degrees, and varus of the distal femur of 15 degrees. (**C**) Prediction of the result of perfect correction of the mechanical axis by tibial osteotomy only. The knee is left in 15 degrees of lateral downward tilt, which is the deformity present in the unoperated femur. This is not acceptable. (**D**) Prediction of the result of perfect correction of the mechanical axis by femoral osteotomy only. The knee is left in 25 degrees of medial downward tilt, which is the deformity present in the unoperated tibia. This is not acceptable. (**E**) Prediction of the result of perfect correction of the mechanical axis by combined distal femoral and proximal tibial osteotomies. The knee is perfectly perpendicular to the mechanical axis. The surgeon should not be misled by the fact that Blount disease is a tibial disease into performing only a tibial osteotomy.

reliable approach is simply to make the distal osteotomy cut exactly perpendicular to the mechanical axis of the distal segment in two planes and the proximal cut exactly perpendicular to the mechanical axis of the proximal segment. In a proximal tibial osteotomy, the proximal segment for alignment includes the proximal tibial segment above the level of the osteotomy and the entire femur to the hip with the knee fully extended. The distal segment for alignment is the tibia from the level of the osteotomy to the ankle (see Fig. 22-42). When the wedge of bone is removed and the two cut surfaces opposed, the leg is perfectly aligned in both planes. It is not necessary to make reference to the tilt of the knee joint in single bone correction, only to a location of its center.

In the case of two-bone corrections, a different strategy must be employed. The goal of the first osteotomy is to correct the deformity in that bone, to make its mechanical axis exactly perpendicular to the knee joint. To accomplish this, reference to the knee joint needs to be made. Passing a K-wire through the joint has been recommended but is not very dependable. A better method is to see the knee joint under fluoroscopy and make the nearest osteotomy cut exactly parallel to it. After correcting the deformity in that single

bone, the goal of the osteotomy of the second bone is the same as it would be in the single-bone correction: to make the mechanical axis of the two bones colinear. I prefer to perform the tibial correction first because it allows a sterile tourniquet to be placed on the thigh, minimizing blood loss and allowing the first osteotomy to be performed in a bloodless field. The tourniquet can be removed for the femoral osteotomy, if necessary.

Gradual and Acute Correction

The relative advantages and disadvantages of gradual and acute correction have been discussed earlier. The selection of type of correction is made on the basis of surgeon's preference, because there is no clear advantage of either technique in terms of the final outcome.

If gradual correction using a ring fixator is chosen, then correct hinge placement is critical. If the deformity exists in both the sagittal and coronal planes, the hinge must be placed in the correct axis to correct both deformities simultaneously. This can be estimated using geometric techniques from anteroposterior and lateral radiographs. Then the hinge must be

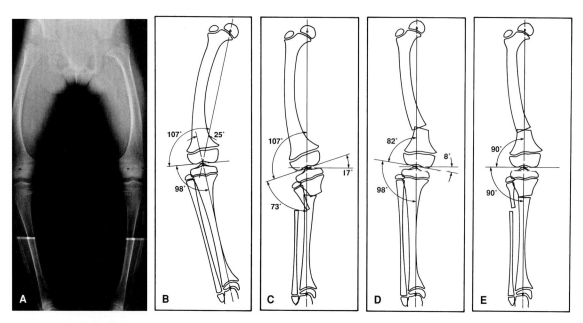

FIGURE 22-44.   Severe deformity in hypophosphatemic rickets. **(A)** Standing anteroposterior radiograph of a boy with hypophosphatemic rickets. **(B)** Measurement of a composite tracing shows a total deviation of the mechanical axis of 25 degrees, varus of the proximal tibia of 8 degrees, and varus of the distal femur of 17 degrees. **(C)** Prediction of the result of perfect correction of the mechanical axis by tibial osteotomy only. The knee is left in 17 degrees of lateral downward tilt, which is the deformity present in the unoperated femur. This is unacceptable. **(D)** Prediction of the result of perfect correction of the mechanical axis by femoral osteotomy only. The knee is left in 8 degrees of medial downward tilt, which is the deformity present in the unoperated tibia. The decision on whether or not to accept this degree of tilt depends on the threshold adopted by the surgeon. **(E)** Prediction of the result of perfect correction of the mechanical axis by combined distal femoral and proximal tibial osteotomies. The knee is perfectly perpendicular to the mechanical axis. The surgeon must decide whether the addition of the tibial osteotomy would be worthwhile to avoid a knee tilt of 8 degrees.

placed with its axis through the bone if angular correction without lengthening is desired; it can be placed eccentric from the bone for combined correction of angular and shortened deformities. An element of translation also can be introduced into the correction by placing the hinge above or below the level of the osteotomy. These decisions can be made accurately preoperatively by relatively simple geometric techniques.

Gradual angular correction, unlike lengthening, involves a differential rate of elongation for the tissues depending on their distances from the hinge. Those tissues farthest from the hinge elongate more rapidly than those close to the hinge. This must be taken into account in calculating the amount of lengthening in the lengthening rods that is to be accomplished each day, and a goal of the fastest lengthening of any tissue of 1 mm per day should be set.

SUMMARY

There are certain problems in orthopaedic surgery that appear simple, even trivial, at first glance but present difficulties in practice and can produce less

than desirable results for reasons that are not entirely clear. The correction of angular deformity falls into this category, particularly deformity in more than one plane or more than one bone. The surgeon can expect and ensure good results by an understanding of the biomechanical and geometric concepts involved, careful evaluation and preoperative planning, and the adoption of a surgical technique that ensures that the biomechanical and geometric goals are met.

References

1. Aaron A, Weinstein D, Thickman D, Eilert R. Comparison of orthoroentgenography and computed tomography in the measurement of limb-length discrepancy. J Bone Joint Surg [Am] 1992;74:897.

2. Acheson RM. The Oxford method of assessing skeletal maturity. Clin Orthop 1957;10:19.

3. Agerholm J. The zig-zag osteotomy. Acta Orthop Scand 1959;29:63.

4. Ahmadi B, Akbarnia BA, Ghobadi F, et al. Experience with 141 tibial lengthenings in poliomyelitis and comparison of 3 different methods. Clin Orthop 1979;145:150.

5. Aitken A, Blackett CW, Ciacotti JJ. Overgrowth of the femoral shaft following fractures in childhood. J Bone Joint Surg 1939;21:334.

6. Altongy J, Harcke H, Bowen J. Measurement of leg length

inequalities by micro-dose digital radiographs. J Pediatr Orthop 1987;7(3):311.

7. Anders G, Stachon I. Experience with temporary epiphyseodesis after Blount. Z Orthop 1979;117:922.

8. Anderson L, Westin GW, Oppenheim WL. Syme amputation in children: indications, results, and long-term follow-up. J Pediatr Orthop 1984;4:550.

9. Anderson M, Green W, Messner M. Growth and predictions of growth in the lower extremities. J Bone Joint Surg [Am] 1963;45:1.

10. Anderson M, Green WT. Lengths of the femur and tibia: norms derived from orthoroentgenograms of children from five years of age until epiphyseal closure. Am J Dis Child 1948;75:279.

11. Anderson M, Messner M, Green W. Distribution of lengths of the normal femur and tibia in children from one to eighteen years of age. J Bone Joint Surg [Am] 1964;46(6):1197.

12. Anderson WV. Leg lengthening. J Bone Joint Surg [Br] 1952;34:150.

13. Arkin AM, Katz JF. The effects of pressure on epiphyseal growth. The mechanism of plasticity of growing bone. J Bone Joint Surg [Am] 1956;38:1056.

14. Armstrong P. Attempts to accelerate longitudinal bone growth. In: Uhthoff H, Wiley J, eds. Behaviour of the growth plate. New York: Raven, 1988:237.

15. Askins G, Ger E. Congenital constriction band syndrome. J Pediatr Orthop 1988;8:461.

16. Atar D, Lehman W, Grant A, Strongwater A. Percutaneous epiphysiodesis. J Bone Joint Surg [Br] 991;73:173.

17. Axer A, Elkon A, Eliahu H. Hypertension as a complication of limb lengthening. J Bone Joint Surg [Am] 1966;48:520.

18. Barry K, McManus F, O'Brien T. Leg lengthening by the transiliac method. J Bone Joint Surg [Br] 1992;74:275.

19. Bayley N. Individual patterns of development. Child Develop 1956;27:45.

20. Beals R, Lovrein E. Diffuse capillary hemangiomas associated with skeletal hypotrophy. J Pediatr Orthop 1992;12:401.

21. Beals RK. Hemihypertophy and hemiatrophy. Clin Orthop 1982;166:199.

22. Bell D. The effect of limb lengthening on articular cartilage: an experimental study. Presented at the Annual Meeting of the Pediatric Orthopaedic Society of North America, Newport, RI, 1992.

23. Bell JS, Thompson WAL. Modified spot scanography. Am J Roentgenol 1950;63:915.

24. Bellier G, Carlioz H. The prediction of growth in long bones in poliomyelitis. Rev Chir Orthop 1979;65:373.

25. Bensahel H, Huguenin P, Briard JL. Transepiphyseal lengthening of the tibia. Rev Chir Orthop 1983;69:245.

26. Bianco AJ Jr. Femoral shortening. Clin Orthop 1978;136:49.

27. Bisgard JD. Longitudinal bone growth, the influence of sympathetic deinnervation. Ann Surg 1973;97:374.

28. Bjerkreim I, Hellum C. Femur lengthening using the Wagner technique. Acta Orthop Scand 1983;54:263.

29. Blair V, Walker S, Sheridan J, Schoenecker P. Epiphysiodesis: a problem of timing. J Pediatr Orthop 1982;2:281.

30. Blount WP. A mature look at epiphyseal stapling. Clin Orthop 1971;77:149.

31. Blount WP, Clarke GR. Control of bone growth by epiphyseal stapling. A preliminary report. J Bone Joint Surg 1949;31:464.

32. Bohlman HR. Experiments with foreign materials in the region of the epiphyseal cartilage plate of growing bones to increase their longitudinal growth. J Bone Joint Surg 1929; 11:365.

33. Bost FC, Larson LJ. Experiences with lengthening of the femur over an intramedullary rod. J Bone Joint Surg [Am] 1956; 38:567.

34. Bowen J, Levy E, Donohue M. Comparison of knee motion and callous formation in femoral lengthening with the Wagner or monolateral-ring device. J Pediatr Orthop 1993;13:467.

35. Brockway A, Craig WA, Cockrell BRJ. End result of 62 stapling operations. J Bone Joint Surg [Am] 1954;36:1063.

36. Brockway A, Fowler SB. Experience with 105 leg-lengthening operations. Surg Gynecol Obstet 1942;75:252.

37. Bylander B, Hansson LI, Selvik G. Pattern of growth retardation after Blount stapling: a roentgen stereophotogrammetric analysis. J Pediatr Orthop 1983;3:63.

38. Canale S, Christian C. Techniques for epiphysiodesis about the knee. Clin Orthop 1990;255:81.

39. Canale S, Russell T, Holcomb R. Percutaneous epiphysiodesis. experimental study and preliminary clinical results. J Pediatr Orthop 1986;6:150.

40. Carpenter C, Lester E. Skeletal age determination in young children: analysis of three regions of the hand/wrist film. J Pediatr Orthop 1993;13:76.

41. Carroll N, Grant C, Hudson R, et al. Experimental observations on the effects of leg lengthening by the Wagner method. Clin Orthop 1981;160:250.

42. Cauchoix J, Morel G. One stage femoral lengthening. Clin Orthop 1978;136:66.

43. Chandler D, King J, Bernstein S, et al. Results of 21 Wagner limb lengthenings in 20 patients. Clin Orthop 1988;230:214.

44. Chapman M, Duwelius P, Bray T, Gordon J. Closed intramedullary femoral osteotomy. Shortening and derotation procedures. Clin Orthop 1993;287:245.

45. Cleveland R, Kushner D, Ogden M, et al. Determination of leg length discrepancy. A comparison of weight-bearing and supine imaging. Invest Radiol 1988;23:301.

46. Codivilla A. On the means of lengthening in the lower limbs the muscles and tissues which are shortened through deformity. Am J Orthop Surg 1905;2:353.

47. Coleman S. Simultaneous femoral and tibial lengthening for limb length discrepancies. Arch Orthop Trauma Surg 1985; 103:359.

48. Coleman S, Stevens P. Tibial lengthening. Clin Orthop 1978; 136:92.

49. Compere E. Indications for and against the leg lengthening operation. J Bone Joint Surg 1936;18:692.

50. Compete E, Adams C. Studies of the longitudinal growth of long bones: the influence of trauma to the diaphysis. J Bone Joint Surg 1937;19:922.

51. Connolly J, Huurman W, Lippiello L, Pankaj R. Epiphyseal traction to correct acquired growth deformities. An animal and clinical investigation. Clin Orthop 1986;202:258.

52. De Bastiani G, Aldegheri R, Renzi-Brivio L, Trivella G. Chondrodiatasis—controlled symmetrical distraction os the epiphyseal plate. Limb lengthening in children. J Bone Joint Surg [Br] 1986;68:550.

53. De Bastiani G, Aldegheri R, Renzi-Brivio L, Trivella G. Limb lengthening by callus distraction (callotasis). J Pediatr Orthop 1987;7:129.

54. Delpech J. De l'orthomorphie, par rapport a l'espece humaine. Paris: Gabon; 1829.

55. Doyle J. Stimulation of bone growth by short-wave diathermy. J Bone Joint Surg [Am] 1963;45:15.

56. Dutkowsky J, Kasser J, Kaplan L. Leg length discrepancy associated with vivid cutis marmorata. J Pediatr Orthop 1993; 13:456.

57. Edwards K, Cummings R. Fat embolism as a complication of closed femoral shortening. J Pediatr Orthop 1992;2:542.

58. Frantz C. Epiphyseal stapling. Clin Orthop 1971;77:149.

59. Fries J. Growth following epiphyseal arrest. A simple method of calculation. Clin Orthop 1976;114:316.

60. Froh R, Yong-Hing K, Cassidy J, Houston C. The relationship between leg length discrepancy and lumbar facet orientation. Spine 1988;13:325.

61. Garbarino J, Clancy M, Harcke H, et al. Congenital diastasis of the inferior tibiofibular joint: a review of the literature and report of two cases. J Pediatr Orthop 1985;5:225.

62. Gekeler J, Dietz J, Schuler T. Prognosis of leg length difference in congenital fibula defect. Z Orthop 1982;120:729.

63. Gibson P, Papaioannou T, Kenwright J. The influence on the spine of leg length discrepancy after femoral fracture. J Bone Joint Surg 1983;65B:584.

64. Gillespie R, Torode I. Classification and management of congenital abnormalities of the femur. J Bone Joint Surg [Br] 1983;65:557.

65. Gillis J. Too tall, too small. Champagne, IL: Institute for Personality and Ability Testing, 1982.

66. Glass R, Poznanski A. Leg length determination with biplanar CT scanograms. Radiology 1985;156:833.

67. Gofton J. Persistent low back pain and leg length disparity. J Rheumatol 1985;12:747.

68. Gofton J, Trueman G. Studies in osteoarthritis of the hip. II. Osteoarthritis of the hip and leg length disparity. Can Med Assoc J 1971;104:791.

69. Gotz J, Schellerman W. Continuous lengthening of the femur with intramedullary stabilisation. Arch Orthop Unfallchir 1975;82:305.

70. Green N, Griffin P. Hip dysplasia associated with abduction contracture of the contralateral hip. J Bone Joint Surg [Am] 1982;64:1273.

71. Green W, Anderson M. Experiences with epiphyseal arrest in correcting discrepancies in length of the lower extremities in infantile paralysis. J Bone Joint Surg 1947;29:659.

72. Green W, Anderson M. Skeletal age and the control of bone growth. Instr Course Lect 1960;17:199.

73. Green W, Wyatt G, Anderson M. Orthoroentgenography as a method of measuring the bones of the lower extremity. J Bone Joint Surg 1946;28:60.

74. Greulich W, Pyle S. Radiographic atlas of the skeletal development of the hand and wrist. 2nd ed. Stanford, CA: Stanford University Press, 1959.

75. Grimes J, Blair V, Gilula L. Roentgen rounds #81. Posteromedial bowing of the tibia. Orthop Rev 1986;15:249.

76. Gross R. Leg length discrepancy—How much is too much? Presented at Annual Meeting of the American Academy of Orthopaedic Surgeons, Dallas, TX, 1978.

77. Groves E. Stimulation of bone growth. J Surg 1958;95:125.

78. Grumbach M. Growth hormone therapy and the short end of the stick. N Engl J Med 1988;319(4):238.

79. Grundy P, Roberts C. Does unequal leg length cause back pain? A case-control study. Lancet 1984;2(8397):256.

80. Guidera K, Hess W, Highhouse K, Ogden J. Extremity lengthening: results and complications with the Orthofix system. J Pediatr Orthop 1991;11:90.

81. Hamanishi C, Tanaka S, Tamura K. Early physeal closure after femoral chondrodiatasis. Loss of length gain in 5 cases. Acta Orthop Scand 1992;63:146.

82. Harper M, Canale S. Angulation osteotomy. A trigonometric analysis. Clin Orthop 1982;166:173.

83. Harris R, McDonald J. The effect of lumbar sympathectomy upon the growth of legs paralysed by anterior poliomyelitis. J Bone Joint Surg 1936;18:35.

84. Hass S. Mechanical retardation of bone growth. J Bone Joint Surg [Am] 1948;30:506.

85. Heim M, Horszowski H, Martinowitz U. Leg length inequality in hemophilia. An interesting case report. Clin Pediatr 1985; 24:600.

86. Helms C, McCarthy S. CT scanograms for measuring leg length discrepancy. Radiology 1984;151:802.

87. Hemborg J, Nilsson B. The natural course of untreated osteoarthritis of the knee. Clin Orthop 1977;123:130.

88. Herring J, Moseley C. Posttraumatic valgus deformity of the tibia. J Pediatr Orthop 1981;1:435.

89. Herron L, Amstutz H, Sakai D. One stage femoral lengthening in the adult. Clin Orthop 1978;136:74.

90. Herzenberg J, Waanders N. Calculating rate and duration of distraction for deformity correction with the Ilizarov technique. Orthop Clin North Am 1991;22(4):601.

91. Heuter C. Anatomische studien an den extremitatengelenken neugeborener und erwachsener. Virchows Arch 1862;25:572.

92. Hofmann A, Wenger D. Posteromedial bowing of the tibia. Progression of discrepancy in leg lengths. J Bone Joint Surg [Am] 1981;63:384.

93. Holschneider A, Vogl D, Dietz H. Differences in leg length following femoral shaft fractures in childhood. Z Kinderchir 1985;40:341.

94. Hood R, Riseborough E. Lengthening of the lower extremity by the Wagner method. J Bone Joint Surg [Am] 1981;63(7):1122.

95. Hootnick D, Boyd N, Fixsen J, Lloyd-Roberts G. The natural history and management of congenital short tibia with dysplasia or absence of the fibula. J Bone Joint Surg [Br] 1977;59:267.

96. Hsu RW, Himeno S, Coventry MB, Chao EY. Normal axial alignment of the lower extremity and load-bearing distribution at the knee. Clin Orthop 1990;255:215.

97. Hughes T, Maffulli N, Fixsen J. Ultrasonographic appearance of regenerate bone in limb lengthening. J R Soc Med 1993; 86:18.

98. Huurman W, Jacobsen F, Anderson J, Chu W-K. Limb-length discrepancy measured with computerized axial tomographic equipment. J Bone Joint Surg [Am] 1987;69(5):699.

99. Ilizarov G, Deviatov A. Surgical lengthening of the shin with simultaneous correction of deformities. Ortop Travmatol Protez 1969;30:32.

100. Ilizarov G, Deviatov A. Surgical elongation of the leg. Ortop Travmatol Protez 1971;32:20.

101. Ilizarov G, Deviatov A, Trokhova V. Surgical lengthening of the shortened lower extremities. Vestn Khir Im I I Ghek 1972; 107:100.

102. Ilizarov G, Irianov I, Migalkin N, Petrovskaia N. Ultrastructural characteristics of elastogenesis in the major arteries of the canine hindlimb during lengthening. Arkh Anat Gistol Embriol 1987;93:94.

103. Ilizarov G, Palienko L, Shreiner A. Bone marrow hematopoietic function and its relationship to osteogenesis activity during reparative regeneration in leg lengthening in the dog. Ontogenez 1984;15:146.

104. Ilizarov G, Trokhova V. Surgical lengthening of the femur. Ortop Travmatol Protez 1973;34:73.

105. Ingelmark B, Lindstrom J. Acta Morph Scand 1954;16(Suppl).

106. Ireland J, Kessel L. Hip adduction/abduction deformity and apparent leg length inequality. Clin Orthop 1980;153:156.

107. Jackson D, Cozen L. Genu valgum as a complication of proximal tibial metaphyseal fractures in children. J Bone Joint Surg [Am] 1971;53:1571.

108. Jenkins D, Cheng D, Hodgson A. Stimulation of growth by periosteal stripping. A clinical study. J Bone Joint Surg [Br] 1975;57:482.

109. Johansson E, Aparisi T. Missing cruciate ligament in congenital short femur. J Bone Joint Surg [Am] 1983;65:1109.

110. Jones D, Moseley C. Subluxation of the knee as a complication of femoral lengthening by the Wagner technique. J Bone Joint Surg [Br] 1985;67:33.

111. Kaelin A, Hulin P, Carlioz H. Congenital aplasia of the cruciate ligaments. A report of six cases. J Bone Joint Surg [Br] 1986; 68:827.

112. Kalamchi A, Cowell H, Kim K. Congenital deficiency of the femur. J Pediatr Orthop 1985;5:129.

113. Karger C, Guille J, Bowen J. Lengthening of congenital lower limb deficiencies. Clin Orthop 1993;291:236.
114. Kawamura B. Limb lengthening. Orthop Clin North Am 1978;9:155.
115. Kawamura B, Mosona S, Takahashi T, et al. Limb lengthening by means of subcutaneous osteotomy. J Bone Joint Surg [Am] 1968;50:851.
116. Kempf I, Grosse A, Abalo C. Locked intramedullary nailing. Its application to femoral and tibial axial, rotational, lengthening and shortening osteotomies. Clin Orthop 1986;212:165.
117. Kenwright J, Albinana J. Problems encountered in leg shortening. J Bone Joint Surg [Br] 1991;73:671.
118. Kettlekamp D, Hillberry B, Murrish D, Heck D. Degenerative arthritis of the knee secondary to fracture malunion. Clin Orthop 1988;234:159.
119. Khoury S, Silberman F, Cabrine R. Stimulation of the longitudinal growth of long bones by periosteal stripping. J Bone Joint Surg [Am] 1963;45:1679.
120. Kohan L, Cumming W. Femoral shaft fractures in children: the effect of initial shortening on subsequent limb overgrowth. Aust N Z J Surg 1982;52:141.
121. Koman L, Meyer L, Warren F. Proximal femoral focal deficiency: a 50-year experience. Dev Med Child Neurol 1982;24:344.
122. Kujala U, Friberg. O, Aalto T, et al. Lower limb asymmetry and patellofemoral joint incongruence in the etiology of knee exertion injuries in athletes. Int J Sports Med 1987;8:214.
123. Lee D, Choi I, Ahn J, Steel H. Triple innominate osteotomy for hip stabilisation and transiliac leg lengthening after poliomyelitis. J Bone Joint Surg [Br] 1993;75:858.
124. Lokietek W, Legaye J, Lokietek J-C. Contributing factors for osteogenesis in children's limb lengthening. J Pediatr Orthop 1991;11:452.
125. Lorenzi G, Rossi P, Quaglia F, et al. Growth disturbances following fractures of the femur and tibia in children. Ital J Orthop Traumatol 1985;11:133.
126. Luke D, Schoenecker P, Blair V, Capelli A. Fractures after Wagner Limb Lengthening. J Pediatr Orthop 1992;12:20.
127. Lynch M, Taylor J. Periosteal division and longitudinal growht in the tibia of the rat. J Bone Joint Surg [Br] 1987;69:812.
128. Maffulli N, Hughes T, Fixen J. Ultrasonographic monitoring of limb lengthening. J Bone Joint Surg [Br] 1992;74(1):130.
129. Magnuson P. Lengthening of shortened bones of the leg by operation. Ivory screws with removable heads as a means of holding the two bone fragments. Surg Gynecol Obstet 1913;16:63.
130. Mahar R, Kirby R, MacLeod D. Simulated leg length discrepancy: its effect on mean center-of-pressure position and postural sway. Arch Phys Med Rehabil 1985;66:822.
131. Malhis T, Bowen J. Tibial and femoral lengthening. A report of 54 cases. J Pediatr Orthop 1982;2:487.
132. Mallet J, Rigault P, Padovani J, et al. Braces for congenital leg length inequality in children. Rev Chir Orthop 1986;72:63.
133. Manning C. Leg lengthening. Clin Orthop 1978;136:105.
134. Mayer-Bahlburg H, Psychosocial management of short stature, In: Shaffer D, Ehrhardt A, Greenhill L, eds. The clinical guide to child psychiatry. New York: Free Press, 1985:110.
135. McCarroll H. Trials and tribulations in attempted femoral lengthening. J Bone Joint Surg [Am] 1950;32:132.
136. McGibbon K, Deacon A, Raisbeck C. Experiences in growth retardation with heavy Vitallium staples. J Bone Joint Surg [Br] 1962;44:86.
137. Meals R. Overgrowth of the femur following fractures in children: influence of handedness. J Bone Joint Surg [Am] 1979;61:381.
138. Mears T, Vesely D, Kennedy H. Effect of surgically induced arteriovenous fistula on leg length inequality. Clin Orthop 1963;30:152.
139. Menelaus M. Correction of leg length discrepancy by epiphyseal arrest. J Bone Joint Surg [Br] 1966;48:336.
140. Merchant T, Dietz F. Long-term follow-up after fractures of the tibial and fibular shafts. J Bone Joint Surg [Am] 1989;71:599.
141. Merle D'Aubigne R, Dubousset J. Surgical correction of large length discrepancies in the lower extremities of children and adults. J Bone Joint Surg [Am] 1971;53:411.
142. Miller A, Rosman M. Hypertensive encephalopathy as a complication of femoral lengthening. Can Med Assoc J 1981;124:296.
143. Millis M, Hall J. Transiliac lengthening of the lower extremity. A modified innominate osteotomy for the treatment of postural imbalance. J Bone Joint Surg [Am] 1979;61:1182.
144. Monticelli G, Spinelli R. Distraction epiphyseolysis as a method of limb lengthening. II. Morphologic investigations. Clin Orthop 1981;154:262.
145. Monticelli G, Spinelli R. Distraction epiphyseolysis as a method of limb lengthening. III. Clinical applications. Clin Orthop 1981;154:274.
146. Monticelli G, Spinelli R. Distraction epiphysiolysis as a method of limb lengthening. I. Experimental study. Clin Orthop 1981;154:254.
147. Monticelli G, Spinelli R. Limb lengthening by epiphyseal distraction. Int Orthop 1981;5:85.
148. Monticelli G, Spinelli R. Leg lengthening by closed metaphyseal corticotomy. Ital J Orthop Traumatol 1983;9:139.
149. Morel G, Morin C. Simplified technique of extemporaneous lengthening of the femur in children 1986;27:326.
150. Morel G, Servant J, Valle A, et al. Extemporaneous femoral lengthening by the Cauchoix technic in children and adolescents. Rev Chir Orthop 1983;69:195.
151. Moreland JR, Bassett LW, Hanker GJ. Radiographic analysis of the axial alignment of the lower extremity. J Bone Joint Surg [Am] 1987;69(5):745.
152. Mosca V, Moseley C. Results of limb lengthening using the Wagner device. Orthop Trans 1987;11:52.
153. Moseley C. A straight-line graph for leg-length discrepancies. J Bone Joint Surg [Am] 1977;59(2):174.
154. Moseley C. A straight-line graph for leg length discrepancies. Clin Orthop 1978;136:33.
155. Mosca V, Moseley C. Results of limb lengthening using the Wagner device. Orthop Trans 1987;11:52.
156. Murrell P, Cornwall M, Doucet S. Leg length discrepancy: effect on the amplitude of postural sway. Arch Phys Med Rehabil 1992;73:401.
157. O'Connor K, Grady J, Hollander M. CT scanography for limb length determination. Clin Podiatr Med Surg 1988;5:267.
158. Ogilvie J. Epiphysiodesis: evaluation of a new technique. J Pediatr Orthop 1986;6:147.
159. Paley D. Current techniques of limb lengthening. J Pediatr Orthop 1988;8:73.
160. Papaioannou T, Stokes I, Kenwright J. Scoliosis associated with limb-length inequality. J Bone Joint Surg [Am] 1982;64:59.
161. Pappas A. Congenital abnormalities of the femur and related lower extremity malformations: classification and treatment. J Pediatr Orthop 1983;3:45.
162. Pappas A. Congenital posteromedial bowing of the tibia and fibula. J Pediatr Orthop 1984;4:525.
163. Pappas A, Nehme A. Leg length discrepancy associated with hypertrophy. Clin Orthop 1979;144:198.
164. Parrini L, Paleari M, Biggi F. Growth disturbances following fractures of the femur and tibia in children. Ital J Orthop Traumatol 1985;11:139.

165. Peixinho M, Arakaki T, Toledo C. Correction of leg inequality in the Klippel-Trenaunay-Weber syndrome. Int Orthop 1982; 6:45.

166. Peterson H. Premature physeal arrest of the distal tibia associated with temporary arterial insufficiency. J Pediatr Orthop 1993;13:672.

167. Petty W, Winter R, Felder D. Arteriovenous fistula for treatment of discrepancy in leg length. J Bone Joint Surg [Am] 1974;56:581.

168. Phemister D. Operative arrestment of longitudinal growth of bones in the treatment of deformities. J Bone Joint Surg 1933;15:1.

169. Porat S, Peyser A, Robin G. Equalization of lower limbs by epiphysiodesis: Results of treatment. J Pediatr Orthop 1991; 11:442.

170. Price C. Unilateral fixators and mechanical axis realignment. Orthop Clin North Am 1994;25(3):499.

171. Raschke M, Mann J, Oedekoven G, Claudi B. Segmental transport after unreamed intramedullary nailing. Preliminary report of a monorail system. Clin Orthop 1992;282:233.

172. Rezaian S. Tibial lengthening using a new external extension device. Report of thirty-two cases. J Bone Joint Surg [Am] 1976;58:239.

173. Rezaian S, Abtahi M. A simple and safe technique for tibial lengthening. Clin Orthop 1986;207:216.

174. Rigault P, Dolz G, Padovani J, et al. Progressive tibial lengthening in children. Rev Chir Orthop 1981;67:461.

175. Ring P. Experimental bone lengthening by epiphyseal distraction. Br J Surg 1958;46:169.

176. Robert H, Moulies D, Longis B, et al. Traumatic seperation of the lower end of the femur. Rev Chir Orthop 1988;74:69.

177. Roberts P. Disturbed epiphyseal growth at the knee after osteomyelitis in infancy. J Bone Joint Surg [Br] 1970;52:692.

178. Robertson W, Butler M, D'Angio G, Rate W. Leg length discrepancy following irradiation for childhood tumors. J Pediatr Orthop 1991;11:284.

179. Rooker G. The effect of division of the periosteum on the rate of longitudinal bone growth: an experimental study in the rabbit. Orthop Trans 1980;4(3):400.

180. Rosenthal A, Anderson M, Thomson S, et al. Superficial femoral artery catheterization. Effect on extremity length. Am J Dis Child 1972;124:240.

181. Rush W, Steiner H. A study of lower extremity length inequality. Am J Roentgen 1946;56:616.

182. Salai M, Chechick A, Ganel A, et al. Subluxation of the hip joint during femoral lengthening. J Pediatr Orthop 1985;5:642.

183. Salter R, Best T. Pathogenesis and prevention of valgus deformity following fractures of the proximal metaphyseal region of the tibia in children. J Bone Joint Surg [Br] 1972;54:767.

184. Salter R, Harris W. Injuries involving the epiphyseal plate. J Bone Joint Surg [Am] 1963;45:587.

185. Sandberg D, Brook A, Campos S. Short stature: a psychosocial burden requiring growth hormone therapy? J Pediatr 1994; 94(6):832.

186. Scheller M, Uber den Einfluss der Beinverkurzung auf die Wirbelsaule. Koln: Inaug Diss, 1964.

187. Seitz D, Yancey H. A review of tibial lengthening procedures. South Med J 1976;69:1349.

188. Setoguchi Y. Comparison of gait patterns and energy efficiency of unilateral PFFD in patients treated by Symes amputation and by knee fusion and rotational osteotomy. Presented at the Association of Children's Prosthetic and Orthotic Clinics Annual Meeting, Minneapolis, MN, 1994.

189. Shannak A. Tibial fractures in children: follow-up study. J Pediatr Orthop 1988;8:306.

190. Shapiro F. Developmental patterns in lower-extremity length discrepancies. J Bone Joint Surg [Am] 1982;64(5):639.

191. Shapiro F. Legg-Calve-Perthes disease: a study of lower extremity length discrepancies and skeletal maturation. Acta Orthop Scand 1982;53:437.

192. Shapiro F. Ollier's disease. An assessment of angular deformity, shortening, and pathological fractures in twenty-one patients. J Bone Joint Surg [Am] 1982;64:95.

193. Shapiro F. Longitudinal growth of the femur and tibia after diaphyseal lengthening. J Bone Joint Surg [Am] 1987;69:684.

194. Silver R, de la Garza J, Rang M. The myth of muscle balance. J Bone Joint Surg [Br] 1985;67:432.

195. Simon S, Whiffen J, Shapiro F. Leg length discrepancies in monoarticular and pauciarticular juvenile rheumatoid arthritis. J Bone Joint Surg [Am] 1981;63:209.

196. Sola C, Silberman F, Cabrini R. Stimulation of the longitudinal growth of long bones by periosteal stripping. J Bone Joint Surg [Am] 1963;45:1679.

197. Soukka A, Alaranta H, Tallroth K, Helliovaara M. Leg length inequality in people of working age. The association between mild inequality and low-back pain is questionable. Spine 1991;16:429.

198. Stephens D. Femoral and tibial lengthening. J Pediatr Orthop 1983;3:424.

199. Stephens D, Herrick W, MacEwen G. Epiphyseodesis for limb length inequality: results and indicatons. Clin Orthop 1978; 136:41.

200. Straub L, Thompson T, Wilson P. The results of epiphyseodesis and femoral shortening in relation to equalization of leg length. J Bone Joint Surg 1945;27:254.

201. Sugi M, Cole W. Early plaster treatment for fractures of the femoral shaft in childhood. J Bone Joint Surg [Br] 1987;69:743.

202. Taillard W, Morscher E. Beinlangenunterschiede. Basel: Karger, 1965.

203. Tanner J, Whitehouse R, Marshall W, et al. Assessment of skeletal maturity and prediction of adult height (TW2 method). London: Academic Press, 1975.

204. Taylor J, Warrell E, Evans R. Response of the growth plates to tibial osteotomy in rats. J Bone Joint Surg [Br] 1987;69:664.

205. Taylor S. Tibial overgrowth. A cause of genu valgum. J Bone Joint Surg [Am] 1963;45:659.

206. Temme J, Chu W, Anderson J. CT scanograms compared with conventional orthoroentgenograms in long bone measurement. Skeletal Radiol 1987;16:442.

207. Thomas C, Gage J, Ogden J. Treatment concepts for proximal femoral ischemic necrosis complicating congenital hip disease. J Bone Joint Surg [Am] 1982;64:817.

208. Timperlake R, Bowen J, Guille J, Choi I. Prospective evaluation of fifty-three consecutive percutaneous epiphysiodeses of the distal femur and proximal tibia and fibula. J Pediatr Orthop 1991;11:350.

209. Todd T, Atlas of skeletal maturation. St Louis: CV Mosby, 1973.

210. Torode I, Gillespie R. Anteroposterior instability of the knee: a sign of congenital limb deficiency. J Pediatr Orthop 1983; 3:467.

211. Torode I, Gillespie R. The classification and treatment of proximal femoral deficiencies. Prosthet Orthop Int 1991;15:117.

212. Trueta J. Stimulation of bone growth by redistribution of the intra-osseous circulation. J Bone Joint Surg [Br] 1951;33:476.

213. Tupman G. Treatment of inequality of the lower limbs. The results of operations for stimulation of growth. J Bone Joint Surg [Br] 1960;42:489.

214. Volkmann R. Chirurgische erfahrungen uber knochenverbiegungen und knochenwachsthum. Arch F Pathol Anat 1862; 24:512.

215. Vostrejs M, Hollister J. Muscle atrophy and leg length discrepancies in pauciarticular juvenile rheumatoid arthritis. Am J Dis Child 1988;142:343.

216. Wagner H. Operative Beinverlangerung (surgical leg prolongation). Chirurgie 1971;42:260.

217. Wagner H. Operative correction of leg length discrepancy. Langenbecks Arch Chir 1977;345:147.

218. Wagner H. Surgical lengthening or shortening of femur and tibia; technique and indications. Prog Orthop Surg 1977;1:71.

219. Wagner H. Operative lengthening of the femur. Clin Orthop 1978;136:125.

220. Wagner H. Surgical lengthening of the femur. Report of fifty-eight cases. Ann Chir 1980;34:263.

221. Wagner H. Radiation injuries of the locomotor system. Langenbecks Arch Chir 1981;355:181.

222. Wasserstein I, Correll J, Niethard F. Closed distraction epiphyseolysis for leg lengthening and axis correction of the leg in children. Z Orthop 1986;124:743.

223. Westh R, Menelaus M. A simple calculation for the timing of epiphyseal arrest: a further report. J Bone Joint Surg [Br] 1981;63:117.

224. Westin G. Femoral lengthening using a periosteal sleeve. Report of twenty-six cases. J Bone Joint Surg [Am] 1967;49:836.

225. Westin G, Sakai D, Wood W. Congenital longitudinal deficiency of the fibula: follow-up of treatment by Syme amputation. J Bone Joint Surg [Am] 1976;58:492.

226. White J, Stubbins SJ. Growth arrest for equalizing leg lengths. JAMA 1944;126:1146.

227. Wilde G, Baker G. Circumferential periosteal release in the treatment of children with leg length inequality. J Bone Joint Surg [Br] 1987;69:817.

228. Winquist R. Closed intramedullary osteotomies of the femur. Clin Orthop 1986;212:155.

229. Winquist R, Hansen S, Pearson R. Closed inramedullary shortening of the femur. Clin Orthop 1978;136:54.

230. Winter R, Pinto W. Pelvic obliquity. Its causes and its treatment. Spine 1986;11:225.

231. Yabsley R, Harris W. The effect of shaft fractures and periosteal stripping on the vascular supply to epiphyseal plates. J Bone Joint Surg [Am] 1965;47:551.

232. Yadav S. Double oblique diaphyseal osteotomy. A new technique for lengthening deformed and short lower limbs. J Bone Joint Surg [Br] 1993;75:962.

233. Yosipovich Z, Palti Y. Alterations in blood pressure during leg lengthening. A clinical and experimental investigation. J Bone Joint Surg [Am] 1967;49:1352.

234. Young N, Davis R, Bell D, Redmond D. Electromyographic and nerve conduction changes after tibial lengthening by the Ilizarov method. J Pediatr Orthop 1993;13:473.

235. Zanasi R. Surgical equalisation of leg length: shortening of the long femur and lengthening of the short in one operation. Ital J Orthop Traumatol 1982;8:265.

Lovell & Winter's Pediatric Orthopaedics, fourth edition,
edited by Raymond T. Morrissy and Stuart L. Weinstein.
Lippincott–Raven Publishers, Philadelphia © 1996.

Chapter 23

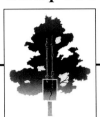

Developmental Hip Dysplasia and Dislocation

Stuart L. Weinstein

In the pediatric orthopaedic literature, the long-standing terminology of *congenital dysplasia* or *dislocation of the hip* (CDH) has been progressively replaced by the use of *developmental dysplasia* or *dislocation of the hip* (DDH). The *CDH* term is attributed to Hippocrates. The term *congenital* implies that a condition existed at birth. The American Academy of Orthopaedic Surgeons,[340] the Pediatric Orthopaedic Society of North America, and the American Academy of Pediatrics have endorsed the name change of this entity from CDH to DDH to be more representative of the wide range of abnormalities seen in this condition.[187]

The term *developmental* is more encompassing and is taken in the literal sense of organ growth and differentiation, which includes embryonic, fetal, and infantile periods. This terminology includes all cases that are clearly congenital and those that are developmental, and it incorporates subluxation, dislocation, and dysplasia of the hip. Because this change in terminology has not yet been incorporated into the International Classification of Disease, the term *CDH*, which has existed in the literature for years, will continue to be used in many publications.

One of the most confusing areas in DDH is the terminology used to the discuss the condition. What different investigators mean by *instability, dysplasia, subluxation,* and *dislocation* varies considerably. In this chapter, the term *DDH* means developmental dysplasia of the hip and encompasses all the variations of the condition described. Within this spectrum are two entities: subluxation and dislocation. For the newborn, the term *dysplasia* refers to any hip with a positive Ortolani sign, which is a hip that may be provoked to subluxation (i.e., partial contact between the femoral head and acetabulum), provoked to dislocation (i.e., no contact between the femoral head and the acetabulum), or reduced from either of these positions. The distinction between these two entities is often difficult, especially because of the subtleties of arthrographic and ultrasonographic classifications.

903

Because further subclassification bears no influence on treatment, I prefer to use the term *dysplasia* to encompass these entities and other variations. I use *developmental dislocation* only to refer to complete unreducible dislocations.

NORMAL GROWTH AND DEVELOPMENT OF THE HIP JOINT

For normal hip joint growth and development to occur, there must be a genetically determined balance of growth of the acetabular and triradiate cartilages and a well-located and centered femoral head. Embryologically, the components of the hip joint, the acetabulum and the femoral head, develop from the same primitive mesenchymal cells (Fig. 23-1).[118,205,337,338] A cleft develops in the precartilaginous cells at about the seventh week of gestation. This cleft defines the acetabulum and the femoral head. By the 11th week of intrauterine life, the hip joint is fully formed.[337,338,375] Theoretically, the 11th week is the earliest time at which a dislocation could develop, although this rarely happens.[375] Acetabular development continues throughout intrauterine life, particularly by means of growth and development of the labrum.[118,338]

In the normal hip at birth, the femoral head is deeply seated in the acetabulum and held within the confines of the acetabulum by the surface tension of the synovial fluid. It is extremely difficult to dislocate a normal infant's hip by incising the hip joint capsule.[86,284] The retaining force is similar to that of a suction cup. Hips in newborns with DDH are not merely normal hips with capsular laxity; they are pathologic entities.

After birth, continued growth of the proximal femur and the acetabular cartilage complex are ex-tremely important to continuing the development of the hip joint.[118,146,285,375] The growth of these two members of the hip joint is interdependent.

Acetabular Growth and Development

The acetabular cartilage complex (Fig. 23-2) is a three-dimensional structure with three limbs (triradiate) medially and a cup-shaped structure laterally. The acetabular cartilage complex is interposed between the ilium above, the ischium below, and the pubis anteriorly. Acetabular cartilage forms the outer two thirds of the acetabular cavity, and the nonarticular medial wall of the acetabulum is formed by a portion of the ilium above, the ischium below, and portions of the triradiate cartilage.

Thick cartilage from which a secondary ossification center, the os acetabulum, develops in early adolescence, separates the acetabular cavity from the pubic bone.[285] The fibrocartilaginous labrum is at the margin of the acetabular cartilage, and the joint capsule inserts just above its rim (Fig. 23-3).[374]

The triradiate cartilage is a triphalanged structure. One phalange is oriented horizontally between the ilium and ischium. One phalange is oriented vertically and interposed between the pubis and ischium. The third phalange is located anteriorly and slanted superiorly between the ilium and the pubis (Fig. 23-4).

The entire acetabular cartilage complex is composed of very cellular hyaline cartilage (see Fig. 23-3). The lateral portion of the acetabular cartilage is homologous with other epiphyseal cartilages of the skeleton.[145] This is important in understanding normal growth and development and the shape of the acetabulum in skeletal dysplasias and in injury. The labrum or fibrocartilaginous edge of the acetabulum is at the margin of the acetabular cartilage. The hip joint capsule inserts just above the labrum. The capsule inser-

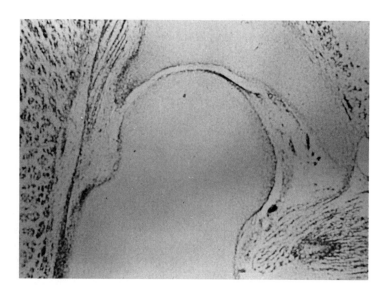

FIGURE 23-1. Embryonic hip. The components of the hip joint, the acetabulum, and the femoral head develop from the same primitive mesenchymal cells. A cleft develops in the precartilaginous cells at about the seventh week of gestation, defining the acetabulum and the femoral head.

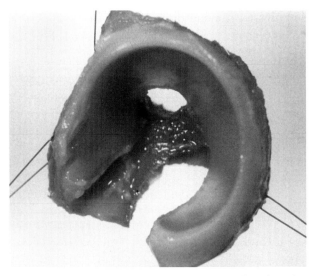

FIGURE 23-2. Normal acetabular cartilage complex of a 1-day-old infant. The ilium, ischium, and pubis have been removed with a curet. The lateral view shows the cup-shaped acetabulum. (From Ponseti IV. Growth and development of the acetabulum in the normal child. J Bone Joint Surg [Am] 1978;60:575.)

tion is continuous with the labrum below and the periosteum of the pelvic bones above.

Articular cartilage covers the acetabular cartilage on the side that articulates with the femoral head. On the opposite side is a growth plate, with its degenerating cells facing toward the pelvic bone it opposes. New bone formation occurs in the metaphysis adjacent to the degenerating cartilage cells. Growth of the acetabular cartilage occurs through interstitial growth within the cartilage and appositional growth under the perichondrium. This fact is most important when considering various inominate bone osteotomies, because surgical injury to this important area may jeopardize further acetabular growth.

Each phalange of the triradiate cartilage is composed of very cellular hyaline cartilage. This cartilage contains many canals. Each side of each limb of the triradiate cartilage has a growth plate. Interstitial growth within the triradiate cartilage causes the hip joint to expand its diameter during growth.

Growth of the Proximal Femur

In the infant, the entire proximal end of the femur, including the greater trochanter, intertrochanteric zone, and proximal femur, is composed of cartilage. Between the fourth and seventh month of life, the proximal femoral ossification center appears. This bony centrum continues to enlarge, although with a slowly decreasing rate, along with its cartilaginous anlage until adult life, when only a thin layer of articular cartilage remains over it. The proximal femur and the trochanter enlarge by appositional cartilage cell proliferation.[322]

The three main growth areas in the proximal femur are the physeal plate, the growth plate of the greater trochanter, and the femoral neck isthmus (Fig. 23-5).[322] A balance among the growth rates of these centers accounts for the normal configuration of the proximal femur, the relation between the proximal femur and the greater trochanter, and the overall femoral neck width. The growth of the proximal femur is affected by muscle pull, the forces transmitted across the hip joint by weight bearing, normal joint nutrition, circulation, and muscle tone.[112,272,317] Any alterations in these factors may cause profound changes in development of the proximal femur.

During infancy, a small cartilaginous isthmus connects the trochanteric and femoral growth plates along the lateral border of the femoral neck and is a reflection of their previous common origin. This

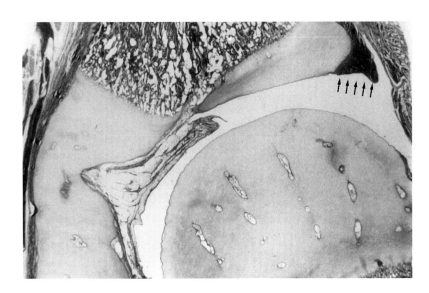

FIGURE 23-3. Coronal section through the center of the acetabulum in a full-term infant. Notice the fibrocartilaginous edge of the acetabulum, the labrum (arrows), at the peripheral edge of the acetabular cartilage. The hip capsule inserts just above the labrum.

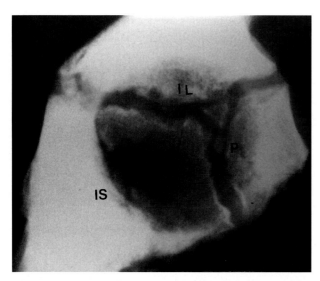

FIGURE 23-4. Lateral roentgenogram of the acetabulum in a 9-year-old girl. Two centers of ossification are seen within the cartilage adjoining the pubis (P) and appear to be developing within the vertical phalange of the triradiate cartilage. The position of the ischium (IS) and the ilium (IL) are indicated. (From Ponseti IV. Growth and development of the acetabulum in the normal child. J Bone Joint Surg [Am] 1978; 60:575.)

growth cartilage contributes to the lateral width of the femoral neck and remains active until maturity.

It is the normal growth of these three physes that determines adult femoral neck configuration. Disturbances in growth in any of these three growth plates by whatever mechanism alter the shape of the proximal femur. Hyperemia secondary to surgery or inflammatory conditions may stimulate growth in any or all of these growth plates.[322]

The proximal femoral physeal plate contributes approximately 30% of the growth of the overall length of the femur. Any disruptions to the blood supply or damage to the proximal physeal plate results in a varus deformity because of continued growth of the trochanter and the growth plate along the femoral neck.[167,322] Partial physeal arrest patterns may be caused by damage to portions of the proximal femoral physeal plate. The relation between growth of the trochanter and the physis of the proximal femur should remain constant, and it is measured by the articular trochanteric distance, which is the distance between the tip of the greater trochanter and superior articular surface of femoral head. The greater trochanter usually is classified as a traction epiphysis, depending on normal abductor pull for growth stimulation. The trochanter, like the proximal femur, grows by appositional growth.

Determinants of Acetabulum Shape and Depth

Experimental studies and clinical findings in humans with unreduced dislocations suggest that the main stimulus for the concave shape of the acetabulum is the presence of a spherical femoral head.[60,145,146,325,326] Harrison determined that the acetabulum failed to develop in area and depth after femoral head excision in rats.[145] He also demonstrated atrophy and degeneration of the acetabular cartilage, although the growth plates of the triradiate cartilage remained histologically normal, as did the length of the inominate bones. These experimental findings are characteristic of humans who have had untreated hip dislocations (Fig. 23-6).

For the normal depth of the acetabulum to increase during development, several factors must act in concert. There must be a reduced spherical femoral head. There also must be normal interstitial and appositional growth within the acetabular cartilage, and periosteal new bone formation must occur in the adjacent pelvic bones.[146,285] The depth of the acetabulum is further enhanced at puberty by the development of three secondary centers of ossification (Fig. 23-7). These three secondary centers of ossification are homologous with other epiphyses in the skeleton.[145,285] The os acetabulum develops in the thick cartilage that separates the acetabular cavity from the pubis bone.

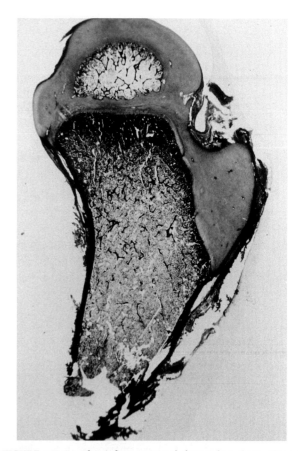

FIGURE 23-5. The infant proximal femur has three physeal plates: the growth plate of the greater trochanter, the growth plate of the proximal femoral physeal plate, and the growth plate of the femoral neck isthmus connecting the other two plates.

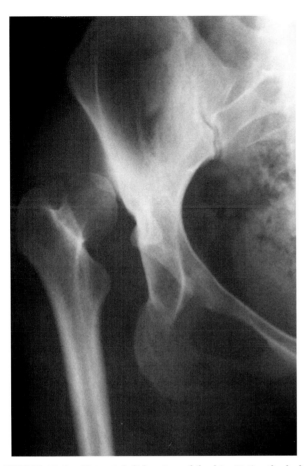

FIGURE 23-6. Untreated dislocation of the hip. Notice the lack of the concave shape and shallowness of the acetabulum.

The os acetabulum is the epiphysis of the pubis and forms the anterior wall of the acetabulum. The epiphysis of the ilium, the acetabular epiphysis, forms a major portion of the superior edge of the acetabulum. A third small epiphysis also forms in the ischial region.[145,285,384]

Normal acetabular growth and development occur through balanced growth of the proximal femur, the acetabular and triradiate cartilages, and the adjacent bones. This balance, which is probably genetically determined, may be at fault in DDH. There is ample evidence to suggest that an adverse intrauterine environment also plays an important role in the pathogenesis of hip dysplasia.[46,47,59,285,324,398]

PATHOANATOMY

Dislocations in Newborns

In the newborn with DDH, the tight fit between the femoral head and the acetabulum is lost. The femoral head can be made to glide in and out of the acetabulum, with a palpable sensation known clinically as the Ortolani sign.[166,271,272,285] DDH in the newborn refers to a spectrum of anatomic abnormalities, from mild dys-

plastic changes to the severe pathoanatomic changes that are found in the rare idiopathic teratologic dislocation and more commonly in teratologic dislocations associated with conditions such as as myelomeningocele and arthrogryposis.

The most common pathologic change in the newborn with DDH is a hypertrophied ridge of acetabular cartilage in the superior, posterior, and inferior aspects of the acetabulum. This ridge was referred to by Ortolani as the "neolimbus."[271,272] The neolimbus is composed of hypertrophied acetabular cartilage (Fig. 23-8).[166,284] There often is a trough or groove in the acetabular cartilage, caused by secondary pressure of the femoral head or neck. It is over this ridge of acetabular cartilage that the femoral head glides in and out of acetabulum, with the palpable sensation referred to as the Ortolani sign.[271,272,284]

In the typical newborn with DDH, there is empiric evidence that the pathologic changes are reversible, because there is a 95% success rate of treatment using simple devices such as the Pavlik harness and the von Rosen splint.[246] These changes are typical of 98% of DDH cases that occur at or around birth. However, about 2% of newborns have teratologic (antenatal) dislocations not associated with a syndrome or neuromuscular condition.[59,384] In these rare cases, the patho-

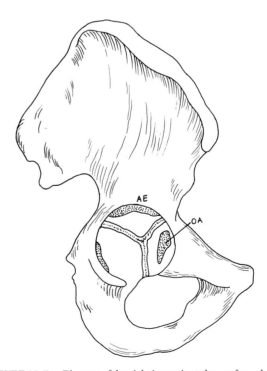

FIGURE 23-7. Diagram of the right innominate bone of an adolescent. The os acetabuli (OA) is shown within the acetabular cartilage adjoining the pubic bone. The acetabular epiphysis (AE) is within the acetabular cartilage adjoining the iliac bone, and another small epiphysis is within the acetabular cartilage adjoining the ischium (left). (Adapted from Ponseti IV. Growth and development of the acetabulum in the normal child. J Bone Joint Surg [Am] 1978; 60:575.)

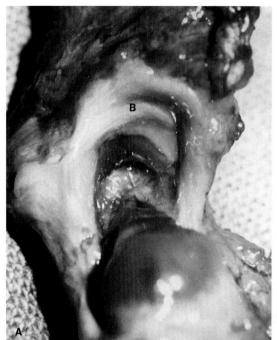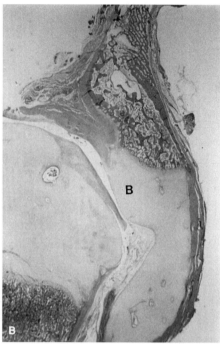

FIGURE 23-8. (A) Right acetabular cavity and femoral head of a newborn baby with bilateral congenital hip dysplasia. There is an acetabular bulge (**B**) or neolimbus along the upper acetabular cartilage, and the acetabular cavity is small. (**B**) Frontal section of the same hip. The femoral head is very large in relation to the acetabular cavity. Notice how the labrum is everted and adheres to the joint capsule above. The neolimbus (**B**) is composed of hypertrophied acetabular cartilage. (From Ishii Y, Weinstein SL, Ponseti IV. Correlation between arthrogram and operative findings in congenital dislocation of the hip. Clin Orthop 1980;153:138.)

logic and clinical findings are similar to those seen in late-diagnosed DDH, which is described later.

Acetabular Development in Developmental Hip Dysplasia

Acetabular development in treated DDH cases may be different from that described for the normal hip. This is particularly true for the late-diagnosed case. The primary stimulus for normal growth and development comes from the femoral head within the acetabulum.[146,325,326] When there is a delay in diagnosis and treatment, some aspects of normal growth and development are lost. The femoral head must be reduced as soon as possible, and the reduction must be maintained to provide the stimulus for acetabular development. If concentric reduction is maintained, the acetabulum has the potential for recovery and resumption of normal growth and development for many years.[140,144,209]

The age at which a dysplastic hip can still return to "normal" after reduction remains controversial.[140,141,209,223,279,305,318,329,382,387] The resumption and adequacy of acetabular development is a multifactorial problem that depends on the age at which the reduction is obtained and on whether the growth potential of the acetabular cartilage and the proximal femur is normal. The capacity of the acetabular cartilage to

resume normal growth depends on its intrinsic growth potential, whether it has been damaged by the subluxated or dislocated femoral head, and whether it has been damaged by various attempts at reduction.

In the treated DDH patient, especially in late-diagnosed cases, accessory centers of ossification contribute to acetabular development (Fig. 23-9). Accessory centers of ossification in the acetabulum are seen in only 2% to 3% of normal hips, and they rarely appear before 11 years of age. However, among patients treated for DDH, the centers may be present in as many as 60% of hips, usually appearing from 6 months to 10 years after the reduction (see Fig. 23-9).[140,141,209,391] In treated DDH cases, these accessory centers of ossification should be sought on every sequential radiograph to determine if acetabular development is progressing. This is an important factor to consider in deciding if surgical intervention is necessary to correct residual acetabular dysplasia.

ETIOLOGY, EPIDEMIOLOGY, AND DIAGNOSIS

Causes of Developmental Dysplasia of the Hip

Many factors contribute to DDH. Genetic and ethnic factors play a key role, with the incidence of DDH as

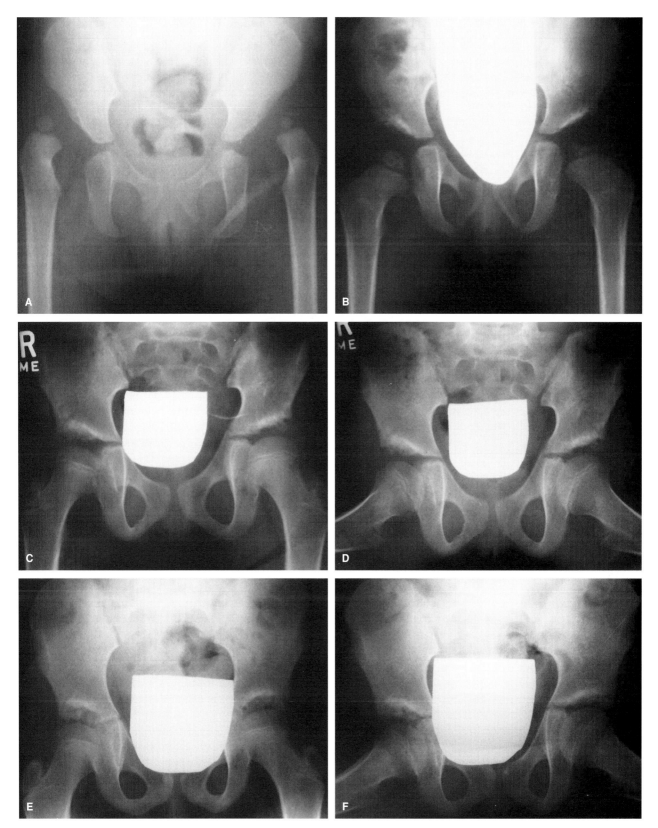

FIGURE 23-9. (A) An 18-month-old girl with bilateral high dislocations. Notice the poorly developed acetabula with well-developed secondary acetabula. (B) At 33 months of age, the irregular ossification centers in the left and right hip have coalesced, with a slight improvement in the acetabular index. (C) When the girl was 7 years of age, an anteroposterior (AP) view shows the appearance of the accessory centers of ossification in the periphery of the acetabulum. (D) The accessory centers of ossification are somewhat better appreciated in the abduction view at 7 years of age. (E) An AP view at 8 years of age shows the coalescence of the accessory centers of ossification, increasing the depth of the acetabulum. Notice the excellent sourcil formation. (F) The accessory centers of the ossification are well demonstrated in an abduction view at 8 years of age.

high as 25 to 50 cases per 1000 live births among Lapps or Native Americans and a very low rate among the southern Chinese population and persons of African descent.[30,31,61,62,72,89,122,148,160,161,282,291,324,377]

A positive family history for DDH may be garnered in 12% to 33% of affected patients.[30,273,398] One study reported 10-fold increase among the parents of index patients and a 7-fold increase among siblings compared with the general population.[30] There is some suggestion that femoral neck or acetabular anteversion may be an etiologic factor.[94,141,166,203,324,379]

The genetic effects on the hip joint in patients with DDH are revealed in primary acetabular dysplasia, various degrees of joint laxity, or a combination of both. Intrauterine mechanical factors, such as breech position or oligohydramnios, and neuromuscular mechanisms, such as myelomeningocele, can profoundly influence genetically determined intrauterine growth.[337,338,372,373] The first-born child is more likely to be affected than subsequent children. Any of the factors providing an "adverse" intrauterine environment may influence the development of the hip joint, and postnatal influences may also contribute to the development of DDH.[274,337,378,398,400]

Risk Factors and Incidence

Caucasian infants have an increased incidence of DDH among first-born children.[4,46,47,14,15,86,87] The unstretched abdominal muscles and the primigravida uterus may subject the fetus to prolonged periods of abnormal positioning, forcing the fetus against the mother's spine. This restraint limits fetal mobility, especially hip abduction. The high rate of association of DDH with other intrauterine molding abnormalities, such as torticollis and metatarsus adductus, lends some support to the theory that the "crowding phenomenon" plays a role in the pathogenesis.[86,87,192,380] Oligohydramnios, which is associated with limited fetal mobility is associated with DDH.[86,87] The left hip is the most commonly affected hip; in the most common lie, this is the hip that is usually forced into an adduction against the mother's sacrum.[61,86,87]

DDH is more common among female patients (80% of cases) and children born breech. In the general population, breech presentations occur in about 2% to 4% of vaginal deliveries; for children with DDH, the reported incidence is higher, with Carter and Wilkinson reporting 17% and Salter reporting 23%. Twice as many girls as boys are born breech.[394] Fifty-nine percent of breech presentations are first-born children.[46,47,394] Ramsey and MacEwen demonstrated that 1 of 15 girls born breech have evidence of hip instability. In animal studies, the prolonged maintenance of an abnormal position, such as the breech position, is associated with the production of DDH.[325,326]

The postnatal extrauterine environment may significantly influence the development of DDH. In socie-ties using swaddling (i.e., hips forced into adduction and extension) in the postnatal period, the incidence of DDH is high and may be a result of the forceful positioning of the legs in extension and adduction in the face of normal newborn hip flexion and hamstring contractures.[1,61,194,288,377,379,398–400]

The influence of hip capsular laxity on the development of DDH has been addressed by many investigators. Newborns with DDH may have capsular laxity. Hip capsular laxity has been implicated in the pathogenesis of DDH, because the diagnostic test for DDH, the Ortolani sign, depends on the head gliding in and out of the dysplastic acetabulum over a ridge of abnormal acetabular cartilage. Proponents argue that, because reversible dysplasia can be produced in animals by producing ligamentous laxity, the acetabular dysplasia seen in DDH is a secondary phenomenon.[166,293,307,325,326,398] LeDamany demonstrated that the acetabulum is shallowest at birth.[203] Râlis and McKibbin confirmed LeDamany's anatomic work on a small number of cases.[293] They too demonstrated that the acetabulum was shallowest at birth and that this combined with normal joint laxity of the infant makes the time around delivery a high-risk period for dislocation.[228,293] These anatomic experiments were repeated by Skirving and Scadden in African neonates. In the African neonate, the acetabulum was deeper more frequently and in a narrower range, possibly explaining why DDH is almost nonexistent among persons of African descent.[324] This finding also provided indirect evidence of acetabular dysplasia as a primary cause of DDH.

Laxity of the hip joint capsule is often seen in newborn infants and has been documented by ultrasonography.[85] The laxity may allow some instability without a positive Ortolani sign. In postmortem examination of seven stillborns, the hips demonstrated instability with a negative Ortolani sign; arthrograms demonstrated a slight pooling of the contrast media medially. On gross examination, the hip capsules were stretched, and the femoral heads could be pulled slightly away from the acetabula. However, the hips were anatomically and histologically normal, unlike the postmortem findings reported for all specimens with positive Ortolani signs.[270,271,273,282,284,285] In addition to the normal physiologic capsular laxity expected in the newborn, DDH is not a feature of conditions characterized by hyperlaxity such as Down, Ehlers-Danlos, and Marfan syndromes.[271]

Combining the epidemiologic and etiologic factors, a high-risk group of patients can be identified. This group includes any patient who has a combination of the factors listed in Table 23-1. For an infant manifesting any combination of these factors, the physician should be alert to the possibility of DDH.

The incidence of DDH is influenced by geographic and ethnic factors and by the diagnostic criteria used

TABLE 23-1   High-Risk Factors for Developmental Dysplasia or Dislocation of the Hip

Breech position
Female gender
Positive family history or ethnic background (e.g., Native
    American, Laplander)
Lower limb deformity
Torticollis
Metatarsus adductus
Oligohydramnios
Significant persistent hip asymmetry (e.g., abducted hip
    on one side, adducted hip on the other)
Other significant musculoskeletal abnormalities

by the examining physician. Another important factor is the diagnostic acumen of the examiner. The age of the patient at the time of diagnosis must be taken into account, because the physical findings and manifestations of the condition change with increasing delay in diagnosis.[20,77,85,86,87,157,218,270,271,273,282,284,285,398]

Most DDH cases are detectable at birth.[133,136] Despite newborn screening programs, some cases are not detected, and there is some evidence to suggest that a few cases may arise after birth.[77,164,165,170,217,257,370,398] Moreover, the problem of whether acetabular dysplasia is primary or secondary to an unrecognized dislocation or subluxation that has spontaneously reduced remains unanswered. The results of newborn screening programs estimate that 1 of 100 newborns examined has evidence of some hip instability (i.e., positive Ortolani or Barlow sign), although the true incidence of dislocation is reported to be between 1 and 1.5 cases per 1000 live births.[20,55,108,109,170,217,257,284,366,370,382,382]

Diagnosis

The clinical diagnostic test for DDH was originally described by LeDamany in 1912.[203] LeDamany referred to the palpable sensation of the hip gliding in and out of the acetabulum as the "signe de ressaut." In 1936, Ortolani, an Italian pediatrician, described the pathogenesis of this diagnostic sign.[270,271] Ortolani called the palpable sensation the "segno dello scotto." Fellander and colleagues likened this diagnostic sign to the femoral head gliding in and out of the acetabulum over a ridge and referred to this palpable sensation as the "ridge phenomenon."[99] This ridge was named the neolimbus by Ortolani. This ridge over which the femoral head glides in and out of the acetabulum is composed of hypertrophied acetabular cartilage (see Fig. 23-8).[166,270,271,284]

Unfortunately, inadequate translation of LeDamany's and Ortolani's works into English resulted in the use of the term "click" to describe this diagnostic sign.

High-pitched soft tissue clicks are often elicited in the hip examination of newborns. These clicks are usually transmitted from the trochanteric region or the knee and have no diagnostic significance.[99] This poor understanding of the pathoanatomy of the primary diagnostic sign of DDH in the newborn has no doubt led to overdiagnosis and overtreatment of infants.[73,74,109,171]

Another diagnostic test, the Barlow maneuver, is often referred to as the "click of exit." The Barlow maneuver is a provocative maneuver in which the hip is flexed and adducted and the femoral head is palpated to exit the acetabulum partially or completely over a ridge of the acetabulum.[20] Many physicians refer to the Ortolani sign as the "click of entry," caused when the hip is abducted, the trochanter is elevated, and the femoral head glides back into the acetabulum. Because Ortolani and LeDamany described the palpable sensation as the femoral head exits or enters the acetabulum, I prefer to use the Ortolani sign to refer to the palpable sensation of subluxating or dislocating the hip and to reducing a subluxated or dislocated hip.

Complete unreducible dislocations are extremely rare in newborns and are usually associated with other generalized conditions, such as arthrogryposis, myelodysplasia, or other syndromes. These perinatal teratologic dislocations are at the extreme end of the DDH pathologic spectrum and account for only 2% of cases in newborn examination series.[61,62,147,284,333] They are usually manifested by the secondary adaptive changes more characteristic of the late-diagnosed case.

Although the clinical examination remains the gold standard, ultrasonography has gained popularity worldwide as a screening tool. Its cost effectiveness has yet to be documented for wholesale screening of DDH.

Late Diagnosis

If the diagnosis of DDH is not made early, preferably in the newborn nursery, secondary adaptive changes develop.[31] The most reliable physical finding in the late-diagnosed DDH is limitation of abduction (Fig. 23-10). Limited abduction is a clinical manifestation of the various degrees of adductor longus shortening associated with hip subluxation or dislocation.[62] Other manifestations of late-diagnosed DDH may include apparent femoral shortening, also called the Galeazzi sign (Fig. 23-11); asymmetry of the gluteal,[23] thigh, or labial folds[11]; and limb length inequality (Fig. 23-12). In patients with bilateral dislocations, clinical findings include a waddling gait and hyperlordosis of the lumbar spine (Fig. 23-13).

If DDH goes undetected, normal hip joint growth and development is impaired. With increasing age at detection and reduction, particularly for children older than 6 months of age, the obstacles, intraar-

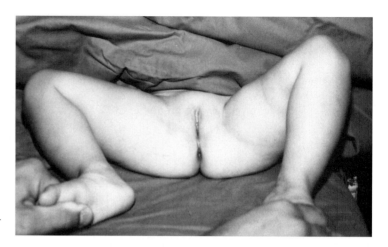

FIGURE 23-10. A 15-month-old child wih left hip dislocation. Notice the limited abduction of the hip.

ticular and extraarticular, to concentric reduction become increasingly difficult to overcome by simple treatment methods, such as the Pavlik harness or von Rosen splint, and closed or open reduction usually must be performed under a general anesthetic. Restoration of normal acetabulum development is less likely as age at detection increases.[166,382–386]

In the late-diagnosed case, the extraarticular obstacles to reduction include the contracted adductor longus and the iliopsoas. These muscles are shortened because of the hip being in the subluxated or dislocated position, allowing secondary muscle shortening.

The intraarticular obstacles to reduction in the late-diagnosed DDH include the ligamentum teres, the transverse acetabular ligament, the constricted anteromedial joint capsule, and rarely, an inverted and hypertrophied labrum.[166] In the late-diagnosed case, the most significant intraarticular obstacle to reduction is some degree of anteromedial hip capsular constriction.[100,166,208,215,226,244] The ligamentum teres may be thickened and it may become the primary obstacle to reduction in some cases. In children of walking or crawling age, the ligamentum teres may be signifi-

cantly elongated and enlarged. Its sheer bulk precludes concentric reduction without excision of the ligament. The transverse acetabular ligamentum may hypertrophy secondary to the constant pull of the ligamentum teres on its attachment at the base of the acetabulum.[166,244] This effect decreases the diameter of the acetabulum.

A rare finding in other than teratologic dislocations is a true inverted labrum or limbus (i.e., hypertrophied labrum; Fig. 23-14).[208] The acetabular labrum may be iatrogenically inverted and be an obstacle to

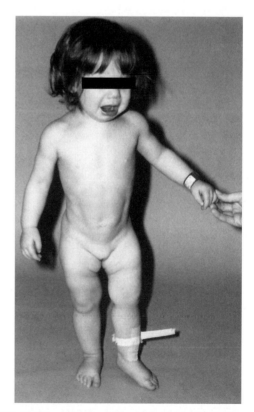

FIGURE 23-12. A 1-year-old Caucasian girl with developmental dislocation of the left hip was referred for toe walking. Notice the apparent limb length inequality and asymmetry of the thigh and labial folds.

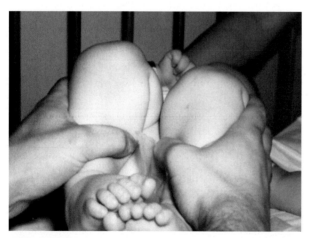

FIGURE 23-11. A 15-month-old girl with developmental dislocation of the left hip. Notice the apparent femoral shortening.

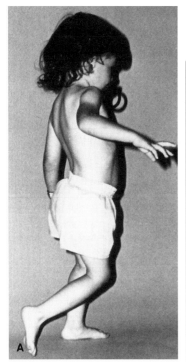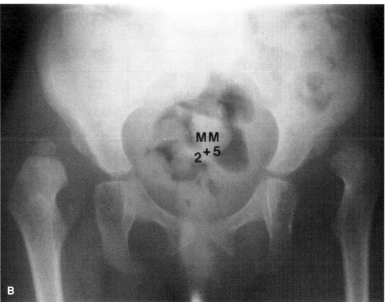

FIGURE 23-13. A 2-year, 5-month-old Caucasian girl with bilateral hip dislocations. (**A**) Notice the waddling gait and hyperlordosis. (**B**) Radiograph shows high bilateral dislocations and poorly developed acetabula with well-developed secondary acetabula where the femoral heads articulate with the ilia.

reduction in patients previously treated by unsuccessful closed reductions. Arthrograms are often misinterpreted as showing an inverted labrum,[319] although the shadow thought to be the inverted labrum or limbus is instead the neolimbus described by Ortolani (Fig. 23-15).[166,204,284,382] This neolimbus is epiphyseal cartilage and is almost never an obstacle to reduction. It must not be removed, because removal impairs acetabular development.[284,269]

The cartilage of the neolimbus may be primarily abnormal or be damaged by a traumatic open or closed reduction. A response to this damage may be responsible for the appearance of the previously discussed accessory centers of ossification seen in treated cases of DDH (see Fig. 23-9).[284]

Diagnostic Imaging and Radiography

The use of ultrasound in the diagnosis and management of children with DDH remains controversial.[27,28,33,36,49,56–58,75,76,90,119,120,124,125,137,138,139,153,224,243,281,336,346–349,362] Many proponents strongly recommend that ultrasonography be used as a routine screening tool in the newborn nursery and used extensively in the management of all DDH problems. The use of ultrasonography in orthopaedic practice was pioneered by Graf in Austria in the 1970s.[124,125] Harcke in the United States,[137–139] and Terjesen in Norway[346–349] have been the prime mo-

tivators in evaluating this tool for the diagnosis of DDH and other hip disorders.

Ultrasonography can be used in two basic ways to evaluate the child with DDH: morphologic assessment and dynamic assessment. The morphologic assessment, as pioneered by Graf, focuses primarily on critical evaluation of anatomic characteristics of the hip joint. This is accomplished by measuring two angles on the ultrasound image: the α angle, which is a measurement of the slope of the superior aspect of the bony acetabulum, and the β angle, which evaluates the cartilaginous component of the acetabulum. The hip is classified, according to Graf, into four types and several subtypes according to various factors.[124,125] In Terjesen's evaluation, the percentage of acetabular coverage of the femoral head (i.e., percent coverage) is a key measurement.[346–349]

The morphologic approach to ultrasonography is widely practiced in Europe. This approach has been criticized because of substantial interobserver and intraobserver variations in the measurement of various angles, particularly the β angle.[138]

The availability of real-time equipment by which motion can be observed in multiple planes provides a means of seeing what occurs during the Ortolani or Barlow maneuver. The use of the dynamic ultrasonography, as popularized by Harcke, is criticized for being excessively operator dependent and requiring a subjective assessment of the findings.[137–139]

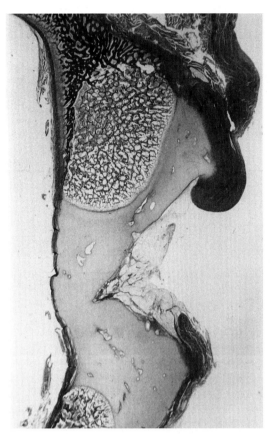

FIGURE 23-14. A coronal section of the acetabulum demonstrates the hypertrophic labrum (limbus) extending over the margin of a slightly thickened acetabular cartilage. The thick capsule extends upward above the inverted labrum, from which it is separated by a shallow groove. In this section thorugh the ilium, the growth plate is slanted upward laterally, but endochondral ossification is normal. At the margin of the roof, periosteal bone growth is retarded. (From Ponseti IV. Morphology of the acetabulum in congenital dislocation of the hip. J Bone Joint Surg [Am] 1978; 60:586.)

The indications for ultrasound in the diagnosis and treatment of DDH are not universally established. Because there are many controversies yet to be resolved, ultrasonography cannot be advocated as a routine screening tool.[138] Although it is used as such in Europe, prospective longitudinal studies documenting the outcome of minor anatomic abnormalities found in ultrasonographic examinations need to be completed.[301] Its routine use in newborn nurseries has resulted in overdiagnosis, above the expected incidence of DDII, and could not be considered cost effective.[153] Its use for only high-risk infants (see Table 23-1) may eventually prove cost effective. However, Clarke and colleagues showed that screening all high-risk infants and all infants who had any abnormality on physical examination did not reduce the prevalence of late-diagnosed cases.[33,57,58]

Some centers advocate the use of ultrasonography for all Ortolani-positive infants to assess stability at the completion of treatment.[138] An ideal indication for ultrasonography is for guided reduction of a dislocated hip in an infant. Ultrasonography can be used to check the reduction of the hip and its stability during Pavlik harness treatment at 7- to 10-day intervals. This may temporarily obviate the need for radiographic evaluation. Other uses for ultrasonography in the treatment of DDH include monitoring of the hip position while the patient is in traction before attempts at reduction and evaluating closed reductions in the operating room. The distinct advantage of ultrasonography is that it provides some anatomic evaluation of the hip joint without exposing the infant to radiation.

Debate continues about the appropriate planes for evaluation and whether an orthopaedic surgeon, the treating physician, or the radiologist with expertise in ultrasonography should do the evaluation. In the newborn, DDH is not a radiographic diagnosis; the diagnosis should be made by clinical evaluation, which may be enhanced by ultrasonography if the examination results are questionable. Some groups have used vibration arthrometry.[182-184]

After the newborn period, the diagnosis of DDH should be confirmed by a radiograph. Many radiographic measurements can be made, but there are wide interobserver and intraobserver variations in these measurements.[39] Because it is difficult to standardize radiographic positioning of infants, many centers use positioning frames.[262]

When monitoring the treatment of children with DDH, it is essential to notice changes in the radiographic measurements over time and not to make significant decisions based on a single radiograph. The classic radiographic features of the late-diagnosed DDH include an increased acetabular index,[8-10,59,121,351,356] disruption of the Shenton line, a widened pelvic floor,[275] an absent teardrop figure,[6,189,311,327,363] delayed appearance of the femoral ossific nucleus on the involved side or dissimilar sizes of the ossific nuclei, abnormality in Smith centering ratios,[209,325,326] decreased femoral head coverage, and failure of the medial metaphyseal beak of the proximal femur and subsequently the secondary ossification center to be located in the lower inner quadrant, as defined by the Hilgenreiner and Perkins lines (Fig. 23-16A).[25,157,280] When the triradiate cartilage is closed, the acetabular angle of Sharp (i.e., inferior edge of teardrop figure to the edge of the acetabulum) is a useful measurement of acetabular dysplasia.[320]

In children younger than 8 years of age, the acetabular index is a reasonable method to measure acetabular development.[39] The center edge (CE) angle only becomes useful after 5 years of age and is most useful in the adult patient (Fig. 23-16B).[391] Radiographs show only the ossified portion of the pelvic bones and the proximal femur. Excellent acetabular coverage of the femoral head may be found, albeit by unossified carti-

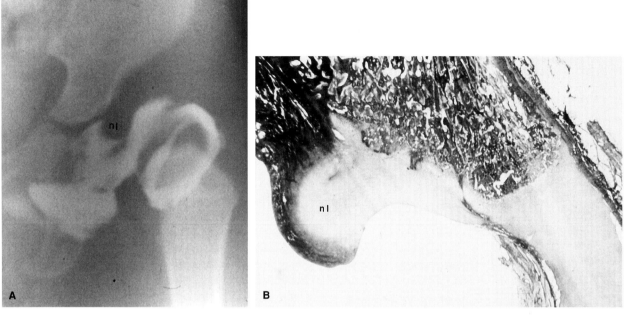

FIGURE 23-15. (A) Arthrogram of the left hip in a 15-month-old child with complete dislocation. Notice the shadow of the neolimbus (nl). (B) A histologic specimen demonstrates hypertrophied acetabular cartilage of the neolimbus (nl), consistent with the arthrographic appearance in **A**.

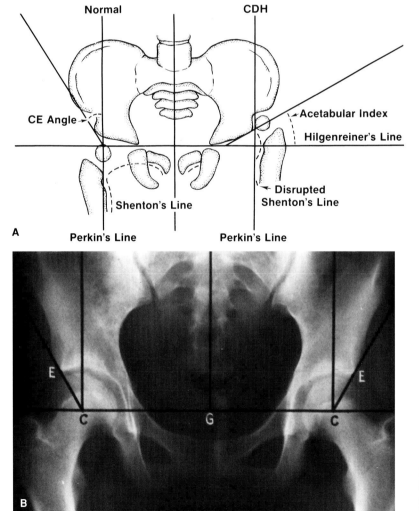

FIGURE 23-16. (A) Radiographic parameters. (B) Center-edge (CE) angle of Wiberg. (C, center of the femoral head; E, boney edge of acetabulum; G, gravity line.)

915

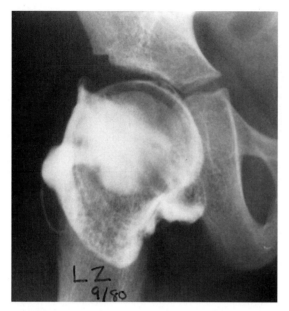

FIGURE 23-17. Arthrogram of a 5-year-old Caucasian girl 3 years after open reduction. Notice the excellent coverage of the femoral head by unossified acetabular cartilage.

lage (Fig. 23-17). If this cartilage does not ossify, the residual dysplasia may eventually lead to subluxation and degenerative joint disease.

The Shenton line during the first few years of life provides only a qualitative estimate of dysplasia. After 3 or 4 years of age, the Shenton line should be intact on all views of the hip; thereafter, any disruption of the Shenton line indicates an abnormality in the relation between the proximal femur and acetabulum. This relation must be restored to prevent degenerative joint disease in later life.[377,379,384,386,391]

Magnetic resonance imaging has been used for DDH diagnosis and evaluation.[35] With advances in software, this modality will no doubt provide useful information in the future. The need for anesthesia for pediatric patients limits the utility of this modality.[104,127,130,169]

NATURAL HISTORY

Course in Newborns

The natural history of untreated DDH in the newborn is quite variable. Yamamuro and Doi followed 52 hips with positive Ortolani signs over a 2 year period without treatment for the first 5 months. Of the 12 they called "dislocated" hips, 3 (25%) were radiographically normal at 5 months of age. Of the 42 of what they called "subluxable" hips, 24 (57%) were normal at 5 months.[399]

Barlow reported that 1 of 60 infants born has instability (i.e., positive Barlow sign) of one or both hips. More than 60% of these stabilize during the first week of life, and 88% stabilize during the first 2 months

without treatment. The remaining 12% become true congenital dislocations and persist without treatment. Pratt and colleagues followed 18 "dysplastic" hips in patients younger than 3 months of age who were diagnosed by clinical and radiographic parameters for an average of 11.2 years and found that 15 were roentgenographically normal.[288]

Coleman followed 23 untreated DDH patients younger than 3 months of age who were diagnosed by clinical and radiographic criteria. He found that 26% of the femoral heads became completely dislocated, 13% had partial contact of the femoral head with the acetabulum, 39% remained located but retain dysplastic features, and 22% were normal.[61]

Most of the unstable hips in these newborns stabilize shortly after birth, some may go on to subluxation or dislocation, and some may remain correctly located but retain anatomic dysplastic features. Because it is not possible to predict the outcome of unstable hips in newborns, all newborns with clinical hip instability, as manifested by a positive Ortolani or Barlow sign, should be treated.

Course in Adults

In adults, the natural history of untreated complete dislocations varies and is affected by societal considerations.[70,230,371,377,378] Despite a complete dislocation, there may be little or no functional disability.

The natural history of complete dislocations depends on two factors: the presence or absence of a well-developed false acetabulum and bilaterality.[151,365,377,378,384,386] Wedge and Wasylenko demonstrated only a 24% chance of a good clinical result with a well-developed false acetabulum, but with a moderately developed or absent false acetabulum, the patients had a 52% chance of a good clinical result.[377,378] Of 42 complete dislocations, 13 had roentgenographically confirmed degenerative joint disease, such as a loss of joint space, cyst formation, sclerosis, osteophyte formation, and flattening of the femoral head. Of these 13 cases, 10 (76%) had poor clinical results.

Milgram reported the gross and histologic features of a case of bilateral DDH discovered at postmortem examination. This 74-year-old man had no hip or thigh pain and only mild backache for 5 years before his death. His femoral head had no articulation with any portion of the ilium. The femoral head was covered with a thickened, markedly elongated hip joint capsule. The only degenerative changes occurred where the lesser trochanter abutted the overhanging superior acetabular rim.[233] In the absence of a false acetabulum, most patients with complete dislocations do well, maintaining a good range of motion with little functional disability (Fig. 23-18). Completely dislocated hips with well-developed false acetabula are more

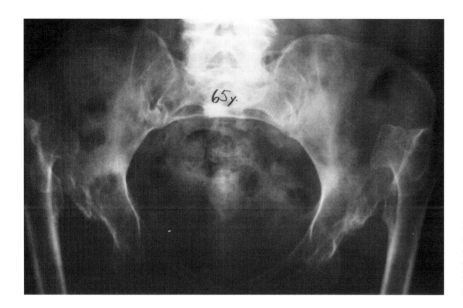

FIGURE 23-18. A 55-year-old Caucasian woman with bilateral, untreated developmental dislocations of the hips complained of some low back pain but had no hip pain. She had a waddling gait and hyperlordosis.

likely to develop roentgenographic degenerative joint disease changes and have poor clinical results (Fig. 23-19). Factors that lead to the formation or lack of formation of a false acetabulum remain unknown.[384]

Back pain may occur in patients with bilateral dislocations. It is thought that this pain is secondary to the hyperlordosis of the lumbar spine that is associated with bilateral dislocations (Fig. 23-20).[51,70,230,233,377,378,384]

In unilateral complete dislocations, secondary problems of limb length inequality, ipsilateral knee deformity and pain, scoliosis, and gait disturbance are common. Limb length inequalities of as much as 10 cm have been reported in patients with unilateral dislocations. These patients acquire flexion adduction deformities of the hip, which may lead to valgus deformities of the knee. The valgus knee deformity is often associated with attenuation of the medial collateral ligament and lateral compartment degenerative joint disease, although some medial compartment disease has been described.[230,365,377,378,384,386] The same factors concerning the development of secondary degenerative disease in the false acetabulum and with associated clinical disability in bilateral cases affect unilateral dislocations.

Course of Dysplasia and Subluxation

The natural history of dysplasia and subluxation in untreated patients is important because of the likelihood that we can extrapolate these findings to residual dysplasia and subluxation after treatment.[98,220,321,386]

After the neonatal period, the term dysplasia has an anatomic and radiographic definition. Anatomic

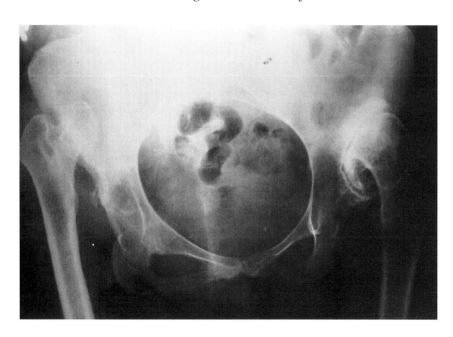

FIGURE 23-19. Roentgenogram of a 43-year-old woman with complete dislocation of both hips. She is asymptomatic on the right but has disabling symptoms from the left hip. She has no false acetabulum on the right but has a well-developed false acetabulum on the left, with secondary degenerative changes. (From Weinstein SL. Natural history of congenital hip dislocation [CDH] and hip dysplasia. Clin Orthop Rel Res 1987; 225:52.)

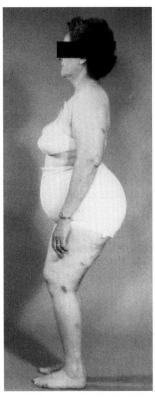

FIGURE 23-20. A 45-year-old Caucasian women with bilateral complete dislocations, hip flexion deformity, and marked hyperlodosis. The patient's only complaints were referable to her back.

dysplasia refers to inadequate development of the acetabulum, femoral head, or both.[62] All subluxated hips (i.e., those in which there is some contact between the femoral head and the acetabulum) are by definition anatomically dysplastic. Radiographically, the major difference between dysplasia and subluxation is determined by the integrity of the Shenton line. In hip subluxation, the Shenton line is disrupted and the femoral head is superiorly, laterally, or superolaterally displaced from the medial wall of the acetabulum. In radiographic dysplasia, the normal Shenton line relation is intact (Fig. 23-21).[24,69,377,378] In the literature describing the natural history of DDH, these two roentgenographic and clinical entities often are not separated. Moreover, secondary degenerative changes may convert a radiographically dysplastic hip into a subluxated hip (Figs. 23-22 and 23-23).[34,69,220,339]

Anatomic abnormalities are seen roentgenographically in subluxation and dysplasia, but the natural history of these two radiographic entities is different. Residual radiographic subluxation after treatment for DDH invariably leads to degenerative joint disease and clinical disability.[69,220,377,378,384,386] The rate of deterioration is directly related to the severity of the subluxation and the age of the patient.[69,220]

There is considerable evidence that residual radiographic acetabular dysplasia leads to secondary de-

generative joint disease, especially in female patients, although there are no predictive radiographic parameters.[69,143,220,339] The reasons for degenerative changes in radiographically dysplastic hips are probably mechanical in nature and related to increased contact stress with time. A certain "overpressure"[132] may correlate with long-term outcome. Aspherical femoral heads (e.g., secondary to aseptic necrosis) tend to experience even more severe degrees of overpressure. It appears that radiographic degenerative joint disease correlates with the magnitude of the overpressure and the time of exposure.[132]

Because the physical signs of radiographic hip dysplasia are usually lacking, cases are often diagnosed only incidentally on the basis of roentgenograms taken for other reasons or only after the patient develops symptoms.[46,47,339,391,394] Stulberg and Harris found that 50% of their patients with radiographic dysplasia and degenerative joint disease had radiographic evidence of dysplasia in the opposite hip.[339] Melvin and associates, in their unpublished 30- to 50-year follow-up of DDH, demonstrated that 40% of the patients with DDH had roentgenographic evidence of dysplasia in the opposite hip.[230]

It has been estimated that 20% to 50% of degenerative joint disease of the hip is secondary to subluxation or residual radiographic acetabular dysplasia.[69,143,210,249,328,339,377,391] Wiberg suggested that there was direct correlation between the onset of roentgenographic degenerative joint disease and the amount of dysplasia as measured by the decrease in the CE angle (see Fig. 23-16).[391]

Cooperman and colleagues, in a roentgenographic study of degenerative joint disease and its relation to the severity of radiographic acetabular dysplasia, reviewed the 17 cases on which Wiberg based his conclusions. They concluded that 7 of 17 hips were actually subluxated. These subluxated hips were the most anatomically dysplastic; their CE angles averaged 2 degrees, and all 7 had roentgenographic degenerative changes by 42 years of age. The other 10 hips in Wiberg's series were radiographically dysplastic. They had an intact Shenton line and an average CE angle of 10 degrees. None of these patients developed radiographic degenerative joint disease before 39 years of age; however, degenerative changes became apparent roentgenographically by 57 years of age. In this review of Wiberg's series, the decrease in CE angle was associated with an increase in anatomic acetabular dysplasia and the increased likelihood that the hip was subluxated. Subluxation was the primary factor in the development of degenerative joint disease in this group. Subluxation predictably leads to degenerative joint disease and clinical disability over time.[69]

Cooperman and associates described 32 hips (28 patients) with radiographic evidence of acetabular dys-

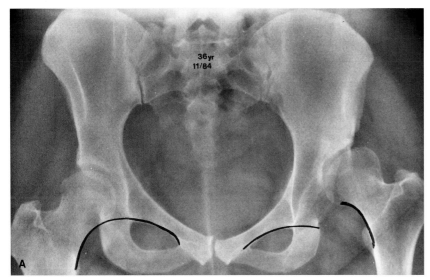

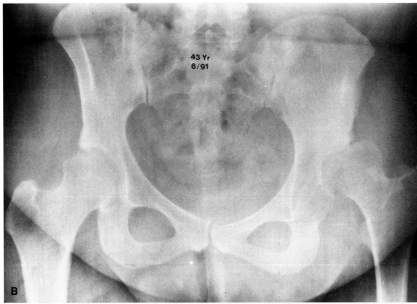

FIGURE 23-21. Radiographic subluxation and dysplasia. (**A**) A 36-year-old woman with bilateral anatomically abnormal (dysplastic) hips. The left hip is radiographically subluxated, with the Sheton line disrupted, and the right hip is radiographically dysplastic, with the Sheton line intact. (**B**) Seven years later, notice the marked loss of joint space in the secondary acetabulum of the left hip and very early disruption of the Shenton line on the right. The right hip is asymptomatic, and the left hip is about to undergo total hip arthroplasty.

plasia (i.e., CE angle less than 20 degrees but without subluxation and the Shenton line intact) at an average follow-up of 22 years. All patients eventually developed radiographic evidence of degenerative joint disease. There was, however, no linear correlation between the CE angle and the rate of development of degenerative joint disease, as had been previously suggested by Wiberg. A decreased CE angle was associated solely with increasing radiographic evidence of acetabular dysplasia and not with subluxation, because patients with subluxation had been excluded in this series. Cooperman and colleagues demonstrated that radiographic evidence of acetabular dysplasia leads to radiographically detectable degenerative joint disease, but the process may take decades. This study also demonstrated that conventional radiographic parameters used to describe dysplasia (e.g., CE angle, acetabular index of Sharp, percent coverage, depth, inclina-

tion) could not predict the rate at which a radiographically confirmed dysplastic hip joint would develop roentgenographic evidence of degenerative joint disease.[69]

Stulberg and Harris demonstrated that there is no roentgenographic picture of degenerative joint disease uniquely associated with preexisting acetabular dysplasia.[339] In 80% of patients with dysplasia, the CE angle is usually less than 20 degrees, but acetabular shallowness, as measured by acetabular depth, affects all of these patients. The investigators also demonstrated that the CE angle, the criterion most commonly used to quantitate dysplasia, could be affected by many parameters, including roentgenographic positioning and the changes accompanying the normal development of degenerative joint disease. The secondary degenerative changes in a dysplastic acetabulum may give the

(text continues on p. 922)

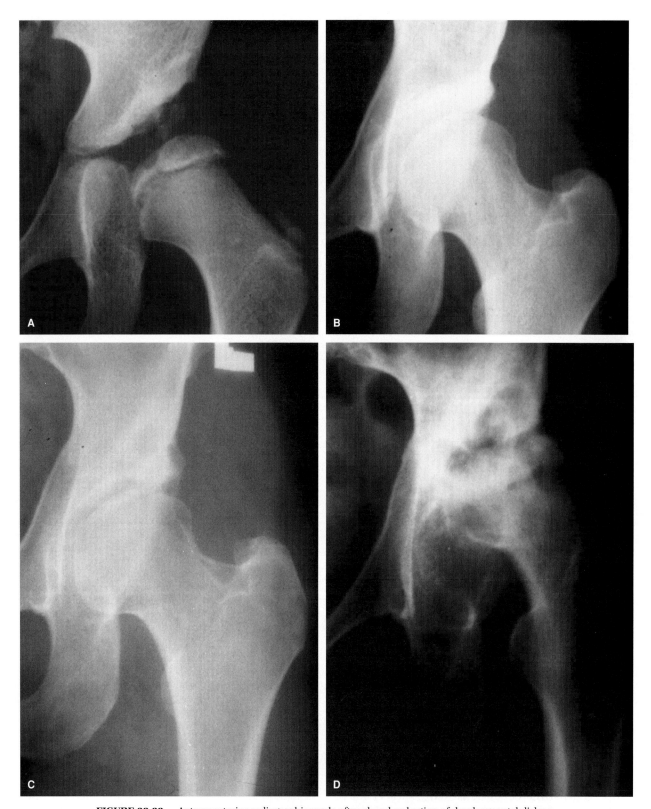

FIGURE 23-22.   Anteroposterior radiographic made after closed reduction of developmental dislocation of the hip that had been performed when the patient was 2 years, 4 months of age. (**A**) Thirty-nine
months after reduction, when the patient was 5 years, 7 months of age, the accessory centers of
ossification are visible in the acetabular cartilage. (**B**) Fifteen years after reduction, when the patient
was 17 years of age, the Shenton line is intact, and there is mild, acetabular dysplasia. (**C**) Forty-two
years after reduction, when the patient was 44 years of age, degenerative changes are present. (**D**) Fifty-
one years after the reduction, when the patient was 53 years of age, the hip is subluxed and has severe
degenerative changes (Iowa Hip Rating 48 of 100 points). The patient subsequently had a total hip
replacement. (From Malvitz TA, Weinstein SL. Closed reduction for congenital dysplasia of the hip:
functional and radiographic results after an average of 30 years. J Bone Joint Surg [Am] 1994; 76:1777.)

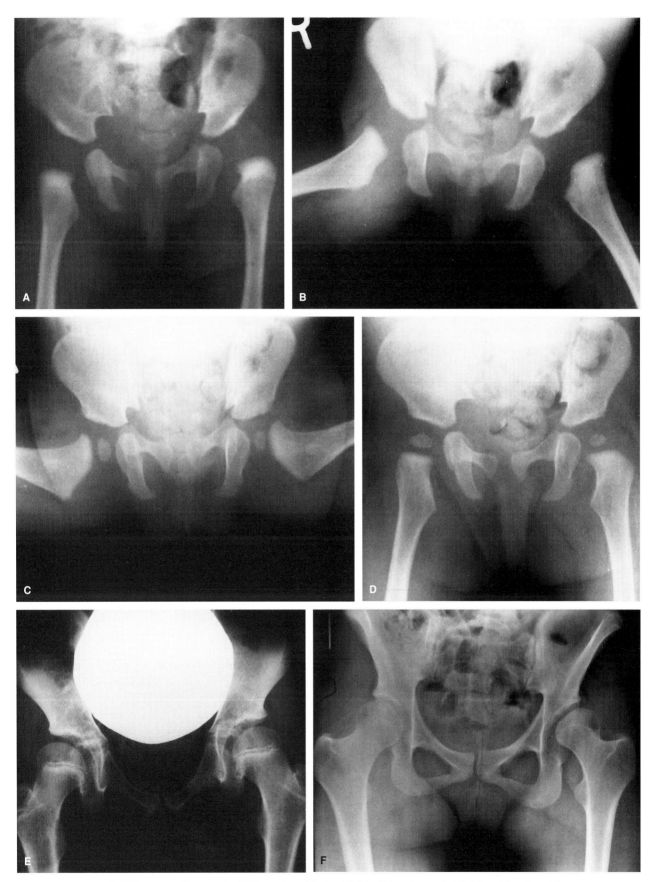

FIGURE 23-23. A 4-month-old Caucasian girl with left hip dislocation and right hip subluxation. (**A**) Anteroposterior (AP) view. (**B**) Abduction view. (**C**) Abduction view at 7 months of age, 3 months after closed treatment. (**D**) AP view at 7 months of age, 3 months after closed treatment. (**E**) AP view at 7 years of age. Notice the mild anatomic dysplasia of both hips. (**F**) AP view at 15 years of age. Notice the bilateral anatomic dysplasia. The right hip is radiographically dysplastic, and the left hip is radiographically subluxated.

hip a normal-appearing CE angle. In their series of 130 patients with primary or idiopathic degenerative joint disease, Stulberg and Harris were able to demonstrate that 48% had evidence of primary acetabular dysplasia and that acetabular dysplasia frequently occurred in females with degenerative joint disease.[339]

Further evidence for the association between radiographic evidence of acetabular dysplasia and degenerative joint disease comes from the southern Chinese population. In an epidemiologic study from Hong Kong, where the incidence of childhood hip disease is low, the incidence of adult osteoarthritis (nontraumatic) is also low.[160,161]

Wedge and Wasylenko reported three peak incidences of pain in subluxation, depending on the severity of the subluxation. Patients with the most severe subluxations usually had the onset of symptoms during the second decade of life. Those with moderate subluxation presented during their third and fourth decades, and those with minimal subluxation experienced the onset of symptoms usually around menopause.[377,378]

Patients who present soon after symptom onset rarely have the classic signs of degenerative joint disease, such as decreased joint space, cyst formation, double acetabular floor, and inferomedial femoral head osteophytes. The only radiographic feature present at symptom onset may be increased sclerosis in the weight-bearing area. This increased sclerosis is secondary to increasing osteoblastic stimulation in response to the decreased width of the weight-bearing surface; the increase of the normal per unit load strains the bone. The mechanism of pain in these instances is purely speculative (see Fig. 23-22).

In cases of subluxation, the mean age at symptom onset is 36.6 years for women and 54 years for men. Severe degenerative roentgenographic changes become evident approximately 10 years later, by 46.4 years of age for women and 69.6 years of age for men.

Patients with subluxated hips usually have symptom onset at a younger age than those with complete dislocations. After pain and radiographically evident degenerative disease starts, it progresses rapidly. Harris reported that symptoms of degenerative joint disease associated with radiographic evidence of acetabular dysplasia occurred early in life and that almost 50% of the patients in his series with acetabular dysplasia had their first reconstructive procedure before 60 years of age, with fewer than 5% having their first reconstruction after 60 years of age.[143]

TREATMENT

Treatment of Hip Dislocation

Newborns and Infants Younger Than 6 Months of Age

Based on the understanding of normal growth and development of the hip, the fundamental treatment goals in DDH are the same regardless of the age. The first goal is to obtain a reduction and maintain that reduction to provide an optimal environment for femoral head and acetabular development.[385] As has been demonstrated by many follow-up studies of treated DDH, the acetabulum has the potential for development for many years after reduction as long as the reduction is maintained.[140,141,209,382] A series of patients treated by closed or open reduction showed that the femoral head and femoral anteversion can remodel if the reduction is maintained.[82,220] Further intervention is necessary only to alter an otherwise adverse natural history, as in the treatment of residual dysplasia and the prevention or treatment of subluxation. The later the diagnosis of DDH is made, the more difficult it is to achieve these goals, the less potential there is for acetabular and proximal femoral remodeling, and the more complex are the required treatments. With increasing age and complexity of treatment, the risk of complications is greater, and the patient is more likely to develop degenerative joint disease.

The diagnosis of DDH ideally should be made in the newborn nursery.[360] If the diagnosis is made in the nursery, treatment should be initiated immediately.[88] Triple diapers or abduction diapers have no place in the treatment of DDH in the newborn. They give the family a false sense of security and are generally ineffective. Any success with the use of triple diapers or abduction diapers could be attributed to the natural resolution of the disorder.

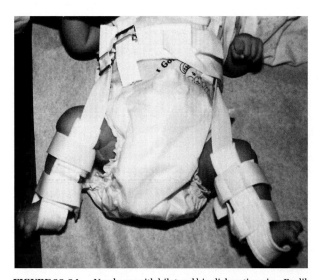

FIGURE 23-24. Newborn with bilateral hip dislocations in a Pavlik harness. Appropriately applied, the harness prevents hip extension and adduction, which can lead to redislocation, but allows further flexion and abduction, which lead to reduction and stabilization.

The most commonly used device for the treatment of DDH in the newborn is the Pavlik harness (Fig. 23-24). Although other devices are available (e.g., von Rosen splint, Frejka Pillow), the Pavlik harness remains the most commonly used device worldwide.[17,43,102,129,144,149,158,163,168,207,228,276,277] When appropriately applied, the Pavlik harness prevents hip extension and adduction, which can lead to redislocation, but it allows further flexion and abduction, which lead to reduction and stabilization. By maintaining the Ortolani-positive hip in a Pavlik harness on a full-time basis for 6 weeks, hip instability resolves in 95% of cases.

The Pavlik harness may be used effectively up to 6 months of age for any child with residual dysplasia, subluxation, or complete dislocation. After 6 months of age, the failure rate for the Pavlik harness is greater than 50%, because it is difficult to maintain the increasingly active and crawling child in the harness. It may also be used to achieve a reduction in a dislocated hip of a child in this age group. Ideally, the harness should be applied as soon after birth as the diagnosis is made.

Mubarak and colleagues and others outlined the pitfalls associated with the use of the Pavlik harness for the treatment of DDH. They pointed out that failures of treatment most often result from problems related to the physician, orthotic, or patient.[246,364]

Physician-related errors fall into two categories: inappropriate indications and persistence of inadequate treatment. The Pavlik harness is contraindicated in patients with significant muscle imbalance, such as those with myelodysplasia or cerebral palsy. It is also contraindicated for patients who have significant joint stiffness, such as children with arthrogryposis. The harness will fail if it is applied in a child with excessive ligamentous laxity, as seen in Ehlers-Danlos syndrome.[246]

Persistence of inadequate treatment is a multifactoral problem. Physicians using the harness must be well versed in the appropriate application and the adjustments that are necessary throughout the course of treatment if treatment is to be successful. It is important that the physician treating the patient understands when a treatment failure has occurred so as not to prolong treatment with the harness and cause secondary pathologic changes, called "Pavlik harness disease."[172] Persistence of treatment may damage the femoral head, injure the acetabular cartilage, and impair bone growth. An inappropriately applied harness is a physician failure, not an orthotic failure.[245,364]

Another major Pavlik harness pitfall is related to the specific orthotic device. Not all Pavlik harnesses are the same; the strap attachment sites vary. However, since the article by Mubarak and colleagues, most harnesses on the market do meet the requisite standards they outlined.[246,364]

Some problems are patient related. Certain family, social, and educational situations make compliance impossible. In these situations, the Pavlik harness would be inappropriate, and closed reduction and casting may be the more judicious approach. The family must be educated about the importance of the harness, its care and maintenance, how the child should be bathed while wearing the harness, and the consequences of failure to achieve success. Family noncompliance can lead to failure, and the use of a visiting nurse may be helpful in these situations.

Application of the harness (see Fig. 23-24) should be demonstrated for the family members. The chest halter strap should be positioned at the nipple line, and the shoulder straps are set to hold the cross strap at this level. The leg and foot stirrups must have their anterior and posterior straps oriented anteriorly and posteriorly to the child's knees. Hip flexion should be set at 100 to 110 degrees. These straps should be in the anterior axillary line. The posterior abduction strap should be at the level of the child's scapula and adjusted to allow comfortable abduction within the "safe zone."[294] The safe zone is defined as the arc of abduction and adduction that is between redislocation and comfortable, unforced abduction. The posterior strap acts as a check rein to prevent the hip from adducting to the point of redislocation. Ultrasonography is a useful way to document relocation of the Ortolani-positive hip.

There is great variability in the treatment regimens for the Pavlik harness. If the Pavlik harness is used to stabilize an unstable hip (i.e., an Ortolani- or Barlow-positive hip), the harness is used full time for 6 to 12 weeks after clinical stability is achieved. Most hips stabilize in days to weeks. The harness is checked at 7- to 10-day intervals to assess hip stability and to adjust the flexion and abduction straps to allow for growth of the infant. Clinical examination is usually sufficient to check the progress at each visit; ultrasonography may be used, but radiographs are unnecessary.

In a child younger than 6 months of age with a complete dislocation, the Pavlik harness may be used in a trial of guided reduction. In this case, the harness must be applied with enough hyperflexion and abduction to point the femoral head toward the triradiate cartilage. This situation is the ideal indication for the use of ultrasonography to follow the reduction. When the harness is used for a guided reduction, the infant should be checked at 7 to 10 days to assess whether the reduction is being accomplished. Clinical examination alone may be adequate, but initial radiographs should be obtained in the harness to document adequate flexion and redirection of the femoral neck toward the triradiate cartilage in the harness. After clinical stability is obtained, a radiograph is not indicated until about 3 months of age to assess acetabular development (Fig. 23-25). Ultrasonography is an excellent way to document progress toward and completion of a successful reduction.[343]

Although the Pavlik harness has provided a 95% overall success rate for treatment of the Ortolani-positive hip, the success rate for using the harness to guide the reduction of a subluxated or dislocated hip in a child younger than 6 months of age is 85%.[7,22,246]

The use of the Pavlik harness can be associated with complications; most of these complications are iatrogenic and can be avoided. Inferior dislocations may occur with prolonged excessive hip flexion.[299]

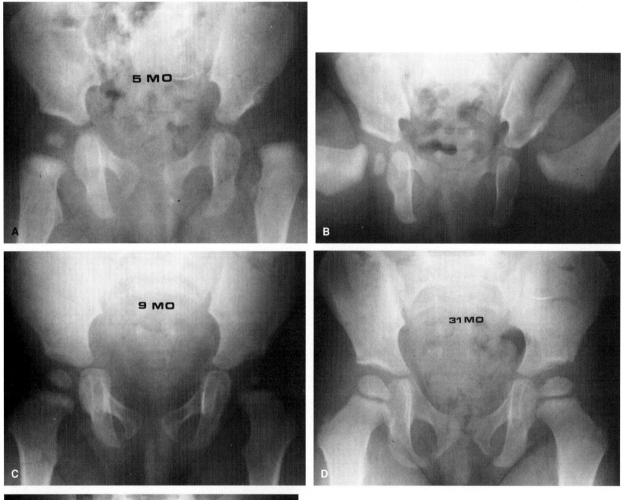

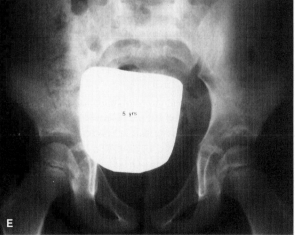

FIGURE 23-25. A 5-month-old child with left developmental dislocation of the hip. (**A**) Anteroposterior (AP) view of the pelvis at diagnosis. The acetabular index is increased, the medial floor of the acetabulum is widened, and the acetabular teardrop figure is absent. There is a well-developed secondary acetabulum, the Shenton line is disrupted, and the femoral ossific nucleus is decreased in size. The femoral head is located in the upper outer quadrant, as defined by Hilgenreiner and Perkins lines. (**B**) AP view of the pelvis with a hip Pavlik harness in place to demonstrate an excellent reduction. Notice the hyperflexed position. (**C**) AP view of the pelvis at 9 months of age shows reduction, early appearance of the teardrop figure, and improvement in the acetabular index. (**D**) AP view of the pelvis at 31 months of age. There is marked improvement in the acetabular teardrop figure and acetabular development. (**E**) AP view of the pelvis at 5 years of age. There has been continued improvement in acetabular and femoral head development.

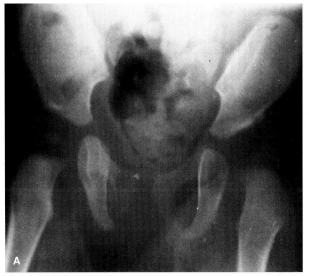

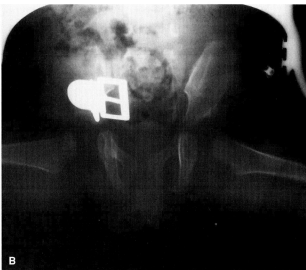

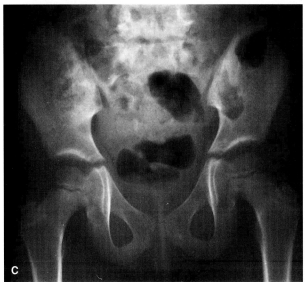

FIGURE 23-26. A 6-month-old girl with apparent left hip subluxation and acetabular dysplasia secondary to excessive anteversion. (**A**) Diagnostic anteroposterior (AP) view of the pelvis. Notice the increased acetabular index, poorly developed teardrop figure, and small ossific nucleus. (**B**) AP view of the pelvis in the fixed abduction brace. Excellent reduction of the hip has been achieved. (**C**) AP view of the pelvis at 5 years of age. The left hip appears normal.

Hyperflexion may also induce a femoral nerve compression neuropathy; these generally resolve after the harness is removed. It is important during each examination to make certain the patient has active quadriceps function. Brachial plexus palsy may occur from compression by the shoulder straps, and knee subluxations may occur from improperly positioned straps.

Skin breakdown may occur in the groin creases and in the popliteal fossa if great care is not taken in keeping these areas clean and dry. Instruction on bathing and skin care is essential.

The most disastrous consequence of Pavlik harness treatment is damage to the cartilaginous femoral head and physeal plate.[342] This is usually secondary to forced abduction in the harness or persistent use of the harness despite failure of the guided reduction in a complete dislocation.

Children 6 Months to 2 Years of Age

It is difficult to maintain a child older than 6 months of age in a Pavlik harness because of the child's activity levels. In this age group, subluxated or dislocated hips should be treated by closed or open means, as necessary, because success rates using the Pavlik harness are less than 50%.

In the late-diagnosed case or the case that fails treatment with the Pavlik harness, the obstacles to reduction are different, treatment has greater risks, and the results are far less predictable. The principal goals in the treatment of late-diagnosed patient are similar to those for the newborn. The goal is to obtain a reduction, to maintain that reduction to provide an adequate environment for femoral head and acetabular development, and to avoid proximal femoral growth disturbance.

For patients older than 6 months of age at diagnosis and those who have failed a trial of Pavlik harness reduction, closed reduction is indicated. In most centers, closed reduction and spica cast immobilization usually is preceded by a period of skin or skeletal traction (Fig. 23-27).[41,78,79,111,191,200,206,242,381,401] The theoretic purpose of the traction is to facilitate reduction by allowing gradual stretching of the soft tissue structures impeding reduction and stretching of the neurovascular bundle to avoid inciting aseptic necrosis of the proximal femur by a sudden reduction. Generally, 1 to 2 weeks of skin or skeletal traction is thought to be sufficient. Skin traction is the most commonly used method, although some physicians recommend skeletal traction.[41] Skin tapes should be applied above the knee to distribute the traction over a large area (see Fig. 23-27). I prefer to wrap Elastoplast tape loosely over tincture of Benzoin from the ankle to the upper thigh. It is important not to stretch the Elastoplast tape at all; it should merely lie on the skin in a circumferential fashion, with each edge directly opposing the preceding edge. Buck traction tapes are then applied from above the ankle to the thigh and then applied to the foot plate; weights may be added to both legs such that the buttocks "lightly" touch the bed. I have used this method for a number of years without adverse consequences. The direction of application of the traction forces (e.g., overhead, longitudinal, divarication) and duration of traction vary worldwide from days to months.

The use of prereduction traction, although still employed by most treating physicians, is a somewhat controversial topic. Traction theoretically stretches contracted muscles, allows reduction without excessive force, and decreases the need for open reduction. These ideas are lacking the support of scientifically valid studies. The assessment of the adequacy of closed reduction and the need for open reduction vary and are subjective. Fish and colleagues surveyed the members of the Pediatric Orthopaedic Society of North America on this topic.[103] Most pediatric orthopaedic surgeons thought that traction did reduce the incidence of necrosis in the treatment of DDH. Only 5% of responders did not employ traction in their practice. The purpose of traction is to allow gradual relaxation of secondarily contracted muscles, such as the iliopsoas and adductor longus; this theoretically allows reduction without creating excessive joint forces, but the relevant reports on this subject are subjective. Several articles on open and closed reduction without the use of preliminary traction report incidences of proximal femoral damage comparable to those series in which prereduction traction was used.[63,174,289,382] These researchers think the main obstacles to reduction are intraarticular and therefore would not be affected by the use of traction. Controversy also exists about the amount of weight applied, direction of the force application, and duration of applied traction. There are no clinical or experimental studies of the direct effects of traction, and there are no well-controlled studies that analyze the effect of traction as a single variable.

The complications of traction include skin loss and ischemia to the lower extremities due to inappropriate application. Neurocirculatory checks must be done frequently, and traction must be applied in a carefully supervised fashion.

In appropriate circumstances, traction may be used at home.[173,247,367] This markedly decreases the costs associated with hospitalization. Patients usually are hospitalized for 24 hours to allow their parents to become familiar with the traction apparatus, to learn how to monitor neurocirculatory status, and to become totally familiar with the potential risks and danger signs. The patient and family must be cooperative; a visiting nurse is often helpful in instituting this program.

Closed reductions are performed in the operating room. Gentle reduction must be done under general anesthesia. The hip is gently manipulated into the acetabulum by flexion, traction, and abduction. An open or percutaneous adductor tenotomy usually is necessary in these cases because of secondary adduction contracture and to increase the safe zone, which lessens the incidence of proximal femoral growth disturbance. The reduction must be documented (Fig. 23-28).[84,110,156,166] Because large portions of the femoral head and acetabulum are cartilaginous, arthrography is a useful tool in assessing the obstacles to and adequacy

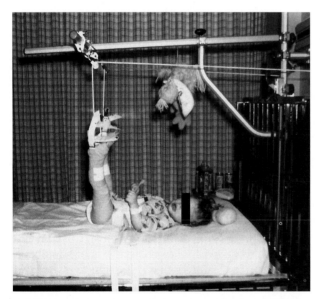

FIGURE 23-27. A 1-year-old child with bilateral hip dislocations in traction. Closed reduction and spica cast immobilization usually is preceded by a period of skin or skeletal traction.

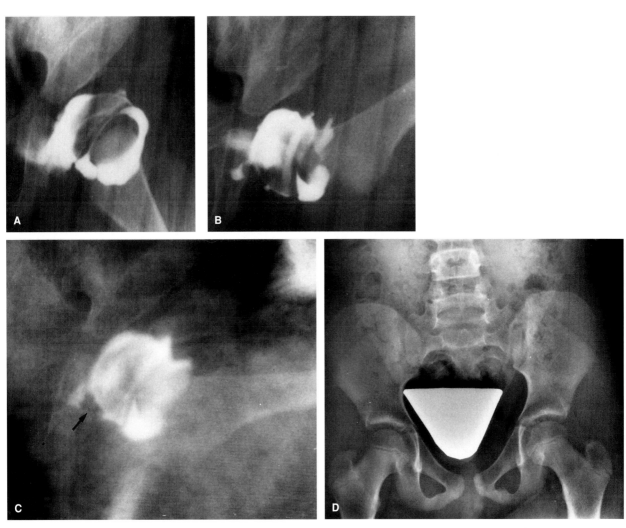

FIGURE 23-28.   Arthrograms demonstrate closed reduction of developmental dysplasia of the left hip in an 8-month-old infant. (**A**) Untreated. (**B**) Reduced. There is no pooling of dye medially. The acetabular cartilage completely covers the femoral head. (**C**) Reduction in a plaster cast. Notice the arthrographic shadow of transverse acetabular ligament (*arrow*). (**D**) Nine years after reduction. Notice the symmetric acetabular and proximal femoral development.

of reduction.[12,107,297] Dynamic arthrography using fluoroscopy helps to achieve both of these goals. Intraoperative ultrasonography may also be used.

The reduction is maintained in a well-molded plaster cast. The plaster must be well molded dorsal to the greater trochanters to prevent redislocation (Fig. 23-29). The "human position" of hyperflexion and limited abduction is the preferred position (Fig. 23-30).[106,308] The amount of apparent hip flexion during cast application is often greater than the flexion seen on x-ray films. Wide, forced abduction or forced abduction with internal rotation should be avoided, because these approaches are associated with an increased incidence of proximal femoral growth disturbance (Fig. 23-31).

I prefer to use plaster of Paris because of its moldability, but some surgeons prefer to use synthetic materials. The time of maintenance of reduction in the plaster cast varies considerably. I prefer to maintain the plaster below the knee on the involved side and above the knee on the uninvolved side for approximately 6 weeks, regardless of the patient's age. At that time, the plaster on the involved side (or sides) is cut to above the knee to allow some hip rotation and knee range of motion for an additional 6 weeks.

Twelve weeks after closed reduction, the plaster cast is removed and replaced by an abduction orthoses to be used on a full-time basis for 2 months, except during bathing, and then at nap time and nighttime until acetabular development is normal. The greatest rate of improvement in acetabular development occurs during the first 18 months after reduction. Reduction after casting should be documented by x-ray film, single-cut tomography, computed tomography scanning, or ultrasonography (see Fig. 23-29).[152,153] The adequacy of closed reduction is somewhat subjective. In

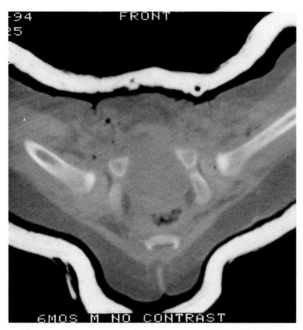

FIGURE 23-29. The computed tomography scan documents a successful closed reduction of a right hip dislocation. The plaster cast is molded dorsal to the greater trochanters to help prevent redislocation.

my opinion, "anatomic reduction" is the only acceptable reduction (see Fig. 23-28C). The use of the femoral head as a "dilating sound" to overcome the intra-articular obstacles to reduction may cause damage to the femoral head and may make open reduction more difficult.[172,315,304]

In patients 6 months to 2 years of age, open reduction is indicated if there is failure of closed treatment, persistent subluxation, soft tissue interposition, and reducible but unstable reductions other than in extreme positions of abduction.

The goals of open treatment are to obtain reduction, maintain the reduction, avoid damage to the femoral head, and provide an optimal environment for acetabular and proximal femoral development. Open reduction of a DDH may be accomplished with a variety of surgical approaches.[2,81,100,215,221,226,227,244,294,305,306,309,310,356,382]

The most commonly used surgical approach to open reduction is the anterolateral Smith-Petersen approach with a modified "bikini" incision, as described by Salter.[309] This is a standard approach to the hip joint and is familiar to most surgeons. In the late-diagnosed DDH patient, any associated capsular laxity can be plicated through this approach. If the surgeon thinks that a secondary procedure, such as pelvic osteotomy, is necessary, it also can be accomplished through the same surgical approach.[305,306,309,310]

One of the advantages of the anterior Smith-Petersen approach is that the hip is immobilized in a functional position, with minimal hip flexion and some degree of abduction. If this approach is used in conjunction with a capsular plication, the postoperative immobilization period usually is 6 to 8 weeks.

The disadvantages may include greater blood loss than with the various medial and anteromedial ap-

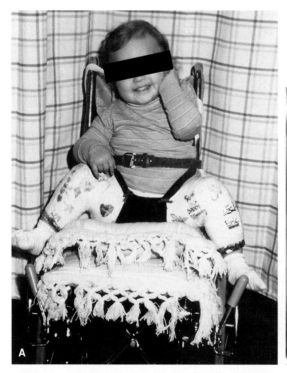

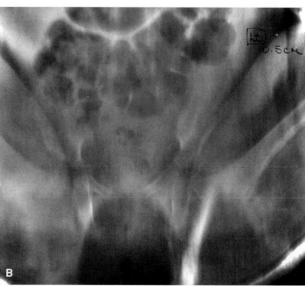

FIGURE 23-30. (A) The "human position" of hyperflexion and limited abduction is the preferred position after closed reduction. The patient in the picture had bilateral reductions. (B) Single-cut tomogram documents the hyperflexed, minimal abduction position.

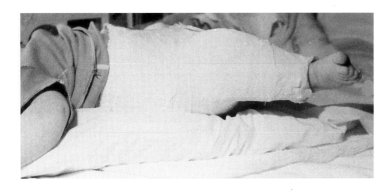

FIGURE 23-31. Wide abduction should be condemned. This position is associated with a high incidence of damage to the proximal femoral epiphysis and physeal plate.

proaches, possible damage to the iliac crest apophysis and the hip abductors, and postoperative stiffness. If this approach is used in bilateral cases, the procedures usually are staged at 2- to 6-week intervals.

The various medial approaches have the advantage of approaching the hip joint directly over the site of the obstacles to reduction.[100,180,215,221,226,232,241,244,268,300,382] The medial approach described by Ferguson is in the plane between the adductor brevis and the adductor magnus.[100] Advocates of this particular approach think that its advantages include minimal soft tissue dissection, direct access to the medial joint capsule and the iliopsoas tendon, avoidance of damage to the iliac apophysis and adductor muscles, minimal blood loss, and excellent cosmesis. It is, however, is a less familiar approach to most surgeons, and visualization is somewhat impaired. Capsular repair cannot be accomplished through this approach. The stability of the reduction is maintained only by the postoperative cast. The approach is somewhat difficult to use in older patients, and no concomitant surgical procedures can be done through the same incision. Questions have been raised about a higher incidence of proximal femoral growth disturbance after using this approach.

A third approach to open reduction in this age group is the anteromedial approach originally described by Ludloff and modified by Weinstein and Ponseti.[48,50,95,215,313,330,382,383,385] The approach is made in the interval between the femoral neurovascular bundle and the pectineus muscle. The advocates of this particular approach cite minimal blood loss (i.e., transfusion is never necessary), and it is the most direct approach to the obstacles to reduction. There is minimal muscle dissection in this approach; only the iliopsoas and the adductor longus are sectioned. Both hips can be done at the same operative sitting, the scar is extremely cosmetic, and there is no damage to hip abductor muscles or the iliac apophysis. Postoperative stiffness is not a problem.

The disadvantages of the anteromedial approach is that it is not a familiar approach to most surgeons. Only open reduction can be accomplished; no secondary procedures can be done through this incision. It is difficult to use in older patients because of the depth of the hip joint and difficulty with visualization.

If the surgeon thinks that capsular plication should be done, it cannot be done through this approach. The medial femoral circumflex vessels (i.e., primary blood supply to the proximal femur) are in the operative field. Moreover, visualization is claimed by some to be poor, and the approach is associated with a higher incidence of aseptic necrosis.[105,323] In my experience of more than 200 cases, visualization is excellent (Fig. 23-32), and the incidence of aseptic necrosis with a minimum 4-year follow-up is approximately 10%, which is well in line with the results of other series of open reductions.[244] Capsular plication appears to be unnecessary in this age group, because in a successful closed reduction, the capsule tightens, and the scar induced by the surgical procedure helps to provide capsular stability. This approach, however, depends on the placement of a well-molded cast. The approach to casting after reduction is the same as previously described for closed reduction. A certain degree of capsular stability is gained through the prolonged postoperative immobilization that is necessary. No residual stiffness has been experienced.

Most physicians use abduction orthoses for some period after cast removal. Some use them on a full-time bases for several months and then part time, usually during the night and napping hours, until acetabular development has caught up to the opposite, normal side. It is important in assessing acetabular development after open or closed reduction to look for accessory ossification centers. These give the treating physician an idea of whether the cartilage in the region of the neolimbus in the periphery of the acetabulum has the potential for ossification.

In the patients younger than 2 years of age, a secondary acetabular or femoral procedure is rarely required. The potential for acetabular development after closed and or open reduction is excellent and continues for 4 to 8 years after the procedure.[52,141,209,258,382] The most rapid improvement in acetabular development, as measured by parameters such as the acetabular index, development of the teardrop figure, and thinning of the medial floor, occurs in the first 18 months after surgery.[37,52,140,141,209,238,382] Femoral anteversion and any coxa valga associated with the untreated condition have an excellent chance to

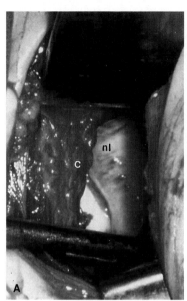
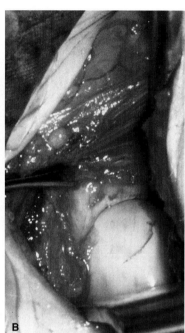

FIGURE 23-32. (A) Open reduction through an anteromedial approach in a 14-month-old child. Notice the anterior joint capsular edge (c) and the neolimbus (nl). (B) The hip is reduced under direct view. The femoral head is well seated in the acetabulum, and the anterior edge of the hip capsule is everted by a hemostat.

resolve during this time. However, some surgeons think every child older than 18 months of age should have a hip osteotomy accompanying open reduction because of the poor acetabular development potential.[305,306,309,113]

Children Older Than 2 Years of Age

In a child older than 2 years of age at the time of diagnosis of DDH, open reduction is usually necessary. In this age group, the treating surgeon must also consider whether to do a concomitant femoral shortening in conjunction with the open reduction. In children older than 3 years of age, femoral shortening to avoid excessive pressure on the proximal femur gives far lower rates of proximal femoral growth disturbance (e.g., aseptic necrosis) than does preliminary traction followed by open reduction (Fig. 23-33).[186,316] Schoenecher and Strecker reported a 54% incidence of aseptic necrosis, with a 32% incidence of redislocation by the use of skeletal traction in patients older than 3 years of age.[316]

The age range of 2 to 3 years is considered a "gray zone," with some surgeons advocating preliminary traction before open reduction and others doing concomitant femoral shortening.[114,150,188] In this age range, because the potential for acetabular development is markedly diminished, many surgeons recommend a concomitant acetabular procedure in conjunction with the open reduction or 6 to 8 weeks after the open reduction. The decision about whether to do a secondary acetabular procedure is subjective. I prefer to judge stability at the time of open reduction. If

good stability is evident, I prefer to observe acetabular development over the next few years, and if acetabular development is not improving by radiographic criteria (e.g., acetabular index, improvement in teardrop appearance and shape), I consider secondary acetabular procedures.

The most common accompanying procedure done in this age group in conjunction with open reduction is an innominate osteotomy as described by Salter[305,376] or by Pemberton.[64,65,96,279] Anatomic deficiency of the acetabulum in this age group usually is anterior, and the Salter innominate osteotomy gives anterior coverage, although at the expense of posterior coverage. The Pemberton osteotomy provides coverage anteriorly and various degrees of lateral coverage, depending on the direction of the osteotomy cuts.

In this age group, the standard anterolateral approach described by Smith-Petersen through the Salter modification is the ideal approach, because it enables capsular plication, immobilization of the hip joint in a more functional position, and an innominate osteotomy at the same time through the same incision.

A theoretic advantage of open reduction accompanied by femoral shortening is that it can be used to correct any anatomic abnormality, such as excessive femoral anteversion. The disadvantages of femoral shortening include the need for a second incision and internal fixation for the osteotomy, requiring another operation for hardware removal.

After 3 years of age, open reduction of the hip should be accompanied by femoral shortening and possibly by a concomitant acetabular procedure, depending on hip stability at the time of surgery.[40,188,388]

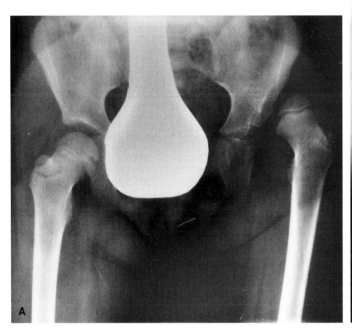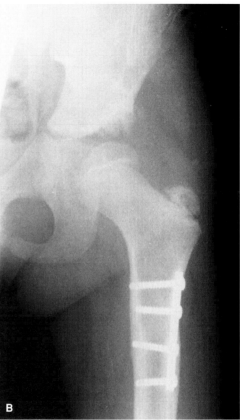

FIGURE 23-33. (A) A preoperative anteroposterior roentgenogram of a 4-year-old girl with developmental dislocation of the left hip. (B) Eighteen months after reduction and femoral shortening accessory centers of ossification are appearing in the lateral portion of the acetabular cartilage.

The acetabular procedure may be done at the time of open reduction, 6 weeks later or at a later date, depending on acetabular development.

Treatment of Acetabular Dysplasia in Children 6 Months to 2 Years of Age

In children between 6 months and 2 years of age, acetabular dysplasia diagnosed incidentally or as a residual result after Pavlik harness, open reduction, or closed reduction is often treated with a fixed abduction orthosis. The theory behind use of the fixed abduction orthosis is that dysplasia is associated with mild hip instability, and the orthosis can correct that instability. These devices can only be used if the hip is well reduced, as verified on a radiograph taken in the orthosis (see Fig. 23-26). The abduction orthosis usually is worn full time for several months and then worn on at night and during nap time until acetabular development is normal, as measured by the acetabular index.

The complications of a fixed abduction orthosis include skin breakdown and proximal femoral growth disturbance. It is important in positioning the fixed abduction orthosis that the hip not be placed in extreme positions of abduction to avoid interruption of the vascular supply to the proximal femur.

SEQUELAE AND COMPLICATIONS

Residual Femoral and Acetabular Dysplasia

Based on natural history studies, it is the goal of treatment to have a radiographically normal hip at maturity to prevent degenerative joint disease in the future. Hip subluxations must be corrected. The evidence demonstrates that residual acetabular dysplasia, even in the absence of subluxation, eventually leads to degenerative joint disease, and this also should be corrected. The goal of treatment of DDH is to have a hip as anatomically normal as possible by the end of skeletal growth.

When evaluating the patient with persistent dysplasia, the relation between the acetabulum and the femur must be assessed. The anatomic dysplasia can involve the acetabulum, the proximal femur, or both. In DDH cases, the deficiency is most commonly on the acetabular side, or the dysplasia is significantly greater on the acetabular side. If there has been disturbance of the proximal femoral growth secondary to previous treatment, the femoral side may be more dysplastic.

Dysplasias of hip joint can be evaluated by plain radiographs taken in the standing position when possible and with standard evaluations of acetabular development determined by the acetabular index, acetabular angle of Sharp, and CE angle. In young children with DDH, most cases of acetabular deficiency are anterior, and in adolescents and adults with DDH, the acetabular deficiencies can be anterior, posterior, or global.[21,211,248,305,306,307,393] Excessive femoral anteversion can be ascertained clinically but is best measured by a CT scan.[303] There has been an increased interest in evaluating dysplasia by the use of three-dimensional CT scans.[321,235] However, CT scanning cannot show the cartilaginous component of the proximal femur or the acetabulum, and it is therefore most useful for the patient at or close to maturity.

Deformities of the femoral neck assume significance only if they lead to subluxation of the joint: lateral subluxation with extreme coxa valga or anterior subluxation with excessive anteversion.[356] In general, patients with DDH usually have a normal neck-shaft angle. They may have persistent anteversion that gives a radiologic appearance of subluxation.

If acetabular dysplasia persists for 2 to 3 years after closed or open reduction and the patient has residual anteversion, a proximal femoral rotational osteotomy should be considered. Excessive anteversion or valgus of the proximal femur may contribute to hip joint instability and failure of normalization of acetabular growth. Varus derotation osteotomies are indicated in children with hip dysplasia, because it is assumed that the femoral head directed toward the center of the acetabulum stimulates normal acetabular development.[51,179,240,356] This approach may also be indicated to correct residual deformity from a partial physeal arrest as a result of aseptic necrosis. Intertrochanteric osteotomies can provide adequate medialization of the femoral shaft and prevent further varus deformity of the proximal femur.[252,395]

Before doing a varus derotation osteotomy, the surgeon must be certain that the femoral head can be concentrically reduced; if not, this procedure must be accompanied by open reduction. An anteroposterior pelvic film of the hip with apparent coxa valga and anteversion shows lateralization and subluxation of the femoral head (Fig. 23-34). Before surgery, the surgeon must document that the femoral head is concentrically reduced on an anteroposterior pelvic radiograph with the patient's legs abducted 30 degrees and maximally internally rotated (see Fig. 23-34). This position allows visualization of the actual femoral neck angle.

When the Shenton line is disrupted, the proper relation of the proximal femur usually can be restored by derotation osteotomies with or without various degrees of varus. After reduction is obtained in most cases of DDH, the femoral neck anteversion that exists in most patients corrects spontaneously.[83] The varus derotation osteotomy is used alone in such cases by surgeons who think that redirection of the femoral head toward the center of the acetabulum stimulates normal acetabular development.[32,54,57,67,179,212,296,344] The proximal femoral varus derotation osteotomy, if used to "stimulate" more normal acetabular development, must be used for children younger than 4 years of age.[179] After 8 years of age, no improvement in acetabular dysplasia can result from the procedure. These osteotomies must be done in the intertrochanteric region to provide adequate medialization of the femoral shaft. Doing the osteotomy in the intertrochanteric area avoids posterior displacement of the lesser trochanter, and it prevents excessive varus deformity of the femur, which can lead to mechanical abnormalities at the knee.

In small children, any leg length discrepancy resulting from varus osteotomy should resolve by growth stimulation and restoration of the normal neck shaft angle.[178] In teenagers, however, more than a 15-degree correction of varus deformity may result in limb shortening. The varus osteotomy, if excessive, can cause lateralization of the shaft, shifting the mechanical axis medial to the knee joint. This is an undesirable effect; a varus osteotomy should be accompanied by shaft medialization. If the osteotomy is transfixed with smooth wires, they can be removed after 6 to 8 weeks. Internal fixation devices are usually removed 12 to 18 months postoperatively; if they are not removed in young children, they become encased within the proximal femur, which could pose problems if future operations become necessary.

In the adolescent or adult patient with residual dysplasia in whom there is no potential for acetabular growth and remodeling, changing the orientation of the proximal femur does not increase the weight-bearing area but does shift the weight-bearing area to another portion on the femoral head.[278] Proximal femoral osteotomies in the adolescent or adult group are indicated only as adjuncts to pelvic operations and in extreme cases of coxa valga and subluxation (Fig. 23-35).[356]

Indications for treatment of residual radiographic acetabular dysplasia depend on the age of the child and whether or not the patient has symptoms.[222] The goal of treatment is to restore the anatomy to as near normal as possible by skeletal maturity. After a concentric reduction is obtained and maintained, the potential for acetabular development continues for many years.[140,141,209,220,382] However, after 4 years of age, this potential for restoration of normal anatomy decreases. For minimal residual dysplasias in children younger than 4 years of age, observation can be continued, but

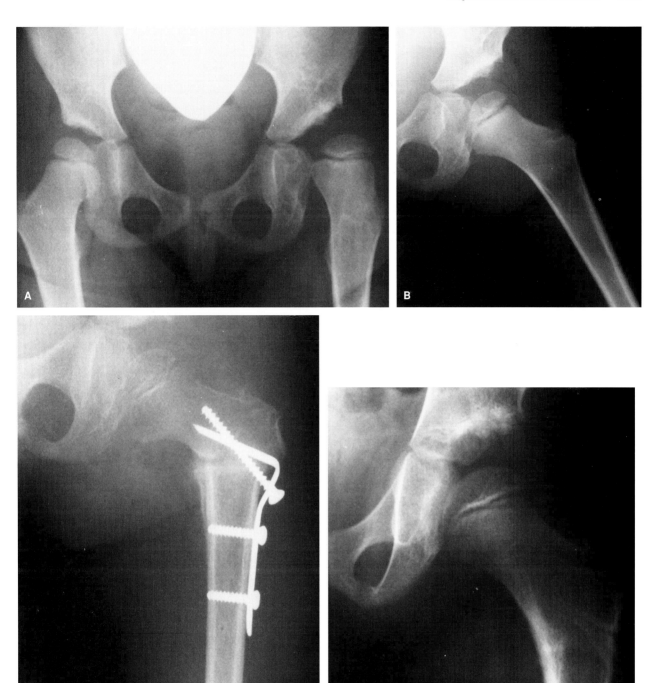

FIGURE 23-34. A 3-year-old Caucasian girl, 2 years after closed reduction. (**A**) Anteroposterior (AP) view of the pelvis. Notice the persistent acetabular dysplasia and apparent coxa valga. (**B**) The radiograph shows the leg is abducted approximately 30 degrees and is maximally internally rotated. The femoral head is seated well within the acetabulum, and the Shenton line is restored. (**C**) AP view of the left hip 6 weeks after varus derotation osteotomy. (**D**) AP view of the left hip 18 months after varus derotation osteotomy, with hardware removal. The Shenton line has been restored, there is improved teardrop figure development, and accessory centers of ossification appear in periphery of the acetabular cartilage.

for significant dysplasia, surgical intervention should be entertained.

The treatment options for acetabular dysplasia traditionally are divided into four groups. The first group consists of osteotomies of the pelvis that redirect the entire acetabulum. This redirection of the entire acetabulum provides coverage of the femoral head by acetabular articular cartilage. These osteotomies include the Salter innominate (Fig. 23-36) osteotomy,[177,234,305–307,309,310] the Sutherland double innominate osteotomy,[341] the triple innominate osteotomies of Tonnis,[353–357,359] Steel,[97,131,193,334,335] and Ganz,[117,185] the spherical osteotomies of Wagner[368,369,236] and Eppright,[91] and others.[250,253,254] These procedures involve complete

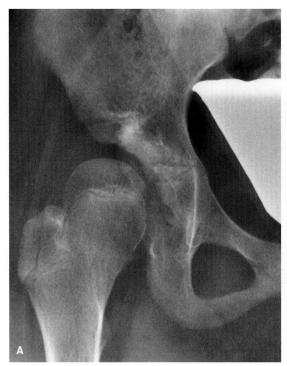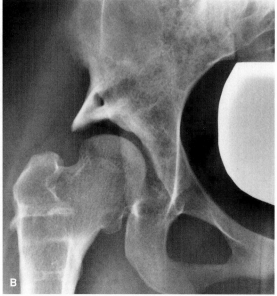

FIGURE 23-35. A 10-year-old girl with a diagnosis of developmental dysplasia of the hip made at 5 years of age. She had previously undergone open reduction but had residual proximal femoral and acetabular deformities. (**A**) Preoperative anteroposterior radiograph of the pelvis. (**B**) Three years after varus derotation osteotomy and Staheli slotted acetabular augmentation.

cuts through various pelvic bones and rotation of the acetabulum.

Other acetabuloplasties that involve incomplete cuts and hinge on different aspects of the triradiate cartilage include the acetabular procedures described Pemberton[64,93,96,279] and Dega.[195,213,345] These procedures can decrease the "volume" of the acetabulum because they depend on the triradiate cartilage as the fulcrum.

One group of acetabular reconstructive procedures places bone over the hip joint capsule on the uncovered portion of the femoral head. These provide coverage of the femoral head by capsular fibrous metaplasia.[3,159] They include the various shelf procedures[134,202,214,390,392,331,332] and the medial displacement osteotomy described by Chiari.[19,53,66,396,397]

Correction of residual dysplasia theoretically provides for a better weight-bearing surface for the femoral head, restores normal biomechanics of the hip, and may increase the longevity of the hip by prevention of degenerative joint disease. Unfortunately, only prospective long-term follow-up studies of these procedures can provide unambiguous answers.

Shelf procedures were described before 1900 and were used widely until the mid-1950s, when Chiari described his medial displacement osteotomy.[53] Later, Salter, Pemberton, and others described various pelvic osteotomies used to redirect the acetabulum and cover the femoral head by articular cartilage. In 1981,

Staheli introduced a modification of a previously described shelf arthroplasty, which gained widespread popularity used alone for significant anatomic dysplasia and in conjunction with various rotational procedures as an augmentation to provide increased femoral head coverage (see Fig. 23-35).[332]

Although intuitively it seems better to cover the femoral head with articular cartilage than to rely on fibrous metaplasia, it is impossible to to be certain about the long-term results of shelf arthroplasties because no such results exist.

In the young child, acetabular deficiencies generally are assessed by arthrography and by inspection at the time of the open reduction. For reduced hips with residual dysplasia, I have found that the problem is not one of deficiency of the acetabulum but a failure of the peripheral acetabular cartilage to ossify (see Fig. 23-36). In most cases, an arthrogram at the time of surgery shows excellent coverage of the femoral head by the unossified acetabular cartilage. This cartilage fails to undergo normal development because it is intrinsically abnormal or because it was damaged by the femoral head in the unreduced position, causing pressure necrosis. Given enough time, some of this acetabular cartilage may resume normal ossification and correct a large amount of the dysplasia. However, in my experience of a large number of cases treated by open and closed reduction, this does not happen

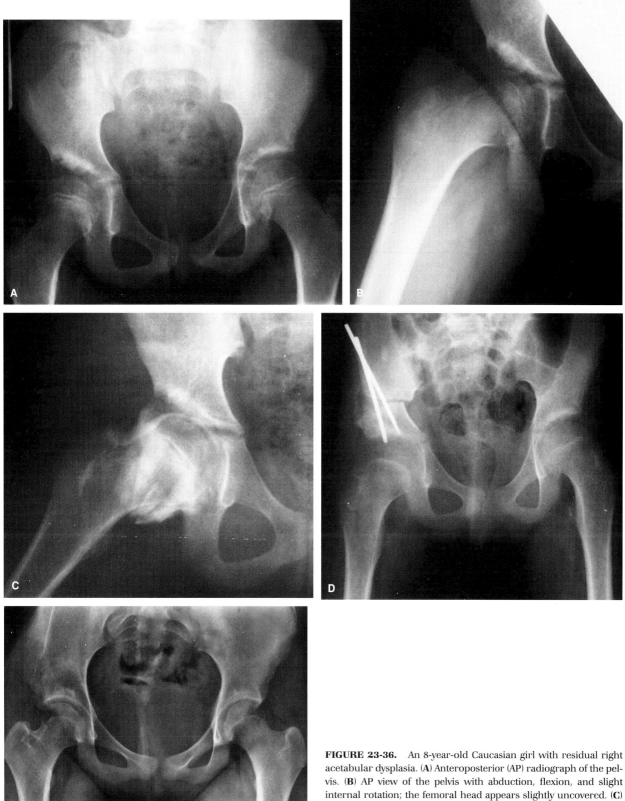

FIGURE 23-36. An 8-year-old Caucasian girl with residual right acetabular dysplasia. (**A**) Anteroposterior (AP) radiograph of the pelvis. (**B**) AP view of the pelvis with abduction, flexion, and slight internal rotation; the femoral head appears slightly uncovered. (**C**) Similar view with the addition of an arthrographic dye. Notice the excellent coverage of the proximal femur by unossified acetabular cartilage. (**D**) Immediately after the innominate osteotomy. (**E**) Four years after the innominate osteotomy.

in many cases, and intervention should be undertaken after the acetabulum has had a reasonable chance to develop on its own.[5,220,244] The osteotomy of the iliac bone and the neovascularity stimulated in healing may increase the ossification of the otherwise unossified acetabular cartilage. In any case, the redirection of the acetabulum restores more normal bony anatomy and normal biomechanics, which also may be a factor in stimulating ossification.[245]

The best means for evaluating acetabular dysplasia in the mature patient include the three-dimensional CT scan,[16,18,198,197,204,231,263] the false profile view, and plain x-ray films.[190] For young, immature patients, CT scanning does not provide adequate assessment of the deficiencies, because it does not show the acetabular cartilage.

Concentric reduction is an absolute requirement for all osteotomies other than the shelf or Chiari procedures. All osteotomies that depend on the triradiate cartilage as the fulcrum must obviously be done in patients with an open triradiate cartilage. The Salter innominate osteotomy, which hinges on the symphysis pubis, is better performed in the infant, child, and adolescent because of the flexibility of the symphysis pubis. However, this osteotomy can be performed in adults. The procedure is more likely to succeed when the CE angle is greater than 10 degrees.

An important factor to be considered when planning correction of acetabular dysplasia is the amount of dysplasia the needs to be corrected. The amount of coverage obtained by osteotomies such as the Salter procedure is limited, but osteotomies that cut all three pelvic bones provide the ability to obtain greater coverage.[290,135] The closer the osteotomies are placed to the acetabulum, the greater is the femoral head coverage. The triple innominate osteotomies described by Tonnis and Ganz provide greater rotational possibilities than that described by Steel. The osteotomies that are closest to the acetabulum (e.g., Eppright, Wagner) provide for the greatest potential for redirection, but these require significant technical expertise and have higher rates of complications.

The shelf arthroplasty and the Chiari osteotomy may be performed for well-reduced hips, but they usually are reserved for hips that lack significant femoral head coverage that could not be otherwise obtained through one of the other previously mentioned articular cartilage-covering procedures.[116,239] Many of these procedures can be done in patients with early degenerative changes in the hope of delaying the onset of arthroplasty or fusion. Further discussion of these issues is beyond the scope of the chapter.

The procedures that involve hinging on the triradiate cartilage, such as the Pemberton, have the potential to injure the triradiate cartilage and cause premature closure, but these complications are not common.[256] Procedures that must cross the triradiate cartilage, such as the Ganz osteotomy, and would induce closure cannot be done in patients with an open triradiate cartilage. In shelf arthroplasties done in immature patients, it is important to avoid cutting the ilium in the region of the groove of Ranvier, because this may severely impair acetabular development. Acetabular rotational procedures that depend on hinging on the cartilage of the symphysis pubis or various portions of the triradiate cartilage are better performed in younger patients. Rotational pelvic osteotomies in the face of subluxation may lead to severe damage to the femoral head.

The general prerequisites for rotational osteotomies include complete concentric reduction and release of muscle contractures, including the iliopsoas and hip adductors; a congruous joint; and a good range of motion. These procedures are best performed before 6 years of age, but the age limits vary considerably, depending on the surgeon.

The double innominate osteotomy of Sutherland aims to allow greater rotation of the pelvic fragment by cutting through the pubis instead of hinging only on the symphysis pubis.[341] Complications of this procedure can involve injury to the spermatic cords, bladder, and urethra. The triple innominate osteotomy allows even greater coverage by osteotomies of all three hip bones.

The Chiari medial displacement osteotomy hinges on the symphysis pubis, with the distal fragment displacing medially and upward (Figs. 23-37 and 23-38). This medialization results in reduction of the lever arm to reduce joint loading. Abductor muscle function is theoretically improved. Patients may limp for as long as 1 year. There is some concern that bilateral Chiari osteotomies may interfere with a woman's ability to deliver children. This is one of the few procedures for which long-term results exist, and these show that, in the absence of subluxation and degenerative joint disease, good long-term results may persist for many years.[23,26,44,80,126,162,196,237,295,298,302,396,402]

Decision making is somewhat difficult for the asymptomatic, mature patient. For the asymptomatic adolescent with minimal radiographic dysplasia, because degenerative arthritis is a probability but not a certainty, I prefer to inform the family about the potential for an adverse natural history and recommend surgery only at the onset of symptoms. There usually is a long interval between symptom onset and radiographic degenerative joint disease.[378] The patient can be reassured that, if symptoms develop, surgical treatment can help to avoid long-term degenerative joint disease. However, faced with an adolescent with radiographic evidence of subluxation, regardless of the

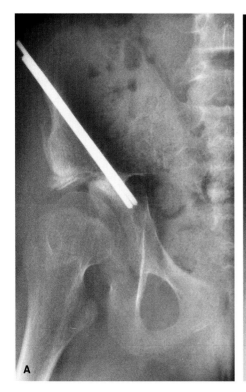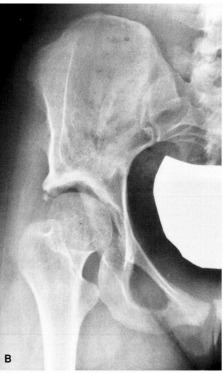

FIGURE 23-37. An 11-year-old Caucasian girl with pain and residual right hip subluxation with severe acetabular dysplasia. (**A**) Immediately after the right Chiari osteotomy. Notice the additional graft placed anteriorly. (**B**) Eight years postoperatively, there is excellent remodeling of the acetabulum with sourcil development.

symptoms, I recommend surgical correction, because an adverse natural history is certain without treatment.

Growth Disturbance of the Proximal Femur

The most disastrous complication associated with the treatment of DDH are various degrees of growth dis-

turbance of the proximal femur, including the epiphysis and physeal plate. This is commonly referred to by the term aseptic necrosis. Because there has never been a study of a pathologic specimen of what is called aseptic necrosis, I prefer to use the term proximal femoral growth disturbance.[220] These growth disturbances can be precipitated by experimental vascular injuries in animals and resemble the growth

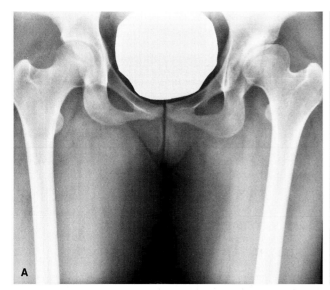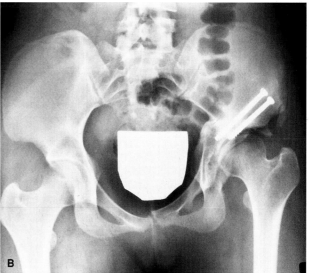

FIGURE 23-38. A Caucasian girl had an open reduction of the left dysplastic hip at 18 months of age. She presented at 17 years of age with subluxation, as seen on the radiograph. (**A**) Preoperative anteroposterior view of the pelvis. (**B**) Eight weeks after Chiari osteotomy. Notice the additional graft placed anteriorly.

disturbances seen in humans with treated DDH. The disturbance may be caused by vascular insults to the epiphysis or physeal plate or by pressure injury to the epiphyseal cartilage or physeal plate.[38,42,45,68,123,128,175,181,201,251,264–267,304,314,315,361] The blood supply to the proximal femur is described in Chapter 24.

Growth disturbance of the proximal femur in DDH occurs only in patients who have been treated. This may also occur in the opposite normal hip in a patient who has been treated.[154,155] The reported incidence of proximal femoral growth disturbance varies from none to 73%.[24,71,176,220] Different opinions exist about the reasons for this variation.[286,350] The use of prereduction traction,[24,41,71,111,175,220,389] adductor tenotomy,[251,292,308] open or closed reduction,[100,175,225,287,312,319,323,382] the force of reduction,[71,92,216,292] postoperative immobilization,[41,111,251,265,266,283,308,314,315] and the age at reduction[41,111,251,381] have been implicated as etiologic factors. Others think that the incidence may be much less variable than the means by which it is assessed.[220,350]

In an extensive study of the development of ischemic necrosis published by the German Society for Orthopaedics and Traumatology, 3316 conservatively treated hips and 730 operatively treated hips were evaluated to find the factors associated with the development of ischemic necrosis. The factors associated with necrosis included high dislocations and dislocations with inversion of the labrum, narrowing of the introitus between the superior labrum and the transverse ligament in the position of reduction, inadequate depth of reduction of the femoral head (>3 mm from the acetabular floor), older patients (>12 months), immobilization in 60 or more degrees of abduction for joint instability, and adductor tonotomy.[356]

Westin thought that the marked variation of the reported incidence indicated a lack of definition of terms.[389] Thomas and associates concluded that there was some association between the reported incidence in a given series and the rigor with which the diagnosis had been sought.[350] Buchanan thought that, if signs of growth disturbance were not present within 12 months of reduction, they were highly unlikely to appear.[41]

Bucholz and Ogdon[42] and Kalamchi and MacEwen[175] identified a lateral physeal arrest pattern that may not be evident until a patient is older than 12.5 years of age (mean, 9 years; Fig. 23-39). This is the most common pattern of growth disturbance reported. Kalamchi and MacEwen stressed that it may be difficult to identify this group early, and studies reporting growth disturbances with follow-up periods of less than 12 years must be regarded as preliminary and may not reflect the actual incidence of proximal growth disturbance.[175]

The incidence of proximal femoral growth disturbance increases with delay in reduction.[111,381] The younger patients have a lower rate of growth disturbance. Kalamchi and MacEwen, however, documented an increase the incidence of the severe form (type IV) in younger patients.[175] Salter[308] and Ogden[265,266] proposed that the femoral head in DDH is most vulnerable to ischemic changes during the first 12 to 18 months of life when it is composed mostly of cartilage. According to some orthopaedic specialists, the risk of total head involvement becomes somewhat less after the appearance of the femoral ossific nucleus.[381]

Prereduction traction to bring the proximal femur epiphysis to the level of the triradiate cartilage is considered essential by many surgeons to decrease the incidence of proximal femoral growth disturbance. Gage and Winter thought that there was a direct correlation between inadequate traction and the incidence of growth disturbance. They studied a group of patients to quantify prereduction hip positions.[112] Weiner found that, in patients younger than 1 year of age, traction for longer than 21 days substantially reduced the rate of growth disturbance.[381] Buchanan recommended a minimum of 2 weeks of traction, until achievement of a 2+ traction station using the Gage and Winter Scale. Skeletal traction gradually increased over several weeks, and an average of 39% of body weight usually was required to achieve this position.[41] In contrast, Cooperman studied 30 DDH hips with aseptic necrosis and 30 hips without necrosis and found at an average 39-year follow-up that the degree of initial displacement that had to be overcome to obtain reduction was comparable in both groups and that it was not a factor in the development of proximal femoral growth disturbance.[68] Some of the worst results were seen in patients with minimal superior dislocation. Schoenecker demonstrated that results of traction were not as good as femoral shortening in older patients with DDH.[316] Gibson and Benson thought that, although preliminary traction protects against growth disturbance, there was no relation between the original degree of displacement of the proximal femur and the final result.[316]

Several factors associated with an increased incidence of proximal femoral growth disturbance have been documented in the clinical setting and in experimental studies. These include extremes in positioning of the proximal femur in abduction and abduction with extreme medial rotation. Extremes in position can cause compression of the medial femoral circumflex vessel as it goes around the iliopsoas tendon and compression of the terminal branch between the lateral femoral neck and the acetabular margin.[265,266,308] Anatomic and experimental investigations have persistently shown that strong medial rotation with concomitant abduction and extreme abduction alone (i.e., Lorenz position) can compromise the blood flow to the capital femoral epiphysis. If the hip is maximally ab-

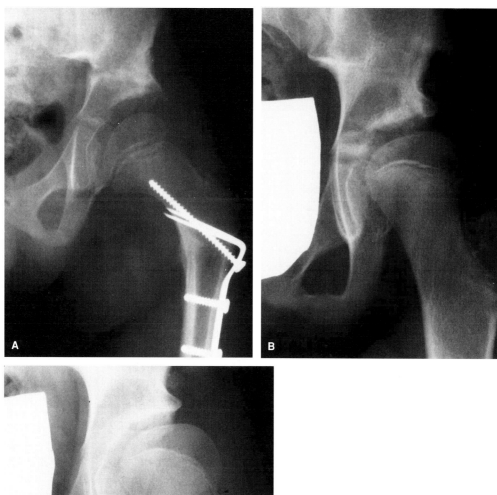

FIGURE 23-39. A 5-year-old girl who underwent varus derotation osteotomy, an innominate osteotomy for residual dysplasia 3 years after open reduction. (**A**) An anteroposterior (AP) view 3 months postoperatively. (**B**) AP view at 9 years of age. Note the valgus tilt to the proximal femur. (**C**) AP view at 11 years of age. Notice the lateral tether, a typical type II physeal plate tether, and how the tether produces hip subluxation. A physeal growth arrest pattern may not be evident until a patient is 9 years of age or older.

ducted against firm resistance, the blood flow can be completely or almost completely arrested. The same is true in forced medial rotation. The blood vessels and blood supply to the proximal femur can be occluded outside the femoral head by compression or as the vessels cross through the epiphyseal cartilage.[304,308,361] Schoenecker showed a diminution of epiphyseal profusion by increased pressure, which was relieved after the external fixation device was removed.[314,315]

The extreme positions of abduction, frequently called the frog-leg position (see Fig. 23-31) and used in cases of unrelieved adduction contracture as seen in dislocations, uniformly result in severe growth disturbances of the epiphysis.[106,308,314]

Extreme positions can also cause pressure necrosis of the vulnerable epiphyseal cartilage and the physeal plate. This has been experimentally shown by Law and colleagues[201] and by Schoenecker and associates.[314] These studies and others demonstrated the severe effects of cartilage necrosis.[304,308,356] These effects can also be precipitated by circumscribed pressure, such as the use of the vulnerable femoral head as a "dilating sound" to overcome the intraarticular obstacles to reduction.

Severin advocated the use of the femoral head placed in close apposition to the acetabulum to induce regression of the obstacles to reduction. The idea is that sustained pressure from the femoral head causes the labrum to adapt itself to the spherical contour of the head.[319] This maneuver can be used to obtain reduction, but the price is an increased incidence of necrosis.[292,356] Although the use of prereduction traction has been implicated as a factor in reducing the incidence of necrosis, the German Orthopaedic Study Group did not find this to be the case.[356]

The persistence of using closed techniques in an attempt to have the femoral head overcome the intraarticular obstacles to reduction can lead to severe necrosis.[356] If closed reduction is attempted, in my opinion, the only acceptable reduction is an "anatomically perfect" reduction; otherwise, the hip must be reduced openly to prevent damage to the vulnerable femoral head.[352,356,358]

The most widely used classification of proximal femoral growth disturbance is that of Salter and colleagues (Table 23-2).[308] I disagree with the inclusion of coxa magna, because coxa magna is often seen after open reductions as the result of stimulation of blood flow to the proximal femur.[115,259] It is also often difficult to ascertain if some of the residual deformities seen after treatment of DDH are alterations in the proximal femur secondary to disturbances that occurred before the reduction or are the result of complications associated with the reduction. One of the most common deformities seen is flattening of the medial aspect of the proximal femur, which occurs because of pressure of the femoral head lying against the ilium before reduction.

Another area of uncertainty is the issue of "temporary irregular ossification" of the femoral epiphysis and whether this represents damage to the epiphyseal cartilage or merely multiple ossification centers that eventually coalesce. These areas may be analogous to the accessory centers of ossification seen in the periphery of the acetabulum. This pattern usually does not result in growth disturbance of the proximal femur. Only long-term follow-up studies of this entity can resolve this issue.

Kalamchi and MacEwen developed a classification of necrosis that emphasized the growth disturbances associated with various degrees of physeal arrest. This classification (Fig. 23-40) puts all the growth disturbances seen in the ossific nucleus into one category if they are not associated with physeal involvement.[175] Bucholz and Ogdon provided an additional classification based on patterns of vascular supply resulting in partial or total ischemia.[42] There are few studies documenting interobserver or intraobserver reliability of these classifications of growth disturbance. As many as 25% of hips may not fit into a particular classification.

O'Brien and associates discussed the importance of identification of growth disturbance lines to predict future deformity of the proximal femur.[260,261] These growth arrest lines may provide the physician with early evidence of a future problem. However, the utility of this approach must await long-term follow-up studies.

Long-term follow-up studies exist of patients suffering from proximal femoral growth disturbance.[68,356] The results indicate that any alteration of proximal femoral growth disturbance shortens the longevity of the hip.

In the treatment of the residual effects of necrosis, reduction must be maintained by corrective femoral and or acetabular procedures. With arrest of the proximal femoral physeal plate, trochanteric overgrowth ensues, producing an abductor lurch. If identified, greater trochanteric physeal plate arrest may maintain articular trochanteric distance (ATD) if performed in children younger than 8 years of age[13,167,199]; otherwise, distal transfer of the greater trochanter may be necessary.[29,101,213,219]

The painful hip in the teenager with residual proximal femoral growth disturbance and dysplasia may be caused by a torn labrum.[142,255] The diagnosis can be made using contrast-enhanced CT or magnetic resonance scans, and treatment may require open repair or excision. Another cause of pain includes early degenerative joint disease, which should be treated by the previously described methods to correct residual subluxation and dysplasia. In extreme cases, hip fusion or early total joint arthroplasty may be the only alternatives available. These circumstances are rare among patients younger than 30 years of age.

The key to the diagnosis and management of DDH is early detection. This results in a 95% success rate

---

TABLE 23-2 *Classification of the Femoral Head*

SALTER CLASS	FEATURES
1	Failure of the appearance of the ossific nucleus of the femoral head within 1 year after reduction
2	Failure of growth of an existing ossific nucleus within 1 year after reduction
3	Broadening of the femoral neck within 1 year after reduction
4	Increased radiographic bone density, followed by fragmentation of the femoral head
5	Residual deformity of the femoral head and neck when reossification is complete; these deformities include coxa magna, coxa plana, coxa vara, and a short, broad femoral neck

From Salter RB, Kostiuk J, Dallas S. Avascular necrosis of the femoral head as a complication of treatment for congenital dislocation of the hip in young children: a clinical and experimental investigation. Can J Surg 1969;12:44.

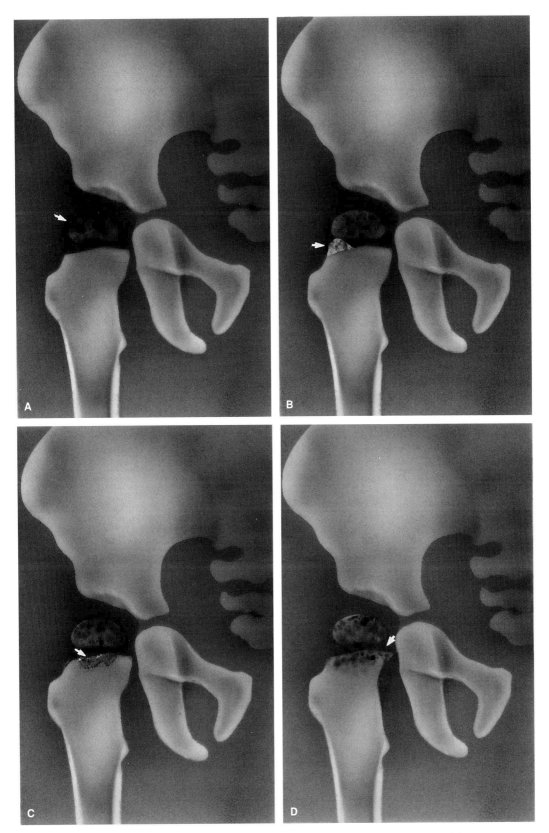

FIGURE 23-40. Classification of proximal femoral growth disturbances. (**A**) Group I. (**B**) Group II. (**C**) Group III. (**D**) Group IV. (Adapted from Kalamchi A, MacEwen GD. Avascular necrosis following treatment of congenital dislocation of the hip. J Bone Joint Surg [Am] 1980;62:876.)

of treatment, with a low risk of complications. It is the initial treating physician who has the greatest chance of success in obtaining a normal hip. Orthopaedic surgeons must educate primary care colleagues in making the diagnosis early and initiating prompt referral.

References

1. Abd-el-Kader-Shaheen M. Mehad: the Saudi tradition of infant wrapping as a possible aetiological factor in congenital dislocation of the hip. J R Coll Surg Edinb 1989;34:85.

2. Akazawa H, Tanabe G, Miyake Y. A new open reduction treatment for congenital hip dislocation: long-term follow-up of the extensive anterolateral approach. Acta Med Okayama 1990;44:223.

3. Albee FH. The bone graft wedge. NY Med J 1915;52:433.

4. Albinana J, Quesada JA, Certucha JA. Children at high risk for congenital dislocation of the hip: late presentation. J Pediatr Orthop 1993;13:268.

5. Albinana J, Weinstein SL, Morcuende JA, Dolan L, Meyer M. DDH acetabular remodeling after open or closed reduction; timing for secondary procedures. 1995 (in press).

6. Albinana J, Morcuende JA, Weinstein SL. Predictive value of the teardrop figure in congenital dislocation of the hip: a quantitative study. 1995 (in press).

7. Almby B, Hjelmstedt A, Lonnerholm T. Neonatal hip instability. Reason for failure of early abduction treatment. Acta Orthop Scand 1979;50:315.

8. Almby B, Lonnerholm T. Hip joint instability after the neonatal period. I. Value of measuring the acetabular angle. Acta Radiol Diagn 1979;20:200.

9. Anda S, Terjesen T, Kvistad KA, Svenningsen S. Acetabular angles and femoral anteversion in dysplastic hips in adults: CT investigation. J Comput Assist Tomogr 1991;15:115.

10. Anda S, Terjesen T, Kvistad KA. Computed tomography measurements of the acetabulum in adult dysplastic hips: which level is appropriate? Skeletal Radiol 1991;20:267.

11. Ando M, Gotoh E. Significance of inguinal folds for diagnosis of congenital dislocation of the hip in infants aged three to four months. J Pediatr Orthop 1990;10:331.

12. Ando M, Gotoh E, Matsuura J. Tangential view arthrogram at closed reduction in congenital dislocation of the hip. J Pediatr Orthop 1992;12:390.

13. Andrisano A, Marchiodi L, Preitano M. Epiphyseodesis of the great trochanter. Ital J Orthop Traumatol 1986;12:217.

14. Asher MA. Orthopedic screening: especially congenital dislocation of the hip and spinal deformity. Pediatr Clin North Am 1977;24:713.

15. Asher MA. Screening for congenital dislocation of the hip, scoliosis, and other abnormalities affecting the musculoskeletal system. Pediatr Clin North Am 1986;33:1335.

16. Atar D, Lehman WB, Grant AD. 2-D and 3-D computed tomography and magnetic resonance imaging in developmental dysplasia of the hip. Orthop Rev 1992;21:1189.

17. Atar D, Lehman WB, Tenenbaum Y, Grant AD. Pavlik harness versus Frejka splint in treatment of developmental dysplasia of the hip: bicenter study. J Pediatr Orthop 1993;13:311.

18. Azuma H, Taneda H, Igarashi H. Evaluation of acetabular coverage: three-dimensional CT imaging and modified pelvic inlet view. J Pediatr Orthop 1991;11:765.

19. Bailey TE Jr, Hall JE. Chiari medial displacement osteotomy. J Pediatr Orthop 1985;5:635.

20. Barlow TG. Early diagnosis and treatment of congenital dislocation of the hip. J Bone Joint Surg [Br] 1962;44:292.

21. Barrett WP, Staheli LT, Chew DE. The effectiveness of the Salter innominate osteotomy in the treatment of congenital dislocation of the hip. J Bone Joint Surg [Am] 1986;68:79.

22. Bensahel GF, Canadell J, Dungl PTM, Vizkelety T. The Pavlik harness in the treatment of congenital dislocating hip: report on a multicenter study of the European Paediatric Orthopaedic Society. J Pediatr Orthop 1988;8:1.

23. Benson MKD, Evans JDC. The pelvic osteotomy of Chiari: an anatomical study of the hazards and misleading radiographic appearance. J Bone Joint Surg [Br] 1976;58:163.

24. Berkeley ME, Dickson JH, Cain TE, Donovan MM. Surgical therapy for congenital dislocation of the hip in patients who are twelve to thirty-six months old. J Bone Joint Surg [Am] 1984;66:412.

25. Bertol P, Macnicol MF, Mitchell GP. Radiographic features of neonatal congenital dislocation of the hip. J Bone Joint Surg [Br] 1982;64:176.

26. Betz RR, Kumar SJ, Palmer CT, MacEwen GD. Chiari pelvic osteotomy in children and young adults. J Bone Joint Surg [Am] 1988;70:182.

27. Bialik V, Reuveni A, Pery M, Fishman J. Ultrasonography in developmental displacement of the hip: A critical analysis of our results. J Pediatr Orthop 1989;9:154.

28. Bialik V, Wiener F. Sonography in suspected developmental dysplasia of the hip. J Pediatr Orthop [B] 1993;2:000.

29. Bialik V, Rosenberg N. Transfer of greater trochanter. J Pediatr Orthop, Part B 1994;3:30.

30. Bjerkreim I, Arseth PH. Congenital dislocation of the hip in Norway. Late diagnosis CDH in the years 1970 to 1974. Acta Paediatr Scand 1978;67:329.

31. Bjerkreim I, Johansen J. Late diagnosed congenital dislocation of the hip. Acta Orthop Scand 1987;58:504.

32. Blockey NJ. Derotation osteotomy in the management of congenital dislocation of the hip. J Bone Joint Surg [Br] 1984;66:485.

33. Boeree NR, Clarke NMP. Ultrasound imaging and secondary screening for congenital dislocation of the hip. J Bone Joint Surg [Br] 1994;76:525.

34. Bombelli R. Osteoarthritis of the hip. Heidelberg: Springer-Verlag, 1983.

35. Bos CF, Bloem JL, Verbout AJ. Magnetic resonance imaging in acetabular residual dysplasia. Clin Orthop 1991;265:207.

36. Bradley J, Wetherill M, Benson MK. Splintage for congenital dislocation of the hip. Is it safe and reliable? J Bone Joint Surg [Br] 1987;69:257.

37. Brougham DI, Broughton NS, Cole WG, Menelaus MB. The predictability of acetabular development after closed reduction for congenital dislocation of the hip. J Bone Joint Surg [Br] 1988;70:733.

38. Brougham DI, Broughton NS, Cole WG, Menelaus MB. Avascular necrosis following closed reduction of congenital dislocation of the hip. Review of influencing factors and long-term follow-up. J Bone Joint Surg [Br] 1990;72:557.

39. Broughton NS, Brougham DI, Cole WG, Menelaus MB. Reliability of radiological measurements in the assessment of the child's hip. J Bone Joint Surg [Br] 1989;71:6.

40. Browne RS. The management of late diagnosed congenital dislocation and subluxation of the hip-with special reference to femoral shortening. J Bone Joint Surg [Br] 1979;61:7.

41. Buchanan JR, Greer RB III, Cotler JM. Management strategy for prevention of avascular necrosis during treatment of congenital dislocation of the hip. J Bone Joint Surg [Am] 1981;63:140.

42. Bucholz R, Ogden J. Patterns of ischemic necrosis of the proximal femur in nonoperatively treated congenital hip disease. In: The hip: proceedings of the sixth open scientific meeting of the Hip Society. St. Louis: CV Mosby, 1978.

43. Burger BJ, Burger JD, Bos CF, et al. Frejka pillow and Becker device for congenital dislocation of the hip. Prospective 6-year study of 104 late-diagnosed cases. Acta Orthop Scand 1993;64:305.

44. Calvert PT, August AC, Albert JS, et al. The Chiari pelvic osteotomy. A review of the long-term results. J Bone Joint Surg [Br] 1987;69:551.

45. Campbell P, Tarlow SD. Lateral tethering of the proximal femoral physis complicating the treatment of congenital hip dysplasia. J Pediatr Orthop 1990;10:6.

46. Carter CO, Wilkinson J. Congenital dislocation of the hip. J Bone Joint Surg [Br] 1960;42:669.

47. Carter CO, Wilkinson JA. Genetic and environmental factors in the etiology of congenital dislocation of the hip. Clin Orthop 1964;33:119.

48. Castillo R, Sherman FC. Medial adductor open reduction for congenital dislocation of the hip. J Pediatr Orthop 1990;10:335.

49. Catterall A. The early diagnosis of congenital dislocation of the hip (editorial). J Bone Joint Surg [Br] 1994;76:515.

50. Cech O, Sosna A, Vavra J. Indications and surgical technique for open reposition of congenital dislocation of the hip after Ludloff (author's translation). Acta Chir Orthop Traumatol Cech 1976;43:233.

51. Chapchal GJ. The intertrochanteric osteotomy in the treatment of congenital dysplasia. Clin Orthop 1976;119:54.

52. Cherney DL, Westin GW. Acetabular development in the infant's dislocated hips. Clin Orthop 1989;242:98.

53. Chiari K. Medial displacement osteotomy of the pelvis. Clin Orthop 1974;98:55.

54. Chuinard EG. Femoral osteotomy in the treatment of congenital dysplasia of the hip. Orthop Clin North Am 1972;3:157.

55. Churgay CA, Caruthers BS. Diagnosis and treatment of congenital dislocation of the hip. Am Fam Physician 1992;45:1217.

56. Clarke NM, Harcke HT, McHugh P, et al. Real-time ultrasound in the diagnosis of congenital dislocation and dysplasia of the hip. J Bone Joint Surg [Br] 1985;67:406.

57. Clarke NMP, Clegg J, Al-Chalabi AN. Ultrasound screening of hips at risk for CDH. Failure to reduce the incidence of late cases. J Bone Joint Surg [Br] 1989;71:9.

58. Clarke NM. Diagnosing congenital dislocation of the hip (editorial). Br Med J 1992;305:435.

59. Coleman SS. Diagnosis of congenital dysplasia of the hip in the newborn infant. J Bone Joint Surg [Am] 1956;162:548.

60. Coleman CR, Slager RF, Smith WS. The effect of environmental influence on acetabular development. Surg Forum 1958;9:775.

61. Coleman SS. Congenital dysplasia of the hip in the Navajo infant. Clin Orthop 1968;56:179.

62. Coleman SS. Congenital dysplasia and dislocation of the hip. St. Louis: CV Mosby, 1978.

63. Coleman S. A critical analysis of the value of preliminary traction in the treatment of CDH. Orthop Trans 1987;13:180.

64. Coleman SS. The pericapsular (Pemberton) pelvic osteotomy and the redirectional (Salter) pelvic osteotomy. Mapfre Med 1992;3(Suppl 1):124.

65. Coleman S. Prevention of developmental dislocation of the hip: practices and problems in the United States. J Pediatr Orthop [B] 1993;2:000.

66. Colton CL. Chiari osteotomy for acetabular dysplasia in young subjects. J Bone Joint Surg [Br] 1972;54:578.

67. Conforty B. Femoral osteotomy for correction of sequelae of conservative treatment of congenital dislocation of the hip. Isr J Med Sci 1980;16:284.

68. Cooperman DR, Wallensten R, Stulberg SD. Post-reduction avascular necrosis in congenital dislocation of the hip. J Bone Joint Surg [Am] 1980;62:247.

69. Cooperman DR, Wallensten R, Stulberg SD. Acetabular dysplasia in the adult. Clin Orthop 1983;175:79.

70. Crawford AW, Slovek RW. Fate of the untreated congenitally dislocated hip. Orthop Trans 1978;2:73.

71. Crego CH Jr, Schwartzmann JR. Medial adductor open reduction for congenital dislocation of the hip. J Bone Joint Surg [Am] 1948;30:428.

72. Czeizel A, Szentpetery J, Kellermann M. Incidence of congenital dislocation of the hip in Hungary. Br J Prev Soc Med 1974;28:265.

73. Czeizel A, Tusnady G, Vaczo G, Vizkelety T. The mechanism of genetic predisposition in congenital dislocation of the hip. J Med Genet 1975;12:121.

74. Czeizel AE, Intody Z, Modell B. What proportion of congenital abnormalities can be prevented? Br Med J 1993;306:499.

75. Dahlstrom H, Oberg L, Friberg S. Sonography in congenital dislocation of the hip. Acta Orthop Scand 1986;57:402.

76. Dahlstrom H, Friberg S, Oberg L. Current role of sonography in late CDH. Acta Orthop Scand 1988;59(Suppl 227):94.

77. Danielsson LG, Nilsson BE. Attitudes to CDH (guest editorial). Acta Orthop Scand 1984;55:244.

78. Danzhou S, Hongzhi I, Weinmin Y, Desheng D. Preoperative intermittent manual traction in congenital dislocation of the hip. J Pediatr Orthop 1989;9:205.

79. DeRosa GP, Feller N. Treatment of congenital dislocation of the hip. Management before walking age. Clin Orthop 1987;225:77.

80. Dewaal Malefijt MC, Hodgland T, Nielsen HKL. Chiari osteotomy in the treatment of the congenital dislocation and subluxation of the hip. J Bone Joint Surg [Am] 1982;64:996.

81. Dhar S, Taylor JF, Jones WA, Owen R. Early open reduction for congenital dislocation of the hip. J Bone Joint Surg [Br] 1990;72:175.

82. Dimitriou JK, Cavadias AX. One-stage surgical procedure for congenital dislocation of the hip in older children. Long-term results. Clin Orthop 1989;246:30.

83. Doudoulakis JK, Cavadias A. Open reduction of CDH before one year of age: 69 hips followed for 13 (10–19) years. Acta Orthop Scand 1993;64:188.

84. Drummond DS, ODonnell J, Breed A, et al. Arthrography in the evaluation of congenital dislocation of the hip. Clin Orthop 1989;243:148.

85. Dunn PM. Congenital dislocation of the hip (CDH): necropsy studies at birth. J R Soc Med 1969;62:1035.

86. Dunn PM. The anatomy and pathology of congenital dislocation of the hip. Clin Orthop 1976;119:23.

87. Dunn PM. Prenatal observation on the etiology of congenital dislocation of the hip. Clin Orthop 1976;119:11.

88. Dyson PH, Lynskey TG, Catterall A. Congenital hip dysplasia: problems in the diagnosis and management in the first year of life. J Pediatr Orthop 1987;7:568.

89. Edlestein J. Congenital dislocation of the hip in the Bantu. J Bone Joint Surg [Br] 1966;48:397.

90. Engesaeter LB, Wilson DJ, Nag D, Benson MK. Ultrasound and congenital dislocation of the hip. The importance of dynamic assessment. J Bone Joint Surg [Br] 1990;72:197.

91. Eppright RH. Dial osteotomy of the acetabulum in the treatment of dysplasia of the hip. J Bone Joint Surg [Am] 1976;58:726.

92. Esteve R. Congenital dislocation of the hip. A review and assessment of results of treatment with special reference to frame reduction as compared with manipulative reduction. J Bone Joint Surg [Br] 1960;42:253.

93. Eyre-Brook AL, Jones DA, Harris FC. Pemberton's acetabuloplasty for congenital dislocation or subluxation of the hip. J Bone Joint Surg [Br] 1978;60:18.

94. Fabry G, MacEwen GD, Shands AR Jr. Torsion of the femur. A follow-up study in normal and abnormal conditions. J Bone Joint Surg [Am] 1973;55:1726.

95. Fabry G. Open reduction by the Ludloff approach to congenital dislocation of the hip under the age of two. Acta Orthop Belg 1990;56:233.

96. Faciszewski T, Kiefer GN, Coleman SS. Pemberton osteotomy for residual acetabular dysplasia in children who have congenital dislocation of the hip. J Bone Joint Surg [Am] 1993;75:643.

97. Faciszewski T, Coleman S. Triple innominate osteotomy in the treatment of acetabular dysplasia. J Pediatr Orthop 1993;13:426.

98. Fairbank JC, Howell P, Nockler I, Lloyd-Roberts GC. Relationship of pain to the radiological anatomy of the hip joint in adults treated for congenital dislocation of the hip as infants: a long-term follow-up of patients treated by three methods. J Pediatr Orthop 1986;6:539.

99. Fellander M, Gladnikoff H, Jacobsson E. Instability of the hip in the newborn. Acta Orthop Scand Suppl 1970;130:36.

100. Ferguson AB Jr. Treatment of congenital dislocation of the hip in infancy using the medial approach. In: Tachdjian MO, ed. Congenital dislocation of the hip. New York: Churchill Livingstone, 1982.

101. Fernbach SK, Poznanski AKK, Kelikian AS, et al. Greater trochanteric overgrowth: development and surgical correction. Radiology 1954;3:661.

102. Filipe G, Carlioz H. Use of the Pavlik harness in treating congenital dislocation of the hip. J Pediatr Orthop 1982;2:357.

103. Fish DN, Herzenberg JE, Hensinger RN. Current practice in use of prereduction traction for congenital dislocation of the hip. J Pediatr Orthop 1991;11:149.

104. Fisher R, OBrien TS, Davis KM. Magnetic resonance imaging in congenital dysplasia of the hip. J Pediatr Orthop 1991;11:617.

105. Fisher EHI, Beck PA, Hoffer MM. Necrosis of the capital femoral epiphysis and medial approaches to the hip in piglets. J Orthop Res 1991;9:203.

106. Fogarty EE, Accardo NY. Incidence of avascular necrosis of the femoral head in congenital hip dislocation related of the degree of abduction during preliminary traction. J Pediatr Orthop 1981;1:307.

107. Forlin E, Choi IH, Guille JT, et al. Prognostic factors in congenital dislocation of the hip treated with closed reduction. The importance of arthrographic evaluation. J Bone Joint Surg [Am] 1992;74:1140.

108. Frankenburg WK. To screen or not to screen: congenital dislocation of the hip (editorial). Am J Public Health 1981;71:1311.

109. Fredensborg N, Nilsson BE. Overdiagnosis of congenital dislocation of the hip. Clin Orthop 1976;119:89.

110. Gabuzda GM, Renshaw TS. Reduction of congenital dislocation of the hip. J Bone Joint Surg [Am] 1992;74:624.

111. Gage JR, Winter RB. Avascular necrosis of the capital femoral epiphysis as a complication of closed reduction of congenital dislocation of the hip. J Bone Joint Surg [Am] 1972;54:373.

112. Gage JR, Camy JM. The effects of trochanteric epiphysiodesis on growth of the proximal end of the femur following necrosis of the capital femoral epiphysis. J Bone Joint Surg [Am] 1980;62:785.

113. Gallien R, Bertin D, Lirette R. Salter procedure in congenital dislocation of the hip. J Pediatr Orthop 1984;4:427.

114. Galpin RD, Roach JW, Wenger DR, et al. One-stage treatment of congenital dislocation of the hip in older children, including femoral shortening. J Bone Joint Surg [Am] 1989;71:734.

115. Gamble JG, Mochizuki C, Bleck EE, Rinsky LA. Coxa magna following surgical treatment of congenital hip dislocation. J Pediatr Orthop 1985;5:528.

116. Gangloff S, Onimus M. Chiari pelvic osteotomy: technique and indications. J Pediatr Orthop 1994;3:68.

117. Ganz R, Vinh TS, Mast JW. A new periacetabular osteotomy for the treatment of hip dysplasias. Technique and preliminary results. Clin Orthop Rel Res 1988;232:26.

118. Gardiner HM, Dunn PM. Controlled trial of immediate splinting versus ultrasonographic surveillance in congenitally dislocatable hips. Lancet 1990;336:1553.

119. Gardiner HM, Clarke NM, Dunn PM. A sonographic study of the morphology of the preterm neonatal hip. J Pediatr Orthop 1990;10:633.

120. Gardner E, Gray D. Prenatal development of the human hip joint. Am J Anat 1950;87:163.

121. Garvey M, Donoghue VB, Gorman WA, et al. Radiographic screening at four months of infants at risk for congenital hip dislocation. J Bone Joint Surg [Br] 1992;74:704.

122. Getz B. The hip in Lapps and its bearing on the problem of congenital dislocation. Acta Orthop Scand Suppl 1955;22:

123. Gotoh E, Ando M. The pathogenesis of femoral head deformity in congenital dislocation of the hip. Experimental study of the effects of articular interpositions in pigs. Clin Orthop 1993;288:303.

124. Graf R. The diagnosis of congenital hip-joint dislocation by the ultrasonic compound treatment. Arch Orthop Traumatol Surg 1980;97:117.

125. Graf R. Hip sonography in infancy. Procedure and clinical significance. Fortschr Med 1985;103:62.

126. Graham S, Westin GW, Dawson E, Oppenheim WL. The Chiari osteotomy. A review of 58 cases. Clin Orthop 1986;208:249.

127. Greenhill BJ, Hugosson C, Jacobsson B, Ellis RD. Magnetic resonance imaging study of acetabular morphology in developmental dysplasia of the hip. J Pediatr Orthop 1993;13:314.

128. Gregosiewicz A, Wosko I. Risk factors of avascular necrosis in the treatment of congenital dislocation of the hip. J Pediatr Orthop 1988;8:17.

129. Grill F, Bensahel H, Canadell J, et al. The Pavlik harness in the treatment of congenital dislocating hip: report on a multicenter study of the European Paediatric Orthopaedic Society. J Pediatr Orthop 1988;8:1.

130. Guidera KJ, Einbecker ME, Berman CG, et al. Magnetic resonance imaging evaluation of congenital dislocation of the hips. Clin Orthop 1990;261:96.

131. Guille JT, Forlin E, Kumar SJ, MacEwen GD. Triple osteotomy of the innominate bone in treatment of developmental dysplasia of the hip. J Pediatr Orthop 1992;12:718.

132. Hadley NA, Brown TD, Weinstein SL. The effect of contact pressure elevations and aseptic necrosis on the long-term outcome of congenital hip dislocation. J Orthop Res 1990;8:504.

133. Hadlow V. Neonatal screening for congenital dislocation of the hip. A prospective 21-year survey. J Bone Joint Surg [Br] 1988;70:740.

134. Hamanishi C, Tanaka S, Yamamuro T. The Spitzy shelf operation for the dysplastic hip. Retrospective 10 (5–25) year study of 124 cases. Acta Orthop Scand 1992;63:273.

135. Hansson LI, Olsson TH, Selvik G, Sunden G. A roentgen stereophotogrammetric investigation of innominate osteotomy (Salter). Acta Orthop Scand 1978;49:68.

136. Hansson G, Nachemson A, Palmen K. Screening of children with congenital dislocation of the hip joint on the maternity wards in Sweden. J Pediatr Orthop 1983;3:271.

137. Harcke HT, Lee MS, Sinning L, et al. Ossification center of the infant hip: sonographic and radiographic correlation. AJR 1986;147:317.

138. Harcke HT, Kumar SJ. The role of ultrasound in the diagnosis and management of congenital dislocation and dysplasia of the hip. J Bone Joint Surg [Am] 1991;73:622.

139. Harcke HT. Imaging in congenital dislocation and dysplasia of the hip. Clin Orthop 1992;281:22.

140. Harris NH, Lloyd-Roberts GC, Gallien R. Acetabular development in congenital dislocation of the hip with special reference to the indications for acetabuloplasty and pelvic or femoral realignment osteotomy. J Bone Joint Surg [Br] 1975;57:46.

141. Harris NH. Acetabular growth potential in congenital dislocation of the hip and some factors upon which it may depend. Clin Orthop 1976;119:99.

142. Harris WH, Bourne RB, Oh I. Intra-articular acetabular labrum: a possible etiological factor in certain cases of osteoarthritis of the hip. J Bone Joint Surg [Am] 1979;61:510.

143. Harris WH. Etiology of osteoarthritis of the hip. Clin Orthop 1986;213:20.

144. Harris IE, Dickens R, Menelaus MB. Use of the Pavlik harness for hip displacements. Clin Orthop 1992;281:29.

145. Harrison TJ. The growth of the pelvis in the rat—a mensoral and morphological study. J Anat 1958;92:236.

146. Harrison TJ. The influence of the femoral head on pelvic growth and acetabular form in the rat. J Anat 1961;95:127.

147. Hass J. Congenital dislocation of the hip. Springfield, IL: Charles C Thomas, 1951.

148. Heikkila E. Congenital dislocation of the hip in Finland. An epidemiologic analysis of 1035 cases. Acta Orthop Scand 1984;55:125.

149. Heikkila E. Comparison of the Frejka pillow and the von Rosen splint in treatment of congenital dislocation of the hip. J Pediatr Orthop 1988;8:20.

150. Heinrich SD, Missinne LH, MacEwen GD. The conservative management of congenital dislocation of the hip after walking age. Clin Orthop 1992;281:34.

151. Henderson RS. Osteotomy for unreduced congenital dislocation of the hip in adults. J Bone Joint Surg [Br] 1970;52:468.

152. Hernandez RJ. Concentric reduction of the dislocated hip. Computed-tomographic evaluation. Radiology 1984;150:266.

153. Hernandez RJ, Cornell RG, Hensinger RN. Ultrasound diagnosis of neonatal congenital dislocation of the hip. J Bone Joint Surg [Br] 1994;76:539.

154. Herold HZ. Avascular necrosis of the femoral head in children under the age of three. Clin Orthop 1977;126:193.

155. Herold HZ. Unilateral congenital hip dislocation with contralateral avascular necrosis. Clin Orthop 1980;148:196.

156. Herring JA. Inadequate reduction of congenital dislocation of the hip (letter). J Bone Joint Surg [Am] 1982;64:153.

157. Hilgenreiner H. Aur Fruhdiagnose und Fruhbehandlungder angeborenen Huftgelenkuerrenkung. Med Klin 1925;21:1385.

158. Hinderaker T, Rygh M, Uden A. The von Rosen splint compared with Frejka pillow. A study of 408 neonatally unstable hip. Acta Orthop Scand 1992;63:389.

159. Hiranuma S, Higuchi F, Inoue A. Miyazaki M. Changes in the interposed capsule after Chiari osteotomy. An experimental study on rabbits with acetabular dysplasia. J Bone Joint Surg [Br] 1992;74:463.

160. Hoagland FT, Yau AC, Wong WL. Osteoarthritis of the hip and other joints in Southern Chinese in Hong Kong. J Bone Joint Surg [Am] 1973;55:545.

161. Hoaglund FT, Healey JH. Osteoarthrosis and congenital dysplasia of the hip in family members of children who have congenital dysplasia of the hip [published erratum appears in J Bone Joint Surg [Am] 1991;73:293]. J Bone Joint Surg [Am] 1990;72:1510.

162. Hogh J, MacNicol MF. The Chiari pelvic osteotomy. A long term review of clinical and radiographic results. J Bone Joint Surg [Br] 1987;69:365.

163. Ilfeld FW, Makin M. Damage to the capital femoral epiphysis due to Frejka pillow treatment. J Bone Joint Surg [Am] 1977;59:654.

164. Ilfeld FW, Westin GW. "Missed" or late-diagnosed congenital dislocation of the hip. A clinical entity. Isr J Med Sci 1980;16:260.

165. Ilfeld FW, Westin GW, Makin M. Missed or developmental dislocation of the hip. Clin Orthop 1986;203:276.

166. Ishii Y, Weinstein SL, Ponseti IV. Correlation between arthrograms and operative findings in congenital dislocation of the hip. Clin Orthop 1980;153:138.

167. Iverson LJ, Kalea V, Eberle C. Relative trochanteric overgrowth after ischemic necrosis in congenital dislocation of the hip. J Pediatr Orthop 1989;9:391.

168. Iwasaki K. Treatment of congenital dislocation of the hip by the Pavlik harness. Mechanism of reduction and usage. J Bone Joint Surg [Am] 1983;65:760.

169. Johnson ND, Wood BP, Jackman KV. Complex infantile and congenital hip dislocation: assessment with MR imaging. Radiology 1988;168:151.

170. Jones D. An assessment of the value of examination of the hip in the newborn. J Bone Joint Surg [Br] 1977;59:318.

171. Jones DA. Neonatal hip stability and the Barlow test. A study in stillborn babies. J Bone Joint Surg [Br] 1991;73:216.

172. Jones GT, Schoenecker PL, Dias LS. Developmental hip dysplasia potentiated by inappropriate use of the Pavlik harness. J Pediatr Orthop 1992;12:722.

173. Joseph K, MacEwen GD, Boos ML. Home traction in the management of congenital dislocation of the hip. Clin Orthop 1982;165:83.

174. Kahle WK, Anderson MB, Alpert J, et al. The value of preliminary traction in the treatment of congenital dislocation of the hip. J Bone Joint Surg [Am] 1990;72:1043.

175. Kalamchi A, MacEwen GD. Avascular necrosis following treatment of congenital dislocation of the hip. J Bone Joint Surg [Am] 1980;62:876.

176. Kalamchi A, Schmidt TL, MacEwen GD. Congenital dislocation of the hip. Open reduction by the medial approach. Clin Orthop 1982;169:127.

177. Kalamchi A. Modified Salter osteotomy. J Bone Joint Surg [Am] 1982;64:183.

178. Karadimas JE, Holloway GM, Waugh W. Growth of the proximal femur after varus-derotation osteotomy in the treatment of congenital dislocation of the hip. Clin Orthop 1982;162:61.

179. Kasser JR, Bowen JR, MacEwen GD. Varus derotation osteotomy in the treatment of persistent dysplasia in congenital dislocation of the hip. J Bone Joint Surg [Am] 1985;67:195.

180. Katz K, Yosipovitch Z. Medial approach open reduction without preliminary traction for congenital dislocation of the hip. J Pediatr Orthop [B] 1994;3:82.

181. Keret D, MacEwen GD. Growth disturbance of the proximal part of the femur after treatment for congenital dislocation of the hip. J Bone Joint Surg [Am] 1991;73:410.

182. Kernohan WG, Beverland DE, McCoy GF, et al. Vibration arthrometry. A preview. Acta Orthop Scand 1990;61:70.

183. Kernohan WG, Cowie GH, Mollan RA. Vibration arthrometry in congenital dislocation of the hip. Clin Orthop 1991;272:167.

184. Kernohan WG, Trainor B, Nugent G, et al. Low-frequency vibration emitted from unstable hip in human neonate. Clin Orthop 1993;288:214.

185. Klaue K, Sherman M, Perren SM, et al. Extra-articular augmentation for residual hip dysplasia. J Bone Joint Surg [Br] 1993;75:750.

186. Klisic P, Jankovic L. Combined procedure of open reduction and shortening of the femur in treatment of congenital dislocation of the hips in older children. Clin Orthop 1976;119:60.

187. Klisic P, Jankovic L, Basara V. Long-term results of combined operative reduction of the hip in older children. J Pediatr Orthop 1988;8:532.

188. Klisic PJ. Congenital dislocation of the hip—a misleading term: brief report. J Bone Joint Surg [Br] 1989;71:136.

189. Kohler A. The borderlands of the normal and early pathological in the Skiagram. In: Roentgenology. London: Bailliere, Tindall, & Cox, 1935.

190. Konishi N, Nagoya MD, Mieno T. Determination of acetabular coverage of the femoral head with use of a single anteroposterior radiograph. A new computerized technique. J Bone Joint Surg [Am] 1993;75:1318.

191. Kramer J, Schleberger R, Steffen R. Closed reduction by two-phase skin traction and functional splinting in mitigated abduction for treatment of congenital dislocation of the hip. Clin Orthop 1990;258:27.

192. Kumar SJ, MacEwen GD. The incidence of hip dysplasia with metatarsus adductus. Clin Orthop 1982;164:234.

193. Kumar SJ, MacEwen GD, Jaykumar AS. Triple osteotomy of the innominate bone for the treatment of congenital hip dysplasia. J Pediatr Orthop 1986;6:393.

194. Kutlu A, Memik R, Mutlu M, et al. Congenital dislocation of the hip and its relation to swaddling used in Turkey. J Pediatr Orthop 1992;12:598.

195. Labaziewicz L, Grudziak JS, Kruczynski J, et al. Combined one stage open reduction femoral osteotomy and Dega pelvic osteotomy for DDH. Presented at the American Academy of Orthopaedic Surgeons annual meeting, San Francisco, 1993.

196. Lack W, Windhager R, Kutschera H, Engel A. Chiari pelvic osteotomy for osteoarthritis secondary to hip dysplasia. J Bone Joint Surg [Br] 1991;73:229.

197. Lafferty CM, Sartoris DJ, Tyson R, et al. Acetabular alterations in untreated congenital dysplasia of the hip: computed tomography with multiplanar re-formation and three-dimensional analysis. J Comput Assist Tomogr 1986;10:84.

198. Lang P, Genant H, Steiger P, et al. Three-dimensional digital displays in congenital dislocation of the hip: preliminary experience. J Pediatr Orthop 1989;9:532.

199. Langenskjold A, Salenius P. Epiphysiodesis of the greater trochanter. Acta Orthop Scand 1967;38:199.

200. Langenskjold A, Paavilainen T. The effect of traction treatment on the results of closed or open reduction for congenital dislocation of the hip: a preliminary report. In: Tachdjian MO, ed. Congenital dislocation of the hip. New York: Churchill Livingstone, 1982.

201. Law EG, Heistad DD, Marcus ML, Mickelson MR. Effect of hip position on blood flow to the femur in puppies. J Pediatr Orthop 1982;2:133.

202. Le-Saout J, Kerboul B, Lefevre C, et al. Results of 56 acetabular shelf operations—with a long follow-up. Acta Orthop Belg 1985;51:955.

203. LeDamany P. La Luxation Congenitale de la Hanche. In: Etudes d'Anatomie Comparee d'Anthropogenie Normale et Pathologique, Deductions Therapeutique. Paris: Feliz Alcan, 1912.

204. Lee DY, Choi IH, Lee CK, Cho TJ. Assessment of complex hip deformity using three-dimensional CT image. J Pediatr Orthop 1991;11:13.

205. Lee J, Jarvis J, Uhthoff HK, Avruch L. The fetal acetabulum. A histomorphometric study of acetabular anteversion and femoral head coverage. Clin Orthop 1992;281:48.

206. Lehman WB, Grant AD, Nelson J, et al. Hospital for Joint Diseases' traction system for preliminary treatment of congenital dislocation of the hip. J Pediatr Orthop 1983;3:104.

207. Lempicki A, Wierusz-Kozlowska M, Kruczynski J. Abduction treatment in late diagnosed congenital dislocation of the hip. Follow-up of 1,010 hips treated with the Frejka pillow 1967–76. Acta Orthop Scand Suppl 1990;236:1.

208. Leveuf J. Results of open reduction of "true" congenital luxation of the hip. J Bone Joint Surg [Am] 1948;30:875.

209. Lindstrom JR, Ponseti IV, Wenger DR. Acetabular development after reduction in congenital dislocation of the hip. J Bone Joint Surg [Am] 1979;61:112.

210. Lloyd-Roberts GC. Osteoarthritis of the hip: a study of the clinical pathology. J Bone Joint Surg [Br] 1955;37:8.

211. Lloyd-Roberts GC, Harris NH, Chrispin AR. Anteversion of the acetabulum in congenital dislocation of the hip: a preliminary report. Orthop Clin North Am 1978;9:89.

212. Lloyd-Roberts GC. The role of femoral osteotomy in the treatment of congenital dislocation of the hip. In: Tachdjian MO, ed. Congenital dislocation of the hip. New York: Churchill Livingstone, 1982.

213. Lloyd-Roberts GC, Wetherill MH, Fraser M. Trochanteric advancement for premature arrest of the femoral capital growth plate. J Bone Joint Surg [Br] 1985;67:21.

214. Love BR, Stevens PM, Williams PF. A long-term review of shelf arthroplasty. J Bone Joint Surg [Br] 1980;62:321.

215. Ludloff K. The open reduction of the congenital hip dislocation by an anterior incision. Am J Orthrop Surg 1913;10:438.

216. MacKenzie IG, Seddon HJ, Trevor D. Congenital dislocation of the hip. J Bone Joint Surg [Br] 1960;42:689.

217. MacKenzie IG, Wilson JG. Problems encountered in the early diagnosis and management of congenital dislocation of the hip. J Bone Joint Surg [Br] 1981;38.

218. MacNicol MF. Results of a 25-year screening programme for neonatal hip instability. J Bone Joint Surg [Br] 1990;72:1057.

219. MacNicol MF, Makris D. Distal transfer of the greater trochanter. J Bone Joint Surg [Br] 1991;73:838.

220. Malvitz TA, Weinstein SL. Closed reduction for congenital dysplasia of the hip. Functional and radiographic results after an average of thirty years. J Bone Joint Surg [Am] 1994;76:1777.

221. Mankey MG, Arntz CT, Staheli LT. Open reduction through a medial approach for congenital dislocation of the hip. A critical review of the Ludloff approach in sixty-six hips. J Bone Joint Surg [Am] 1993;75:1334.

222. Marafioti RL, Westin GW. Factors influencing the results of acetabuloplasty in children. J Bone Joint Surg [Am] 1980;62:765.

223. Mardam-Bey TH, MacEwen GD. Congenital hip dislocation after walking age. J Pediatr Orthop 1982;2:478.

224. Marks DS, Clegg J, Al-Chalabi AN. Routine ultrasound screening for neonatal hip instability. Can it abolish late-presenting congenital dislocation of the hip? J Bone Joint Surg [Br] 1994;76:534.

225. Massie WK. Vascular epiphyseal changes in congenital dislocation of the hip. Results in adults compared with results in coxa plana and in congenital dislocation without vascular changes. J Bone Joint Surg [Am] 1951;33:284.

226. Mau H, Dorr WM, Henkel L, Lutsche J. Open reduction of congenital dislocation of the hip by Ludloff's method. J Bone Joint Surg [Br] 1971;53:1281.

227. McCluskey WP, Bassett GS, Mora-Garcia G, MacEwen GD. Treatment of failed open reduction for congenital dislocation of the hip. J Pediatr Orthop 1989;9:633.

228. McKibbin B. Anatomical factors in the stability of the hip joint in the newborn. J Bone Joint Surg [Br] 1970;63:148.

229. McKibbin B, Freedman L, Howard C, Williams LA. The management of congenital dislocation of the hip in the newborn. J Bone Joint Surg [Br] 1988;70:423.

230. Mclvin P, Johnston R, Ponseti IV. Untreated CDH: long-term follow-up. 1970;.

231. Mendes DG. The role of computerized tomography scan in preoperative evaluation of the adult dislocated hip. Clin Orthop 1981;161:198.

232. Mergen E, Adyaman S, Omeroglu H, et al. Medial approach open reduction for congenital dislocation of the hip using the Ferguson procedure. A review of 31 hips. Arch Orthop Trauma Surg 1991;110:169.

233. Milgram JW. Morphology of untreated bilateral congenital dislocation of the hips in a seventy-four-year-old man. Clin Orthop 1976;119:112.

234. Millis MB, Hall JE. Transiliac lengthening of the lower extremity. A modified innominate osteotomy for the treatment of postural imbalance. J Bone Joint Surg [Am] 1979;61:1182.

235. Millis MB, Murphy SB. Use of computed tomographic reconstruction in planning osteotomies of the hip. Clin Orthop 1992;274:154.

236. Millis MB, Kaelin AJ, Schluntz K, et al. Spherical acetabular osteotomy for treatment of acetabular dysplasia in adolescents and young adults. J Pediatr Orthop [B] 1994;3;47.

237. Mitchell GP. Chiari medial displacement osteotomy. Clin Orthop 1974;98:146.

238. Molina-Guerrero JA, Munuera-Martinez L, Esteban-Mugica B. Acetabular development in congenital dislocation on the hip. Acta Orthop Belg 1990;56:293.

239. Moll FK Jr. Capsular change following Chiari innominate osteotomy. J Pediatr Orthop 1982;2:573.

240. Monticelli G. Intertrochanteric femoral osteotomy with concentric reduction of the femoral head in treatment of residual congenital acetabular dysplasia. Clin Orthop 1976;119:48.

241. Monticelli G, Milella PP. Indications for treatment of congenital dislocation of the hip by the surgical medial approach. In: Tachdjian MO, ed. Congenital dislocation of the hip. New York: Churchill Livingstone, 1982.

242. Morel G. The treatment of congenital dislocation and subluxation of the hip in the older child. Acta Orthop Scand 1975;46:364.

243. Morin C, Harcke HT, MacEwen GD. The infant hip: real-time US assessment of acetabular development. Radiology 1985;157:673.

244. Morquende JA, Weinstein SL, Dolan L, Meyer M. DDH: results of treatment after reduction by an anteromedial surgical approach at a minimum four year follow-up. 1995 (in press).

245. Moseley CF. The biomechanics of the pediatric hip. Orthop Clin North Am 1980;11:3.

246. Mubarak S, Garfin S, Vance R, et al. Pitfalls in the use of the Pavlik harness for treatment of congenital dysplasia, subluxation and dislocation of the hip. J Bone Joint Surg [Am] 1981;63:1239.

247. Mubarak SJ, Beck LR, Sutherland D. Home traction in the management of congenital dislocation of the hips. J Pediatr Orthop 1986;6:721.

248. Murphy SB, Kijewski PK, Millis MB, Harless A. Acetabular dysplasia in the adolescent and young adult. Clin Orthop 1990;261:214.

249. Murray RO. The aetiology of primary osteoarthritis of the hip. Br J Radiol 1965;38:810.

250. Nakamura T, Yamaura M, Nakamitu S, Suzuki K. The displacement of the femoral head by rotational acetabular osteotomy. A radiographic study of 97 subluxated hips. Acta Orthop Scand 1992;63:33.

251. Nicholson JT, Kopell HP, Mattei FA. Regional stress angiography of the hip. A preliminary report. J Bone Joint Surg [Am] 1954;36:503.

252. Niethard FU, Carstens C. Results of intertrochanteric osteotomy in infant and adolescent hip dysplasia. J Pediatr Orthop, Part B 1994;3:9.

253. Ninomiya S, Tagawa H. Rotational acetabular osteotomy for the dysplastic hip. Clin Orthop 1984;247:127.

254. Ninomiya S. Rotational acetabular osteotomy for the severely dysplastic hip in the adolescent and adult. Clin Orthop 1989;247:127.

255. Nishina T, Saito S, Ohzono K, et al. Chiari pelvic osteotomy for osteoarthritis. The influence of the torn and detached acetabular labrum. J Bone Joint Surg [Br] 1990;72:765.

256. Nishiyama K, Sakamaki T, Okinaga A. Complications of Pemberton's pericapsular osteotomy. A report of two cases. Clin Orthop Rel Res 1990;254:205.

257. Noble TC, Pullan CR, Craft AW, Leonard MA. Difficulties in diagnosing and managing congenital dislocation of the hip. Br Med J 1978;2:620.

258. Noritake K, Yoshihashi Y, Hattori TTM. Acetabular development after closed reduction of congenital dislocation of the hip. J Bone Joint Surg [Br] 1993;75:737.

259. O'Brien T, Salter RB. Femoral head size in congenital dislocation of the hip. J Pediatr Orthop 1985;5:299.

260. O'Brien T. Growth-disturbance lines in congenital dislocation of the hip. J Bone Joint Surg [Am] 1985;67:626.

261. O'Brien T, Millis MB, Griffin PP. The early identification and classification of growth disturbances of the proximal end of the femur. J Bone Joint Surg [Am] 1986;68:970.

262. O'Brien T, Barry C. The importance of standardised radiographs when assessing hip dysplasia. Ir Med J 1990;83:159.

263. O'Sullivan GS, Goodman SB, Jones HH. Computerized tomographic evaluation of acetabular anatomy. Clin Orthop Rel Res 1992;277:175.

264. Ogden JA, Southwick WO. A possible cause of avascular necrosis complicating the treatment of congenital dislocation of the hip. J Bone Joint Surg [Am] 1973;55:1770.

265. Ogden JA. Anatomic and histologic study of factors affecting development and evolution of avascular necrosis in congenital hip dislocation. In: The hip: proceedings of the second annual meeting of the Hip Society. St. Louis: CV Mosby, 1974.

266. Ogden JA. Changing patterns of proximal femoral vascularity. J Bone Joint Surg [Am] 1974;56:941.

267. Ogden JA. Normal and abnormal circulation. In: Tachdjian MO, ed. Congenital dislocation of the hip. New York: Churchill Livingstone, 1982.

268. OHara JN, Bernard AA, Dwyer NS. Early results of medial approach open reduction in congenital dislocation of the hip: use before walking age. J Pediatr Orthop 1988;8:288.

269. OHara JN. Congenital dislocation of the hip: acetabular deficiency in adolescence (absence of the lateral acetabular epiphysis) after limbectomy in infancy. J Pediatr Orthop 1989;9:640.

270. Ortolani M. Nuovi Criteri Diagnostici Profilattico Correttvi. Bologna: Cappelli, 1948.

271. Ortolani M. Congenital hip dysplasia in the light of early and very early diagnosis. Clin Orthop 1976;119:6.

272. Osborne D, Effmann E, Broda K, Harrelson J. The development of the upper end of the femur with special reference to its internal architecture. Radiology 1980;137:71.

273. Palmen K. Preluxation of the hip joint: diagnosis and treatment in the newborn and the diagnosis of congenital dislocation of the hip joint in Sweden during the years 1948–1960. Acta Paediatr Scand Suppl 1961;129:1.

274. Palmen K. Prevention of congenital dislocation of the hip. The Swedish experience of neonatal treatment of hip joint instability. Acta Orthop Scand Suppl 1984;208:1.

275. Papavasiliou VA, Piggott H. Acetabular floor thickening and femoral head enlargement in congenital dislocation of the hip: lateral displacement of femoral head. J Pediatr Orthop 1983;3:22.

276. Pavlik A. Stirrups as an aid in the treatment of congenital dysplasias of the hip in children. J Pediatr Orthop 1989;9:157.

277. Pavlik A. The functional method of treatment using a harness with stirrups as the primary method of conservative therapy for infants with congenital dislocation of the hip, 1957 (classical article). Clin Orthop 1992;281:4.

278. Pellicci PM, Hu S, Garvin KL, et al. Varus rotational femoral osteotomies in adults with hip dysplasia. Clin Orthop 1991;272:162.

279. Pemberton PA. Pericapsular osteotomy of the ilium for treat-

ment of congenital subluxation and dislocation of the hip. J Bone Joint Surg [Am] 1965;87:65.

280. Perkins G. Signs by which to diagnose congenital dislocation of the hip, 1928 (classical article). Clin Orthop 1992;274:3.

281. Polanuer PA, Harcke HT, Bowen JR. Effective use of ultrasound in the management of congenital dislocation and/or dysplasia of the hip. Clin Orthop 1990;252:176.

282. Pompe Van Meerdervoort HF. Congenital musculoskeletal disorders in the South African Negro. J Bone Joint Surg [Br] 1977;59:257.

283. Ponseti IV, Frigerio ER. Results of treatment of congenital dislocation of the hip. J Bone Joint Surg [Am] 1959;41:823.

284. Ponseti IV. Morphology of the acetabulum in congenital dislocation of the hip. Gross, histological and roentgenographic studies. J Bone Joint Surg [Am] 1978;60:586.

285. Ponseti IV. Growth and development of the acetabulum in the normal child. Anatomical, histological and roentgenographic studies. J Bone Joint Surg [Am] 1978;60:575.

286. Pous JG, Camous JY, el-Blidi S. Cause and prevention of osteochondritis in congenital dislocation of the hip. Clin Orthop 1992;281:56.

287. Powell EN, Gerratana FJ, Gage JR. Open reduction for congenital hip dislocation: the risk of avascular necrosis with three different approaches. J Bone Joint Surg [Am] 1986;58:1000.

288. Pratt WB, Freiberger RH, Arnold WD. Untreated congenital hip dysplasia in the Navajo. Clin Orthop 1982;162:69.

289. Quinn RH, Renshaw TS, DeLuca PA. Preliminary traction in the treatment of developmental dislocation of the hip. J Pediatr Orthop 1994;14:636.

290. Rab GT. Preoperative roentgenographic evaluation for osteotomies about the hip in children. J Bone Joint Surg [Am] 1981;63:306.

291. Rabin DL, Barnett CR, Arnold WD, et al. Untreated congenital hip disease. A study of the epidemiology, natural history and social aspects of the disease in a Navajo population. Am J Public Health 1965;55:1.

292. Race C, Herring JA. Congenital dislocation of the hip: an evaluation of closed reduction. J Pediatr Orthop 1983;3:166.

293. Rális A, McKibbin B. Changes in shape of the human hip joint during its development and their relation to its stability. J Bone Joint Surg [Br] 1973;55:780.

294. Ramsey PS, Lasser S, MacEwen GD. Congenital dislocation of the hip: use of the child during the first 6 months of life. J Bone Joint Surg [Am] 1976;58:1000.

295. Rejholec M, Stryhal F, Rybka V, Popelka S. Chiari osteotomy of the pelvis: a long-term study. J Pediatr Orthop 1990;10:21.

296. Rejholec M, Stryhal F. Behavior of the proximal femur during the treatment of congenital dysplasia of the hip: a clinical long-term study. J Pediatr Orthop 1991;11:506.

297. Renshaw TS. Inadequate reduction of congenital dislocation of the hip. J Bone Joint Surg [Am] 1981;63:1114.

298. Reynolds DA. Chiari innominate osteotomy in adults. Technique, indications and contraindications. J Bone Joint Surg [Br] 1986;68:45.

299. Rombouts JJ, Kaelin A. Inferior (obturator) dislocation of the hip in neonates. A complication of treatment by the Pavlik harness. J Bone Joint Surg [Br] 1992;74:708.

300. Roose PE, Chingren GL, Klaaren HE, Broock G. Open reduction for congenital dislocation of the hip using the Ferguson procedure. A review of twenty-six cases. J Bone Joint Surg [Am] 1979;61:915.

301. Rosendahl K, Markestad T, Lie RT. Congenital dislocation of the hip: a prospective study comparing ultrasound and clinical examination. Acta Paediatr 1992;81:177.

302. Rush J. Chiari osteotomy in the adult: a long-term follow-up study. Aust N Z J Surg 1991;61:761.

303. Ruwi PA, Gage JR, Ozonoff MB, DeLuca PA. Clinical determi-

nation of femoral anteversion. J Bone Joint Surg [Am] 1992;74:820.

304. Salter RB, Field P. The effects of continuous compression on living articular cartilage. J Bone Joint Surg [Am] 1960;42:31.

305. Salter RB. Innominate osteotomy in treatment of congenital dislocation of the hip. J Bone Joint Surg [Br] 1961;43:72.

306. Salter RB. Role of innominate osteotomy in the treatment of congenital dislocation and subluxation of the hip in the older child. J Bone Joint Surg [Am] 1966;48:1413.

307. Salter R. Etiology, pathogenesis, and possible prevention of congenital dislocation of the hip. Can Med Assoc J 1968;98:933.

308. Salter RB, Kostiuk J, Dallas S. Avascular necrosis of the femoral head as a complication of treatment for congenital dislocation of the hip in young children: a clinical and experimental investigation. Can J Surg 1969;12:44.

309. Salter RB, Dubos J-P. The first fifteen years' personal experience with innominate osteotomy in the treatment of congenital dislocation and subluxation of the hip. Clin Orthop 1974;98:72.

310. Salter RB, Hansson G, Thompson GA. Innominate osteotomy in the management of residual congenital subluxation of the hip in young adults. Clin Orthop 1984;182:53.

311. Samani DJ, Weinstein SL. The pelvic tear-figure: a three-dimensional analysis of the anatomy and effects of rotation. J Pediatr Orthop 1994;14:650.

312. Scaglietti O, Calandriello B. Open reduction of congenital dislocation of the hip. J Bone Joint Surg [Br] 1962;44:257.

313. Scapinelli R, Ortolani M Jr. Open reduction (Ludloff approach) of congenital dislocation of the hip before the age of two years. Isr J Med Sci 1980;16:276.

314. Schoenecker PL, Bitz DM, Whiteside LA. The acute effect of position of immobilization on capital femoral epiphyseal blood flow. A quantitative study using the hydrogen washout technique. J Bone Joint Surg [Am] 1978;60:899.

315. Schoenecker PL, Lesker PA, Ogata K. A dynamic canine model of experimental hip dysplasia. Gross and histological pathology, and the effect of position of immobilization on capital femoral epiphyseal blood flow. J Bone Joint Surg [Am] 1984;66:1281.

316. Schoenecker PL, Strecker WB. Congenital dislocation of the hip in children. Comparison of the effects of femoral shortening and of skeletal traction in treatment. J Bone Joint Surg [Am] 1984;66:21.

317. Schofield CB, Smibert JG. Trochanteric growth disturbance after upper femoral osteotomy for congenital dislocation of the hip. J Bone Joint Surg [Br] 1990;72:32.

318. Schwartz D. Acetabular development after reduction of congenital dislocation of the hip—a follow-up study of fifty hips. J Bone Joint Surg [Am] 1965;47:705.

319. Severin E. Contribution to the knowledge of congenital dislocation of the hip. Acta Scand Chir [Suppl] 1941;63:84.

320. Sharp IK. Acetabular dysplasia. The acetabular angle. J Bone Joint Surg [Br] 1961;43:269.

321. Sherlock DA, Gibson PH, Benson MK. Congenital subluxation of the hip. A long-term review. J Bone Joint Surg [Br] 1985;67:390.

322. Siffert RS. Patterns of deformity of the developing hip. Clin Orthop Rel Res 1981;160:14.

323. Simons GW. A comparative evaluation of the current methods for open reduction of the congenitally displaced hip. Orthop Clin North Am 1980;11:161.

324. Skirving AP, Scadden WJ. The African neonatal hip and its immunity from congenital dislocation. J Bone Joint Surg [Br] 1979;339.

325. Smith WS, Ireton RJ, Coleman CR. Sequelae of experimental dislocation of a weight-bearing ball-and-socket joint in a young growing animal. J Bone Joint Surg [Am] 1958;40:1121.

326. Smith WS, Coleman CR, Olix ML, Slager RF. Etiology of congenital dislocation of the hip. J Bone Joint Surg [Am] 1963;45:491.

327. Smith JT, Matan S, Coleman SS, et al. The predictive value of the development of the acetabular teardrop figure in developmental dysplasia of the hip. Presented at the American Academy of Orthopaedic Surgeons annual meeting, San Francisco, 1993.

328. Solomon L. Patterns of osteoarthritis of the hip. J Bone Joint Surg [Br] 1976;58:176.

329. Somerville EW. A long-term follow-up of congenital dislocation of the hip. J Bone Joint Surg [Br] 1978;60:25.

330. Sosna A, Rejholec M, Rybka V, et al. Long-term results of Ludloff's repositioning method. Acta Chir Orthop Traumatol Cech 1990;57:213.

331. Staheli LT. Surgical management of acetabular dysplasia. Clin Orthop Rel Res 1991;264:111.

332. Staheli LT, Chew DE. Slotted acetabular augmentation in childhood and adolescence. J Pediatr Orthop 1992;12:569.

333. Stanisavljevic S. Diagnosis and treatment of congenital hip pathology in the newborn. Baltimore: Williams & Wilkins, 1964.

334. Steel HH. Triple osteotomy of the innominate bone. J Bone Joint Surg [Am] 1973;55:343.

335. Steel HH. Triple osteotomy of the innominate bone. Clin Orthop 1977;122:116.

336. Stone MH, Clarke NM, Campbell MJ, et al. Comparison of audible sound transmission with ultrasound in screening for congenital dislocation of the hip. Lancet 1990;336:421.

337. Strayer LM. Embryology of the human hip joint. Yale J Biol Med 1943;16:13.

338. Strayer LM Jr. Embryology of the human hip joint. Clin Orthop 1971;74:221.

339. Stulberg SD, Harris WH. Acetabular dysplasia and development of osteoarthritis of the hip. In: The hip: proceedings of the second open meeting of the Hip Society. St. Louis: CV Mosby, 1974.

340. Surgeons Advisory Statement, American Academy of Orthopaedic Surgeons. ''CDH'' should be ''DDH.'' Park Ridge, IL: American Academy of Orthopaedic Surgeons, 1991.

341. Sutherland DH, Moore M. Clinical and radiographic outcome of patients treated with double innominate osteotomy for congenital hip dysplasia. J Pediatr Orthop 1991;11:143.

342. Suzuki S, Yamamuro T. Avascular necrosis in patients treated with the Pavlik harness for congenital dislocation of the hip. J Bone Joint Surg [Am] 1990;72:1048.

343. Suzuki S. Ultrasound and the Pavlik harness in CDH. J Bone Joint Surg [Br] 1993;75:483.

344. Swenningsen S, Apalset K, Terjesen T. Osteotomy for femoral anteversion. Complications in 95 children. Acta Orthop Scand 1989;60:401.

345. Synder M, Zwierzchowski H. One-stage hip reconstruction with Dega's transiliacal osteotomy in the treatment of congenital hip dislocation in children. Beitr Orthop Traumatol 1990;37:571.

346. Terjesen T, Bredland T, Berg V. Ultrasound screening of the hip joints. Acta Orthop Scand 1988;59(Suppl 227):93.

347. Terjesen T, Runden T, Tangerud A. Ultrasonography and radiography of the hip in infants. Acta Orthop Scand 1989;60:651.

348. Terjesen T, Bredland T, Berg V. Ultrasound for hip assessment in the newborn. J Bone Joint Surg [Br] 1989;71:767.

349. Terjesen T. Femoral head coverage evaluated by ultrasonography in infants and children. Mapfre Med 1992;3(Suppl 1):41.

350. Thomas IH, Dunin AJ, Cole WG, Menelaus MB. Avascular necrosis after open reduction for congenital dislocation of the hip: analysis of causative factors and natural history. J Pediatr Orthop 1989;9:525.

351. Tonnis D. Normal values of the hip joint for the evaluation of x-rays in children and adults. Clin Orthop 1976;119:39.

352. Tonnis D. An evaluation of conservative and operative methods in the treatment of congenital hip dislocation. Clin Orthop 1976;119:76.

353. Tonnis D. A new technique of triple osteotomy for acetabular dysplasia in older children and adults. In: Abstracts of the 14th world congress of the Society of International Chirurgiae Orthopaedicae et Traumatologiae, Kyoto, 1978.

354. Tonnis D, Behrens K, Tscharani F. A modified technique of the triple pelvic osteotomy: early results. J Pediatr Orthop 1981;1:241.

355. Tonnis D. Triple osteotomy close to the hip joint. In: Tachdjian MO, ed. Congenital dislocation of the hip. New York: Livingstone, 1982:555.

356. Tonnis D, ed. Congenital dysplasia and dislocation of the hip in children and adults. New York: Springer-Verlag, 1987.

357. Tonnis D, Kasperczyk WJ. Acetabuloplasty and acetabular rotation. In: Freeman M, Reynolds D, eds. Osteoarthritis in the young adult hip. Edinburgh: Churchill Livingstone, 1988.

358. Tonnis D. Surgical treatment of congenital dislocation of the hip. Clin Orthop 1990;258:33.

359. Tonnis D, Arning A, Bloch M, et al. Triple pelvic osteotomy. J Pediatr Orthop 1994;3:54.

360. Tredwell SJ. Neonatal screening for hip joint instability. Its clinical and economic relevance. Clin Orthop 1992;281:63.

361. Trueta RJ, ed. Studies of the development and decay of the human frame. Philadelphia: WB Saunders, 1988.

362. Uden A, Lindberg H, Josefsson PO, et al. Sonography in the diagnosis of neonatal hip instability. Acta Orthop Scand 1988;59(Suppl 227):94.

363. Vare VB. The anatomy of the pelvic tear figure. J Bone Joint Surg [Am] 1952;34:167.

364. Viere RG, Birch JG, Herring JA, et al. Use of the Pavlik harness in congenital dislocation of the hip. An analysis of failures of treatment. J Bone Joint Surg [Am] 1990;72:238.

365. Visser JD. Functional treatment of congenital dislocation of the hip. Acta Orthop Scand Suppl 1984;206:1.

366. von Rosen S. Diagnosis and treatment of congenital dislocation of the hip in the newborn. J Bone Joint Surg [Br] 1962;44:284.

367. Voutsinas SA, MacEwen GD, Boos ML. Home traction in the management of congenital dislocation of the hip. Arch Orthop Trauma Surg 1984;102:135.

368. Wagner H. The hip: proceedings of the fourth open scientific meeting of the Hip Society. St. Louis: CV Mosby, 1976.

369. Wagner H. Spherical acetabular osteotomy: long-term results. In: Fourth Harvard medical school course on osteotomy of the hip and knee. Boston: Harvard University Press, 1992.

370. Walker G. Problems in the early recognition of congenital hip dislocation. Br Med J 1971;3:147.

371. Walker JM. Congenital hip disease in Cree-Ojibwa population: a retrospective study. Can Med Assoc J 1977;116:501.

372. Walker JM. Morphological variants in the human fetal hip joint. Their significance in congenital hip disease. J Bone Joint Surg [Am] 1980;62:1073.

373. Walker JM, Goldsmith CH. Morphometric study of the fetal development of the human hip joint: significance for congenital hip disease. Yale J Biol Med 1981;54:411.

374. Walker JM. Histological study of the fetal development of the human acetabulum and labrum: significance in congenital hip disease. Yale J Biol Med 1981;54:255.

375. Watanabe RS. Embryology of the human hip. Clin Orthop 1974;98:8.

376. Waters P, Kurica K, Hall J, Micheli LJ. Salter innominate osteotomies in congenital dislocation of the hip. J Pediatr Orthop 1988;8:650.

377. Wedge JH, Wasylenko MJ. The natural history of congenital dislocation of the hip: a critical review. Clin Orthop 1978;137:154.

378. Wedge JH, Wasylenko MJ. The natural history of congenital disease of the hip. J Bone Joint Surg [Br] 1979;334.

379. Wedge JH, Munkacsi I, Loback D. Anteversion of the femur and idiopathic osteoarthorosis of the hip. J Bone Joint Surg [Am] 1989;71:1040.

380. Weiner DS. Congenital dislocation of the hip associated with congenital muscular torticollis. Clin Orthop 1976;121:163.

381. Weiner DS, Hoyt WA Jr, Odell HW. Congenital dislocation of the hip. The relationship of premanipulation traction and age to avascular necrosis of the femoral head. J Bone Joint Surg [Am] 1977;59:306.

382. Weinstein SL, Ponseti IV. Congenital dislocation of the hip. J Bone Joint Surg [Am] 1979;61:119.

383. Weinstein SL. The medial approach in congenital dislocation of the hip. Isr J Med Sci 1980;16:272.

384. Weinstein SL. Natural history of congenital hip dislocation [CDH] and hip dysplasia. Clin Orthop 1987;225:62.

385. Weinstein SL. Closed versus open reduction of congenital hip dislocation in patients under 2 years of age. Orthopedics 1990;13:221.

386. Weinstein SL. Congenital hip dislocation. Long-range problems, residual signs, and symptoms after successful treatment. Clin Orthop 1992;281:69.

387. Weintroub S, Green I, Terdiman R, Weissman SL. Growth and development of congenitally dislocated hips reduced in early infancy. J Bone Joint Surg [Am] 1979;61:125.

388. Wenger DR. Congenital hip dislocation: techniques for primary open reduction including femoral shortening. Instr Course Lect 1989;38:343.

389. Westin GW, Ilfeld FW, Provost J. Total avascular necrosis of the capital femoral epiphysis in congenital dislocated hips. Clin Orthop 1976;119:93.

390. White RE Jr, Sherman FC. The hip-shelf procedure. A long-term evaluation. J Bone Joint Surg [Am] 1980;62:928.

391. Wiberg G. Studies on dysplastic acetabula and congenital subluxation of the hip joint. Acta Chir Scand 1939;83(Suppl 58):1.

392. Wiberg G. Shelf operation in congenital dysplasia of the acetabulum and in subluxation and dislocation of the hip. J Bone Joint Surg [Am] 1953;35:65.

393. Wientroub S, Boyde A, Chrispin AR, Lloyd-Roberts GC. The use of stereophotogrammetry to measure acetabular and femoral anteversion. J Bone Joint Surg [Br] 1981;209.

394. Wilkinson JA. A postnatal survey for the congenital displacement of the hip. J Bone Joint Surg [Br] 1972;54:40.

395. Williamson DM, Glover SD, Benson MK. Congenital dislocation of the hip presenting after the age of three years. A long-term review. J Bone Joint Surg [Br] 1989;71:745.

396. Windhager R, Pongracz N, Schonecker W, Kotz R. Chiari osteotomy for congenital dislocation and subluxation of the hip. Results after 20 to 34 years follow-up. J Bone Joint Surg [Br] 1991;73:890.

397. Winkler W, Weber A. Osteotomy of the pelvis (Chiari) [author's translation]. Z Orthop 1977;115:167.

398. Wynne-Davies R. Acetabular dysplasia and familial joint laxity: two etiological factors in congenital dislocations of the hip. J Med Genet 1970;7:315.

399. Yamamuro T, Doi H. Diagnosis and treatment of congenital dislocation of the hip in newborns. J Jpn Orthop Assoc 1965;39:492.

400. Yamamuro T, Ishida K. Recent advances in the prevention, early diagnosis, and treatment of congenital dislocation of the hip in Japan. Clin Orthop 1984;184:34.

401. Zionts LE, MacEwen GD. Treatment of congenital dislocation of the hip in children between the ages of one and three years. J Bone Joint Surg [Am] 1986;68:829.

402. Zlati M, Radojevi B, Lazovi D, Lupulovi I. Late results of Chiari's pelvic osteotomy. A follow-up of 171 adult hips. Int Orthop 1988;12:149.

Lovell & Winter's Pediatric Orthopaedics, fourth edition,
edited by Raymond T. Morrissy and Stuart L. Weinstein.
Lippincott–Raven Publishers, Philadelphia © 1996.

Chapter

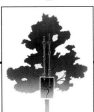

24

Legg-Calvé-Perthes Syndrome

Stuart L. Weinstein

HISTORY

Legg-Calvé-Perthes syndrome is a disorder of the hip in young children. The condition was described independently, in 1910, by Legg,[225] Calvé,[42] Perthes,[292] and Waldenström.[381,382] In the late 19th century, however, Hugh Owen Thomas,[370] Baker[6] and Wright[405] described patients with supposed hip joint infections that resolved without surgery whose histories were consistent with Legg-Calvé-Perthes syndrome. Maydl,[252] in 1897, reported this condition and thought it was a related condition of congenitally dislocated hip.[132]

In 1909, Arthur Legg presented a paper on five children with a limp after injury. This paper was published in 1910. He called this condition an "obscure affectation of the hip" and postulated that pressure secondary to injury caused flattening of the femoral head.[225] In that same year, Calvé reported 10 cases of a noninflammatory self-limiting condition that healed with flattening of the weight-bearing surface. He postulated that the cause of this condition was an abnormal or delayed osteogenesis. He reported coxa vara and increased femoral head size in these patients, and on physical examination, all of the patients had decreased abduction.[42] Perthes simultaneously re-

ported six cases of what he termed "arthritis deformans juveniles." He postulated that this was an inflammatory condition.[292] In his description of the condition, Waldenström postulated that the disease was a form of tuberculosis.[381,382]

Perthes was the first to describe the pathologic and histologic description of the disorder.[293] He reported on a 9-year-old boy with the symptoms for 2 years. Examination of the portion of the excised head revealed numerous cartilage islands throughout and "strings" connecting the joint cartilage and the physeal plate. Perthes noted the marrow spaces to be widened with fatty infiltration; he saw no evidence of inflammation. He believed that the cartilage islands were new and that this was an osteochondritis, not a tubercular, process.[293] Schwartz,[345] an associate of Perthes, described the pathologic changes in a 7-year-old boy with a 2-year history of symptoms and reported similar findings. Waldenström[383] suggested the use of the term *coxa plana* to make the description of the disease consistent with other hip deformities, such as coxa vara and coxa valga. Sundt[362,363] published the first monograph on Legg-Calvé-Perthes syndrome, reporting on 66 cases and the pathology of the condition. The essential feature in all of his cases was the cartilaginous islands in the epiphysis. Sundt attributed the disease to a "osteodystrophy due to dysendocrinia of a hereditary disposition." He believed that those people so predisposed would get Legg-Perthes disease after they had an injury to the hip (i.e., infection or trauma). Sundt was the first person to introduce the modern concept of the "susceptible child."

Phemister,[298] reporting on the curettage findings of a 10-year-old child with an 8-month history of symptoms, described areas of bone necrosis, granulation tissue, old bone with new bone formation, and osteoclasts. He interpreted these findings as an inflammatory and infectious process. In 1922, Riedel[321] reported on two cases and presented the histology. He described the thickening of the articular cartilage and noted that the junction between the bone and the articular cartilage was filled with blood. He also noted that the physeal plate was destroyed and that there were many cartilage rests. Dead bone was surrounded by a rich granulation tissue, and many giant cells were present. He also noted that farther away from the main disease process the marrow was fibrotic with inflammatory infiltrates. Riedel was the first to notice that there were blastic and clastic changes at the same time working on the same bone trabeculae. In his second specimen he found regeneration of the cartilage in the subchondral area, cell atrophy, and some inflammatory cells. That same year Waldenström[384] proposed the first radiographic classification of the disease process, based on 22 patients followed until the completion of growth. Since then, most of the orthopaedic literature has centered on the etiologic and epidemiologic and prognostic factors in Legg-Calvé-Perthes syndrome and follow-up of various treatment modalities.[398]

EPIDEMIOLOGY AND ETIOLOGY

Legg-Calvé-Perthes syndrome occurs most commonly in the age range of 4 to 8 years,[406] but cases have been reported in children from 2 years of age to the late teenage years. It is more common in boys than girls by a ratio of 4 or 5 to 1.[8] The incidence of bilaterality has been reported as 10% to 12%.[406] Although the incidence of a positive family history in patients with Legg-Calvé-Perthes syndrome ranges from 1.6% to 20%[113,132,139,143,284,379,387,406,407] there is no evidence that Legg-Calvé-Perthes syndrome is an inherited condition.[149]

Wynne-Davies and Gormley[406] reported on a series of 310 index patients with Legg-Calvé-Perthes syndrome. They noted that of the children of affected index patients, only 2% had Legg-Calvé-Perthes syndrome. In this series all twins were discordant, including one monozygotic pair. Eleven percent had abnormal birth presentations, including breech and

transverse lie compared with the 2% to 4% incidence that would be expected in the general population. There is an increased incidence of Legg-Calvé-Perthes syndrome in later born children, particularly the third to the sixth child, and a higher percentage in lower socioeconomic groups.[144,146] Parental age of affected patients is higher than in the general population.[142,406,407]

Legg-Calvé-Perthes syndrome is more common in certain geographic areas, particularly in urban rather than rural communities, giving rise to the suspicion of a nutritional cause, possibly a trace element deficiency.[7,62,64,142,144–146,290] There is also a recently reported strong association (33% of affected patients) of Legg-Calvé-Perthes disease with the psychological profiles associated with attention deficit hyperactivity disorder.[236] Malloy and colleagues[243,244] noted that the birth weight was lower in affected children. Harrison reported that children with Legg-Calvé-Perthes syndrome lagged behind their chronologic age, and 89% of the involved individuals had delayed bone age.[152] Ralston demonstrated that this delay in skeletal maturation averaged 21 months, but that during the healing stages of the disease there would be recovery of height and weight through increased growth velocity.[48,108,314] There may be certain racial factors in that there is increased frequency of Legg-Calvé-Perthes syndrome in Japanese people, other Asians, Eskimos, and central Europeans and a decreased frequency in native Australians, Americans Indians, Polynesians, and blacks.[64,131,132,307]

There is considerable evidence of anthropometric abnormalities in children with Legg-Calvé-Perthes syndrome. Cameron and Izatt[44] reported that affected boys were 1 inch shorter and affected girls 3 inches shorter compared with normal nonaffected children. Burwell and colleagues[34,35,37] and others[144,214] demonstrated that affected children are smaller in all dimensions except for head circumference and shorter in the distal portions of the extremities as opposed to the proximal. The short stature of the patient affected with the disorder at a young age tends to correct during adolescence, whereas those affected at an older age tend to be small throughout life.[407] Burwell and colleagues demonstrated an abnormality of growth hormone–dependent somatomedin in boys with Legg-Calvé-Perthes syndrome, whereas Tanaka and colleagues,[368] Fisher and associates,[113] and Kitsugi and colleagues[206] reported contrary results.

Growth hormone regulates postnatal skeletal development. The effects of growth hormone on postnatal skeletal development are mediated, in part, by the somatomedins (insulin-like growth factors).[277] Somatomedin C (IGF1) is the principle somatomedin responsible for postnatal skeletal bone maturation.[277] Plasma IGF1 levels have been reported to be significantly reduced in affected children during the first 2 years after the diagnosis of Perthes disease. These alterations were accompanied by a tendency toward growth arrest and impaired weight gain. This is accompanied by an acceleration in growth and weight gain during the healing stages of the disease. In plasma, nearly all IGF1 is bound to specific binding proteins. However, the major binding protein (IGFBP3) levels are normal during the first 2 years after the diagnosis of Perthes disease.[278,280] Low levels of circulating IGF1 and failure of IGF1 to increase normally during the prepubertal years in patients with Perthes disease in conjunction with reportedly normal growth hormone levels raise the possibility of decreased responsiveness of growth plate chondrocytes and hepatocytes.[277] The combination of moderately reduced IGF1 levels with normal IGFBP3 has been reported in normal variant short stature children. The skeletal maturation delay and retarded bone age reported in patients with Perthes disease in conjunction with the findings listed earlier could be considered a retention of the infantile hormone pattern.[280] Malnutrition is one factor that leads to low IGF levels, and this could interrelate to the reportedly increased incidence of Perthes disease in low-income families. The disproportionate skeletal development affecting the distal portions of the body is a tendency toward infantile body proportions. This correlates with the reduced IGF1 levels in the face of normal binding proteins.[279]

There is increased incidence of hernia in patients with Legg-Calvé-Perthes syndrome and their first-degree relatives. There is also an increased incidence of minor congenital abnormalities in affected patients.[50,55,139,140]

The etiology of Legg-Calvé-Perthes syndrome remains unknown. Many etiologic theories have been proposed. In the early part of this century most investigators thought that it was a disease of an inflammatory or infectious nature.[5,111,212,292,381,382] Phemister[297,298] believed the disease was an infectious process, although cultures were negative. Axhausen[5] believed it was caused by bacillary embolism in which the infection either was not manifested or was too weak and healed quickly. As late as 1975, Matsoukas[250] demonstrated an association between Legg-Calvé-Perthes syndrome and prenatal rubella.

Until the 1950s, trauma was considered by many investigators to be the cause of or a significant contributing factor in Perthes disease.[15,30,78,79,161,225,228,230] As with most childhood orthopaedic conditions a significant number of patients may relate an episode of trauma to the onset of symptoms.

Many authors, particularly eastern European investigators, thought that Legg-Calvé-Perthes syndrome was of congenital origin and that there was a relation between this disease and congenitally dislocated hips.[32,41,47,126,167,182,350] Glimcher[129] proposed that cytotoxic

agents of external or endogenous origin may be responsible for bone cell death. At one time, Perthes disease was believed to be related to hypothyroidism[63,102,127]; this has since been disapproved.[194,304] Recent reports demonstrate moderately increased plasma concentrations of free thyroxin and free triiodothyronine in Perthes disease patients compared with controls.[279] The aforementioned findings and the reduced levels of IGF1 reported in the early disease stages and their causative effect on Perthes disease is yet to be determined. They do, however, provide additional evidence that growth-related systemic abnormalities exist in patients with Legg-Calvé-Perthes syndrome.[279]

Transient synovitis has been thought by many investigators to be a precursor to the condition. Gershuni[121] reported that 25% of children with benign transient synovitis developed Legg-Calvé-Perthes disease, whereas Jacobs reported three cases of Legg-Calvé-Perthes disease out of 25 patients with acute transient synovitis. Review of the literature reveals that an average of 1% to 3% of patients with a history of transient synovitis later develops Legg-Calvé-Perthes syndrome.[156,189,190,273,401,402] Chuinard[67] and Craig and colleagues[78,79] have proposed that excessive femoral neck anteversion is a causative factor in the development of Legg-Calvé-Perthes syndrome.

Most current etiologic theories involve vascular embarrassment. The blood supply to the proximal femur has been elucidated by many authors. The terminology used in the literature varies. However, there are three main sources of blood to the proximal femur: an extracapsular arterial ring, the ascending cervical (retinacular branches) vessels, and the artery of the ligamentum teres (Fig. 24-1).[68] The extracapsular ring is formed mostly by the medial and lateral femoral circumflex vessels. This ring gives rise to the ascending cervical branches, which are extracapsular, and these in turn give rise to the metaphyseal and epiphyseal branches. The anterior portion of the extracapsular ring is formed primarily by the lateral femoral circumflex artery. The posterior, lateral, and medial aspects of the ring are formed by the medial femoral circumflex artery. Chung found that the greatest volume of blood flow to the femoral head comes through the lateral ascending cervical vessel (the termination of the medial femoral circumflex artery), which crosses the capsule in the posterior trochanteric fossa. Both Trueta and Pinto de Lima[373,374] and Chung[68] demonstrated that the anterior vascular anastomotic network (see Fig. 24-1) is much less extensive than the posterior anastomotic network, particularly in specimens from patients aged 3 to 10 years, which correlates with the age range of Legg-Calvé-Perthes syndrome. Chung also demonstrated that the anterior anastomotic network was incomplete more often in boys, which correlates with male gender predominance in Legg-Calvé-Per-

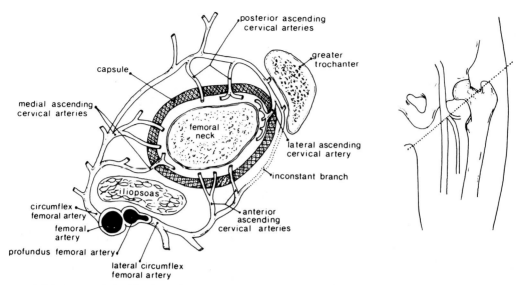

FIGURE 24-1. The blood supply to the normal proximal femur in a child. (Adapted from Chung SMK. The arterial supply of the developing proximal end of the human femur. J Bone Joint Surg [Am] 1976;58:961.

thes syndrome. Ogden[285] found vessels crossing the physeal plate in some of his specimens, but Chung disagreed, believing that the vessels did not actually cross the plate but passed through the peripheral perichondral fibrocartilaginous complex.

Interruption of the blood supply to the femoral head in Perthes disease was first demonstrated in 1926, when Konjetzny[212] showed obliterative vascular thickening in a pathologic specimen. Théron[369] used selective angiograms to demonstrate obstruction of the superior retinacular artery in patients with Legg-Calvé-Perthes syndrome. In 1973, Sanches and colleagues[340] proposed the second infarction theory. They experimentally infarcted the femoral head of animals labeled with tetracycline. They were unable to produce a typical histologic picture of Legg-Calvé-Perthes syndrome with only a single infarction. With a second infarction, however, they were able to show a more characteristic histologic picture of Legg-Calvé-Perthes syndrome. Inoue and colleagues[178] later correlated this double infarction theory with human histologic material. Clinical correlation for this theory is supported by reports of recurrent Perthes disease (Fig. 24-2).[196,248] Salter and Thompson[335,337] proposed that Legg-Calvé-Perthes syndrome is a complication of aseptic necrosis and that a fracture manifested radiographically by a subchondral radiolucent zone initiates the resorptive phase. Kleinman and Bleck[207] demonstrated increased blood viscosity in a group of patients with Legg-Calvé-Perthes syndrome, possibly leading to decreased blood flow to the femoral epiphysis. Vascular embarrassment caused by intraosseous venous hypertension and venous obstruction has been demonstrated by several authors.[149,159,366]

PATHOGENESIS

Histologically, changes seen in Legg-Calvé-Perthes syndrome must be put in perspective. Few human specimens have been studied, and each specimen studied only represents a stage in the disease process. Most specimens are from curettage or core biopsies, which show only one portion of the involved head at a time.

In the developing normal human femoral head, the secondary center of ossification is covered by cartilage that is composed of three zones (Fig. 24-3). The superficial zone has the morphologic properties of adult articular cartilage. Beneath this is the zone of epiphyseal cartilage, which is histochemically different. The zone becomes thinner as the skeleton matures and the epiphyseal bone enlarges in size. Underneath the epiphyseal cartilage is a thin zone, formed by small clusters of cartilage cells that hypertrophy and degenerate. Capillaries penetrate this zone from below, and bone forms at a much slower rate than in the metaphysis.[305]

Histologic changes of the epiphyseal and physeal cartilage of patients with Legg-Calvé-Perthes syndrome (Figs. 24-4 and 24-5) were described as early as 1913. These and current studies demonstrate that the superficial zone of the epiphyseal cartilage covering the affected femoral head is normal but thickened. In the middle layer of the epiphyseal cartilage, however, two types of abnormalities are seen: areas of extreme hypercellularity with the cells varying in size and shape and often arranged in clusters, and areas containing a loose fibrocartilaginous-like matrix. These abnormal areas in the epiphyseal cartilage have

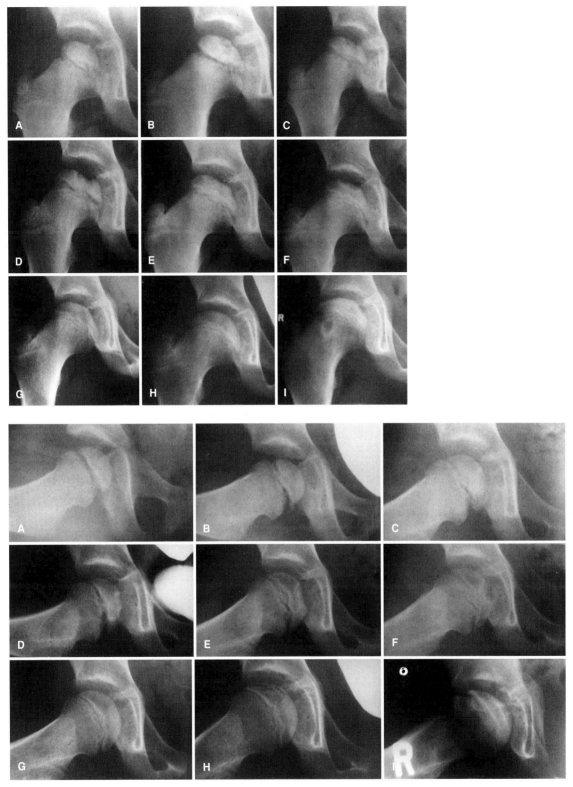

FIGURE 24-2. A 4-year, 8-month-old girl was treated for left hip Perthes disease (late fragmentation phase) beginning in January 1983. Anteroposterior (*top*) and Lauenstein (*bottom*) views of the right hip at different stages. January 1983 to December 1987. (**A**) View of the right hip at the time of initial presentation with no signs of involvement (January 1983). (**B**) Early involvement, patient still asymptomatic (September 1983). **C,D,E,F:** Progressive healing of the right femoral epiphysis at May 1984, August 1984, May 1985, and November 1985, respectively. (**G**) Femoral head was completely healed by December 1986. (**H**) Recurrent changes in the density of the femoral head and a subchondral fracture that involves less than 50% of the head (Catterall type II) was seen in June 1987. (**I**) Complete involvement of the ossific nucleus (Catterall type IV) with diffuse metaphyseal reaction and cysts in December 1987. (From Martinez AG, Weinstein SL. Recurrent Legg-Calvé-Perthes disease. Case report and review of the literature. J Bone and Joint Surg [Am] 1991;73:1081.)

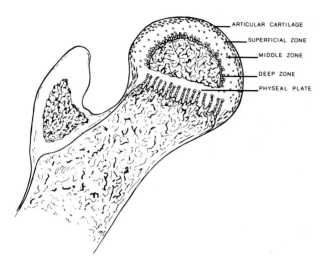

ARTICULAR CARTILAGE

SUPERFICIAL ZONE

MIDDLE ZONE

DEEP ZONE

PHYSEAL PLATE

FIGURE 24-3. Proximal femur in a child.

different histochemical and ultrastructural properties from normal cartilage and fibrocartilage. Areas of small secondary ossification centers are evident with bony trabeculae of uneven thickness forming directly on the abnormal cartilage matrix.[59,57,93,184,303,305] The superficial and middle layers of epiphyseal cartilage are nourished by synovial fluid and continue to proliferate, whereas only the deepest layer of the epiphyseal cartilage is dependent on epiphyseal blood supply and is affected by the ischemic process.[16,17,23,57,218,255,257,305,342]

The physeal plate in Legg-Calvé-Perthes syndrome shows evidence of cleft formation with amorphis debris and extravasation of blood. In the metaphyseal region endochondral ossification is normal in some areas, but in others the proliferating cells are separated by a fibrillated cartilaginous matrix that does not calcify (see Fig. 24-5). The cells in these areas do not degenerate but continue to proliferate without endochondral ossification leading to tongues of cartilage extending into the metaphysis as bone growth proceeds in adjoining areas.[56,169,184,303,305,352]

Catterall has demonstrated thickening, abnormal staining, sporadic calcification, and diminished evidence of ossification in the deep zone of the articular cartilage of the unaffected hip. He also demonstrated the physeal plate in these unaffected hips to be thinner than normal with irregular cell columns and cartilage masses remaining unossified in the primary spongiosa.[56]

Some of the preceding cartilage changes have been seen in other epiphyseal plates, such as the greater trochanter and the acetabulum.[119] In the human specimens described by Ponseti[303] the physeal plate lesions were long standing in view of the fact there was only necrotic bone in the femoral head and no evidence of repair. Catterall and colleagues reported similar cartilaginous lesions in a patient with

Catterall group 1 disease, in which there is no sequestrum formation (Fig. 24-6).[57,184] The various reported physeal plate and epiphyseal plate lesions resemble those lesions produced by Ponseti in rats by the administration of aminonitrils.[302] These epiphyseal, as well as physeal, plate changes in conjunction with the unusual and precarious blood supply of the proximal femur make the femoral head vulnerable to the effects of physeal plate disruption.

Skeletal surveys of patients with Legg-Calvé-Perthes syndrome confirm the histologic abnormalities by demonstrating irregularities of ossification in other epiphyses, especially Köhlers disease of the navicular.[5,303,351] Harrison and Blakemore,[153] studying 153 consecutive patients with unilateral Legg-Calvé-Perthes disease, found that 48% had contour irregularities in the contralateral normal capital epiphysis compared with 10% of matched controls. Aire and colleagues[2] demonstrated that the unaffected hip showed anterior and lateral flattening at the time of diagnosis of the affected hip. These data suggest that Legg-Calvé-Perthes disease is a generalized process affecting other epiphyses, and therefore should not be referred to as a disease but should be called Legg-Calvé-Perthes syndrome.

Disorganization of the physeal plate together with minimal trauma may interrupt the continuity of retinacular vessels causing necrosis.[303,305] This, in conjunction with the aforementioned epidemiologic, histologic, and radiologic data, supports the belief that Legg-Calvé-Perthes syndrome may be a localized manifestation of a generalized disorder of epiphyseal cartilage in the susceptible child.[48,58,55,132,149,155,214,305]

Radiographic Stages

Radiographically, Legg-Calvé-Perthes syndrome can be classified into four stages: initial, fragmentation, reossification, and healed. In the initial stage[185,384] one of the first signs of this condition is failure of the femoral ossific nucleus to increase in size because of lack of blood supply (Fig. 24-7). The affected femoral head appears smaller than the opposite unaffected ossific nucleus. Widening of the medial joint space, as initially described by Waldenström (see Fig. 24-7),[384,385] is another early radiographic finding. Widening has been theorized by some to be caused by synovitis. Others have proposed that this finding is secondary to decreased head volume because of necrosis and collapse and secondary increase in blood flow to the soft tissue parts, such as the ligamentum teres and pulvinar causing the head to displace laterally.[185,191] Synovitis may be present in patients with Perthes disease, but the medial joint space widening is probably an apparent radiographic phenomenon secondary to epiphyseal cartilage hypertrophy (Fig. 24-8).

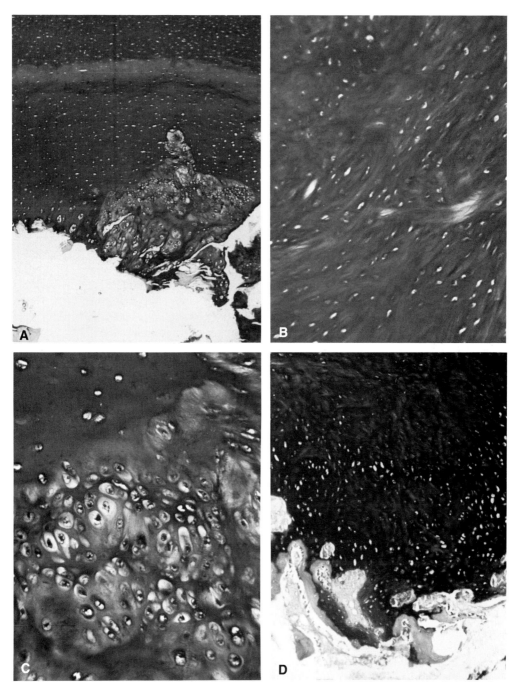

FIGURE 24-4.   (A) Superficial-zone cartilage and epiphyseal cartilage of the femoral head. The superficial-zone cartilage is normal and is alcian-blue–positive. The epiphyseal cartilage stains with periodic acid–Schiff; but only the perilacunar rims stain with alcian-blue. In the epiphyseal cartilage, there is an area of disorganized abnormal alcian-blue–positive cartilage. (Alcian-blue with 0.6-molar magnesium chloride; Original magnification ×25). (B) Abnormal area of epiphyseal cartilage. The matrix has a fibrillated appearance and is strongly alcian-blue–positive. (Alcian-blue with 0.6-molar magnesium chloride; Original magnification ×100). (C) Junction between the normal and abnormal epiphyseal cartilage. Normal cartilage is periodic acid–Schiff–positive, whereas the abnormal cartilage is very cellular and retains alcian-blue positivity at high concentrations of magnesium chloride. (Alcian blue with 0.7-molar magnesium chloride; Original magnification ×165). (D) Extensive area of abnormal epiphyseal cartilage in the femoral head. Bone seems to form directly on th abnormal cartilage. Abnormal cartilage retains intense alcian-blue positivity at a high concentration of magnesium chloride but loses the alcianophilia and becomes strongly positive to periodic acid–Schiff at the bone–cartilage junction (Alcian blue with 0.7-molar magnesium chloride, periodic acid–Schiff, and Weigert hematoxylin stains; original magnification ×40; From Ponseti IV, Maynard JA, Weinstein SL et al. Legg-Calvé-Perthes disease. Histochemical and ultrastructural observations of the epiphyseal cartilage and physis. J Bone Joint Surg [Am] 1983;65:797.)

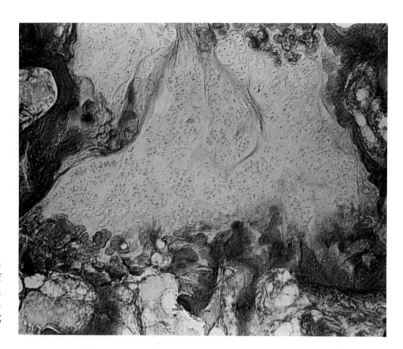

FIGURE 24-5. Photomicrograph showing a large area of cartilage in between the bone trabeculae of the femoral neck. (Original magnification ×80; from Ponseti IV. Legg-Perthes disease. Observations on pathological changes in two cases. J Bone Joint Surg [Am] 1956;38:739.)

The subchondral radiolucent zone (i.e., crescent sign) first described by Waldenström[385,386] and later popularized by Caffey[38] is the third of the early signs of Legg-Calvé-Perthes syndrome (Fig. 24-9; see Fig. 24-2). According to Salter and associates,[333,337] this radiographic finding results from a subchondral stress fracture, and the extent of this zone determines the extent of the necrotic fragment.

In the initial stage, the physeal plate is irregular and the metaphysis is blurry and radiolucent[126] (Fig. 24-10). The femoral ossific nucleus appears radiodense.[20] This relative increased radiodensity may be caused by osteopenia of the surrounding bone[317,388] or an increase in the mass of bone in the area.

The second radiographic stage is called the fragmentation phase.[185,384] Radiographically the repair aspects of the disease become more prominent (see Fig. 24-10B). The bony epiphysis begins to fragment, and there are areas of increased radiolucency and increased radiodensity. Increased radiodensity at this stage may be caused by new bone forming on old bone[21,199,202,256,299] and thickening of existing trabeculae.[202]

The third radiographic stage is the reparative or reossification phase.[185,384] Roentgenographically normal bone density returns, with radiodensities appearing in areas that were formerly radiolucent. Alternations in the shape of the femoral head and neck become apparent (see Fig. 24-10B).

The final stage is the healed phase. In this stage the proximal femur is left with any residual deformity from the disease and the repair process (see Fig. 24-10B). Legg-Calvé-Perthes syndrome cannot be compared with aseptic necrosis following fracture of the neck of the femur or traumatic dislocations of the hip in the young child. In this situation, the vascular insult to the femoral head usually heals rapidly without going through the prolonged stages of fragmentation and repair that are seen in children with Legg-Calvé-Perthes disease.[29,138,305]

Pathogenesis of Deformity

The head deformities that occur in Legg-Calvé-Perthes syndrome come about in many ways. First, there is growth disturbance in the epiphyseal and physeal plates. In the physeal plate this may result in premature closure with resultant deformity, such as a central physeal arrest, causing a shortened neck and trochanteric overgrowth (Fig. 24-11).[9,28] The repair process itself may cause physical compaction resulting from structural failure and displacement of tissue elements.[129] During the healing process the femoral head will deform according to the asymmetric repair process and the applied stresses. The molding action of the acetabulum during new bone formation also may be a factor.[74,203] With deformity of the femoral head, the acetabulum, particularly its lateral aspect, is deformed secondarily.

The articular cartilage of the femoral head shows changes in shape secondary to the disease process itself. The deepest layer of the articular cartilage is nourished by the subchondral blood supply. This layer is often devitalized in Legg-Calvé-Perthes syndrome.[16,17,23,57,218,257] The superficial layers that are nourished by synovial fluid continue to proliferate, causing an increase in the thickness of the articular cartilage. With trabecular collapse and fracture and articular

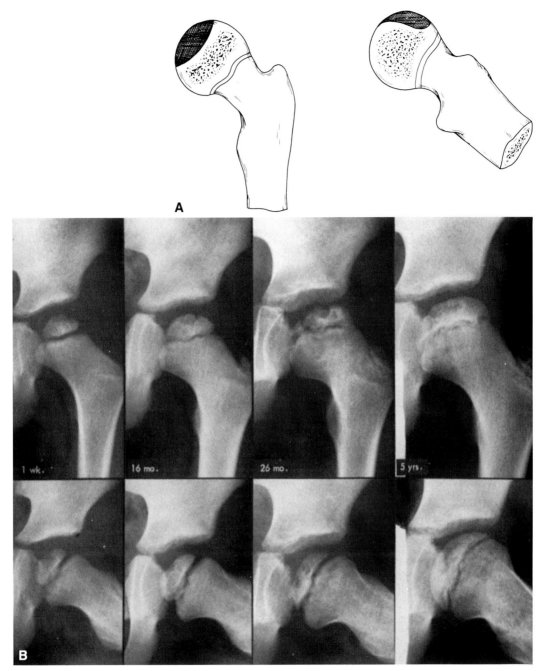

FIGURE 24-6. (A) Catterall group 1 disease shows anterior head involvement with no evidence of sequestrum or of a subchondral fracture line or metaphyseal abnormalities. (B) Catterall group 1 disease 1 week to 5 years after symptom onset.

cartilage overgrowth significant head deformities develop that are manifested clinically by loss of abduction and rotation (see Fig. 24-8).

The source of vessel ingrowth is under debate. Many investigators[16,17,160] demonstrated that the new blood vessels arise from the metaphysis and the metaphyseal periosteum and penetrate between the epiphysis and the joint cartilage into the epiphysis. Other investigators have shown metaphyseal vessels penetrating the physeal plate into the epiphysis.[24,285] When the blood supply of the subchondral area is restored, it generally comes from the periphery and moves to the center, restoring endochondral ossification at the periphery first and causing asymmetric growth (Fig. 24-12).[257] In addition, there is abnormal ossification of the disorganized matrix of the epiphyseal cartilage. Finally, there is periosteal bone growth and reactivation of the physeal plate along the femoral

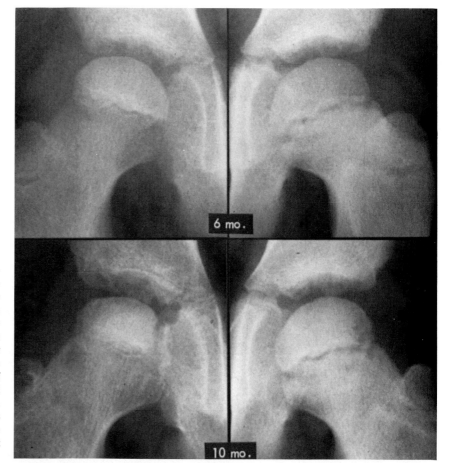

FIGURE 24-7. Anteroposterior roentgenogram of a hip in a patient who developed Legg-Calvé-Perthes disease. On the initial film, taken 6 months after symptom onset, the right ossific nucleus is smaller than the left, and the medial joint space is widened. Note also the retained density of the ossific nucleus compared with the normal hip and the relative osteopenia of the viable bone of the proximal femur and pelvis. Ten months after symptom onset, the evolution of the radiographic changes are seen. (From Weinstein SL. Legg-Calvé-Perthes disease. Instr Course Lect 1983;32:272.)

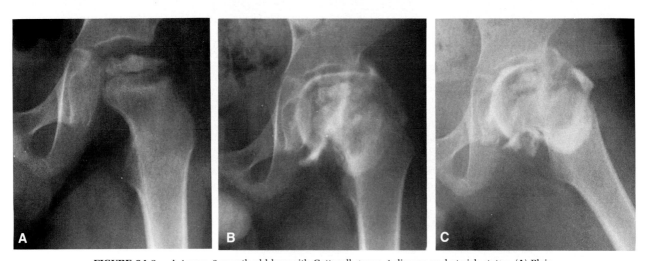

FIGURE 24-8. A 4-year, 9-month-old boy with Catterall group 4 disease and at risk status. (**A**) Plain x-ray film. (**B**) Arthrogram in neutral abduction, adduction, and rotation. There is enlargement and flattening of cartilaginous femoral head, and the lateral margin of the acetabulum is deformed by the femoral head. (**C**) Arthrogram in abduction and slight external rotation. The femoral head hinges on the lateral edge of the acetabulum, further deforming the lateral acetabulum. Slight pooling of dye is seen medially.

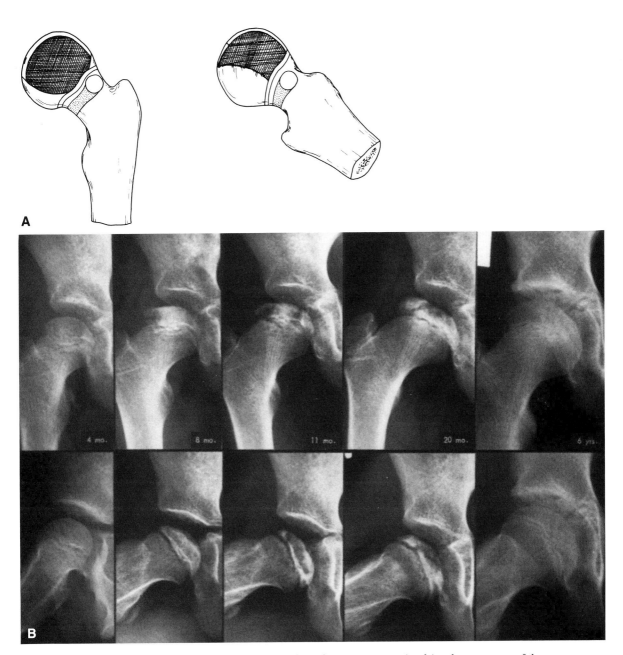

FIGURE 24-9. (A) Catterall group 3 disease shows large sequestrum involving three quarters of the head. The junction between the involved and the uninvolved portions is sclerotic. Metaphyseal lesions are diffuse, particularly anterolaterally, and the subchondral fracture line extends to the posterior half of the epiphysis. The lateral column is involved. (B) Catterall group 3 disease 4 months to 6 years after symptom onset. Note involvement of the lateral pillar as well as subchondral radiolucent zone on the radiograph taken 8 months after onset of symptoms.

neck with abnormally long cartilage columns leading to coxa magna and a widened femoral neck.[303,305]

The actual deformity that develops is profoundly influenced by the duration of the disease. This in turn is proportional to the extent of the epiphyseal involvement, the age of disease onset, the remodeling potential of the patient, and the stage of disease when treatment is initiated. An additional factor is the type of treatment.[391,394,395,397]

Patterns of Deformity

Four patterns of a residual deformity result from Legg-Calvé-Perthes syndrome: coxa magna, premature physeal arrest patterns, irregular head formation, and osteochondritis dissecans.[27,28] Coxa magna (see Fig. 24-10B) develops with ossification of the hypertrophied articular cartilage and also from reactivation of the physeal plate along the femoral neck. This also occurs

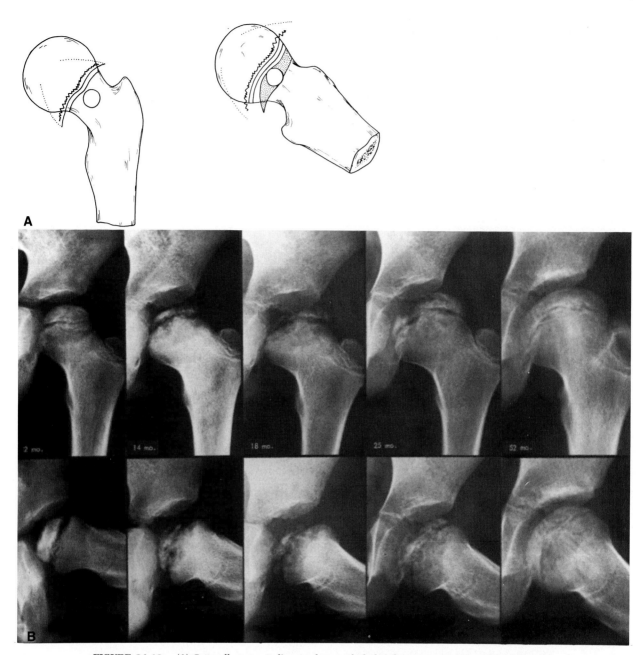

FIGURE 24-10. (A) Catterall group 4 disease shows whole-head movement with either diffuse or central metaphyseal lesions and posterior remodeling of the epiphysis. (B) Catterall group 4 disease 2 months to 52 months following onset of symptoms. Note the stage: 4 months—fragmentation; 18 months—early reossification; 25 months—late reossification; 52 months—healed. Note also the growth arrest line and evidence of reactivation of the growth plate along the femoral neck.

in conjunction with periosteal new bone formation along the femoral neck.

Premature physeal plate closure generally leads to one of two patterns of arrest: central or lateral. In the central arrest pattern the femoral neck is short and the epiphysis is relatively round (see Fig. 24-11). There is trochanteric overgrowth and mild acetabular deformity. In the lateral arrest pattern the femoral head is tilted externally (Fig. 24-13). There is also trochanteric overgrowth. The epiphysis is oval with a corresponding acetabular deformity.[27,28]

The irregular head may occur secondary to certain patterns of physeal arrest but it also may be an iatrogenic deformity from attempts at "containment" of a noncontainable head (Fig. 24-14). After the femoral head becomes deformed and is no longer containable within the acetabulum, the only motion that is allowed is in the flexion and extension plane with abduction leading to hinging on the lateral edge of the acetabulum. This hinge abduction causes acetabular and secondary head deformity (see Fig. 24-8).[54,137]

The fourth and least common (3% incidence) re-

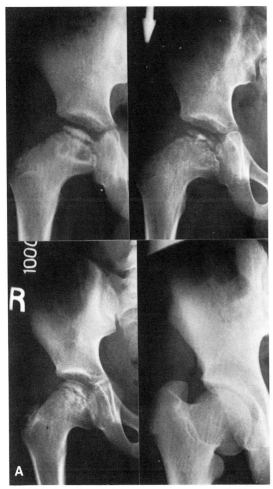

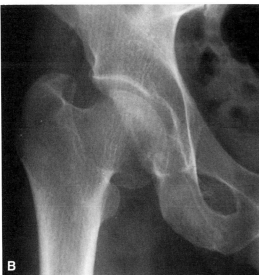

FIGURE 24-11.   (A) A 6-year-old boy with Catterall group 4 disease. Age 6 years, 2 months—fragmentation stage (*Upper left*). Age 6 years, 9 months—early reossification stage (*Upper Right*). Age 8 years, 9 months—healed (*Lower left*). Age 16 years, 2 months—skeletally mature (*Lower right*). Patient healed with central physeal arrest pattern. (B) A 51-year old patient at 45-year follow-up. He is asymptomatic and has a full range of motion (Iowa Hip Rating 95 of 100 points). At maximal fragmentation (*upper right*) the hip is classified as a Catterall group 4, Salter-Thompson type B, and a lateral pillar type C.

sidual deformity that occurs in Legg-Calvé-Perthes syndrome is osteochondritis dissecans (Fig. 24-15). This usually occurs with the late onset of disease and with prolonged ineffectual repair.[27,28,222,229,327]

NATURAL HISTORY

The formulation of disease treatment requires that the treating physician knows what happens to the patient without treatment (natural history) and what prognostic factors lead to an adverse outcome. The treating physician must determine which of these adverse prognostic factors can be affected by treatment. A treatment plan is then initiated, and long-term follow-up determines whether treatment favorably alters the natural history of the disease over the long term. The fundamental problem in developing treatment plans for patients with Legg-Calvé-Perthes syndrome is the paucity of natural history data.[51,55,65,281,361]

Catterall[51] compared 46 untreated hips of Murley and Lloyd-Roberts with a matched control group of 51 hips treated by a weight-relieving caliper. The average age at diagnosis was 4 years and 6 months, and the average follow-up was 10 years and 5 months with a range of 4 to 18 years. The patients were evaluated according to the grading system of Sundt, which requires some subjective assessments.[364] The 10-year average follow-up in this series is too short to determine outcomes of patients and thus the natural history of the disease, because most patients with childhood hip disease do well regardless of radiographic appearance in their early years.[410,179,253,271] In addition, no data are presented on interrater or intrarater reliability of the outcome criteria.

Catterall also reported on 97 untreated patients gathered from around the British isles. The average follow-up in this series was only 6 years, and results were graded according to the system of Sundt.[364] The outcomes of this group of patients (Table 24-1) are widely quoted in the literature as a comparison for outcomes of various treatment modalities. Unfortu-

TABLE 24-1.   Results of 95 Untreated Hips

	GOOD	FAIR	POOR
Group 1	27 ⎤ 92%	1	0
Group 2	25 ⎦	6	2 ⎤
Group 3	4	7	11 ⎥ 91%
Group 4	0	4	10 ⎦
Total	56 (57%)	18 (19%)	23 (24%)

From Catterall A. Legg-Calve-Perthes disease. Edinburgh: Churchill Livingstone, 1982.

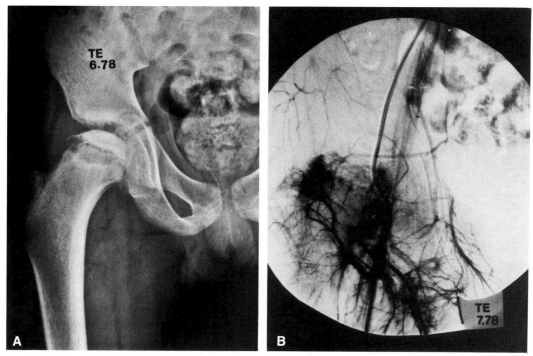

FIGURE 24-12. **(A)** A 12-year-old boy with total head involvement in the early fragmentation stage of the disease. **(B)** Subtraction arteriogram demonstrating the avascularity of the central portion of the head with increased vascularity at the periphery. (Courtesy of J. G. Pous, Montpellier, France.)

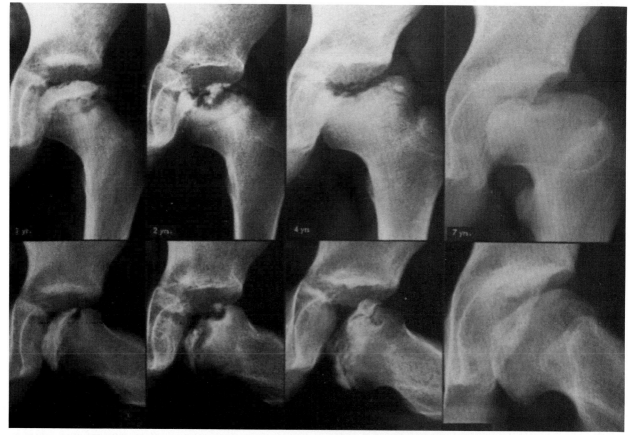

FIGURE 24-13. A 7-year follow-up from presentation in a patient with Catterall group 4 disease who had a lateral growth arrest pattern. At maximal fragmentation the radiographic classification would be Salter Thompson B and Lateral Pillar C. (From Weinstein SL. Perthes disease, an overview. Curr Orthop 1988;2:181.)

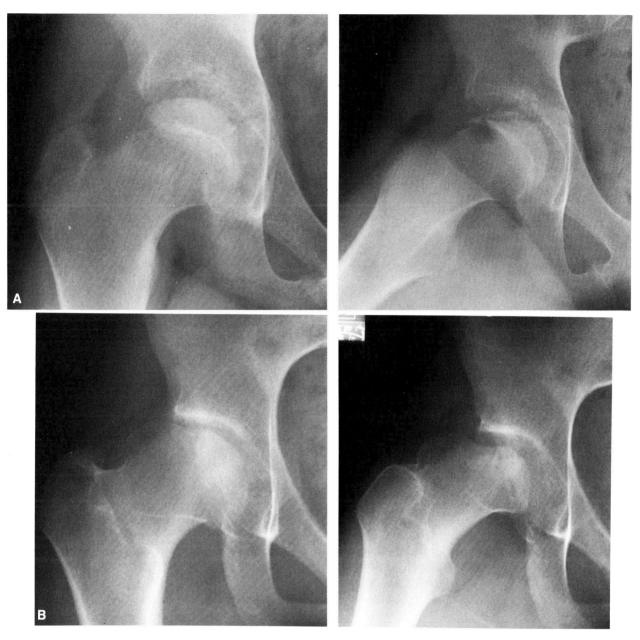

FIGURE 24-14. An 11-year, 3-month-old female with Catterall group 3 disease had a noncontainable head yet was treated for a long time in an abduction brace. (**A**) Anteroposterior radiograph in early fragmentation stage (*left*) and Lauenstein radiograph in early fragmentation stage (*right*). (**B**) At age 14 years, the patient is skeletally mature and has an irregular femoral head. Anteroposterior radiograph (*left*) and Lauenstein radiograph (*right*). (From Weinstein SL: Perthes disease, an overview. Curr Orthop 1988;2:181.)

nately, very few articles in the literature use the same grading system for outcomes, and the follow-up of this group is too short to be defined as natural history.

The only other article on natural history in the literature other than untreated cases included in various series of treated patients[361] is not a natural history study but a study of patients treated by different methods from three centers. The study attempted to establish a relation between residual deformity and degenerative joint disease and to identify clinical and radiographic factors in the active phase of disease

that would be predictive of hip deformity and degenerative joint disease. Decision making with reference to treatment is difficult because of the lack of true long-term natural history data.

Long-Term Follow-Up Results

Although there is little information available on natural history, there are many long-term follow-up studies of patients with Legg-Calvé-Perthes syndrome. The long-term studies that are available suffer from the faults

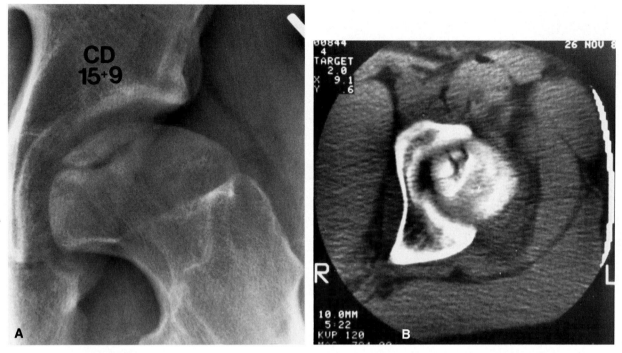

FIGURE 24-15.   (A) A 15-year-old boy with onset of disease at 8.5 years of age returned to the physician with pain and synovitis. Anteroposterior radiographs demonstrate osteochondritis of the femoral head. (B) Computed tomographic scan shows multiple fragments that appear as one on the radiograph.

of retrospective long-term reviews in that most series contain only small numbers of patients with many of the original pool of patients not traced; original radiographs often are not available. Many of the longer series contain patients diagnosed in the years 1910 to 1940, when little was known about the disease, prognostic factors, and radiographic classifications. In most series patients are combined regardless of the extent of epiphyseal involvement, age of disease onset, age at the beginning of treatment, and stage of the disease at treatment initiation. Various treatment modalities are combined in many series, and control groups generally are absent. Because of these inherent problems, different grading systems being used to judge clinical and radiographic end results, and lack of interrater and intrarater reliability data it is difficult to compare and contrast the various reported series. Despite these shortcomings, a great deal has been learned about the prognosis in Legg-Calvé-Perthes syndrome.

In reviewing long-term follow-up studies it is apparent that results can improve with time as remodeling potential continues until the end of growth (see Figs. 24-9 and 24-10).[55,165] Mose wrote that "for a precise prognosis, conclusions from any measurements ought not be made before the patient reaches the age of 16 when growth stops."[271] Reviews of the outcomes of treatment modalities prior to skeletal maturity must be viewed as preliminary reports.

Twenty to 40 years after the onset of symptoms the majority (70%–90%) of patients with Legg-Calvé-Perthes syndrome are active and pain free. Most patients maintain a good range of motion despite the fact that few patients have normal appearing radiographs. Clinical deterioration and symptoms of increasing pain, decreasing range of motion, and loss of function are observed only in those patients with flattened irregular heads at the time of primary healing and in those patients with premature physeal closure, as evidenced by neck shortening, head deformity, and trochanteric overgrowth (see Fig. 24-13).[394]

Danielson and Hernborg[85] reported a 33-year follow-up on 35 patients. Twenty-eight of the 35 patients were free of pain, with 34 of 35 functioning without restrictions. In a 34-year follow-up, Hall[141] reported 71% satisfactory results in 209 cases. Perpich and colleagues[291] reported a 30-year follow-up of 37 patients. The average Iowa Hip Rating was 93 of a possible 100 points. Eighty-five percent of the patients had a good clinical result despite the fact that only 33% had spherical femoral heads, as rated by the Mose Sphericity Scale[271] (Fig. 24-16). Forty-three percent of the patients had a poor Mose rating; however, of these patients 76% had a good clinical result.

Ratliff[315] followed 34 cases for an average of 30 years and noted that 80% were fully active and pain free, whereas only 40% were roentgenographically normal. He followed 16 of these hips an additional 11

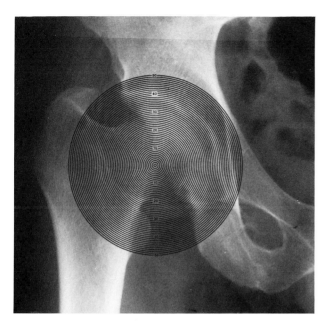

FIGURE 24-16. Mose sphericity scale.

years[316] and noted that despite the fact that only one third had good anatomic results "deterioration rarely occurred and many patients had no pain and normal activity."

Yrjonen followed 96 patients (106 hips), all of whom had noncontainment treatment, for an average of 35 years. At maturity 61% had a poor result by the Mose criteria. In a final follow-up 48% had evidence of degenerative joint disease. However, at an average 35-year follow-up only 4% had had a total hip arthroplasty with an additional 13% having significant clinical

symptoms to warrant arthroplasty.[410] Ippolito and colleagues[179] reported on 61 patients with an average follow-up of 25 years. Only 19% of the patients had a poor result as measured by the Iowa Hip Rating at final follow-up. Cumming and colleagues[82] reported on 82 patients with 95 involved hips treated by prolonged frame recumbency with an average follow-up of 38 years. Only 10% of the patients had required arthroplasty at follow-up with an additional 10% having symptoms significant enough to warrant arthroplasty.

Gower and Johnston[133] reported on 30 nonoperated hips with an average 36-year follow-up. This series is representative of the 20 to 40 year long-term series reported to that time. The average Iowa Hip Rating for these 30 patients was 91 points. The typical patient had minimal shortening, absent or mild hip pain and minimal, and no functional impairment with respect to job and activities of daily living. Ninety-two percent of the patients had Iowa Hip Ratings above 80 points, and only 8% of the patients had undergone arthroplasty.

In follow-up studies beyond 40 years, hip function begins to deteriorate. In another study of the Iowa group of patients at 48-year follow-up, McAndrew and Weinstein[253] reported that only 40% maintained an Iowa Hip Rating of greater than 80 points. Forty percent of the patients had come to arthroplasty, and an additional 10% were suffering from disabling osteoarthritis symptoms but had not yet had an arthroplasty (Fig. 24-17). Thus at 48-year follow-up, 50% of the patients had disabling osteoarthritis and pain with an additional 10% having Iowa Hip Ratings of less than 80 points. The prevalence of osteoarthritis in this group

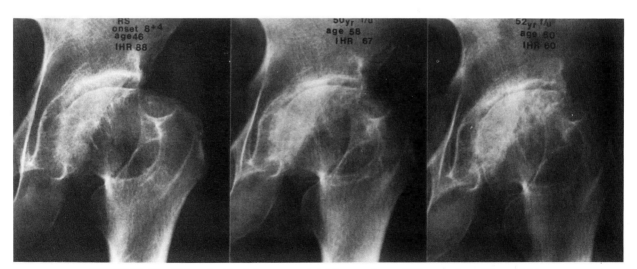

FIGURE 24-17. This patient had disease onset at 8.3 years of age. At 46 years of age (38-year follow-up), the Iowa Hip Rating was 88 points (*left*). At 58 years of age (50-year follow-up) there was a loss of 21 points on the Iowa Hip Rating to 67 (*center*). At 60 years of age, just before arthroplasty, the Iowa Hip Rating was 60 points (*right*). (From Weinstein SL. Legg-Perthes disease. Results of long term follow-up. In: The Hip. Proceedings of the Thirteenth Open Scientific Meeting of the Hip Society. Baltimore: CV Mosby, 1985;28.)

TABLE 24-2. *Prognostic Factors*

Deformity of the femoral head
Hip joint incongruity
Age at disease onset
Extent of epiphyseal involvement
Growth disturbance secondary to premature physeal
  closure
Protracted disease course
Remodeling potential
Type of treatment (?)
Stage at treatment initiation

of patients was 10 times that found in the general population in the age range of the studied patients.[394] Mose followed a group of patients into the seventh decade of life. All of the patients with irregular heads had degenerative arthritis. Of those patients that Mose classified as "normal, ball shaped," no patient had degenerative joint disease by the middle of the fourth decade, but 67% had severe degenerative arthritis by the middle of the seventh decade.[271] Therefore the follow-up studies beyond 40 years demonstrate marked reduction of function, with the overwhelming majority of patients developing degenerative joint disease by the sixth and seventh decades.[179,253,271,361,394]

Prognostic Factors

In reviews of the long-term series of patients with Legg-Calvé-Perthes syndrome, certain clinical and roentgenographic features have been identified that have prognostic value (Table 24-2).[54,164,179,274,392,394,396,410]

The most important prognostic factor in outcome is the residual deformity of the femoral head coupled with hip joint incongruity.[357] Femoral head deformity and joint congruity are multifactoral problems. They are interrelated with all of the other prognostic factors. It must be kept in mind that Legg-Calvé-Perthes syndrome represents a growth disturbance of the proximal femur; the epiphyseal and physeal cartilage is abnormal. Other key factors involved in the development of deformity include the extent of epiphyseal involvement and the varying degrees and patterns of premature physeal closure associated with this condition.[296]

Stulberg and colleagues[361] established a relation between residual deformity and degenerative joint disease. This was accomplished by retrospectively looking at the long-term outcomes of patients from three different centers treated by various methods (e.g., bed rest, spica cast, ischial weight bearing, brace, crutches, cork shoe lift on normal side, combination). They attempted to identify clinical and radiographic factors in the active phase of the disease that were predictive of the development of hip deformity. They proposed a radiographic classification of deformity related to long-term outcome (Table 24-3). The more deformity at maturity (i.e., the higher the Stulberg classification) the worse the long-term outcome. However, as noted from long-term follow-up studies, it is the class 5 hips that deteriorate the earliest, usually having significant symptoms by the end of the fourth decade.[179,253,271,410]

TABLE 24-3. *Stulberg Classification*

CLASS	RADIOGRAPHIC FEATURES	CONGRUENCY
1	Normal hip	Spherical
2 (Figs. 24-9 and 24-18)	Spherical femoral head, same concentric circle on anteroposterior and frog-leg lateral views but with one or more of the following: coxa magna, shorter than normal neck, abnormally steep acetabulum	Spherical
3 (Figs. 24-11 and 24-17)	Ovoid, mushroom-shaped, (but not flat) head, coxa magna, shorter than normal neck, abnormally steep acetabulum	Aspherical
4 (Fig. 24-13)	Flat femoral head and abnormalities of the head, neck, and acetabulum	Aspherical
5 (Fig. 24-14)	Flat head, normal neck and acetabulum	Aspherical incongruency

From Stulbug SD, Cooperman DR, Wallensten R. The natural history of Legg-Calve-Perthes disease. J Bone Joint Surg [Am] 1981;63:1095.

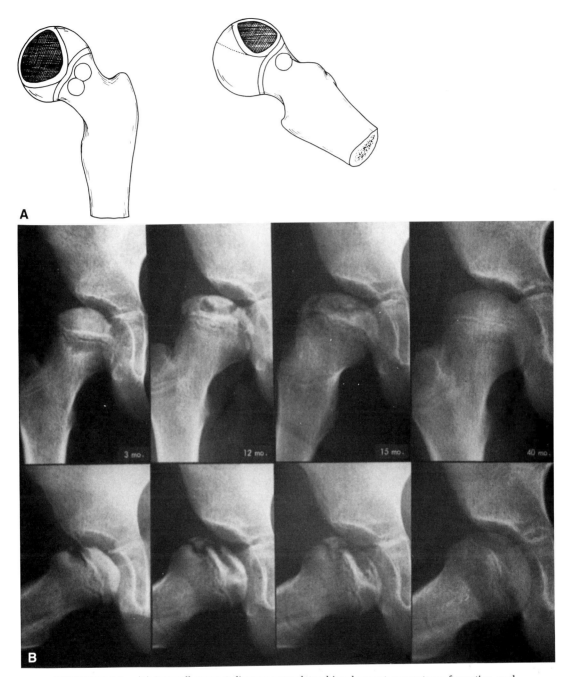

FIGURE 24-18. (**A**) Catterall group 2 disease: anterolateral involvement, sequestrum formation, and a clear junction between the involved and the uninvolved areas. There are anterolateral metaphyseal lesions, and the subchondral fracture line is in the anterior half of the head. The lateral column is intact. (**B**) Catterall group 2 disease: 3 to 40 months after symptom-onset of symptoms the lateral pillar is still intact.

Patients with aspherical congruency (Stulberg types 3 and 4 disease) may have a satisfactory outcome for many years, with most patients undergoing significant functional deterioration in the fifth and sixth decades of life.[179,253,271,410]

O'Garra,[282] Salter and Thompson,[335,337] and others[51,54,55,234,303,304] confirmed Waldenström's original concept that partial or anterior head involvement leads to a more favorable prognosis than whole head involvement. Catterall[51,55,59] demonstrated the impor-

tance of the extent of the epiphyseal involvement relating to prognosis and proposed four groups based on the presence or absence of seven radiographic signs in 97 untreated hips (Fig. 24-18; see Figs. 24-6, 24-9, and 24-10). He compared the final radiograph to the initial radiograph using the clinical grading of Sundt.[364] He reported that 90% of the good results in untreated patients were in groups 1 and 2, whereas 90% of the poor results were in groups 3 and 4. This commonly used classification has been criticized as being difficult to use in that there may be a great deal of interobserver error.[148,164] It also has been criticized as not being sufficiently prospective in that it may take up to 8 months or until the hip is well into the fragmentation phase to determine the extent of epiphyseal involvement.[198,377] Furthermore, it also has been noted that the classification may change when radiographs taken during the initial phase are compared with those taken at maximal fragmentation.[249,377]

Salter and Thompson[337] described a simplified two-group classification based on prognosis and determined by the extent of the subchondral fracture line, which appears early in the course of the disease: group A—less than one half of head involved (Catterall group 1 and 2), and group B—more than one half of head involved (Catterall group 3 and 4). The major determining factor between groups A and B is the presence or absence of a viable lateral column of the epiphysis. This intact lateral column (i.e., Catterall type 2, Salter-Thompson type A) may shield the epiphysis from collapse and subsequent deformity (see Fig. 24-18).

The importance of maintenance of the integrity of the lateral column and the height of the femoral head has been described by several authors.[55,141,164,208,209] Hall[141] reported on the long-term follow-up (34 years) of 209 hips. He considered loss of femoral head height, as seen on the initial radiograph, an important prognostic sign. All of his patients in whom there had been a loss of 2 mm of height or more of the femoral head compared with that of the unaffected hip had a unsatisfactory result in adult life. When the height of the head was within 2 mm of that of the unaffected hip on the initial radiograph all but six hips had done well.

Herring and colleagues[164] proposed a radiographic classification based on the radiolucency of the lateral pillar of the femoral head on anteroposterior x-ray films during the fragmentation phase of the disease (Table 24-4; Fig. 24-19; see Figs. 24-11 and 24-13). The lateral pillar occupies the lateral 15% to 30% of the femoral head width on an anteroposterior radiograph. The central pillar occupies approximately 50% of the head width and the medial pillar 20% to 35% of the medial aspect of the head width on an anteroposterior radiograph.

Herring and colleagues reported on the outcomes of 93 hips in 86 patients with radiographic follow-up to maturity.[164] Intraobserver reliability was reported at a 0.78 level with a good correlation of outcome as measured by the classification of Stulberg and colleagues.[361] The importance of the integrity of the lateral column is seen in other classifications, with Salter-Thompson A and Catterall groups 1 and 2 having intact lateral columns. The results of treatment in long-term outcome studies show this to be an important prognostic factor (Fig. 24-20).[164,179,249,322]

In analyzing the unexpectedly poor results in each category, Catterall[51,52,54,55,61] identified certain radiographic signs, known as at-risk signs, that were associated with poor results (Fig. 24-21). Results in untreated cases show that there were no poor results in patients who did not have 2 or more of the radiologic at-risk signs during the active stage of the disease. Radiographic at-risk signs include Gage sign, which is a radiolucency in the lateral epiphysis and metaphysis, and calcification lateral to the epiphysis. These two signs are indicative of early ossification in the enlarged epiphysis. These are present only when the head is deformed. These signs are present when the changes are reversible with treatment.[55,272] A third at-risk sign is metaphyseal lesions. These metaphyseal radiolucencies may herald the potential for growth disturbance of the physeal plate.[1,49,352] The final two at-risk signs are lateral subluxation and the horizontal growth plate.[124] Lateral subluxation is indicative of a widened head. The horizontal growth plate (adducted hip) is indicative of a developing head deformity that if left untreated will lead to fixed deformity, hinge abduction, and sub-

---

TABLE 24-4.   *Lateral Pillar Classification*

Group A	No involvement of the lateral pillar
	Lateral pillar is radiographically normal
	May be lucency and collapse in the central and medial pillars, but full height of the lateral pillar is maintained
Group B	Greater than 50% of the lateral pillar height is maintained
	Lateral pillar has some radiolucency with maintenance of bone density at a height between 50% and 100% of the original height of the lateral head
Group C	Less than 50% of lateral pillar height is maintained
	Lateral pillar becomes more radiolucent than in Group B, and any preserved bone is at height of <50% of the original height of the lateral pillar

From Herring JA, Neustadt JB, Williams JJ, et al. The lateral pulse classification of Legg-Calvé-Perthes disease. J Pediatr Orthop 1992;12:143.

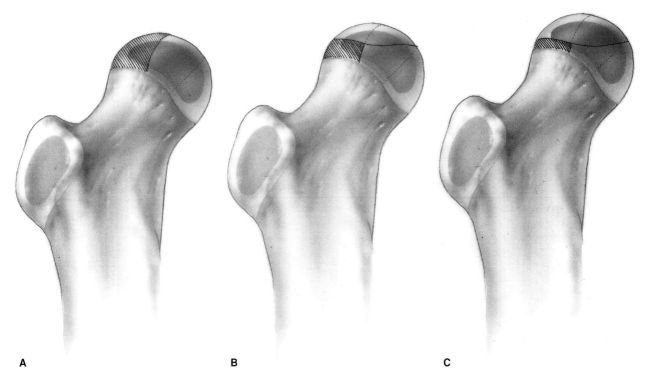

FIGURE 24-19. Lateral pillar classification.

sequent further deformity. These radiographic at-risk signs are manifested clinically by loss of motion and adduction contracture. Catterall reported no poor results in patients not manifesting at-risk signs. The validity of the Catterall classification and the at-risk signs have been confirmed by several series[66,70,91,134,193,263,264,348,377] but questioned by others.[164,179,249]

Stulberg and colleagues[361] identified lateral and superior subluxation, which are indicative of significant growth disturbance and flattening of the femoral head, as the key factors associated with the development of class 3 and 4 hips and poor long-term outcome (i.e., after 40 years). Disease onset after age 9 years and partial head involvement, particularly anterior superior quadrant involvement, was associated with the development of a class 5 hip and the early onset of degenerative joint disease (i.e., third to fifth decade of life).

The duration of the disease is related to the extent of epiphyseal involvement. In general, the greater the extent of epiphyseal involvement the longer the duration and course of the disease. End results are worse with prolonged disease duration.[163–165,235] The gender of the patient also relates to the extent of epiphyseal involvement in that girls affected by Legg-Calvé-Perthes syndrome have a poorer prognosis than boys.[239] This may be explained by the fact that there are more girls, who tend to be more skeletally mature than comparably aged boys, with Catterall groups 3 and 4 disease, which have a less favorable prognosis.[58]

Age of disease onset is the most significant factor related to outcome, second only to deformity. Eight years seems to be the watershed age in most long-term series[253,394]; however, some authors believe the prognosis is markedly worse for long-term outcome in patients over 6 years of age at disease onset.[179] Cumming and colleagues[82] estimated that 45% of patients with onset of Perthes disease after the age of 6 years have undergone arthroplasty by age 60 years. Patients over age 11 or 12 years, even with Catterall group 2 or Salter-Thompson type A disease may get a poor anatomic and clinical result even with treatment.[76] Age at healing, however, is probably a more important factor (see Fig. 24-11). The overall skeletal maturation delay[314] in patients with Legg-Calvé-Perthes syndrome and the usual compensation for this delay during the pubertal growth spurt[48] contributes to the favorable prognosis in the young patient. The more immature the patient at the time of entering the reossification stage the greater the potential for remodeling. At-risk signs are also less likely to occur in younger patients, particularly those younger than 5 years of age. The shape of the acetabulum is dependent on the geometric pattern within it during growth.[12,74,192] In addition, the acetabulum continues to have significant potential for development up to age 8 or 9 years.[41,230,390] If a young patient develops a deformity, the immature acetabulum conforms to the altered femoral head shape. This may lead to the development of aspherical congruency

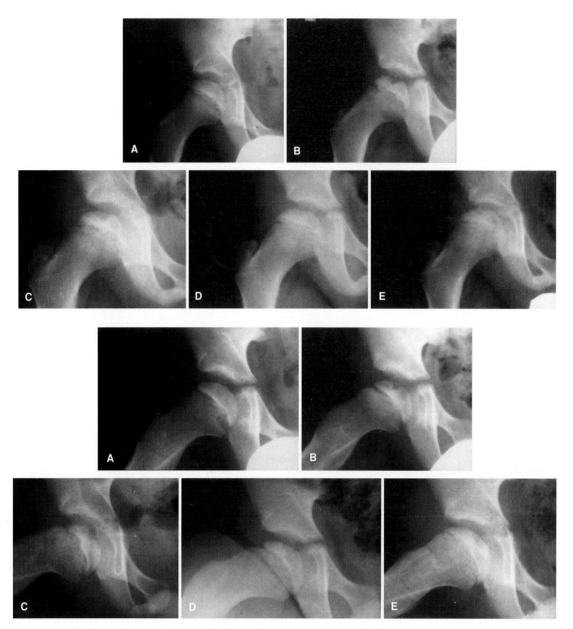

FIGURE 24-20. Anteroposterior (*top*) and lateral (*bottom*) views of a 7-year-old boy who presented with hip pain and a limp. (**A**) At presentation he was in the initial radiographic stage of the disease; his prognosis was indeterminant. (**B**) Six months after presentation he has minimal loss of height of the lateral pillar and some radiolucency in that region as well as significant bone resorption centrally. Note how the lateral pillar maintains its height throughout the course of the disease. (**C**) One year, (**D**) 18 months, and (**E**) 3 years after onset of disease. The patient had only mild symptoms on occasion and maintained good range of motion throughout the disease course. Only symptomatic treatment was provided.

(Stulberg classes 3 and 4) that may be compatible with normal function for many years.[179,192,253,271,361,410]

The importance of premature physeal arrest secondary to the disease process cannot be overemphasized. Keret and colleagues,[203] in a study of 80 patients with Legg-Calvé-Perthes syndrome, showed that 90% had interference with physeal growth, with 25% having premature physeal closure. They demonstrated a direct correlation between severity of physeal involve-

ment and deformity of the head. Clarke and Harrison[71] reported that 47% of the 31 patients who presented with painful hips after Legg-Calvé-Perthes syndrome at an average age of 27 years had evidence of premature physeal closure.

Various methods have been used to measure sphericity of the femoral head and congruency at healing. Goff[130–132] used a transparent protractor with concentric circles drawn at 2 mm of radial difference to

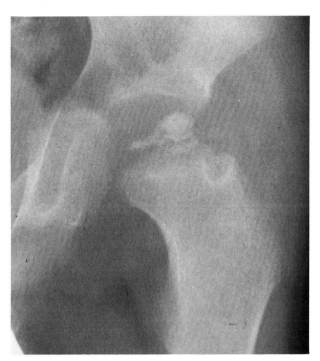

FIGURE 24-21. A 6-year, 5-month-old boy with Catterall group 4 disease demonstrates all the at-risk signs.

evaluate femoral head shape. Mose further developed Goff's method and applied it clinically. This is the most commonly used method of measuring sphericity (see Fig. 24-16).[186-189] It is not clear from the criteria of Mose whether the measurement under consideration is the difference between the outline of the femoral head on the anteroposterior, and lateral radiographs or the deviation from a given circle, measured in millimeters, on either the anteroposterior or lateral radiograph or a combination of these two parameters. This variability in the application of the method of Mose and colleagues is evident in the literature on Legg-Calvé-Perthes syndrome.[83,91,134,194,205,294,308] In general, the template with concentric circles is superimposed on the anteroposterior and lateral roentgenograms. In our practice, if the outline of the femoral head is a perfect circle in both projections it is rated good; less than 2 mm of deviation is rated fair, and greater than 2 mm of deviation from a circle in the anteroposterior, or lateral projection is rated poor. Regardless of measurements used it is important to realize that with growth and remodeling of the femoral head and acetabulum the various parameters used to measure head deformity and congruency may change, and the shape of the head and its congruency as measured at skeletal maturity are probably the most reliable indicators of prognosis and the development of degenerative joint disease. Catterall[55] showed, in a follow-up of untreated patients, that 33% of the patients improved in anatomic grade. Twenty percent of these cases improved two anatomic grades; all of these patients were younger than 5 years of age at disease onset. However, it also must be remembered that the various deformities of the femoral head and acetabulum congruency are three-dimensional parameters that cannot be measured adequately by two-dimensional radiographs. Thus far the only existing radiographic parameter that correlates with good clinical outcome is a perfectly spherical head. Loss of sphericity, however, in and by itself does not necessarily lead to a poor long-term result.[253,394]

Thompson and Westin[371] confirmed the work of Ferguson and Howarth,[111] which demonstrated that after the femoral head is in the reossification stage of the disease it will not deform further. For any treatment to influence head deformity it must be instituted early in the course of the disease, that is, in the initial or fragmentation stage.

CLINICAL PRESENTATION

Patients with Legg-Calvé-Perthes syndrome most commonly present with a history of the insidious onset of a limp. Most patients do not complain of much discomfort unless specifically questioned about this aspect. Pain, when present, is usually activity related and relieved by rest. Because of its mild nature most patients do not present for medical attention until weeks or months after the clinical onset of disease. The pain the patients experience generally is localized to the groin or referred to the anteromedial thigh or knee region. Failure to recognize that thigh or knee pain in the child may be secondary to hip pathology may cause further delay in the diagnosis. Some children present with more acute symptom onset. Seventeen percent of patients with Legg-Calvé-Perthes syndrome may give a history of related trauma.[33,113,406]

PHYSICAL EXAMINATION

The child with Legg-Calvé-Perthes syndrome usually presents with limited hip motion, particularly abduction and medial rotation. Early in the course of the disease the limited abduction is secondary to synovitis and muscle spasm in the adductor group; however, with time and the subsequent deformities that may develop, limitation of abduction may become permanent. Long-standing adductor spasm occasionally leads to adductor contracture. The Trendelenburg test in patients with Legg-Calvé-Perthes syndrome is often positive. These children most commonly have evidence of thigh, calf, and buttock atrophy from disuse secondary to pain. This is additional evidence of the long-standing nature of the condition prior to detection.[42,130,225,292,381,382,391] Limb length should be measured; inequality is indicative of significant head collapse and a poor prognosis. Evaluation of the patient's overall height and weight and bone age may be helpful in the ruling out of skeletal dysplasias or growth disorders in the differential diagnosis and may provide confirmatory evidence of the disorder. Laboratory studies generally are not helpful in Legg-Calvé-Perthes syndrome, although they may be necessary to rule out other conditions.

IMAGING

In Legg-Calvé-Perthes syndrome the diagnosis is made and the clinical course assessed by plain radiographs taken in the anteroposterior and frog-leg lateral position. These radiographs are generally sufficient for the assessment of the patient and subsequent follow-up evaluations. From the plain radiographs the extent of epiphyseal involvement (e.g., Catterall groups 1–4; Salter-Thompson type A or B; lateral pillar types A, B, or C) and the stage of the disease (initial, fragmentation, or reossification) can be determined. According to Salter and Thompson, if appropriate radiographs are taken within 4 months of the clinical onset of the disease, the subchondral radiolucent zone will be detectable.[337] Catterall, however, states that this sign is helpful in only 25% of cases because it is only present transiently in the early phases of the disease.[55] It is most important in following the course of the disease that all radiographs be viewed sequentially and compared with previous radiographs to assess the stage of the reparative process and determine the constancy of the extent of epiphyseal involvement. Additional radiographic or imaging studies are rarely necessary but may be helpful in the initial assessment and follow-up of the condition.[223,276,403]

Radionuclide bone scanning with technetium and pinhole columnation (Fig. 24-22) may be helpful in the early stages of the disease when the diagnosis is in question, particularly if the differential diagnosis is between transient synovitis and Perthes disease. Some investigators consider scintigraphy helpful in determining the extent of the epiphyseal involvement and prognosis.[43,86,87,90,114,210,365]

Magnetic resonance imaging is widely available in many medical centers. It appears to be sensitive in detecting infarction, but cannot yet accurately portray the stages of healing. Its role in the management of Perthes syndrome has yet to be defined. In the future, magnetic resonance imaging may not only help the clinician in the diagnosis but shed additional light on the underlying pathology of the condition (Fig. 24-23).

Arthrography is useful primarily in demonstrating any flattening of the femoral head that may not be seen on plain radiographs (Fig. 24-24). It can be used to demonstrate the hinge abduction (see Fig. 24-8) phenomenon with abduction of the leg.[54,137,191,324] Arthrography in conjunction with plain films or computed tomography scan also may be useful in the diagnosis of osteochondritis dissecans following Perthes disease. Arthrography is most useful for assessing head shape and the relation to the acetabulum that would be necessary for treatment decisions (Fig. 24-25). With severe flattening of the femoral head, arthrography is helpful in determining containability before any treatment, whether Pietrie casts, bracing, or surgery. It is also useful in determining the best position of containment, such as internal or external rotation and abduction or adduction if surgical management is considered.

DIFFERENTIAL DIAGNOSIS

The patient history, physical examination, and plain radiographs are usually sufficient to make a diagnosis of Legg-Calvé-Perthes syndrome (Table 24-5). Diagnosis early in the initial phase of the disease must be differentiated from conditions, such as septic arthritis, primary or secondary to proximal femoral osteomyelitis, and toxic synovitis.[18,118,240] A complete blood count, including white cell differential, erythrocyte sedimentation rate, and hip joint aspiration and analysis of the fluid may be necessary to rule out infection. All laboratory studies of Legg-Calvé-Perthes syndrome generally are normal, although the erythrocyte sedimentation rate may be slightly elevated. In early cases, if all the laboratory and plain radiographic studies

---

TABLE 24-5.   *Differential Diagnosis*

Chondrolysis
Gaucher disease
Hemophilia
Hypothyroidism
Juvenile rheumatoid arthritis
Lymphoma
Muccopolysacharridosis
Multiple epiphyseal dysplasia
Myer dysplasia
Neoplasm
Old congenital dysplasia of the hip residuals
Osteomyelitis of proximal femur
Septic arthritis
Sickle cell disease
Spondyloepiphyseal dysplasia
Toxic synovitis
Traumatic aseptic necrosis

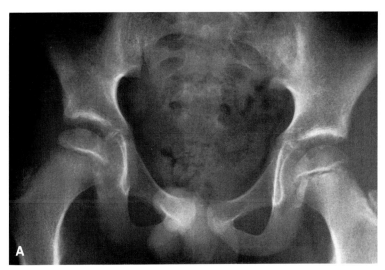

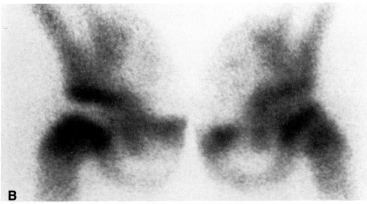

FIGURE 24-22. An 8-year-old boy with right hip pain. (**A**) Anteroposterior radiograph demonstrates slight increase in width and medial joint space, femoral ossific-nucleus is slightly smaller than the opposite side. (**B**) Technetium 99 radionuclide scan demonstrates decreased uptake in entire right femoral head with increased vascularity in the neck.

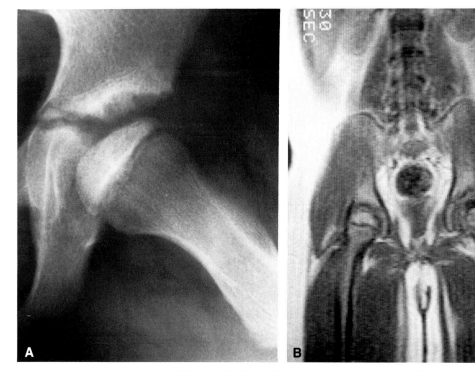

FIGURE 24-23. A 6-year-old boy with Catterall group 3 disease in the early fragmentation stage. (**A**) Plain radiograph shows apparent sparing of the posterior head. (**B**) Magnetic resonance imaging demonstrates complete absence of signal on affected side. (Courtesy of Peter Scoles, M.D., Case Western Reserve Medical School, Cleveland.)

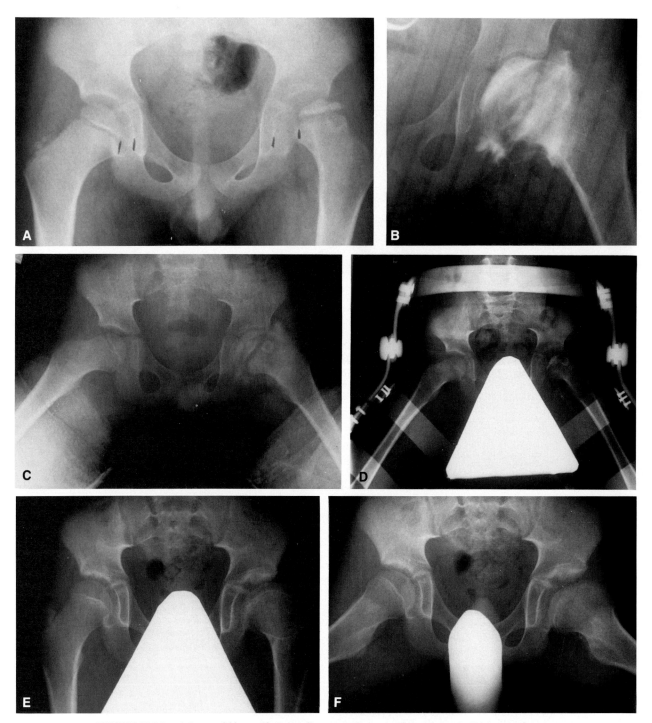

FIGURE 24-24. A 5-year-old boy with Catterall group 4 disease and at-risk status. (**A**) Anteroposterior radiograph on presentation. (**B**) Anteroposterior arthrogram in the same position as **C** after 10 days of traction. Note the relation between the lateral acetabular margin and the lateral margin of cartilaginous femoral head as well as the severe flattening of the femoral head. (**C**) Anteroposterior roentgenogram in Pietrie "broomstick" abduction plasters. The patient was maintained in casts for 6 weeks. (**D**) Anteroposterior radiograph with pelvis abduction orthosis (weight-bearing). (**E**) Anteroposterior radiograph at age 13 years. Note residual deformity. (**F**) Lauenstein radiograph age 13 years.

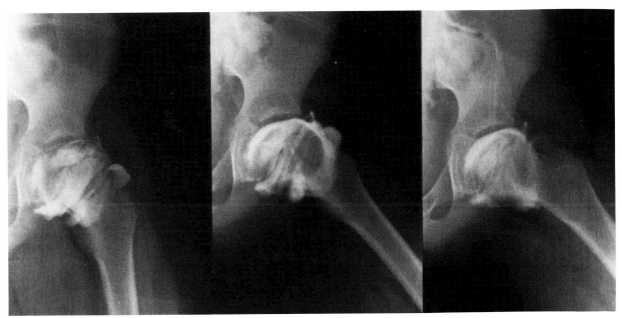

FIGURE 24-25. Arthrogram of a 6-year-old boy with Catterall group 4 disease. (**A**) Neutral position; (**B**) abduction, external rotation, and slight flexion (position that would be maintained by an abduction Scottish Rite–type orthosis); and (**C**) abduction internal rotation (position that would be maintained by a varus derotation osteotomy). On the basis of the arthrogram, the hip can be contained either by the position as would be maintained by bracing (**B**) or by surgery (**C**).

are normal and doubt as to the diagnosis persists, radionuclide scanning may be helpful.

In patients with bilateral hip involvement, generalized disorders, such as hypothyroidism and multiple epiphyseal dysplasia, must be considered.[3,176] Patients with bilateral involvement, particularly those with atypical radiographic features, must have a careful family history obtained, measurements of height and weight, and a bone survey to rule out a metabolic or a genetic condition (see Chaps. 6 and 7). Meyer dysplasia, a benign resolving condition, must be considered in children younger than 4 years of age.[180]

TREATMENT

Throughout the past 70 years, considerable therapeutic nihilism has been expressed by many authors.[29,226,361–364] Sundt[364] believed that treatment could not prevent degenerative joint disease. Because there is a paucity of long-term natural history data available, the question must be raised as to whether the outcome of Legg-Calvé-Perthes syndrome can be altered by any particular treatment. As previously mentioned, long-term series of treated patients are difficult to evaluate. Long-term series of patients with uniform treatment and matched for age, gender, stage, and extent of epiphyseal involvement are necessary to determine the most effective treatment of Perthes syndrome.

Most patients (60%) with Legg-Calvé-Perthes dis-

ease do not need treatment.[19,51,55,198,272,337] Treatment must be considered for only those patients who have an otherwise known poor prognosis based on prognostic factors gleaned from long-term follow-ups. It is difficult to formulate specific treatments for patients because natural history is not well known and most studies of current treatment methods lack interrater and intrarater reliability of classifications of extent of epiphyseal involvement and outcome measures, and all lack control groups. These factors and other variables examined in most series make it difficult to support a "best" method of treatment.

No treatment is warranted in patients with a good prognosis (i.e., those with Catterall group 1, Salter-Thompson type A or lateral pillar type A disease; Table 24-6). Those patients with a poor prognosis should be considered for treatment, such as patients with Catterall groups 3 and 4 disease, Salter-Thompson type B disease, and lateral pillar type C disease. There is another large group of patients whose prognosis is indeterminate; these patients require careful follow-up because they may need treatment. The group includes patients with Catterall group 2 disease (good prognosis in 90% of cases) and those with lateral pillar B disease. All patients should be treated if they manifest clinical at-risk signs (i.e., they lose range of motion and have pain) or if they demonstrate several of the radiographic at-risk signs regardless of their extent of epiphyseal involvement. If the patient is already in the reossification or healing stage of the disease, little

---

TABLE 24-6.   Treatment of Legg-Calvé-Perthes Disease

Poor Prognostic Group: Treatment Indicated
Catterall 3 and 4
Salter-Thompson B
Lateral pillar C
At-risk clinically
At-risk radiographically regardless of the disease extent

Good Prognosis: No Treatment Necessary
Catterall 1 and 2 (generally good prognosis in 90% of
    cases)
Salter-Thompson A
Lateral pillar A

Indeterminate Prognoses: May Require Treatment
Catterall 2
Lateral pillar B

In Reossification Stage: No Treatment Warranted

---

deformity ensues and no treatment is indicated (see Treatment Options in the Noncontainable Hip and the Late-Presenting Case).

The earliest treatment methods employed weight relief until the head was reossified. These methods were based on the premise that weight relief would prevent the mechanical deformation of the head and prevent early degenerative joint disease.[84,109,126,172] These modalities included prolonged, strict bed rest, often in the hospital, and bed rest with or without various periods of traction on special frames or in spica casts. These methods of treatment were associated with disuse atrophy of muscles, osteopenia, shortening of the involved extremity, loss of thoracic kyphosis, urinary calculi, social and emotional problems, and high hospital costs.[10,83,96,106,105,155,150,166,315,316,319,347]

The concept of weight relief as a treatment for Legg-Calvé-Perthes syndrome was challenged as early as 1927, when Legg stated that "while the process suggesting weakness of bone structure is going on it is theoretically sound to allow no weight bearing but in practice relief from weight bearing in no way affects the end results."[226] In addition, prolonged immobilization and bed rest do not influence the radiographic course of the disease[13,198,262-264,354] Harrison[150] pointed out, as had Pauwels,[150,151,155,289] that even at rest, significant forces act on the femoral head with minimal activity.

The cornerstone of treatment for Legg-Calvé-Perthes syndrome is referred to as "containment." This concept was originally described by Parker[150] and Eyre-Brook[109] The rationale for this concept has been defined further by Harrison and Menon[150] Petrie and Bitenc,[294] Salter,[332,335] and others.[31,89,195,197,311,312] The essence of containment is that to prevent deformities

of the diseased epiphysis, the femoral head must be contained within the depths of acetabulum to equalize the pressure on the head and subject it to the molding action of the acetabulum. Containment is an attempt to reduce the forces through the hip joint by actual or relative varus positioning.[25] Containment may be achieved by nonoperative or operative methods. Considering all the methods of containment, the femoral head represents over three-fourths of the sphere and the acetabulum only half of the sphere. No method of containment can provide for a totally contained femoral head within the acetabulum during all portions of the gait cycle.[257,311-313]

Patient Management

The primary goals in the treatment of Legg-Calvé-Perthes syndrome are to prevent deformity (Stulberg classes 3, 4, and 5), alter growth disturbance, and thus prevent degenerative joint disease. To obtain this goal each patient must be assessed clinically and radiographically. Clinically, the patient is evaluated for clinical at-risk signs of loss of motion, joint contracture, and pain. Radiographically, anteroposterior and frog-leg lateral radiographs are evaluated to determine the radiographic stage of the disease, the extent of epiphyseal involvement, and the presence of radiographic at-risk signs. For treatment to have any effect on subsequent deformity it must be initiated in the initial or fragmentation phase of the disease.[111,371]

Treatment is not indicated if the child demonstrates none of the clinical or radiographic at-risk signs, if it is Catterall type 1 or 2, Salter-Thompson type A, or lateral pillar type A disease, or if the disease is already in the reossification stage. A child who demonstrates clinical or radiographic at-risk signs regardless of the extent of epiphyseal involvement should receive treatment.[391] Even patients with Catterall 2 disease (or lateral pillar B disease) who are at risk may end up with a poor result without treatment.[55,82,230]

The first principle of treatment, regardless of the definitive method of treatment chosen, is restoration of motion. Joint motion enhances synovial nutrition and cartilage nutrition.[100,247] This tenet of treatment cannot be overemphasized. The most successful reported series of patients treated for extensively involved femoral heads is that of Brotherton and McKibbon.[31] These patients were treated by bed rest and containment. End results in these patients were superior to another long-term follow-up[315,316] of patients treated by bed rest and containment on a frame. The only difference between the two treatment regimens was that in the former series motion was always maintained. Restoration of motion can be accomplished by bed rest with skin traction and progressive abduction to relieve the muscle spasms. Occasionally surgical release of the contracted adductors may be necessary.

Restoration of motion allows abduction of the hip, which reduces the forces on the hip joint and allows positioning of the uncovered anterolateral aspect of the femoral head in the acetabulum. Mobilization of the hip joint also can be obtained by rest followed by the use of progressive abduction plasters to stretch the hip adductor muscles while allowing hip flexion and extension. A full or almost full range of motion is usually obtainable within 7 to 10 days of treatment. Because of early deformity complete abduction and internal rotation may not always be obtainable. Persistence of an adduction contracture is always associated with a serious femoral head deformity and will not respond to traction.[60]

Arthrography is a useful adjunct in determining whether the head actually can be contained and if so in what position this is best accomplished[122] (see Fig. 24-25). Arthrography can reveal any flattening of the femoral head that may not be seen on plain radiographs. More importantly, it can demonstrate the hinge abduction phenomenon[54,137] (see Fig. 24-8). Demonstration of the hinge abduction phenomenon, or the inability to contain the hip, is a contraindication to any type of containment treatment. Serious damage to the femoral head and acetabulum may result from trying to contain a noncontainable head (see Fig. 24-14). Arthrography should be performed under general anesthesia. This also provides an opportunity to examine whether muscle spasm, contracture, or mechanical deformity is responsible for any apparent fixed deformities.

The treatment of Legg-Calvé-Perthes disease remains controversial, and there is lack of agreement regarding whether operative or nonoperative treatment is beneficial. The shortage of natural history studies for comparison of results of different modalities of treatment is another reason why it is difficult to resolve this controversy. In addition, the variability of criteria for inclusion of patients in studies and the use of different measurements to assess outcomes of treatment, lack of interrater and intrarater reliability data, and lack of untreated control groups make comparisons difficult. The three most widely used methods to maintain containment are an abduction orthosis, femoral osteotomy, and innominate osteotomy. Interest has grown in combined femoral and innominate surgical procedures as well as the use of procedures originally thought of as salvage procedures in the primary treatment of Perthes disease.

Nonoperative Treatment

In 1971, Petrie and Bitenc[294] reported excellent results applying the principles of containment using broomstick abduction long-leg plasters (see Fig. 24-24C). This series proved that weight bearing with the head contained was not harmful. This method of treatment allows for weight bearing and maintenance of hip range of motion in the contained position. Successful treatment results using this technique have been reported.[320] Pietrie casts are used following muscle release procedures and capsulotomies for reducing heads that are deformed and subluxated[336] to maintain containment prior to bracing or surgical treatment or as definitive nonsurgical treatment in a situation in which bracing compliance is in question.

To avoid the repeated hospitalizations necessary to regain knee and ankle motion, as well as to avoid the occasional flattening of the femoral condyles seen in patients treated with broomstick plasters, attention turned to the use of removal abduction orthoses, as typified by the Newington abduction brace,[83] the Robert orthosis,[323] the Houston A-frame brace,[94] and the Toronto Legg-Calvé-Perthes orthosis.[21,22] These devices provided for containment in the abducted internal rotation position.

The most widely used abduction orthosis is the Atlanta Scottish Rite orthosis or a modification thereof (Fig. 24-26). These devices provide for containment solely by abduction without fixed internal rotation.[110,205,238,308] These orthotic devices allow free motion of the knee and ankle. Containment is provided for by the abduction of the brace and the hip flexion required to walk with the legs in abduction. These devices are less cumbersome than other braces and are well tolerated by patients. On arthrography the position of containment that would be maintained by an abduction orthosis of this variety would be demonstrated by abduction, slight flexion, and external rotation (see Fig. 24-25). Patients must demonstrate containment on a radiograph in the weight-bearing position while in the brace (see Fig. 24-24). At each subsequent visit the patient must be examined out of the orthosis to be certain that range of motion is maintained. If the range of motion is not adequate, traction should be initiated to restore range of motion, and containability should be reassessed. The brace is worn on a full-time basis until the head is in the reossification stage, when there is no further risk of collapse. Full-time bracing ranges from 6 to 18 months. The negative aspects of bracing include prolonged treatment times and the necessity of having a compliant patient. Some patients may not tolerate the brace for psychological reasons.[306] This type of treatment also may be difficult for girls and older patients to accept.[241]

Although early radiographic anatomic results were reported comparable with previously used containment weight-bearing methods[238,308] recent reports question the efficacy of this method of management.[249,258]

Martinez and colleagues[249] reported on 31 patients with 34 hips who had severe Perthes disease (Catterall groups 3 and 4) who had been treated with a weight-

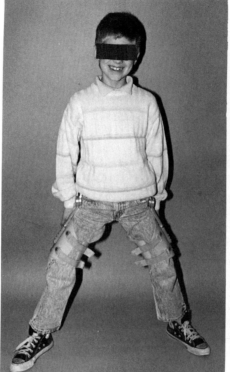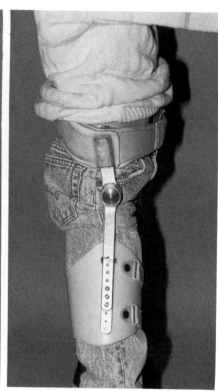

FIGURE 24-26. An abduction orthosis.

bearing abduction orthosis. The mean age of the patients when first seen was 6 years, and the mean duration of follow-up was 7 years. According to the Mose criteria, at follow-up no hip had a good result, 35% had a fair result, and 65% had a poor result. On the basis of the classification of Stulberg and colleagues there were 41% class 2 results, 53% class 3 and 4 results, and 6% class 5 results. With respect to the lateral column, of the 20 hips in which collapse occurred, only 10% had a Stulberg class 2 result, 35% class 3, 45% class 4, and 10% class 5. By comparison, in the 14 hips in which collapse of the lateral column did not occur, 86% had a Stulberg class 2 result and only 14% had a class 3 result. No hip in which collapse did not occur had a class 4 or 5 result. The authors concluded that although containment is the most widely accepted principle of treatment of Legg-Calvé-Perthes disease, little clinical information supports the contention that bracing in abduction and external rotation as provided by the Atlanta Scottish Rite Orthosis and its modifications is effective.

Meehan and colleagues[258] reported on 34 patients with Catterall group 3 and 4 disease with the average age at diagnosis of 8 years. The average follow-up in this series was 6 years and 9 months. At follow-up there were no Stulberg class 1, 3 class 2, 24 class 3, 6 class 4, and 1 class 5 result. These authors also arrived at a similar conclusion concerning the use of this orthotic device in the treatment of Perthes disease. In both of these studies the issue of compliance is not documented, and as with all studies of Perthes disease in the literature, control groups other than historic are absent. Because the radiographic outcomes in both of these studies was poor it is questionable whether the orthosis itself adds anything to the treatment other than maintenance of range of motion. As expected, the majority of patients in both series were doing well clinically as do most patients who have Perthes disease over the short-term regardless of the extent of the deformity. The long-term prognosis for all but the Stulberg class 1 and 2 hips is guarded.

Because of these results many physicians have begun treating patients only with maintenance of range of motion programs, including stretching exercises, nighttime abduction splinting, home traction, and other combinations. Long-term follow-up studies of these nonoperative range of motion regimes are needed to determine their efficacy.

Surgical Treatment

Surgical methods of providing or maintaining containment have been advocated by many investigators. Surgical containment methods offer the advantage of early mobilization and the avoidance of prolonged bracing or cast treatment. In addition, no end point for discontinuing treatment is required, and any improved containment is permanent.[336] Surgical containment may be approached either from the femoral side, the acetabular side, or both sides of the hip joint. Procedures used to obtain or maintain containment in Legg-Calvé-Perthes syndrome are those that originally were used in the treatment of problems associated with developmental hip dysplasia and dislocation.

Varus Osteotomy

Varus osteotomy with or without associated derotation offers the theoretical advantage of deep seating of the femoral head and positioning of the vulnerable anterolateral portion of the head away from the deforming influences of the acetabular edge.[4,60,158,170,224,272] The varus position reduces the joint forces on the femoral head.[4,25] This procedure also relieves the intraosseous venous hypertension and improves the disturbed intraosseous venous drainage reported in Legg-Calvé-Perthes syndrome and thus speeds the healing process.[4,23,135,158,159,366] This belief, however, has been disproved.[69,201,246]

Prerequisites for varus derotation osteotomy include a full range of motion, congruency between the femoral head and the acetabulum, and the ability to contain the femoral head in the acetabulum in abduction and internal rotation (see Fig. 24-25).[73,336] This assessment may require arthrography if the femoral head is well into the fragmentation phase. As with nonoperative treatment the procedure must be performed early in the initial or fragmentation stage of the disease to have any effect on head deformity.[4,9,234]

The negative aspects of this treatment modality must be considered. Varus osteotomy with or without derotation usually requires the use of internal fixation and external mobilization in plaster for 6 weeks. The patient must incur the inherent risks and cost associated with at least one surgical procedure and most likely a second surgical procedure for hardware removal. The limb is temporarily shortened by the procedure. The varus angle must not exceed a neck shaft angle of less than 110 degrees. The varus angle generally decreases with growth[54,265,355]; however, if there has been physeal plate damage secondary to the disease this remodeling potential may be lost, and the patient may have permanent shortening and temporary or permanent weakness of the hip abductors.[46,23,107,355,356,389] The proponents of varus osteotomy with or without derotation report 70% to 90% satisfactory anatomic results using this method.[4,23,46,72,77,158,234,356]

Innominate Osteotomy

Innominate osteotomy provides for containment by redirection of the acetabulum, providing better coverage for the anterolateral portion of the femoral head. The head is placed in relative flexion, abduction, and internal rotation with respect to the acetabulum in the weight-bearing position. Any shortening caused by the disease can be corrected, and the need for bracing is eliminated.[45,73,88,334–336,338,356] Prerequisites for innominate osteotomy include restoration of a full range of motion, a round or almost round femoral head, and joint congruency demonstrated arthrographically. Treatment must be performed early in the course of the disease, and the head must be well seated in flexion, abduction, and internal rotation.

Innominate osteotomy is performed in a similar fashion as for residual hip subluxation. The tendinous portion of the iliopsoas muscle is always released at the musculotendinous junction, and any residual contractures of the adductor muscles are released by subcutaneous adductor tenotomy.[335,336] The osteotomy is fixed by two or three threaded pins for internal fixation. Partial weight bearing may be resumed in a cooperative child several days following surgery; however, in an uncooperative patient, immobilization in a spica cast for 6 weeks is required.

The disadvantages of innominate osteotomy are the associated risks and cost factors of the surgical procedure and the procedure for pin removal. Secondly, the operation is performed on the normal side of the joint. This procedure may increase the forces on the femoral head by lateralizing the acetabulum and increasing the lever arm of the abductors,[4] although this supposition has thus far not been substantiated. Innominate osteotomy also may cause a persistent acetabular configuration change in the face of a previously normal acetabulum, leading to the loss of motion, particularly flexion.[75] Satisfactory anatomic results from this procedure range from 69% to 94%.[45,88,177,288,325,336,356,358]

There is significant biomechanical evidence to show that neither method of surgical containment, innominate nor femoral osteotomy, may effectively stress shield an extensively necrotic segment of the femoral head; the same may also apply for patients treated with a brace.[125,310–312] Wenger[397] reported a high incidence of complications in surgically treated patients in which the accepted methods and prerequisites were met.

Varus Osteotomy Plus Innominate Osteotomy

Several short-term results of combined varus osteotomy plus innominate osteotomy have been reported in severely involved Catterall group 3 or 4 disease. This combined procedure has a theoretical advantage of maximizing femoral head containment while avoiding the complications of either procedure alone. The femoral osteotomy directs the femoral head into the acetabulum while theoretically reducing any increasing joint pressure or stiffness that would result from the pelvic osteotomy. The coverage provided by the innominate osteotomy reduces the degree of correction needed from the femoral osteotomy, thereby minimizing the complications of excessive neck shaft varus, associated abductor weakness, and limb shortening. Advocates of this procedure also believe that permanent correction of the deformity, early weight bearing, and shortened treatment time are obtained. The disadvantages of the procedure include those mentioned for varus osteotomy and innominate osteotomy alone. Surgical time is increased, potential blood loss is magnified, and the combined procedures are technically more difficult. Satisfactory anatomic results from this combined procedure are reported in up to 78% of cases. As would be expected in short-term follow-up, clinical results are excellent.[80,81,286] The prerequisites for this operation include those for the varus and innominate osteotomies alone in a patient who probably would not get satisfactory coverage from either procedure alone.

Shelf Arthroplasty

Shelf arthroplasty formerly was used as a salvage procedure. However, it recently has been proposed as a primary method of management in children over age 8 years with Catterall group 3 and 4 disease.[400] Only short-term follow-up studies exist, but proponents believe that containment of the femoral head before significant deformity develops improves femoral head remodeling. The shelf procedure may cover the anterolateral portion of the head preventing subluxation and lateral overgrowth of the epiphysis. Other indications include lateral subluxation of the femoral head, inadequate coverage of the femoral head, or hinge abduction associated with severe Legg-Calvé-Perthes disease.[14,215]

Regardless of the method of containment chosen, any episode indicative of loss of containment, such as recurrent pain and loss of range of motion, must be treated aggressively by rest, traction, and reassessment of containment.

Treatment Options in the Noncontainable Hip and the Late-Presenting Case

Patients presenting in the later stages (reossification) of the disease, those with noncontainable deformities, and those who have lost containment after either surgical or nonsurgical containment present a problem. These patients usually demonstrate hinge abduction on arthrography and have an extremely poor prognosis without additional treatment.[61,253,270,309,336,394] These patients generally present with persisting pain, shortening of the involved extremity with a fixed deformity, generally 10 to 15 degrees of fixed flexion and 15 to

20 degrees of fixed adduction.[61,309] The salvage procedures to be considered at this point include Chiari osteotomy, shelf procedure, cheilectomy, and abduction extension osteotomy.[61,254,309,336,341,378] These procedures must be viewed as salvage procedures with each having specific limited aims that may include pain relief, correction of limb length inequality, increasing head coverage, and improvement of movement and abductor weakness.[309]

Chiari osteotomy improves the lateral coverage of the deformed femoral head but does not reduce the lateral impingement in abduction and may exacerbate any existing abductor weakness.[61,309] Chiari osteotomy may be useful in the enlarged poorly covered femoral head that is beginning to develop symptoms of early degenerative joint disease. Although good preliminary results have been reported,[14,39,147,341,378] the role of Chiari osteotomy in the treatment of Legg-Calvé-Perthes syndrome is yet to be defined.

Cheilectomy removes the anterolateral portion of the femoral head that is impinging on the acetabulum in abduction (Fig. 24-27). It is indicated only for functionally limiting restricted range of motion. The procedure must be done only after the physis is closed, otherwise a slipped capital femoral epiphysis may ensue.[120,254] Although cheilectomy may produce gratifying results concerning improved range of motion, in some cases increasing stiffness may occur secondary to capsular adhesions at the osteotomy site.[336] In addition, shortening associated with the femoral head deformity is not corrected.

In patients in the active stage of the disease with a noncontainable hip or those with a painful hip after healing who demonstrate hinge abduction, abduction extension osteotomy should be considered. Abduction extension osteotomy of the femur is indicated when arthrography demonstrates joint congruency improved by the extended adducted position. The preliminary results with this modality of treatment indicate improvement in the limb length, decrease in limp, and improvement in function and range of motion.[309] This procedure may be applied either in the active or late stages of the disease when arthrography demonstrates joint congruency improved by the extended adducted position. This modality of treatment allows for realignment of the congruent position of the hip in the neutral weight-bearing position.[309,336]

Osteochondritis dissecans after Perthes syndrome may or may not be symptomatic. If symptomatic the pain may be intermittent. In patients with pain, several treatment options are available. Symptomatic treatment with antiinflammatories and protective weight bearing may be used in order to promote healing. Persistent pain may warrant attempts at revascularization. This may include drilling of the fragment via the femoral neck, drilling, and internal fixation, either

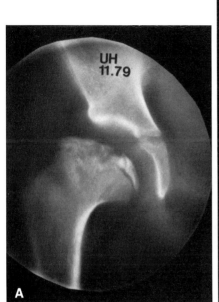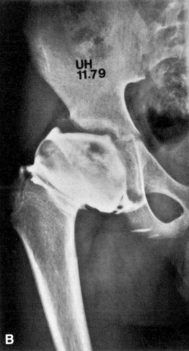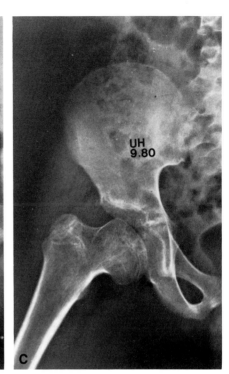

FIGURE 24-27.   An 8-year, 6-month-old male with Catterall group 4 disease. Hip range of motion included flexion of 140 degrees, extension of 0 degrees, abduction of 20 degrees, adduction of 30 degrees, internal rotation of 10 degrees, and external rotation of 30 degrees. (**A**) Polytome indicating superolateral growth arrest. (**B**) Arthrogram demonstrating femoral head flattening and enlargement and deformation of the peripheral acetabulum. (**C**) Abduction radiograph 7 months after cheilectomy. Range of motion at this time was flexion, 130 degrees; extension, 20 degrees; abduction, 50 degrees; adduction, 50 degrees; internal rotation, 45 degrees; and external rotation, 40 degrees. (Courtesy of J. G. Pous, M.D. Montpellier, France.)

percutaneously with pins or open with devices such as the Herbert screw. If the fragment becomes detached and cannot be reattached and causes mechanical catching symptoms it may require removal.[137] There is a paucity of information on the natural history of the condition and the results of treatment.

In patients with Legg-Calvé-Perthes syndrome who have premature physeal arrest, trochanteric overgrowth may ensue.[27,28] Such patients may develop a Trendelenburg gait and pain secondary to muscle fatigue. This rarely has been a significant problem in long-term reviews.[394] However, distal and lateral advancement of the greater trochanter may be necessary.[242]

FUTURE DEVELOPMENTS

Long-term series of patients with the uniform treatment matched for age, gender, degree of epiphyseal involvement, and other diagnostic factors compared with an untreated control group will no doubt be required to determine the most effective treatment for Perthes syndrome. As our fundamental understanding

of Legg-Calvé-Perthes syndrome increases so does our understanding of how various treatment modalities influence this complex growth disturbance.

References

1. Aguirre M, Pellise F, Castellote A. Metaphyseal cysts in Legg-Calvé-Perthes disease (letter; comment). J Pediatr Orthop 1992;12:404.
2. Aire E, Johnson F, Harrison MHM, et al. Femoral head shape in Perthes' disease. Is the contralateral hip abnormal? Clin Orthop 1986;209:77.
3. Andersen PE Jr, Schantz K, Bollerslev J, Justesen P. Bilateral femoral head dysplasia and osteochondritis. Multiple epiphyseal dysplasia tarda, spondylo-epiphyseal dysplasia tarda, and bilateral Legg-Perthes disease. Acta Radiol 1988;29:705.
4. Axer A, Gershuni DH, Hendel D, Mirovski Y. Indications for femoral osteotomy in Legg-Calvé-Perthes disease. Clin Orthop 1980;150:78.
5. Axhausen G. Kohler's disease and Perthes' disease. Zentralbl Chir 1923;50:553.
6. Baker WM. Epiphyseal necrosis and its consequences. Br Med J 1883;2:416.
7. Barker DJP, Dixon E, Taylor JF. Perthes' disease of the hip in three regions of England. J Bone Joint Surg [Br] 1978;60:478.
8. Barker DJP, Hall AJ. The epidemiology of Perthes' disease. Clin Orthop 1986;209:89.

9. Barnes JM. Premature epiphyseal closure in Perthes' disease. J Bone Joint Surg [Br] 1980;62:432.

10. Barranco SD, Traver RC, Friedman FM, Chiroff RT. A comparative study of Legg-Perthes Disease. Clin Orthop 1973;96:304.

11. Beaty JH. Legg-Calvé-Perthes disease: diagnostic and prognostic techniques. Instr Course Lect 1989;38:291.

12. Bellyei A, Mike G. Acetabular development in Legg-Calvé-Perthes disease. Orthopedics 1988;11:407.

13. Bellyei A, Mike G. Weight bearing in Perthes' disease. Orthopedics 1991;14:19.

14. Bennett JT, Mazurek RT, Cash JD. Chiari's osteotomy in the treatment of Perthes' disease. J Bone Joint Surg [Br] 1991;73:225.

15. Bentzon PGK. Experimental studies on the pathogenesis of coxa plana and other manifestations of "local dyschondroplasia." Acta Radiol 1926;6:155.

16. Bernbeck R. Kritischenzum Perthes-Problem der Hufte. Arch Orthop UnfallChir 1950;44:445.

17. Bernbeck R. Zur Pathogenese der jugendlichen Huftkopfnekrose. Arch Orthop UnfallChir 1950;44:164.

18. Bickerstaff D, Neill L, Booth A, et al. Ultrasound examination of the irritable hip. J Bone Joint Surg [Br] 1990;7(4):549.

19. Blakemore ME, Harrison MHM. A prospective study of children with untreated Catterall group I Perthes disease. J Bone Joint Surg [Br] 1979;61:329.

20. Bobechko WP, Harris WR. The radiographic density of avascular bone. J Bone Joint Surg [Br] 1960;42:626.

21. Bobechko WP, McLaurin CA, Motloch WM. Toronto orthosis for Legg-Perthes disease. Artif Limbs 1968;12:36.

22. Bobechko WP. The Toronto brace for Legg-Perthes Disease. Clin Orthop 1974;102:115.

23. Bohr H, Baadsgaard K, Sager P. The vascular supply to the femoral head following dislocation of the hip joint: an experimental study in new-born rabbits. Acta Orthop Scand 1965;35:264.

24. Bohr HH. On the development and course of Legg-Calvé-Perthes disease (LCPD). Clin Orthop 1980;150:30.

25. Bombelli R. Osteoarthritis of the hip. Berlin: Springer-Verlag, 1983.

26. Bos CF, Bloem JL, Bloem RM. Sequential magnetic resonance imaging in Perthes' disease. J Bone Joint Surg [Br] 1991;73:219.

27. Bowen JR, Schreiber FC, Foster BK, Wein BK. Premature femoral neck physeal closure in Perthes disease. Clin Orthop 1982;171:24.

28. Bowen JR, Foster BK, Hartzell CR. Legg-Calvé-Perthes Disease. Clin Orthop 1985;185:97.

29. Brailsford JF. Avascular necrosis of bone. J Bone Joint Surg 1943;25:249.

30. Broder H. The late results in Legg-Perthes disease and factors influencing them: a study of one hundred and two cases. Bull Hosp Joint Dis 1953;14:194.

31. Brotherton BJ, McKibbin B. Perthes' disease treated by prolonged recumbency and femoral head containment: a long-term appraisal. J Bone Joint Surg [Br] 1977;59:8.

32. Bunger C, Solund K, Joyce F, Jonson OM. Carrageenan-induced coxities in puppies. Acta Orthop Scand 1988;59:249.

33. Bunnell WP. Legg-Calvé-Perthes disease. Pediatr Rev 1986;7:299.

34. Burwell RG, Coates CL, Vernon CL, et. al. Anthropometry and Perthes' disease: a preliminary report. J Bone Joint Surg [Br] 1976;58:254.

35. Burwell RG, Dangerfield PH, Hall DJ, et al. Perthes' disease: an anthropometric study revealing impaired and disproportionate growth. J Bone Joint Surg [Br] 1978;60:461.

36. Burwell RG, Vernon CL, Dangerfield PH, et al. Raised somatomedin activity in the serum of young boys with Perthes disease revealed by bioassay: a disease of growth transition? Clin Ortho Rel Res 1986;209:129.

37. Burwell RG. Perthes' disease: growth and aetiology. Arch Dis Child 1988;63:1408.

38. Caffey J. The early roentgenographic changes in essential coxa plana: their significance in pathogenesis. Am J Roentgenol 1968;103:620.

39. Cahuzac JP, Onimus M, Trottmann F, Clement JL, Laurain JM, Lebarbier P. Chiari pelvic osteotomy in Perthes disease. J Pediatr Orthop 1990;10:163.

40. Cahuzac JP, de-Gauzy JS, Vidal H, Gaubert J. The acetabular opening angle in Perthes' disease. Radiographic study of 62 unilateral cases. Acta Orthop Scand 1992;63:278.

41. Calot F. Uber Neuere Anschauungen in der Pathologie der Hufte auf Grund der Arbeiten der letzen Jahre. Z Orthop Chir 1929;51:134.

42. Calvé J. Sur une forme particuliere de coxalgie greffe sur des deformations caracteristiques de l'extremite superieure de femur. Rev Chir 1910;42:54.

43. Calvér R, Venugopal V, Dorgan J, et al. Radionuclide scanning in the early diagnosis of Perthes' disease. J Bone Joint Surg [Br] 1981;63:379.

44. Cameron J, Izatt MM. Legg-Calvé-Perthes disease. Scott Med J 1960;5:148.

45. Canale ST, D'Anca AF, Cotler JM, Snedden HE. Innominate osteotomy in Legg-Calvé-Perthes disease. J Bone Joint Surg [Am] 1972;54:25.

46. Canario AT, Williams L, Weintraub S, et al. A controlled study of the results of femoral osteotomy in severe Perthes' disease. J Bone Joint Surg [Br] 1980;62:348.

47. Canestri G, Monzali GL. Osteocondrite postridut Lattante iva nella L.C.A. L'osteochondrite apre reduction de la luxation congenitale de la hanche. Lattante 1957;28:537.

48. Cannon SR, Pozo JL, Catterall A. Elevated growth velocity in children with Perthes' disease. J Pediatr Orthop 1989;9(3):285.

49. Carroll NC, Donaldson J. Metaphyseal cysts in Legg-Calvé-Perthes disease (letter; comment). J Pediatr Orthop 1992;12:405.

50. Catterall A, Lloyd-Roberts GC, Wynne-Davies R. Association of Perthes' disease with congenital anomalies of genitourinary tract and inguinal region. Lancet 1971;1:996.

51. Catterall A. The natural history of Perthes' disease. J Bone Joint Surg [Br] 1971;53:37.

52. Catterall A. Coxa plana. In: Apley AP, ed. Modern trends in orthopaedics. London: Butterworths, 1972.

53. Catterall A. Perthes' disease. Br Med J 1977;1:1145.

54. Catterall A. Legg-Calvé-Perthes syndrome. Clin Orthop 1981;158:41.

55. Catterall A. Legg-Calvé-Perthes Disease. Edinburgh: Churchill Livingstone, 1982.

56. Catterall A, Pringle J, Byers PD, et al. Perthes' disease: is the epiphyseal infarction complete? A study of 2 cases. J Bone Joint Surg [Br] 1982;64:276.

57. Catterall A, Pringle J, Byers PD, et. al. A review of the morphology of Perthes disease. J Bone Joint Surg [Br] 1982;64:269.

58. Catterall A. Thoughts on the etiology of Perthes Disease. Iowa Orthop J 1984;4:34.

59. Catterall A. Legg-Calvé-Perthes disease. Classification and pathology. In: Fitzgerald RH Jr, ed. The hip. Proceedings of the thirteenth open scientific meeting of The Hip Society. St. Louis: CV Mosby, 1985.

60. Catterall A. The place of femoral osteotomy in the management of Legg-Calvé-Perthes disease. In: Fitzgerald RH Jr, ed. The Hip: Proceedings of the thirteenth open scientific meeting of The Hip Society. St. Louis: CV Mosby, 1985.

61. Catterall A. Adolescent hip pain after Perthes' disease. Clin Orthop 1986;209:65.

62. Catterall A. Legg-Calvé-Perthes disease. Instr Course Lect 1989;38:297.

63. Cavanaugh LA, Shelton EK, Sutherland R. Metabolic studies in osteochondritis of the capital femoral epiphysis. J Bone Joint Surg [Br] 1936;18:957.

64. Chacko V, Joseph B, Seetharam B. Perthes' disease in South India. Clin Orthop 1986;209:95.

65. Chigwanda PC. Early natural history of untreated Perthes' disease. Cent Afr J Med 1992;38:334.

66. Christensen FKS, Ejsted R, Luxiji T. The Catterall classification of Perthes. An assessment of reliability. J Bone Joint Surg [Br] 1978;60:166.

67. Chuinard EG. Femoral osteotomy in treatment of Legg-Calvé-Perthes syndrome. Orthop Rev 1979;8:113.

68. Chung SMK. The arterial supply of the developing proximal end of the human femur. J Bone Joint Surg [Am] 1976;58:961.

69. Clancy M, Steel HH. The effect of an incomplete intertrochanteric osteotomy on Legg-Calvé-Perthes disease. J Bone Joint Surg [Am] 1985;67:213.

70. Clarke TE, Finnegan TL, Fisher RL, et al. Legg-Perthes disease in children less than four years old. J Bone Joint Surg [Am] 1978;60:166.

71. Clarke NMP, Harrison MHM. Painful sequelae of coxa plana. J Bone Joint Surg [Am] 1983;65:13.

72. Coates CJ, Paterson JM, Woods KR, et al. Femoral osteotomy in Perthes' disease. Results at maturity. J Bone Joint Surg [Br] 1990;72:581.

73. Coleman SS. Observations on proximal femoral osteotomy and pelvic osteotomy. Orthop Rev 1979;8:139.

74. Coleman RC, Slager RF, Smith WS. The effect of environmental influences on acetabular development. Surg Forum 1958;9:775.

75. Coleman S, Kehl D. An evaluation of Perthes' disease: Comparison of non-surgical and surgical means. Presented at the American Academy of Orthopaedic Surgeons Meeting, Las Vegas, 1981.

76. Cooperman DR, Stulberg SD. Ambulatory containment treatment in Legg-Calvé-Perthes disease. In: Fitzgerald RH Jr, ed. The hip. Proceedings of the thirteenth open scientific meeting of The Hip Society. St. Louis: CV Mosby, 1985.

77. Cordeiro EN. Femoral osteotomy in Legg-Calvé-Perthes disease. Clin Orthop 1980;150:69.

78. Craig WA, Kramer WG, Watanabe R. Etiology and treatment of Legg-Calvé-Perthes syndrome. J Bone Joint Surg [Am] 1963;45:1325.

79. Craig WA. Course of Legg-Calvé-Perthes: natural history, pathomechanics. Orthop Rev 1979;8:29.

80. Craig WA KW. Combined Iliac and femoral osteotomies in Legg-Calvé-Perthes syndrome. J Bone Joint Surg [Am] 1974;56:1314.

81. Crutcher JP, Staheli LT. Combined osteotomy as a salvage procedure for severe Legg-Calvé-Perthes disease. J Pediatr Orthop 1992;12:151.

82. Cumming WJ. Personal communication. 1993.

83. Curtis BH, Gunther SF, Gossling HR, Paul SW. Treatment for Legg-Perthes disease with the Newington ambulation-abduction brace. J Bone Joint Surg [Am] 1974;56:1135.

84. Danforth MS. The treatment of Legg-Calvé-Perthes disease without weight bearing. J Bone Joint Surg [Br] 1934;16:516.

85. Danielsson LG, Hernborg J. Late results in Perthes' disease. Acta Orthop Scand 1965;36:70.

86. Danigelis JA, Fisher RL, Ozonoff MB, Sziklas JJ. 99m Tc-polyphosphate bone imaging in Legg-Perthes disease. Radiology 1975;115:407.

87. Danigelis JA. Pinhole imaging in Legg-Perthes disease: further observations. Semin Nucl Med 1976;6:69.

88. Dekker M, VanRens TJG, Sloff TJJH. Salter's pelvic osteotomy in the treatment of Perthes disease. J Bone Joint Surg [Br] 1981;68:282.

89. Denton J. Experience with Legg-Calvé-Perthes disease (LCPD), 1968–1974, at the New York Orthopaedic Hospital. Clin Orthop 1980;150:36.

90. Deutsch SD, Gandsman E, Spraragen SC. Quantitative radioscintigraphy in the evaluation of hip pain in children. Trans Orthop Res Soc 1979;4:187.

91. Dickens DRV, Menelaus MB. The assessment of the prognosis of Perthes' disease. J Bone Joint Surg [Br] 1978;60:189.

92. Dmitrienkov BN, Fedin AV, Zhvaniia TG, Subbotina EN. The diagnostic importance of a quantitative evaluation of gamma scintigraphy in Perthes' disease in children. Med Radiol 1989;34:19.

93. Dolman CL, Bell HM. The pathology of Legg-Calvé-Perthes disease. J Bone Joint Surg [Am] 1973;55:184.

94. Donovan MM, Urquhart BA. Treatment with ambulatory abduction brace. Orthop Rev 1979;8:147.

95. Doudoulakis JK. Trochanteric advancement for premature arrest of the femoral-head growth plate. 6-year review of 30 hips. Acta Orthop Scand 1991;62:92.

96. Eaton GO. Long-term results of treatment in coxa plana: a follow-up study of eighty-eight patients. J Bone Joint Surg [Am] 1967;49:1031.

97. Edberg E. Studien uber die sog: Osteochondritis coxae juvenilis. Zentralbl Chur 1919;11:206.

98. Edvardsen P, Slordahl J, Svenningsen S. Operative versus conservative treatment of Calvé-Legg-Perthes disease. Acta Orthop Scand 1981;52:553.

99. Egund N, Wingstrand H. Legg-Calvé-Perthes disease: imaging with MR. Radiology 1991;179:89.

100. Ekholm R. Nutrition of articular cartilage. Acta Anat 1955;24:329.

101. Elsig JP, Exner GU, von-Schulthess GK, Weitzel M. False-negative magnetic resonance imaging in early stage of Legg-Calvé-Perthes disease. J Pediatr Orthop 1989;9:231.

102. Emerick RW, Corrigan KF, Joistad AH Jr, Holly LE. Thyroid function in Legg-Calvé-Perthes disease: a new approach to an old problem. Clin Orthop 1954;4:160.

103. Englehardt P. Die Spatprognose des Morbus Perthes: Welche Faktoren festimmen das Arthroserisiko? Zeitschrift fur Orthopadie 1985;123:168.

104. Erken EH, Katz K. Irritable hip and Perthes' disease. J Pediatr Orthop 1990;10:322.

105. Evans DL, Lloyd-Roberts GC. Treatment in Legg-Calvé-Perthes disease. J Bone Joint Surg [Br] 1958;40:182.

106. Evans DL. Legg-Calvé-Perthes disease: a study of late results. J Bone Joint Surg [Br] 1958;40:168.

107. Evans IK, Deluca PA, Gage JR. A comparative study of ambulation-abduction bracing and varus derotation osteotomy in the treatment of severe Legg-Calvé-Perthes disease in children over 6 years of age. J Pediatr Orthop 1988;8:676.

108. Exner GU. Elevated growth velocity in children with Perthes' disease (letter; comment). J Pediatr Orthop 1989;9:732.

109. Eyre-Brooke AI. Osteochondritis deformans coxae juvenalis, or Perthes' disease: the results of treatment by traction in recumbency. Br J Surg 1936;24:166.

110. Fackler CD. Nonsurgical treatment of Legg-Calvé-Perthes disease. Instr Course Lect 1989;38:305.

111. Ferguson AB, Howorth MB. Coxa plana and related conditions at the hip. J Bone Joint Surg [Br] 1934;16:781.

112. Ferguson AB Jr. Synovitis of the hip and Legg-Perthes disease. Clin Orthop 1954;4:180.

113. Fisher RI. An epidemiological study of Legg-Perthes disease. J Bone Joint Surg [Am] 1972;54:769.

114. Fisher RL, Roderique JW, Brown DC, et al. The relationship of isotopic bone imaging findings to prognosis in Legg-Perthes disease. Clin Orthop 1980;150:23.

115. Fox KW, Griffin LL. Transient synovitis of the hip joint in children. Tex J Med 1956;52:15.

116. Frankel VH, Nordin M. Basic biometric of the skeletal system. Philadelphia: Lea & Febiger, 1980.

117. Fulford GE, Lunn PG, Macnicol MF. A prospective study of nonoperative and operative management for Perthes' disease. J Pediatr Orthop 1993;13:281.

118. Futami T, Kasahara Y, Suzuki S, et al. Ultrasonography in transient synovitis and early Perthes' disease. J Bone Joint Surg [Br] 1991;73:635.

119. Gall EA, Bennett GA. Osteochondritis deformans of the hip (Legg-Perthes disease) and renal osteitis fibrosa cystica: report of a case with anatomic studies. Arch Pathol 1942;33:866.

120. Garceau GJ. Surgical treatment of coxa plana. Presented at the Joint Meeting of the Orthopaedic Associations of the English Speaking World. J Bone Joint Surg [Br] 1964;46:779.

121. Gershuni DH. Etiology of Legg-Calvé-Perthes syndrome. Orthop Rev 1979;8:49.

122. Gershuni DH, Axer A, Handel D. Arthrography as an aid to the diagnosis and therapy in Legg-Calvé-Perthes disease. Acta Orthop Scand 1980;51:505.

123. Gershuni DH. Preliminary evaluation and prognosis in Legg-Calvé-Perthes disease. Clin Orthop 1980;150:16.

124. Gershuni DH. Subluxation of the femoral head in coxa plana (letter). J Bone Joint Surg [Am] 1988;70:950.

125. Ghaida HI, Hull ML, Rab GT. An instrumented brace for study of Legg-Calvé-Perthes disease. Biomaterials, Medical Devices, and Artificial Organs 1987;15:719.

126. Gill AB. Legg-Perthes disease of the hip: its early roentgeno-graphic manifestations and its clinical course. J Bone Joint Surg [Br] 1940;22:1043.

127. Gill AB. Relationship of Legg-Perthes disease to the function of the thyroid gland. J Bone Joint Surg [Br] 1943;25:892.

128. Gledhill RB, McIntyre JM. Transient synovitis and Legg-Calvé-Perthes disease. Can Med Assoc J 1969;7:311.

129. Glimcher MJ. Legg-Calvé-Perthes syndrome: biological and mechanical considerations in the genesis of clinical abnormalities. Orthop Rev 1979;8:33.

130. Goff CW. Legg-Calvé-Perthes syndrome and related osteochondroses of youth. Springfield, II: Charles C. Thomas, 1954.

131. Goff CW. Recumbency versus nonrecumbency treatment of Legg-Perthes disease. Clin Orthop 1959;14:50.

132. Goff CW. Legg-Calvé-Perthes syndrome (L.C.P.S.). Clin Orthop 1962;22:93.

133. Gower WE, Johnston RC. Legg-Perthes disease, long-term follow-up of thirty-six patients. J Bone Joint Surg [Am] 1971;53:759.

134. Green NE, Beauchamp RD, Griffen PP. Epiphyseal extrusion as a prognostic index in Legg-Calvé-Perthes disease. J Bone Joint Surg [Am] 1981;63:900.

135. Green NE, Griffen PP. Intra osseous venous hypertension in Legg-Perthes disease. J Bone Joint Surg [Am] 1982;64:666.

136. Gregosiewicz A, Okonski M, Stoecka D, et al. Ischemia of the femoral head in Perthes' disease: is the cause intra- or extravascular? J Pediatr Orthop 1989;9:160.

137. Grossbard GD. Hip pain in adolescence after Perthes disease. J Bone Joint Surg [Br] 1981;63:572.

138. Haliburton RA, Brockenshire FA, Barber JR. Avascular necrosis of the femoral capital epiphysis after traumatic dislocation of the hip in children. J Bone Joint Surg [Br] 1961;43:43.

139. Hall D, Harrison MHM. An association between congenital abnormalities and Perthes' disease of the hip. J Bone Joint Surg [Br] 1978;60:138.

140. Hall DJ, Harrison MHM, Burwell RG. Congenital abnormalities and Perthes disease. Clinical evidence that children with Perthes disease may have a major congenital defect. J Bone Joint Surg [Br] 1979;61:18.

141. Hall G. Some long-term observations of Perthes' disease. J Bone Joint Surg [Br] 1981;63:631.

142. Hall AJ, Barker DJ, Dangerfield PH, Taylor JF. Perthes' disease of the hip in Liverpool. Br Med J (Clin Res) 1983;287:1757.

143. Hall DJ. Genetic aspects of Perthes disease. A critical review. Clin Orthop 1986;209:100.

144. Hall AJ, Barker DJ, Dangerfield PH, et al. Small feet and Perthes' disease. A survey in Liverpool. J Bone Joint Surg [Br] 1988;70:611.

145. Hall AJ, Margetts BM, Barker DJ, et al. Low blood manganese levels in Liverpool children with Perthes' disease. Paediatr Perinat Epidemiol 1989;3:131.

146. Hall AJ, Barker DJ. Perthes' disease in Yorkshire. J Bone Joint Surg [Br] 1989;71:229.

147. Handlesmann JE. The Chiari pelvic shelving osteotomy. Orthop Clin North Am 1980;11:105.

148. Hardcastle PH, Ross R, Hamalainen M, Mata A. Catterall grouping of Perthes' disease: an assessment of observer error and prognosis using the Catterall classification. J Bone Joint Surg [Br] 1980;62:428.

149. Harper PS, Brotherton BJ, Cochlin D. Genetic risks in Perthes' disease. Clin Genet 1976;10:178.

150. Harrison MHM, Menon MPA. Legg-Calvé-Perthes disease: the value of x-ray measurement in clinical practice with special reference to the broomstick plaster method. J Bone Joint Surg [Am] 1966;48:1301.

151. Harrison MHM, Turner MH, Nicholson FJ. Coxa plana: results of a new form of splinting. J Bone Joint Surg [Am] 1969;51:1057.

152. Harrison MHM, Turner MH, Jacobs P. Skeletal immaturity in Perthes' disease. J Bone Joint Surg [Br] 1976;58:37.

153. Harrison MHM, Blakemore ME. A study of the "normal" hip in children with unilateral Perthes disease. J Bone Joint Surg [Br] 1980;62:36.

154. Harrison MHM, Burwell RG. Perthes' disease: a concept of pathogenesis. Clin Orthop 1981;156:115.

155. Harrison MHM, Turner MH, Smith DN. Perthes disease treatment with the Birmingham splint. J Bone Joint Surg [Br] 1982;64:3.

156. Haueisen DC, Weiner DS, Weiner SD. The characterization of transient synovitis of the hip in children. J Pediatr Orthop 1986;6:11.

157. Haythorn SR. Pathological changes found in material removed at operation in Legg-Calvé-Perthes disease. J Bone Joint Surg [Am] 1949;31:599.

158. Heikkinen E, Puranen J. Evaluation of femoral osteotomy in the treatment of Legg-Calvé-Perthes disease. Clin Orthop 1980;150:60.

159. Heikkinen E, Lanning P, Suramo I, Puranen J. The venous drainage of the femoral neck as a prognostic sign of Perthes' disease. Acta Orthop Scand 1980;51:501.

160. Heitzman O. Epiphysenerkrankungen im Wachstumsalter. Klin Webnschr 1923;327.

161. Helbo S. Morbus Calvé Perthes. Odense, Denmark: Fyna Tidendes Bogtrykkeri, 1954.

162. Henderson RC, Renner JB, Sturdivant MC, Greene WB. Evaluation of magnetic resonance imaging in Legg-Perthes disease: a prospective, blinded study. J Pediatr Orthop 1990;10:289.

163. Herring JA. Legg-Calvé-Perthes disease: a review of current knowledge. Instr Course Lect 1989;38:309.

164. Herring JA, Neustadt JB, Williams JJ, et al. The lateral pillar classification of Legg-Calvé-Perthes disease. J Pediatr Orthop 1992;12:143.

165. Herring JA, Williams JJ, Neustadt JN, Early JS. Evolution of femoral head deformity during the healing phase of Legg-Calvé-Perthes disease. J Pediatr Orthop 1993;13:41.

166. Heyman CH, Herndon CH. Legg-Perthes disease: method for measurement of roentgenographic result. J Bone Joint Surg [Am] 1950;32:767.

167. Hilgenreiner H. Beitrag zur atiologie der osteochondritis coxae juvenilis. Med Klin 1933;29:234.

168. Hoffinger SA, Rab GT, Salamon PB. "Metaphyseal" cysts in Legg-Calvé-Perthes' disease. J Pediatr Orthop 1991;11:301.

169. Hoffinger SA, Henderson RC, Renner JB, et al. Magnetic resonance evaluation of "metaphyseal" changes in Legg-Calvé-Perthes disease. J Pediatr Orthop 1993;13:602.

170. Hoikka V, Poussa M, Yrjonen T, Osterman K. Intertrochanteric varus osteotomy for Perthes' disease. Radiographic changes after 2–16-year follow-up of 126 hips. Acta Orthop Scand 1991;62(6):549.

171. Holdsworth FW. Epiphyseal growth: speculations on the nature of Perthes's disease. Ann R Coll Surg Engl 1966;39:1.

172. Howarth B. Coxa plana. Arch Pediatr 1959;76:1.

173. Howell FR, Newman RJ, Wang HL, et al. The three-dimensional anatomy of the proximal femur in Perthes' disease. J Bone Joint Surg [Br] 1989;71:408.

174. Hulth A. The vessel anatomy of the upper femur end with special regard to the mechanism of origin of different vascular disorders. Acta Orthop Scand 1958;27:192.

175. Hulth A. The femoral head—dead or alive! Acta Orthop Scand 1985;56:193.

176. Ikegawa S, Nagano A, Nakamura K. A case of multiple epiphyseal dysplasia complicated by unilateral Perthes' disease. Acta Orthop Scand 1991;62:606.

177. Ingman AM, Paterson DC, Sutherland AD. A comparison between innominate osteotomy and hip spica in the treatment of Legg Perthes disease. Clin Orthop 1982;163:141.

178. Inoue A, Freeman MAR, Vernon-Roberts B, Mizuno S. The pathogenesis of Perthes' disease. J Bone Joint Surg [Br] 1976;58:483.

179. Ippolito D, Tudisco C, Farsetti P. The long-term prognosis of unilateral Perthes' disease. J Bone Joint Surg [Br] 1987;69:243.

180. Iwasaki K. The role of blood vessels within the ligamentum teres in Perthes disease. Clin Orthop 1981;159:248.

181. Jacobs BW. Early recognition of osteochondrosis of capital epiphysis of femur. JAMA 1960;172:527.

182. Jansen M. Platte huftpfanne und ihre folgen coxa plana. Valga, vara and malum coxae. Z Orthop Chir 1925;46:234.

183. Jantzen PM. Hueftkoptnckrosen nach lateralen: Schenkelhalstrakturch. Z Orthop 1959;92:50.

184. Jensen OM, Lauritzen J. Legg-Calvé-Perthes disease. J Bone Joint Surg [Br] 1976;58:332.

185. Jonsater A. Coxa plana, a histopathologic and arthrographic study. Acta Orthop Scand 1953;12(suppl):1.

186. Joseph B, Chacko V, Rao BS, Hall AJ. The epidemiology of Perthes' disease in south India. Int J Epidemiol 1988;173:603.

187. Joseph B. Morphological changes in the acetabulum in Perthes' disease. J Bone Joint Surg [Br] 1989;71:756.

188. Kahle WK, Coleman SS. The value of the acetabular teardrop figure in assessing pediatric hip disorders. J Pediatr Orthop 1992;12:586.

189. Kallio P, Ryoppy S. Hyperpressure in juvenile hip disease. Acta Orthop Scand 1985;56:211.

190. Kallio P, Ryoppy S, Kunnamo I. Transient synovitis and Perthes: is there an etiologic connection. J Bone Joint Surg [Br] 1986;68:608.

191. Kamegaya M, Moriya H, Tsuchiya K, et al. Arthrography of early Perthes' disease. Swelling of the ligamentum teres as a cause of subluxation. J Bone Joint Surg [Br] 1989;71:413.

192. Kamegaya M, Shinada Y, Moriya H, et al. Acetabular remodelling in Perthes' disease after primary healing. J Pediatr Orthop 1992;12:308.

193. Kamhi E, MacEwen D. Treatment of Legg-Calvé-Perthes disease. J Bone Joint Surg [Am] 1975;57:651.

194. Katz JF. Protein-bound iodine in Legg-Calvé-Perthes disease. J Bone Joint Surg [Am] 1955;37:842.

195. Katz JF. Conservative treatment of Legg-Calvé-Perthes disease. J Bone Joint Surg [Am] 1967;49:1043.

196. Katz JF. Recurrent Legg-Calvé-Perthes disease. J Bone Joint Surg [Am] 1973;55:833.

197. Katz JF. Nonoperative therapy in Legg-Calvé-Perthes disease. Orthop Rev 1979;8:69.

198. Kelly FP, Canale ST, Jones RR. Legg-Calvé-Perthes disease: long-term evaluation of noncontainment treatment. J Bone Joint Surg [Am] 1980;62:400.

199. Kemp HBS, Boldero JL. Radiological changes in Perthes' disease. Br J Radiol 1966;39:744.

200. Kemp HBS. Experimental Perthes' disease. J Bone Joint Surg [Br] 1969;51:178.

201. Kendig RJ, Evans GA. Biologic osteotomy in Perthes Disease. J Pediatr Orthop 1986;6:278.

202. Kenzora JE, Steele RE, Yosipovitch ZH, Glimcher MJ. Experimental osteonecrosis of the femoral head in adult rabbits. Clin Orthop 1978;130:8.

203. Keret D, Harrison MHM, Clarke NMP, Hall DJ. Coxa plana: the fate of the physis. J Bone Joint Surg [Am] 1984;66:870.

204. Kiepurska A. Late results of treatment in Perthes' disease by a functional method. Clin Orthop 1991;272:76.

205. King EW, Fisher RL, Gage JR, Gossling HR. Ambulation-abduction treatment in Legg-Calvé-Perthes disease (LCPD). Clin Orthop 1980;150:43.

206. Kitsugi T, Kasahara Y, Seto Y, Komai S. Normal somatomedin-C activity measured by radioimmunoassay in Perthes' disease. Clin Orthop 1989;244:217.

207. Kleinman RG, Bleck EE. Increased blood viscosity in patients with Legg-Perthes disease: a preliminary report. J Pediatr Orthop 1981;1:131.

208. Klisic P, Seferovic O, Blazevic U. Perthes syndrome, classification and indications for treatment. Orthop Rev 1979; 8:81.

209. Klisic P, Blazevic U, Seferovic O. Approach to treatment of Legg Perthes disease. Clin Orthop 1980;150:54.

210. Kohler R, Seringe R, Borgi R. Osteochondrite de la hanche. Paris: Expansion Scientific Francais, 1981.

211. Kohler R, Michel CR, Chauvot P, et al. La-Scintigraphic osseuse dans la maladie de Legg Perthes-Calvé technique resultats, indications. Rev Chir Orthop 1984;(suppl 2): 70.

212. Konjetzny GE. Zur Pathologie und pathologischen anatomie der Perthes-Calvé schen krankheit. Acta Chir Scand 1943;74:361.

213. Krauspe R. Splint treatment of Perthes disease. Z Orthop 1990;128:411.

214. Kristmundsdottir F, Burwell RG, Harrison MHM. Delayed skeletal maturation in Perthes' disease. Acta Orthop Scand 1987;58:277.

215. Kruse RW, Guille JT, Bowen JR. Shelf arthroplasty in patients who have Legg-Calvé-Perthes disease. A study of long-term results. J Bone Joint Surg [Am] 1991;73:1338.

216. Kumasaka Y, Harada K, Watanabe H, et al. Modified epiphyseal index for MRI in Legg-Calvé-Perthes disease (LCPD). Pediatr Radiol 1991;21:208.

217. Lack W, Feldner-Busztin H, Ritschl P, Ramach W. The results of surgical treatment for Perthes' disease. J Pediatr Orthop 1989;9:197.

218. Larsen FH, Reiman I. Calvé-Perthes disease. Acta Orthop Scand 1973;44:426.

219. Laurent LE, Poussa M. Intertrochanteric varus osteotomy in the treatment of Perthes disease. Clin Orthop 1980;150:73.

220. Lauritzen J. The arterial supply to the femoral head in children. Acta Orthop Scand 1974;45:724.

221. Lauritzen J. Legg-Calvé-Perthes disease: a comparative study. Acta Orthop Scand 1975;159(suppl):1.

222. Lecuire F, Rebouillat J. Long-term development of primary osteochondritis of the hip (Legg-Perthes-Calvé). Apropos of 60 hips with a follow-up of more than 30 years. Rev Chir Orthop 1987;73:561.

223. Lee DY, Choi IH, Lee CK, Cho TJ. Assessment of complex hip deformity using three-dimensional CT image. J Pediatr Orthop 1991;11:13.

224. Lee DY, Seong SC, Choi IH, et al. Changes of blood flow of the femoral head after subtrochanteric osteotomy in Legg-Perthes' disease: a serial scintigraphic study. J Pediatr Orthop 1992;12:731.

225. Legg AT. An obscure affection of the hip joint. Boston Med Surg J 1910;162:202.

226. Legg AT. The end results of coxa plana. J Bone Joint Surg [Br] 1927;25:26.

227. Leitch JM, Paterson DC, Foster BK. Growth disturbance in Legg-Calvé-Perthes disease and the consequences of surgical treatment. Clin Orthop 1991;262:178.

228. Leriche R. Recherches experimentales sur le me canisme de formation de l'osteochondrite de la hanche. Lyon Chir 1934;31:610.

229. Levine B, Kanat IO. Subchondral bone cysts, osteochondritis dissecans, and Legg-Calvé-Perthes disease: a correlation and proposal of their possible common etiology and pathogenesis. J Foot Surg 1988;27:75.

230. Lindstrom JR, Ponseti IV, Wenger DR. Acetabular development after reduction in congenital dislocation of the hip. J Bone Joint Surg [Am] 1979;61:112.

231. Lippmann RK. The pathogenesis of Legg-Calvé-Perthes disease based upon the pathologic findings in a case. Am J Surg 1929;6:785.

232. Liu SL, He TQ. Mechanism of femoral head necrosis in Legg-Perthes disease. Chung Hua Wai Ko Tsa Chih 1987;25:643.

233. Liu SL, Ho TC. The role of venous hypertension in the pathogenesis of Legg-Perthes disease. A clinical and experimental study. J Bone Joint Surg [Am] 1991;73:194.

234. Lloyd-Roberts GC, Catterall A, Salamon PB. A controlled study of the indications for the results of femoral osteotomy in Perthes' disease. J Bone Joint Surg [Br] 1976;58:31.

235. Lloyd-Roberts GC. The management of Perthes disease. J Bone Joint Surg [Br] 1982;64:1.

236. Loder RT, Schwartz EM, Hensinger RN. Behavioral characteristics of children with Legg-Calvé-Perthes disease. J Pediatr Orthop 1993;13:598.

237. Lohmander LS, Wingstrand H, Heinegard D. Transient synovitis of the hip in the child: increased levels of proteoglycan fragments in joint fluid. J Orthop Res 1988;6:420.

238. Lovell WW, Hopper WC, Purvis JM. The Scottish Rite orthosis for Legg-Perthes disease. Exhibited at the annual meeting of the American Academy of Orthopaedic Surgeons, Dallas, Texas, 1978.

239. Lovell WW, MacEwen GD, Stewart WR, et al. Legg-Perthes disease in girls. J Bone Joint Surg [Br] 1982;64:637.

240. Lucht U, Bunger C, Krebs B, et al. Blood flow in the juvenile hip in relation to changes of the intraarticular pressure. An experimental investigation in dogs. Acta Orthop Scand 1983;54:182.

241. MacEwen GD. Conservative treatment of Legg-Calvé-Perthes condition. In: Fitzgerald RH Jr, ed. The hip. Proceedings of the thirteenth open scientific meeting of The Hip Society. St. Louis: CV Mosby, 1985.

242. Macnicol MF, Makris D. Distal transfer of the greater trochanter. J Bone Joint Surg [Br] 1991;73:838.

243. Malloy MK, MacMahon B. Incidence of Legg-Calvé-Perthes disease (osteochondritis deformans). N Engl J Med 1966;275:998.

244. Malloy MK, MacMahon B. Birth weight and Legg-Perthes disease. J Bone Joint Surg [Am] 1967;49:498.

245. Mandell GA, Harcke HT, Kumar SJ. Avascular necrosis and related conditions. Top Magn Reson Imaging 1991;4:31.

246. Marklund T, Tillberg G. Coxa plana: a radiological comparison of the rate of healing with conservative measures and after osteotomy. J Bone Joint Surg [Br] 1976;58:25.

247. Maroudas A, Bullough P, Swanson SAV, Freeman MAR. The permeability of articular cartilage. J Bone Joint Surg [Br] 1968;50:166.

248. Martinez AG, Weinstein SL. Recurrent Legg-Calvé-Perthes disease. Case report and review of the literature. J Bone Joint Surg [Am] 1991;73:1081.

249. Martinez AG, Weinstein SL, Dietz FR. The weight-bearing abduction brace for the treatment of Legg-Perthes disease. J Bone Joint Surg [Am] 1992;74:12.

250. Matsoukas J. Viral antibody titers to rubella in coxa plana or Perthes' disease. Acta Scand Orthop 1975;46:957.

251. Mau H. Juvenile osteochondroses endochondral dysostoses. Clin Orthop 1958;11:154.

252. Maydl K. Coxa vara arthritis deformans coxae. Wien Klin Rudsch 1897;10:153.

253. McAndrew MP, Weinstein SL. A long term follow-up of Legg-Calvé-Perthes disease. J Bone Joint Surg [Am] 1984;66:860.

254. McKay DW. Cheilectomy of the hip. Orthop Clin North Am 1980;11:141.

255. McKibbin B, Holdsworth FW. The nutrition of immature joint cartilage in the lamb. J Bone Joint Surg [Br] 1966;48:793.

256. McKibbin B, Rails Z. Pathological changes in a case of Perthes' disease. J Bone Joint Surg [Br] 1974;56:438.

257. McKibbin B. Recent advances in Perthes' disease. In: McKibbin B, ed. Recent advances in Perthes' disease. Edinburgh: Churchill Livingstone, 1975.

258. Meehan PL, Angel D, Nelson JM. The Scottish Rite abduction orthosis for the treatment of Legg-Perthes disease. A radiographic analysis. J Bone Joint Surg [Am] 1992;74:2.

259. Meyer J. Dysplasia epiphysealis capitus femoris: a clinical-radiological syndrome and its relationship to Legg-Calvé-Perthes Disease. Acta Orthop Scand 1964;34:183.

260. Meyer J. Treatment of Legg-Calvé-Perthes disease. Acta Orthop Scand 1966;86(suppl):9.

261. Millis MB, Poss R, Murphy SB. Osteotomies of the hip in the prevention and treatment of osteoarthritis. Instr Course Lect 1992;41:145.

262. Mindell ER, Sherman MS. Late results in Legg-Perthes disease. J Bone Joint Surg [Am] 1951;33:1.

263. Mintowt-Czyz WJ, Tayton KJ. The role of weight relief in Catterall group IV Perthes disease. J Bone Joint Surg [Br] 1982;64:247.

264. Mintowt-Czyz WJ, Tayton KJ. Indication for weight relief and containment in the treatment of Perthes disease. Acta Orthop Scand 1983;54:439.

265. Mirovski Y, Axer A, Hendel D. Residual shortening after osteotomy for Perthes disease. J Bone Joint Surg [Br] 1984;66:184.

266. Moberg A, Rehnberg L. Incidence of Perthes' disease in Uppsala, Sweden. Acta Orthop Scand 1992;63:157.

267. Moberg A RLaKC. Magnetic resonance imaging not indicated in healed Perthes disease. Comparison with radiography in 10 cases. Acta Orthop Scand 1993;64:537.

268. Mose K. Legg-Calvé-Perthes disease: a comparison among

three methods of conservative treatment. Arthus, Denmark: Universitesforlaget, 1964.

269. Mose K. Legg-Calvé-Perthes disease. Acta Orthop Scand 1966;86(suppl):1.

270. Mose K, Hjorth J, Ulfeldt M, et al. Legg-Calvé-Perthes disease: the late occurrence of coxarthrosis. Acta Orthop Scand 1977;169(suppl):1.

271. Mose K. Methods of measuring in Legg-Calvé-Perthes disease with special regard to the prognosis. Clin Orthop 1980;150:103.

272. Muirhead-Allwood W, Catterall A. The treatment of Perthes disease. The results of a trial of management. J Bone Joint Surg [Br] 1982;64:282.

273. Mukamel M, Litmanovitch M, Yosipovitch Z, et al. Legg Calvé Perthes disease following transient synovitis. How often. Clin Pediatr 1985;24:629.

274. Mukherjee A, Fabry G. Evaluation of the prognostic indices in Legg-Calvé-Perthes disease. J Pediatr Orthop 1990;10:153.

275. Naito M, Schoenecker PL, Owen JH, Sugioka Y. Acute effect of traction, compression, and hip joint tamponade on blood flow of the femoral head: an experimental model. J Orthop Res 1992;10:800.

276. Naumann T, Kollmannsberger A, Fischer M, Puhl W. Ultrasonographic evaluation of Legg-Calvé-Perthes disease based on sonoanatomic criteria and the application of new measuring techniques. Eur J Radiol 1992;15:101.

277. Neidel J, Zander D, Hackenbroch MH. Low plasma levels of insulin-like growth factor I in Perthes' disease. A controlled study of 59 consecutive children. Acta Orthop Scand 1992;63:393.

278. Neidel J, Zander D, Hackenbroch MH. No physiologic age-related increase of circulating somatomedin-C during early stage of Perthes' disease: a longitudinal study in 21 boys. Arch Orthop Trauma Surg 1992;111:171.

279. Neidel J, Boddenberg B, Zander D, et al. Thyroid function in Legg-Calvé-Perthes disease: cross-sectional and longitudinal study. J Pediatr Orthop 1993;13:592.

280. Neidel JSE, Zander D, Rutt J, Hackenbroch MH. Normal plasma levels of IGF binding protein in Perthes disease. Follow up of a previous report. Acta Orthop Scand 1993;64:540.

281. Norlin R, Hammerby S, Tkaczuk H. The natural history of Perthes' disease. Int Orthop 1991;15:13.

282. O'Garra JA. The radiographic changes in Perthes' disease. J Bone Joint Surg [Br] 1959;41:465.

283. O'Hara JP, Davis ND, Gage JR, et al. Long-term follow-up of Perthes' disease treated nonoperatively. Clin Orthop 1977;125:49.

284. O'Sullivan M, O'Rourke SK, MacAuley P. Legg-Calvé-Perthes disease in a family: genetic or environmental. Clin Orthop 1985;199:179.

285. Ogden JA. Changing patterns of proximal femoral vascularity. J Bone Joint Surg [Am] 1974;56:941.

286. Olney BW, Asher MA. Combined innominate and femoral osteotomy for the treatment of severe Legg-Calvé-Perthes disease. J Pediatr Orthop 1985;5;645.

287. Oshima M, Yoshihasi Y, Ito K, et al. Initial stage of Legg-Calvé-Perthes disease: comparison of three-phase bone scintigraphy and SPECT with MR imaging. Eur J Radiol 1992;15:107.

288. Paterson DC, Leitch JM, Foster BK. Results of innominate osteotomy in the treatment of Legg-Calvé-Perthes disease. Clin Orthop 1991;266:96.

289. Pauwels F. Des affections de la hanche d'origine mecanique et de laur traitement par l'osteotomie d'adduction. Rev Chir Orthop 1951;37:22.

290. Peic S. Contribution to Perthes disease. Z Orthop 1962;96:276.

291. Perpich M, McBeath A, Kruse D. Long term follow-up of Perthes disease treated with spica casts. J Pediatr Orthop 1983;3:160.

292. Perthes G. Uber arthritis deformans juvenilis. Dtsch Z Chir 1910;10:111.

293. Perthes G. Osteochondritis deformans juvenilis. Arch Klin Chir 1913;101:779.

294. Petrie JG, Bitenc I. The abduction weight bearing treatment in Legg-Perthes disease. J Bone Joint Surg [Br] 1971;53:54.

295. Pettersson H, Wingstrand H, Thambert C, et al. Legg-Calvé-Perthes disease in hemophilia: incidence and etiologic considerations. J Pediatr Orthop 1990;10:28.

296. Moller PF. The clinical observations after healing of Calvé Perthes disease compared with final deformities left by that disease and the bearing of those final deformities on ultimate prognosis. Acta Radiol 1926;5:1.

297. Phemister DB. Operation for epiphysitis of the head of the femur (Perthes' disease). Arch Surg 1921;2:221.

298. Phemister DB. Perthes' disease. Surg Gynecol Obstet 1921;33:87.

299. Phemister DB. Bone growth and repair. Ann Surg 1935;102:261.

300. Pinto MR, Peterson HA, Berquist TH. Magnetic resonance imaging in early diagnosis of Legg-Calvé-Perthes disease. J Pediatr Orthop 1989;9:19.

301. Pirescle CF, Macielde GR Jr, Tovo R. Angiography in Perthes disease. Clin Orthop 1984;191:216.

302. Ponseti IV, Shepard RS. Lesions of the skeleton and of other mesodermal tissues in rats fed sweet-pea (Lathyrus odoratus) seeds. J Bone Joint Surg [Am] 1954;36:1031.

303. Ponseti IV. Legg-Perthes disease. J Bone Joint Surg [Am] 1956;38:739.

304. Ponseti IV, Cotton RL. Legg-Calvé-Perthes disease: pathogenesis and evaluation. J Bone Joint Surg [Am] 1961;43:261.

305. Ponseti IV, Maynard JA, Weinstein SL, et al. Legg-Calvé-Perthes disease. Histochemical and ultrastructural observations of the epiphyseal cartilage and the physis. J Bone Joint Surg [Am] 1983;65:797.

306. Price CT, Day DD, Flynn JC. Behavioral sequelae of bracing versus surgery for Legg-Calvé-Perthes disease. J Pediatr Orthop 1988;8:285.

307. Purry NA. The incidence of Perthes disease in the population groups in the Eastern Cape region of South Africa. J Bone Joint Surg [Br] 1982;64:286.

308. Purvis JM, Dimon JH III, Meehan PL, Lovell WW. Preliminary experience with the Scottish Rite Hospital abduction orthosis for Legg-Perthes disease. Clin Orthop 1980;150:49.

309. Quain S, Catterall A. Hinge abduction of the hip. Diagnosis and treatment. J Bone Joint Surg [Br] 1986;68:61.

310. Rab GT. Containment of the hip: a theoretical comparison of osteotomies. Clin Orthop 1981;154:191.

311. Rab GT, DeNatale JS, Herrmann LR. Three dimensional finite element analysis of Legg-Calvé-Perthes disease. J Pediatr Orthop 1982;2:39.

312. Rab GT. Determination of femoral head containment during gait. Biomaterials, Medical Devices, and Artificial Organs 1983;11:31.

313. Ralis Z, McKibbin B. Changes in shape of the human hip joint during its development and their relation to its stability. J Bone Joint Surg [Br] 1973;55:780.

314. Ralston EL. Legg-Perthes disease and physical development. J Bone Joint Surg [Am] 1955;37:647.

315. Ratliff AHC. Perthes' disease: a study of 34 hips observed for 30 years. J Bone Joint Surg [Br] 1967;49:108.

316. Ratliff AHC. Perthes' disease: a study of 16 patients followed up for 40 years. J Bone Joint Surg [Br] 1977;59:248.

317. Ray RD, LaViolette D, Buckley HD, Mosiman RS. Studies of bone metabolism. I. A comparison of the metabolism of strontium in living and dead bone. J Bone Joint Surg [Am] 1955;37:143.

318. Rayner PHW, Schwalbe SL, Hall DJ. An assessment of endocrine function in boys with Perthes disease. Clin Orthop 1986;209:124.

319. Remvig Q, Mose K. Perthes' disease. J Bone Joint Surg [Br] 1961;43:855.

320. Richards BS, Coleman SS. Subluxation of the femoral head in coxa plana. J Bone Joint Surg [Am] 1987;69:1312.

321. Riedel G. Pathologic anatomy of osteochondritis deformans coxae juvenilis. Zentralbl Chir 1922;49:1447.

322. Ritterbusch JF, Shantharam SS, Gelinas C. Comparison of lateral pillar classification and Catterall classification of Legg-Calvé-Perthes' disease. J Pediatr Orthop 1993;13:200.

323. Roberts JM, Meehan P, Counts G, Counts W. Ambulatory abduction brace for Legg-Perthes disease. Exhibited at the annual session of the American Academy of Orthopaedic Surgeons, Dallas, Texas, 1974.

324. Roberts JM, Zink WP. Arthrographic classification of Legg-Perthes disease. Exhibited at the annual meeting of the American Academy of Orthopaedic Surgeons, Las Vegas, Nevada, 1981.

325. Robinson HJ Jr, Putter H, Sigmond MB, et al. Innominate osteotomy in Perthes disease. J Pediatr Orthop 1988;8:426.

326. Rockemer K. Zur histopathogenese der Perthesschen drankheit, an der hand eines Fruhfalles. Frankfurt Z Path 1927;35:1.

327. Rowe SM, Kim HS, Yoon TR. Osteochondritis dissecans in Perthes' disease. Report of 7 cases. Acta Orthop Scand 1989;60:545.

328. Royle SG, Galasko CSB. The irritable hip. Scintigraphy in 192 children. Acta Orthop Scand 1992;63:25.

329. Rush BH, Bramson RT, Ogden JA. Legg-Calvé-Perthes disease: detection of cartilaginous and synovial change with MR imaging. Radiology 1988;167:473.

330. Ryder CT, Lebouvier JD, Kane R. Coxa plana. Pediatrics 1957;19:979.

331. Saito STK, Ono K, Minobe Y, Inoue A. Residual deformities related to arthritic change after Perthes disease: a long term follow up of fifty one cases. Arch Orthop Trauma Surg 1985;104:7.

332. Salter RB. Experimental and clinical aspects of Perthes' disease. J Bone Joint Surg [Br] 1966;48:393.

333. Salter RB, Bell M. The pathogenesis of deformity in Legg-Perthes disease: an experimental investigation. J Bone Joint Surg [Br] 1968;50:436.

334. Salter RB. Perthes' disease: treatment by innominate osteotomy. Instr Course Lect 1973;22:309.

335. Salter RB. Legg-Perthes disease: the scientific basis for the methods of treatment and their indications. Clin Orthop 1980;150:8.

336. Salter RB. The present status of surgical treatment of Legg-Perthes disease: current concept review. J Bone Joint Surg [Am] 1984;66:961.

337. Salter RB, Thompson GH. Legg-Calvé-Perthes disease. The prognostic significance of the subchondral fracture and a two group classification of the femoral head involvement. J Bone Joint Surg [Am] 1984;66:479.

338. Salter RB. The scientific basis for innominate osteotomy for Legg-Calvé-Perthes disease and the results in children with a bad prognosis. Orthop Trans 1985;9:203.

339. Salvo-Legarre JC. Confrontacion de los resultados operatorios y concervadores en la entermeded de L.C.P. M Clin 1957;28:380.

340. Sanchis M, Freeman MAR, Zahir A. Experimental stimulation of the blood supply to the capital epiphysis in the puppy. J Bone Joint Surg [Am] 1973;55:335.

341. Schepers A, VonBormann PFB, Craig JJG. Coxa magna in Perthes disease: treatment by Chiari pelvic osteotomy. J Bone Joint Surg [Br] 1978;60:297.

342. Schiller MG, Axer A. Hypertrophy of the femoral head in Legg-Calvé-Perthes syndrome (LCPS). Acta Orthop Scand 1972;43:45.

343. Schlesinger I, Crider RJ. Gage's sign—revisited! J Pediatr Orthop 1988;8:201.

344. Schoen. Legg-Perthes disease in children under 6 years old. Orthop Rev 1993;22:201.

345. Schwartz E. Eine typische Erkrankung der oberen femurepiphyse. Beitr Klin Chir 1914;93:127.

346. Scoles PV, Yoon YS, Makley JT, Kalamachi A. Nuclear magnetic resonance imaging in Legg-Calvé-Perthes disease. J Bone Joint Surg [Am] 1984;66:1357.

347. Siffert RS. Osteochondritis of the proximal femoral epiphysis. Instr Course Lect 1973;22:270.

348. Simmons ED, Graham HK, Szalai JP. Interobserver variability in grading Perthes' disease. J Bone Joint Surg [Br] 1990;72:202.

349. Sjovall H. Zur frage der behandlung der coxa plana mit besondererberucksichtigung der primarerfolge bei konsequenter ruhigstellung. Acta Orthop Scand 1942;13:324.

350. Slavik J. Coxa plana: morbus maydl-Calvé-Legg-Perthes. Prague: Albertova Sbirka, 1956.

351. Smith RB, Nevelos AB. Osteochondritis occurring at multiple sites. Acta Orthop Scand 1980;51:449.

352. Smith RB, Ions GK, Gregg PJ. The radiological features of the metaphysis in Perthes disease. J Pediatr Orthop 1982;2:401.

353. Snow SW, Keret D, Scarangella S, Bowen JR. Anterior impingement of the Legg-Calvé-Perthes' disease. J Pediatr Orthop 1993;13:286.

354. Snyder CF. A sling for use in Legg-Perthes disease. J Bone Joint Surg [Br] 1947;29:524.

355. Somerville EW. Osteotomy in treatment of Perthes' disease of the hip. Orthop Rev 1979;8:61.

356. Sponseller PD, Desai SS, Millis MB. Comparison of femoral and innominate osteotomies for the treatment of Legg-Calvé-Perthes disease. J Bone Joint Surg [Am] 1988;70:1131.

357. Sponseller PD, Desai SS, Millis MB. Abnormalities of proximal femoral disease. J Bone Joint Surg [Br] 1989;71:610.

358. Stevens P, Williams P, Menelaus M. Innominate osteotomy for Perthes' disease. J Pediatr Orthop 1981;1:47.

359. Stulberg SD, Salter RB. The natural course of Legg-Perthes disease and its relationship to degenerative arthritis of the hip: long-term follow-up study. Orthop Trans 1977;1:105.

360. Stulberg SD. Legg-Calvé-Perthes disease: update. In: The hip. Proceedings of the sixth open scientific meeting of The Hip Society. St. Louis: CV Mosby, 1978.

361. Stulberg SD, Cooperman DR, Wallensten R. The natural history of Legg-Calvé-Perthes disease. J Bone Joint Surg [Am] 1981;63:1095.

362. Sundt H. Malum coxae: Calvé-Legg-Perthes. Zentralbl Chir 1920;22:538.

363. Sundt H. Malum coxae Calvé-Legg-Perthes. Kristiania: Monographie, 1920.

364. Sundt H. Malum coxae Calvé-Legg Perthes. Acta Chir Scand 1949;148(suppl):1.

365. Suramo I, Puranen J, Heikkinen E, Vuorinen P. Disturbed patterns of venous drainage of the femoral neck in Perthes disease. J Bone Joint Surg [Br] 1974;56:448.

366. Sutherland AD, Savage JP, Patterson DC, Foster BK. The nuclide bone scan in the diagnosis and management of Perthes disease. J Bone Joint Surg [Br] 1980;63:300.

367. Tachdjian MO, Grana L. Response of the hip joint to increased intra-articular hydrostatic pressure. Clin Orthop 1968;61:199.

368. Tanaka H, Tamura K, Takano K, et al. Serum somatomedin A in Perthes disease. Acta Orthop Scand 1984;55:135.

369. Theron J. Angiography in Legg-Calvé-Perthes disease. Radiology 1980;135:81.

370. Thomas HO. Contributions to surgery and medicine. Part II. Principles of the treatment of diseased joints. London: H.K. Lewis, 1883.

371. Thompson G, Westin GW. Legg-Calvé-Perthes disease: results discontinuing treatment in the early reossification stage. Clin Orthop 1979;139:70.

372. Trueta J, Harrison MHM. The normal vascular anatomy of the femoral head in adult man. J Bone Joint Surg [Br] 1953;35:442.

373. Trueta J. The normal vascular anatomy of the human femoral head during growth. J Bone Joint Surg [Br] 1957;39:358.

374. Trueta J, Pinto de Lima CS. Studies of osteochondritis of the femoral head or Legg-Calvé-Perthes disease. Rev Orthop Traum Lat Am 1959;4:115.

375. Trueta J, Little K, Amato VP. The vascular contribution to osteogenesis. II. Studies with the electron microscope. III. Changes in the growth cartilage caused by experimentally induced ischaemia. J Bone Joint Surg [Br] 1960;42:367.

376. Tucker FR. Arterial supply to the femoral head and its clinical importance. J Bone Joint Surg [Br] 1949;31:82.

377. Van Dam BE, Crider RJ, Noyes JD, Larsen LJ. Determination of the Catterall classification in Legg-Calvé-Perthes disease. J Bone Joint Surg [Am] 1981;63:906.

378. Van der Hayden AM, Van Tongerloo RB. Shelf operations in Perthes disease. J Bone Joint Surg [Br] 1981;63:282.

379. Vasseur PB, Foley P, Stevenson S, Heitter D. Mode of inheritance of Perthes' disease in Manchester terriers. Clin Orthop 1989;244:281.

380. Vila-Verde VM. Magnetic resonance imaging in early diagnosis of Legg-Calvé-Perthes disease (letter; comment). J Pediatr Orthop 1989;9:630.

381. Waldenstrom H. Der obere Tuberkulose collumnerd. Z Orthop Chir 1909;24:487.

382. Waldenstrom H. Die Tuberkulose des Collum Femoris im Kindersalte ihre Beziehungen zur Huftgelenkentzundung. Stockholm: 1910.

383. Waldenstrom H. Coxa plana, osteochondritis deformans coxae, Calvé-Perthes'schen krankheit, Legg's disease. Zentralbl Chir 1920;17:539.

384. Waldenstrom H. The definitive forms of coxa plana. Acta Radiol 1922;1:384.

385. Waldenstrom H. The first stages of coxa plana. Acta Orthop Scand 1934;5:1.

386. Waldenstrom H. The first stages of coxa plana. J Bone Joint Surg [Br] 1938;20:559.

387. Wansborough RM, Carrie AW, Walker NF, Ruckerbauer G. Coxa plana: its genetic aspects and results of treatment with long Taylor walking caliper. J Bone Joint Surg [Am] 1959;41:1959.

388. Watson-Jones R, Roberts RE. Calcifications, decalcification and ossification. Br J Surg 1934;21:461.

389. Weiner SD, Weiner DS, Riley PM. Pitfalls in treatment of Legg-Calvé-Perthes disease using proximal femoral varus osteotomy. J Pediatr Orthop 1991;11:20.

390. Weinstein SL, Ponseti IV. Congenital dislocation of the hip: open reduction through a medial approach. J Bone Joint Surg [Am] 1979;61:119.

391. Weinstein SL. Legg-Calvé-Perthes disease. St. Louis: CV Mosby, 1983.

392. Weinstein SL. Improving the prognosis in Legg-Calvé-Perthes disease. J Musculoskeletal Medicine 1984;11:22.

393. Weinstein SL. Long-term follow-up of patients with Legg-Calvé-Perthes disease. Orthop Trans 1985;9:204.

394. Weinstein SL. Legg-Calvé-Perthes disease: results of long-term follow-up. In: Fitzgerald RH Jr, ed. The hip. Proceedings of the thirteenth open scientific meeting of The Hip Society. St. Louis: CV Mosby, 1985.

395. Weinstein SL. The pathogenesis of deformity in Legg-Calvé-Perthes' disease. In: Uhthoff H, Wiley J, eds. Behavior of the growth plate. New York: Raven, 1988.

396. Weinstein SL. Perthes disease: an overview. Curr Orthop 1988;2:181.

397. Wenger DR. Selective surgical containment for Legg Perthes disease: recognition and management of complications. J Pediatr Orthop 1981;1:153.

398. Wenger DR, Ward WT, Herring JA. Legg-Calvé-Perthes disease. J Bone Joint Surg [Am] 1991;73(5):778.

399. Wiberg G. Studies on dysplastic acetabula and congenital subluxation of the hip joint. Acta Chir Scand 1939;83(suppl 58):1.

400. Willett K, Hudson I, Catterall A. Lateral shelf acetabuloplasty: an operation for older children with Perthes' disease. J Pediatr Orthop 1992;12:563.

401. Wingstrand H, Bauer G, Brimar J, et al. Transient ischemia of the proximal femoral epiphysis in the child. Interpretation of bone scintimetry for diagnosis in hip pain. Acta Orthop Scand 1985;56:197.

402. Wingstrand H, Egund N, Carlin NO, et al. Intracapsular pressure in transient synovitis of the hip. Acta Orthop Scand 1985;56:204.

403. Wirth T, LeQuesne GW, Paterson DC. Ultrasonography in Legg-Calvé-Perthes disease. Pediatr Radiol 1992;22:498.

404. Wolcott WE. The evolution of the circulation in the developing femoral head and neck: an anatomic study. Surg Gynecol Obstet 1943;77:61.

405. Wright GA. The value of determining the primary lesion in joint disease as an indication for treatment. Br Med J 1883;2:419.

406. Wynne-Davies R, Gormley J. The aetiology of Perthes' disease. J Bone Joint Surg [Br] 1978;60:6.

407. Wynne-Davies R. Some etiologic factors in Perthes' disease. Clin Orthop 1980;150:12.

408. Yamaguchi M. A histological study of the neck of the femur in Perthes' disease. Igaku Kenkyu 1959;29:317.

409. Yrjonen T, Hoikka V, Poussa M, Osterman K. Leg-length inequality and low-back pain after Perthes' disease: a 28–47-year follow-up of 96 patients. J Spinal Disord 1992;5:443.

410. Yrjonen T. Prognosis in Perthes' disease after noncontainment treatment. 106 hips followed for 28–47 years. Acta Orthop Scand 1992;63:523.

411. Yrjonen T, Poussa M, Hoikka V, Osterman K. Poor prognosis in atypical Perthes' disease. Radiographic analysis of 19 hips after 35 years. Acta Orthop Scand 1992;63:399.

412. Zemansky AP. The pathology and pathogenesis of Legg-Calvé-Perthes disease (osteochondritis juvenilis deformans coxae). Am J Surg 1928;4:169.

Lovell & Winter's Pediatric Orthopaedics, fourth edition,
edited by Raymond T. Morrissy and Stuart L. Weinstein.
Lippincott–Raven Publishers, Philadelphia © 1996.

Chapter

25

Slipped Capital Femoral Epiphysis

Douglas K. Kehl

Slipped capital femoral epiphysis (SCFE) remains one of the most common disorders affecting the hip during adolescence. The condition is characterized by a displacement of the capital femoral epiphysis from the femoral neck through the physeal plate. The femoral head is held securely in the acetabulum, whereas the femoral neck displaces mainly in an anterior direction creating an apparent varus deformity at the proximal femur. Rarely, femoral neck displacement can be in a posterior direction creating a proximal femoral valgus deformity.[144] The physiolysis in SCFE differs from that seen in traumatic physeal fracture. Histologic studies have shown that the separation in SCFE is through a widened zone of hypertrophy, which has become weakened by alterations in chondrocyte maturation and endochondral ossification.[18,62]

EPIDEMIOLOGY

The annual incidence of SCFE has been reported to average 2 per 100,000 in the general population. Minomiya and colleagues have reported an incidence as low as 0.2 per 100,000 in the eastern half of Japan,[144] whereas Kelsey and colleagues have reported an inci-

dence as high as 10.08 per 100,000 in certain regions of the United States.[70]

SCFE is related to puberty, as evidenced by 78% of cases of SCFE occurring during the adolescent growth phase.[125] The age range at presentation in boys is most often between 10 and 16 years of age (average, 13.5 years), and in girls it is between 10 and 14 years of age (average, 11.5 years).[55,70] When a patient with SCFE presents at an age outside of these ranges, the treating physician should strongly consider an underlying endocrine or systemic disorder to include primary and secondary hypothyroidism, panhypopituitarism, hypogonadal conditions, and renal osteodystrophy.

A delay in skeletal maturation commonly is seen in patients with SCFE. In some studies, skeletal age has been found to be as much as 20 months behind chronologic age in up to 70% of affected individuals.[98,125]

A male predilection for SCFE has been reported at 2.4 to 1, with the left hip being affected twice as often.[146] An increased incidence of SCFE has been reported in African-American people.[70]

Obesity definitely is associated with the development of SCFE. Kelsey and colleagues have reported weight for age profiles over the 95th percentile in 49% of affected individuals.[69] Brenkel and colleagues have reported weight for height profiles over the 90th percentile in 73% of affected boys and 52% of affected girls.[17] Clinically obese patients acquiring SCFE also tend to present at a younger age.[78]

Bilateral symptomatic involvement with SCFE averages 25% during adolescence (range, 21%–37%).[22,49,78,122,146] Approximately 50% of these patients present with bilateral involvement, and the remaining 50% show sequential onset.[22,78,122,146] Long-term follow-up studies, however, identify changes of bilateral involvement in as much as 60% to 80% of patients with known unilateral SCFE.[14,49] This implies that many sequential SCFEs occur asymptomatically, prior to the end of growth. When bilateral symptomatic involvement occurs sequentially, Loder and colleagues have shown the second slip to present by 12 months in 77% of patients and 18 months in 80% of patients.[78] Bilateral involvement also is reported to have a higher incidence in males, African-American patients, and obese patients with younger age at initial presentation.[78,146]

PATHOANATOMY

Historically the femoral head was believed to displace mainly in a medial direction off of the femoral neck in SCFE, creating a radiographic varus deformity at the proximal femur.[47] Nguyen and Morrissy have demonstrated that the displacement in SCFE occurs mainly in a posterior direction as the femoral head rotates around the axis of the femoral neck with the apparent proximal femoral varus deformity being secondary to radiographic parallax.[102] Some cephalad displacement of the femoral neck can occur in chronic SCFE but only after the femoral head has slipped to the posterior aspect of the femoral neck (Fig. 25-1). This knowledge becomes extremely important when considering surgical stabilization of a slip.

Histologic examination of the hip joint and physeal plate in patients with SCFE has shown several abnormalities. The synovium demonstrates a hyperplasia with increased vascularity and round cell infiltration indicative of an inflammatory response.[40,96] The physeal plate is noted to be widened. Ippolito and colleagues have shown that this increase in physeal plate width can be as much as twice normal.[62] The majority of the change in the physeal plate occurs in the zone of hypertrophy. The hypertrophic zone normally constitutes 15% to 30% of the width of the normal physeal plate. In SCFE, this zone can increase to as much as 80% of the width of the physeal plate.[62,144] Abnormal cartilage maturation and subsequent endochondral ossification are implied by the microscopic identification of disruption of the normal columnar pattern of the cartilage columns into cartilage cell clusters and

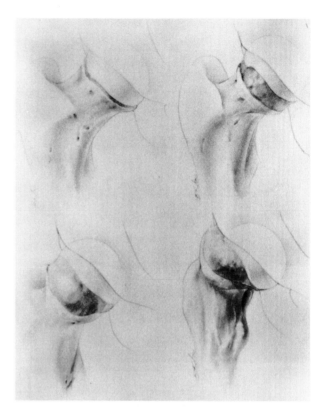

FIGURE 25-1. In the early displacement of chronic slipped capital femoral epiphysis, the femoral head is held securely in the acetabulum while the femoral neck initially migrates in an anterior direction (*top left, top right*). The resultant posterior displacement of the femoral head around the axis of the femoral neck continues until the femoral head contacts the posterior aspect of the femoral neck (*bottom left*). In this later stage of displacement, the femoral neck may begin to additionally migrate cephalad in relation to the femoral head (*bottom right*). (From Morrissy RT. Principles of in situ fixation in chronic slipped capital femoral epiphysis. Instr Course Lect 1989;38:259.)

the presence of cartilage cell islands extending into the adjacent femoral metaphysis[3,62,91] (Fig. 25-2). The slip cleft is noted to traverse mainly the zone of hypertrophy.[62,91,108]

Electron microscopic studies demonstrate disorganized collagen fibrils in the physeal plate with abnormal accumulations of proteoglycans and glycoproteins particularly adjacent to the slip cleft.[4,62,91]

Although several abnormalities in the hip joint synovium and proximal femoral physeal plate have been documented histologically, it remains undetermined whether these changes are primary abnormalities or, more likely, responses secondary to minimal physeal slippage.

ETIOLOGY

The true etiology of SCFE remains unknown. It is unlikely that it is the result of a single factor but rather

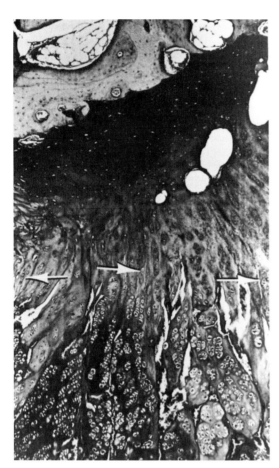

FIGURE 25-2. Photomicrograph of the proximal femoral growth plate of a 13-year-old boy with slipped capital femoral epiphysis. The resting zone is noted to be thinned and accounts for much less than its normal 60% to 70% of the thickness of the physeal plate. The proliferating zone (*arrows*) demonstrates short columns of chondrocytes enveloped in a compact matrix. The hypertrophic zone is greatly thickened. Large clusters of chondrocytes separated by deep clefts containing matrix debris replace the orderly columnar pattern normally seen in this zone. (From Ippolito E, Mickelson M, Ponseti I. A histochemical study of slipped capital femoral epiphysis. J Bone Joint Surg [Am] 1981;63:1110.

is more likely secondary to multiple factors resulting in a weakened physeal plate that is loaded with a higher than normal shear stress resulting in a failure of the proximal femoral physeal plate.[46,59,72,88,110]

Local trauma to the proximal femur frequently is reported as a possible contributing etiologic factor in SCFE.[107,146] Wilson and colleagues reported 26% of the patients in their review to have had a history of antecedent trauma.[146] Trauma was reported much more frequently in slips that presented with an acute onset and a short duration of symptoms. Although traumatic transphyseal fracture of the proximal femur and SCFE share a similar gender and peak incidence, the amount of force required to cause physiolysis and the region of the physis through which the slip cleft traverses differ in the two conditions.[18,62] The majority of traumatic transphyseal fractures of the proximal

femur are the result of high-energy injuries, such as motor vehicle accidents and falls from a height. SCFE presenting with an acute onset, on the other hand, usually follows a minor torsional or low energy injury.

Mechanical factors affecting the proximal femoral physis also have been proposed. Obesity, a decrease in normal femoral anteversion, or an actual retroversion of the femoral neck and a more oblique orientation of the physeal plate during adolescence have been shown to be associated with increased shear force generation at the proximal femoral physeal plate and could be factors associated with physeal plate fatigue.[46,72,110] The physeal perichondrial ring, which functions as a stabilizer of the physeal plate, decreases in strength during the growth years. Chung and colleagues have shown experimentally that physiologic forces at the proximal femur generated by normal activities in obese patients can be of adequate magnitude to cause physeal fatigue if the perichondrial ring is adequately weakened.[26]

Inflammatory factors that weaken the physeal plate must be considered in any proposed etiology of SCFE, as evidenced by the almost universal association of synovitis of the hip with SCFE.[59] It remains unknown, however, whether the synovitis precedes or is a secondary response to the physeal slippage. Eisenstein and Rothchild proposed the etiology of SCFE to be a systemic immunologic condition with a local manifestation at the hip.[35] Their work demonstrated an increase in immunoglobulins and C3 component of complement in the serum as well as the synovium of the hip joint in patients with SCFE. Other authors disagree and propose a local immunologic disorder confined to the hip joint. Morrissy and colleagues have shown no serum abnormalities but did find increased plasma cells, IgG, and C3 component of complement in the hip joint synovium of patients with SCFE.[96] Morrissy and colleagues also have demonstrated the presence of immune complexes in the synovial fluid of the hip in 10 of 12 patients with SCFE but not in the synovial fluid of other conditions associated with synovitis.[97]

Endocrine imbalance is known to change physeal plate physiology and must therefore be considered as a possible etiologic factor in SCFE.[88] An association between endocrine function and SCFE is suggested by the majority of SCFE occurring during the adolescent growth phase. This is a period of significant hormonal change, in which SCFE occurs prior to menarche in girls[125] and is more common in boys who are known to have a longer, more accelerated growth phase and a frequent association with obesity, which may have an underlying hormonal basis. Additional evidence for an association with endocrine dysfunction is suggested by the frequent association of SCFE with primary and secondary hypothyroidism,[57,58,92,148] panhypopituitarism,[52,54,92] hypogonadal conditions,[109] renal osteodystrophy,[121] and during growth hormone therapy.[41,114]

Experimental data have confirmed that various hormonal changes affect physeal strength by altering physeal cartilage collagen and matrix production. Estrogens have been shown to thin the physis and increase physeal strength,[52] whereas oophorectomy leads to a decrease in physeal strength.[52,105] Growth hormone therapy is known to be associated with the development of SCFE.[41] Growth hormone through somatomedin increases the width of the physis by increasing cell activity and matrix production, which in turn decreases the physeal strength.[52,114] Testosterone in low levels has been shown to weaken the physeal plate, whereas high levels for long durations leads to physeal plate narrowing.[98] In spite of this association between hormonal alternations and physeal plate physiology, numerous clinical reports have shown no reproducible laboratory endocrine abnormalities in patient with SCFE.[17,35,84,112] A recent report by Wilcox and colleagues[145] did show significant changes in the levels of thyroid hormone (T_3), testosterone, and growth hormone in a group of patients with SCFE. T_3 levels were significantly decreased in 25% of 80 patients reviewed. In 64 patients tested, the levels of testosterone and growth hormone were depressed in 76% and 87%, respectively.[145]

Although a definite hereditary pattern in SCFE has never been established, there is some evidence that inheritance can be an etiologic factor. Wilson and colleagues reported a 5% incidence of SCFE in family members of 240 patients with SCFE.[146] Rennie proposed an autosomal dominant inheritance pattern with incomplete penetrance in SCFE and reported a 7.1% risk of SCFE to a second family member.[113]

CLINICAL PRESENTATION

Patients with SCFE usually present with complaints of pain in the affected hip or groin, a change in hip range of motion, and a gait abnormality. A patient can present with pain perceived in the medial thigh and knee region of the affected limb. This phenomenon represents referred pain along the sensory distribution of the obturator nerve and commonly is seen in association with hip pathology. If not recognized as referred pain it can lead to a significantly delayed or even missed diagnosis. The intensity and duration of symptoms traditionally have been used to classify SCFE into four patterns of presentation: preslip, acute, chronic, and acute-on-chronic.

The true preslip or prodromal stage of SCFE theoretically occurs prior to any actual slippage through the physeal plate. Whether preslip is an actual phase in SCFE or is secondary to a mild synovitis induced by minimal slippage through the physeal plate remains controversial. The patient provides history of an episodic limp and limb weakness associated with intermittent mild pain in the groin, medial thigh, or knee region, particularly with exertion. On physical examination, the patient may show mild pain with rotation of the affected hip and a minimal decrease in internal rotation. Plain radiographs may show osteopenia and a minor widening and fuzziness of the physeal plate; however, the physeal plate–femoral neck relation appears normal. The preslip stage in SCFE most likely is not a true prodromal phase but represents early symptomatology associated with mild physeal slippage that cannot be detected on plain radiographs.

An acute presentation in SCFE occurs in approximately 10% of patients.[16,22] It is manifest by the sudden onset of severe pain and hip dysfunction in a patient who was previously asymptomatic. A few patients may describe prodromal symptoms for a short time preceding the acute onset of pain, which is frequently associated with minimal trauma. Although the literature varies with respect to the duration of painful symptoms prior to presentation for a SCFE to be classified as acute, most reviews stipulate that the painful symptoms be present for no longer than a 3-week duration.[1,16,23,38,144] Physical examination demonstrates the affected limb externally rotated and shortened with the patient refusing to bear weight. Active motion of the affected hip is severely limited by muscle spasm, and the patient complains of intense pain with any attempt at passive hip motion. Radiographs document the epiphyseal displacement and show no evidence of bone healing or remodeling[6,139] (Fig. 25-3).

The most frequent pattern of presentation is a chronic SCFE. The patient describes intermittent pain in the groin, the medial thigh, or the anterior suprapatellar region of the knee for longer than 3 weeks. The patient remains ambulatory but does show an antalgic gait with associated limp. The affected limb positions itself in an externally rotated and mildly shortened position. Range of hip motion shows a decrease mainly in internal rotation and abduction with the amount of limitation being dependent of the severity of the slip. Mild to moderate pain is noted with motion of the hip, particularly at the extremes of motion. There may be some thigh and gluteal muscle atrophy secondary to long standing symptoms and disuse. A frequently seen sign associated with SCFE can be demonstrated during passive flexion of the affected hip. As flexion is increased from an extended position, the thigh of the affected limb abducts and externally rotates. Radiographs frequently show attempts at bony healing and remodeling along the posterior and medial femoral neck (Fig. 25-4).

The acute-on-chronic presentation in SCFE occurs when a patient with an extended history of symp-

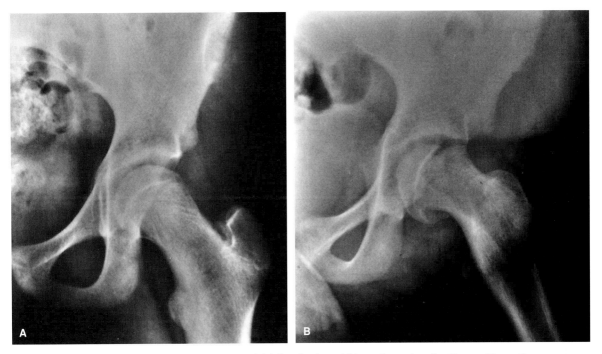

FIGURE 25-3. (A) Anteroposterior and (B) frog-leg lateral hip radiographs of a 12-year, 10-month-old girl demonstrate acute epiphyseal displacement. There is no evidence of bone healing or remodeling at the femoral neck.

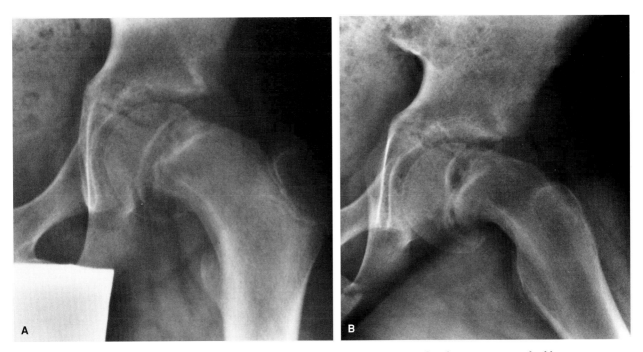

FIGURE 25-4. (A) Anteroposterior and (B) frog-leg lateral hip radiographs of a 13-year, 4-month-old boy demonstrate chronic epiphyseal displacement. The bony resorption on the superior and anterior femoral neck and the new bone formation on the inferior and posterior femoral neck indicate a more prolonged process.

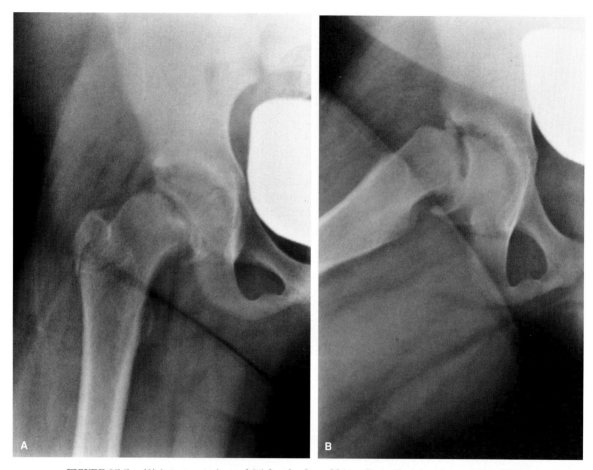

FIGURE 25-5. (A) Anteroposterior and (B) frog-leg lateral hip radiographs of a 12-year, 4-month-old girl demonstrate an acute-on-chronic epiphyseal displacement. Both radiographic views demonstrate increased displacement of the femoral head from a previous, more chronic position of displacement.

toms and signs of chronic SCFE presents with an acute increase in pain and loss of motion at the affected hip. This presentation is associated with an acute increase in slip severity from a previous more mild chronically displaced pattern (Fig. 25-5).

Loder and colleagues proposed a new simplified classification system determined by the degree of physeal stability.[79] A slip is classified as unstable if the patient has such severe pain that walking is not possible even with crutches regardless of the duration of symptoms. A slip is classified as *stable* if walking and weight bearing are still possible with or without crutches.

Classification systems are only useful to the treating physician if they assist in the planning of treatment or relate to the outcome of a specific disease process. In SCFE, the classification system of acute, chronic, or acute-on-chronic with respect to patterns of presentation traditionally has been used. Recently, the simplified classification system proposed by Loder and colleagues and based on physeal plate stability at the time of presentation has been introduced. Both classification systems in SCFE have been shown to be of assistance in the planning of treatment and the projec-

tion of outcome. The more simplified system, in which slips are classified as stable or unstable, seems to be more objective in its method of classification and has the potential to be more useful not only in determining treatment but also predicting outcome. Loder and colleagues have shown that not all slips classified as acute are unstable, and not all slips classified as chronic are stable. They have also shown that slips treated by the same technique and classified as stable have a higher rate of satisfactory results from treatment when compared with unstable slips, which show a lower rate of satisfactory results primarily because of higher rates of osteonecrosis.[79] As more experience with the more simplified system of classification is acquired, it will most likely become the more useful form of classification in SCFE.

RADIOGRAPHIC FEATURES

The actual diagnosis of SCFE is confirmed by radiographic examination of the affected hip. The anteroposterior radiograph is usually diagnostic of SCFE with the possible exception of the early presentation with minimal slipping. Physeal plate widening, irregularity and a decrease in epiphyseal height in the center of the acetabulum usually are noted. A crescent-shaped area of increased density frequently can be identified in the proximal portion of the femoral neck and is known as the *blanch sign of Steel*.[131] This radiographic finding is created by the double density of the posteriorly displaced femoral head on the femoral neck. The femoral metaphysis of the affected hip also appears to be more laterally displaced from the medial acetabular wall compared with the unaffected hip (Fig. 25-6). A positive Klein line is identified as the amount of slip increases. Klein line is defined as a straight line drawn along the superior basal margin of the femoral neck on the anteroposterior radiograph.[74] Normally this line intersects the lateral aspect of the epiphysis. The amount of femoral head intersected is dependent on the degree of hip rotation and is greatest when the hip is in maximum internal rotation. As progressive displacement of the epiphysis occurs, the amount of Klein line that intersects the epiphysis decreases compared with the uninvolved hip. Eventually the line fully misses intersection with the proximal femoral epiphysis (Fig. 25-7).

A true lateral or cross-table lateral radiographic view of the hip better defines the extent of posterior

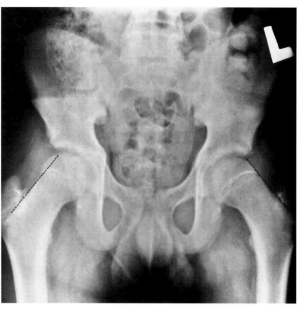

FIGURE 25-7. Anteroposterior pelvic radiograph of a 15-year, 6-month-old boy demonstrates a positive Klein line measurement. A line drawn along the superior basal margin of the femoral neck (i.e., Klein line) intersects the lateral aspect of the right femoral head but essentially misses intersection with the left femoral head. This finding indicates displacement of the left femoral head–femoral neck relation and indicates a slipped capital femoral epiphysis at the left hip.

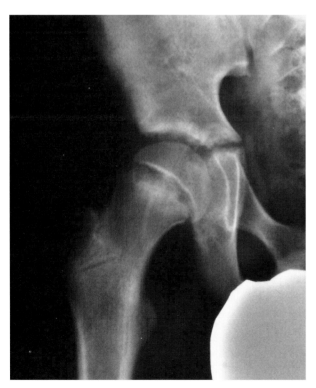

FIGURE 25-6. Anteroposterior hip radiograph demonstrates the classic radiographic findings in slipped capital femoral epiphysis, which include physeal plate widening and irregularity, a decrease in epiphyseal height, and a lateral displacement of the femoral neck from the medial acetabular wall. Also of note is a crescentic area of increased density in the proximal portion of the femoral neck adjacent to the physeal plate known as the blanch sign of Steel.

displacement of the femoral epiphysis (Fig. 25-8). This view can be of assistance in diagnosing minimal slips because it better elucidates the posterior displacement. This view, however, remains difficult to obtain in the extremely obese patient.

A frog-leg lateral radiographic view demonstrates the posterior displacement and step-off of the epiphysis on the femoral neck (Fig. 25-9). Although the frog-leg lateral view assists in confirming the diagnosis, it should be avoided in the acute presentation because of the potential of increasing the physeal displacement during positioning for the radiograph.

Two radiographic images of the affected hip in SCFE taken in orthogonal planes should be obtained when possible to assist in diagnosis and planning of treatment. The anteroposterior and true lateral radiographic views of the affected hip are preferred.

Ultrasonography recently has been proposed in the diagnosis and evaluation of SCFE. Kallio and colleagues used ultrasonography in 26 hips of patients with SCFE to confirm diagnosis and degree of slip by evaluating the step-off in the anterior physeal outline and by measuring the amount of posterior epiphyseal displacement.[67] Although ultrasonography can confirm the diagnosis of SCFE it offers little if any information over conventional radiography in SCFE and has no additional use in treatment.

Computed tomography scan has been shown to be of assistance in both the diagnosis and treatment

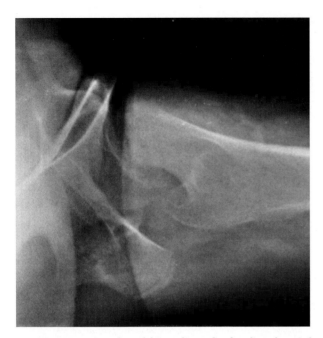

FIGURE 25-8. True lateral hip radiograph of a slipped capital femoral epiphysis demonstrates the posteriorly displaced femoral head remaining in close contact with the femoral neck. Early secondary resorption and rounding of the posterior femoral neck region are noted.

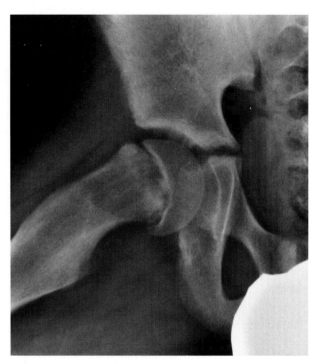

FIGURE 25-9. Frog-leg lateral hip radiograph of a slipped capital femoral epiphysis demonstrates an epiphyseal step-off and posterior displacement of the femoral head on the femoral neck classically seen in slipped capital femoral epiphysis.

of SCFE.[25] Computed tomography scan can be used to confirm epiphyseal displacement and accurately measure the amount of displacement in patients with symptoms suggestive of a SCFE but without documentation on plain radiographs (Fig. 25-10). It also has been shown to be of assistance in better evaluating the relation between the femoral head and neck as well as in assessing early physeal plate closure in severe slips, in which positioning for standard radiographic views can be difficult.

Reports of the use of magnetic resonance imaging studies in hips affected with SCFE remain rare.[132] Although confirmation of physeal displacement can be made, these studies offer no additional information in the diagnosis and classification of SCFE.

A radiographic classification system based on the maximum anatomic displacement of the femoral head on the femoral neck as seen on any of the radiographic views of the hip in a patient with SCFE has been described.[64] In this classification system, a minimal slip is defined as epiphyseal displacement of less than one third of the width of the femoral neck; moderate slip is defined as displacement of one third to one half of the width of the femoral neck; and severe slip is defined as displacement greater than half of the width of the femoral neck. Southwick has recommended displacement be measured by the angle subtended between the femoral head and the femoral shaft on the anteroposterior and lateral radiographic views.[126] Boyer and colleagues have proposed measurement of the maximum difference in the Southwick angles between the involved and uninvolved hip in SCFE as a radiographic classification system.[16] These authors define a mild slip as a head-shaft angle difference of 30 degrees or less, a moderate slip as a 30- to 50-degree difference, and a severe slip as a difference of more than 50 degrees. These radiographic classification systems are shown to be of assistance in planning treatment but more importantly will help in determining outcome in SCFE with respect to the severity of slip and the future development of degenerative joint disease.

NATURAL HISTORY

The complete natural history of the hip in SCFE remains unknown. Very few long-term studies with untreated patients exist in the current literature, and the studies that do exist deal only with small numbers of patients.[22,50,65,106,117]

The current literature shows that not all hips affected with SCFE are symptomatic during slippage. In fact, the second slip can be asymptomatic in 30% to 40% of patients. In most of these patients, the slip shows a very slow progression with ongoing remodel-

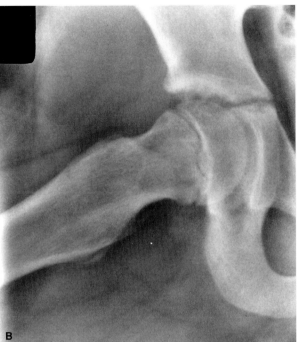

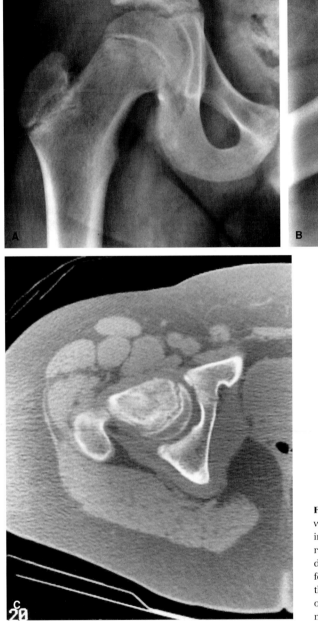

FIGURE 25-10. Radiographs of a 12-year, 2-month-old girl with recent onset of hip pain and a physical examination showing early findings of slipped capital femoral epiphysis. (**A**) Anteroposterior and (**B**) frog-leg lateral hip radiographs do not demonstrate definite radiographic findings of slipped capital femoral epiphysis. (**C**) Computed tomography (CT) image of the same hip demonstrates minimal posterior displacement of the femoral head on the femoral neck, consistent with a mild slipped capital femoral epiphysis.

ing during the adolescent growth phase.[14,49,73] Symptomatic slips, on the other hand, usually show more rapid progressive displacement. Jacobs has shown that the longer the duration of symptoms the more likely the slip will have a greater severity of displacement.[64]

Howorth stated that SCFE during adolescence frequently is associated with degenerative joint disease of the hip during middle life.[60] Although not all authors agree, long-term studies of patients with SCFE do indicate a definite relation between SCFE during adolescence and the subsequent development of degenerative joint disease.[16,22]

The incidence of degenerative joint disease at the hip associated with previous SCFE remains unknown. Murray reported on 200 patients with degenerative joint disease at the hip and described the tilt deformity, a sign of femoral neck remodeling believed to be associated with previous SCFE, in 40% of the patients.[101] Stulberg and colleagues have reported a pistol grip deformity at the proximal femur believed to be secondary to previous SCFE or Perthes disease in 40% of patients with assumed primary osteoarthritis undergoing total hip arthroplasty.[133] Solomon, however, reviewed 327 patients with degenerative joint disease at the hip and found only six patients with a history of previous SCFE.[124] Resnick refuted the association of the radiographic tilt deformity with previous SCFE by showing that the remodeling process at the femoral neck was not the result of SCFE but rather solely related to the osteoarthritis.[115]

Long-term studies have confirmed that the prognosis for subsequent development of degenerative joint disease and deteriorating function at the hip affected with SCFE are dependent on the severity of the slip and increasing patient age at follow-up.[22,65,106,117] Oram has demonstrated that severe slips develop earlier degenerative joint disease and poorer hip function than do moderate slips.[106] Jerre[65] and Ross and colleagues[117] reported an increase in symptoms and a deterioration in hip function associated with increasing patient age at follow-up in patients with SCFE. Jerre also noted that the clinical symptoms do not always correlate with the changes seen radiographically.[65] Carney and colleagues recently reported long-term follow-up on 155 hips in 124 patients affected with SCFE with a mean follow-up of 41 years from symptom onset.[22] Their work represents continued follow-up on the patients previously reported by Boyer and colleagues.[16] Carney reported a continued deterioration in Iowa hip-rating scores with increasing time of follow-up. This deterioration in hip-rating scores was shown to occur in all of the grades of slip severity. An accompanying deterioration in the radiographic grade for degenerative joint disease also was documented.

The current literature suggests that the onset of both symptoms and degenerative joint disease at the hip will be accelerated in most cases of SCFE. This accelerated onset of degenerative joint disease has been shown to be directly related to the severity of the slip. Treatment therefore can influence positively the natural history of SCFE if early recognition and subsequent intervention to prevent progressive deformity are achieved.

TREATMENT

The treatment in SCFE is designed to improve on the natural history of the untreated condition as it is currently understood. The goals of treatment include the prevention of further slipping by stabilizing the diseased physis and thereby reducing the incidence and

onset of osteoarthritis at the affected hip and the avoidance of iatrogenically induced osteonecrosis of the femoral head and chondrolysis.

Treatment can be divided into three categories: treatment to prevent further slippage, treatment to reduce the degree of slippage, and salvage treatment.

Treatment to Prevent Further Slippage

After slipping of the proximal femoral epiphysis has been documented, treatment should be directed at prevention of further slippage. This can be accomplished by spica cast immobilization, in situ metallic pin and screw fixation, and bone peg epiphyseodesis.

The treatment rationale for the use of spica cast immobilization in SCFE is based on the following assumptions—not all of which have been proven to be true. The slippage in SCFE is short lived and will heal spontaneously if immobilized for a long enough period. Further slipping can be prevented by external immobilization. The treatment process is associated with a low complication rate because there is no violation of the proximal femur or hip joint. Prolonged joint immobilization in adolescence is without increased complications.[13,22,47]

Treatment by spica cast immobilization has been reported mainly in chronic and acute-on-chronic SCFE. The use of spica cast immobilization in acute SCFE has been reported in only a limited number of patients.[13,89] Previous authors[13,89] have standardized the method of treatment, which includes an initial phase of bed rest with split Russell or Buck skin traction until joint irritability has lessened. Traction averages 10 days but has been reported to last as long as 30 days.[13] A one-and-a-half or double-spica cast is then applied without any attempt at epiphyseal reduction. The hip is positioned at the midpoint of comfortable internal and external rotation. Radiographs of the hip are obtained every 4 weeks to document that no additional progression of slip has occurred and to evaluate healing. Adequate physeal plate healing to allow for discontinuation of the immobilization is determined radiographically and is present when either physeal plate closure is identified or the metaphyseal juxtaphyseal lucency (i.e., a radiolucent zone on the metaphyseal side of the physis)[113] is no longer seen on radiographs of the affected hip. The immobilization averages 12 weeks with a range of 8 to 16 weeks. After cast removal, gentle range of motion and muscle strengthening exercises are initiated.

The results of treatment with spica cast immobilization in SCFE have been reported by several authors.[13,22,87,89] Successful prevention of further slippage by spica cast immobilization is reported at 82 to 97 percent.[13,89] Associated with this high rate of success in preventing further slippage, Betz and colleagues reported 14 of 17 hips (82%) treated by spica cast immobilization to show premature physeal closure at the affected physis in comparison with the contralateral uninvolved hip.[13]

Complications associated with spica cast immobilization include recurrent slip after cast removal in as high as 18% of patients.[89] Betz and colleagues reported only a 3% rate of recurrent slip if the spica cast is maintained until full resolution of the metaphyseal juxtaphyseal radiolucent zone radiographically has been documented.[13] Osteonecrosis of the femoral head has been reported by Carney and colleagues to be associated with spica cast immobilization without reduction in 2 of 27 hips (7%).[22] Meier and colleagues reported full-thickness skin pressure ulcers in 2 of 13 patients (16%).[89] The development of psychosocial complications during prolonged treatment with a spica cast in these generally obese patients also must be considered. The most frequent and serious complication associated with spica cast immobilization in SCFE remains chondrolysis. This complication is reported to occur in 19% to 67% of affected hips treated by spica cast immobilization and has been shown to have a higher occurrence rate with more severe degrees of slippage at the time of spica cast placement.[13,22,87,89]

Although treatment with spica cast immobilization to prevent further slippage has been considered as an alternative in patients with chronic SCFE, I recommend abandoning its use secondary to the high rate of associated serious long-term complications.

In situ fixation of the displaced femoral head with metallic pins or screws historically has been and remains the most commonly used method of stabilization in SCFE. The rationale behind the use of metallic fixation is that the fixation device, by crossing the diseased physeal plate, provides mechanical support to prevent further slippage, whereas its violation of the physeal plate can induce early physeal closure. Historically, in situ fixation has been associated with some technical difficulties arising from poor imaging obtained from biplane plain radiographs and inadequate internal fixation. Currently available surgical techniques, fixation devices, and fluoroscopic equipment, as well as a better understanding of the actual pathoanatomy found in SCFE, have greatly improved and simplified the performance of the procedure. When in situ fixation is performed percutaneously or through a minimal incision, it has the advantages of minimal blood loss, avoidance of opening of the hip joint, and minimal requirement for postoperative hospitalization and rehabilitation.[139] Certain disadvantages, however, are inherent with the technique and include the possibility of penetration of the hip joint by the fixation device,[12] increased technical difficulty in more severe slips, and the need for subsequent hardware removal,

although recent reports have questioned the need for routine hardware removal.[37,139]

Review of the historical literature on metallic fixation in SCFE demonstrates previous complication rates as high as 20% to 40% with the majority of the complications related to hardware placement and hip joint violation leading to osteonecrosis and chondrolysis. Proximal femoral fracture, unsuccessful stabilization, and hardware breakage also were reported complications.[48,116] The use of multiple pins and screws, improper starting position for the hardware, and inadequate radiography were shown to be associated with this higher incidence of complications.[15,93,102] With experience and a better understanding of the actual pathoanatomy found in SCFE, the principles of safe and successful in situ metallic fixation have been developed and have been shown to significantly lower the incidence of complications previously associated with metallic fixation in SCFE.

In situ fixation remains a surgical technique dependent on biplane fluoroscopy to properly perform. With the advent of current fluoroscopic equipment and patient positioning devices, adequate visualization of the femoral head and proximal femur, even in obese patients, is possible and has greatly improved the simplicity and safety of in situ fixation. The proper technique of percutaneous in situ fixation in SCFE to include patient positioning, hardware start point determination, hardware placement, and postoperative care has been described by Aronson and Carlson[6] and Morrissy.[95]

The principles of successful in situ fixation in SCFE warrant reemphasis. It is imperative that the outline of the femoral head be seen on both the anteroposterior and true lateral (not frog-leg lateral) radiographic projections prior to any attempt at fixation placement.

The central axis of the femoral head remains the only safe position for the fixation device. The farther off the central axis the fixation is, the more likely penetration of the femoral head is to occur. Walters and Simon,[138] through the use of mathematical models, have demonstrated what is called the blind spot of the femoral head. In the use of biplane radiography it was shown that there is always an area where a pin can violate the femoral head and not be seen radiographically. This blind spot is small in the central axis of the femoral head; however, it increases greatly the farther the position of the fixation device is off of the femoral head central axis (Fig. 25-11). Only by positioning the fixation device centrally and at least 5 mm from the margin of the femoral head can avoidance of penetration be assured (Fig. 25-12). Because there is only one central axis in the femoral head, the use of multiple pins and screws must position some of the devices off the central axis and increase the incidence of potential

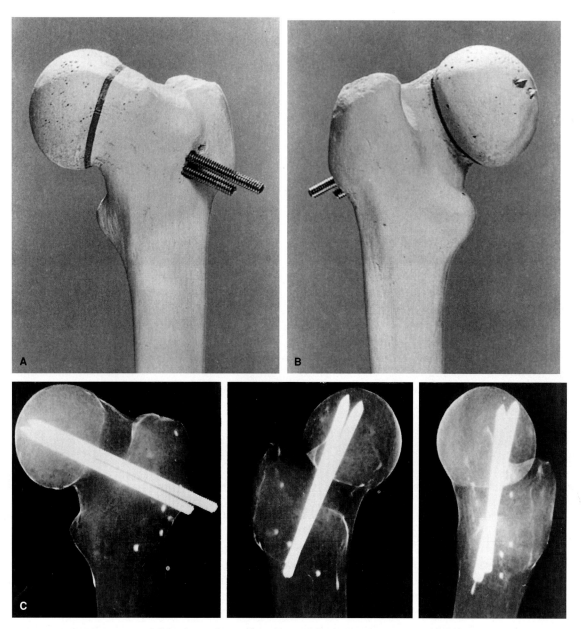

FIGURE 25-11.   Models of a moderate slipped capital femoral epiphysis stabilized in situ with two threaded pins demonstrate the concept of the radiographic blind spot of the femoral head. This concept proposes that there will always be an area in the femoral head where a pin may violate the head itself and yet not be seen on plain radiographs. The blind spot is smallest in the central axis of the femoral head and increases greatly the farther the fixation device position is off the central axis. Only by positioning the fixation device centrally and at least 5 mm from the margin of the femoral head can avoidance of penetration be assured.

femoral head penetration. Blanco and colleagues validated this concept in their report of 114 hips in 80 patients treated with single, double, or multiple pins.[15] The authors reported a decrease in pin-related complications from 36% in hips stabilized by multiple pins to 4.6% in hips stabilized by a single pin.

The metaphysis of the femoral neck displaces anteriorly from the femoral head as the femoral head rotates posteriorly around the axis of the femoral neck. For the fixation device to enter and stay central in the femoral head, it must be placed perpendicular to the plane of the femoral head. This only can be accomplished if the starting position for the fixation is on the anterior femoral neck and not the lateral cortex of the proximal femur[31,93,102] (Fig. 25-13). The proper starting point on the femoral neck is determined by the severity of displacement of the femoral head. In hips with minimal displacement the starting point is anterolateral at the base of the femoral neck. In hips with more severe femoral head displacement the start-

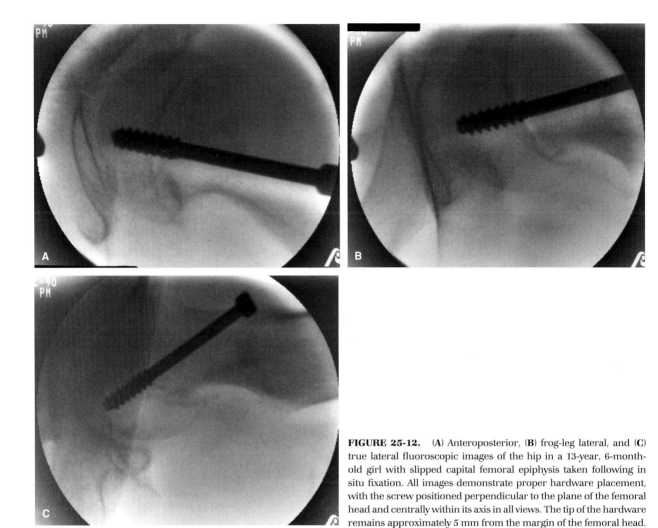

FIGURE 25-12. (A) Anteroposterior, (B) frog-leg lateral, and (C) true lateral fluoroscopic images of the hip in a 13-year, 6-month-old girl with slipped capital femoral epiphysis taken following in situ fixation. All images demonstrate proper hardware placement, with the screw positioned perpendicular to the plane of the femoral head and centrally within its axis in all views. The tip of the hardware remains approximately 5 mm from the margin of the femoral head.

ing point moves progressively more medial on the femoral neck (Fig. 25-14).

The internal fixation device should always avoid the superior and anterior quadrant of the femoral head. The terminal branches of the lateral ascending cervical artery traverse this quadrant[27] (Fig. 25-15). These intraosseous vessels are at high risk for injury leading to segmental osteonecrosis of the femoral head if the fixation device is placed in the superior quadrant of the femoral head, as has been shown by Brodetti[19] and Stambough and colleagues[129] (Fig. 25-16).

Following fixation, radiographic confirmation that the fixation device has not penetrated the joint space is mandatory. This can be accomplished by removing the affected limb from the holding device on the fracture table and moving the hip through a full range of motion under fluoroscopic examination. The "approach-withdraw" technique of Moseley has been proposed to radiographically confirm avoidance of femoral head penetration.[99] This technique employs visualization of the femoral head fluoroscopically

while the fully extended limb is rotated from maximum internal rotation to maximum external rotation. As the hip is ranged, the tip of the fixation device in the femoral head is observed to approach the subchondral outline of the femoral head and then withdraw without ever violating the subchondral bone. If violation of the subchondral bone is noted, then femoral head penetration has occurred.

The metallic device used for femoral head stabilization must be of appropriate strength to avoid failure prior to physeal plate closure. It should also be of such strength to avoid the need for multiple devices that increase the prevalence of penetration and the volume of metal occupying the femoral head. The device should be of a cannulated design to facilitate placement and have back-cutting threads for ease of removal. Doane and colleagues, through the use of biomechanical analysis of bovine proximal slipped femoral epiphyses, reported that a single 5.5-mm-diameter screw provided approximately the structural stiffness of two 4.5-mm-diameter screws and that a single centrally placed 7.5-mm-diameter screw ap-

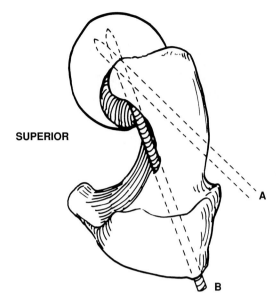

SUPERIOR

FIGURE 25-13. The metaphysis of the femoral neck displaces anteriorly from the femoral head as the femoral head rotates posteriorly in slipped capital femoral epiphysis. For the fixation device to enter and stay central in the femoral head, it must be placed perpendicular to the plane of the femoral head. This approach necessitates a starting point along the anterior femoral neck (A). The more traditional starting point on the lateral cortex of the femur (B) is associated with penetration of the cortex of the posterior femoral neck before reentering the femoral head. This route can lead to damage of the posterior retinacular vessels, which provide the major blood supply to the femoral head, and direct the hardware into the more vulnerable anterior femoral head quadrant. (From Riley PM, Weiner DS, Gillespie R, Weiner SD. Hazards of internal fixation in the treatment of slipped capital femoral epiphysis. J Bone Joint Surg [Am] 1990;72:1505.)

proached the stiffness of an unslipped epiphysis.[33] Karol and colleagues, using mechanical force analysis in cannulated screw fixation of slipped proximal femoral epiphyses in bovine models, reported only a 33% increase in stiffness to failure in specimens secured with double screw fixation over single screw fixation.[68] They concluded that the small gain in fixation stiffness seen with a second screw does not offset the potential increase in complications associated with its placement to warrant its routine use.

By adhering to these treatment guidelines and principles, almost all slipped proximal femoral epiphyses should be able to be stabilized with percutaneous placement of a single 6.5- to 7.0-mm cannulated screw. One possible exception is the severe SCFE in the extremely obese patient, in whom adequate radiographic images cannot be obtained and in which case percutaneous metallic fixation should not be attempted. Another possible exception is the acute unstable slip in a very obese and unreliable patient, in whom the need for a second screw to control femoral head rotation has been proposed by Koval and colleagues.[75] The need for a second screw remains controversial, with recent

reports implying that it is not needed. Aronson and Carlson[6] reported on single screw fixation in SCFE in 58 hips. Eight of these 58 hips were classified as acute slips with only 1 of the 8 hips showing loss of fixation. Ward and colleagues[139] reported on fixation with a single screw in SCFE in 53 hips. Five of the 53 hips were acute slips with none of the 5 hips showing loss of fixation.

Reports confirm the safety, reliability, and efficacy of the in situ single centrally positioned cannulated screw fixation technique for the stabilization of acute and chronic SCFE.[6,75,139] If these series are combined, 171 hips of acute, acute-on-chronic, and chronic patterns were stabilized by a single screw, of which 13 hips were classified as acute or acute-on-chronic presentations. Following stabilization there was only 1 case of osteonecrosis that was identified in a patient with an acute slip and no cases of chondrolysis. Five hips were reported to have had transient femoral head penetration all of which were recognized and adjusted and none of which developed any complications related to the penetration. There were no reported cases of hardware breakage. Two hips developed fractures in the proximal femur following treatment related to the hardware.[11] Two cases of increased slippage around the fixation were reported. One case occurred in a hip in which the fixation was placed outside of the central quadrant of the femoral head, and the other case was following single screw fixation of an acute slip.

Reports suggest that in situ pin and screw fixation of SCFE can be associated with an accelerated closure of the affected physeal plate. Ward and colleagues, in review of 53 SCFE hips, reported 49 hips (92%) to have undergone closure following single screw fixation.[139] The time to closure was analyzed in 29 of the 49 hips. Physeal plate closure averaged 13 months (range, 2–34 months) and showed no correlation to age at the time of fixation, race, or gender. A longer time to physeal closure was noted in hips with more severe displacement and increasingly eccentric screw placement. Premature closure of the physeal plate in the treated hip compared with the contralateral normal hip was demonstrated in 19 of 20 patients treated by single screw fixation. Stanton and Shelton reported on 26 SCFE hips treated with in situ fixation and demonstrated the pinned physes to close an average of 10.2 months earlier than the unpinned physes.[130] The average time to closure was 12 months in the pinned physes and 22.2 months in the nonpinned physes. Although accelerated physeal plate closure in SCFE treated with in situ metallic fixation has been demonstrated, the reason for the early closure has not been established. Physeal damage from placement of the fixation device and physeal damage secondary to the slip itself could be considered as possible etiologies.

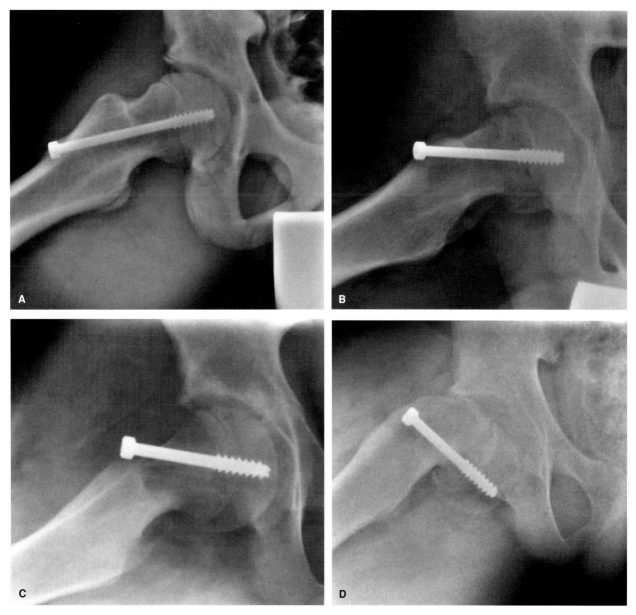

FIGURE 25-14.   Series of frog-leg lateral hip radiographs in slipped capital femoral epiphysis following in situ fixation. Each radiograph demonstrates progressive posterior displacement of the femoral head. For the fixation device to stay central in the femoral head, its starting position progressively moves more proximal on the anterior femoral neck as the femoral head displacement becomes more severe.

In patients whose age at the onset of SCFE is at least 1 year earlier than the reported mean for the disorder (boys younger than 12.5 years old and girls younger than 10.5 years old) premature closure of the proximal femoral physis induced by metallic stabilization can lead to growth disturbances in the proximal femur to include relative greater trochanteric overgrowth, coxa vara, and coxa breva.[120] These authors demonstrated radiographic sequelae about the proximal femur in 64% of 33 hips in these younger patients at follow-up who had been stabilized by metallic fixation for SCFE. The authors concluded that stabilization

in younger patients with SCFE should be by fixation devices that will not induce early physeal closure but rather will allow continued proximal physeal plate growth. Hansson has proposed a similar concept for stabilization in SCFE.[51] He has recommended the use of the hook pin as the fixation device of choice and has shown continued growth of the femoral neck along the pin of as much as 15 mm. In spite of the large number of patients showing radiographic changes at the proximal femur[120] only two patients demonstrated limb length discrepancy, both of which measured 1 cm or less, and three patients demonstrated a Trendelen-

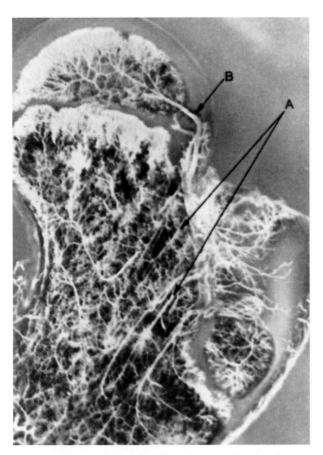

FIGURE 25-15.   The blood supply to the femoral neck and proximal femoral epiphysis. (**A**) The lateral ascending cervical artery gives off metaphyseal branches into the femoral neck and (**B**) then continues on to form epiphyseal branches that provide a segmental blood supply to the superior quadrant of the femoral head. Fixation placed into the superior quadrant of the femoral head could damage this blood supply, leading to osteonecrosis. (From Chung SM. The arterial supply of the developing proximal end of the human femur. J Bone Joint Surg [Am] 1976;58:966.)

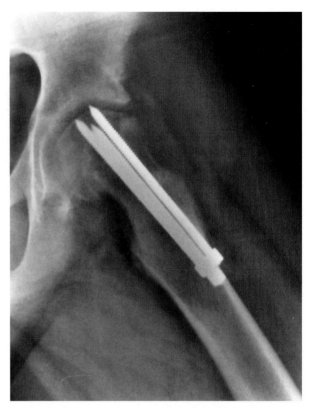

FIGURE 25-16.   Frog-leg lateral hip radiograph in patient with slipped capital femoral epiphysis demonstrates multiple pin fixation from a lateral starting position. The hardware is not maintained in the center of the femoral head but rather is confined to the vulnerable anterosuperior quadrant. Penetration of the femoral head and early segmental osteonecrosis are demonstrated.

burg gait. The true clinical significance of these radiographic findings remains in doubt.

In hips in which physeal closure is not induced, femoral head overgrowth off of the fixation device is possible. This was reported by Ward and colleagues in 3 of 53 hips treated by single screw fixation.[139] No slip progression or detrimental consequences were noted in these patients.

Carney and colleagues reported long-term follow-up of SCFE patients treated by various techniques and with a mean follow-up of 41 years after onset of symptoms.[22] They concluded that regardless of the slip severity in SCFE, pinning in situ "provides the best long-term function with a low risk of complications and most effectively delays the development of degenerative arthritis."[22] Other recent studies have also demonstrated that fixation with a single 6.5- to 7.0-mm screw provides safe and reliable epiphyseal stabilization and

promotes premature physeal fusion in patients with SCFE while decreasing the rate of complications historically associated with multiple pin fixation.[6,15,75,139]

The use of open bone peg epiphyseodesis for stabilization in SCFE was first described by Ferguson and Howorth in 1931.[40] The rationale behind the use of this technique in the stabilization of SCFE is based on the assumption that open bone grafting of the proximal femoral physis should lead to a more rapid physeal closure and a lower rate of complications as a result of direct visualization of the femoral neck and head. The procedure has the advantages of being a direct approach to the deformity and makes violation of the articular surface of the femoral head less likely, particularly in more severe slips. The intracapsular approach and visualization of the femoral neck also allows for the simultaneous removal of any superior femoral neck bony prominence that can impinge on the acetabulum and restrict hip motion.[29,56,90] Open bone grafting in SCFE should lead to more predictable and rapid closure of the proximal femoral physeal plate as a result of the curetting of a large portion of the physeal plate with subsequent placement of bone graft bridging the physeal plate. The procedure also has the advantage of not using metal fixation, which could require later removal.

The disadvantages associated with open bone peg epiphyseodesis include its more demanding and extensive surgical approach, longer operative times, increased blood loss, and the potential for continued femoral head displacement prior to physeal plate closure. Ward and Wood reported operative times averaging 3 hours (range, 2–5 hours) and blood loss averaging 800 mL (range, 250–2400 mL) in association with 17 hips treated by bone peg epiphyseodesis.[140] Irani and colleagues reported an average operative time of 3 hours and 40 minutes and average blood loss of 750 mL in 48 hips treated by open bone grafting.[63] Longer hospitalization times and the need for more extensive postoperative rehabilitation seen in bone peg epiphyseodesis make it a more costly form of treatment. The minimal stability created by the bone graft itself makes the potential for continued femoral head displacement prior to physeal plate closure a definite risk. This potential instability necessitates the additional inconvenience and requirement for spica cast immobilization in most patients, particularly in slips with an acute or unstable presentation. It also necessitates the need for extended limited weight bearing on the affected hip until physeal plate closure has occurred.[142]

The recommended surgical technique used in bone peg epiphyseodesis has been described.[140,142] Historically, an anterior iliofemoral approach to the hip joint has been used, but Weiner and colleagues have recommended an anterolateral approach, which they report is associated with reduced operative time, less blood loss, and improved wound healing compared with the anterior iliofemoral approach.[141] After the hip capsule is opened, a tunnel is created between the femoral neck and the central femoral head with drills and curettes. Corticocancellous iliac bone graft is then obtained and packed tightly into the tunnel (Fig. 25-17). Unfortunately, no standardized dimensions or cross-sectional area for the size of the bone graft needed to avoid graft failure have been documented. Weiner and colleagues recommended sandwiching multiple corticocancellous slips into the bone tunnel to a width of approximately 1 cm.[142] Ward and Wood recommended using a single rectangular bone graft measuring 5 cm in length and 6 mm in height by 6 mm in width, which is impacted tightly across the physis.[140] Postoperatively a spica cast is placed on all patients with acute slips as well as any chronic slip demonstrating physeal instability at the time of surgery.

A limited number of reports concerning the use of bone peg epiphyseodesis in SCFE is available.[1,90,140,142] Osteonecrosis and chondrolysis rarely are reported in association with this form of treatment. Weiner and colleagues reviewed 185 hips treated with bone peg epiphyseodesis, including 26 acute slips and 159 chronic slips.[142] A total of only three cases of osteonecrosis and 1 case of chondrolysis were reported. Other reported complications associated with bone peg epiphyseodesis include failure to achieve physeal fusion, bone graft insufficiency with continued slippage, myositis ossificans, and lateral femoral cutaneous nerve dysesthesia.

The time to physeal plate closure following bone peg epiphyseodesis averaged 2.5 months, as reported by Weiner and colleagues,[142] and 4.8 months (range, 3–15 months), as reported by Irani and colleagues.[63] Ward and Wood reported physeal closure in 12 of 17 hips treated by bone peg epiphyseodesis.[140] Eight of the 12 hips achieving physeal closure did so by 16 weeks. Two hips, however, required between 24 and 36 weeks for closure.

Bone graft insufficiency defined as bone graft breakage, displacement, or resorption was noted in 8 of the 17 hips (47%) reported by Ward and Wood.[140] Three of these hips went onto physeal closure, whereas five hips required additional stabilization by metallic pin fixation. Continued radiographic displacement of the femoral head after bone graft epiphyseodesis but prior to physeal closure was reported in all patients demonstrating bone graft insufficiency but also was noted in three of nine hips in which no insufficiency was noted.

The more extensive surgical approach, greater blood loss, longer hospitalization, and reported problems with bone graft insufficiency and continued femoral head displacement associated with bone peg epiphyseodesis preclude this technique from being the procedure of choice for stabilization of the physeal plate in SCFE.

Treatment to Reduce the Degree of Slippage

Natural history studies have shown a direct relation between the degree of displacement in SCFE and the affected hips' final outcome to include the development of degenerative joint disease.[22,106] Treatment methods that reduce the degree of slip and create a more anatomic relation of the femoral head with the remainder of the femur should lead to improved function and motion as well as delay the onset of degenerative joint disease. To truly have a beneficial effect on the natural history, however, these treatment methods must not be associated with a significant increase in complications, in particular, osteonecrosis and chondrolysis of the femoral head. Techniques to reduce the degree of slip include closed manipulation prior to physeal plate stabilization and osteotomies of the proximal femur performed either

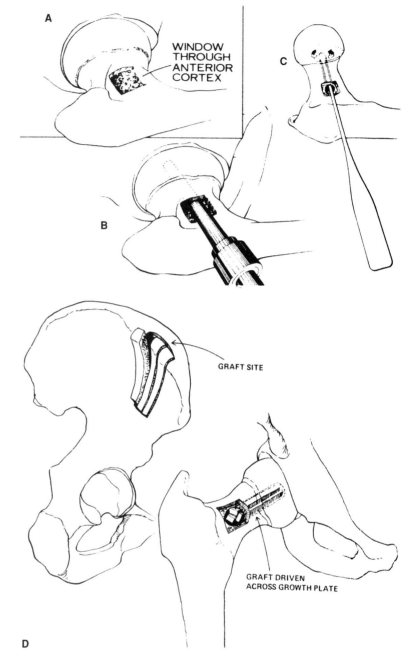

FIGURE 25-17. Technique used in open bone-peg epiphysiodesis in slipped capital femoral epiphysis. (**A**) Using an anterolateral approach to the hip, the hip capsule is opened and the proximal femoral physis is identified. A small anterior metaphyseal cortical window is formed in the femoral neck immediately distal to the physis. (**B**) A 1-cm hollow mill drill is then passed through the window into the center of the femoral head under flouroscopic image intensification. (**C**) The physeal plate is throughly curretted adjacent to the cylindrical bone tunnel. (**D**) Cortical cancellous grafts are obtained from the adjacent ilium and packed tightly into the bone tunnel bridging the physeal plate. The cortical window of bone from the anterior femoral neck is replaced. (From Weiner DS. Bone graft epiphysiodesis in the treatment of slipped capital femoral epiphysis. Instr Course Lect 1989;38:266.)

concurrently with physeal stabilization or after physeal closure.

The potential need for closed manipulation of femoral head displacement in SCFE is based on the concept that spontaneous remodeling at the proximal femur following physeal stabilization will not be adequate to restore femoral head and femoral neck and femoral head and femoral shaft relations to near-normal alignment. Several authors have implied that remodeling following in situ fixation in SCFE has the ability to correct proximal femoral deformity and secondarily improve hip motion. Key[72] and Billing and Severin[14] have reported on bony remodeling of the contour of the proximal femur that occurs in SCFE. These authors defined remodeling as the radiographic appearance of new bone formation between the overhanging femoral head and the posteroinferior femoral neck in association with a rounding off of the prominent anterosuperior margin of the femoral neck. Lacroix and Verbrugge have demonstrated histologically that these radiographic changes are secondary to appositional new bone formation on the inferior margin and osteoclastic resorption on the superior margin of the femoral neck.[77] O'Brien and Fahey, in a review of 12 hips of moderate to severe displacement in SCFE treated by in situ fixation, suggested that femoral neck remodeling leads to an associated improvement in hip motion to essentially normal values, except for a mild residual loss of internal rotation.[104] They reported the probability of sufficient femoral neck remodeling to increase with an open triradiate cartilage but to decrease with greater severity of slip.[66,104]

Siegel and colleagues recently have confirmed that hip motion significantly improves following in situ fixation in SCFE, but remodeling at the proximal femur is insufficient to restore normal hip alignment.[122] Their study employed a quantitative evaluation of hip motion and proximal femoral remodeling following in situ fixation in 39 patients with SCFE with 2 or more years follow-up. Hip motion was found to improve most rapidly in the first 6 months after treatment, mainly as a result of resolving muscle spasm, pain, and synovitis. Although hip motion continued to show improvement over the entire period of follow-up related to continued soft tissue stretching and bone resorption from the anterolateral femoral neck, it never approached the motion of the unaffected hip. Plain radiography and computed tomography demonstrated femoral neck remodeling, which produced an apparent improvement in the displaced femoral head and femoral neck relation but did not confirm any significant change in the more critical relation between the displaced femoral head and the femoral shaft. The authors concluded that the improvement in hip motion seen following in situ fixation in SCFE was not directly related to significant osseous remodeling.

Although motion at the affected hip in SCFE after in situ fixation can be expected to improve as synovitis and protective spasm resolve, the bony deformity created by the slip shows little if any true realignment through remodeling. Closed manipulation to reduce the degree of displacement prior to stabilization in SCFE therefore has a potentially beneficial effect on the natural history if it can be performed without increased complications. The major complication seen in association with closed manipulation in SCFE remains osteonecrosis of the femoral head, which leads to rapid deterioration in hip function. Although the incidence of osteonecrosis following closed manipulation in SCFE varies, most studies confirm an increase in the incidence in manipulated hips over nonmanipulated hips.[14,22,80] Carney and colleagues reported that osteonecrosis developed in 12 of 39 hips (31%) in which reduction of the slippage was attempted, whereas osteonecrosis occurred in only 6 of 116 hips (6%) in which no reduction had been attempted.[22] Vigorous reductions, multiple attempts at reduction, and overreduction have all been associated with an increased incidence of osteonecrosis.[23,39]

Closed manipulation can be considered in patients presenting with acute or acute-on-chronic presentations with severe displacement in which the risk of significant limitation in range of motion and accelerated degenerative arthritis associated with fixation in situ outweighs the risk of potential complications from reduction. It is never indicated in patients presenting with chronic or stable slips or in slips with displacement of a mild to moderate degree.

If closed manipulation is to be attempted, it can be performed by either slow reduction with skeletal traction through a distal femoral pin over a period of days prior to stabilization or by a gentle reduction performed at the time of surgical stabilization. Neither method, properly performed, has been proven to be safer or more beneficial than the other.[23,39]

If traction is employed, it is applied through longitudinal skeletal traction, allowing for slow reduction of the femoral head over a few days. The use of skeletal traction is necessitated by the generally larger body weights of these patients, which require the generation of greater forces than can be safely achieved through skin traction. The addition of an internal rotation force applied to the lateral aspect of the femoral pin to assist in reduction also can be used.

If reduction under anesthesia is performed it should be done without force or repeated attempts. The accepted reduction is what is obtained when the patient is placed onto the fracture table and the affected limb is rotated to neutral while the hip is maintained in extension. No forced internal rotation or flexion should be performed at the affected hip because of the increased potential for vascular injury associated with these maneuvers.[39]

Osteotomies about the proximal femur in SCFE are designed as realignment procedures through which restoration of a more normal relation among the femoral head, the femoral neck and shaft, and the acetabulum can be achieved. The various osteotomies accomplish this goal by creating a compensatory deformity through which the primary deformity created by the original femoral head displacement is realigned. Realignment of the proximal femur by osteotomy, when indicated, should result in an improved range of hip motion and a delay in the development of degenerative joint disease. The complications of femoral head osteonecrosis and chondrolysis must be avoided. Osteotomies in SCFE can be performed at the time of physeal stabilization, although most are performed as delayed procedures in patients in whom residual hip function remains inadequate.

Several osteotomies performed at various levels along the femoral neck and proximal femur have been described in SCFE.[2,9,10,28,34,42–45,103,111,118,126,134] In general, as the location of the osteotomy proceeds distally along the proximal femur, the amount of correction achieved at the primary site of deformity decreases. Conversely, as the location of the osteotomy proceeds proximally along the proximal femur, the risk of osteotomy-induced osteonecrosis of the femoral head increases. Procedures performed in the proximal femoral neck can achieve almost anatomic correction of the primary deformity; however, they are associated with a high incidence of osteonecrosis of the femoral head. More distal osteotomies performed at the intertrochanteric region have a very low incidence of osteonecrosis of the femoral head but are limited in the amount of correction of the primary deformity that they can achieve. The use of osteotomies in SCFE is limited to patients with displacement of the femoral head in the severe range in whom motion at the affected hip after initial treatment remains significantly limited and restricts activities of daily living. The needs of the patient must be weighed against the potential complications when realignment osteotomies are considered. The osteotomy that fulfills the patient's needs at the lowest potential risk should always be chosen.

The use of cuneiform osteotomy of the femoral neck in SCFE has been described by several authors.[9,34,42,43,45,103] Cuneiform osteotomy at the level of the proximal femoral physis is the only procedure that has the ability to restore an anatomic relation of the femoral head with the femoral neck as well as the femoral shaft. The procedure should be performed only in patients with an open proximal femoral physeal plate.[34,42,43] Cuneiform osteotomy performed by the method reported by Fish is preferred.[42,43] The hip capsule is opened anteriorly, and the procedure is performed under direct visualization. The physeal plate is removed in conjunction with a wedge resection of bone from the juxtaphyseal femoral neck. The size of the wedge to be removed is determined by the severity of the displacement being corrected. The wedge resection shortens the femoral neck, which allows for reduction of the femoral neck onto the femoral head without excessive tension. Care must be taken throughout the procedure not to damage the periosteum and the vasculature running along the posterior femoral neck (Fig. 25-18). The reduced femoral head is then stabilized with pin or screw fixation.

Although anatomic correction of the deformity is possible, a high incidence of femoral head osteonecrosis remains associated with this procedure. Gage and colleagues reviewed the literature and reported the average incidence of femoral head osteonecrosis in association with cuneiform osteotomy to be 21%.[45] Some series demonstrate the rate of femoral head osteonecrosis following cuneiform osteotomy to be between 12% and 35%.[34,45,50,146] More recently, a lower incidence of osteonecrosis of the femoral head has been reported following cuneiform osteotomy performed by the subcapital wedge resection technique. Fish reported osteonecrosis of the femoral head in 3 of 66 hips (4.5%),[43] and Nishiyama and colleagues reported osteonecrosis in 1 of 18 hips (5.5%) treated by

the technique of cuneiform osteotomy.[103] Chondrolysis also has been reported in association with cuneiform osteotomy but usually is in association with osteonecrosis.[45] Fish reported an 11% incidence of pin-related complications due to hardware violation of the hip joint in cuneiform osteotomy.[43]

Realignment of the femoral head by cuneiform osteotomy remains a technically demanding procedure, and although a lower incidence of osteonecrosis recently has been reported the potential for severe complications remains very high.

Osteotomy at the base of the femoral neck has been described by several authors.[2,10,45,76] Intracapsular[45,76] and extracapsular[2,10] techniques have been reported. The base of the femoral neck is exposed, and an anterosuperior-based wedge of bone is removed. Care is taken not to place retractors posterior to the femoral neck. The posterior cortex of the femoral neck and its periosteum are not cut but are "greensticked" during closure of the osteotomy. This avoids injury to the vasculature running along the posterior femoral neck. The osteotomy is stabilized by pins or screws (Fig. 25-19). The procedure has a lower reported incidence of osteonecrosis of the femoral head than is found in cuneiform osteotomy but is limited to a greater extent in its ability to fully correct the more proximal femoral deformity. A maximum correction of 35 to 55 degrees is reported with base of neck osteotomies.[2,30] The osteotomy secondarily creates a coxa breva, which can cause the greater trochanter to impinge on the acetabulum during hip motion.[76]

Transtrochanteric rotational osteotomy originally was described by Sugioka.[134] This osteotomy represents a transtrochanteric osteotomy proximal to the abductor insertion on the greater trochanter. Rotational correction of severe deformities of the proximal femur is possible with this procedure without disturbing abductor muscle mechanics or limb length. Reports of the use of the procedure in SCFE, however, are limited. Sugioka reported osteonecrosis in 1 of 9 hips (11%) treated with this procedure.[134] Masuda and colleagues reported osteonecrosis in 1 of 5 hips (20%) treated by transtrochanteric osteotomy.[86] The use of transtrochanteric rotational osteotomy has rarely been reported in SCFE and is not recommended for routine use.

Intertrochanteric osteotomies remain the most frequently used procedures for realignment in SCFE. The surgical technique was originally described by Southwick[126] and has since been slightly modified by several authors.[28,44,111,118] Intertrochanteric osteotomy can be performed in a single-plane, biplane, or multiplane technique. A derotational osteotomy of the proximal femur represents a single-plane intertrochanteric osteotomy and serves only to adjust internal and external rotation at the affected hip. The biplane

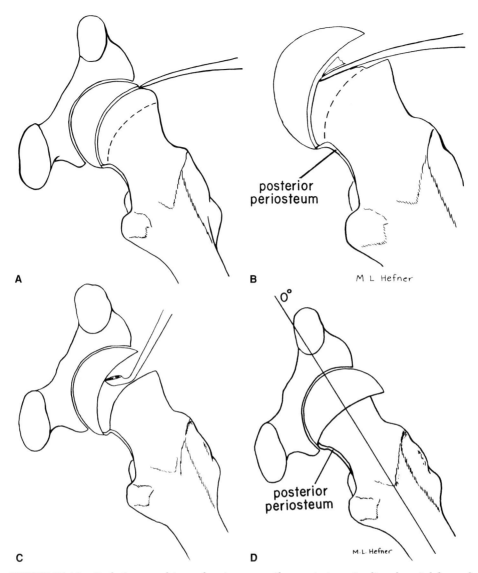

FIGURE 25-18. Technique used in performing a cuneiform osteotomy in slipped capital femoral epiphysis. (**A**) The hip capsule is opened anteriorly, and the location of the physeal plate is carefully identified. (**B**) A wedge of bone of predetermined size is removed in small pieces from the juxtaphyseal femoral neck. The physeal plate cartilage continuously is identified as the bone wedge is resected. Extreme care is taken not to damage the posterior periosteum. (**C**) After the bone wedge has been removed, the physeal plate cartilage is curetted. Adequate bone must be excised from the posterior corner to allow for reduction of the femoral head without tension on the posterior periosteum and vasculature. (**D**) The femoral neck is reduced onto the femoral head, re-creating more normal proximal femoral alignment. The reduction is stabilized with pin or screw fixation. (From Fish JB. Cuneiform osteotomy of the femoral neck in the treatment of slipped capital femoral epiphysis. J Bone Joint Surg [Am] 1984;66:1156.

and multiplane intertrochanteric osteotomies remove a wedge of bone of varying size from the anterior and lateral cortices of the affected femur at the level of the lesser trochanter. When this osteotomy is reduced and coupled with internal rotation of the femoral shaft, a realignment of the proximal femoral deformity occurs as a secondary deformity in the intertrochanteric region is created (Fig. 25-20). The correction achieved by osteotomy at this level is limited to deformities equal to or less than 45 degrees on the anteroposterior

radiograph and 60 degrees on the lateral radiograph as measured by the Southwick method.[111,118,126]

Intertrochanteric osteotomy enjoys a very low incidence of osteonecrosis of the femoral head compared with femoral neck osteotomies. This is secondary to the intertrochanteric osteotomy being performed in an area of the proximal femur that is not in direct proximity to the blood supply of the femoral head. An increased incidence of chondrolysis with joint space narrowing and stiffness, however, has been

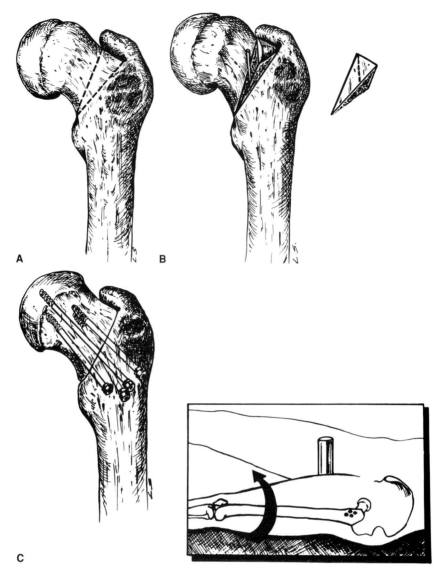

FIGURE 25-19.   Technique for performing a base of the neck osteotomy in slipped capital femoral epiphysis. (**A**) The base of the femoral neck is exposed through an anterolateral approach to the hip. The outline of an anterosuperior-based wedge of bone of predetermining size is marked on the base of the femoral neck. (**B**) The bony wedge is then cut and excised in such a manner that a triangular segment is created that contacts but does not penetrate through the posterior cortex. This avoids injury to the vasculature running along the posterior femoral neck. (**C**) The gap in the femoral neck is closed by internally rotating the limb while maintaining traction, which "greensticks" the posterior cortex of the femoral neck. The reduction is stabilized by pins or screws. (From Abraham E, Garst J, Barmada R. Treatment of moderate to severe slipped capital femoral epiphysis with extracapsular base-of-neck osteotomy. J Pediatr Orthop 1993;13:299.)

reported to be associated with intertrochanteric oste- otomy. Southwick, in his original description of the procedure, noted 6 of 55 hips (11%) that showed the development of chondrolysis.[126] More recent series have reported the development of chondrolysis of the hip in SCFE following corrective intertrochanteric os- teotomy to range from 6% to 56%.[44,111,118] The reason for the increase in chondrolysis seen in association with intertrochanteric osteotomy in SCFE remains un-

known. I believe that the development of chondrolysis is related to increased pressure at the femoral head, which is created as the osteotomy is closed and the limb is lengthened. A simple femoral shortening from the distal segment of the femur at the osteotomy site should relieve femoral head pressure and thereby re- duce the incidence of chondrolysis. The deformity created in the intertrochanteric region of the proximal femur by this osteotomy also can have a potentially

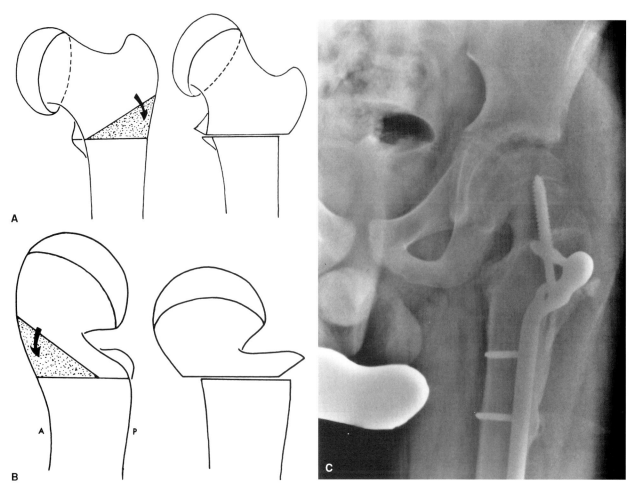

FIGURE 25-20. Technique used in performing a biplane intertrochanteric osteotomy in slipped capital femoral epiphysis as described by Southwick. Following surgical exposure of the proximal femur, a transverse line is marked on the (**A**) anterior and (**B**) lateral surfaces of the proximal femur at the level of the lesser trochanter. This line acts as the base of the subsequent bony wedge resections. The predetermined size of the anterior and lateral wedges to be removed are marked on the respective femoral surfaces. The biplane wedge of bone created is excised, and the transverse osteotomy at the level of the lesser trochanter is completed. The distal femoral segment is de-rotated, and the osteotomy is closed into the corrected position as demonstrated. The osteotomy is stabilized with a plate and screws. (**A** and **B** from Clark CR, Southwick WO, Ogden JA. Anatomic aspects of slipped capital femoral epiphysis and correction by biplane osteotomy. Instr Course Lect 1980;29:90.) (**C**) Anteroposterior hip radiograph of a 14.5-year-old boy following biplane intertrochanteric osteotomy for correction of residual deformity in slipped capital femoral epiphysis.

deleterious effect on later total hip arthroplasty.[123] The wedge resections of bone create an angular deformity in the intertrochanteric region that results in a tortuous proximal femoral canal. This could necessitate the need for excessive bone resection from the femoral neck calcar and make for difficult passage and seating of the femoral component during future total hip arthroplasty.

Salvage Procedures

If the femoral head in SCFE becomes severely deformed and the joint becomes stiff and painful as a result of osteonecrosis or chondrolysis, salvage proce-

dures are indicated to relieve pain and improve function. The procedure of choice in adolescents and young adults remains arthrodesis. Sponseller and colleagues reported on 53 patients who had had a hip arthrodesis and who had been under 35 years of age at the time of the procedure.[128] At an average follow-up of 38 years, 78% of the patients remained satisfied with the arthrodesis, and all remained employable. Only 13% had had the arthrodesis converted to a total hip arthroplasty. Callaghan and colleagues reviewed 28 patients who had had a hip arthrodesis as an adolescent or young adult.[20] At an average 35-year follow-up, some pain in the ipsilateral knee, the lower back, or the contralateral hip frequently was reported but had not become symptomatic until an average 20 years or longer following the procedure. Only one patient (4%) was unemployed because of pain, and only six patients (21%) had undergone conversion to a total hip arthroplasty. Hip arthrodesis, therefore, remains a very successful salvage procedure for relief of severe pain in young patients who develop complications in SCFE.

The procedure relieves pain and allows the patient a high level of activity and employment at most occupations. Some pain at the ipsilateral knee, the lower back, or the contralateral hip commonly occurs but usually only many years following the procedure. Proper positioning of the femur in relation to the pelvis is extremely important to function as well as avoidance of future back and knee pain. The proper position for the hip during arthrodesis is 20 degrees flexion with neutral rotation and neutral to slight adduction. Abduction at the hip is to be avoided secondary to it being associated with accelerated ipsilateral knee pain.[20] A take-down of the arthrodesis and conversion to a total

hip replacement is possible if painful back and knee symptoms become too severe.[5,20,82,128] Also the abductor muscles should not be injured in order to facilitate future hip function following total hip arthroplasty. The method of arthrodesis described by Mowery and colleagues is preferred.[100] This technique offers many advantages, which include a familiar anterior approach to the hip, a large surface area for fusion, a relatively simple technique of compression arthrodesis using minimal hardware, no disturbance of the greater trochanter and abductor muscles, no additional loss of limb length, and an upper femoral osteotomy that reduces the lever arm force on the fusion area and allows for adjustment of limb position postoperatively (Fig. 25-21). The main disadvantage associated with this technique remains the need for postoperative immobilization in a spica cast for 6 to 8 weeks.

Arthroplasty of the affected hip is not recommended for most adolescents and young adults, with severe unilateral hip osteoarthritis associated with SCFE.[8,24] The potential for early component loosening

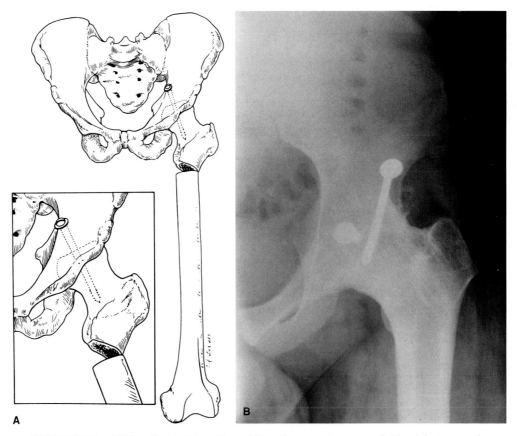

FIGURE 25-21. (A) Hip arthrodesis is performed through an anterior approach. The abductor muscles are not disturbed. Compression arthrodesis is achieved with minimal hardware. A proximal femoral osteotomy reduces force on the fusion area and allows for adjustment in limb position postoperatively. (From Mowery CA, Houkom JA, Roach JW, Sutherland DH. A simple method of hip arthrodesis. J Pediatr Orthop 1986;6:10.) (B) Anteroposterior hip radiograph of a 16-year, 4-month-old boy demonstrates a solid hip arthrodesis performed by the previously described technique. Femoral head osteonecrosis had occurred following treatment for slipped capital femoral epiphysis.

and wear in active young adults remains very high. The need for several revisions over the patient's lifetime and the subsequent risk of chronic infection preclude total hip arthroplasty as the recommended procedure in these younger patients. Chandler and colleagues reported on 29 patients who had been treated with a total hip arthroplasty at an average age of 23 years (range, 14–30 years).[24] At 5-year follow-up, 57% of the patients showed evidence of loosening of at least one of the components of the implant. Seven patients (24%) had already undergone revision surgery. The factors of associated osteonecrosis of the femoral head, heavy activity, and excessive weight, all commonly seen in patients with SCFE, were associated with poorer results from arthroplasty. One exception in SCFE is the patient with bilateral disease. Although no universally good method of treatment for bilateral disease has been documented, one option is an arthrodesis of one hip and an arthroplasty of the contralateral hip, which would provide a better balance of function and durability.

Osteoplasty of the femoral neck has been reported as a means of improving function in hips with severe displacement of the femoral head and secondary deformity.[56,143] The prominent bony projection on the superior and anterior segments of the femoral neck can be excised to eliminate the mechanical block to motion between the bony prominence and the acetabulum. Although early improved motion has been documented, mainly in abduction and internal rotation, the long-term results of this procedure remain unpublished. Remodeling of the femoral neck can have a similar result on motion over time. Osteoplasty also leaves a large area of denuded bone surface in the weight-bearing area of the hip, which can lead to accelerated degenerative joint disease.

PROPHYLACTIC PINNING OF THE CONTRALATERAL HIP

The controversy over prophylactic pinning of the uninvolved hip in SCFE remains unanswered. Proponents of prophylactic pinning emphasize the rate of bilateral disease and the higher risk of osteoarthritis associated with increasing slip severity.[49] Opponents of prophylactic pinning stress the fact that in situ pinning can be associated with severe complications that can be more devastating to hip function than the slip itself.[93] Symptomatic bilateral SCFE averages 25% (range, 21%–37%) during growth.[22,49,78,122,146] One half of these patients (12.5%) develop the second symptomatic slip prior to skeletal maturity.[22,78,122,146] Asymptomatic slipping of the contralateral hip prior to maturity has been proposed in as high as 40% of patients.[14,49] If all contralateral hips in SCFE were pinned prophylac-

tically, 50% to 80% of contralateral hips would be treated unnecessarily.

After a patient has had treatment for unilateral SCFE, the patient is under established medical follow-up until maturity. The patient also is aware of the prodromal symptoms of a second slip, and should they develop, the patient is instructed to return immediately for evaluation and treatment. In this situation, only acute unstable slips should have the potential for significant initial displacement. With acute slips representing only 10% of SCFE, 90% of symptomatic slips should be able to be treated prior to the development of more significant displacement.

Observation of the unaffected hip rather than prophylactic pinning remains the most appropriate treatment in patients presenting with unilateral SCFE.[73,93] Exceptions to this treatment include patients with an inability to obtain appropriate and timely follow-up due to personal or family circumstances and patients who have SCFE associated with known metabolic or endocrine disorders in which the risk of a contralateral slip is extremely high. In these situations, prophylactic pinning of the contralateral hip is appropriate.

COMPLICATIONS

The two major complications in SCFE that are associated with the development of accelerated degenerative joint disease and motion loss at the affected hip are osteonecrosis of the femoral head and chondrolysis.

Osteonecrosis of the femoral head has been reported to occur in 10% to 15% of patients with SCFE.[16,21,22,50] More recent reviews of in situ fixation in SCFE using cannulated screws and strict attention to technical detail report a much lower incidence of osteonecrosis, 0% to 5%.[7,75,127,139] Osteonecrosis of the femoral head is believed to be a complication of treatment because it is reported only rarely in untreated SCFE.[16,22] Osteonecrosis of the femoral head remains more frequently identified with acute and unstable slips[22,79] (Fig. 25-22).

The etiology of osteonecrosis is related to vascular injury to the extraosseous or intraosseous circulation of the femoral head. An increased incidence of osteonecrosis of the femoral head has been reported with increasing severity of the slip.[16,22] Carney and colleagues, in a review of 155 hips, reported an incidence of femoral head osteonecrosis of 12%.[22] Osteonecrosis was noted in 2% of 65 mild slips, 20% of 50 moderate slips, and 20% of 40 severe slips. Acute slips have a higher incidence of femoral head osteonecrosis, which is secondary to the rapid and excessive stretch of the extraosseous epiphyseal vessels that can occur during the acute displacement.[16,22] Iatrogenic injury to the extraosseous epiphyseal vessels can occur during

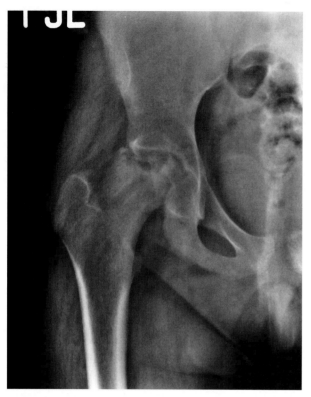

FIGURE 25-22. Anteroposterior hip radiograph of a 14-year, 4-month-old girl with osteonecrosis of the femoral head following treatment for slipped capital femoral epiphysis.

manipulation of the femoral head, stabilization of the femoral head if the fixation device violates the posterior cortex of the femoral neck, and realignment of the femoral head through osteotomy of the femoral neck.[22] Iatrogenic injury to the intraosseous circulation of the femoral head usually is related to hardware placement into the vulnerable superior quadrant of the femoral head, as previously discussed.[19]

After osteonecrosis of the femoral head has been established, treatment must be directed at maintaining motion and preventing collapse by decreasing the magnitude of the forces at the affected hip through relieved weight bearing until healing occurs. Any hardware in the zone of collapse of the femoral head must be withdrawn and replaced to avoid joint injury. The use of vascularized bone graft and redirectional intertrochanteric osteotomy with bone grafting to the femoral head has been proposed to improve outcome in osteonecrosis of the femoral head.[119] No large report directly addressing treatment of osteonecrosis associated with SCFE has been published.

Long-term reviews of SCFE show that hips affected with osteonecrosis have a poorer outcome that continues to deteriorate over time.[16,22]

Acute cartilage necrosis of the femoral head or chondrolysis was first described by Elmslie, in 1913,[53] and was later reported in association with SCFE by

Waldenstrom.[137] Chondrolysis is defined as an acute dissolution of articular cartilage in association with rapid progressive joint stiffness and pain.

The etiology of chondrolysis in association with SCFE remains unknown. Historically, the condition was believed to be a result of synovial malnutrition,[137] ischemic injury of articular cartilage,[50] or excessive cartilage pressure.[81] Modern theory suggests an etiology associated with an immunologic and an autoimmune disorder within the hip joint.[35,85,96] A genetic factor is implied by the increased incidence of chondrolysis in female patients in spite of SCFE being more prevalent in males patients.

The incidence of chondrolysis of the hip in SCFE has been reported in the literature to average 16% to 20% (range, 1.8%–55%).[22,53,61] Recent reviews of the association of chondrolysis with treatment of SCFE by in situ stabilization with a single cannulated screw have been reported.[75,139] Ward and colleagues reported no chondrolysis in 53 treated hips with at least 24-month follow-up.[139] Koval and colleagues reported no cases of chondrolysis to have developed postoperatively in any of 60 hips with at least 2 years follow-up.[75] Modern techniques of stabilization and attention to detail during treatment seem to be associated with a lower incidence of chondrolysis than has been previously reported.

Ingram and colleagues have reported on 79 hips in SCFE affected by chondrolysis.[61] The authors found the incidence of chondrolysis to be higher in female patients, patients with acute slips, and patients with slips with increased severity of displacement. Similar results have been reported by additional authors.[22,53,87] Historically, African-American patients and patients of Hawaiian ancestry have been reported to have a higher incidence of chondrolysis of the hip in association with treatment of SCFE.[32,61,87,135,146] Recent reports of treatment in SCFE by modern techniques of in situ stabilization have shown the incidence of chondrolysis in the African-American population to be no higher than in the general population. Kennedy and Weiner reported on in situ stabilization of SCFE in 44 African-American children with an incidence of chondrolysis of 2.3%.[71] Spero and colleagues reported an incidence of chondrolysis of 6.8% in 44 hips in 29 African-American patients treated by in situ pinning.[127] Aronson and Loder reviewed in situ stabilization of 97 SCFE hips in 74 African-American children, and reported the development of chondrolysis in only 3%.[7]

Although chondrolysis of the hip in SCFE can occur in the untreated hip,[22,136] the majority of chondrolysis in SCFE has been reported to follow treatment. The treatment modalities shown to be associated with an increased incidence of chondrolysis include manipulative reduction,[22] prolonged immobilization,[13,89] and realignment osteotomies of the proximal femur.[22,45,118] Persistent pin penetration of the femoral head has been shown to be associated with the development of chondrolysis.[136,138] Transient penetration of the hip joint in SCFE by stabilizing hardware also was believed to be associated with the induction of chondrolysis. Zionts and colleagues,[147] Koval and colleagues,[75] and Vrettos and Hoffman[136] have shown that a single episode of transient penetration of the hip joint by a pin or screw with immediate recognition and removal is not associated with an increased incidence in the development of chondrolysis.

The diagnosis of chondrolysis is confirmed in a patient with clinical symptoms of progressive hip stiffness and pain by radiographic confirmation of joint space narrowing at the hip to 3 mm or less.[36,61] If chondrolysis does develop it usually appears within the first year following the SCFE. If chondrolysis follows surgical treatment of SCFE, a septic process mimicking chondrolysis must always be ruled out by hip aspiration. Mandell and colleagues have reported radiographic premature closure of the greater trochanteric physis to be a predictive sign of chondrolysis.[83] The authors demonstrated that decreased activity on bone scintigraphy at the greater trochanteric physis was associated with concurrent or developing chondrolysis in 16 patients with SCFE.

The recommended early treatment of chondrolysis in SCFE has not been standardized but should include elements of relieved weight bearing, antiinflammatory medication, and passive as well as active hip motion.[64] In the early stages of chondrolysis and during recurrent episodes of synovitis and pain, therapeutic doses of nonsteroidal antiinflammatory medications should be initiated and maintained. Periodic hospitalization for enforced bed rest, traction, and frequent physical therapy can be used during episodes of increased pain and motion loss. Physical therapy consisting of aggressive passive and active motion to the affected hip should be initiated early. The use of continuous passive motion equipment can be of assistance in maintaining reacquired motion. If pain during physical therapy remains excessive, continuous epidural anesthesia can be of benefit. Ambulation should remain protected with non–weight-bearing and limited–weight-bearing crutch use continued until pain has resolved and joint space narrowing radiographically has ceased.

A fibrous ankylosis of the hip joint often can be the final outcome in hips affected by chondrolysis.[94,146] However, spontaneous partial cartilage recovery from chondrolysis following SCFE has been reported.[81] The prognosis for the hip developing chondrolysis following SCFE is not invariably bad, as had been supposed. Hartman and Gates reported partial restoration of the cartilage space at the hip joint and hip motion in 9 of 28 hips (32%) with chondrolysis.[53] At follow-up of 2 to 5 years, 6 of the 9 hips showing recovery were classified as good results. Vrettos and Hoffman confirmed partial reconstitution of the joint space to average of 2.6 mm (range, 1–5 mm) in 14 hips with chondrolysis following SCFE.[136] This reconstitution of joint space occurred as late as 3 years after maximum joint involvement. At an average follow-up of 13.3 years, a good functional outcome was reported in 64% of the patients with chondrolysis. Although this information allows for a more optimistic attitude in reference to the early outcome of chondrolysis associated with SCFE, Carney and colleagues at a mean follow-up of 41 years, have reported that the hip affected by chondrolysis in SCFE eventually shows a continued deterioration in hip function over time.[22]

References

1. Aadelen R, Weiner D, Hoyt W, Herndon C. Acute slipped capital femoral epiphysis. J Bone Joint Surg [Am] 1974;56:1473.
2. Abraham E, Garst J, Barmada R. Treatment of moderate to severe slipped capital femoral epiphysis with extracapsular base-of-neck osteotomy. J Pediatr Orthop 1993;13:294.
3. Agamanolis DP, Weiner DS, Lloyd JK. Slipped capital femoral epiphysis: a pathological study. I. A light microscopic and histochemical study of 21 cases. J Pediatr Orthop 1985;5:40.
4. Agamanolis DP, Weiner DS, Lloyd JK. Slipped capital femoral epiphysis: a pathological study II. An ultrastructural study of 23 cases. J Pediatr Orthop 1985;5:47.
5. Amstutz HC, Sakai DN. Total joint replacement for ankylosed hips—indications, technique and preliminary results. J Bone Joint Surg [Am] 1975;57:619.
6. Aronson DD, Carlson WE. Slipped capital femoral epiphysis. A prospective study of fixation with a single screw. J Bone Joint Surg [Am] 1992;74:810.
7. Aronson DD, Loder RT. Slipped capital femoral epiphysis in black children. J Pediatr Orthop 1992;12:74.
8. Aronson J. Osteoarthritis of the young adult hip: etiology and treatment. Instr Course Lect 1986;35:119.
9. Badgley E, Isaacson A, Wolgamot J, Miller J. Operative therapy for slipped capital femoral epiphysis. J Bone Joint Surg [Am] 1948;30:19.
10. Barmada R, Bruch RF, Gimbel JS, Ray RD. Base of neck extracapsular osteotomy for correction of deformity in slipped capital femoral epiphysis. Clin Orthop 1978;132:98.
11. Baynham GC, Lucie RS, Cummings RJ. Femoral neck fracture secondary to in situ pinning of slipped capital femoral epiphysis. A previously unreported complication. J Pediatr Orthop 1991;11:187.
12. Bennet GC, Koreska J, Rang M. Pin placement in slipped capital femoral epiphysis. J Pediatr Orthop 1984;4:574.
13. Betz RR, Steel HH, Emper WD, et al. Treatment of slipped capital femoral epiphysis—spica cast immobilization. J Bone Joint Surg [Am] 1990;72:587.
14. Billing L, Severin E. Slipping epiphysis of the hip: a roentgenological and clinical study based on a new roentgen technique. Acta Radiol 1959;(Suppl):174:1.
15. Blanco JS, Taylor B, Johnston, CE. Comparison of single pin versus multiple pin fixation in treatment of slipped capital femoral epiphysis. J Pediatr Orthop 1992;12:384.
16. Boyer D, Mickelson M, Ponseti T. Slipped capital femoral epiphysis: long-term follow up and study of one hundred and twenty-one patients. J Bone Joint Surg [Am] 1981;63:85.

17. Brenkel IJ, Dias JJ, Davies TG, et al. Hormone status in patients with slipped capital femoral epiphysis. J Bone Joint Surg [Br] 1989;71:33.

18. Bright R, Burstein A, Elmore S. Epiphyseal plate cartilage: a biomechanical and histological analysis of failure modes. J Bone Joint Surg [Am] 1974;56:688.

19. Brodetti A. The blood supply of the femoral neck and head in relation to the damaging effects of nails and screws. J Bone Joint Surg [Br] 1960;42:794.

20. Callaghan JJ, Brand RA, Pedersen DR. Hip arthrodesis. A long-term follow-up. J Bone Joint Surg [Am] 1985;67:1328.

21. Canale ST. Problems and complications of slipped capital femoral epiphysis. Instr Course Lect 1989;38:281.

22. Carney BT, Weinstein SL, Noble J. Long-term follow-up of slipped capital femoral epiphysis. J Bone Joint Surg [Am] 1991;73:667.

23. Casey B, Hamilton H, Bobechko W. Reduction of acutely slipped upper femoral epiphysis. J Bone Joint Surg [Br] 1972;54:607.

24. Chandler HP, Reineck FT, Wilson RL, McCarthy JC. Total hip replacement in patients younger than thirty years old. J Bone Joint Surg [Am] 1981;63:1426.

25. Cohen MS, Gelberman RH, Griffin PP, Kasser JR, et al. Slipped capital femoral epiphysis: assessment of epiphyseal displacement and angulation. J Pediatr Orthop 1986;6:259.

26. Chung S, Batterman S, Brighton C. Shear strength of the human femoral capital epiphyseal plate. J Bone Joint Surg [Am] 1976;58:94.

27. Chung SM. The arterial supply of the developing proximal end of the human femur. J Bone Joint Surg [Am] 1976;58:961.

28. Clark CR, Southwick WO, Ogden JA. Anatomic aspects of slipped capital femoral epiphysis and correction by biplane osteotomy. Instr Course Lect 1980;29:90.

29. Crawford AH. Slipped capital femoral epiphysis. J Bone Joint Surg [Am] 1988;70:1422.

30. Crawford AH. The role of osteotomy in the treatment of slipped capital femoral epiphysis. Instr Course Lect 1989; 38:273.

31. Crider RJ, Kroll T, McGuire M, et al. Anterolateral approach for moderate to severe slipped capital femoral epiphysis. J Pediatr Orthop 1988;8:661.

32. Cruess RL. The pathology of acute necrosis of cartilage in slipping of the capital femoral epiphysis. J Bone Joint Surg [Am] 1963;45:1013.

33. Doane RM, Haut RC, Karol L, Manoli A. Biomechanical analysis of the slipped capital femoral epiphysis with single and double screw fixation. Trans Orthop Res Soc 1990;15:430.

34. Dunn DM, Angel JC. Replacement of the femoral head by open operation in severe adolescent slipping of the upper femoral epiphysis. J Bone Joint Surg [Br] 1978;60:394.

35. Eisenstein A, Rothschild S. Biochemical abnormalities in patients with slipped capital femoral epiphysis and chondrolysis. J Bone Joint Surg [Am] 1976;58:459.

36. El-Khoury G, Mickelson M. Chondrolysis following slipped capital femoral epiphysis. Radiology 1977;123:327.

37. England SP, Morrissy RT. Metal removal following in-situ fixation for slipped capital femoral epiphysis: a cost/benefit analysis. American Academy of Orthopaedic Surgeons 61st Annual Meeting Final Program 1994:296.

38. Fahey J, O'Brien E. Acute slipped capital femoral epiphysis. J Bone Joint Surg [Am] 1965;47:1105.

39. Fairbank JT. Manipulative reduction in slipped upper femoral epiphysis. J Bone Joint Surg [Br] 1969;51:252.

40. Ferguson AB, Howorth MB. Slipping of the upper femoral epiphysis: a study of seventy cases. JAMA 1931;97:1867.

41. Fidler M, Brook C. Slipped upper femoral epiphysis following treatment with human growth hormone. J Bone Joint Surg [Am] 1974;56:1719.

42. Fish JB. Cuneiform osteotomy of the femoral neck in the treatment of slipped capital femoral epiphysis. J Bone Joint Surg [Am] 1984;66:1153.

43. Fish JB. Cuneiform osteotomy of the femoral neck in the treatment of slipped capital femoral epiphysis. A follow-up note. J Bone Joint Surg [Am] 1994;76:46.

44. Frymover J. Chondrolysis of the hip following Southwick osteotomy for severe slipped capital femoral epiphysis. Clin Orthop 1974;99:120.

45. Gage J, Sundberg A, Nolan D, et al. Complications after cuneiform osteotomy for moderately of severely slipped capital femoral epiphysis. J Bone Joint Surg [Am] 1978;60:157.

46. Gelberman R, Cohen M, Shaw B, et al. The association of femoral retroversion with slipped capital femoral epiphysis. J Bone Joint Surg [Am] 1986;68:1000.

47. Green WT. Slipping of the upper femoral epiphysis: diagnostic and therapeutic considerations. Arch Surg 1945;50:19.

48. Greenough CG, Bromage JD, Jackson AM. Pinning of the slipped upper femoral epiphysis—a trouble-free procedure? J Pediatr Orthop 1985;5:657.

49. Hagglund G, Hansson LI, Ordeberg G, Sandstrom S. Bilaterality in slipped upper femoral epiphysis. J Bone Joint Surg [Br] 1988;70:179.

50. Hall JE. The results of treatment of slipped femoral epiphysis. J Bone Joint Surg [Br] 1957;39:659.

51. Hansson LI. Osteosynthesis with the hook-pin in slipped capital femoral epiphysis. Acta Orthop Scand 1982;53:87.

52. Harris WR. The endocrine basis for slipping of the femoral epiphysis. J Bone Joint Surg [Br] 1950;32:5.

53. Hartman J, Gates D. Recovery from cartilage necrosis following slipped capital femoral epiphysis. Orthop Rev 1972;1:33.

54. Heatley FW, Greenwood RH, Boase DL. Slipping of the upper femoral epiphysis in patients with intracranial tumors causing hypopituitarism and chiasmal compression. J Bone Joint Surg [Br] 1976;58:169.

55. Henrickson B. The incidence of slipped capital femoral epiphysis. Acta Orthop Scand 1969;40:365.

56. Herndon CH, Heyman CH, Bell DM. Treatment of slipped capital femoral epiphysis by epiphyseodesis and osteoplasty of femoral neck. J Bone Joint Surg [Am] 1963;45:999.

57. Heyerman W, Weiner D. Slipped epiphysis associated with hypothyroidism. J Pediatr Orthop 1984;4:569.

58. Hirano T, Stamelos S, Harris V, Dumbovich N. Association of primary hypothyroidism and slipped capital femoral epiphysis. J Pediatr 1978;93:262.

59. Howorth MB. Slipping of the upper femoral epiphysis. J Bone Joint Surg [Am] 1949;31:734.

60. Howorth MB. Treatment and slipping of the upper femoral epiphysis. Clin Orthop 1966;48:53.

61. Ingram AJ, Clarke MS, Clarke CS, Marshall RW. Chondrolysis complicating slipped capital femoral epiphysis. Clin Orthop 1982;165:99.

62. Ippolito E, Mickelson M, Ponseti I. A histochemical study of slipped capital femoral epiphysis. J Bone Joint Surg [Am] 1981;63:1109.

63. Irani RN, Rosenzweig AH, Cotler HB, Schwentker EP. Epiphysiodesis in slipped capital femoral epiphysis. A comparison of various surgical modalities. J Pediatr Orthop 1985;5:661.

64. Jacobs B. Diagnosis and natural history of slipped capital femoral epiphysis. Instr Course Lect 1972;21:167.

65. Jerre T. A study in slipped upper femoral epiphysis with special reference to late functional and roentgenological results and the value of closed reduction. Acta Orthop Scand 1950;6(Suppl):1.

66. Jones JR, Paterson DC, Hillier TM, Foster BK. Remodelling

after pinning for slipped capital femoral epiphysis. J Bone Joint Surg [Br] 1990;72:568.

67. Kallio P, Lequesne GW, Paterson DC, Foster BK. Ultrasonography in slipped capital femoral epiphysis. Diagnosis and assessment of severity. J Bone Joint Surg [Br] 1991;73:884.

68. Karol LA, Doane RM, Cornicelli SF, et al. Single versus double screw fixation for treatment of slipped capital femoral epiphysis: a biomechanical analysis. J Pediatr Orthop 1992;12:741.

69. Kelsey J, Acheson R, Keggi K. The body builds of patients with slipped capital femoral epiphysis. Am J Dis Child 1972;124:276.

70. Kelsey J, Keggi K, Southwick W. The incidence and distribution of slipped capital femoral epiphysis in Connecticut and the Southwestern United States. J Bone Joint Surg [Am] 1970;52:1203.

71. Kennedy JP, Weiner DS. Results of slipped capital femoral epiphysis in the black population. J Pediatr Orthop 1990;10:224.

72. Key J. Epiphyseal coxa vara or displacement of the capital epiphysis of the femur in adolescence. J Bone Joint Surg 1926;8:53.

73. Klein A, Joplin RJ, Reidy JA, Hanelin J. Management of the contralateral hip in slipped capital femoral epiphysis. J Bone Joint Surg [Am] 1953;35:81.

74. Klein A, Joplin RJ, Reidy JA, Hanelin J. Roentgenographic features of slipped capital femoral epiphysis. AJR 1951;66:361.

75. Koval KJ, Lehman WB, Rose D, et al. Treatment of slipped capital femoral epiphysis with a cannulated-screw technique. J Bone Joint Surg [Am] 1989;71:1370.

76. Kramer WG, Craig WA, Noel S. Compensating osteotomy at the base of the femoral neck for slipped capital femoral epiphysis. J Bone Joint Surg [Am] 1976;58:796.

77. Lacroix P, Verbrugge J. Slipping of the upper femoral epiphysis: a pathological study. J Bone Joint Surg [Am] 1951;33:371.

78. Loder RT, Aronson DD, Greenfield ML. The epidemiology of bilateral slipped capital femoral epiphysis. J Bone Joint Surg [Am] 1993;75:1141.

79. Loder RT, Richards BS, Shapiro PS, Reznick LR, Aronson DD. Acute slipped capital femoral epiphysis: the importance of physeal stability. J Bone Joint Surg [Am] 1993;75:1134.

80. Lowe HG. Avascular necrosis after slipping of the upper femoral epiphysis. J Bone Joint Surg [Br] 1961;43:688.

81. Lowe HG. Necrosis of articular cartilage after slipping of the capital femoral epiphysis. Report of six cases with recovery. J Bone Joint Surg [Br] 1970;52:108.

82. Lubahn JD, Evarts CM, Feltner JB. Conversion of ankylosed hips to total hip arthroplasty. Clin Orthop 1980;153:146.

83. Mandell GA, Keret D, Harcke HT, Bowen JR. Chondrolysis: detection by bone scintigraphy. J Pediatr Orthop 1992;12:80.

84. Mann DC, Weddington J, Richton S. Hormonal studies in patients with slipped capital femoral epiphysis without evidence of endocrinopathy. J Pediatr Orthop 1988;8:543.

85. Mankin HJ, Sledge CB, Rothschild S, Eisenstein A. Chondrolysis of the hip. In: The hip: proceedings of the Third Open Scientific Meeting of the Hip Society. St Louis: CV Mosby, 1975:127.

86. Masuda T, Matsuno T, Hasegawa I, et al. Transtrochanteric anterior rotational osteotomy for slipped capital femoral epiphysis: a report of five cases. J Pediatr Orthop 1986;6:18.

87. Maurer R, Larsen I. Acute necrosis of cartilage in slipped capital femoral epiphysis. J Bone Joint Surg [Am] 1970;52:39.

88. McAfee P, Cady R. Endocrinologic and metabolic factors in atypical presentations of slipped capital femoral epiphysis. Clin Orthop 1983;180:188.

89. Meier MC, Meyer LC, Ferguson RL. Treatment of slipped capital femoral epiphysis with a spica cast. J Bone Joint Surg [Am] 1992;74:1522.

90. Melby A, Hoyt W, Weiner D. Treatment of chronic slipped capital femoral epiphysis by bone-graft epiphysiodesis. J Bone Joint Surg [Am] 1980;62:119.

91. Mickelson MR, Ponseti IV, Cooper RR, Maynard JA. The ultrastructure of the growth plate in slipped capital femoral epiphysis. J Bone Joint Surg [Am] 1977;59:1076.

92. Moorefield WG, Urbaniak JR, Ogden WS, Frank JL. Acquired hypothyroidism and slipped capital femoral epiphysis. J Bone Joint Surg [Am] 1976;58:705.

93. Morrissy RT. Principles of in situ fixation in chronic slipped capital femoral epiphysis. Instr Course Lect 1989;38:257.

94. Morissy RT. Slipped capital femoral epiphysis—natural history and etiology in treatment. Instr Course Lect 1980;29:81.

95. Morrissy RT. Slipped capital femoral epiphysis technique of percutaneous in situ fixation. J Pediatr Orthop 1990;10:347.

96. Morrissy RT, Kalderon AE, Gerdes MH. Synovial immunofluorescence in patients with slipped capital femoral epiphysis. J Pediatr Orthop 1981;1:55.

97. Morrissy RT, Steele RW, Gerdes MH. Localized immune complexes and slipped capital femoral epiphysis. J Bone Joint Surg [Br] 1983;65:574.

98. Morsher E. Strength and morphology of growth cartilage under hormonal influence of puberty. Reconstr Surg Traumatol 1968;10:3.

99. Moseley C. The "approach-withdraw" phenomenon in the pinning of slipped capital femoral epiphysis. Orthop Trans 1985;9:497.

100. Mowery CA, Houkom JA, Roach JW, Sutherland DH. A simple method of hip arthrodesis. J Pediatr Orthop 1986;6:7.

101. Murray RO. The etiology of primary osteoarthritis of the hip. Br J Radiol 1965;38:810.

102. Nguyen D, Morrissy RT. Slipped capital femoral epiphysis: rationale for the technique of percutaneous in situ fixation. J Pediatr Orthop 1990;10:341.

103. Nishiyama K, Sakamaki T, Ishii Y. Follow-up study of the subcapital wedge osteotomy for severe chronic slipped capital femoral epiphysis. J Pediatr Orthop 1989;9:412.

104. O'Brien E, Fahey J. Remodeling of the femoral neck after in situ pinning for slipped capital femoral epiphysis. J Bone Joint Surg [Am] 1977;59:62.

105. Oka M, Miki T, Hama H, Yamamuro T. The mechanical strength of the growth plate under the influence of sex hormones. Clin Orthop 1979;145:264.

106. Oram V. Epiphysiolysis of the head of the femur. Acta Orthop Scand 1953;23:100.

107. Peterson CA, Peterson HA. Analysis of the incidence of injuries to the epiphyseal growth plate. J Trauma 1972;12:275.

108. Ponseti IV, McClintock R. The pathology of slipping of the upper femoral epiphysis. J Bone Joint Surg [Am] 1956;38:71.

109. Primiano GA, Hughston JC. Slipped capital femoral epiphysis in a true hypogonadal male (Klinefelter's mosaic XY/XXY). J Bone Joint Surg [Am] 1971;53:597.

110. Pritchett JW, Perdue KD. Mechanical factors in slipped capital femoral epiphysis. J Pediatr Orthop 1988;8:385.

111. Rao J, Francis A, Siwek C. The treatment of chronic slipped capital femoral epiphysis by biplane osteotomy. J Bone Joint Surg [Am] 1984;66:1169.

112. Razzano CD, Nelson C, Eversman J. Growth hormone levels in slipped capital femoral epiphysis. J Bone Joint Surg [Am] 1972;54:1224.

113. Rennie AM. The inheritance of slipped upper femoral epiphysis. J Bone Joint Surg [Br] 1982;64:180.

114. Rennie W, Mitchell N. Slipped capital femoral epiphysis occurring during growth hormone therapy. Report of a case. J Bone Joint Surg [Br] 1974;56:703.

115. Resnick D. The "tilt deformity" of the femoral head in osteoarthritis of the hip, a poor indicator of previous epiphysiolysis. Clin Radiol 1976;27:355.

116. Riley PM, Weiner DS, Gillespie R, Weiner SD. Hazards of internal fixation in the treatment of slipped capital femoral epiphysis. J Bone Joint Surg [Am] 1990;72:1500.

117. Ross P, Lyne E, Morawa L. Slipped capital femoral epiphysis: long-term results after 10–38 years. Clin Orthop 1979;141:176.

118. Salvati E, Robinson H, O'Dowd T. Southwick osteotomy for severe chronic slipped capital femoral epiphysis. Results and complications. J Bone Joint Surg [Am] 1980;62:561.

119. Scher MA, Jakim I. Intertrochanteric osteotomy and autogenous bone-grafting for avascular necrosis of the femoral head. J Bone Joint Surg [Am] 1993;75:1119.

120. Segal LS, Davidson RS, Robertson WW, Drummond DS. Growth disturbances of the proximal femur after pinning of juvenile slipped capital femoral epiphysis. J Pediatr Orthop 1991;11:631.

121. Shea D, Mankin HJ. Slipped capital femoral epiphysis in renal rickets: report of three cases. J Bone Joint Surg [Am] 1966; 48:349.

122. Siegel DB, Kasser JR, Sponseller P, Gelberman RH. Slipped capital femoral epiphysis. A quantitative analysis of motion, gait and femoral remodeling after in situ fixation. J Bone Joint Surg [Am] 1991;73:659.

123. Soballe K, Boll KL, Kofod S, et al. Total hip replacement after medial-displacement osteotomy of the proximal part of the femur. J Bone Joint Surg [Am] 1989;71:692.

124. Solomon L. Patterns of osteoarthritis of the hip. J Bone Joint Surg [Br] 1976;58:176.

125. Sorenson K. Slipped upper femoral epiphysis: clinical study on etiology. Acta Orthop Scand 1968;39:499.

126. Southwick W. Osteotomy through the lesser trochanter for slipped capital femoral epiphysis. J Bone Joint Surg [Am] 1967;49:807.

127. Spero CR, Masciale JP, Tornetta P, et al. Slipped capital femoral epiphysis in black children: incidence of chondrolysis. J Pediatr Orthop 1992;12:444.

128. Sponseller PD, McBeath AA, Perpich M. Hip arthrodesis in young patients. A long-term follow-up study. J Bone Joint Surg [Am] 1984;66:853.

129. Stambough JL, Davidson RS, Ellis RD, Gregg JR. Slipped capital femoral epiphysis: an analysis of 80 patients as to pin placement and number. J Pediatr Orthop 1986;6:265.

130. Stanton RP, Shelton YA. Closure of the physis after pinning of slipped capital femoral epiphysis. Orthopedics 1993;16:1099.

131. Steel HH. The metaphyseal blanch sign of slipped capital femoral epiphysis. J Bone Joint Surg [Am] 1986;68:920.

132. Stoller DW. Magnetic resonance imaging in orthopaedics and sports medicine. Philadelphia: JB Lippincott, 1993:83.

133. Stulberg SD, Cordell LD, Harris WH, et al. Unrecognized childhood hip diseases: a major cause of idiopathic osteoarthritis of the hip. In: The hip: proceedings of the Third Open Scientific Meeting of the Hip Society. St Louis: CV Mosby, 1975:212.

134. Sugioka Y. Transtrochametric rotational osteotomy of the femoral head. In: Riley LH Jr, ed. The hip. Proceedings of the Eighth Open Scientific Meeting of the Hip Society. St Louis: CV Mosby, 1980:3.

135. Tillema D, Golding J. Chondrolysis following slipped capital femoral epiphysis in Jamaica. J Bone Joint Surg [Am] 1971;53:1528.

136. Vrettos BC, Hoffman EB. Chondrolysis in slipped upper femoral epiphysis. J Bone Joint Surg [Br] 1993;75:956.

137. Waldenstrom H. On necrosis of the joint cartilage by epiphyseolysis capitis femoris. Acta Chir Scand 1930;67:936.

138. Walters R, Simon S. Joint destruction—a sequel of unrecognized pin penetration in patients with slipped capital femoral epiphysis. In: Riley LH Jr, ed. The hip: proceedings of the Eighth Open Scientific Meeting of the Hip Society. St Louis: CV Mosby, 1980:145.

139. Ward WT, Stefko J, Wood KB, Stanitski CL. Fixation with a single screw for slipped capital femoral epiphysis. J Bone Joint Surg [Am] 1992;74:799.

140. Ward WT, Wood K. Open bone graft epiphyseodesis for slipped capital femoral epiphysis. J Pediatr Orthop 1990;10:14.

141. Weiner DS, Weiner SD, Melby A. Anterolateral approach to the hip for bone graft epiphysiodesis in the treatment of slipped capital femoral epiphysis. J Pediatr Orthop 1988;8:349.

142. Weiner DS, Weiner S, Melby A, Hoyt WA. A 30-year experience with bone graft epiphysiodesis in the treatment of slipped capital femoral epiphysis. J Pediatr Orthop 1984;4:145.

143. Whitesides LA, Schoenecker PL. Combined valgus derotation osteotomy and cervical osteoplasy for severely slipped capital femoral epiphysis. Clin Orthop 1978;132:88.

144. Weinstein SL. Background on slipped capital femoral epiphysis. Instr Course Lect 1984;33:310.

145. Wilcox PG, Weiner DS, Leighley B. Maturation factors in slipped capital femoral epiphysis. J Pediatr Orthop 1988;8:196.

146. Wilson P, Jacobs B, Schector L. Slipped upper femoral epiphysis: an end result study. J Bone Joint Surg [Am] 1965;47:1128.

147. Zionts LE, Simonian PT, Harvey JP. Transient penetration of the hip joint during in situ cannulated-screw fixation of slipped capital femoral epiphysis. J Bone Joint Surg [Am] 1991;73:1054.

148. Zubrow A, Lane J, Parks J. Slipped capital femoral epiphysis occurring during treatment for hypothyroidism. J Bone Joint Surg [Am] 1978;60:256.

Lovell & Winter's Pediatric Orthopaedics, fourth edition,
edited by Raymond T. Morrissy and Stuart L. Weinstein.
Lippincott–Raven Publishers, Philadelphia © 1996.

Chapter

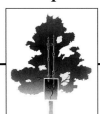

26

Developmental Coxa Vara; Transient Synovitis; and Idiopathic Chondiolysis of the Hip

Douglas K. Kehl

This chapter addresses three conditions affecting the juvenile and adolescent hip: developmental coxa vara, transient synovitis, and idiopathic chondrolysis of the hip. Developmental coxa vara and idiopathic chondrolysis of the hip remain relatively uncommon but continue to present challenging dilemmas in diagnosis and treatment. Transient synovitis remains the most common condition causing hip pain in childhood. A knowledge of this condition's presentation, diagnosis, and treatment is crucial for any physician treating musculoskeletal problems in pediatric patients.

DEVELOPMENTAL COXA VARA

Coxa vara is defined as any decrease below the normal values of the neck-shaft angle of the proximal femur, which is the angle subtended by the femoral neck and shaft in the coronal plane (Fig. 26-1). However, instead of referring to a specific clinical disease entity, coxa vara comprises a group of conditions occurring during childhood with different causes and natural histories that ultimately produce a specific deformity in the proximal femur.

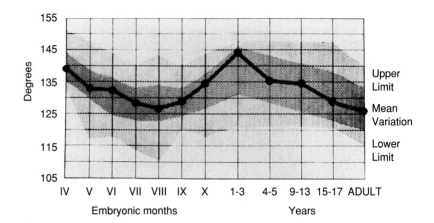

FIGURE 26-1. Variation of the normal neck-shaft angle with age. (From von Lanz T. Mayet A. Die gelenkorper Des Menschlichen Hufgelenkes In Der Progredienten Phase Iherer umwegigen Ausforming. Z Anat 1953;117:317.)

Elmslie[13] proposed a classification system for coxa vara that was later expanded by Fairbank.[14] This classification system of coxa vara groups was based on the proposed causes and included the congenital, rachitic, infantile or cervical, adolescent (i.e., slipped capital femoral epiphysis), traumatic, inflammatory, and metabolic types. These multiple categories have subsequently been condensed into three: congenital coxa vara, acquired coxa vara, and developmental coxa vara.

Congenital coxa vara is present at birth and is assumed to be caused by an embryonic limb bud abnormality. Significant proximal femoral varus is present at birth but usually shows minimal progression in the degree of varus during growth. Associated congenital musculoskeletal abnormalities and significant limb length inequality secondary to femoral segment shortening are common. This category includes cases of proximal femoral focal deficiency, congenital short femur, and congenital bowed femur (Fig. 26-2).

Acquired coxa vara includes all clinical entities in which the deformity of the proximal femur is secondary to an underlying metabolic, tumorous, or traumatic condition. This classification includes coxa vara secondary to rickets, fibrous dysplasia, and early traumatic proximal femoral epiphyseal plate closure (Fig. 26-3).

Developmental coxa vara, also known as cervical or infantile coxa vara, represents coxa vara not present at birth but that develops in early childhood and produces progressive deterioration of the proximal femoral neck-shaft angle during growth. Classic radiographic changes accompany the physical findings. There is no significant increase in associated musculoskeletal anomalies. A minimal limb length inequality develops secondary to the progressive varus deformity of the proximal femur but not because of a significant true decrease in the femoral segment length (Fig. 26-4).

More complete discussions on the various forms of congenital and acquired coxa vara are reviewed in other chapters in this textbook. The remainder of this section is devoted to a review of developmental coxa vara.

Developmental coxa vara is a specific deformity of the proximal femur, manifesting in the pediatric patient with characteristic behavior during growth and associated radiographic findings that differentiate it from other forms of childhood coxa vara.

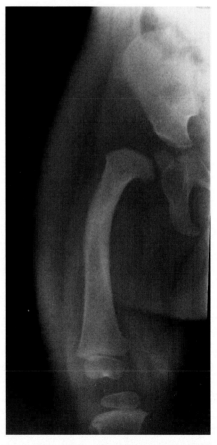

FIGURE 26-2. The radiographic appearance of congenital coxa vara in a 14-month-old girl with a congenital short femur.

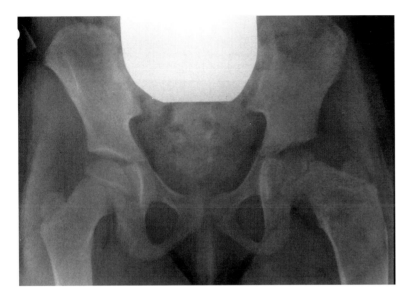

FIGURE 26-3. The radiographic appearance of acquired coxa vara in a girl 7 years, 2 months of age who had fibrous dysplasia and a shepherd crook deformity of the proximal femur.

Historical Review

The initial clinical description of coxa vara was presented in 1881 by Fiorani, who described a "bending of the femoral neck" in adult patients.[34] In 1888, Muller[3] confirmed Fiorani's description by anatomic dissection. The first radiographic confirmation of a decreased neck-shaft angle was described by Hofmeister in 1894.[34] He has also been credited with first using the term "coxa vara" in the clinical description of this entity. In 1905, Hoffa[3] was the first to report the microscopic pathologic findings associated with coxa vara.

Coxa vara occurring during childhood was first described by Kredel in 1896.[34] He proposed that childhood coxa vara had a congenital origin. In 1907,

Elmslie[13] proposed the childhood form of coxa vara to be a separate entity from that seen in the adult and recommended the term "infantile coxa vara." A progressive tendency to the proximal femoral deformity during growth was described in childhood coxa vara by Fairbank in 1928.[14] In 1938, Duncan[12] disagreed with Kredel's congenital origin theory and proposed that progressive childhood coxa vara represented a deformity that appeared during the early years of growth. He coined the term "developmental coxa vara."

Despite Duncan's developmental theory for progressive coxa vara of childhood being well documented by his series, his theory was not generally accepted. It was not until 1970 that the confusion about the developmental theory was clarified by Amstutz,[1]

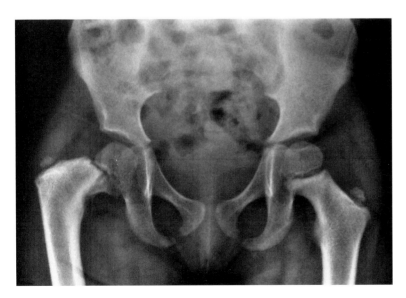

FIGURE 26-4. Radiographic appearance of developmental coxa vara in a girl 3 years, 9 months of age.

when he reported two patients with documented normal hip radiographs during the first year of life who subsequently developed typical clinical and radiographic manifestations of developmental coxa vara by 2 and 3 years of age, respectively. Amstutz documented the presence of a childhood developmental form of coxa vara and drew attention to the differentiation of this form of coxa vara from the true congenital and acquired varieties.

Incidence

Developmental coxa vara is a rare entity with a reported incidence of 1 in 25,000 live births worldwide.[17] Compared with developmental hip dislocation, this represents a ratio of approximately one developmental coxa vara case for every 20 developmental hip dislocations. The reported rates of male to female and right to left involvement are essentially equal. Bilateral involvement occurs in 30% to 50% of patients.[19,23,26] Although previous reports have shown developmental coxa vara to occur among Caucasians and those of African descent, later reports demonstrated a preference for the latter group.[12,19] Although most investigators have not been able to prove a definite hereditary inheritance pattern for developmental coxa vara, reports by Fisher and Waskowitz[15] and Say and colleagues[27] demonstrated a familial pattern in a limited number of cases, which they propose follows an autosomal dominant pattern of genetic transmission.

Etiology

The cause of developmental coxa vara remains unknown. Several investigators have proposed hypotheses about the cause of the varus deformity. A metabolic abnormality causing a deficient production of or a delay in the normal ossification process of the proximal end of the femur has been proposed.[34] Hoffa and Alsberg proposed a mechanical abnormality occurring during hip development in which excessive intrauterine pressure on the developing hip results in a depression in the neck of the femur.[34] A partial vascular insult causing an arrest in the early development of the femoral head and neck has been proposed by Nillsone.[24] Duncan proposed the varus deformity occurred secondary to a developmental error, resulting in faulty maturation of the cartilage and metaphyseal bone of the femoral neck.[12]

Biopsies of the proximal femoral growth plate and femoral neck in patients with developmental coxa vara have been reported by Pylkkanen,[26] Chung and Riser,[9] and Bos and colleagues.[7] Histopathologically confirmed abnormalities exist in cartilage production and secondary metaphyseal bone formation in the inferior portion of the proximal femoral physeal plate and adjacent femoral neck. Biopsies of the involved segment of the femoral neck have shown an increase in the width of the true growth plate, with irregularly distributed germinal cells in the resting zone, an absence of normal orderly progression of the cartilage columns, and a poorly defined or absent zone of provisional calcification. Associated nests of cartilage have been found to extend deeply into the metaphyseal region. The metaphyseal bone is osteoporotic, with an increased vascularized fibrous element between bony spicules (Fig. 26-5). There was no evidence of aseptic necrosis in the reported biopsy specimens. These histopathologic findings are similar to those previously reported from biopsy specimens of the proximal tibias

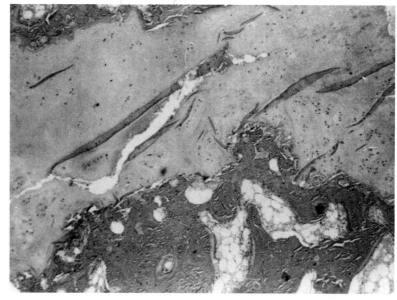

FIGURE 26-5. Photomicrograph of a biopsy specimen of the proximal femoral physeal plate from a patient with developmental coxa vara demonstrates irregularly distributed germinal cells in the resting zone; an absence of normal, orderly progression of the cartilage columns; and a poorly defined zone of provisional calcification. Nests of cartilage cells reside at the margin of the metaphyseal bone. (From Bos CFA, Sakkers RJB, Bloem JL, et al. Histological, biochemical and MRI studies of the growth plate in congenital coxa vara. J Pediatr Orthop 1989;9:662.)

of patients with Blount disease[20,33] and biopsy specimens of the proximal femoral physeal plates of patients with metaphyseal chondrodysplasia (Schmid type).[7] The significance of these histopathologic similarities and of any possible association between the cause or pathogenesis of developmental coxa vara and infantile Blount disease or metaphyseal chondrodysplasia remains undetermined.

In 1960, Pylkkanen[26] proposed what remains as the most widely accepted theory about the cause of developmental coxa vara. He postulated that the deformity in the proximal femur is the result of a primary ossification defect in the inferior femoral neck, on which physiologic shearing stresses applied during weight bearing cause fatigue of the local dystrophic bone, resulting in the progressive varus deformity seen clinically. Bos and associates,[7] after reviewing biopsy specimens and magnetic resonance imaging studies of hips affected by developmental coxa vara, concurred with Pylkkanen's theory. In particular, their studies found no evidence of slippage of the proximal femoral physeal plate as the cause of the progressive proximal femoral varus deformity.

Clinical Presentation

Most patients affected with developmental coxa vara present sometime between the initiation of ambulation and 6 years of age.[19,25] Their most frequent complaint is a progressive gait abnormality; pain is rarely reported. In patients with unilateral involvement, the gait abnormality is caused by combined abductor muscle weakness and limb length inequality. As the neck-shaft angle of the proximal femur decreases in developmental coxa vara, the articulotrochanteric distance between the femoral head and greater trochanter also decreases, which affects normal hip joint mechanics. As the articulotrochanteric distance decreases, the normal length-tension relation of the abductor muscles is lessened, and the abductor muscles ability to control the pelvis in one-legged stance is weakened. The functionally weaker abductor muscles produce the gait abnormality seen in patients with developmental coxa vara. Patients with bilateral involvement present with a waddling gait pattern associated with increased lumbar lordosis, similar to that seen in bilateral developmental hip dislocation.[5,12,14,19,21,22]

Physical examination usually reveals a somewhat prominent and elevated greater trochanter, which is often associated with an abductor muscle weakness and positive Trendelenburg testing. An associated limb length inequality is commonly identified, but this is usually mild and averages only 2.5 cm.[19,26] The range of motion of the affected hip is usually restricted in all planes of motion, with the most significant limitations

occurring in abduction and internal rotation.[19,26] The loss of abduction is associated with a decrease in the neck-shaft angle of the proximal femur. The loss of internal rotation is secondary to the progressive decrease in femoral anteversion seen in developmental coxa vara.[19,29] An associated hip flexion contracture is often identified. Associated musculoskeletal anomalies are rare.[3]

Radiographic Findings

The diagnosis of developmental coxa vara and its differentiation from other forms of coxa vara depends on the identification of certain classic radiographic findings. These radiographic features include a decreased femoral neck-shaft angle, often to values below 90 degrees; a more vertical position of the physeal plate; a triangular metaphyseal fragment in the inferior femoral neck surrounded by an inverted radiolucent Y pattern; a decrease in normal anteversion of the proximal femur, which may become true retroversion; coxa brevia; and in some patients, mild acetabular dysplasia (Fig. 26-6).[12,14,25,28,29,34]

The more vertical position of the physeal plate is measured by the Hilgenreiner physeal angle, which is defined by the angle subtended by the planes of the physeal plate and the Hilgenreiner line (Fig. 26-7).[32] This angle is normally 25 degrees or less, but in developmental coxa vara, it is usually in the range of 40 to 70 degrees.[19]

The inverted Y pattern seen in the inferior femoral neck remains the sine qua non of this condition. The inverted Y radiolucency was once postulated to be a true double physeal plate. Biopsy specimens and magnetic resonance imaging studies, however, have shown that the radiolucent area actually represents a zone of widening of the inferior portion of the physeal plate, with associated abnormal ossification and an interposed triangular segment of dystrophic bone.[7,9]

Natural History

Historically, untreated developmental coxa vara was viewed as a condition in which a pattern of progressive varus deformity of the proximal femur ultimately resulted in the development of a stress fracture–related nonunion of the femoral neck and premature degenerative arthritic changes within the hip joint.[3] These changes led to progressive pain and disability for the patient and were thought to occur universally after the condition was established. Weinstein and colleagues[32] and Serafin and Szulc[29] showed that not all patients with developmental coxa vara follow such a progressive course. Their studies demonstrated that the determining factor for progression of the varus deformity was the Hilgenreiner physeal angle. Patients demon-

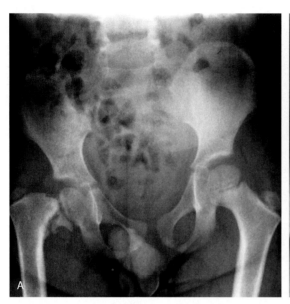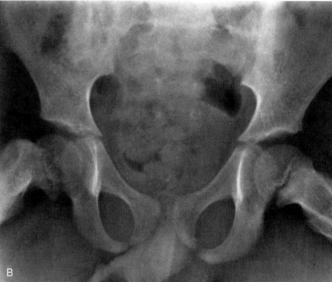

FIGURE 26-6. **(A)** Anteroposterior pelvic radiograph demonstrates the classic radiographic findings in developmental coxa vara, which include a decreased femoral neck-shaft angle, a more vertical physeal plate, an inferior triangular metaphyseal fragment surrounded by an inverted radiolucent Y, and coxa brevia. **(B)** Lateral pelvic radiograph demonstrates changes in the posterior segment of the proximal femoral neck.

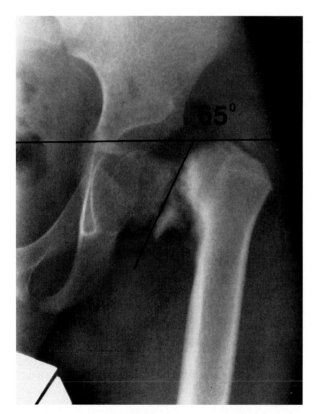

FIGURE 26-7. The anteroposterior view of a hip affected with developmental coxa vara demonstrates the method of measurement of the Hilgenreiner physeal angle. The physeal angle represents the angle subtended between the planes of the Hilgenreiner line and the physeal plate, which measures 65 degrees in this example.

strating a physeal angle that remained less than 45 degrees more commonly had spontaneous healing of the femoral neck defect and an associated arrest in progression of the varus deformity. Patients with a physeal angle greater than this value were found to more commonly manifest the more classic progressive pattern.

Treatment

As long as the actual cause of developmental coxa vara remains unknown, treatment of the condition must continue to concentrate on prevention of the secondary deformities of the proximal femur created by the condition's natural history instead of on prevention of the disease itself. Borden[6] identified the main objectives of current treatment to include correction of the varus angulation into a more normal physiologic range, changing the loading characteristics seen by the abnormal femoral neck from shear to compression, correction of limb length inequality, and reestablishment of a proper abductor muscle length-tension relation.

Nonoperative treatment during childhood has historically been unsuccessful in achieving the objectives of proper treatment. Jones and Lovett[14] and Barr[4] previously proposed spica cast immobilization, with the affected limb in abduction for 6 to 12 months. Although Barr was able to demonstrate closure of the femoral neck defect, neither group found any improvement in the neck-shaft angle of the proximal femur with this form of treatment. Nillsonne[24] and Le Mesurier[22] investigated the use of heavy skeletal traction and bed rest, but they could not identify any beneficial effects from such treatment. Zadek,[34] in a review of conservative treatment of developmental coxa vara, concluded that the previously attempted nonoperative methods had universally poor or no value.

Surgical derotational valgus producing proximal femoral osteotomy has been shown to be the most effective form of treatment in the restoration of more normal hip joint mechanics in developmental coxa vara.[2,6,14,16,19,22,26,31] Historically, femoral osteotomies at the level of the neck and intertrochanteric and subtrochanteric regions have been proposed. Brackett[8] recommended a femoral neck procedure in which the dysplastic neck was resected, with the remaining proximal shaft inserted into the femoral head, coupled with advancement of the greater trochanter. In general,

this and other femoral neck procedures have higher morbidity rates and poorer clinical results than the intertrochanteric-subtrochanteric osteotomies, which remain the treatment of choice.[23] Pauwels' Y-shaped osteotomy[10,30] and Langenskiold's valgus producing osteotomy[26] are examples of intertrochanteric corrective osteotomies that have produced good results. Unfortunately, Pauwels' Y-shaped osteotomy does not allow rotational correction of the upper femur. Subtrochanteric valgus-producing osteotomies as described by Fairbanks,[14] Borden,[6] and Amstutz and Wilson[2] also remain well-proven forms of successful therapy in achieving the goals of surgical treatment (Fig. 26-8).

Additional principles of proper surgical treatment include a concomitantly performed adductor tenotomy that allows less forceful correction of the bony deformity and improved stability at the osteotomy site when the femur is put into valgus.[31] A proximal femoral shortening procedure at the level of the osteotomy

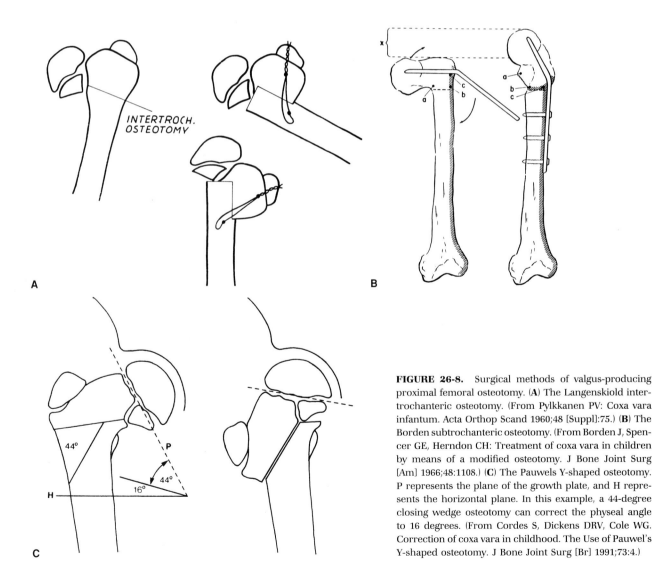

FIGURE 26-8. Surgical methods of valgus-producing proximal femoral osteotomy. (**A**) The Langenskiold intertrochanteric osteotomy. (From Pylkkanen PV: Coxa vara infantum. Acta Orthop Scand 1960;48 [Suppl]:75.) (**B**) The Borden subtrochanteric osteotomy. (From Borden J, Spencer GE, Herndon CH: Treatment of coxa vara in children by means of a modified osteotomy. J Bone Joint Surg [Am] 1966;48:1108.) (**C**) The Pauwels Y-shaped osteotomy. P represents the plane of the growth plate, and H represents the horizontal plane. In this example, a 44-degree closing wedge osteotomy can correct the physeal angle to 16 degrees. (From Cordes S, Dickens DRV, Cole WG. Correction of coxa vara in childhood. The Use of Pauwel's Y-shaped osteotomy. J Bone Joint Surg [Br] 1991;73:4.)

can be employed to facilitate correction of the varus deformity and unload the femoral head in situations in which difficulty in reduction of the osteotomy and excessive femoral head pressure are realized as proximal femoral valgus is recreated.[18] To prevent loss of the surgical correction achieved before healing of the osteotomy, firm internal fixation by a tension band technique, blade plate, or nail-plate system is recommended. Violation of the physeal plate by the internal fixation device should be avoided if possible. A spica cast may or may not be applied, depending on the stability of the internal fixation and patient compliance.

It is important to include internal rotation of the distal segment at the time of osteotomy to correct the loss of internal rotation seen in developmental coxa vara and reestablish more normal rotational arcs at the hip postoperatively. The goal of surgical treatment is to produce a valgus overcorrection of the neck-shaft angle of the proximal femur, regardless of the patient's age. Several researchers have demonstrated that the neck-shaft angle of the proximal femur should be corrected to a value of 160 degrees or greater and that the Hilgenreiner physeal angle should be corrected to 30 to 40 degrees or less at the time of osteotomy to significantly decrease the potential for varus deformity recurrence (Fig. 26-9).[10,11,19,32]

The criteria for surgical intervention in a patient with developmental coxa vara include one or more of the following clinical and radiographic findings: the proximal femoral Hilgenreiner physeal angle is greater than 45 to 60 degrees, the proximal femoral neck-shaft angle is progressively decreasing or measures less than or equal to 90 to 100 degrees, or the patient with developmental coxa vara develops a Trendelenburg gait.[2,19,32]

Duncan[12] and Weinstein and colleagues[32] recommended delaying surgical intervention until after the patient is 5 to 6 years of age. Weighill[31] proposed performing surgery on all patients after 18 months of age, as soon as the proper diagnosis has been made. Pylkkanen[26] and Serafin and Szulc[29] demonstrated improved results from surgery in younger patients. Corrective osteotomy is best performed not at a particular age, but as soon as the criteria for surgical intervention are apparent. If the proper indications are unambiguous, a delay in surgical intervention until an older age in hope of achieving better internal fixation is not justified. The progressive proximal femoral deformity and dysplastic changes at the femoral head, neck, and acetabulum that occur with time make complete and lasting correction much more difficult or impossible to achieve.

Results

Zadek[34] and Le Mesurier[22] proposed drilling and supplemental bone grafting of the femoral neck at the

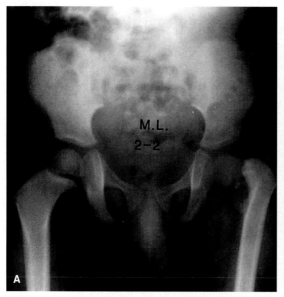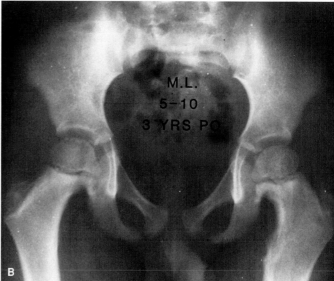

FIGURE 26-9. Anteroposterior pelvic radiograph of a boy 2 years, 2 months of age with developmental coxa vara. (**A**) Preoperative radiograph. (**B**) Postoperative radiograph. A subtrochanteric derotational proximal femoral osteotomy successfully achieved the objectives of surgical correction, including correction of the varus angulation into a physiologic range, changing the loading characteristics of the femoral neck from shear to compression by achieving a physeal angle of 30 degrees or less, and reestablishing a proper abductor muscle length-tension relation.

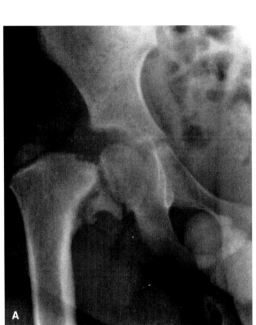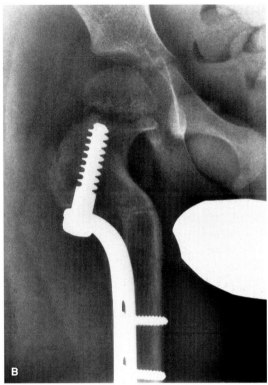

FIGURE 26-10. Anteroposterior radiograph of a hip affected with developmental coxa vara. (**A**) The preoperative radiograph demonstrates a classic inferior femoral neck triangular fragment. (**B**) Three months postoperatively, the radiograph demonstrate correction of the physeal angle, with spontaneous closure of the femoral neck triangular metaphyseal fragment.

time of osteotomy to facilitate healing of the femoral neck defect and to restrain recurrent deformity. The need for these additional procedures at the time of osteotomy has subsequently been shown to be unnecessary. The triangular metaphyseal defect in the femoral neck spontaneously closes by 3 to 6 months postoperatively in virtually all cases of developmental coxa vara if adequate valgus has been created (Fig. 26-10).[19] Between 50% and 89% of operated hips demonstrate a premature closure of the proximal femoral physeal plate. This usually occurs within 12 to 24 months after surgery (Fig. 26-11).[19,28]

This premature physeal plate closure is not related to surgical trauma, patient age, or degree of valgus correction. It more likely represents a possible surgically induced acceleration of natural physeal plate closure. Premature physeal plate closure may also be a manifestation of an inherently abnormal proximal femoral physis in developmental coxa vara that is stimulated to undergo closure as the stresses across the plate change from shear to compression after surgical realignment of the proximal femur. If premature closure of the proximal femoral physeal plate occurs, the patient must be monitored closely for the development of a growth-related recurrent

varus deformity of the proximal femur and for development of a significant limb length inequality secondary to the proximal femoral physis, accounting for approximately 13% of the growth of the lower limb.

Historically, recurrence of the proximal femoral varus after surgical correction was a frequent complication as patient growth continued. This recurrence of the varus deformity was thought to be secondary to the underlying pathologic process associated with developmental coxa vara. However, Weighill,[31] Weinstein and colleagues,[32] Kehl and associates,[19] Desai and Johnson,[11] and Cordes' group[10] have all demonstrated that true varus recurrence secondary to the underlying pathologic process is rare if adequate proximal femoral valgus is reestablished and maintained by stable internal fixation and if there is no early closure of the proximal femoral physeal plate.

The proximal femoral physeal angle must be corrected to 30 to 40 degrees or less to facilitate the conversion of shear to compression forces on the proximal femoral growth plate. It is equally important that stable internal fixation be used to maintain the valgus correction until full osseous healing has occurred and that the internal fixation device does not violate the physeal plate. If premature proximal femoral epiphy-

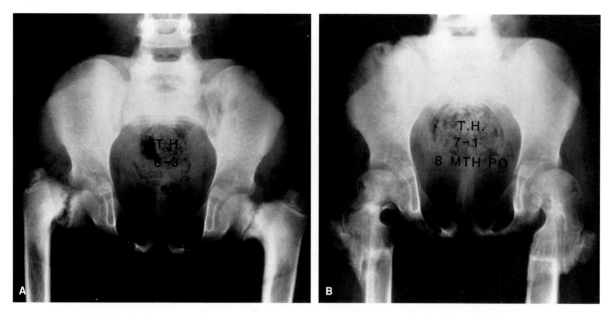

FIGURE 26-11. The anteroposterior pelvic radiograph of a boy 6 years, 3 months of age demonstrates bilateral developmental coxa vara. (**A**) Preoperative radiograph. (**B**) The postoperative radiograph 8 months after the subtrochanteric proximal femoral derotational osteotomies demonstrates bilateral spontaneous closure of the proximal femoral epiphyseal plates, and the greater trochanteric apophyses remain open. (From Kehl DK: Developmental coxa vara. Lesson 36. Orthop Surg Update Series 1983;2:1.)

seal plate closure occurs, it creates a situation of unbalanced growth about the proximal femur, with secondary trochanteric overgrowth and recurrent coxa vara and coxa brevia (Fig. 26-12). To prevent this recurrent deformity, it is recommended that, after premature closure of the proximal femoral epiphyseal plate has been documented, greater trochanteric apophysseodesis or advancement be performed before the development of a recurrent deformity.[19] If the varus deformity does recur, a repeat valgus-producing femoral osteotomy can be performed.

Proper and timely treatment of developmental coxa vara can result in a hip joint that is painless,

has a functional range of motion, and demonstrates a negative Trendelenburg gait at maturity. Although most patients continue to show a mild residual limb length inequality, it rarely is significant enough to require a shoe lift.[19,26]

Through compliance with the outlined surgical indications and proper technique, the objectives of treatment of developmental coxa vara can be accomplished with a predictable conversion of the condition's natural history—development of degenerative arthritis and pain in late adolescence or early maturity—to a hip joint that is painless and has a much-improved long-term functional outcome.[10,11,19]

FIGURE 26-12. Illustration of recurrent coxa vara secondary to premature proximal femoral epiphyseal plate closure and secondary greater trochanteric overgrowth. (**A**) Preoperatively, the proximal femoral physeal plate is open. (**B**) Postoperatively, adequate surgical correction has been achieved. (**C**) Premature closure of the proximal femoral physeal plate, with the greater trochanteric apophyseal plate remaining open. (**D**) Recurrent coxa vara secondary to unbalanced growth about the proximal femur. (From Kehl DK: Developmental coxa vara. Lesson 36. Orthop Surg Update Series 1983; 2:1.)

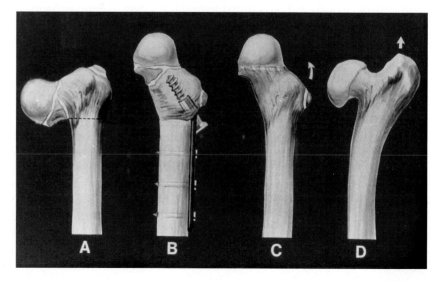

TRANSIENT SYNOVITIS OF THE HIP

Transient synovitis of the hip represents the most common cause of hip pain in childhood.[60,67] Although the condition's true cause remains unknown, the associated signs and symptoms, natural history, and ultimate patient outcome have been well documented. Transient synovitis is usually characterized by the acute onset of monarticular hip pain, limp, and restricted hip motion in a patient who is otherwise not systemically ill. The symptoms generally show a gradual but complete resolution over several days to weeks and are rarely associated with recurrences or late sequelae.

This clinical entity has been previously described by numerous names because of confusion about its cause. Some of the previously used terms include transitory synovitis, transitory coxitis, acute transient epiphysitis, coxitis fugax, coxitis serosa seu simplex, phantom hip, toxic synovitis, and observation hip. Transient synovitis is most commonly used to describe this clinical condition. Transient synovitis also remains the most descriptive term because of its reference to the condition's short duration and associated pathology.

Historical Review

In 1892, Lovett and Morse[61] first described transient synovitis of the hip and differentiated it from tuberculous synovitis when they referred to the condition as "a short-lived and ephemeral form of hip disease that presents at first the characteristics of common hip disease, but the symptoms of which disappear within a few weeks or months instead of continuing for years." Bradford and Lovett,[38] Todd,[69] Fairbank,[45] and Belmonte[52] subsequently described a similar painful condition of the hip that was characterized by a transient course of symptoms with rapid resolution and permanent recovery. In 1933, Butler[40] described children admitted to the hospital with painful hip symptoms but normal radiographs who subsequently demonstrated a self-limiting and rapidly resolving clinical course. He coined the term "observation hip" for this condition. In 1936, Finder[46] confirmed through biopsy specimens that the condition was characterized by a nonpyogenic inflammatory response of the synovium of the hip joint.

Etiology

Although the cause of transient synovitis of the hip remains undefined, the more popular hypotheses proposed imply an association between transient synovitis and one or more of the following: active or recent infection, trauma, or allergic hypersensitivity.[40,43,45,48,62,64,65,67,69]

The concept of a possible infectious cause is given credence by the frequent association of transient synovitis with current or antecedent illness. A nonspecific upper respiratory infection, pharyngitis, or otitis media have been associated with the occurrence of transient synovitis in as many as 70% of cases.[48,67] Fairbank,[45] Miller,[62] Butler,[40] and Spock[67] have proposed a definite causal association between transient synovitis and a concomitant viral or bacterial infection. Spock reported isolating an increased incidence of β-hemolytic streptococci from the nose and throat of patients with transient synovitis compared with asymptomatic pediatric patients. He also found elevated vital titers in 50% of the patients tested.[67] Hardinge,[49] however, could find no definite correlation between infectious sources and transient synovitis when comparing parameters of infection found in involved patients with age-matched controls. Blockey and Porter[37] were unable to confirm any correlation with viral infections through detailed virologic studies of patients with transient synovitis.

A history of preceding local trauma to the involved hip in transient synovitis has been reported in 17% to 30% of patients.[52,67] In 1925, Todd[69] proposed that trauma was a frequent factor associated with transient synovitis of the hip and thought that the condition was nothing more than a simple "contusion of the hip." Rauch[64] proposed injury to be the leading cause of transient synovitis, and Gledhill and McIntyre[48] also found trauma frequently was associated with the condition.

An association between an allergic predisposition and the development of transient synovitis of the hip has been reported for 16% to 25% of symptomatic patients.[52,67] Edwards thought the condition represented an allergic hypersensitivity response manifesting itself within the hip joint, as evidenced by the dramatic clinical improvement seen in symptomatic patients given antihistamines.[43] Rothschild, Russ, and Wasserman[65] supported an allergic cause based on the rapid clinical improvement seen in their patients with transient synovitis when given intramuscular steroid injections. Nachemson and Scheller[63] reported on 12 patients (16.4%) of a 73-patient study group with transient synovitis of the hip who demonstrated an association between a hyperallergic state and a history of transient synovitis of the hip. This association, however, was also discredited when the investigators demonstrated that the percentage of patients in the general population reporting allergic hypersensitivity was essentially equal to that found in patients with previous transient synovitis.

Spock[67] proposed that body size in the child may predispose to the development of transient synovitis. He demonstrated a three times greater incidence of the condition in patients of a stocky and obese physique than in a randomly selected group of children with similar ages.

Biopsy specimens from hip joints of patients with transient synovitis have universally demonstrated synovial hypertrophy secondary to a nonspecific nonpyogenic inflammatory reaction.[35,46,55] Hip joint aspiration has shown an associated culture-negative synovial effusion, usually measuring 1 to 3 mL.[51,56]

Incidence

Transient synovitis has been reported to be the most common cause of hip pain in children. The diagnosis of transient synovitis has historically accounted for 0.4% to 0.9% of annual pediatric hospital admissions.[60,67] The actual incidence of the condition, however, is likely to be higher than that reported, because many patients with the condition never seek medical attention. Landin and colleagues[60] reported that the risk for a child to have at least one episode of transient synovitis of the hip is 3%. A seasonal preference for the condition has not been demonstrated other than by Landin and associates,[60] who showed a slightly higher rate of occurrence during the autumn months.

Right and left involvement is essentially equal, with simultaneous bilateral involvement never having been reported. There is an approximately 2 : 1 male to female ratio and a much lower incidence among African Americans.[51]

Clinical Presentation

The condition has been reported in patients as young as 9 months of age through adolescence. The average age of symptom onset is 6 years, with most cases occurring between 3 and 8 years of age.[48,51,52,66] The most frequent presenting complaint is the acute onset of unilateral hip pain in an otherwise healthy patient. The pain is usually confined to the ipsilateral groin and hip area; however, it may present as anterior thigh or knee pain. An associated limp and antalgic gait are usually seen, with some patients refusing to bear weight on the involved extremity. The involved extremity is held in a flexed and externally rotated position and has a restricted range of hip motion, especially abduction and internal rotation. Protective muscle spasm and an associated flexion contracture are frequently identified. The patient may have a low-grade temperature that is rarely greater than 38°C.[51,52,67] Ipsilateral muscle atrophy is rarely seen, but when present, it usually implies a long-standing duration of symptoms, and a diagnosis other than transient synovitis should be considered.

Laboratory values are nonspecific and are usually within normal limits despite the wide range of values that have been reported. The peripheral blood smear includes a white blood cell count averaging 10,000 to 14,000 cells/mm³ (range, 3000–28,000 cells/mm³) and a Westergren erythrocyte sedimentation rate averaging 20 mm/hour (range, 1–63 mm/hour).[51] Urinalysis, blood culture, febrile agglutinins, serum electrophoresis, rheumatoid factor, and tuberculin skin test results are usually within normal limits.

The diagnosis of transient synovitis of the hip remains a diagnosis of exclusion. Although routine laboratory and radiographic studies have not been of specific value in making the diagnosis, they do assist in eliminating other conditions of the hip that may have features similar to those of transient synovitis. The differential diagnosis of transient synovitis includes pyogenic arthritis, osteomyelitis in the adjacent femoral neck or pelvis, tuberculous arthritis, juvenile rheumatoid arthritis, acute rheumatic fever, Perthes disease, tumor, and slipped capital femoral epiphysis.

Pyogenic arthritis of the hip with or without associated osteomyelitis of the femoral neck differs from transient synovitis of the hip in that the patient is usually systemically ill with a high fever. Pain at the affected hip is usually more intense than is seen in transient synovitis, with voluntary guarding allowing little or no hip motion. Unlike transient synovitis, the symptoms of pyogenic arthritis do not improve significantly with rest and are progressive. Laboratory studies of pyogenic arthritis show a higher elevation in the white blood cell count, usually with a left shift; a higher elevation of the erythrocyte sedimentation rate; and purulent fluid on aspiration of the hip joint.

The synovitis associated with acute rheumatic fever usually occurs 2 to 4 weeks after a streptococcal infection. The affected joint is warm, erythematous, and exquisitely tender to any attempt at motion. Unlike transient synovitis, the joint symptoms in acute rheumatic fever may be migratory and can be associated with a transient rash.

The pain and synovitis associated with juvenile rheumatoid arthritis, tuberculous arthritis, and Perthes disease usually are more insidious in onset and more protracted in duration than is seen in transient synovitis. Hip motion at the onset of symptoms tends be limited to a lesser degree than is seen in transient synovitis. Skin testing results are positive in tuberculous arthritis, and radiographic changes subsequently develop in Perthes disease and tuberculous arthritis.

Radiographic Findings

Radiographs of the pelvis and hip of a patient with transient synovitis are usually normal. Their main purpose is to exclude other diseases that may involve the hip joint. Drey[42] and Hermel and Sklaroff[53] previously proposed the use of plain radiographs in diagnosing hip joint effusion in transient synovitis. They proposed that capsular distention resulted in measurable displacement of the muscle shadows of the iliopsoas, obturator internus, and gluteus minimus. They also proposed that local inflammation could lead to the loss of the intermuscular fat planes lateral to the hip joint. Subsequent investigators have reported demonstrating these soft tissue changes in as many as 60% of patients with transient synovitis.[48] In 1975, Brown[39] refuted this finding by showing that the previously reported soft tissue changes lateral to the hip on plain radiographs were unreliable in determining true hip joint effusion. He demonstrated that the displacement of the muscle planes was related to positioning of the limb and was not the result of true capsular distention.

Wingstrand,[70] Bickerstaff and colleagues,[36] Futami and associates,[47] and Terjesen and Osthus[68] have used ultrasound for patients with transient synovitis to document the presence of a hip joint effusion and determine its natural history (Fig. 26-13). Bickerstaff and colleagues used ultrasound to document joint effusions in 71% of 111 patients presenting with an acutely irritable hip. Serial ultrasound studies showed the effusions to decrease steadily in size, with resolution in a mean time of 9 days. Symptoms resolved in these same patients in a mean period of 5 days. Larger effusions at presentation were associated with a longer duration of symptoms and a longer time to effusion resolution. Thirty-two (29%) symptomatic patients had no evidence of a joint effusion at presentation or at follow-up, indicating that the joint effusion in transient synovitis is not always the source of symptoms. Although ultrasound can be useful in documenting and following a hip joint effusion in transient synovitis, it is not in and of itself diagnostic of the condition and is not routinely required in making the diagnosis.

Wingstrand and colleagues,[71] Kloiber and associates,[59] and Hasegawa, Wingstrand, and Gustafson[50] evaluated pin-hole collimation scintigraphy of the hip involved with transient synovitis and showed a variety of possible patterns of isotope uptake. Hasegawa and colleagues demonstrated that 49% of femoral heads of 55 patients involved with transient synovitis appeared normal on the scan. Twenty-four percent of femoral heads demonstrated decreased activity, and increased regional activity about the femoral head was found in 27%. It was observed that the patients with decreased femoral head activity on scintigraphy had an average of 5 days from the onset of symptoms, and the patients with increased femoral head activity averaged 23 days. When follow-up scintigraphy was performed on 5 of the patients initially demonstrating decreased uptake in the femoral head, all 5 patients demonstrated normalization or increased isotope activity in the femoral head.

These findings demonstrate that there can be a transient decrease in vascular perfusion of the femoral head during the early stages of transient synovitis. The decrease in perfusion, however, was never severe and seemed to resolve spontaneously, with femoral head perfusion subsequently returning to a normal or increased pattern.[50,62] The role of bone scanning in transient synovitis remains undetermined, and until the proposed therapeutic benefits afforded by early bone scintigraphy in the patient with transient synovitis have been documented, its routine use is not recommended.

Natural History

As its name implies, transient synovitis usually demonstrates a limited duration of symptoms. The average

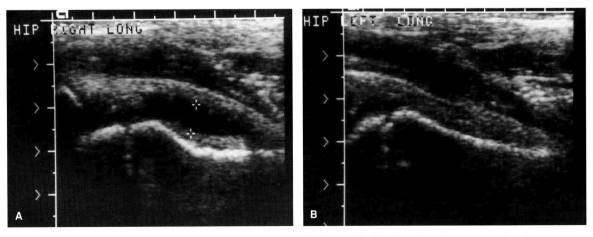

FIGURE 26-13.   Longitudinal linear ultrasonographic view of the hips in a boy 5 years, 4 months of age who had transient synovitis of the right hip. (**A**) Ultrasound scan of the symptomatic right hip demonstrates a large joint effusion, as indicated between the cursor markings. (**B**) Ultrasound scan of the asymptomatic left hip for comparison demonstrates no joint effusion.

duration of symptoms is 10 days, but some patients have remained symptomatic for as long as 8 weeks.[48,51] Haueisen and colleagues,[51] in reviewing a large number of cases, reported the duration of symptoms to be less than 1 week for 67% of patients and less than 4 weeks for 88% of patients. Although most episodes of transient synovitis are isolated to a single event, recurrence of the symptoms in the same or contralateral hip has been reported for approximately 4% to 17% of patients.[51,54] Illingworth has shown that recurrences can develop at any time but are most likely to occur within the first 6 months after the initial episode.[54]

Most short-term retrospective reviews on transient synovitis report complete resolution of all signs and symptoms in the affected hip, with no immediate residual clinical or radiographic abnormalities.[45,52,67] Although most patients remain asymptomatic, long-term studies have demonstrated mild radiographic changes in the involved hip.

Kallio reported asymptomatic coxa magna of 2 mm or greater in 32% of 109 patients with transient synovitis of the hip after a follow-up period of 1 year.[56] He questioned if this high frequency of coxa magna seen after transient synovitis could play a role in the development of degenerative joint disease in adulthood. De Valderrama[41] reported 23 patients who had had transient synovitis and were reviewed at an average of 21 years later. He reported a 50% incidence of radiographic changes in the involved hip, consisting of various degrees of coxa magna, degenerative joint disease, and femoral neck widening. He thought these changes were secondary to the local hypervascularization of the hip that had been associated with the initial inflammatory synovitis. Nachemson and Scheller[63] described 73 patients with 20- to 22-year follow-up periods. When the clinical and radiographic sequelae of transient synovitis occurred, they were described as "few and mild." Although the researchers described a few patients with mild decreases in hip motion, the change was not associated with any functional disability. Coxa magna and femoral neck density changes were increased over normal values, but these changes were unassociated with functional limitations. Nachemson and Scheller[63] found no radiographic changes of degenerative joint disease in their patients at follow-up.

The full importance of these radiographic changes occurring about the hip previously involved with transient synovitis remains unknown. Although very few of the patients whose radiographs showed mild changes have been found to be symptomatic, with longer follow-up, it is possible that the incidence of symptoms may change.

Several investigators have reported cases of Legg-Calve-Perthes disease developing several months after an episode of transient synovitis.[36,44,48,60,67,68] Jacobs[55] and

Bickerstaff and colleagues[36] thought that there was a definite correlation between the two conditions and that patients with transient synovitis who had a more slowly resolving or recurrent clinical pattern were much more likely to develop Legg-Calve-Perthes disease. Spock's survey of the modern literature demonstrates an association of the two conditions for an average of 1.5% of patients (range, 0%–17%).[55,58,67] Gledhill and McIntyre[48] reported an association for 0.9% of patients with transient synovitis. A direct causative correlation, however, between transient synovitis and the subsequent development of Legg-Calve-Perthes disease secondary to an induced vascular insult to the femoral head has never been documented. It is more reasonable to conclude that that the small percentage of patients demonstrating this association were patients with Legg-Calve-Perthes disease who manifested an early synovitis that was indistinguishable from that seen in transient synovitis.

Treatment

Treatment of transient synovitis of the hip is directed at rapidly resolving the underlying inflammatory synovitis with its associated symptomatology. Bed rest and full relief of weight bearing on the involved joint until pain resolves and full motion returns is the initial treatment of choice.[48,51,52,67] This is followed by a period of continued cessation of all strenuous activities involving the hip. If an asymptomatic limp persists, continued bed rest for younger patients or partially relieved weight bearing for patients capable of crutch ambulation should be used until a normal gait pattern has returned. Failure to enforce joint rest and a too-early return to activities were shown by Hermel and Albert to result in a doubling of the time required for initial symptomatic relief and an increased rate of symptom recurrence.[52]

During the initial treatment of transient synovitis, the routine use of skin traction on the involved limb is no longer recommended. Skin traction is mainly used in patients with recalcitrant or recurrent symptoms. It can also be of assistance for the younger child in whom enforcement of bed rest cannot otherwise be easily achieved. If traction is to be employed, the position of the involved limb and hip during traction has potential significance. Wingstrand and associates[72] and Kallio and Ryoppy,[57] through the use of ultrasound scanning and intraarticular pressure measurements of patients with transient synovitis and an associated joint effusion, demonstrated that hip joint pressure measurements are at a maximum when the hip is positioned in extension and can reach potentially critical values with respect to capillary blood flow. Minimum pressure measurements are recorded when the hip is placed in 30 to 45 degrees of flexion. To avoid potential vascular complications, the involved limb and hip should not be positioned in extension when skin traction is used during bed rest; the limb and hip should be placed in 30 to 45 degrees of flexion and subsequently lowered as determined by patient comfort.

To aid in resolution of the inflammatory synovitis, oral nonsteroidal antiinflammatory medication given in therapeutic doses can be used. The use of aspirin is avoided in the child with an active viral infection because of the association of aspirin and Reye syndrome in children with acute viral illnesses. The routine use of antibiotics and systemic steroid preparations is not indicated.

Routine aspiration of the hip joint is of no therapeutic value in transient synovitis and is recommended only to assist in diagnosis.[44,58] Wingstrand and colleagues[72] and Terjesen and Osthus[68] demonstrated by ultrasound scans that intracapsular hip joint effusions in this condition are only minimally evacuated by aspiration and that they recur rapidly after aspiration.

IDIOPATHIC CHONDROLYSIS OF THE HIP

Chondrolysis represents a process characterized by progressive destruction of the articular cartilage, resulting in secondary joint space narrowing and stiffness. Chondrolysis involving the hip joint has followed infection, trauma, prolonged immobilization,[80] and severe burns about the lower extremities.[92] It is most frequently reported as a complication associated with the treatment of slipped capital femoral epiphysis.[74,80,87] An acute form of rapidly progressive chondrolysis occurring most frequently during adolescence, with isolated involvement of the hip joint but without a demonstrable cause, has also been reported. This condition is referred to as idiopathic chondrolysis of the hip. The rapid dissolution of articular cartilage from the femoral head and the acetabulum in this condition is unique and differs from that usually seen in other noninfectious inflammatory conditions affecting the hip joint in this same age group.

Historical Review

Chondrolysis involving the hip joint was originally referred to by Elmslie[87] in 1913 as a potential complication after the treatment of slipped capital femoral epiphysis. The association between chondrolysis and slipped capital femoral epiphysis was documented by Waldenstrom in 1930.[97] In 1971, Jones[85] reported a series of nine adolescent black African girls who had no clinical or radiographic evidence of slipped capital femoral epiphysis or hip joint infection who spontane-ously developed the symptoms and signs of classic chondrolysis of the hip. Jones' series represents the first clinical description of idiopathic chondrolysis of the hip joint. Several articles since that time have documented the condition's existence, clinical presentation, suggested treatment, and prognosis.[73,75–77,79,80,99]

Etiology

As the name implies, the cause of idiopathic chondrolysis of the hip remains unknown. Previously proposed theories about the cause of idiopathic chondrolysis of the hip include nutritional abnormalities,[74,97] mechanical injury,[84] ischemia,[78] abnormal intracapsular pressure,[78] and an inherent abnormal chondrocyte metabolism within the articular cartilage.[86] Waldenström[97] proposed that an alteration in the normal synovial supply of nutrition to the articular cartilage led to chondrolysis. Cruess[74] agreed with this theory and proposed that a fibrosis of the synovial membrane led to a decrease in synovial fluid production within the hip joint that resulted in inadequate nutritional support of the articular cartilage, with subsequent chondrocyte death and secondary cartilage resorption. Jacobs[84] proposed that chondrolysis was the result of a mechanical insult to the articular cartilage or synovium that resulted in a release of lysosomal chondrolytic enzymes that led to cartilage destruction. Kozlowski and Scougall[86] proposed that idiopathic chondrolysis represents a form of articular cartilage dysplasia in which the chondrocytes of articular cartilage have an inherent abnormality in metabolism that can be triggered into a disease state by an unknown environmental event in susceptible individuals.

The most plausible theory concerning the cause of chondrolysis remains that proposed by Golding in 1973,[79] Mankin, Sledge, Rothchild and Eisenstein in 1975,[89] and Eisenstein and Rothchild in 1976,[78] in which they postulated articular cartilage resorption to be secondary to an autoimmune response within the hip joint in genetically susceptible individuals. Microscopic evaluation of the synovial tissue from hip joints involved with idiopathic chondrolysis give credence to the autoimmune theory by routinely demonstrating an increase in chronic inflammatory cells consisting of lymphocytes, plasma cells, and monocytes concentrated in a perivascular pattern.[77,83,85,90]

Eisenstein and Rothchild[78] demonstrated significant elevations of serum and synovial fluid immunoglobulins and of the C3 component of complement in patients with slipped capital femoral epiphysis and associated chondrolysis. In particular, the levels of the IgM fraction of the serum immunoglobulins showed the greatest elevations in patients with associated chondrolysis. Morrissy, Kalderon, and Gerdes[90] evaluated 16 patients with slipped capital femoral epiphysis.

Although they did not demonstrate an increase in the serum immunoglobulin levels above normal values, they did document 3 of the 16 patients to have positive immunofluorescence for immunoglobulin G (IgG) and the C3 component of complement in the synovial tissue of the hip, with two of these patients subsequently developing chondrolysis. Van der Hoeven and colleagues[96] demonstrated immunocomplex deposition of IgM and the C3 component of complement in the synovium of 3 of 4 patients with idiopathic chondrolysis.

Minimal information has been reported concerning similar evaluations of the serum or synovial factors of the autoimmune system in patients with idiopathic chondrolysis of the hip. Bleck reviewed nine patients with idiopathic chondrolysis of the hip and reported normal levels of serum immunoglobulins in all.[73] In 1983, a case report by Smith, Ninin, and Keays[94] demonstrated normal immunofluorescence studies of the synovium and cartilage in a single patient with idiopathic chondrolysis of the hip.

Incidence

The incidence of chondrolysis of the hip associated with the treatment of slipped capital femoral epiphysis is 8.2%.[77] The incidence of idiopathic chondrolysis of the hip remains unreported. The condition, however, is relatively uncommon, with only 42 patients having been recorded in the literature through 1989.[75]

Clinical Presentation

Idiopathic chondrolysis of the hip occurs five times more frequently in female patients than in male patients. The reported age at the onset of symptoms averages 12.5 years for girls (range, 9–18 years) and 14.8 years for boys (range, 13–20 years). The right hip is involved at a slightly higher frequency than the left.[81] Bilateral hip involvement has been reported for five patients.[73,75,76] Following Jones' original description of idiopathic chondrolysis of the hip in nine adolescent black African females, the condition was regarded as an affliction primarily of persons of African descent. Since that time, idiopathic chondrolysis has been recorded in Caucasian, Hispanic, and American Indian patients. As of 1989, 52% of the recorded patients were of African descent, and 38% were Caucasian.[75]

The most frequent presenting complaint is the insidious onset of pain in the anterior or medial side of the affected hip in an afebrile patient. The pain is associated with progressive joint stiffness and a limp. Patients often complain of the development of a limb length inequality secondary to contractures about the affected hip with secondary pelvic obliquity. Examination of the involved hip demonstrates significant restriction of motion in all planes and associated muscle spasm. Variable patterns of contracture about the affected joint in idiopathic chondrolysis of the hip have been reported; the most common presenting pattern is that of a fixed flexion, abduction, and externally rotated position.[73,75,79,81,85]

Laboratory values for complete blood count, urinalysis, rheumatoid factor, antinuclear antibody, HLA-B27 marker, blood culture, and tuberculin skin testing are usually within normal limits. The Westergren erythrocyte sedimentation rate is also usually within normal limits. It can be slightly elevated but rarely exceeds 30 mm/hour.[81,96]

The differential diagnosis for idiopathic chondrolysis of the hip includes such entities as pyogenic arthritis, tuberculous arthritis, juvenile rheumatoid arthritis, seronegative spondyloarthropathy, and pigmented villonodular synovitis. Pyogenic arthritis of the hip differs from idiopathic chondrolysis in that the patient is systemically ill with high fever. Hip pain is usually of a more acute onset and is associated with intense guarding against hip motion. Laboratory studies in pyogenic arthritis show a significant elevation in the white blood cell count and erythrocyte sedimentation rate, which are usually not seen in idiopathic chondrolysis.

The chondrolysis associated with juvenile rheumatoid arthritis and tuberculous arthritis occurs only after an extended period of symptoms. Although hip motion is limited in these conditions, it rarely reaches the degree of restriction seen in idiopathic chondrolysis. Skin testing is positive in tuberculous arthritis.

Seronegative spondyloarthropathy can present as isolated involvement at the hip but usually has additional joint involvement later in the course of the disease. Unlike idiopathic chondrolysis of the hip, seronegative spondyloarthropathy has a male predominance and is frequently seen in patients who are positive for the HLA-B27 marker.

Pigmented villonodular synovitis of the hip has an insidious onset, with progressive motion loss as in idiopathic chondrolysis. The course of the disease leading to chondrolysis in pigmented villonodular synovitis tends to be more chronic and prolonged than in idiopathic chondrolysis. Radiographs of the hip in pigmented villonodular synovitis show more cystic erosions in the subchondral bone on both sides of the joint. Aspiration of the hip of a patient with pigmented villonodular synovitis usually produces a moderate amount of bloody fluid.

Radiographic Findings

The recognition of certain abnormalities on the plain radiographs of the affected hip in conjunction with the presence of appropriate clinical findings establishes the correct diagnosis of idiopathic chondrolysis. The radiographic hallmark of the condition remains a narrowing of the joint space of the involved hip from its normal 3 to 5 mm to a value less than 3 mm.[73,75] Complete obliteration of the joint space rarely or never occurs. There is usually associated osteopenia of the periarticular osseous structures, an irregular blurring of the subchondral sclerotic lines at the femoral and acetabular joint surfaces, and an enlargement of the fovea capitis femori. With time, the involved femoral head develops a mild coxa magna, and the femoral neck widens slightly (Fig. 26-14).[73,75,79,81,85,91] Moule and Golding reported that the femoral neck may occasionally demonstrate a limited area of periosteal new bone formation (Fig. 26-15).[91]

With time, the hip involved with idiopathic chondrolysis frequently demonstrates a premature closure of the proximal femoral physis and the trochanteric apophysis. This rarely results in any major growth

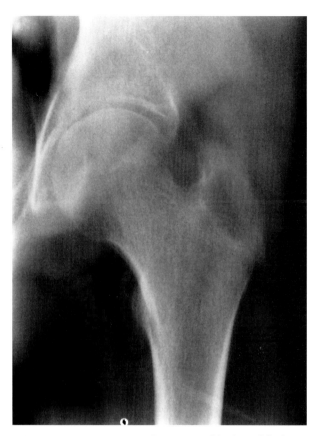

FIGURE 26-15. Anteroposterior tomographic view of the hip in a girl 12 years, 3 months of age with idiopathic chondrolysis demonstrates a limited area of periosteal new bone formation along the inferior femoral neck.

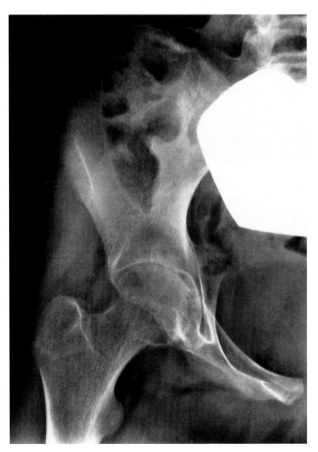

FIGURE 26-14. Anteroposterior hip radiograph of a girl 14 years, 2 months of age. The classic radiographic findings in this case of idiopathic chondrolysis of the hip include a narrowing of the joint space to less than 3 mm, diffuse osteopenia, blurring of the subchondral sclerotic lines on both sides of the joint, and an enlargement of the fovea capitis femori. The hip is also in a position of abduction, which is commonly seen in this condition.

abnormality or significant architectural change at the proximal femur because of the limited growth remaining at these growth centers. A mild protrusio acetabuli and a buttressing osteophyte at the lateral margin of the acetabulum have been seen in some patients.[73,75,81]

Arthrography of the hip of a patient with idiopathic chondrolysis can be used to document the cartilage resorption and secondary joint space narrowing (Fig. 26-16). Moule and Golding[91] have described a "dappled" pattern of contrast outlining the femoral head in idiopathic chondrolysis secondary to the patchy loss of articular cartilage that is associated with the condition.

Scintigraphic evaluation of the hip in the active stage of idiopathic chondrolysis demonstrates a generalized increase in uptake on both sides of the affected joint. This is secondary to the local inflammatory and hyperemic response associated with the early stage of the condition (Fig. 26-17). Mandell and colleagues[88] have shown that decreased activity on bone scintigraphy around the physis of the greater trochanter in patients with slipped capital femoral epiphysis is frequently associated with concurrent or developing

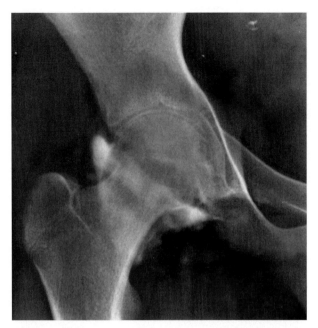

FIGURE 26-16. Arthrographic appearance of a hip involved with idiopathic chondrolysis, demonstrating articular cartilage loss on the femoral head and acetabulum.

chondrolysis. Whether this scintigraphic finding is of prognostic value in idiopathic chondrolysis has not yet been determined.

Axial computed tomography scans of the pelvis can be used to document local changes in the subchondral bone, cartilage resorption, and secondary narrowing of the joint space at the involved hip (Fig. 26-18). The use of magnetic resonance imaging as a method of assessing the local bone and cartilage changes at the hip may also be of benefit, but no large volume of experience has been recorded.

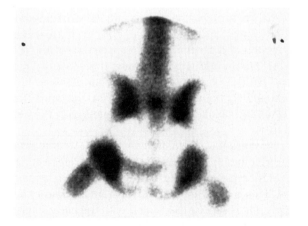

FIGURE 26-17. The scintigraphic appearance of a technetium 99m bone scan of a hip with idiopathic chondrolysis demonstrates a diffuse increased uptake of the isotope by both sides of the affected hip.

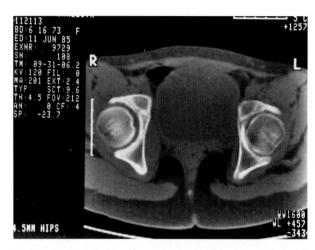

FIGURE 26-18. Axial computed tomographic view of the pelvis and hips in a patient with idiopathic chondrolysis demonstrates osteopenia and narrowing of the involved joint space of the affected hip.

Pathology

Exploration of the hip joint involved with idiopathic chondrolysis demonstrates numerous abnormalities. The capsule is routinely thickened. The quantity of synovial fluid is decreased, producing a "dry joint."[94] The synovial tissue can be edematous and hypertrophic in the early stages of the disease, but with more prolonged involvement, the synovium becomes thinned and fibrotic. The articular cartilage shows changes on both sides of the joint, with the more significant alterations occurring on the femoral head. The cartilage has a lusterless appearance, with irregular thinning, fibrillation, and fragmentation seen in the surface layers. Areas of erosion in the articular cartilage of various sizes tapering down to subchondral bone are identified mainly in the weight-bearing region of the femoral head (Fig. 26-19).[77,78,81,83,85,91,94]

Microscopic review of biopsy specimens of the synovium consistently demonstrates a nonspecific chronic inflammation. An increased infiltration of plasma cells, lymphocytes, and monocytes is interspersed throughout a stroma, exhibiting an increased vascular and fibrotic pattern. Specimens of the involved articular cartilage demonstrate frayed and fragmented superficial layers with areas of necrotic chondrocytes. The more basal layers of chondrocytes are usually viable, which may be important in the subsequent regeneration of articular cartilage. The subchondral bone is histologically normal and often demonstrates a mild increase in vascularity. No evidence of bone necrosis has been identified (Fig. 26-20).[75,76,77,81,83,85,87,96]

Ippolito and associates[82] reported the ultrastructural findings in the articular cartilage from the femo-

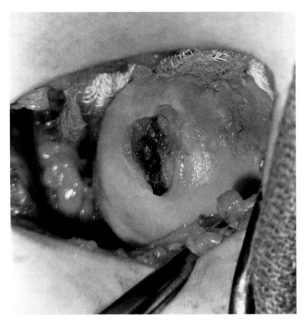

FIGURE 26-19. The clinical photograph of the femoral head of a girl 12 years, 3 months of age with idiopathic chondrolysis demonstrates the lusterless appearance of the articular cartilage and areas of irregular erosion, fibrillation, and fragmentation.

ral head of a patient with idiopathic chondrolysis, as demonstrated on electron microscopy. The superficial zone I of normal articular cartilage was found to be missing.[98] The normally deeper zone II had become the most superficial layer. The collagen fibrils of this zone showed abnormalities in alignment and architecture. Degenerated chondrocytes and debris were found to be interspersed among viable chondrocytes within the extracellular matrix of this layer.

Natural History

At one time, idiopathic chondrolysis of the hip was viewed as a universally progressive disorder with an inevitable outcome of joint destruction, pain, and stiffness. Additional information concerning the condition's natural history changed this pessimistic point of view. In 1971, Jones,[85] in his original description of idiopathic chondrolysis of the hip, recorded a very poor prognosis for the condition. All nine patients he described ultimately developed significantly stiffened hips, with most also showing significant dysfunction secondary to hip pain and joint malposition. In 1982, Sparks and Dall[95] reexamined six of Jones' original nine patients and found no significant change in their conditions. They concluded that idiopathic chondrolysis inevitably results in the development of a malpositioned fibrous ankylosis of the involved hip joint.

In 1970, Lowe[87] reported six cases of chondrolysis complicating slipped capital femoral epiphysis. Before

his review, the prognosis for this form of chondrolysis was also poor. Lowe demonstrated that after 2 to 9 years, all six patients showed improved function, range of motion, and radiographic widening of the involved joint space. He therefore concluded that, at least in some cases of chondrolysis of the hip, the articular cartilage has the ability to recover partially with time. In 1983, Bleck[73] demonstrated a similarly favorable outcome for patients affected with idiopathic chondrolysis of the hip. At a mean follow-up of 6.2 years, 6 of the 9 patients had become essentially asymptomatic, with an improved range of hip motion and a partial restoration of joint space width. In 1989, Daluga and Millar[75] reported 14 patients (16 hips) with idiopathic chondrolysis of the hip after a mean follow-up period of 84 months. Although no patient showed full restoration of the joint space, eight hips showed partial joint space restoration up to 2 mm. Nine hips demonstrated improved range of motion, and five of these hips had a full return of motion.

Idiopathic chondrolysis of the hip appears to have two separate stages. The acute stage is initiated at the

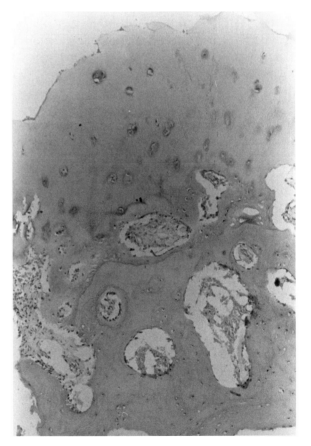

FIGURE 26-20. The photomicrograph of a biopsy specimen of the femoral head from a patient with idiopathic chondrolysis demonstrates a frayed and fragmented superficial layer of articular cartilage, with viable chondrocytes remaining in the more basal layers. The subchondral bone appears histologically normal.

condition's onset and lasts for 6 to 16 months. This stage is characterized by an inflammatory response within the affected hip joint, leading to a painful hip with a decreasing range of motion and loss of articular cartilage. During the latter portion of this stage, the degree of synovial inflammation decreases, with the synovium showing an increase in fibrous tissue deposition. The acute stage is followed by the chronic stage, which may last for 3 to 5 years. During this stage, the hip joint manifests one of three possible outcomes. The involved hip may continue to deteriorate to an ultimately painful and malpositioned ankylosis. The involved hip may become painlessly ankylosed in a position that causes limitation of hip function for the patient. Alternatively, the involved hip may have a resolution of pain with a partial or complete return of motion and improved joint space width shown on radiographs (Fig. 26-21).

Although this new information concerning idiopathic chondrolysis of the hip allows a more optimistic prognosis, the full understanding of the condition's natural history and outcomes awaits further investigation. Questions about the condition's cause, variable severity of involvement, and inherent factors such as race, age, and gender and how they may influence outcome need to be answered before the optimum recommendations for treatment can be determined.

Treatment

As knowledge about the natural history of idiopathic chondrolysis is gained, a change in philosophy concerning the condition's treatment will follow. Pre-

viously, the prognosis of idiopathic chondrolysis was viewed as universally poor, with ultimate hip joint function rapidly declining and symptoms rapidly increasing. Recommended treatment included early definitive intervention with corrective osteotomy, bony fusion, or joint arthroplasty for the involved hip. As knowledge has been gained, a less pessimistic treatment approach was developed. As many as 50% to 60% of involved hip joints have the potential to achieve satisfactory function and motion.[73,75,81]

In 1979, Duncan, Nasca, and Schrantz[76] reviewed eight patients with idiopathic chondrolysis of the hip. Assuming that the hip involved with idiopathic chondrolysis would inevitably undergo ankylosis and that many previously reported patients who had been treated with range of motion had undergone ankylosis of the hip in a nonfunctional position, the investigators proposed early and prolonged spica cast treatment, with the affected hip held in a functional position until fibrous ankylosis was achieved. They reported that all patients so treated were functioning well with an ankylosed pain-free hip and satisfactory gait at last evaluation. Treatment to attempt to maintain motion was only recommended for patients with hip involvement of a "milder degree."[76]

In the 1980s, Bleck[73] and Daluga and Millar[75] reported a much more favorable prognosis for idiopathic chondrolysis of the hip with respect to ultimate function, persistent joint pain, partial restoration of the radiographic joint space, and range of motion of the involved joint. The researchers employed a treatment protocol that included therapeutic doses of nonsteroidal antiinflammatory medications, aggressive physical therapy, periodic traction and bed rest, and

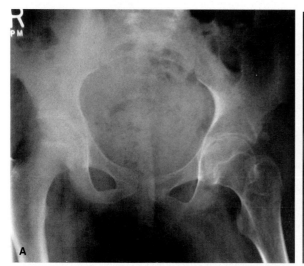
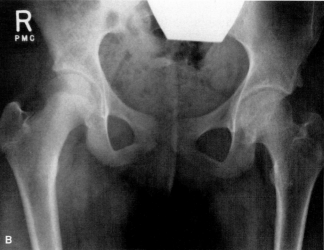

FIGURE 26-21. Anteroposterior pelvic radiograph of a girl 12 years, 3 months of age with idiopathic chondrolysis of the hip. (**A**) A radiograph made at the time of diagnosis demonstrates significant joint space narrowing at the involved hip. (**B**) A radiograph of the same patient 2 years after diagnosis demonstrates partial regeneration of the joint space width at the affected hip.

prolonged non–weight-bearing or limited weight-bearing crutch activities for the involved hip. In 1985, Hughes[81] reported the use of continuous passive motion in the acute stage of idiopathic chondrolysis of the hip for one patient who demonstrated the maintenance of an improved range of hip motion throughout early treatment.

The potential benefit of aggressive surgical treatment within the first year after the onset of symptoms of idiopathic chondrolysis of the hip has only recently been investigated. Bleck reported one patient who underwent surgical release of tendon contractures and a limited anterior capsulotomy. This patient at follow-up was asymptomatic, with a functional range of motion and an improved radiographic joint space width. In 1988, Roy and Crawford[93] reported three patients with idiopathic chondrolysis of the hip who were treated with a subtotal circumferential capsulectomy and release of tendons at the involved hip. The surgical procedure was followed by a period of traction, continuous passive motion, and an aggressive program of physical therapy. The patients were subsequently allowed crutch ambulation with partial weight relief for a prolonged period. At an average follow-up time of 3 years, the investigators reported all patients to be asymptomatic, with a full return of hip motion and an improved joint space width on radiograph.

Although these limited reports demonstrate favorable outcomes for aggressive surgical release, many questions remain unanswered. What are the specific clinical indications for an aggressive surgical release to be considered for an individual patient? Does the degree of radiographically demonstrated involvement affect outcome? Is the procedure best performed early or late within the actively evolving pathophysiology of the disease process? Were the favorable results attributable to the surgical intervention or to the aggressive joint motion and prolonged joint unloading after surgery? The answers to these questions can only be obtained through further investigations.

The current recommendations for treatment of idiopathic chondrolysis of the hip embrace the philosophy of a more favorable long-term prognosis for improved motion and function in most patients. The principles of early treatment include control of synovial inflammation, maintenance of hip motion, and prolonged relief of weight bearing on the involved joint. For most patients, these principles are achieved through the administration of nonsteroidal antiinflammatory medications at therapeutic doses, the periodic use of skin traction and bed rest during periods of acute exacerbation of joint pain and motion loss, surgical release of unresolving contractures, and an aggressive program of passive and active physical therapy for the involved joint. The patient is also maintained on non–weight-bearing or limited weight-bearing crutch ambulation for the involved hip until all pain has resolved and progressive loss of joint space radiographically has ceased. The use of prolonged spica casting with the hip in a position of function should only be considered for patients who do not respond to the described protocol. Although the early reports on the use of aggressive subtotal capsulectomy and tendon release indicated very favorable initial results, the routine use of this procedure cannot not yet be recommended.

References

Developmental Coxa Vara

1. Amstutz HC. Developmental (infantile) coxa vara—a distinct entity. Clin Orthop 1970;72:242.
2. Amstutz HC, Wilson PD Jr. Dysgenesis of the proximal femur (coxa vara) and its surgical management. J Bone Joint Surg [Am] 1962;44:1.
3. Babb FS, Ghormley RK, Chatterton CC. Congenital coxa vara. J Bone Joint Surg [Am] 1949;31:115.
4. Barr JS. Congenital coxa vara. Arch Surg 1929;18:1909.
5. Blockey NJ. Observations on infantile coxa vara. J Bone Joint Surg [Br] 1969;51:106.
6. Borden J, Spencer GE, Herndon CH. Treatment of coxa vara in children by means of a modified osteotomy. J Bone Joint Surg [Am] 1966;48:1106.
7. Bos CFA, Sakkers RJB, Bloem JL, et al. Histological, biochemical and MRI studies of the growth plate in congenital coxa vara. J Pediatr Orthop 1989;9:660.
8. Brackett EG, New MS. Treatment of old ununited fracture of the neck of the femur by transplantation of the head of the femur to the trochanter. Boston Med Surg 1917;177:351.
9. Chung SMK, Riser WH. The histological characteristics of congenital coxa vara. Clin Orthop 1978;132:71.
10. Cordes S, Dickens DRV, Cole WG. Correction of coxa vara in childhood. The use of Pauwels' Y-shaped osteotomy. J Bone Joint Surg [Br] 1991;73:3.
11. Desai S, Johnson L. Long-term results of valgus osteotomy for congenital coxa vara. Clin Orthop 1993;294:204.
12. Duncan GA. Congenital and developmental coxa vara. Surgery 1938;3:741.
13. Elmslie RC. Injury and deformity of the epiphysis of the head of the femur-coxa vara. Lancet 1907;1:410.
14. Fairbank HAT. Infantile or cervical coxa vara. In: The Robert Jones birthday volume, a collection of surgical essays. London: Oxford University Press, 1928:225.
15. Fisher RL, Waskowitz WJ. Familial developmental coxa vara. Clin Orthop 1972;86:2.
16. Horwitz T. The treatment of congenital (or developmental) coxa vara. Surg Gynecol Obstet 1948;87:71.
17. Johanning K. Coxa vara infantum—clinical appearance and aetiological problem. Acta Orthop Scand 1951;21:273.
18. Kehl DK. Developmental coxa vara. Lesson 36. Orthop Surg Update Series 1983;2:1.
19. Kehl DK, LaGrone M, Lovell WW. Developmental coxa vara. Orthop Trans 1983;7:475.
20. Langenskiold A, Riska EB. Tibia vara (osteochondrosis deformans tibiae). J Bone Joint Surg [Am] 1964;46:1405.
21. Langenskiold F. On pseudarthrosis of the femoral neck in congenital coxa vara. Acta Chir Scand 1949;98:568.
22. Le Mesurier AB. Developmental coxa vara. J Bone Joint Surg [Br] 1948;30:595.

23. Magnusson R. Coxa vara infantum. Acta Orthop Scand 1954;23:284.

24. Nillsone H. On congenital coxa vara. Acta Chir Scand 1929;64:217.

25. Pavlov H, Goldman B, Freiberger RH. Infantile coxa vara. Pediatr Radiol 1980;135:631.

26. Pylkkanen PV. Coxa vara infantum. Acta Orthop Scand 1960;48(Suppl):1.

27. Say B, Taysi K, Pirnar T, et al. Dominant congenital coxa vara. J Bone Joint Surg [Br] 1974;56:78.

28. Schmidt TL, Kalamchi A. The fate of the capital femoral physis and acetabular development in developmental coxa vara. J Pediatr Orthop 1982;2:534.

29. Serafin J, Szulc W. Coxa vara infantum, hip growth disturbances, etiopathogenesis and long-term results of treatment. Clin Orthop 1991;272:103.

30. Von Bormann PFB, Erken EHW. Pauwels' osteotomy for coxa vara in childhood. J Bone Joint Surg [Br] 1982;64:144.

31. Weighill FJ. The treatment of developmental coxa vara by abduction subtrochanteric and intertrochanteric femoral osteotomy with special reference to the role of adductor tenotomy. Clin Orthop 1976;116:116.

32. Weinstein JN, Kuo KN, Millar EA. Congenital coxa vara. A retrospective review. J Pediatr Orthop 1984;4:70.

33. Wenger DR, Mickelson M, Maynard JA. The evolution and histopathology of adolescent tibia vara. J Pediatr Orthop 1984;4:78.

34. Zadek I. Congenital coxa vara. Arch Surg 1935;30:62.

Transient Synovitis of the Hip

35. Adams AJ. Transient synovitis of the hip joint in children. J Bone Joint Surg [Br] 1963;45:471.

36. Bickerstaff DR, Neal LM, Booth AJ, et al. Ultrasound examination of the irritable hip. J Bone Joint Surg [Br] 1990;72:549.

37. Blockey NJ, Porter BB. Transient synovitis of hip. A virological investigation. Br Med J 1968;4:557.

38. Bradford EH, Lovett RW. Treatment of hip disease. Am J Orthop Surg 1911;9:354.

39. Brown I. A study of the "capsular" shadow in disorders of the hip in children. J Bone Joint Surg [Br] 1975;57:175.

40. Butler RW. Transitory arthritis of the hip joint in childhood. Br Med J 1933;1:951.

41. De Valderrama JAF. The "observation hip" syndrome and its late sequelae. J Bone Joint Surg [Br] 1963;45:462.

42. Drey L. A radiographic study of transient synovitis of the hip joint. Radiology 1953;60:588.

43. Edwards EG. Transient synovitis of hip joint in children. JAMA 1952;148:30.

44. Erken EHW, Katz K. Irritable hip and Perthes' disease. J Pediatr Orthop 1990;10:322.

45. Fairbank HAT. Discussion on non-tuberculous coxitis in the young. Br Med J 1926;2:828.

46. Finder JG. Transitory synovitis of the hip joint in children. JAMA 1936;107:3.

47. Futami T, Kasahara Y, Suzuki S, et al. Ultrasonography in transient synovitis and early Perthes' disease. J Bone Joint Surg [Br] 1991;73:635.

48. Gledhill RB, McIntyre JM. Transient synovitis and Legg-Calve-Perthes disease. A comparative study. Can Med Assoc J 1969;100:311.

49. Hardinge K. The etiology of transient synovitis of the hip in childhood. J Bone Joint Surg [Br] 1970;52:100.

50. Hasegawa Y, Wingstrand H, Gustafson T. Scintimetry in transient synovitis of the hip. Acta Orthop Scand 1988;59:520.

51. Haueisen DC, Weiner DS, Weiner SD. The characterization of "transient synovitis of the hip" in children. J Pediatr Orthop 1986;6:11.

52. Hermel MB, Albert SM. Transient synovitis of the hip. Clin Orthop 1962;20:21.

53. Hermel MB, Sklaroff DM. Roentgen changes in transient synovitis of the hip joint. Arch Surg 1954;68:364.

54. Illingworth CM. Recurrences of transient synovitis of the hip. Arch Dis Child 1983;58:620.

55. Jacobs BW. Synovitis of the hip in children and its significance. Pediatrics 1971;47:558.

56. Kallio P. Coxa magna following transient synovitis of the hip. Clin Orthop 1988;228:49.

57. Kallio P, Ryoppy S. Hyperpressure in juvenile hip disease. Acta Orthop Scand 1985;56:211.

58. Kallio P, Ryoppy S, Kunnamo I. Transient synovitis and Perthes disease. J Bone Joint Surg [Br] 1986;68:808.

59. Kloiber R, Pavlosky W, Portner O, Gartke K. Bone scintigraphy of hip joint effusions in children. AJR 1983;140:995.

60. Landin LA, Danielsson LG, Wattsgard C. Transient synovitis of the hip. Its incidence, epidemiology and relation to Perthes disease. J Bone Joint Surg [Br] 1987;69:238.

61. Lovett RW, Morse JL. A transient or ephemeral form of hip disease. Boston Med Surg J 1892;127:161.

62. Miller OL. Acute transient synovitis of the hip joint. JAMA 1931;96:575.

63. Nachemson A, Scheller S. A clinical and radiological follow-up study of transient synovitis of the hip. Acta Orthop Scand 1969;40:479.

64. Rauch S. Transitory synovitis of the hip joint in children. Am J Dis Child 1940;59:1245.

65. Rothschild HB, Russ JD, Wasserman CF. Corticotropins in treatment of transient synovitis of the hip in children. J Pediatr 1956;49:33.

66. Sharwood PF. The irritable hip syndrome in children. Acta Orthop Scand 1981;52:633.

67. Spock A. Transient synovitis of the hip joint in children. Pediatrics 1959;24:1042.

68. Terjesen T, Osthus P. Ultrasound in the diagnosis and follow-up of transient synovitis of the hip. J Pediatr Orthop 1991;11:608.

69. Todd AH. Discussion on the differential diagnosis of nontuberculous coxitis in children and adolescents. Proc R Soc Med 1925;18:31.

70. Wingstrand H. Transient synovitis of the hip in the child. Acta Orthop Scand 1986;57(Suppl):1.

71. Wingstrand H, Bauer G, Brismar J, et al. Transient ischaemia of the proximal femoral epiphysis in the child. Acta Orthop Scand 1985;56:197.

72. Wingstrand H, Egund N, Carlin NO, et al. Intracapsular pressure in transient synovitis of the hip. Acta Orthop Scand 1985;56:204.

Idiopathic Chondrolysis of the Hip

73. Bleck EE. Idiopathic chondrolysis of the hip. J Bone Joint Surg [Am] 1983;65:1266.

74. Cruess RL. The pathology of acute necrosis of cartilage in slipping of the capital femoral epiphysis. J Bone Joint Surg [Am] 1963;45:1013.

75. Daluga DJ, Millar EA. Idiopathic chondrolysis of the hip. J Pediatr Orthop 1989;9:405.

76. Duncan JW, Nasca R, Schrantz J. Idiopathic chondrolysis of the hip. J Bone Joint Surg [Am] 1979;61:1024.

77. Duncan JW, Schrantz JL, Nasca RJ. The bizarre stiff hip—possible idiopathic chondrolysis. JAMA 1975;231:382.

78. Eisenstein A, Rothschild S. Biochemical abnormalities in pa-

tients with slipped capital femoral epiphysis and chondrolysis. J Bone Joint Surg [Am] 1976;58:459.

79. Golding JSR. Chondrolysis of the hip. J Bone Joint Surg [Br] 1973;55:214.

80. Heppenstall RB, Marvel JP, Chung SMK, Brighton CT. Chondrolysis of the hip joint—usual and unusual presentations. J Bone Joint Surg [Am] 1973;55:1308.

81. Hughes AW. Idiopathic chondrolysis of the hip. A case report and review of the literature. Ann Rheum Dis 1985;44:268.

82. Ippolito E, Bellocci M, Santori FS, Ghera S. Idiopathic chondrolysis of the hip. An ultrastructural study of the articular cartilage of the femoral head. Orthopedics 1986;9:1383.

83. Ippolito E, Ricciardi-Pollini PT. Chondrolysis of the hip—idiopathic and secondary forms. Ital J Orthop Traumatol 1981;7:335.

84. Jacobs B. Chondrolysis after epiphyseolysis. Instr Course Lect 1972;21:224.

85. Jones BS. Adolescent chondrolysis of the hip joint. S Afr Med J 1971;45:196.

86. Kozlowski K, Scougall J. Idiopathic chondrolysis—diagnostic difficulties. Pediatr Radiol 1984;14:314.

87. Lowe HG. Necrosis of articular cartilage after slipping of the capital femoral epiphysis. J Bone Joint Surg [Br] 1970;52:108.

88. Mandell GA, Keret D, Harcke HT, Bowen JR. Chondrolysis: detection by bone scintigraphy. J Pediatr Orthop 1992;12:80.

89. Mankin HJ, Sledge CB, Rothschild S, Eisenstein A. Chondrolysis of the hip. In: The hip. Proceedings of the third open scientific meeting of The Hip Society. St. Louis: CV Mosby, 1975:126.

90. Morrissy RT, Kalderon AE, Gerdes MH. Synovial immunofluorescence in patients with slipped capital femoral epiphysis. J Pediatr Orthop 1981;1:55.

91. Moule NJ, Golding JSR. Idiopathic chondrolysis of the hip. Clin Radiol 1974;25:247.

92. Pellicci PM, Wilson PD. Chondrolysis of the hips associated with severe burns. J Bone Joint Surg [Am] 1979;61:592.

93. Roy DR, Crawford AH. Idiopathic chondrolysis of the hip. Management by subtotal capsulectomy and aggressive rehabilitation. J Pediatr Orthop 1988;8:203.

94. Smith EJ, Ninin DT, Keays AC. Idiopathic chondrolysis of the hip. S Afr Med J 1983;63:88.

95. Sparks LT, Dall G. Idiopathic chondrolysis of the hip joint in adolescents. S Afr Med J 1982;61:883.

96. Van der Hoeven H, Keessen W, Kuis W. Idiopathic chondrolysis of the hip. Acta Orthop Scand 1989;60:661.

97. Waldenström H. On necrosis of the joint cartilage by epiphyseolysis capitis femoris. Acta Chir Scand 1930;67:936.

98. Weiss C, Rosenberg L, Helfet AJ. An ultrastructural study of normal young adult human articular cartilage. J Bone Joint Surg [Am] 1968;50:663.

99. Wenger DR, Mickelson MR, Ponseti IV. Idiopathic chondrolysis of the hip. J Bone Joint Surg [Am] 1975;57:268.

Lovell & Winter's Pediatric Orthopaedics, fourth edition,
edited by Raymond T. Morrissy and Stuart L. Weinstein.
Lippincott–Raven Publishers, Philadelphia © 1996.

Chapter

27

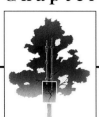

The Lower Extremity

Vernon T. Tolo

IN-TOEING AND OUT-TOEING

No orthopaedic surgeon escapes the need to evaluate a child with feet that are turned in or out. The child may be a patient or an infant relative. Overtreatment with braces or special footwear is common, and because many of the ubiquitous rotational "disorders" are a part of normal lower extremity development in the first few years of life, active treatment usually is unnecessary. However, the orthopaedist needs to know how to best evaluate these conditions and when to consider treatment, based on the natural history of the condition that is expected with continued growth.

The terms associated with conditions leading to in-toeing or out-toeing can be confusing. "Torsion" is defined as a twisting of a part on its axis and is used synonymously with "rotation."[128] Internal tibial torsion and internal tibial rotation describe the same physical or imaging finding.

"Version" was originally used in obstetrics to describe the turning or position of the uterus; "antever-sion" implied a forward tilting or inclination of the entire uterus without bending on itself. Orthopaedists pirated the term version in referring to the femur, and anteversion is used to describe the forward inclination of the femoral neck relative to the bicondylar coronal plane axis of the distal femur. In the strict sense, the femoral neck inclination in anteversion occurs at the base of the femoral neck, and antetorsion involves twisting of the bone anywhere along its long axis. Although the words "torsion" and "version" differ etymologically, in clinical practice, they are used as equivalent to rotation within a long bone. Anteversion and retroversion are used to describe internal and external rotation of the femur, and internal torsion and external torsion are used to describe internal and external rotation in the tibia.

The rotation of the femur and the tibia can be normal or abnormal, and these values differ in various age groups. Abnormal values are usually described as more than two standard deviations from the mean for a given age (Fig. 27-1).[127]

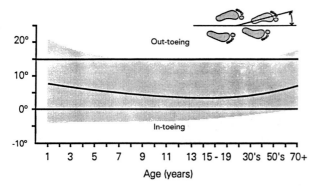

FIGURE 27-1.   The foot progression angle changes with age, with a tendency toward in-toeing which is greatest in the preadolescent period. Out-toeing in toddlers is more common than in-toeing. (From Staheli LT. Rotational problems in children. J Bone Joint Surg [Am] 1993;75:939.)

Etiology

In normal fetal development, the limb bud begins to form at the midpoint of the first trimester. Shortly after limb bud development begins, medial rotation positions the foot near the midline. External tibial rotation then begins and persists until at least 30 weeks of gestation.[3,68] Between 30 weeks of gestation and birth, external or internal rotation of the tibia occurs, presumably because of a combination of genetic factors and intrauterine position. Intrauterine position appears to have more effect on tibial rotation than on the development of femoral anteversion, which is 30 and 40 degrees at birth, regardless of intrauterine position.

Coexisting conditions can affect the natural history of tibial and femoral rotation. For example, in a child with a developmental hip dislocation and in children with cerebral palsy, femoral anteversion remains greater than in a normal child of the same age. Premature infants who have spent several weeks in the neonatal intensive care unit after delivery and have been cared for in the prone position usually have an out-toed gait until 6 years of age because of external tibial rotation.[67]

Clinical Features

Because the child seen for rotational concerns commonly is the first born, the parents have not had the opportunity to witness the natural rotational and angular changes that occur as the child grows. Tripping and falling may be noticed by the parent, but the primary concern remains the appearance of the child's legs while walking or running. Pain is rare, and limping has not been reported.

Knowledge of the child's birth history and of any family history of in-toeing or out-toeing is pertinent to the initial evaluation. The birth history is primarily helpful to determine whether there was prematurity, neonatal distress, or low Apgar scores. The length of time the infant was in the hospital may provide a subtle clue to neurologic problems, such as mild cerebral palsy. Knowledge of other "packaging" conditions, such as metatarsus adductus and torticollis, may be an indicator of the effect of intrauterine position on tibial rotation. If a similar condition affected a parent, it becomes easier for the orthopaedist to explain the generally benign nature of these rotational conditions.

The physical examination for in-toeing and out-toeing should include an assessment from the hips to the toes. If the child is ambulatory, visual evaluation of the child's gait demonstrates the problem that concerns the parents. While the child is walking, the examiner should check for a heel-toe gait and a limp. Absence of a heel-toe gait may be the initial sign of an underlying neurologic disorder such as cerebral palsy. A limp may help explain the rotational position of the extremity, because the child may be positioning the limb in a more comfortable position to avoid pain with walking. Unilateral developmental dysplasia of the hip may present as in-toeing associated with a limp.

An important feature is the foot-progression angle, the angular difference between the long axis of the foot and the line of progression the child is moving along.[126,127] The normal foot-progression angle is slightly externally rotated (positive value). In-toeing of more than 5 degrees is outside the normal range and is recorded in the medical record as a negative value. For example, a normal foot-progression angle could be +10 degrees, and −15 degrees would indicate 15 degrees of in-toeing. A foot-progression angle of +40 degrees would indicate excessive external limb rotation. Increased femoral rotation can be deduced from observing the patellar position to be medially directed during stance phase and from the outward kicking of the lower leg during the swing phase while running.

Before specific assessment for rotational malalignment, the hips need to be examined for hip instability. The child is then placed prone to evaluate hip rotation and tibial torsion (Fig. 27-2). This puts the hips in an extended position, which allows a more accurate representation of the hip position when the child is standing than if the rotation examination is performed with the hip flexed. Because of the obliquity of the fibers in the hip capsule, the volume of the hip joint is least when the hip is extended and internally rotated; examination in this position simulates the extended hip position during walking and detects limited hip internal rotation secondary to fluid (e.g., pus, effusion, blood) within the hip joint that may interfere with normal motion. The knees are flexed, and the legs are then rotated medially and laterally. The pelvis must

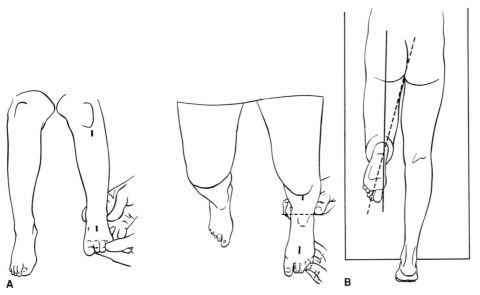

FIGURE 27-2. (A) Tibial torsion can be assessed by comparing the bimalleolar axis at the ankle to the position of the tibial tubercle. (B) The thigh-foot angle is measured with the child in the prone position and is the preferred method for estimating tibial torsion.

be observed to remain level and stationary during this leg rotation. As a rough guide, the amount of external and internal hip rotation in this position should be approximately equal in the older child and adolescent, with the sum of the two rotational measurements approximating 90 degrees. In the younger children, more internal than external rotation is commonly seen.

A clinical estimate of the amount of femoral anteversion can be gained by palpation of the greater trochanter as internal and external hip rotation is checked. The angle between the vertical axis and the long axis of the leg at the position the greater trochanter is the most prominent becomes the amount of femoral anteversion, a value that coincides closely with those found by radiographic and computed tomography (CT) imaging studies.[113]

Tibial torsion is measured with the child in the same prone position used for femoral and hip rotation evaluation. The knees are placed as close together as possible so the thighs are parallel to each other. The long axis of the foot forms the thigh-foot angle with the long axis of the thigh. Although this angle is a combination of tibial rotation and hindfoot rotation, the thigh-foot angle provides a reasonable approximation of tibial rotation if the foot is normal. If metatarsus adductus exists, the thigh-foot angle must be referenced to the hindfoot. Tibial torsion can also be measured by determining the position of the transmalleolar axis relative to the coronal plane of the proximal tibia. The transmalleolar-axis measurement is particularly useful in the setting of coexisting moderate or severe foot deformity. In a study of 1000 neonates, the value of tibial torsion at birth was a mean of 15 degrees using the thigh-foot angle or the transmalleolar-axis measurement.[120]

Although not discussed in this chapter, the foot shape requires notice. Metatarsus adductus may be the primary cause of in-toeing, particularly in the infant, and marked calcaneovalgus may be an important component of out-toeing. Neuromuscular disease, especially mild cerebral palsy, may be noticed initially because of persistent in-toeing; physical findings of increased lower extremity tone in a child who had some delay in motor milestones should lead to a more complete neurologic evaluation for the coexistence of neuromuscular disorders, especially cerebral palsy.

Imaging Studies

Physical examination usually provides the information needed to formulate a treatment plan, although radiographs are indicated in some instances. If there is asymmetrical limitation of hip abduction or if hip abduction in the toddler is less than 60 degrees, an anteroposterior pelvis radiograph is needed to demonstrate hip dysplasia. Hip dysplasia should be suspected in cases of asymmetrical hip rotation. To obtain this radiograph in a manner proper to obtain reliable measurements, the child should be positioned supine with the hips extended and the knees directed anteriorly. If femoral anteversion is increased, the anteroposterior pelvis radiograph demonstrates apparent coxa valga; if the leg is internally rotated, the true neck-shaft angle is obtained. A simple method for measuring the degree of femoral anteversion with a single radiograph is to obtain an anteroposterior radiograph of the pelvis with the child sitting and the legs abducted 10 to 20 degrees.[65] Radiographs of the tibia are not helpful in assessing tibial torsion.

For the child or teenager, fluoroscopy can be used to quantitate the degree of femoral anteversion. The hip is rotated under fluoroscopy until a true anteroposterior view of the hip is obtained; the amount of internal rotation of the leg in that position is the femoral anteversion.[111] Other radiographic techniques have been reported, but it is necessary to use special positioning techniques or special conversion tables, and the use of these methods has been overshadowed by CT methods.

CT is the most widespread imaging technique used for evaluating femoral rotation. The use of CT is indicated primarily in diagnosing a complex hip deformity or if a rotational osteotomy is being contemplated. The child maintains one position while transverse-plane images are made through the femoral head and neck and through the femoral condyles. The angle formed by the bicondylar axis and a line up the femoral neck is the amount of femoral anteversion. In very young children, the error of measurement increases because of unossified femoral head cartilage, which makes the proximal line construction less precise. CT scans can be used for tibial rotation assessment, but clinical evaluation generally is sufficient.

Ultrasonography can be used to measure the amount of femoral or tibial rotation, and ultrasound measurements closely approximate those of CT scans. Although ultrasound avoids ionizing radiation exposure, even this test may be superfluous because most rotational conditions can be evaluated clinically without the additional expense of imaging studies.

Natural History

Femoral anteversion at birth is approximately 40 degrees. Because of the common intrauterine position of hip external rotation, the infant appears on examination to have more hip external rotation than internal rotation. As the soft tissue external hip rotation contractures decrease over the first year of life, the increased hip internal rotation expected from this amount of femoral anteversion starts to become apparent. Femoral anteversion is the most common cause of in-toeing in children older than 3 years of age.[91] There is a gradual decrease in femoral anteversion from 40 degrees at birth to the adult value of 10 to 15 degrees by early adolescence, with most of this improvement occurring before 8 years of age.[34] Similar studies of retroversion, a much less common condition, have not been reported.

With increasing age and growth, tibial torsion tends toward a normal tibial position, with the lateral malleolus 20 to 30 degrees posterior to the medial malleolus.[124,127] If a child is born with internal tibial torsion, gradual derotation occurs during the first 2 years of life, with weight bearing possibly a factor in this derotation. Although children who sleep on their abdomens with the feet turned inward have had more internal tibial torsion, the significance of this observation is unknown.[59] Virtually all children born with internal tibial torsion have tibial torsion within a normal range by 3 years of age. For children with excessive or asymmetrical tibial torsion after 4 or 5 years of age, derotational tibial osteotomy may be considered.

If a child is born with a "normal" amount of external tibial torsion (often associated with a calcaneovalgus foot position from the intrauterine position), further external tibial rotation does not occur during the first few years of life, and the final tibial torsion stays within the normal range. In children born with excessive external tibial torsion, particularly if it is asymmetrical, spontaneous correction is limited, and a rotational osteotomy may be needed later. Progressive external tibial torsion may develop during childhood and preadolescence with persistent femoral anteversion, particularly in children with cerebral palsy. Recognition of these coexisting conditions is important if surgical treatment is contemplated to improve lower extremity position, because both the tibia and the femur may require derotational osteotomy.[124]

A few specific clinical presentations are worth mentioning, because these scenarios are often brought to the attention of the orthopaedist by the parents.

In some cases, one foot turns out and the other points straight ahead. This usually occurs when the child first stands, and the parents are concerned about the out-turned foot. Because of the external rotation soft tissue contractures at the hip present during the first year of life, the out-turned foot is the normal foot and the other foot has hip external rotation and internal tibial torsion, the net effect being a foot that points straight ahead. No treatment is needed, and the feet gradually move to a symmetrical position.

In some patients, both feet turn out, and the feet look very flat. This is seen when the infant is placed in a standing position by the parents. The positions of the feet reflect the external rotation contractures at the hips. The feet look very flat because of the suppleness of the hindfoot; as the body weight force passes medial to the ankle joint, the supple hindfoot moves into valgus and produces the appearance of a flat foot. No treatment is needed, and the feet gradually move to a straighter position.

Controversy continues about whether rotational conditions of the femur or tibia have an effect on the later development of osteoarthritis in adult life. If an effect were present, the use of osteotomies to correct the rotational position of the femur or tibia would be for more than cosmetic improvement. In the dog model, increased femoral anteversion is associated with the development of acetabular dysplasia and early osteoarthritis.[20] In humans, some studies report no correlation between femoral anteversion and hip osteoarthritis,[33,57,69,145] but others imply that early osteoarthritis of the hip is correlated with increased femoral anteversion.[137] Because decreased femoral anteversion has been correlated with the earlier onset of osteoarthritis of the hip[138] and the knee,[33] as has decreased tibial torsion,[151] out-toeing may present more of a risk factor for the development of arthritis than does in-toeing. Slipped femoral capital epiphysis is more common in obese teenagers with femoral retroversion.[41]

Treatment

Nonsurgical Treatment

Nonsurgical treatment consists primarily of a careful explanation to the parents of the cause of in-toeing or out-toeing in the examined child, because most rotational concerns normalize with time and growth. The offer of annual or biannual observation and examination is useful to document the expected rotational change with growth, particularly if the parents need periodic assurance.

No nonsurgical approach is indicated for femoral anteversion. The use of night splints, twister cables, orthotics, or special shoes has not expedited femoral derotation compared with the untreated, natural course.[34] Shoe modifications, such as heel and sole wedges or medial arch supports, may modify the pattern of shoe wear but do not change the foot-progression angle.[70] These minor shoe adjustments do not influence derotation of the femur or tibia.

It is striking how many parents are aware of the use of night splints (e.g., Denis Browne bar) for tibial torsion in toddlers. Despite the widespread use of these splints, no study has proven the efficacy of these splints compared with the expected course for tibial derotation.[48] In the rabbit tibial model, lateral rotational forces led to angulation of the cells within the zone of hypertrophy of the physis, but no cortical remodeling occurred.[90] In a similar rabbit tibial model, lateral rotation splinting changed the static foot angle but did not demonstrate any change in bone rotation, indicating that the "correction" took place primarily through the ankle joint.[6]

Although it often takes less time to write a prescription for a Denis Browne bar or similar night splint device than to answer the parents' questions, it is better to take the time to explain what to expect from this condition as the child grows. Education of the parents (and often the grandparents) is of paramount importance in managing family concerns about internal tibial torsion. Office brochures explaining the condition and the expected resolution with growth are a useful adjunct to a verbal explanation.

Although most internal tibial torsion resolves by 2 years of age, some children take a little longer, but tibial torsion changes little after the age of 3 years. Despite improvement in internal tibial torsion with growth, the in-toeing may remain static or even appear to worsen at 3 or 4 years of age because of the emergence of internal femoral torsion as the primary cause of in-toeing.

Surgical Treatment

Derotation osteotomy is the only surgical treatment to consider for children with rotational abnormalities.[125] An adequate number of years must pass to allow certainty that the expected natural derotation with increasing age will not continue to correct the rotation abnormality without the help of surgical treatment; derotational osteotomy should not be done on a very young child. In general, tibial rotation osteotomy is seldom needed before 5 years of age, and femoral derotation osteotomy should be put off until the child is at least 8 years of age; these ages are selected to allow natural rotational changes to occur.[127] A conscious modification of foot placement during walking seems to come into play after 8 or 9 years of age, and what appears to be consistently significant in-toeing at 6 years may be accommodated for by 8 years of age. Because children with cerebral palsy more often have excessive femoral anteversion than do normal children, derotational osteotomy may be appropriate at earlier ages, particularly if soft tissue surgery is also planned to aid walking development.

In children with cerebral palsy, deviation of the foot internally or externally makes walking more difficult. Derotational femoral osteotomy positions the foot in a more normal position to allow improved push-off at the end of the stance phase of gait, making walking easier with less energy cost.[39] Children with excessive femoral anteversion but who are otherwise normal may find walking and running more difficult, with frequent tripping and hip or thigh aching during activity. The psychologic impact of a negative body image from persistent, marked in-toeing may be a major concern. Any of these factors in conjunction with the physical finding of excessive femoral rotation are appropriate indications for osteotomy.

Most young people who are candidates for femoral derotation osteotomy have less than 10 degrees of hip external rotation and 80 degrees or more of hip internal rotation with the hip extended. If imaging studies demonstrate femoral anteversion of more than 50 degrees, surgery should be considered. Excessive femoral anteversion is usually asymptomatic, but if anterior groin pain occurs with activity, derotation osteotomy may relieve this pain.

If surgical treatment is indicated, the derotation osteotomy can be done anywhere along the rotated femur. At whatever level the osteotomy is done, the saw cut must be perpendicular to the long axis of the femur to avoid producing angulation when rotational correction takes place.

In children older than 12 years of age, closed femoral derotation osteotomy and femoral intramedullary nailing allow the quickest return to weight bearing without the use of a cast.[149] The intramedullary saw used for femoral shortening procedures can also be used for rotational correction (see Chap. 22). The femur is cut near the isthmus in the proximal diaphysis. Although this technique generally requires later intramedullary rod removal, I prefer the technique for a teenager with rotational deformity. An intramedullary rod should not be inserted from the piriformis fossa region in children younger that 10 years of age because of concern about the blood supply to the femoral head that runs through this region in younger children.

Proximal intertrochanteric osteotomy with blade plate fixation is advocated by some physicians to avoid cast immobilization postoperatively of the older child and teenager, based on a reported lower incidence of complications compared with the supracondylar femoral osteotomy.[106] In the child with cerebral palsy, in whom a coincident hip abnormality requires a change in the proximal femoral neck-shaft angle at the same time, this method is unquestionably advantageous. However, weight bearing is limited for a longer period after blade plate fixation than after an intramedullary rod. If plate and screw removal is performed, additional surgery is needed, with another 4 weeks of limited weight bearing after the hardware removal.

In children younger than 10 years of age, femoral derotation is most easily achieved by distal osteotomy, stabilized with Steinmann pins or staples.[54] The osteotomy is done in the metaphyseal-diaphyseal region under fluoroscopic guidance. If staples are used, at least two are placed almost perpendicular to one another after rotational correction is achieved. A long-leg cast for 6 to 8 weeks is usually sufficient postoperatively, but this cast must be molded well in the supracondylar region and proximally to allow limited weight bearing with crutch assistance.

Return to normal walking and running may take several months after femoral rotation osteotomy. Even after muscle strength has been regained, some patients, particularly teenagers, walk with a "jerky" gait until adaptation of the central nervous system to changes in proprioception occurs, usually within a year of the osteotomy.

Tibial derotation osteotomy is indicated if the thigh-foot angle remains internally rotated 10 degrees or more (i.e., thigh-foot angle -10 or more) or if external tibial rotation is 35 degrees or more. Particularly in the case of excessive external tibial rotation, the knee extension moment is diminished, leading to weaker push-off.[39] This push-off power can be improved by tibial osteotomy to improve centralization of the foot.

Tibial rotation osteotomy can be performed proximally or distally, although there are fewer complications with the distal osteotomy.[73] I include a fibular osteotomy with the tibial rotation osteotomy. Other surgeons report that a distal tibial rotation osteotomy can be safely and effectively completed without a coexistent fibular osteotomy, with fewer complications, especially less later angulation at the osteotomy site.[81,108] Fixation of the proximal or distal tibial osteotomy is usually achieved by Steinmann pins or staples, augmented with a long-leg cast until healing is complete (Fig. 27-3).

Both legs should be prepped and draped into the surgical field when derotation osteotomy is performed, ensuring that the alignment of the lower extremities is the same on both sides at the completion of the procedure. No matter how well planned the operative procedure has been, intraoperative visual confirmation of the final corrected position and symmetry between the lower extremities is extremely valuable for the best result.

Complications

The primary complication of nonoperative treatment is the induction of a new rotational condition while trying to treat another. An example is in the use of the Denis Browne bar for in-toeing, although no efficacy of this treatment has been proven.[48] If the bar used is longer than the shoulder or pelvic width, genu valgum can be induced. If this bar is used to treat in-toeing from excessive femoral anteversion, external tibial torsion may be produced, with no effect on the anteversion.[34]

Potential complications from derotational tibial osteotomy differ for distal or proximal procedures. The distal osteotomy site produces fewer complications. Proximally, the osteotomy must be done 1 to 2 cm below the tibial tubercle to avoid producing

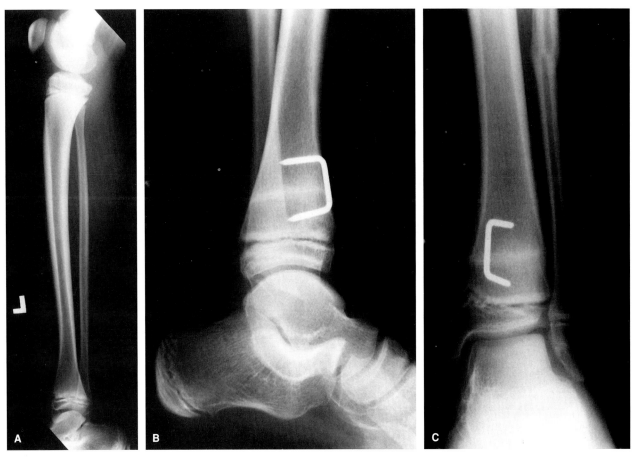

FIGURE 27-3. (A) Preoperative lateral radiograph of the tibia of a 10-year-old boy with unilateral external tibial torsion of 60 degrees. (B) The postoperative lateral radiograph of the ankle after internal rotation osteotomy of the tibia demonstrates the improved ankle alignment. (C) The postoperative anteroposterior radiograph of the ankle demonstrates avoidance of varus or valgus at the time of osteotomy.

recurvatum from injury to the portion of the proximal tibial physis within the tubercle. Osteotomy in the proximal metaphysis also may lead to impingement of the anterior tibial artery as it courses anteriorly from the popliteal region through the interosseous membrane; because this may result in a compartment syndrome postoperatively, a fasciotomy of the anterior and lateral compartments should be done at the time of proximal tibial osteotomy.[85,129] Peroneal palsy may occur.[119] Healing may be a little slower at the distal tibial osteotomy site, but nonunion is rare. Care must be taken to make the saw cut for a rotational osteotomy perpendicular to the long axis of the tibia or tibial varus or valgus will result; I prefer to make this cut using fluoroscopy to determine the bony long, axis because these osteotomies are often made through a rather small skin incision.

A fibular osteotomy should accompany all proximal tibial osteotomies, although it may be unnecessary in all distal tibial rotational osteotomies. The superfi-

cial peroneal nerve should be identified and protected from injury during the fibular osteotomy.[119] Nonunion of the fibular osteotomy is uncommon and can be treated by bone graft and plating if symptomatic or can be ignored if asymptomatic.

The potential complications of femoral rotation osteotomy include angulation, delayed union, and hardware problems. Early angulation can be avoided by ensuring a transverse cut is made at the time of surgery by using fluoroscopy to guide the angle of the cut. Late angulation is avoided by adequate osteotomy fixation. Delayed union may occur with a closed femoral osteotomy stabilized with an interlocking nail, and delayed union in this setting can usually be solved by removing the distal locking screw, allowing compression at the delayed union site with continued weight bearing. Insertion of a reamed intramedullary nail should be limited to children older than 10 years of age to avoid possible femoral head avascular necrosis and injury to the greater trochanter apophysis. If staples are used distally to hold the osteotomy together, care must be taken to place these at about 90 degrees to one another and to not distract the osteotomy site when the staple is seated, or fixation may be lost and union will be delayed.

BOWLEGS AND KNOCK-KNEES

Genu varum (bowlegs) and genu valgum (knock-knees) may be normal or abnormal, depending on the magnitude of the angulation and the age of the child. Because mild bowlegs and knock-knees are common in growing children, the most important role of the examining physician is to recognize those clinical and imaging features that differentiate the unusual pathologic form of bowlegs and knock-knees from the normal.

Normal Development

Almost all infants have some degree of bowlegs. When standing begins, the bowing may seem greater with weight bearing. After walking begins at about 1 year of age, bowing of the thigh and lower leg is commonly noticed. There is gradual improvement in this bowing by 18 months to 2 years of age, and most toddlers no longer have bowlegs after 2 years of age. Knock-knees

begin to appear between 2 and 3 years, developing the greatest amount of valgus at 3 or 4 years, and partial straightening occurs by 6 or 7 years of age, at which point the "adult" position is reached (Fig. 27-4).[114] Although this pattern holds true for most children, ethnic and familial differences occur, and examination of the parents often is useful in explaining differences from this "normal" pattern.

Clinical Features

Parental concern about the appearance of the legs is the most common reason for presentation of these children. Pain should not occur at these young ages from genu varum or valgum, and if pain exists, another cause should be sought.

Medical history is important. A family history of bowlegs, knock-knees, or nutritional problems that required treatment is important. Birth history, percentile for weight at birth and currently, and age of independent walking provide useful information in determining the possible cause of the angulation.

The lower limb angulation is usually apparent during the physical examination. General nutritional status and body proportions are assessed. It is important to evaluate the child for possible rotational abnormalities, because internal tibial torsion tends to accentuate the amount of apparent bowing with standing and walking.

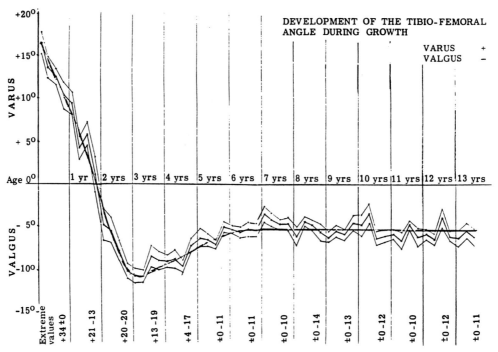

FIGURE 27-4. The graph depicts the expected change in genu varum and genu valgum with age. Children with bowlegs after 2 years of age are outside the normal range and should be thoroughly evaluated. (From Salenius P, Vankka E. The development of the tibiofemoral angle in children. J Bone Joint Surg 1975;57:259.)

The level of bowing or knock-knees is assessed, usually from behind the standing child, to see if the femur and tibia are involved or if only one segment is affected. When the child walks, the presence of a lateral thrust at the knee is identified. The femoral-tibial angle is measured with the child supine and standing. Serial Polaroid photography can document angular changes that occur. The distance between the medial femoral condyles with bowlegs or medial malleoli with knock-knees can be measured sequentially to quantitate the clinical course without radiographs. In a group of 196 Caucasian children, this nonradiographic method confirmed that genu varum was maximal at 6 months of age; neutral alignment was seen by age 18 months; and genu valgum, greatest at 4 years of age, was less than 6 degrees by 11 years of age. In this study, normal children between 2 and 11 years of age had valgus up to 12 degrees and intermalleolar distances of up to 8 cm, but the existence of bowlegs after 2 years of age was not normal. Clinical measurements outside these ranges needed further investigation.[47] If asymmetrical angulation is present, the possibility of a pathologic condition existing is greater than if the legs are symmetrical.

Imaging Studies

Imaging evaluation of bowlegs in children younger than 18 months of age should be reserved for those with asymmetrical bowing or with other physical features not associated with physiologic bowing. Differentiating tibia vara from physiologic bowing is difficult before 2 years of age and is impossible before 18 months of age. For patients with bowlegs or knock-knees, a single anteroposterior radiograph of the lower extremities from hip to ankle, with the child standing, is the most appropriate first imaging study.

Widening of the physes, suggesting rickets, is sought. Delayed ossification of the distal femoral or proximal tibial epiphyses or widening of a portion of the physis may indicate excessive pressure on one side of the knee. Although subject to measurement error, the femoral-tibial angle should be measured serially. In bowed legs, the metaphyseal-diaphyseal angle may be helpful in differentiating tibia vara from physiologic bowing. The mechanical axis is measured between the femoral head and the midpoint of the ankle, with the point of passage through the knee recorded.

Causes and Treatment of Bowlegs

Physiologic Bowing

Bowing of the lower extremities is common when the child begins to walk. The earlier the child walks and the heavier the child, the higher the likelihood that significant bowing will be noticed between 1 and 2 years of age. When the child is standing, the bowing noticeably involves the tibia and the distal femur. Internal tibial torsion may be present.

If a radiograph is obtained, a delay in ossification of the medial side of the distal femoral and proximal tibial epiphyses is usually seen. The medial distal femoral metaphysis may appear flared. The physeal width is normally 1 to 2 mm. The metaphyseal-diaphyseal angle should be less than 11 degrees.[78]

Physiologic bowing always resolves with no treatment. However, at 18 months of age, differentiating physiologic bowing from tibia vara may be impossible. If the diagnosis of physiologic bowing is unambiguous, no treatment should be offered, but follow-up examination of the bowlegs is needed until straightening occurs and physiologic valgus begins to be seen.

Tibia Vara or Blount Disease

In some children, particularly those who are obese and began walking before 1 year of age, bowlegs persist after 2 to 3 years of age. If bowing persists past 2 years of age, tibia vara or Blount disease should be suspected. Because tibia vara is associated with abnormal growth at the medial aspect of the proximal tibial physis, the bowing produced will continue to worsen unless diagnosis and appropriate treatment are accomplished.

Three major types of tibia vara are recognized: infantile, juvenile, and adolescent types.[15] The infantile is the most common type and the late-onset tibia vara, as represented by the juvenile and adolescent types, may represent the later manifestations of a mild infantile type that was not noticed or treated early. However, late-onset tibia vara may occur although a neutral mechanical axis has earlier been demonstrated.[49]

The infantile type is most common in children who are obese and who walked earlier than 1 year of age. Bowing usually was noticed when walking began and has persisted. The parents have seen no improvement over the prior few months. Bowing may be bilateral or may resolve on one side and persist on the other. Just as obesity is a factor in infantile tibia vara development, obesity also appears to be a factor in the development of late-onset tibia vara, which is most common in male African American teenagers.[51] Trauma to the proximal tibial physis medially can present as unilateral tibia vara.[84]

Several studies have attempted to determine the pathogenesis of the progressive bowing of tibia vara. It has long been suspected that the forces on the medial side of the proximal tibial physis when an obese child with bowlegs walks had a detrimental effect on the growth in this portion of the physis. Finite element analysis has demonstrated that the force produced in an obese toddler at the medial proximal tibial physis is sufficient to inhibit physeal growth here at an early age.[23] Histologic evaluation of physes in infantile and late-onset tibia vara demonstrate a disordered columnar arrangement of physeal cells and a suppression of normal endochondral growth, particularly on the medial side.[22,146] This disordered physeal histologic picture is similar in infantile and late-onset tibia vara and in cases of slipped capital femoral epiphysis. Whether repetitive trauma, secondary largely to the obesity, is the primary factor leading to these histologic changes remains an unanswered question.

On physical examination, the obesity and bowing is usually obvious. Bowing may be unilateral or bilateral. When the child walks, if a lateral thrust of the knee or sudden lateral knee movement with weight bearing is noticeable, the child most likely has progressive tibia vara. When the standing child is viewed from behind, the bowing is seen to be below the knee and does not involve the femur. Internal tibial torsion that has not corrected is commonly associated with this bowing.

An anteroposterior radiograph of both legs with the child standing can demonstrate the bowing and an abnormality at the medial aspect of the proximal tibia. In more advanced cases, bowing at both ends of the tibia is seen.[110] A lateral knee radiograph commonly shows a posteriorly directed projection at the proximal tibial metaphyseal level. The femoral-tibial angle confirms the varus position of the leg but is subject to error introduced by coexisting rotational abnormalities in the lower extremity or by positioning of the child when the radiograph is obtained.[131]

Other radiographic measurements have been suggested to be more accurate than the femoral-tibial angle. The metaphyseal-diaphyseal angle is obtained by measuring the angle formed by a line parallel to the top of the proximal tibial metaphysis and a line perpendicular to the long axis of the tibial shaft. If this angle is more than 11 degrees on a standing radiograph, almost all children (29 of 30 in this series) eventually develop tibia vara, and those with measurements less than 11 degrees most likely have physiologic bowing.[78] Others have looked at the error of measurement of the metaphyseal-diaphyseal angle and found standard deviations of ±2.6 degrees and ±4.6 degrees.[38,52] When a group of 106 children with physiologic bowing was compared with a group of 19 children with the established diagnosis of Blount disease, the metaphyseal-diaphyseal angle with physiologic bowing averaged 9 ± 3.9 degrees, and in those with Blount disease, the average was 19 ± 5.7 degrees.[35] It can probably be assumed that all children with a metaphyseal-diaphyseal angle greater than 20 degrees have confirmed tibia vara and that most of those with angles greater

than 15 degrees also have tibia vara. The tibial metaphyseal-metaphyseal angle is larger than the metaphyseal-diaphyseal angle, particularly in the children with the most bowing, and demonstrates that distal tibial bowing occurs in concert with proximal bowing in the more striking cases of tibia vara (Fig. 27-5).[36]

After the diagnosis of tibia vara has been established radiographically, the most common staging classification used is that reported by Langenskiold (Fig. 27-6).[76] Six stages are used to describe the radiologic changes seen with increasing age. Interobserver error in determining the stage is small for the early and late stages but quite large in the intermediate stages.[130] Although many clinicians use this classification to determine what type of treatment is needed, Langenskiold has cautioned that in stages I through IV there is not an intended direct correlation of the stages with prognosis or the type of treatment that is most desirable.[77] Nonetheless, surgical treatment is commonly needed for any child whose radiographs demonstrate any stage III through VI changes.

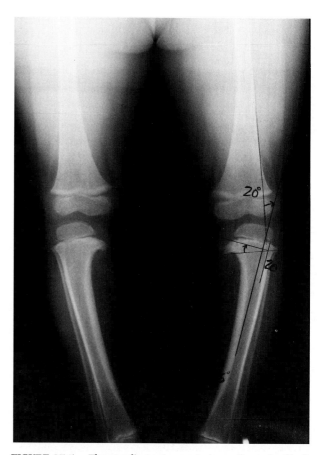

FIGURE 27-5. The standing anteroposterior radiograph of both lower extremities demonstrates bowing in a 2-year-old girl. The femoral-tibial angle is 20 degrees, the metaphyseal-diaphyseal angle is 20 degrees, and the metaphyseal-metaphyseal angle is 25 degrees in the left leg. The diagnosis was Blount disease.

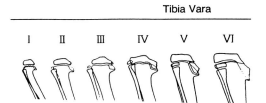

FIGURE 27-6. Depiction of the six stages of radiographic changes seen in Langenskiold's classification of tibia vara. (From Langenskiold A. Tibia vara: a critical review. Clin Orthop Rel Res 1989;246:195.)

In advanced tibia vara or in recurrent tibia vara after valgus osteotomy, a physeal bar may be demonstrated in the medial aspect of the proximal tibial physis. The extent of this physeal bar can be demonstrated by polytomes or by magnetic resonance imaging (MRI) of this region to quantitate the percentage of physeal involvement. I prefer MRI for this evaluation because the physeal cartilage can be directly visualized.

TREATMENT. Nonoperative treatment of tibia vara is appropriate for children younger than 3 years of age with Langenskiold stages I or II.[110] If a child has persistent bowing at 2 years of age with an abnormal metaphyseal-diaphyseal angle, I use a knee-ankle-foot orthosis (KAFO) during the day while the child is walking. The KAFO should be constructed without a knee hinge to obtain the best effect. Night bracing is not needed or recommended.[44]

If the child has no improvement with the brace by 3 years of age or has a Langenskiold stage III or higher condition, proximal tibial valgus osteotomy is needed to correct the tibia vara. If the corrective osteotomy is done before 4 years of age, approximately 85% of these patients are adequately treated with a single osteotomy, which has placed the tibia in about 5 degrees more valgus than on the normal side.[37]

The type of osteotomy used is often a result of surgeon's preference and may include dome osteotomy, oblique osteotomy, closing wedge osteotomy, or spike osteotomy.[30] An attempt to correct the internal rotational deformity should be included with the correction of the varus deformity. The oblique osteotomy allows multiplanar correction with one osteotomy cut.[74,107] Fixation of the osteotomy site may be by long-leg cast, external fixator, internal pins or staples, or compression plate.[74,83,107] If tibia vara recurs after an appropriate valgus osteotomy, evaluation for a medial physeal bar is needed by polytomography or MRI.[6] If a small medial bar is identified, surgical resection with fat interposition is needed with repeat valgus osteotomy to obtain lasting correction (Fig. 27-7). If the proximal tibial physis is still open, lateral tibial hemiepiphyseodesis may be the simplest method to treat some patients with adolescent tibia vara, for

whom the reported complication and malalignment rates are quite high with osteotomy.[50,156]

In patients with Langenskiold stage V or VI conditions, the surgical choices are osteotomy with physeal bar resection using fat interposition or proximal lateral tibial epiphyseodesis to prevent further recurrence. In many of these advanced cases, elevation of the proximal tibial medial plateau and valgus tibial osteotomy is combined with the lateral tibial epiphyseodesis.[45,118] If epiphyseodesis is done, contralateral tibial epiphysiodesis or later tibial leg lengthening may be needed, but control of the tibia vara is achieved. If more than one osteotomy has already been tried to correct the tibia vara, the use of an Ilizarov frame and external hinges allow improved restoration of the normal mechanical axis of the leg by translation, angular correction, and lengthening through the osteotomy site.

COMPLICATIONS. The primary complications of proximal tibial osteotomy for tibia vara are compartment syndrome of the leg, recurrent varus deformity, and recurvatum of the proximal tibia. Proximal tibial osteotomy in the growing child must be done distal to the tibial tubercle; if the osteotomy injures the proximal tibial physis at the tibial tubercle level, proximal tibial recurvatum will result. Regardless of whether a varus or valgus proximal tibial osteotomy is done, there is a greater than 20% risk of anterior and lateral compartment syndrome.[129] This compartment syndrome results during angular correction from a kinking of the anterior tibial artery as it passes through the interosseous membrane in the proximal leg. To avoid the compartment syndrome, fasciotomy of these compartments is carried out at the time of tibial osteotomy, and careful observation postoperatively is essential.

Prevention of recurrent varus deformity may be more difficult. If a recurrence occurs within 1 or 2 years of the original osteotomy, a medial physeal bar usually exists. Although the results of physeal bar resection in this clinical situation are variable in the short term and essentially unknown for the long term, one attempt at resection of the physeal bar with fat interposition is warranted.[6] If varus recurs after physeal bar resection, epiphyseodesis of the lateral half of the proximal tibial physis is used at the time of the final valgus osteotomy to prevent further varus recurrence.

Rickets

Vitamin D–resistant rickets (hypophosphatemic rickets) and nutritional rickets are the most common metabolic conditions that lead to persistent bowlegs

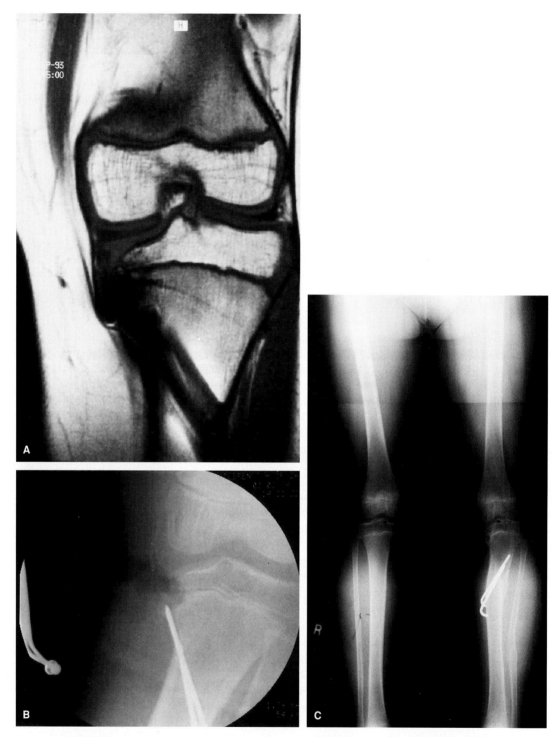

FIGURE 27-7. (A) Magnetic resonance image of the knee demonstrates an asymmetrical growth arrest line, with more growth laterally than medially, in a 5-year-old girl with recurrent bowing 1 year after a proximal tibial valgus osteotomy for unilateral Blount disease. (B) The physeal bar was resected and fat was interposed to prevent repeat bridging. (C) Anteroposterior radiograph of the lower extremity 1 year after repeat tibial osteotomy and medial physeal bridge resection with fat interposition. The deformity has not recurred.

(see Chap. 6). Children with bowing due to rickets are usually in the lower percentiles of height for their age. In hypophosphatemic rickets, a family history of bowed legs may be obtained.

Rickets is usually suspected first by the radiographic finding of a widened physis. The physeal widening, which results from the diminished calcification in the zone of provisional calcification, is seen best at rapidly growing physes, such as the distal femur or distal radius. Serum studies can determine the type of rickets present. A long, standing radiograph of the lower extremities usually shows bowing in the femurs and the tibias. The varus deformity of the distal tibia is often greater in rickets than in other clinical situations.

If the diagnosis of rickets is confirmed, the initial treatment consists of adequate medical control. Remodeling of the bowing to a straight position is more common after treatment of nutritional rickets than hypophosphatemic rickets. Bracing is probably not indicated.

If the bowing worsens or does not improve after medical treatment for several months to a few years, surgical treatment is indicated. In preparing for surgery, it is mandatory that good medical control has been achieved; if not, recurrence is virtually guaranteed. A careful assessment of the standing anteroposterior and lateral radiographs permits an accurate determination of the level or levels of osteotomy needed. Osteotomy of the tibia and femur may be needed, or two osteotomies within the same tibia may be necessary to allow leg realignment and reestablishment of a normal mechanical axis.

Cast immobilization after corrective osteotomies is commonly used until healing occurs. Immobilization-induced hypercalcemia may occur and may require modification of the medical treatment dosages. If medical treatment during osteotomy healing is inadequate, uncalcified osteoid forms at the osteotomy site, and deformity is likely to recur.

Genetic Disorders

Achondroplasia is the most common genetic disorder associated with bowlegs. The bowing occurs below the knee and is a result of the fibula growing longer than the tibia. Although all achondroplastic children have some degree of bowing, surgical treatment is needed in only about 50% of them. Bracing has not been effective in preventing or reversing the bowing.

If the bowing in achondroplasia is progressive and is associated with a lateral thrust of the knee during the stance phase of gait, tibial osteotomy, with removal of a portion of fibula, is curative in most children. Fibular epiphyseodesis may be used to decrease the fibular growth, but correction of the bowing may take

several years. Because not all achondroplastic children need surgery, I prefer the immediate correction provided by a tibial osteotomy in those that do (Fig. 27-8).

A variety of epiphyseal and metaphyseal skeletal dysplasias may be associated with bowing of the legs. In evaluating children with bowlegs, the epiphyses and metaphyses on the standing anteroposterior radiograph should be assessed carefully. If osteotomy is needed for lower extremity alignment in any of the epiphyseal dysplasias, intraoperative arthrograms of the hip, knee, and ankle facilitate the surgical planning for the appropriate osteotomy levels.

Fibrocartilaginous Dysplasia of the Proximal Tibia

Unilateral tibia vara, often presenting before the age that infantile Blount disease is usually diagnosed, may be the result of focal fibrocartilaginous dysplasia of the proximal-medial tibial metaphysis. Although the cause of this unusual condition is unclear, dense fibrous and fibrocartilaginous tissue has been revealed by biopsy of the involved area.[66] Although in some cases this is a self-limited condition, with gradual straightening of the tibia during growth, tibial osteot-

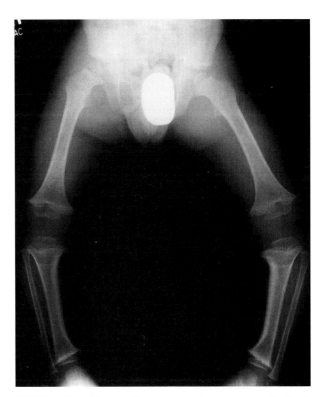

FIGURE 27-8. The standing anteroposterior radiograph of a 4-year-old boy with achondroplasia demonstrates the bowing commonly seen in this skeletal dysplasia as the fibula grows longer than the tibia. Approximately 50% of the bowed legs in achondroplasia require corrective osteotomy.

omy to correct the osteotomy has been recommended by some physicians because the sclerotic medial metaphyseal region becomes diaphyseal.[8,13,99]

The treatment of this condition is initially periodic clinical and radiographic evaluation. Many improve without active treatment. If improvement with age does not occur or if the varus deformity worsens, osteotomy can be performed to correct the residual deformity.[99]

Causes and Treatment of Knock-Knees

Physiologic Knock-Knees

A valgus position of the lower extremities is usually present by 2 years of age.[114] The maximal amount of physiologic valgus occurs between the ages of 3 and 4 years, after which the valgus straightens somewhat to achieve the "adult" position by 6 years of age. There is generally no further change in normal valgus position after this age.[127]

Serial documentation of the degree of valgus positioning can be accomplished by periodic measurement of the intermalleolar distance, by periodic Polaroid photography, or by standing anteroposterior radiographs. If valgus persists after 7 years of age, later consideration of hemiepiphyseodesis, based on growth-remaining data, may be used to produce straight legs by the end of growth.[11]

Rickets

Progressive or marked genu valgum may result from metabolic disorders, particularly rickets. Although genu varum is more common with most types of rickets, genu valgum may result, particularly in the case of renal rickets.[101] A family history of angular leg deformity or a history of renal problems aids in making the appropriate diagnosis.

Clinical considerations are much the same as those for bowlegs associated with rickets. Serum studies should include calcium, phosphate, alkaline phosphatase, urea nitrogen, and creatinine. A standing anteroposterior radiograph of the lower extremities shows the valgus deformity and a widening of the physes of the distal femur and proximal tibia. Lateral widening of the proximal tibial physis in knock-knees associated with renal osteodystrophy has been suggested to be analogous to the medial physeal changes seen in Blount disease.[101]

Bracing as the primary treatment for genu valgum associated with renal rickets has not been effective in preventing or reversing the deformity. If surgical treatment is contemplated, medical control of the renal disease and the serum calcium and phosphate is needed first. As with varus deformity, a single level or multiple levels of osteotomy may be needed to realign

the mechanical axis appropriately. After osteotomy for knock-knees associated with renal osteodystrophy, the lateral physeal widening resolves.[101]

Posttraumatic Tibial Valgus

Valgus deformity of the proximal tibia is not unusual after a fracture of the proximal tibia metaphysis without an associated fracture of the fibula.[23] A variety of theories have been proposed to explain this.[63] The theories include inadequate reduction, early weight bearing, soft tissue imbalance or interposition,[144] and increased growth of the medial physis or decreased lateral physeal growth after injury. In posttraumatic bone scans, increased isotope uptake has been demonstrated in the medial side of the physis compared with the lateral side, lending credence to the theory that valgus is caused by asymmetrical overgrowth of the proximal tibia after this fracture.[64,154]

Whatever the cause, fractures of the proximal metaphysis, even those that appear to be nondisplaced, have a definite predisposition to produce later tibia valga (Fig. 27-9). Although torus fractures here usually do not develop later tibial valgus, more than one half

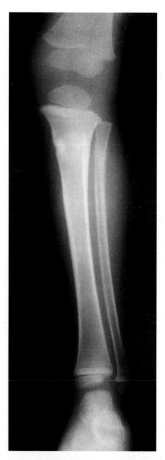

FIGURE 27-9. The anteroposterior radiograph of the tibia in a 5-year-old boy 6 months after a proximal tibial metaphyseal fracture demonstrates a valgus deformity that occurred since the time of injury.

of other fractures in this location do.[109] In one series of 21 patients, the tibial valgus occurring after this fracture ranged from 13 to 25 degrees (mean, 19 degrees) compared with the uninjured tibia.[115] The parents of a child with this injury should be advised at the time of the initial fracture treatment of this possibility. Although the valgus that results from tibial overgrowth (relative to the fibula) cannot be prevented, the orthopaedist should attempt to reduce this fracture fully by using a varus-molding force in a long-leg cast with the knee extended, being careful to avoid leaving even a few degrees of residual valgus at the time of initial reduction. Because the fibula usually is intact, over-reduction into varus is not feasible.

Follow-up of a proximal metaphyseal tibial fracture often should extend for several years after the injury has healed. The tibial valgus may begin to be seen as early as 6 months after injury. Even when the infolded pes anserinus and periosteum in the fracture site was surgically removed, tibial valgus has occurred.[16]

If tibial valgus occurs, early tibial osteotomy should be avoided, because there is a high incidence of recurrence of valgus after attempted corrective osteotomy. In one series of 6 children undergoing corrective osteotomy 12 to 27 months after fracture, all had recurrences of 10 to 25 degrees of valgus in the ensuing 20 to 30 months.[4] Spontaneous improvement over the 3 or 4 years after the initial fracture may occur.[155] If, after prolonged follow-up, an unacceptable degree of tibial valgus remains, the angular deformity can be corrected by proximal tibial hemiepiphyseodesis or varus osteotomy of the tibia. If tibial osteotomy is performed, it is essential to osteotomize the fibula, or valgus recurrence often results. Tibial-fibular osteotomy at skeletal maturity does not produce subsequent valgus deformity.

Genetic Disorders

Although varus deformity is more common in children with skeletal dysplasias, genu valgum may present in patients with epiphyseal or metaphyseal dysplasias. Children with pseudoachondroplasia and metaphyseal dysplasias are particularly likely to develop this deformity. If osteotomy is deemed necessary, as for varus deformity, arthrography of the joints above and below the angulated bone can aid in determining the optimal position at the osteotomy (Fig. 27-10), because the epiphyses commonly are not fully ossified.

Although not a skeletal dysplasia, Morquio syndrome often leads to genu valgum in the young child. If this valgus deformity is progressive, osteotomy may be needed. Because atlantoaxial instability is common in this condition, flexion-extension lateral cervical radiographs are needed before osteotomy surgery. Although the orthopaedist may think that the progressive

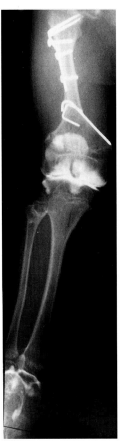

FIGURE 27-10. The anteroposterior radiograph of the right lower extremity in a child with spondyloepiphyseal dysplasia illustrates the use of multijoint arthrography to guide alignment osteotomies in conditions with delayed epiphyseal ossification.

valgus is the cause of decreased ambulatory ability, spinal cord compression at the upper cervical level may be a more important factor and should be evaluated before tibial or femoral osteotomy is undertaken.

KNEE DISORDERS

Recurvatum Deformity

Congenital Knee Dislocation

A recurvatum deformity of the knee at birth may be the result of the intrauterine position or may be a true subluxation or dislocation at the knee level (Fig. 27-11). A breech fetal position predisposes the child to this condition. In the more severe cases, hip dislocation or clubfoot deformities are also present, and the knee recurvatum may be associated with an underlying condition such as arthrogryposis or Larsen syndrome.[25]

At birth, the knee is hyperextended and may have little or no flexion. The spectrum included in the designation of congenital knee dislocation includes knee

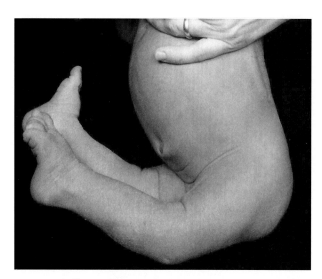

FIGURE 27-11.   A clinical photograph of an infant demonstrates the significant hyperextension of the knee that occurs with congenital knee dislocation associated with a breech position.

dislocation, knee subluxation, and knee recurvatum, in order of decreasing severity. Radiographs allow appropriate classification of the severity of the knee hyperextension. If, on radiographs, the tibia is displaced anterior to the long axis of the femur, actual dislocation exists, but longitudinal contact is at least partially maintained with subluxation.

The pathoanatomy of congenital knee dislocation includes a shortened and often fibrotic quadriceps femoris, a tight anterior joint capsule, and hypoplasia of the suprapatellar pouch. Valgus deformity may result from a failure of medial soft tissue structures, which have been rendered less effective by the anterior displacement of the tibial insertions.[100] It is unclear whether these changes are primary or secondary, but histologic evaluation of a congenital knee dislocation in a 19-week fetus has demonstrated quadriceps fibrosis, absence of a suprapatellar pouch, and incomplete cavitation of the patellofemoral joint.[141] Anterior cruciate ligaments have been described as attenuated and contracted. If no treatment is carried out, the child ends up with a stiff and unstable knee that makes walking difficult.[25,36]

Treatment depends on the severity of the knee hyperextension. Passive stretching of the quadriceps and the anterior knee capsule, combined with splinting the knee in an increasingly flexed position, is sufficient to achieve full knee flexion and knee stability in most without an associated syndrome.[100] The splinting in flexion can be accomplished by a Pavlik harness,[94] by serial long-leg casting, or by rigid splints. Although stretching and splinting is sometimes successful in knee dislocation associated with arthrogryposis or hip and foot deformities and should be tried initially, surgical treatment is more often needed in this group.[100]

If progressive flexion and radiographic evidence of knee reduction is not obtained by nonoperative means, surgery is recommended relatively early, before 2 years of age.[9,32,36,,62,100] Arthrography or MRI is often useful to determine the need for this surgery. The surgical treatment consists primarily of a V-Y lengthening of the quadriceps, with release of the anterior knee retinaculum; the goal is to achieve about 60 degrees of flexion intraoperatively. Reinforcement of the soft tissue medially by posterior transfer of the tibial attachment of the medial collateral ligament has improved the associated valgus deformity.[100] Division of the anterior cruciate ligament may lead to less satisfactory results than quadriceps lengthening alone.[36] Postoperative casting in flexion is used for 3 to 4 weeks after surgery. Later splinting in extension may be needed to balance the need to maintain the newly achieved knee flexion arc while preserving full knee extension. Gradual improvement of the initial extensor lag should occur over the ensuing year. Although it may be argued that the most severe dislocations are the cases that have required surgical treatment, it appears that resultant knee motion is better if nonoperative treatment has been successful in obtaining a reduction than if surgery was needed.[9]

If congenital knee dislocation is associated with a hip dislocation, both conditions can be treated concurrently in a Pavlik harness.[61] However, the Pavlik harness is difficult to apply adequately unless the knee flexion is at least 20 to 30 degrees. If the knee fails to reduce adequately, surgical treatment of the knee dislocation should precede any attempt at surgical treatment of the hip dislocation.[100]

Congenital Dislocation of the Patella

Children born with congenital dislocation of the patella may not have the diagnosis made for several months or years. This condition may be associated with developmental dysplasia of the hip.[86] Normal knee flexion contractures of about 20 degrees are present at birth but disappear before 6 months of age.[120] The knee flexion contracture persists if the patella is dislocated. The patella is positioned laterally, adjacent to a hypoplastic lateral femoral condyle, and adjacent soft tissue contractures exist, including a tight quadriceps and iliotibial band. Although this deformity occurs during fetal development, the cause of its development is unclear.

In infancy, radiographs may show the angular deformity, but the patella has not begun to ossify in the infant. Ultrasonography has been useful in diagnosing a lateral congenital patellar dislocation when it is unossified.[143] MRI can demonstrate the position of the cartilaginous patella at this age. The child has a knee flexion contracture and holds the lower leg externally rotated, with genu valgum noticed later. In untreated cases, the genu valgum persists, and radiographs demonstrate flattened lateral femoral condyles.[40]

Surgical treatment is necessary in this condition; the goal is to realign the entire extensor mechanism of the knee and allow a full range of knee motion. Surgical results in young children are superior to those done at a later age. Surgical treatment generally involves a combination of a lateral release and medial plication, together with lengthening of the quadriceps, especially the vastus intermedius and a portion of the rectus femoris.[7] Using this combined approach, excellent results, including full flexion and no extensor lag, have been reported for almost 90% of the patients.[40]

Quadriceps Fibrosis

Although a quadriceps contracture may be congenital, it may be caused by fibrosis of the quadriceps muscle after multiple intramuscular injections into the thigh. This condition is less common now than in prior decades. Usually, the child has been ill during the first year or two of life and had been given multiple thigh injections. The vastus intermedius is primarily involved, although other portions of the quadriceps muscle may also be affected. As a result of this quadriceps fibrosis, knee flexion is limited, although actual recurvatum deformity is uncommon.

If flexion casting is ineffective in improving knee flexion, surgical treatment is needed. Resection of the fibrotic vastus intermedius (with quadriceps lengthening if needed) allows flexion to 90 degrees. Postoperative casting is used for a few weeks, and then therapy is used, with night splints helping to preserve flexion. Although a continuous passive motion machine may be useful after surgery, the commercially available machines are generally too large to allow adequate passive motion preservation in the young child.

Posttraumatic Knee Recurvatum

Injury to the anterior portion of the proximal tibial physis results in a recurvatum deformity of the proximal tibia. This injury may be noticed initially as a part of other skeletal injuries, but unrecognized tibial tubercle physeal closure may also show up later, even if fractures distant from this location have been initially treated. Placement of a tibial traction pin for femoral fractures must be done in a manner that avoids passage across this physeal region; in most children, a distal femoral traction pin is preferable for the treatment of femoral shaft fractures.

If recurvatum results from premature closure of the anterior part of the proximal tibial physis, the only treatment is surgical. Proximal tibial flexion osteot-

omy, with a closing or an opening wedge, can realign the tibia (Fig. 27-12). An iliac crest bone graft is used if an opening wedge osteotomy is preferred.[117]

Osgood-Schlatter Disease

Thought to be a traction apophysitis of the tibial tubercle, the condition described by Osgood and Schlatter should probably not be called a disease. Ossification of the tibial tubercle begins distally between 7 and 9 years of age. This distal focus of ossification progresses proximally, just as the ossification from the proximal tibial epiphysis proceeds distally.[96] Where the patellar tendon inserts into the tibial tubercle, the unossified cartilage is susceptible to repeated trauma with activity in children between 11 and 14 years of age. Traditionally, the lesion in this condition was thought to be microfractures in the apophyseal cartilage of the tibial tubercle,[98] and there is a often a history of preexisting Osgood-Schlatter disease in adolescents with tibial tuberosity fractures.[150] However, MRI data demonstrate changes in the tendon at the insertion into the tuberosity, suggesting that tendinitis may be as important as apophysitis in the generation of pain at the tibial tuber-

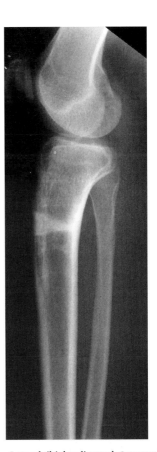

FIGURE 27-12. Lateral tibial radiograph 2 years after an opening wedge osteotomy was performed to correct tibial recurvatum deformity resulting from premature physeal closure at the tibial tubercle in a 13-year-old girl.

cle.[112] HLA antigens are normal in patients with Osgood-Schlatter disease, and this tibial tubercle tenderness should not be confused with an enthesitis associated with an inflammatory arthropathy.[121]

Osgood-Schlatter disease is self-limiting, with pain usually resolving when the tibial tubercle becomes fully ossified and the apophysis closes. The primary clinical feature of this condition is pain and tenderness localized to the tibial tubercle. Knee effusion does not occur if this is the only knee problem of the patient. Prominence or enlargement of the tibial tubercle is evident when compared with the unaffected side, although bilateral involvement affects almost one half of the patients.[72] If point tenderness is not present over the tibial tubercle, attention should be focused on other diagnoses to explain the presence of knee pain.

Imaging studies should be used sparingly in evaluating this condition. An anteroposterior knee radiograph usually appears normal. The lateral knee radiograph may demonstrate one or more areas of calcification in the tibial tubercle region, in addition to the normal ossification pattern expected. In the skeletally mature teenager, a separate ossicle may be seen between the patellar tendon and the bony tibial tubercle. On a sunrise view of the patella, these ossicles in the tibial tubercle area may be misdiagnosed as a loose body within the knee. CT and MRI scans are rarely indicated in the evaluation of Osgood-Schlatter disease.

This diagnosis can generally be accurately made by clinical examination, and radiographs at the initial visit are obtained primarily to rule out the presence of more serious bone pathology. Repeated radiographs during follow-up visits are rarely of clinical use.

Treatment is largely symptomatic.[75] Activity is limited to the degree necessary to control the pain at the tibial tubercle. Complete avoidance of all sports activities is not usually necessary or recommended. Before sports participation, stretching exercises are used, and icing may be helpful after sports activity. A knee immobilizer, in combination with thigh muscle strengthening, may be used for pain relief, but extended periods of casting should be avoided, because muscle atrophy will increase. Corticosteroid injections are not recommended and may aggravate the apophysitis. Because this is a self-limited condition in most cases, conservative treatment, using any or all of the described methods, is generally successful in controlling the pain and allowing continuing sports participation. After skeletal maturity, if tibial tubercle pain with activity persists and the lateral radiograph demonstrates an ossicle between the patellar tendon and the tibial tubercle, surgical excision of the ossicle may ameliorate symptoms,[10,89] although the long-term follow-up results of patients treated with surgical removal of the ossicles is no better as a group than for those treated nonoperatively.[139] The primary continuing problem for both groups seems to be discomfort associated with the prominence of the tibial tubercle.

Complications from Osgood-Schlatter disease are uncommon. Tibial tubercle fractures are more common in teenagers with a history of Osgood-Schlatter disease and usually require open reduction and internal fixation.[150] Premature closure of the tibial tubercle apophysis and resultant recurvatum deformity have been reported.[80,153] Although pain over the tibial tubercle during kneeling is a common adult complaint, this can be managed adequately with avoidance of kneeling or the use of soft knee pads. Patients who had tibial tubercle tenderness and radiographic fragmentation are much more likely to have continued knee pain as adults than those who initially had soft tissue swelling alone, without radiographic evidence of an abnormality.[72]

Larsen-Johansson Disease

When Larsen and Johansson described this condition in the early 1920s, it was thought of as a traction apophysitis at the distal pole of the patella. However, the pathologic change that produces the clinical and radiographic findings of Larsen-Johansson disease is probably secondary to calcification in an avulsed portion of the patellar tendon.[88] Young adolescent athletes are primary affected, because this condition occurs before skeletal maturity is reached. The knee pain is worse with running, climbing stairs, or kneeling. Most often, only one knee is involved. This condition can coexist with Osgood-Schlatter disease.[140]

Tenderness is experienced at the inferior pole of the patella, over the upper portion of the patellar tendon. No knee effusion is present, and local warmth may be noticed.

Radiographs of the knee are the imaging modality of choice to confirm this diagnosis, but ultrasonography also has been effective in diagnosing and following patients with Larsen-Johansson disease.[27] Four radiographic stages have been described. Stage 1 is normal, and in stage 2, discrete calcifications are seen within the patellar tendon. In time, these discrete calcifications coalesce (stage 3) and eventually appear to incorporate into the lower pole of the patella (stage 4A) or form a separate ossicle distinct from the patella (stage 4B).[88] In preadolescents with an acute onset of pain at the inferior patella, the primary condition that must be differentiated from Larsen-Johansson disease is a sleeve fracture of the distal patella. In this fracture, the radiograph may only show a small area of ossification even though the injury is a complete avulsion of the proximal part of the patellar tendon with a portion of patellar articular cartilage; surgical treatment is needed for this sleeve fracture.

The pathoanatomy is thought to consist of a partial tear of the proximal patellar tendon, with resultant calcification within the area of tendon injury. Repetitive, small tears during athletic activity may lead to the several areas of ectopic calcification seen on radiographs.[88]

This condition is self-limiting, and surgery is not advocated. Treatment is much like that used for Osgood-Schlatter disease: relative activity restriction, quadriceps stretching before activity, and icing after sports activity. Full resolution occurs in several months to 1 year. No long-term problems have been reported.

Bipartite Patella

Ossification of the cartilaginous patella begins between 4 and 6 years of age and is completed by adolescence. Secondary ossification centers often occur, beginning around 12 years of age, and are usually located in the superolateral portion of the patella. In about 2% of the population, the secondary ossification centers fail to fuse completely with the primary ossification center.

Most bipartite patellas are asymptomatic, and the diagnosis often is made as a coincidental finding on a radiograph that is obtained for pain in another part of the knee. However, pain may be present directly over the patella after a direct blow to the patella or with repetitive athletic activity. Stair climbing is a particularly painful activity for these teenagers.[12,43]

Although some researchers ascribe the symptoms to a nonunited fracture through the junction of ossification centers,[12] others have shown that an acute cartilage-bone injury to the superolateral pole of the patella may produce this radiographic picture and have equated this condition to Larsen-Johansson disease in the inferior patellar area and Osgood-Schlatter disease in the tibial tubercle.[97] Healing may be somewhat compromised in the superolateral patella, which has less vascular supply than the remainder of the patella.[116] Although the radiographs may demonstrate a lack of osseous union, visual inspection of the articular surface of the patella during arthrotomy usually does not show evidence of discontinuity.

If tenderness exists in the superolateral patella and the radiographs show a bipartite patella at the point of tenderness, immobilization with a knee immobilizer or cast is indicated for 2 to 3 weeks. If symptoms persist for several weeks or months after conservative treatment has been started, excision of the small fragment is indicated.[12] After using a small incision to split the vastus lateralis patellar attachment, returning to sports within 1 to 2 months postoperatively appears feasible.[95] Internal fixation with a screw may be more appropriate than fragment excision if the bipartite pa-

tella region is large and has a significant articular component.

Popliteal Cyst

Popliteal cysts may arise de novo or may be associated with rheumatologic conditions that have associated knee effusions.

In one series, 61% of children with various types of arthritis and clinically detectable knee effusion were shown to have popliteal cysts by ultrasonography.[135] The size of the suprapatellar effusion correlated well with the presence of a popliteal cyst, and all cysts resolved in the children whose arthritis symptoms improved.

The orthopaedist commonly sees a popliteal cyst in a child without a history of arthritis. The cyst is usually painless and has often been noticed by a parent during a bath. On clinical examination, the cyst is a nontender mass that arises between the medial head of the gastrocnemius and the semimembranosus. The cyst commonly transilluminates. If the location of what appears to be a popliteal cyst is not on the medial aspect of the popliteum, other diagnoses should be considered; the foremost is a soft tissue tumor.

Radiographs are normal, unless the child has coexisting, long-standing arthritis. Ultrasound evaluation is excellent in determining the size and location of the cyst and can be used on a serial basis to document changes in size.[135] An MRI evaluation also can outline the cyst and help differentiate a fluid-filled cyst from a solid tumor, but it is indicated primarily when the popliteal mass is not in the classic posteromedial position.

If the popliteal cyst is in the characteristic medial location and there is no coexisting arthritis, no immediate treatment is needed. Periodic follow-up examinations, with documentation of clinical measurement, are appropriate, because many of these cysts resolve within a few years of the initial diagnosis.[30] If the cyst continues to enlarge, is painful, or is located in a position other than the medial posterior knee, further workup with an MR scan is indicated. Surgical excision through a transverse posterior incision should be curative for enlarging or symptomatic cysts.

Osteochondritis Dissecans

Osteochondritis dissecans involves the articular cartilage and a small amount of underlying bone in the distal femur. The bone portion becomes avascular, for reasons that remain unclear, and the overlying cartilage becomes involved secondarily. The involved fragment sometimes displaces from the femoral condyle and becomes a loose body.

Multiple episodes of localized trauma may play a role, particularly in the most commonly involved area, the lateral aspect of the medial femoral condyle, where the tibial spine may abut. The vascular supply in the femoral condyles tends to consist of end arteries, and this lack of collateral circulation is thought to make portions of the femoral condyles susceptible to repetitive trauma or to emboli of erythrocytes or fat.[58] Familial incidence has been reported. A finite element model of forces at the knee has demonstrated that the deformation that occurs during knee flexion, especially with flexion past 60 degrees, leads to more distortion at the lateral side of the medial condyle than in the lateral condyle itself. Because this is the most common site for osteochondritis dissecans, the stress concentration may be important in generating osteochondritis dissecans.[92]

Osteochondritis dissecans may be discovered as an incidental finding or may be found when the child or teenager complains of knee pain after or during activity. If a history of the knee locking or swelling is obtained, a loose body should be suspected.

On physical examination, tenderness may be experienced directly over the femoral condyle when the knee is in a fully flexed position. Quadriceps atrophy is common. Pain may be elicited by flexing the knee fully, internally rotating the leg, and then gradually extending the knee. If pain is present at about 30 degrees of flexion, osteochondritis dissecans is commonly present.[148]

Imaging studies must be interpreted with some caution, because a variety of normal ossification patterns occur in the distal femur of one half of normal children and may masquerade as a pathologic condition.[17] In addition to the normal anteroposterior and lateral radiographs of the knee, a tunnel view, with the knee flexed 20 to 30 degrees, allows the diagnosis of osteochondritis dissecans to be confirmed (Fig. 27-13A). Although the most common location of osteochondritis dissecans is on the lateral portion of the medial femoral condyle, this condition may occur in almost any portion of the posterior one half of either femoral condyle. This condition may appear radiographically bilateral in the distal femurs, even if only one is symptomatic.

Bone scans may be helpful in determining whether treatment is needed. The isotope uptake may localize to the osteochondritic lesion, to the femoral

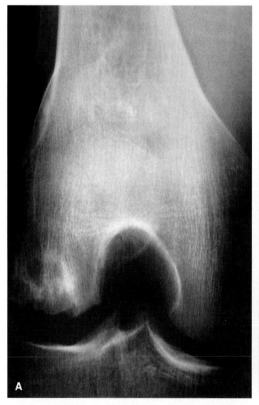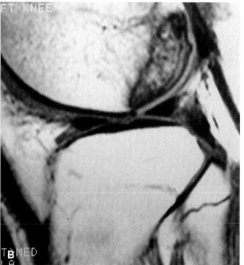

FIGURE 27-13. (A) A tunnel-view anteroposterior radiograph of the knee in a teenager with osteochondritis dissecans demonstrates the advantage of using this view to make the diagnosis, because most of these lesions occur on the posterior half of the femoral condyle. (B) Magnetic resonance imaging demonstrates the cartilage and marrow changes associated with osteochondritis dissecans, as seen in the sagittal plane.

condyle, or to both. Four stages have been described, and increased isotope uptake has been interpreted as a favorable sign for healing.[18] However, it has been suggested that a more accurate method for determining viability of the osteochondritis dissecans fragment is computerized blood flow analysis, using technetium 99m (^{99m}Tc) isotope injection. The information gained allows the clinician to choose continued observation or surgical treatment.[79]

MRI can demonstrate the extent of the area of osteochondritis dissecans involvement most clearly, because changes in the marrow and the cartilage can be seen (Fig. 27-13B). The stability of the lesion, as an indicator for the need of surgical treatment, may be predicted by MRI.[28] The accuracy of the MRI-based diagnosis of osteochondritis dissecans is enhanced by intraarticular injection of gadolinium.[71] MRI also allows evaluation of the menisci and ligaments to help ascertain what the cause of knee pain is, because many of the osteochondritis dissecans lesions are asymptomatic. MRI can be useful postoperatively to assess healing and articular cartilage integrity.[123] Treatment results based on MRI classification have not been reported. The dynamic imaging technique of arthrography is used less often than MRI, but the older technique can demonstrate whether the articular cartilage is intact or if the osteochondritic piece is loose, as evidenced by dye passing deep to the articular surface.

Appropriate treatment methods for osteochondritis dissecans range from simple periodic observation to surgical care. In general, success in obtaining healing of these defects is better before physeal closure in the subgroup classified as juvenile osteochondritis dissecans.[18,19,58] Both knees of a child may demonstrate osteochondritis dissecans on radiographs, although only one may be symptomatic. The larger lesions located on the condylar weight-bearing surface have the poorest prognosis. Although the age of the patient and the location and size of the lesion are important to the prognosis, the primary reason to treat this condition is the amount of pain the child or teenager is experiencing.

If osteochondritis dissecans is discovered as an incidental finding, with no knee pain, the only treatment is the education of the patient and parents to return for evaluation if knee pain or swelling occurs after physical activity. Routine radiographic follow-up is not needed if this area remains asymptomatic. Sports activity is allowed if the knee remains free of pain.

If the knee is painful and the lesion still appears intact on radiographs, limitation of sports activity, isometric quadriceps strengthening exercises, and symptomatic use of a knee immobilizer is prescribed. I do not use a cast for this condition, because the end point to casting is impossible to delineate clearly and more

thigh muscle atrophy occurs with casting than with periodic knee immobilizer use. A graduated return to sports activity is allowed as long as no pain or effusion develops.

If pain or an effusion persists after several weeks or months of activity limitation or if the osteochondritic fragment has separated from the femoral condyle, arthroscopic examination of the knee is indicated. At the time of arthroscopy, the involved region is evaluated for articular cartilage appearance and the presence of fragment movement with instrument probing. Commonly, the articular cartilage appears dull compared with adjacent condylar cartilage. If the fragment is stable or has only minor movement, arthroscopically assisted drilling of the lesion multiple times with a Kirschner wire can accelerate healing and allow an early return to athletic activity.[14] If the fragment can be flapped open, the bony base can be roughened with a bur, and the fragment is anchored in place by buried Kirschner wires or small screws.[2,24,58] The use of tibial bone pegs for this fixation has been suggested as a more physiologic means of fragment fixation.[123] Postoperative activity is limited until early healing is present. If a small loose body has separated from a non–weight-bearing portion of the femoral condyle, the loose body is removed arthroscopically and the lesion base drilled. If a large loose body is found, particularly if this has separated from the weight-bearing aspect of the femoral condyle, drilling the defect base and replacement of the loose body with internal fixation are indicated.

Later degenerative arthritis of the involved femoral condyle is primarily a problem with large osteochondritis dissecans lesions that are present on the weight-bearing portion of the articular cartilage, particularly if flattening of the femoral condyle has occurred or if a large loose body has separated and has not been treated in a timely fashion.

Discoid Lateral Meniscus

The cause for the existence of a pancake-like lateral meniscus, instead of a doughnut-like meniscal ring, is unclear. No embryologic or comparative anatomic studies have demonstrated the normal appearance of a disc-like lateral meniscus in early fetal development, and the youngest reported child with this condition was 6 months of age. Occurrence may be unilateral or bilateral, with an incidence of 1% to 5% in the general population. In a consecutive series of 1000 symptomatic meniscal lesions treated arthroscopically in teenagers and adults, 5% of the lateral meniscal lesions were associated with a discoid meniscus.[26]

The two primary types of discoid lateral meniscus are the complete type and the Wrisberg ligament or Wrisberg variant type.[29] Some classifications include an incomplete type, but this differs from the complete type only in size estimate at the time of arthroscopic examination, and treatment is the same as for the complete type. The complete type is the most common, and the Wrisberg variant type is symptomatic in a larger percentage of cases. A primary differentiating feature is the presence (complete type) or absence (Wrisberg ligament type) of the posterior coronary ligament attachments from the meniscus to the tibial plateau posteriorly and laterally. In the Wrisberg ligament type, the Wrisberg ligament (or the lateral meniscofemoral ligament) pulls the lateral meniscus medially into the intercondylar notch during knee extension, with the meniscus reducing laterally as the knee is flexed. The same symptoms and signs as those of a discoid meniscus are present, even though the lateral meniscus in the Wrisberg variant type is not discoid itself. The Wrisberg variant type has been reported only in children younger than 16 years of age.[29]

The complete type often is asymptomatic and may be noticed during the evaluation for pain in other parts of the knee. If a tear has occurred in this type of discoid meniscus, catching or popping of the knee may be noticed by the patient. This condition may be associated with lateral joint line tenderness. A patient with the Wrisberg ligament type may present with or without pain, but the knee always has an audible click with movement and a palpable snap laterally as the knee nears full extension. With either type, the child may walk with a flexed knee to avoid the pain of full extension. In a series of 68 children and teenagers who underwent knee arthroscopy for knee pain, the preoperative diagnosis most often erroneously made was that of discoid lateral meniscus; the lesson is that other intraarticular abnormalities in this age group should be carefully considered as well.[133]

The knee radiograph may be normal or there may be slight widening of the lateral joint space on the anteroposterior view. Although the diagnosis can be made by arthrography, MR studies are more commonly used to confirm the clinical suspicion, with the coronal cuts at the midcondylar level demonstrating the discoid meniscus (Fig. 27-14).[122]

The absence of a central depression in the discoid lateral meniscus for the lateral femoral condyle to fit may cause no problem. However, the posterolateral quarter of the discoid meniscus in the complete type appears to be more susceptible to tearing with time. In the Wrisberg ligament type, hypertrophy of the posterior horn has been documented, as have articular cartilage changes on the lateral femoral condyle over which the meniscus snaps. Although tears of the complete type are the cause for symptoms, instability of the Wrisberg ligament type may produce symptoms without a meniscal tear.[29]

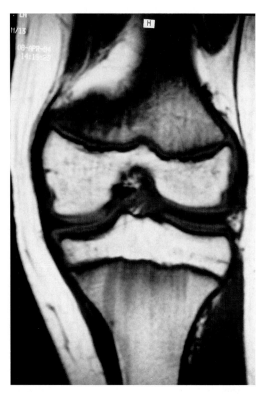

FIGURE 27-14.   A coronal view of a knee in this child demonstrates the findings typical of a discoid lateral meniscus on magnetic resonance imaging.

If an asymptomatic discoid lateral meniscus is found as an incidental finding, no treatment is needed. If symptoms are present in a knee with pain and snapping, nonoperative treatment has little to offer. An arthroscopic examination can detect a meniscal tear and assess possible meniscal stability. Because removal of a nondiscoid lateral meniscus in childhood commonly leads to early osteoarthritis of the lateral knee compartment, partial central meniscectomy appears to be an attractive choice in patients of this age group who have a lateral meniscal tear.[142] However, some reports have demonstrated better short-term results with total or near-total meniscectomy in this situation than those obtained by removing only the central and torn segment.[60] Nonetheless, for a tear of a complete or incomplete type discoid meniscus, arthroscopically assisted partial central meniscectomy, including resection of the torn segment, leaving a 6- to 8-mm rim of normal meniscus peripherally, is preferred to total meniscectomy if the posterior attachment of the discoid meniscus is stable.[1] There is, however, a significant incidence of repeat meniscal tears in the peripheral discoid meniscus rim left after central meniscal removal.[132] If the Wrisberg ligament type of meniscus has a tear, the torn segment requires removal in a total or subtotal manner, as feasible. If this type of discoid meniscus is not torn, reconstruction by suturing the lateral meniscus to the posterolateral capsule at the level of the tibial plateau is preferred and is often successful in avoiding meniscectomy and preventing future tears.[93]

TIBIAL DISORDERS

Toddler's Fracture of the Tibia

A toddler's fracture of the tibia should be suspected as a possible cause of acute limping in a child between 1 and 4 years of age.[87] The injury causing this fracture is often unwitnessed, and the parents may not be aware of an injury having occurred. In one study of 500 acutely limping infants and toddlers, 20% had positive bone scans indicative of fracture, and the most common site was the tibia.[102]

On clinical presentation, the child refuses to walk, or the child limps. Pain from palpation over the fractured area may lead to the child crying or withdrawing the leg from the examiner. The fracture is stable, and a deformity is not seen. Localized edema may be present. Radiographs may be diagnostic, with this middle to distal tibial fracture seen best on the internal oblique view and the anteroposterior view (Fig. 27-15). This fracture is difficult to see on the lateral radiograph.[136] If radiographs are normal, a ^{99m}Tc bone scan can demonstrate the fracture.

The initial step in treatment is to rule out child abuse as the cause of the acute limping. The radiographic pattern seen with toddler's fracture, which is a spiral, nondisplaced fracture of the distal one half of the tibia, is not the most common fracture seen in child abuse; the more common patterns of fracture include a midshaft transverse fracture and a proximal metaphyseal tibial fracture. Nonetheless, a skeletal survey may be indicated, particularly in 1- or 2-year-old children with toddler's fractures.

Treatment is cast immobilization for a few weeks. The child usually begins to walk on the cast within several days of initial immobilization. After cast removal, radiographs demonstrate periosteal callus at the fracture site and can confirm the diagnosis if casting was empirically chosen as treatment for a young child with an acute limp. No long-term sequelae of this injury are expected.

Stress Fracture of the Proximal and Middle Tibia

Stress fractures of the tibia occur primarily in teenagers who are training for a sport or participating actively in a competitive sport situation. It is unusual to see

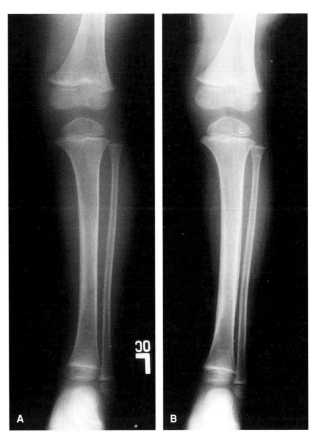

FIGURE 27-15. (**A**) The anteroposterior radiograph of the tibia in a 3-year-old patient with the onset of a limp demonstrates findings typical of a toddler's fracture. (**B**) After 3 weeks of casting, the fracture is healed, and periosteal new bone is evident.

this injury in children who are preadolescent or younger. The physician should consider this condition essentially an overuse syndrome.

Although the controversy about whether bone density must be subnormal to produce a stress fracture remains unanswered, these injuries occur in healthy-appearing teenagers active in athletic activities. Those who participate in volleyball and long-distance running activities are vulnerable to this injury.[46,105] Hip external rotation of more than 65 degrees is a risk factor for tibial stress fractures in young military recruits.[42] Among teenagers, females are most likely to be affected.[109] Bone density in teenage females begins to decrease early naturally in adolescence and is further diminished by exercise-induced amenorrhea, and this may help explain the increased incidence of tibial stress fractures in young females.

The teenager usually presents with leg pain that begins shortly after the running activity commences. This pain usually has existed for several weeks and is interfering with the patient's desired sports activity. Most have already tried stretching before running, and many have tried different shoes before the orthopaedist is consulted. On examination, the tibia may be tender along the proximal to middle tibial region, but often pain is absent in the office. If symptoms have been present for several weeks, a bony prominence without soft tissue mass may be palpated.

Within the first several days, radiographic studies do not usually demonstrate the fracture itself, but later, they clearly show the new bone produced in response to a stress fracture. Thickening of the tibial cortex, particularly in the posterior and medial aspects of the proximal and middle tibia, is almost diagnostic of a stress fracture. Nonunions may happen at the site of stress fractures but are unusual in growing children.

In the initial stages, a ^{99m}Tc bone scan may establish a diagnosis of stress fracture, even if the radiographs are normal, with the increased isotope uptake typically extending through both cortices. Increased isotope uptake at the fracture site can be demonstrated within 1 or 2 days of the initial symptoms. CT scans can help establish the diagnosis of a stress fracture when actual fracture lines are seen.[152] Because the response to a tibial stress fracture may extend throughout a large segment of the bone marrow in the intramedullary canal, MRI may produce images strongly suggestive of a malignancy, especially Ewing sarcoma. MR scans therefore are not as useful for most cases of suspected stress fracture of the tibia as radiographs and bone scans.[56,82]

In cases of running athletes, shin splints should be considered in the differential diagnosis. Shin splints probably result from a mild compartment syndrome in the anterolateral compartments of the leg. Shin splints usually occur in the anterolateral aspect of the leg, and stress fractures tend to occur more proximally. If the diagnosis is difficult to establish, a treadmill test with pressure monitors in the anterior and lateral muscle compartments of the leg may demonstrate increased compartment pressure during running and rule out the possibility of a stress fracture.

If the diagnosis of a tibial stress fracture is confirmed with imaging studies, treatment is directed toward immobilizing the tibia adequately to allow healing. Traditionally, this has been accomplished by a few weeks of long-leg cast immobilization and avoidance of sports activity until pain and tenderness subside. However, success in controlling the pain from a tibial stress fracture and allowing return to athletic training within 1 week was achieved by using a pneumatic leg brace instead of a cast.[147] If the bone density of female teenagers is significantly decreased compared with age-matched controls, daily calcium supplements are recommended. After healing occurs, sports activity can be resumed with no significant limitations.

Posteromedial Bowing of the Tibia

Posteromedial bowing of the tibia and the fibula is an unusual condition. It is recognized at birth by the angulation of the lower leg. The cause remains unknown. The foot is initially in a position of marked dorsiflexion at the ankle and may be confused with a severe example of calcaneovalgus due to fetal positioning (Fig. 27-16). There is no evidence that casting, bracing, manipulation, or stretching exercises have any effect on the natural history of this condition, although casting to improve the foot position in infancy may be appropriate.[55,104] Complete or partial remodeling of the angulation is anticipated as growth occurs.

Unlike anterolateral bowing of the tibia (see Chap. 9), posteromedial bowing does not predispose to fracture of the tibia and is not associated with neurofibromatosis. The primary functional orthopaedic feature associated with posteromedial bowing of the tibia is a leg length discrepancy caused by shortening of the tibia. The greater the bowing at birth, the more tibial shortening will result. In one series of 33 children with this condition, the final leg length discrepancy varied between 3.3 and 6.9 cm.[104] In another group of 13 children, the mean discrepancy was 3.1 cm (range, 1.9–5.6 cm).[55]

The leg length discrepancy may be related to asymmetrical forces across the physis as a result of bowing. Nonetheless, even if the bowing improves, there continues to be a progressive leg length discrepancy with increasing age in most children.[55] Because this leg length discrepancy also occurs in children treated early with realignment osteotomy, the precise cause of the shorter leg remains unclear. Although some degree of muscle atrophy of the posterior muscles of the leg has been associated with smaller calf measurements in these children,[104] muscle strength

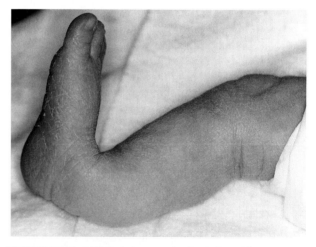

FIGURE 27-16.   Clinical photograph of an infant with posteromedial bowing of the tibia. The foot is in calcaneovalgus.

has been indistinguishable from the uninvolved leg.[55] Although initially the calcaneovalgus foot position gives the appearance of excessive foot dorsiflexion at the ankle, in older children, there appears some limitation of dorsiflexion associated with a smaller foot size.[55]

Radiographs are used to measure the initial degree of angulation and to document the amount of correction that occurs with growth. Scanograms should be periodically obtained, beginning no later than at 5 or 6 years of age, to allow plotting the leg lengths on growth charts to time potential later epiphyseodesis or leg lengthening surgery, depending on the final leg length discrepancy predicted. A shoe lift on the short side may be preferred by some of the children with the larger discrepancies.

The most common surgical procedure used in posteromedial bowing of the tibia is an epiphyseodesis of the contralateral proximal tibia at an appropriate time, predicted by the standard growth charts of Moseley or Green-Anderson.[55,104] Although remodeling may not be complete, the residual angulation usually is not a functional problem. If osteotomy is considered necessary, the valgus is probably more important to correct than the posterior bowing, because the child usually already has some limitation of ankle dorsiflexion. After osteotomy, bone healing appears to be normal in this condition, unlike that seen after osteotomy of a tibia with anterolateral bowing. If the leg length discrepancy is sufficient to recommend tibial lengthening, the residual angular deformity can be corrected at the same time. Long-term functional problems with this condition have not been reported.

IDIOPATHIC TOE WALKING

When a young child first begins to walk, toe walking is common and is considered within the broad range of normal, particularly if the child can stand with the foot flat when not walking. The number of children who are normal toe walkers gradually decreases as age increases. As a part of the development of normal gait, heel strike should occur by 3 years of age,[134] and persistent toe walking past this age is not usually normal. For toe walkers older than 3 years of age, it is important to rule out neurologic causes, particularly mild cerebral palsy. If the neurologic workup is normal and the child continues to toe walk bilaterally, the most likely associated finding with "idiopathic" toe walking is a shortened tendo Achilles.

The child usually presents because of parental concern about persistent toe walking. The medical history is important in this setting. A history of prematurity, low Apgar scores, or delayed motor milestones

should be sought. The family should be quizzed about other family members that walked on their toes until middle childhood, because this condition often is familial.[64]

The physical examination is primarily targeted to detect minor neurologic abnormalities and should include evaluation of stretch responses of the hips and feet to estimate hyperreflexia or the presence of ankle clonus. The calf should be palpated for masses, because intramuscular lesions, such as a hemangioma, can lead to equinus, although this would typically be unilateral. The maximal amount of passive dorsiflexion at the ankle, with the knee flexed and with the knee extended, should be documented with a goniometer. When testing dorsiflexion, the heel should be kept out of valgus to avoid midfoot dorsiflexion.

The initial treatment of idiopathic toe walking is to provide an adequate amount of ankle dorsiflexion to allow a normal heel-toe gait pattern. This requires at least 10 degrees of ankle dorsiflexion. Stretching casts, placing the foot into the maximal dorsiflexion possible, are applied and changed weekly for a few weeks until this range of dorsiflexion is achieved. Night braces, with the foot dorsiflexed at the ankle, may be helpful to maintain this amount of dorsiflexion. As long as this degree of dorsiflexion is maintained, the child may walk during the day without orthotic support. Eventually, most of the children begin to walk with a more normal heel-toe gait, although this may take several years and may be achieved by partial external rotation of the leg. Surgical heel cord lengthening improves ankle motion but should usually be delayed for several years to allow the child to assume a more normal walking pattern, provided the diagnosis of cerebral palsy has been adequately excluded. Extreme care should be exercised to avoid overlengthening the heel cord, which produces a calcaneus gait.

In some instances, computerized gait analysis may be helpful to differentiate an idiopathic toe walker from a child with mild cerebral palsy. The results of dynamic electromyography used alone to differentiate these conditions have been variable. Although some researchers have demonstrated no difference between children with cerebral palsy and idiopathic toe walkers or normal children asked to toe walk,[64] others have demonstrated out-of-phase muscle activity in the gastrocnemius soleus muscle in toe-walking cerebral palsy patients, although the same electromyographic data for toe-walking children with a congenital short tendo Achilles were in phase and normal.[103] Kinematic data demonstrate the lack of heel strike in both groups, but in the cerebral palsy patient, the absence of heel strike is associated with sustained knee flexion at terminal swing phase to a greater degree than is seen in idiopathic toe walkers.[52] The combined kinematic and electromyographic data, as obtained in most computerized gait analysis laboratories, seems to offer a reasonable means to differentiate between these two conditions.

References

1. Aichroth PM, Patel DV, Marx CL. Congenital discoid lateral meniscus in children: a follow-up study and evolution of management. J Bone Joint Surg [Am] 1991;73:932.

2. Anderson AF, Lipscomb AB, Coulam C. Antegrade curettement, bone grafting and pinning of osteochondritis dissecans in the skeletally mature knee. Am J Sports Med 1990;18:254.

3. Badelon O, Bensahel H, Folinais D, Lassale B. Tibiofibular torsion from the fetal period until birth. J Pediatr Orthop 1989;9:169.

4. Balthazar DA, Pappas AM. Acquired valgus deformity of the tibia in children. J Pediatr Orthop 1984;4:538.

5. Barlow DW, Staheli LT. Effects of lateral rotation splinting on lower extremity bone growth: an in vivo study in rabbits. J Pediatr Orthop 1991;11:583.

6. Beck CL, Burke SW, Roberts JM, et al. Physeal bridge resection in infantile Blount disease. J Pediatr Orthop 1987;7:161.

7. Bell MJ, Atkins RM, Sharrard WJ. Irreducible congenital dislocation of the knee. Aetiology and management. J Bone Joint Surg [Br] 1987;69:403.

8. Bell SN, Campbell PE, Cole WG, Menalaus MB. Tibia vara caused by focal fibrocartilaginous dysplasia: three case reports. J Bone Joint Surg [Br] 1985;67:780.

9. Bensahel H, Dal Monte A, Hjelmstedt A, et al. Congenital dislocation of the knee. J Pediatr Orthop 1989;9:174.

10. Binazzi R, Felli L, Vaccare V, Borelli P. Surgical treatment of unresolved Osgood-Schlatter lesion. Clin Orthop Rel Res 1993;289:202.

11. Bowen JR, Torres RR, Forlin E. Partial epiphysiodesis to address genu varum or genu valgum. J Pediatr Orthop 1992;12:359.

12. Bourne MH, Bianco AJ. Bipartite patella in the adolescent: results of surgical excision. J Pediatr Orthop 1990;10:69.

13. Bradish CF, Davies SJM, Malone M. Tibia vara due to focal fibrocartilaginous dysplasia: the natural history. J Bone Joint Surg [Br] 1988;70:106.

14. Bradley J, Dandy DJ. Results of drilling osteochondritis dissecans before skeletal maturity. J Bone Joint Surg [Br] 1989;71:642.

15. Bradway JK, Klassen RA, Peterson HA. Blount disease: a review of the English literature. J Pediatr Orthop 1987;7:472.

16. Brougham DI, Nicol RO. Valgus deformity after proximal tibial fractures in children. J Bone Joint Surg [Br] 1987;69:482.

17. Caffey J, Madell SH, Royer C, et al. Ossification of the distal femoral epiphysis. J Bone Joint Surg 1958;40:647.

18. Cahill BR, Berg BC. 99m-Technetium phosphate compound joint scintigraphy in the management of juvenile osteochondritis dissecans of the femoral condyles. Am J Sports Med 1983;11:329.

19. Cahill BR, Phillips MR, Navarro R. The results of conservative management of juvenile osteochondritis dissecans using joint scintigraphy. A prospective study. Am J Sports Med 1989;17:601.

20. Cahuzac J-P, Autefage A, Fayolle P, et al. Exaggerated femoral anteversion and acetabular development: experimental study in growing dogs. J Pediatr Orthop 1989;9:163.

21. Carter JR, Leeson MC, Thompson GH, et al. Late-onset tibia vara: a histopathologic analysis. A comparative evaluation with infantile tibia vara and slipped capital femoral epiphysis. J Pediatr Orthop 1988;8:187.

22. Cook SD, Lavernia CJ, Burke SW, et al. A biomechanical analysis of the etiology of tibia vara. J Pediatr Orthop 1983;3:449.

23. Cozen L. Fracture of proximal portion of tibia in children followed by valgus deformity. Surg Gynecol Obstet 1953;97:183.

24. Cugat R, Garcia M, Cusco X, et al. Osteochondritis dissecans: a historical review and its treatment with cannulated screws. Arthroscopy 1993;9:675.

25. Curtis BH, Fisher RL. Congenital hyperextension with anterior subluxation of the knee: surgical treatment and long-term observations. J Bone Joint Surg [Am] 1964;51:255.

26. Dandy DJ. The arthroscopic anatomy of symptomatic meniscal lesions. J Bone Joint Surg [Br] 1990;72:628.

27. DeFlaviis L, Nessi R, Scaglione P, et al. Ultrasonic diagnosis of Osgood-Schlatter and Sinding-Larsen-Johansson diseases of the knee. Skeletal Radiol 1989;18:193.

28. DeSmet AA, Fisher DR, Graf BK, Lange RH. Osteochondritis dissecans of the knee: value of MR imaging in determining lesion stability and the presence of articular cartilage defects. AJR 1990;155:549.

29. Dickhaut SC, DeLee JC. The discoid lateral-meniscus syndrome. J Bone Joint Surg [Am] 1982;64:1068.

30. Dietz FR, Weinstein SL. Spike osteotomy for angular deformities of the long bones in children. J Bone Joint Surg [Am] 1988;70:848.

31. Dinham JM. Popliteal cysts in children: the case against surgery. J Bone Joint Surg [Br] 1975;57:69.

32. Drennan JC. Congenital dislocation of the knee and patella. Instr Course Lect 1993;42:517.

33. Eckhoff D, Kramer R, Alongi C, et al. Femoral anteversion and arthritis of the knee. J Pediatr Orthop 1994;14:608.

34. Fabry G, MacEwen GD, Shands AR Jr. Torsion of the femur, a follow-up study in normal and abnormal conditions. J Bone Joint Surg [Am] 1973;55:1726.

35. Feldman MD, Schoenecker PL. Use of the metaphyseal-diaphyseal angle in the evaluation of bowed legs. J Bone Joint Surg [Am] 1993;75:1602.

36. Ferris B, Aichroth P. The treatment of congenital knee dislocation. A review of nineteen knees. Clin Orthop Rel Res 1987;216:135.

37. Ferriter P, Shapiro F. Infantile tibia vara factors affecting outcome following proximal tibial osteotomy. J Pediatr Orthop 1987;7:1.

38. Foreman KA, Robertson WW Jr. Radiographic measurement of infantile tibia vara. J Pediatr Orthop 1985;5:452.

39. Gage JR. Gait analysis in cerebral palsy. London: MacKeith Press, 1991:106.

40. Gao GX, Lee EH, Bose K. Surgical management of congenital and habitual dislocation of the patella. J Pediatr Orthop 1990;10:255.

41. Gelberman RH, Cohen MS, Shaw BA, et al. The association of femoral retroversion with slipped capital femoral epiphysis. J Bone Joint Surg [Am] 1986;68:1000.

42. Giladi M, Milgrom C, Stein M, et al. External rotation of the hip: a predictor of risk for stress fractures. Clin Orthop Rel Res 1987;216:131.

43. Green WT Jr. Painful bipartite patellae. Clin Orthop Rel Res 1975;110:197.

44. Greene WB. Infantile tibia vara. J Bone Joint Surg [Am] 1993;75:130.

45. Gregosiewicz A, Wosko I, Kandzierski G, Drabik Z. Double-elevating osteotomy of tibiae in the treatment of severe cases of Blount's disease. J Pediatr Orthop 1989;9:178.

46. Ha KI, Hahn SH, Chung MY, et al. A clinical study of stress fractures in sports activities. Orthopedics 1991;14:1089.

47. Heath CH, Staheli LT. Normal limits of knee angle in white

children—genu varum and genu valgum. J Pediatr Orthop 1993;13:259.

48. Heinrich SD, Sharps CH. Lower extremity torsional deformities in children: a prospective comparison of two treatment modalities. Orthopedics 1991;14:655.

49. Henderson RC, Greene WB. Etiology of late-onset tibia vara: is varus alignment a prerequisite? J Pediatr Orthop 1994;14:143.

50. Henderson RC, Kemp GJ Jr, Greene WB. Adolescent tibia vara: alternatives for operative treatment. J Bone Joint Surg [Am] 1992;74:342.

51. Henderson RC, Kemp GJ, Hayes PRL. Prevalence of late-onset tibia vara. J Pediatr Orthop 1993;13:255.

52. Henderson RC, Lechner CT, DeMasi RA, Greene WB. Variability in radiographic measurement of bowleg deformity in children. J Pediatr Orthop 1990;10:491.

53. Hicks R, Durinick N, Gage JR. Differentiation of idiopathic toe-walking and cerebral palsy. J Pediatr Orthop 1988;8:160.

54. Hoffer MM, Prietto C, Koffman M. Supracondylar derotational osteotomy of the femur for internal rotation of the thigh in the cerebral palsied child. J Bone Joint Surg [Am] 1981;63:389.

55. Hofmann A, Wenger DR. Posteromedial bowing of the tibia: progression of discrepancy in leg lengths. J Bone Joint Surg [Am] 1981;63:384.

56. Horev G, Korenreich L, Ziv N, Grunebaum M. The enigma of stress fractures in the pediatric age: clarification or confusion through the new imaging modalities. Pediatr Radiol 1990; 20:469.

57. Hubbard DD, Staheli LT, Chew DE, Mosca VS. Medial femoral torsion and osteoarthritis. J Pediatr Orthop 1988;8:540.

58. Hughston JC, Hergenroeder PT, Courtenay BG. Osteochondritis dissecans of the femoral condyle. J Bone Joint Surg [Am] 1984;66:1340.

59. Hutter CG, Scott W. Tibial torsion. J Bone Joint Surg [Am] 1949;31:511.

60. Ikeuchi H. Arthroscopic treatment of the discoid lateral meniscus. Technique and long-term results. Clin Orthop Rel Res 1982;167:19.

61. Iwaya T, Sakaguchi R, Tsuyama N. The treatment of congenital dislocation of the knee with the Pavlik harness. Int Orthop 1983;7:25.

62. Johnson E, Audell R, Oppenheim WL. Congenital dislocation of the knee. J Pediatr Orthop 1987;7:194.

63. Jordan SE, Alonso JE, Cook PF. The etiology of valgus angulation after metaphyseal fractures of the tibia in children. J Pediatr Orthop 1987;7:450.

64. Kalen V, Adler N, Bleck EE. Electromyography of idiopathic toe walking. J Pediatr Orthop 1986;6:31.

65. Kane TJ, Henry G, Furry DL. A simple roentgenographic measurement of femoral anteversion: a short note. J Bone Joint Surg [Am] 1992;74:1540.

66. Kariya Y, Taniguchi K, Yagisawa H, Ooi Y. Focal fibrocartilaginous dysplasia: consideration of healing process. J Pediatr Orthop 1991;11:545.

67. Katz K, Krikler R, Wielunsky E, Merbob P. Effect of neonatal posture on later lower limb rotation and gait in premature infants. J Pediatr Orthop 1991;11:520.

68. Katz K, Naor N, Merlob P, Wielunsky E. Rotational deformities of the tibia and foot in preterm infants. J Pediatr Orthop 1990; 10:483.

69. Kitaoka HB, Weiner DS, Cook AJ, et al. Relationship between femoral anteversion and osteoarthritis of the hip. J Pediatr Orthop 1989;9:396.

70. Knittle G, Staheli LT. The effectiveness of shoe modification for in-toeing. Orthop Clin North Am 1976;7:1019.

71. Kramer J, Stigibauer R, Engel A, et al. MR contrast arthrography (MRA) in osteochondritis dissecans. J Comput Assist Tomogr 1992;16:254.

72. Krause BL, Williams JP, Catterall A. Natural history of Osgood-Schlatter disease. J Pediatr Orthop 1990;10:65.

73. Krengel WF, Staheli LT. Tibial rotational osteotomy for idiopathic torsion. A comparison of the proximal and distal osteotomy levels. Clin Orthop Rel Res 1992;283:285.

74. Kruse RW, Bowen JR, Heithoff S. Oblique tibial osteotomy in the correction of tibial deformity in children. J Pediatr Orthop 1989;9:476.

75. Kujala UM, Kvist M, Heinonen O. Osgood Schlatter's disease in adolescent athletes. Retrospective study of incidence and duration. Am J Sports Med 1985;13:236.

76. Langenskiold A. Tibia vara (osteochondrosis deformans tibiae). A survey of 23 cases. Acta Chir Scand 1952;103:1.

77. Langenskiold A. Tibia vara: a critical review. Clin Orthop Rel Res 1989;246:195.

78. Levine AM, Drennan JC. Physiological bowing and tibia vara. The metaphyseal-diaphyseal angle in the measurement of bowleg deformities. J Bone Joint Surg [Am] 1982;64:1158.

79. Litchman HM, McMullough RW, Bandsman EJ, Schatz SL. Computerized blood flow analysis for decision making in the treatment of osteochondritis dissecans. J Pediatr Orthop 1988;8:208.

80. Lynch MD, Walsh HP. Tibia recurvatum as a complication of Osgood-Schlatter's disease: a report of two cases. J Pediatr Orthop 1991;11:543.

81. Manouel M, Johnson LO. The role of fibular osteotomy in rotational osteotomy of the distal tibia. J Pediatr Orthop 1994;14:611.

82. Martin SD, Healey JH, Horowitz S. Stress fracture MRI. Orthopedics 1993;16:75.

83. Martin SD, Moran MC, Martin TL, Burke SW. Proximal tibial osteotomy with compression plate fixation for tibia vara. J Pediatr Orthop 1994;14:619.

84. Martinez AG, Weinstein SL, Maynard JA. Tibia vara: report of an unusual case. J Bone Joint Surg [Am] 1992;74:1250.

85. Matsen FA, III, Veith RG. Compartmental syndromes in children. J Pediatr Orthop 1981;1:33.

86. McCall RE, Lessenberry HB. Bilateral congenital dislocation of the patella. J Pediatr Orthop 1987;7:100.

87. Mellick LB, Reesor K. Spiral tibial fractures of children: a commonly accidental spiral long bone fracture. Am J Emerg Med 1990;8:234.

88. Medlar RC, Lyne ED. Sinding-Larsen-Johansson disease. Its etiology and natural history. J Bone Joint Surg [Am] 1978; 60:1113.

89. Mital MA, Matza RA, Cohen J. The so-called unresolved Osgood-Schlatter lesions. J Bone Joint Surg [Am] 1980;62:732.

90. Moreland MS. Morphological effects of torsion applied to growing bone: an in vivo study in rabbits. J Bone Joint Surg [Br] 1980;62:230.

91. Murphy SB, Simon SR, Kijewski PK, et al. Femoral anteversion. J Bone Joint Surg [Am] 1987;69:1169.

92. Nambu T, Basser B, Schneider E, et al. Deformation of the distal femur: a contribution towards the pathogenesis of osteochondrosis dissecans in the knee joint. J Biomech 1991; 24:421.

93. Neuschwander DC, Drez D Jr, Finney TP. Lateral meniscal variant with absence of the posterior coronary ligament. J Bone Joint Surg [Am] 1992;74:1186.

94. Nogi J, MacEwen GD. Congenital dislocation of the knee. J Pediatr Orthop 1982;2:509.

95. Ogata K. Pain bipartite patella. J Bone Joint Surg [Am] 1992;76:573.

96. Ogden JA. Radiology of postnatal skeletal development. X. Patella and tibial tuberosity. Skeletal Radiol 1984;11:246.

97. Ogden JA, McCarthy SM, Jokl P. The painful bipartite patella. J Pediatr Orthop 1982;2:263.

98. Ogden JA, Southwick WO. Osgood-Schlatter's disease and tibial tuberosity development. Clin Orthop Rel Res 1976;118:180.

99. Olney BW, Cole WG, Menalaus MB. Three additional cases of focal fibrocartilaginous dysplasia causing tibia vara. J Pediatr Orthop 1990;10:405.

100. Ooishi T, Sugioka Y, Matsumoto S, Fujii T. Congenital dislocation of the knee. Its pathologic features and treatment. Clin Orthop Rel Res 1993;287:187.

101. Oppenheim WL, Shayestehfar S, Salusky IB. Tibial physeal changes in renal osteodystrophy: lateral Blount's disease. J Pediatr Orthop 1992;12:774.

102. Oudjhane K, Newman B, Oh KS, et al. Occult fractures in preschool children. J Trauma 1988;28:858.

103. Papariello SG, Skinner SR. Dynamic electromyography analysis of habitual toe-walkers. J Pediatr Orthop 1985;5:171.

104. Pappas AM. Congenital posteromedial bowing of the tibia and fibula. J Pediatr Orthop 1984;4:525.

105. Paty JG Jr, Swafford D. Adolescent running injuries. J Adolesc Health Care 1984;5:87.

106. Payne LZ, DeLuca PA. Intertrochanteric versus supracondylar osteotomy for severe femoral anteversion. J Pediatr Orthop 1994;14:39.

107. Rab GT. Oblique tibial osteotomy for Blount's disease (tibia vara). J Pediatr Orthop 1988;8:715.

108. Rattey T, Hyndman J. Rotational osteotomies of the leg: tibia alone versus both tibia and fibula. J Pediatr Orthop 1994; 14:615.

109. Robert M, Khouri N, Carlioz H, Alain JL. Fractures of the proximal tibial metaphysis in children: review of a series of 25 cases. J Pediatr Orthop 1987;7:444.

110. Robertson WW Jr. Distal tibial deformity in bowlegs. J Pediatr Orthop 1987;7:324.

111. Rogers SP. A method for determining the angle of torsion of the neck of the femur. J Bone Joint Surg 1931;13:821.

112. Rosenberg ZS, Kawelblum M, Cheung YY, et al. Osgood-Schlatter lesion: fracture or tendinitis? Scintigraphic, CT, and MR imaging features. Radiology 1992;185:853.

113. Ruwe PA, Gage JR, Ozonoff MB, DeLuca PA. Clinical determination of femoral anteversion: a comparison with established techniques. J Bone Joint Surg [Am] 1992;74:820.

114. Salenius P, Vankka E. The development of the tibiofemoral angle in children. J Bone Joint Surg 1975;57:259.

115. Salter RB, Best TN. Pathogenesis of progressive valgus deformity following fractures of the proximal metaphyseal region of the tibia in young children. Instr Course Lect 1992;41:409.

116. Scapinelli R. Blood supply of the human patella. J Bone Joint Surg [Br] 1967;49:563.

117. Scheffer MM, Peterson JA. Opening-wedge osteotomy for angular deformities of long bones in children. J Bone Joint Surg [Am] 1994;76:325.

118. Schoenecker PL, Johnston R, Rich MM, Capelli AM. Elevation of the medial plateau of the tibia in the treatment of Blount disease. J Bone Joint Surg [Am] 1992;74:351.

119. Schrock RD. Peroneal nerve palsy following derotational osteotomies for tibial torsion. Clin Orthop Rel Res 1969;62:172.

120. Schwarze DJ, Denton JR. Normal values of neonatal lower limbs: an evaluation of 1000 neonates. J Pediatr Orthop 1993;13:758.

121. Sherry DD, Petty RE, Tredwell S, Schroeder ML. Histocompatibility antigens in Osgood-Schlatter disease. J Pediatr Orthop 1985;5:302.

122. Silverman JM, Mink JH, Deutsch AL. Discoid menisci of the knee: MR imaging appearance. Radiology 1989;173:351.

123. Slough JA, Noto AM, Schnidt TL. Tibial cortical bone peg fixation in osteochondritis dissecans of the knee. Clin Orthop Rel Res 1991;267:122.

124. Staheli LT. Lower positional deformity in infants and children: a review. J Pediatr Orthop 1990;10:559.

125. Staheli LT, Clawson DK, Hubbard DD. Medial femoral torsion: experience with operative treatment. Clin Orthop Rel Res 1980;146:222.

126. Staheli LT, Corbett M, Wyss C, King H. Lower-extremity rotational problems in children. Normal values to guide management. J Bone Joint Surg [Am] 1985;67:39.

127. Staheli LT. Rotational problems in children. J Bone Joint Surg [Am] 1993;75:939.

128. Stedman's Medical Dictionary. Baltimore: Williams & Wilkins, 1961.

129. Steel HH, Sandrow RE, Sullivan PD. Complications of tibial osteotomy in children for genu varum or valgum. J Bone Joint Surg [Am] 1971;53:1629.

130. Stricker SJ, Edwards PM, Tidwell MA. Langenskiold classification of tibia vara: an assessment of interobserver variability. J Pediatr Orthop 1994;14:152.

131. Stricker SJ, Faustgen JP. Radiographic measurement of bow-leg deformity: variability due to method and limb rotation. J Pediatr Orthop 1994;14:147.

132. Sugawara O, Miyatsu M, Yamashita I, et al. Problems with repeated arthroscopic surgery in the discoid meniscus. Arthroscopy 1991;7:68.

133. Suman RK, Stother IG, Illingworth G. Diagnostic arthroscopy of the knee in children. J Bone Joint Surg [Br] 1984;66:535.

134. Sutherland DH, Olshen R, Cooper L, Woo SLY. The development of mature gait. J Bone Joint Surg 1980;62:336.

135. Szer IS, Klein-Gitelman M, DeNardo BA, McCauley RG. Ultrasonography in the study of prevalence and clinical evolution of popliteal cysts in children with knee effusions. J Rheumatol 1992;19:458.

136. Tenenbein M, Reed MH, Black GB. The toddler's fracture revisited. Am J Emerg Med 1990;8:208.

137. Terjesen T, Benum P, Anda S, Svenningsen S. Increased femoral anteversion and osteoarthritis of the hip joint. Acta Orthop Scand 1982;53:571.

138. Tonnis D, Heinecke A. Diminished femoral antetorsion syndrome: a cause of pain and osteoarthritis. J Pediatr Orthop 1991;11:419.

139. Trail IA. Tibial sequestrectomy in the management of Osgood-Schlatter disease. J Pediatr Orthop 1988;8:554.

140. Traverso A, Beldare A, Cataleni F. The coexistence of Osgood-Schlatter's disease with Sinding-Larsen-Johansson's disease. Case report in an adolescent soccer player. J Sports Med Phys Fitness 1990;30:331.

141. Uhthoff HK, Ogata S. Early intrauterine presence of congenital dislocation of the knee. J Pediatr Orthop 1994;14:254.

142. Vandermeer RD, Cunningham FK. Arthroscopic treatment of the discoid lateral meniscus: results of long-term follow-up. Arthroscopy 1989;5:101.

143. Walker J, Rang M, Daneman A. Ultrasonography of the unossified patella in young children. J Pediatr Orthop 1991;11:100.

144. Weber BG. Fibrous interposition causing valgus deformity after fracture of the upper tibial metaphysis in children. J Bone Joint Surg [Br] 1977;59:290.

145. Wedge JH, Munkacsi I, Loback D. Anteversion of the femur and idiopathic osteoarthrosis of the hip. J Bone Joint Surg [Am] 1989;71:1040.

146. Wenger DR, Mickelson M, Maynard JA. The evolution and histopathology of adolescent tibia vara. J Pediatr Orthop 1984;4:78.

147. Whitelaw GP, Wetzler MJ, Levy AS, et al. A pneumatic leg brace for the treatment of tibial stress fractures. Clin Orthop Rel Res 1991;270:301.

148. Wilson JN. A diagnostic sign of osteochondritis dissecans of the knee. J Bone Joint Surg [Am] 1967;49:477.

149. Winquist RA. Closed intramedullary osteotomies of the femur. Clin Orthop Rel Res 1986;212:155.

150. Wiss DA, Schilz JL, Zionts L. Type III fractures of the tibial tubercle in adolescents. J Orthop Trauma 1991;5:475.

151. Yagi T, Sasaki T. Tibial torsion in patients with medial-type osteoarthritic knee. Clin Orthop Rel Res 1986;213:177.

152. Yousem D, Magid D, Fishman EK, et al. Computed tomography of stress fractures. J Comput Assist Tomogr 1986;10:92.

153. Zimbler S, Merkow S. Genu recurvatum: a possible complica-tion after Osgood-Schlatter disease. J Bone Joint Surg [Am] 1984;66:1129.

154. Zionts LE, Harcke HT, Brooks KM, et al. Posttraumatic tibia valga: a case demonstrating asymmetric activity at the proxi-mal growth plate on technetium bone scan. J Pediatr Or-thop 1987;7:458.

155. Zionts LG, MacEwen GD. Spontaneous improvement in post-traumatic tibia valga. J Bone Joint Surg [Am] 1986;68:680.

156. Zuege RC, Kempken TG, Blount WP. Epiphyseal stapling for angular deformity at the knee. J Bone Joint Surg [Am] 1979;61:320.

Lovell & Winter's Pediatric Orthopaedics, fourth edition,
edited by Raymond T. Morrissy and Stuart L. Weinstein.
Lippincott–Raven Publishers, Philadelphia © 1996.

Chapter

28

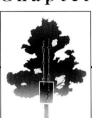

The Child's Foot

J. Andy Sullivan

TERMINOLOGY

In this chapter, several terms are used to describe the parts and motions of the foot (Table 28-1). Varus indicates a deformity or movement toward the midline and valgus away from the midline. To adduct is to draw toward the midline and to abduct is to draw away. Adductus is a noun describing a deformity toward the midline. Equinus denotes that a segment is plantar flexed. Plantigrade indicates walking on the full sole of the foot.

STANDARD RADIOGRAPHY

When evaluating the foot of a child, radiographs should be obtained while the patient bears weight to display the relation of the bones in their functional positions. For patients who are unable to stand or are too young, simulated weight-bearing radiographs can be obtained by placing a plate beneath the foot and applying upward pressure. For a patient who is able to sit, the hips and knees can be flexed 90 degrees and the feet placed in a weight-bearing position on the radiographic plate. The standard initial radiographs should include anteroposterior and lateral projections. The dorsoventral radiograph, commonly referred to as an anteroposterior view, is obtained with the child standing with the legs parallel and the central beam angled 15 degrees toward the heel to eliminate overlap of the lower leg and heel.

The lateral projection is also taken in a weight-bearing or simulated weight-bearing position. It is important, particularly for patients who may have medial deviation of the forefoot (e.g., clubfoot), to align the foot such that the lateral projection is actually of the ankle and hindfoot and not of the forefoot. If it is aligned lateral to the forefoot, the view of the talus is distorted, and the fibula appears posterior to the tibia. Oblique views often are needed to visualize tarsal coalition and traumatic conditions.

The subtalar joint is difficult to visualize radiographically. The sustentaculum does not ossify until after 2 years of age and does not develop until 5 years of age. All plain radiographic techniques that have been used are difficult to interpret because of the wide variability and orientation of the subtalar joint. For most patients who require evaluation of the subtalar joint, computed tomography (CT) can more clearly delineate the anatomy and is more cost effective than multiple radiographic views. Magnetic resonance imaging (MRI) is also useful for viewing the subtalar joint, although the experience with this modality is limited.

NORMAL ALIGNMENT

A variety of lines and angles have been used to describe the foot and delineate normal from abnormal. None of these is universally accepted. In most articles, there are no studies of interobserver and intraobserver error substantiating their interpretation or their use in defining normal. The most usual angles that are measured are the anteroposterior and lateral talocalcaneal angles. The standard anteroposterior midtalar and midcalcaneal lines form an angle of 42 degrees (range, 27–56 degrees) in a newborn. This decreases to an average of 34 degrees by 4 years of age. The lateral talocalcaneal angle is at its highest value at birth and then gradually decreases from a mean of 45 degrees to an average of 33 degrees.[161]

METATARSUS ADDUCTUS

A variety of terms have been used to describe a deformity in which the forepart of the foot is adducted or medially deviated in the transverse plane: metatarsus adductus, metatarsus varus, pes varus, skewfoot, metatarsus internus, and metatarsus adductovarus. Metatarsus adductus and metatarsus varus are the two most frequently used terms, with metatarsus adductus seeming to be the more popular. In addition to forefoot adduction, the heel is in neutral or mild valgus, and there is no other underlying neuromuscular condition. This is the most common foot condition seen by pediatric orthopaedists.[13]

Incidence

The incidence of metatarsus adductus is 1 per 1000 live births.[235] Some investigators think the incidence has been increasing.[118,170]

TABLE 28-1   *Descriptive Terms*

Anatomy

Forefoot	Metatarsals and phalanges
Midfoot	Navicular, cuneiforms, and cuboid
Hindfoot	Calcaneus and talus

Foot Movements

Pronation*	Sole turns outward
Supination*	Sole turns inward
Inversion (varus)	Motion of a segment about the longitudinal axis
Eversion (valgus)	Motion of foot segment about a vertical axis
Abduction	To draw away from the medial plane
Adduction	To draw toward the medial plane

---

* These are combined movements of separate joints.

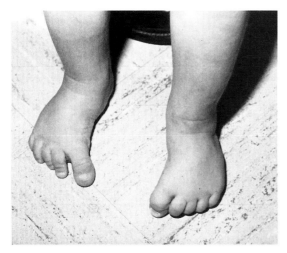

FIGURE 28-1. Clinical photograph of a child with metatarsus adductus. Notice the medial deviation of the toes, particularly the great toe.

An equal male to female ratio or a slight male predominance is reported. In Kite's series, four of the parents of 2818 children had the disorder.[118] In Ponseti's series, 14 of 57 patients had first-degree relatives with metatarsus adductus.[170]

Etiology

The cause of metatarsus adductus remains unknown. There is no association with birth order, gestational age, or maternal age.[170] Kite suggested muscle imbalance as a cause.[118] He suggested that there is a contracture of the medial soft tissues of the tarsometatarsal joints of the foot. The most accepted theory is that metatarsus adductus may be a result of "tight

intrauterine packing" and is associated with hip dysplasia and torticollis. In Jacob's series of 300 patients, there was 10% incidence of associated hip dysplasia.[102] In another series of 720 patients with metatarsus adductus, the incidence of associated hip dysplasia was 1.53%.[123] Although this is higher than the 0.15% reported by Barlow,[7] it is considerably less than the 10% reported by Jacobs.[102] This may be explained by the fact that Jacobs diagnosed acetabular dysplasia if the patient had an acetabular index of more than 30 degrees or a small ossific nucleus radiographically, both of which may resolve and not be true hip dysplasia.

A study by Farsetti and colleagues suggests that the abnormality may result from an anomaly of the medial cuneiform–metatarsal joint.[58] For 21 of 31 patients with metatarsus adductus, radiographs showed an obliquity of the profile of the medial cuneiform joint. This parallels the findings of Reimann and Werner, who found changes in size and shape of the first cuneiform, with a broadened articular surface of the first metatarsal that was medially subluxated.[174]

Clinical Features

The clinical picture is one of adduction of the forefoot, with various degrees of supination. There is a concave medial border of the foot with a convex lateral border and prominence at the base of the fifth metatarsal (Fig. 28-1). The heel is in neutral or slight valgus. There is no equinus or heel varus. An underlying neurologic disorder must be ruled out. The flexibility of the deformity should be assessed. This is accomplished by grasping the heel with one hand and abducting the forefoot with the other (Fig. 28-2).

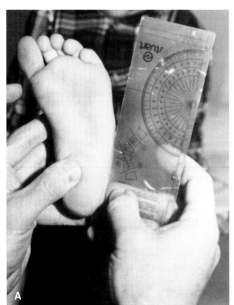
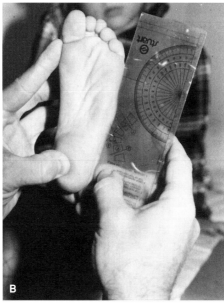

FIGURE 28-2. (A) Metatarsus adductus in a child 4 years of age. (B) Notice the flexibility, even at this age.

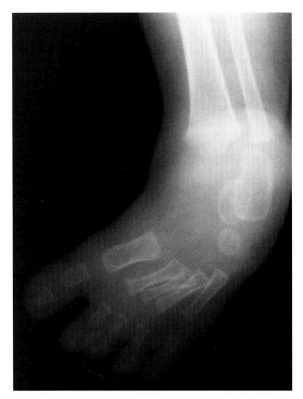

FIGURE 28-3. Radiograph of a patient with metatarsus adductus. Notice the normal talocalcaneal divergence.

Radiographic Evaluation

Radiographic evaluation of most patients is unnecessary. If underlying congenital anomalies are suspected or the foot is unusually stiff, radiographs may be warranted (Fig. 28-3).

Berg suggested a radiographic classification and delineated four configurations of the forefoot.[12] His study suggested that the radiographic classification had prognostic significance. Cook and colleagues attempted to apply Berg's method and found that there was no correlation between the classification system and the length of time required for cast correction.[32] Intraobserver discrepancy in the diagnosis occurred in 26% of the first and second readings, and interobserver disagreements occurred in 36%. The measurement of the talocalcaneal angle was important in Berg's system and was found to be too variable to be reliable. Cook suggested that the best guide to determining treatment and prognosis remains the clinical evaluation of the severity and stiffness of the foot.

Bleck and colleagues' classification system was based on observation of the foot and the heel bisector (Fig. 28-4).[13] In a later study, they suggested that this indicator could be measured accurately and inexpensively using a photocopy machine.[193] Whether it is determined clinically or with a photocopy machine, the method considers the weight-bearing surface of the heel to be an ellipse. By visual examination, the line bisecting the heel is drawn. If this line crosses between the second and third toes, the foot was thought to be normal (i.e., 85% of 1000 children's feet randomly selected). They further classified abnormalities as mild, moderate, or severe, depending on the point at which the heel bisector intersected the toes. Schwartze and Denton, after evaluating 527 girls and 473 boys, determined that the heel bisector normally falls between the second and third toes in neonates.[179]

Natural History

Rushforth performed a prospective study with an average 7-year follow-up of 83 children with 130 affected feet who received no treatment.[176] Eighty-six percent of the feet were normal, 10% were moderately deformed, and only 4% remained stiff and deformed.[176] In Ponseti and Becker's series, 379 patients were examined in crippled children's clinics throughout Iowa from 1953 to 1960.[170] Only 44 of this group required treatment with corrective plaster casts. The remaining 335 received no treatment. In their group, the deformity was passively correctable, often progressed slightly until the 1 or 2 years of age, and then regressed, with the end result of a completely normal foot or mild flatfoot with a minimal amount of metatarsus adductus. Most

FIGURE 28-4. The heel bisector. (Data from Bleck EE, Berzinz UJ. Conservative management of pes valgus with plantar flexed talus, flexible. Clin Orthop 1977;122:85.)

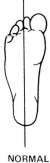 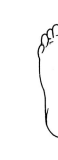 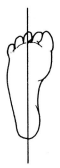 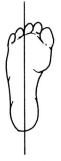 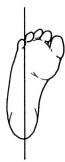

NORMAL　　　VALGUS　　　MILD　　　MODERATE　　　SEVERE

resolved, with only a few requiring treatment. The difficulty is in deciding which ones will resolve.

Treatment

Treatment modalities include simple stretching and observation, plaster casts, corrective shoes, Dennis-Browne bars, and shoes with an adjustable universal joint at the midtarsal level. Ponseti and Becker recommended that manipulation not be done by parents.[170] They did not use reverse-last shoes or Dennis-Browne bars, because they thought the later could accentuate heel valgus. They suggested that mild deformities that are passively correctable need no treatment other than follow-up examinations. Those with rigidity required treatment. The average age at the beginning of plaster treatment was 6 months, at which time the therapy was able to achieve a satisfactory result.[170]

Bleck's study involved 265 feet of 160 children that were prospectively classified by severity and flexibility.[13] Among the 147 patients treated with plaster casts, the only significant predictor of good outcome was the age of the patient. The results were statistically better when treatment was begun between birth and 8 months of age.

Bleck classified the feet as mild, moderate, or severe, based on the heel bisector classification system. This study did not allow prediction with certainty of the cases that should be treated with plaster casts. Mild deformities that were not treated were assessed as normal feet at the time of follow-up, and it appears that these do not progress to severe deformity. He suggested treatment of all cases classified as moderate or severe.

Farsetti, Weinstein, and Ponseti provided the longest follow-up of the outcome of untreated and nonoperatively treated metatarsus adductus.[58] Thirty-one patients (45 feet) were evaluated at average follow-up of 32.5 years. Twenty-nine of the feet were treated by manipulation and plaster casts. The results were good in all of the untreated feet and 90% of the feet treated conservatively. No patient had a poor result. No patient required operative treatment, and hallux valgus was not a long-term problem. The percentage of patients that required treatment in this study closely paralleled the experience of Rushforth.[176] In his series, 10% were moderately deformed but asymptomatic, and 4% remained deformed and stiff.

Most children presenting at birth with metatarsus adductus do not require treatment. If the child has a moderate or severe deformity according to the heel bisector classification and is not passively correctable, casting is indicated. Although some would begin casting at the first visit, I prefer to wait until the child is older than 6 months of age to begin casting, because many feet correct spontaneously. The upper age limit at which casting is successful is unknown, but most series show the best results occur if the casting is done within the first year of life. There are no studies documenting the efficacy of corrective shoes, Dennis-Browne bars, or shoes with adjustable universal joints at the midtarsal level.

Surgical management of metatarsus adductus is less certain. The orthopaedic literature has a noticeable dearth of articles on the operative management of this condition for patients older than 30 years of age. The usual indications are for a child older than 3 to 4 years of age with residual metatarsus adductus. Heyman and colleagues devised a procedure that involved mobilization of the tarsometatarsal and intertarsal joints and claimed success with this procedure.[93] Stark and associates reported a 41% overall failure rate and a 50% incidence of painful dorsal prominence at the surgical scar after using this approach.[197] They reported skin sloughs, avascular necrosis of the second and third cuneiform, dorsal prominence of the base of the first metatarsal, and late degenerative arthritis of the first metatarsocuneiform joint. It is wise to heed the advice of these investigators: "Orthopaedists are specialists in improving function. Cosmesis is of far less concern and such surgical risks as are outlined here are rarely, if ever, justified." Perhaps the most difficult decisions are deciding which patient has significant metatarsus adductus and whether the benefits of surgery outweigh the risks.

Multiple metatarsal osteotomies can correct metatarsus adductus deformity (Fig. 28-5). They can be performed through a single incision or through multiple longitudinal incisions. An additional option is a cuneiform opening wedge osteotomy with a concomitant cuboid closing edge. This had been used in children and adolescents with residual clubfoot deformity and can be used for metatarsus adductus (Fig. 28-6).[144]

One of the complications of surgery is failure to correct the deformity, regardless of the procedure performed. Scars on the dorsum of the foot can become painful, as can the metatarsals themselves, and there can be degenerative tarsometatarsal joint changes.

SKEWFOOT

Skewfoot is a complex foot deformity consisting of forefoot adduction and heel valgus (Fig. 28-7). Synonyms for this abnormality include S-shaped foot, serpentine foot, and Z-foot deformity.[164] Skewfoot has not been recorded at birth and is often first discovered after cast treatment for metatarsus adductus or club-

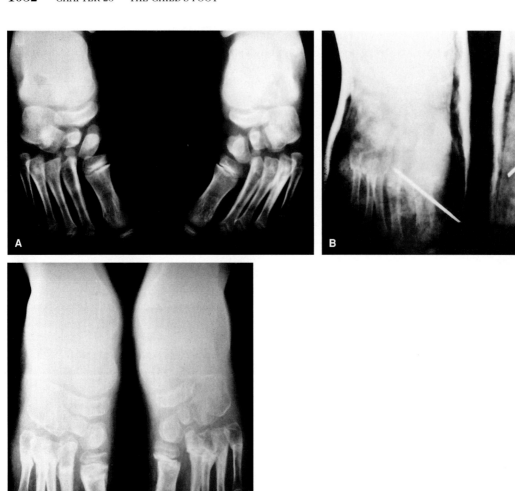

FIGURE 28-5. (**A**) Anteroposterior radiograph of a patient with metatarsus adductus. (**B**) Multiple metatarsal osteotomies, the first of which is fixed with a crossed Kirschner wire. (**C**) Postoperative radiograph.

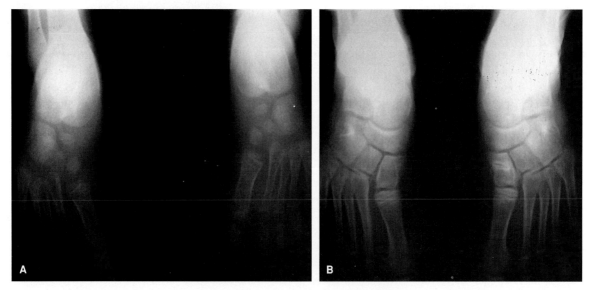

FIGURE 28-6. (**A**) Preoperative radiograph of a patient with resistant metatarsus adductus. (**B**) Postoperative radiograph after lateral cuboid wedge resection and cuneiform open wedge osteotomies.

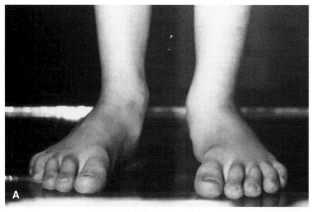

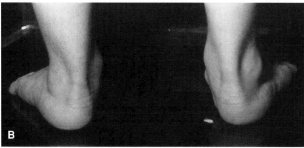

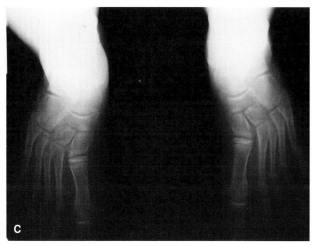

FIGURE 28-7. (A) Standing photograph of a patient with skewfoot. Notice the forefoot adductus. (B) Standing view of heel valgus. (C) Anteroposterior radiograph. Notice the medial deviation of the forefoot and divergence of the talocalcaneal relation, indicating hindfoot valgus.

foot or after ambulation in patients with metatarsus varus.[164]

Incidence

Peterson's literature review revealed only 50 cases, and all the patients were children.[164] McCormick and Blount found more than 20 articles on the subject in the German literature.[143] Kite found 12 cases of skewfoot among 2818 patients with forefoot adduction.[118]

The cause and the natural history of the disorder

are unknown. Some researchers think that it occurs as a result of treatment of metatarsus adductus.

Clinical Features

Shoe wear and abnormal gait are often presenting complaints. The patient is found to have forefoot adduction and increased heel valgus. The patient must be examined while sitting and standing, and the flexibility and correctability of the foot must be assessed. The heel is in valgus, and the Achilles tendon is not contracted. There may be a bursa along the lateral border of the foot over the fifth metatarsal. There is medial heel and sole wear and general problems with the shoes wearing out unevenly.

Radiographic Evaluation

Radiographic evaluation includes standing anteroposterior and lateral radiographs of the foot (see Fig. 28-7C). The talocalcaneal angles are increased, and the navicular bone is located laterally on the head of the talus.

Treatment

Skewfoot is unusual or not seen in the newborn. An older child usually presents with this problem. Berg stated that casts provide a satisfactory method of correction.[12] McCormick thought that manipulation was successful and that casts were unnecessary.[143] Peterson, in his review of literature, found an almost uniform lack of response to nonoperative treatment (Fig. 28-8).[164] He suggested an aggressive approach early in infancy by manipulation and serial casting, with the heel held in varus and lateral pressure on the head of the talus and medial pressure on the navicular with lateral pressure on the metatarsals. The physician must be absolutely certain that the heel is held in neutral or slight varus to avoid accentuating the existing heel valgus deformity. For older children, Peterson recommended surgical realignment of the bones supplemented with hindfoot stabilization.[164]

CONGENITAL CALCANEOVALGUS FOOT

Congenital calcaneovalgus foot is the most common deformity of the foot seen at birth. The reported incidence is 30% to 50%.[228] The condition is thought to result from intrauterine positioning. There are no tarsal dislocations or subluxations. The foot is acutely dorsiflexed, and the dorsum of the foot is in contact with the anterior shin (Fig. 28-9). Heel valgus may be

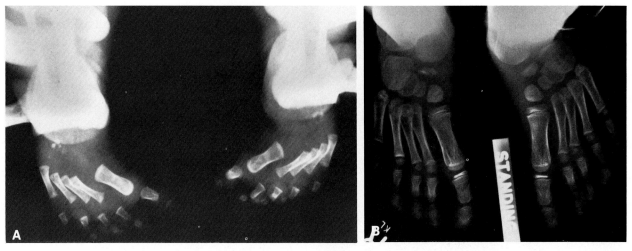

FIGURE 28-8.   (A) Anteroposterior radiograph of a 2-month-old child with marked forefoot adduction caused by skewfoot. The patient was treated with serial casts. (B) At 5 years of age, lateral displacement of the navicular on the head of the talus remains with incomplete correction.

increased. The deformity is usually supple, and the foot can be brought into some plantar flexion and supination.

It requires time and counseling to convince the parents that this is not a fixed deformity. Although they are often encouraged to stretch the foot, the action is probably more for the treatment of the parents, because the deformity resolves without residual sequelae. In an occasional patient, a series of corrective casts can be used to hasten the recovery of a normal position.

Calcaneovalgus feet must be differentiated from congenital vertical talus, in which there is a fixed deformity with a rounded sole (see later section on vertical talus). The heel, rather than being dorsiflexed, is in equinus.

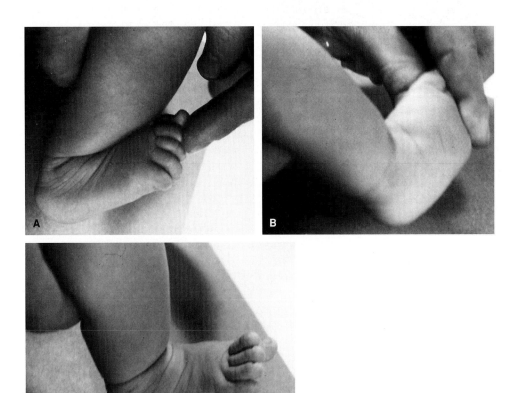

FIGURE 28-9.   (A) Calcaneovalgus foot as it presents at birth. (B) The foot is supple and can be inverted easily. (C) The foot actively come to neutral.

Some investigators think that calcaneovalgus feet predispose the patient to the development of pes planus. Wetzenstein examined 2735 newborn infants and divided those with congenital pes calcaneovalgus into three groups, with the amount of valgus as the determining factor.[228] After short-term follow-up, he thought that the children with severe calcaneovalgus in infancy showed a significantly higher percentage of pes planovalgus at 1 year of age. Larsen and colleagues concluded that this was essentially a benign condition that could be followed clinically and did not require radiographic evaluation nor active treatment.[129]

FLEXIBLE FLATFOOT

A patient with little or no longitudinal arch while standing is said to have a flatfoot. The public associates the absence of a longitudinal arch with undesirable effects in adult life. This idea has been promulgated by the attitude of many physicians who ordered a variety of treatment modalities for asymptomatic children with flexible flatfeet. In most instances, a foot that is flat but flexible and has normal subtalar motion is asymptomatic and is not known to cause disability as an adult. We do not know the natural history of this disorder, but there is a general impression that most remain asymptomatic as adults. These feet must be differentiated from those with pain or stiffness and from those with structural causes for the loss of the arch that may require operative treatment.

Incidence

At birth, most children have a foot that has a minimal longitudinal arch. Staheli confirmed that flatfeet are standard in infants and common in children.[196]

Etiology

Duchenne was able to produce a longitudinal arch in a child with flatfoot by faradization of the peroneus longus, leading some to think that flatfoot had a muscular basis.[52] In a classic study, Basmajian investigated the mechanism of arch support by performing electromyographs on 20 men.[8] He concluded, after studying six muscles in the leg and foot, that only heavy loading elicits muscle activity. In his opinion, the first line of maintenance of the arch is ligamentous, with muscle providing a reserve when the arch was excessively loaded, including during the push-off phase in walking. Smith observed the anterior and posterior tibialis, peroneals, and short plantar muscles during the immobile period of standing.[194] He found that the muscle groups were inactive during the static phase of standing and that the gastrocnemius group performed an

antigravity function. He concluded that, as movement alternates with standing, the mechanism of supporting the arch changes from muscular to the osteoligamentous components.

The conclusion is that the shape of the foot in weight bearing is predominantly related to the bone-ligament complex. Muscle is a dynamic stabilizer. In adults who lose posterior tibial function, flatfoot may develop and become painful.[138] This progression has not been demonstrated in children.

Pathoanatomy

No one has ever performed a large number of dissections on cadaver feet, nor has a large series of operative findings been described. Koutsogiannis described the anatomy of flatfoot as one in which the calcaneus is in valgus, with its superior articular surface tilted medially.[121] The talus is rotated medially and down, with its head producing a prominence medially, just below the navicular bone. In this manner, the medial pilar is lost, and subluxation is produced between the talus and the navicular. In some cases, there is also subluxation between the navicular and the cuneiform bones. These are operative findings that can be observed in patients known to have an absence or flattening of the longitudinal arch with heel valgus.

Natural History

In their review of 3600 recruits, Harris and Beath concluded that flatfoot associated with simple depression of the longitudinal arch is of little consequence as a cause of disability and may be regarded as a normal contour of a strong and stable foot.[84,85] This idea remains the prevailing opinion. Some adolescents and adults require treatment because of excessive pronation, callus formation, and problems with shoes. Multiple studies show that the development of an arch is a natural consequence of growth and development and not related to shoes (Fig. 28-10).[70,173,188,196,215]

Clinical Features

Most flatfeet are variations of normal. In the foot of a young child, the most usual clinical appearance is that of an absence of a longitudinal arch. An arch may exist when sitting but disappear with weight bearing. The arch may reconstitute with tiptoe standing (see Fig. 28-10). The foot should be supple, with normal subtalar motion and normal midtarsal motion. The range of dorsiflexion at the ankle should be checked with the forefoot supinated to lock the subtalar joint. In flatfoot associated with a short tendo Achillis, the supinated foot only comes to neutral or is in mild equinus. When the forefoot is pronated, eversion of

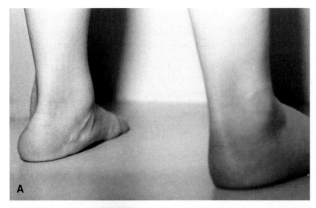

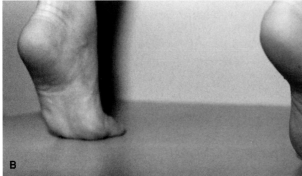

FIGURE 28-10. (A) Photographs of a flexible flatfoot. (B) Standing on tiptoe elevates the arch.

the foot may give a false sense of dorsiflexion that is occurring at the midtarsal joints.

Shephard wrote that the only tarsal joints with mobility other than slight gliding are the subtalar, talonavicular, and calcaneocuboid joints.[187] The subtalar and talonavicular joints form a single functional joint. The combined motion of these joints is very much like a ball-and-socket joint, with the subtalar, talonavicular, and midtarsal joints forming oblique hinged joints. In examining these joints, it is important to try to isolate the various movements. By grasping the heel, more subtalar motion is tested, and in testing the forefoot and everting and inverting the foot, there is also a component of midtarsal joint motion that occurs. The foot should be examined for abnormal callosities or pressure points. The child should be asked to walk normally and then on the toes, heels, and lateral border of the foot. The ability to walk in all of these manners is most often associated with a normal foot. The examination is not complete without manual motor testing of all of the major muscle groups acting on the foot.

The flexible flatfoot must be differentiated from the hypermobile flatfoot associated with a tight tendoachilles. Harris and Beath reviewed 3600 recruits for the Canadian Army.[84,85] They found an association of hypermobile flatfoot with short tendoachilles. These patients had a prolonged history of foot disability starting in childhood that increased during adult life. There seemed to be a hereditary influence. The foot was mobile with a short Achilles tendon that limited dorsiflexion. There was hypermobility at the midtarsal and subtalar joints. The researchers thought this resulted from the unstable architecture of the tarsal bones, which resulted in imperfect support of the head of the talus by the calcaneus.

Examination of the foot is incomplete without an entire torsional evaluation of the lower extremity. Examination of the spine should be performed to look for abnormalities that can be associated with neuromuscular problems of the lower extremity.

Radiography

For most patients, radiographs are indicated only if there is a question of flexibility or findings compatible with the loss of subtalar motion or of a rigid flatfoot. Radiographs should include standing anteroposterior and lateral views. The anteroposterior view is used to assess heel valgus. An anteroposterior talocalcaneal angle greater than 35 degrees is associated with increased heel valgus. On the lateral view, the talocalcaneal angle is measured. A line drawn through the talus, navicular bone, and first metatarsal is ordinarily a straight line. The "relaxed" talus associated with a flexible flatfoot converts this straight line to an angle, with its apex directed plantarly.

Treatment

Nonsurgical Therapy

Most flexible flatfeet require no treatment (Fig. 28-11). No evidence supports the idea that the use of corrective shoes or inserts will lead to permanent formation of a longitudinal arch. It is often difficult to convince parents, well-meaning grandparents, and friends that this is the case.[117]

For many years, children have been treated by a variety of corrective shoes and inserts despite the lack of a scientific basis. The theory was that something inserted on the medial aspect in the shoe, along the counter, or on the sole would push up on the arch and shift the weight bearing to the lateral aspect of the foot. This would lead to some change in the arch and or alleviation of symptoms. Neither of these ideas have been substantiated.

As with lower extremity torsional problems that are variations of normal, it is far more difficult to convince parents that nothing need be done, and the process requires far more time than providing a diagnosis and ordering corrective shoes. This approach is not justifiable, because it is ineffective and costly.

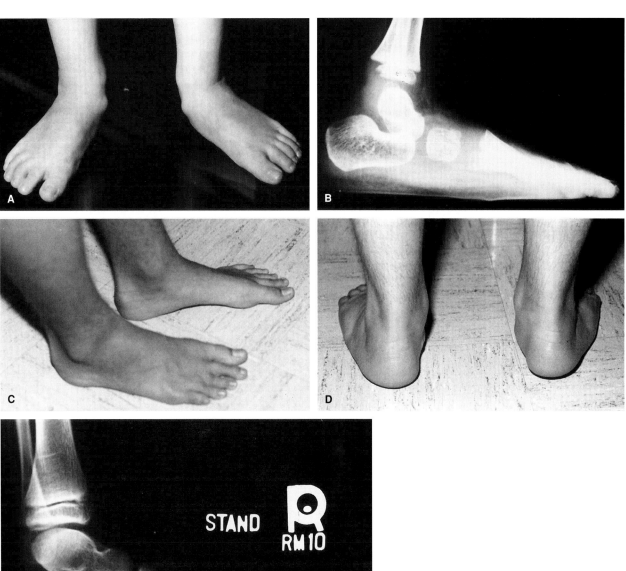

FIGURE 28-11. (A) Clinical appearance of a child who presented for a second opinion regarding the need for surgery for a flexible flatfoot. (B) Radiograph of the 4-year-old child at the time of presentation. (C and D) Clinical appearance of the foot of the patient as a teenager, when the patient returned for an opinion regarding scoliosis. (E) Lateral radiograph of the foot. No treatment had been given for the flatfoot.

Helfet examined the shoe corrections and found them ineffective.[89] He devised a heel-seat and had 500 children use them during a period of 7 years. He was impressed that they provided a sure, simple, and economic method of correcting flatfeet, but documentation for this conviction was lacking.

The most common treatment for pes planus, suggested in 1970, was a ⅛-inch lateral sole wedge and a Thomas heel.[229] Penneau and colleagues evaluated 10 children radiographically who had bilateral pes planus.[163] The radiographs were taken of barefoot children using a Thomas heel, an over-the-counter insert, and two specially molded foot orthoses. No significant radiographic change was seen as an immediate effect of wearing these orthoses.

Bleck prospectively studied the management of flexible pes valgus with a plantar-flexed talus.[14] He defined the flatfeet from clinical parameters, looking at the angle of the heel compared with a straight line of the tibia and a heel bisector drawn along the Achilles tendon and posterior calcaneus. The absence of an arch was not the only criterion for the diagnosis of a flatfoot. Radiographs were used to evaluate the efficacy of treatment.

Patients treated with the Helfet corrective heel-seat or the University of California Berkeley Laboratory (UCBL) insert were followed for a sufficient period to allow evaluation. Bleck stated that the overall results were encouraging, with a mean talar plantar flexion angle of the 71 patients improved from 41.8 to 34.1 degrees. On the basis of this study, they recommended the use of UCBL insert in cases of flexible pes valgus with a plantar-flexed talus if the standard lateral roentgenogram demonstrated the talar plantar flexion angle of 45 degrees. They used different angles for indications for the Helfet heel-seat and the UCBL.

The problem with this study is that the natural history of development of the longitudinal arch is unknown. There are no studies of interobserver or intraobserver error, and the improvements reflected may well be within the range of normal development or error of the method of measurement.

Wenger and colleagues performed a prospective study to determine whether a flexible flatfoot could be influenced by treatment.[225] Patients were assigned to one of four groups: the control group, one treated with corrective shoes prescribed by the prescription footwear association, one using the Helfet heelcup, and one group using a UCBL insert. The patients in the treatment groups had a minimum of 3 years of follow-up, and compliance was ensured. Analysis of the radiographs before treatment and during follow-up examinations showed significant improvement for all groups, including the controls, with no significant difference between controls and treated patients. They concluded that wearing corrective shoes or inserts for 3 years did not influence the course of flexible flatfoot in the child.

Custom-molded inserts can cost $150 to $500 per pair, and they require frequent replacement. There are some moderately priced inserts that can be custom molded from heat-sensitive plastics. They probably should be considered placebos, and it is often the child who ceases using them because of the inconvenience.

Rao and associates analyzed the static footprints of 2300 children who were 4 to 13 years of age to establish the influence of footwear on the prevalence of flatfoot.[173] They found that flatfoot was most common in children who wore closed-toe shoes and less common in those who wore loose slippers or sandals. The researchers postulated that wearing shoes in early childhood is detrimental to the development of a normal longitudinal arch.

Because treatment is not indicated for most cases, it is best to try to convince the family that nothing is indicated or necessary. For the occasional recalcitrant parent who is likely to continue doctor shopping until someone treats the child, an inexpensive option is to use arch supports that can be purchased in most athletic stores or in the foot department of a drug store.

Surgical Management

Surgical management is never indicated for a child. The adolescent nearing skeletal maturity who has a severe, painful flatfoot may require surgery, but surgery is needed only in extreme circumstances.

There are three types of operations for the correction of flexible flatfoot: soft tissue, bone, and implant. Soft tissue procedures described in the first part of this century have not relieved symptoms nor altered the longitudinal arch. An example of a soft tissue procedure is the transfer of the tibialis posterior, which is supposed to give the arch better support. The Durham procedure is a combination of transfer of the posterior tibial tendon with elevation of a long ligamentous and capsular flap from the medial aspect of the foot. The naviculocuneiform joint is fused and the flap inserted into the sustentaculum, with reattachment of the posterior tibialis tendon.[23] There are no long-term studies supporting the use of this procedure.

Crego and Ford reviewed 11 surgical procedures on 102 feet of 53 children performed at Shriners Hospital in St. Louis.[37] They were performed over many years by a variety of surgeons. The operations were done for relief of disabling pain and then only after exhausting every means of conservative treatment. The researchers thought that arthrodesis of the talonavicular and naviculocuneiform joints was fairly satisfactory and that the subtalar joint should be excluded. They stressed that some of the poor results were the result of faulty operative technique or postoperative management.

Among the bony operations offered as remedies, calcaneal displacement osteotomy has been promoted as an effective means of relieving fatigue, improving shape, and preventing abnormal shoe wear for patients with a mobile flatfoot. Nineteen patients had 34 operative procedures, and function was found to be improved in 17 of the 19.[121] It was more successful in correcting the heel deformity but did not improve the longitudinal arch. The operation is performed with the patient supine. The calcaneus is approached on the lateral side. The calcaneus is osteotomized and pried open, and the periosteum is divided along the medial aspect to allow displacement. The fragment is displaced medially until its medial border is in line with the sustentaculum.

Kling looked at calcaneal lengthening for painful pes planus in children.[119] Twenty-four feet of 14 children between the ages of 3 and 16 years (average age,

9 years) were treated by this method. The indications for surgery were daily pain and callosities or ulcerations over the talar head or neck that were unresponsive to orthotics and shoe modifications. Tricorticoiliac crest allograft was internally fixed between the anterior and middle facets of the calcaneus. After an average follow-up of 42 months, (range, 20–64 months), all patients had relief of pain, ambulated without orthotics, used regular shoes, and were pleased with the appearance. Subtalar motion was preserved. Incorporation of the allograft was evident 2 months postoperatively. The anteroposterior talocalcaneal angle was improved, as was the Meary angle and the lateral talocalcaneal angle. These preliminary results indicate that calcaneal lengthening is a safe, effective treatment for painful pes planus after all conservative means fail.

Mosca described his experience with a calcaneal lengthening procedure for children with valgus hindfoot and skewfoot.[153] Thirty-one patients with pain, calluses, or ulceration over the plantar-flexed talus were treated with calcaneal lengthening combined with medial cuneiform opening wedge osteotomy. Because 25 of the 29 flatfeet and 6 skewfeet were secondary to neuromuscular disorders, few operations were for flexible flatfeet. Allograft bone was used in 24 feet. Pain, the need for braces, and shoe intolerance was alleviated for all feet. Subtalar motion was preserved in all, except for two patients who had a concomitant subtalar fusion. A variety of soft tissue procedures were required to release contractures and balance forces. This procedure should rarely be required for flexible flatfoot but may be of use in adolescence as an alternative to triple arthrodesis.

Wenger described a modification of the medial sliding calcaneal osteotomy used in treating cerebral palsy patients with severe heel valgus.[226] The technique includes correction of hindfoot valgus with correction of the forefoot through the calcaneocuboid and talonavicular joints. The heel cord may be lengthened. From his anecdotal experience with approximately 25 children who were 6 to 12 years of age and followed for 8 years, he reported improvement in foot mechanics, decreased foot pain, and increased ability to wear regular shoes. He stressed that the procedure was only for extreme cases with intractable pain and shoe wear problems.

A third class of operative procedures is the insertion of a prosthetic plug in the subtalar joint. Viladot described a procedure to insert a cup-like prosthesis in the subtalar joint, creating an ''arthrorisis . . . an endoprosthesis that limits sliding of the astragalus without suppressing its mobility is made.''[218] He suggests this in place of an arthrodesis. He reported the results of treating 234 children. He indicated that this procedure was only necessary in 1.6% of the cases of flatfoot. A good result was one in which the longitudinal arch was improved on lateral radiographs and on footprints. This article and others in the literature on Silastic plugs suffer the same weaknesses.[48,218] The indication for the surgery is the prediction that the young patients are destined to develop painful, arthritic feet as adults, an assumption that is not supported by the natural history. We also do not know the long-term consequences of this foreign material in the subtalar joint. There are no long-term studies showing the results of these procedures. I think prosthetic devices are never indicated in the patient with a flexible flatfoot.

The risks of all flatfoot surgery must be compared with the benefits. The only complications of nonoperative treatment may be the increased cost of shoes, dealing with possible pain, and perhaps dealing with comments that the child appears different from his peers. Surgical complications include failure to achieve the operative goals, joint stiffness, infection, and the long-term potential for a foreign body reaction that may occur from the prosthesis insertion in the subtalar joint. If surgery is recommended, the goals must be clear and outcomes predictable.

CONGENITAL VERTICAL TALUS

Congenital vertical talus is an uncommonly occurring rigid flatfoot that requires early identification and aggressive treatment. Its various names include congenital convex pes planus, congenital flatfoot with talonavicular dislocation, and congenital rigid rocker-bottom foot. The term congenital vertical talus is easily recognized as descriptive of this condition and is preferred by most orthopaedic specialists.

In their classic article, Lamy and Weissman credit Henken with the first clinical roentgenographic anatomic and pathologic study of the condition, published in 1914.[127] Their article includes an excellent description of pathologic and radiographic findings and a review of the world literature to 1939.

Etiology and Genetics

The cause and incidence of congenital vertical talus are unknown. Stern described the vertical transmission of isolated congenital vertical talus through three generations of a Honduran family.[198] Five of nine family members had the diagnosis confirmed clinically and radiographically. Transmission in this instance was as an autosomal dominant trait with incomplete penetrance. In all series, it has a high association with other congenital anomalies and with disorders of the central nervous system.[51,77,91,127,157] Ten percent of children with myelodysplasia have congenital vertical talus.[51] It can also be associated with congenital dislocation of the hip and with arthrogryposis. This condition also occurs with trisomy 13 through 15 and trisomy 18.[209]

Ogata and Schoenecker studied the familial occurrence in 36 patients with 57 involved feet.[157] Congenital vertical talus occurred as an isolated defect in only 16 patients (44%). It has been stated that this condition occurs predominantly in boys, but in larger groups of patients, such as that reviewed by Ogata and Schoenecker, and in a literature review of 273 cases by Jacobsen and Crawford, boys and girls were affected equally.[103] Ogata and Schoenecker's review revealed a positive family history in first-degree relatives in 10 of their 36 patients, 8 of whom had the primary isolated variety without other underlying conditions. Two had a familial occurrence. Although the cause is unknown, anatomic studies have shown that a neuromuscular imbalance can produce the pathologic findings of this condition.[51]

Clinical Features

The clinical appearance of a foot with congenital vertical talus is diagnostic and easily distinguishable from that of the more common calcaneus foot or flexible flatfoot. The plantar aspect of the foot is convex, giving it the rocker-bottom appearance (Fig. 28-12). The heel is in fixed equinus with a very tight tendoachilles. The head of the talus is prominent and palpable medially in the sole. The hindfoot is in valgus, with the forefoot abducted and in dorsiflexion at the midtarsal joint. The foot does not respond to manipulation, because it is rigidly held in place by the contracted soft tissues. In the calcaneus foot and the hypermobile flatfoot, plantar flexion reduces the navicular bone on the talus, but in congenital vertical talus, the relation of the dorsally displaced talus is not altered by forefoot plantar flexion. The navicular remains dislocated on the dorsum of the talus. With time, the calcaneocuboid joint also displaces, with the cuboid coming to rest more dorsally.

Natural History

If left untreated, these patients develop a rigid, painful flatfoot in adolescence or early adulthood. In the older child of walking age, calluses develop under the prominent head of the talus. Wearing shoes is difficult, and the gait is awkward as the child balances on the talar prominence on the sole of the foot much, as on an end-bearing amputation. The heel does not make contact with the ground.

Radiographic Evaluation

Multiple researchers have described the radiographic findings, but it is difficult to improve on those in the earliest writings of Lamy and Weissman or Coleman and colleagues.[127] The navicular is not ossified until approximately 3 years of age. The diagnosis can be

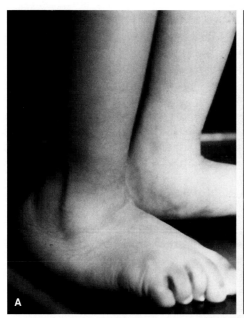
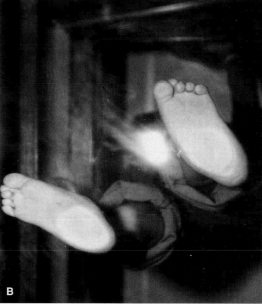

FIGURE 28-12. Photograph of a weight-bearing patient with congenital vertical talus. Notice the rocker-bottom appearance of the foot, with a rounded lateral border, valgus of the heel, and impingement laterally. (**B**) On the plantar surface, most of the weight bearing is on the area of the area of the anterior talus and calcaneus. Clinical radiographs of this patient are shown in Figure 28-13.

confirmed by noticing that there is a talonavicular dislocation, with the forefoot displaced dorsally on the talus. The calcaneus is in fixed equinus. The head of the talus is medial and plantar. Only a small portion of the posterior most aspect of the talus articulates with the tibia. In extreme cases, the talus is parallel to the axis of the tibia. If the navicular is ossified, it rests on the dorsal surface of the talus. There is subluxation of the talocalcaneal joint, with the calcaneus everted and the talus in plantar flexion and medially displaced. The diagnosis can be confirmed by obtaining an extreme plantar-flexion view demonstrating that the relation of the talus to the navicular bone is fixed and rigid (Fig. 28-13). The flexible flatfoot or the flatfoot secondary to a tight tendoachilles is not rigid, and the forefoot and midfoot can be reduced by the plantar-flexion maneuver. The paralytic foot associated with various neuromuscular diseases can usually be differentiated by the same maneuvers.

Pathoanatomy

The pathologic anatomy of congenital vertical talus has been described by several investigators.[30,51,97,183]

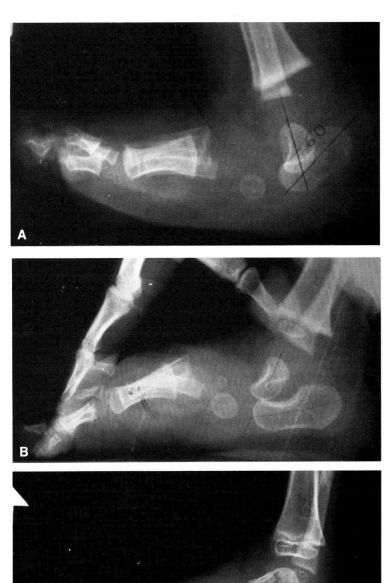

FIGURE 28-13.   (**A**) A lateral radiograph of the right foot shows that the talus is perpendicular to the tibia. The calcaneus and equinus and forefoot are in dorsiflexion. (**B**) Forced plantar flexion views show maintenance of this relation, with the unossified navicular remaining on the dorsum of the talus. (**C**) Radiograph of the patient 1 year after open reduction, pinning, and subtalar arthrodesis with the use of the fibula. These are the radiographs of the patient whose clinical photographs are shown in Figure 28-12.

Drennan and Sharrard performed a postmortem dissection of a baby with myelomeningocele and congenital vertical talus and compared it with dissection of a normal patient of the same age.[51] They observed that the extensor retinaculum was absent and that the calcaneus was everted (in equinus) and laterally displaced. The anterior tibialis tendon ran a straight course and crossed the ankle like a bowstring. All tendons to the dorsum of the foot were tethered medial to the midline of the ankle joint. The peroneal tendons were subluxated anteriorly to the cuboid.

Significant changes were found in the talus and calcaneal head; the talus was hypoplastic and in plantar flexion. The sustentaculum talus was blunted and did not support the head of the talus. There was no anterior talocalcaneal articulation. The sinus tarsi was diminished, and the posterior talocalcaneal facet was tilted. Drennan and Sharrard hypothesized that the triceps had pulled the hindfoot into equinus and that, with decreased function of the posterior tibialis, the dorsiflexors had exerted force on the forefoot and eventually subluxated it dorsolaterally.

Coleman and Stelling commented on the rigid plantar convexity in these patients. They reported the hindfoot to be in valgus and equinus and the forefoot abducted, with midtarsal breakdown. The navicular bone dislocates onto the dorsum of the talar neck.[31]

Seimon presented his concept of the biomechanics of congenital vertical talus in the child younger than 2 years of age and corroborated his theory with dissection of a talus in an arthrogrypotic child who died shortly after birth.[183] He proposed that contracture of the Achilles tendon posteriorly and the extensor digitorum longus anteriorly resulted in increased equinus of the calcaneus and increased verticality of the talus. With dorsal displacement of the navicular bone and eversion of the calcaneus, the talus tilts even farther medially. Seimon considers the extensor digitorum longus to be the major offender anteriorly, pulling the navicular bone dorsally, with the extensor hallucis longus and tibialis anterior involved less often. The cuboid and cuneiform evert, and the forefoot is abducted. The medial structures become redundant with reduction, making section of the talocalcaneal ligament unnecessary.

Treatment

The earliest series recommended a variety of manipulative procedures, often using blocks, wrenches, clamps, and other devices.[127] Later investigators stressed closed manipulation and casting, with limited use of surgical releases.[80,200] The modern literature supports the belief that closed treatment is rarely successful, even if employed early.[103,157,183,221] Most investigators recommend manipulation and casting, starting at birth and extending to the first 3 to 4 months of life, merely as a means to stretch the soft tissues.

Selection of surgical treatment depends on whether the patient's condition has been detected early, is a failure of previous treatment, or is detected during adolescence or adulthood. Although multiple procedures have been described for the early management, three general options exist. The first is to attempt reduction in a single surgical procedure.[120,157,159] Other surgeons have used a two-stage procedure, one on the midfoot and a second on the hindfoot.[91,103,160,221] A third option includes the addition of arthrodesis of the subtalar joint. Talectomy, which was the recommended treatment of Lamy and Weissman, and excision of the navicular, recommended by Eyre-Brook, are no longer accepted as options.[57,127] The original articles should be consulted for details of the operative procedures.

The two-stage method of Coleman and colleagues is a frequently cited procedure.[30] Their initial article described the use of this operation on 28 feet of 19 patients and a follow-up as long as 12 years. They divided the condition into type I, associated with a calcaneocuboid dislocation, and type II, without calcaneocuboid dislocation. Failure to reduce the talocalcaneal dislocation by closed means was the indication for operative treatment. Four to six weeks of casting preceded the surgery. The first operative procedure consisted of tendon lengthenings and midfoot capsulotomies. Their second operative procedure included a posterior capsulotomy of the ankle joint, a tendoachilles lengthening, and transfer of the posterior tibialis to the plantar aspect of the navicular bone. The patients wore casts an additional 6 weeks and were placed in a brace. The investigators reported that earlier treatment produced better results.

Ogata and Schoenecker reviewed the largest series of patients treated in a single institution.[157] In their series, casting was never successful. Using a two-stage procedure had produced a high incidence of complications, including avascular necrosis. They recommended a one-stage open reduction medially of the talonavicular joint, fixing it with a Kirschner wire. Posterior capsulotomy of the talotibial and subtalar joints was performed, sometimes with a delayed subtalar arthrodesis.

Ogata and Schoenecker also suggested a fairly simple classification that is useful in examining results. Patients were divided into three groups. Group I patients had the primary isolated congenital vertical talus without any other underlying condition. Group II patients had an associated congenital anomaly but without neurologic involvement. Group III patients had neurologic impairment. Intuitively, the results should vary in the different groups.

Oppenheim and associates reviewed 15 feet of 12 patients.[159] Casting produced poor results in three of four feet. Eleven surgically treated feet followed for an average of 8 years resulted in four good results, six fair results, and one poor outcome. Their series is unique in that 8 of 11 patients had isolated congenital vertical talus without other underlying conditions. They concluded that a single-stage soft tissue release is the treatment of choice.

Dodge's group reviewed another 36 cases of congenital vertical talus in 21 patients, with an average follow-up of 14 years.[48] In all of these patients, the diagnosis had been made during the first year of life, most at birth. Ten of their patients had another underlying primary diagnosis, and 13 (62%) had at least one other secondary congenital abnormality. Pain did not appear to be an immediate or a long-term problem in their series. Fourteen percent of the feet were painful only during excessive activity, with only 1 foot of 36 reported as symptomatic during the activities of daily living. No surgical procedure was disproportionately associated with these findings. With longer follow-up, no particular operation seemed to be associated with a better outcome. Most feet had restricted subtalar motion. In many of the patients, talotibial motion was also reduced, which could not always be attributed to the underlying primary diagnosis such as arthrogryposis.

The series by Seimon, although small, has the advantage of being done by one surgeon.[183] It demonstrates that correction can be achieved in one stage in the young child before adaptive changes occur and that subtalar fusion is unnecessary.

Kodros and Dias reviewed their long-term follow-up of a single-stage surgical correction of congenital vertical talus in 41 patients (55 feet).[120] Thirty of these feet were associated with neural tube defects, 10 with neuromuscular disorders, and 5 with congenital malformations. None were associated with chromosomal aberrations. Only 10 of the feet were idiopathic. All feet were treated by a single-stage surgical correction using a Cincinnati incision performed by the same surgeon.

Thirty-two patients (42 feet) were available for clinical and radiographic follow-up averaging 7 years (range, 2–12 years). There were cases of no avascular necrosis and no wound complications. Ten feet did require reoperation. All patients and families were satisfied with the results and appearance of the foot. Radiographically, there was improvement in the anteroposterior and lateral talocalcaneal angle and the talar–first metatarsal angle. The surgeons thought that predictable results in this severe condition could be obtained with a low incidence of complications using single-stage surgical correction of the hindfoot and midfoot deformities.

All series in the literature have the same weaknesses. Congenital vertical talus is a rare condition that is seen to a limited extent even in the largest centers. Treatment regimens and surgical procedures have evolved with time, and no one has enough patients treated by one regimen and followed for a sufficient period to give a clear-cut answer. All of the series of congenital vertical talus contain patients with a variety of other underlying medical diagnoses, the most important of which are neurologic abnormalities and myelomeningocele. The results of treating patients who have no other underlying conditions are going to be different from results in those who have such conditions as arthrogryposis or myelomeningocele and therefore do not allow adequate comparison.

For a child younger than 2 years of age, I prefer to perform a single-stage soft tissue release to reduce the talonavicular and subtalar joints, which are held reduced with pins. A subtalar fusion usually is performed at the same time or 6 weeks later if the deformity is severe. Performing a fusion is supported by the review of Dodge and associates, which found that subtalar motion is severely restricted even in feet in which no fusion is performed.[79,115] Subtalar fusion is not easy to obtain in children when so much of the talus and calcaneus is cartilaginous. Parents must be counseled about the high complication rate, including skin slough, loss of reduction, restriction of motion, and avascular necrosis of the talus.

Correction in the adolescent and adult can be accomplished only by triple arthrodesis, usually requiring an excision of a fairly sizable portion of talus to achieve the reduction. Internal fixation until arthrodesis has been obtained may also be beneficial.

TARSAL COALITION

Tarsal coalition is a fibrous, cartilaginous, or bony connection of two or more tarsals. Our understanding of the condition, as with many other orthopaedic diagnoses, has paralleled the development of knowledge in other disciplines, particularly radiology. It is known to have existed since pre-Columbian times, because it was described in the archaeologic remains of several civilizations.[88] Anatomists described the common coalitions in the beginning of the 9th century, and physicians began to describe the clinical syndromes in the latter part of the same century. A comprehensive review by Mosier and Ahser contains details of the major historical contributions.[154]

The definition and management of tarsal coalition have improved with developments in radiographic imaging, starting with the linkage of a clinical radiograph showing calcaneonavicular coalition with the clinical syndrome of peroneal spastic flatfoot by Slomann in

1921 and by Badgley in 1927.[5,191] Talocalcaneal coalition was not linked to the syndrome of peroneal spastic flatfoot until Harris and Beath's description in 1948.[86] The use of CT increased understanding of and improved planning of the operative approach to these conditions.[44,92,158,167,195,202]

Etiology and Incidence

The first etiologic theories suggested that the accessory ossicles became incorporated with the adjacent tarsals, resulting in a coalition.[191] Harris encountered cartilaginous union of the sustentaculum tali with the talus equivalent to the adult talocalcaneal coalition while studying 20 apparently normal feet in embryos.[81] She found that this coalition was bilateral in two and unilateral in two. This finding established that the defect is congenital, resulting from a failure of differentiation and segmentation of the primitive mesenchyme. The ultimate cause of this failure remains to be elucidated.

The condition is associated with other congenital anomalies such as symphalangism, Niervergelt syndrome, and other limb anomalies.[154] Carpal and tarsal coalition can occur together. It has been described in monozygous twins.[66]

The true incidence is not known. Pfitzner's examination of 520 skeletons identified calcaneonavicular coalition in 2.9%.[154] Stormont and Peterson estimated the incidence to be less than 1% in the general population.[201] The most common coalitions involve the calcaneonavicular and the talocalcaneal joints. The first type is bilateral in about 60% of cases, and the second is bilateral in about 50% of cases.[34] Talonavicular, calcaneocuboid, cubonavicular, and naviculocuneiform coalitions are rare.[42,72,178,223]

Tarsal coalition can be fibrous, cartilaginous, or bony. Calcaneonavicular and talocalcaneal coalitions have been described in large enough numbers to delineate their natural history. Family studies have been particularly useful in this regard.

Wray and Herndon studied the occurrence of tarsal coalition in three generations of one family.[232] They were able to rule out autosomal recessive and sex-linked transmission and proposed autosomal dominant inheritance with variable penetrance as the most likely method. Leonard reviewed 31 index patients and 98 first-degree relatives and found that the transmission was compatible with autosomal dominant inheritance with almost full penetrance.[130]

Natural History

Leonard's review provides important insight into the natural history of tarsal coalition.[130] Fourteen percent of the relatives had a coalition, but it was a different type from that in the index patient. Perhaps more important was his findings that clinical evaluation revealed that the first-degree relatives with tarsal coalition were, for the most part, asymptomatic. No ball-and-socket ankles were found. Jayakumar and Cowell also found that many relatives of the index patient were asymptomatic.[106] Although we know that many adults with a coalition are symptomatic and that some of them had symptoms as adolescents, no one has ever studied a large number of patients who, once symptomatic, become asymptomatic with treatment. Scranton reported three adult patients with five involved feet who responded to 3 to 6 weeks of cast immobilization or injection of steroids in the sinus tarsi.[180]

Symptoms usually develop during adolescence. In Scranton's series, the age range was from 11 to 55 years, with some of the adults presenting after a traumatic event that seemed to awaken the latent condition.[180]

In most, the onset of pain seems to correlate with the age at which the bar ossifies. This event begins at about 3 to 5 years of age in talonavicular coalitions, 8 to 12 years in calcaneonavicular coalitions, and 12 to 16 years in talocalcaneal coalitions.[106] With ossification, subtalar motion is progressively decreased, leading to symptoms as the joint is stressed.

Clinical Features

The aching pain is usually vague and insidious in onset. Onset may coincide with trauma or increased activity that would lead to increased stress on the subtalar joint, such as participation in sports. It is worsened by activity and relieved by rest. Because subtalar motion is diminished, activities that require this motion, such as walking over uneven ground, may make the pain worse. The pain usually is localized to the subtalar area, and subtalar motion is diminished or absent. Talocalcaneal coalition is more often associated with a loss of subtalar motion. This loss of motion may increase stress to the ankle joint and increase the number of ankle sprains. Pes planus and ankle valgus may exist to some extent or may not be striking. When present, these conditions may amplify the forces on the subtalar and ankle joint and thereby increase symptoms, although they are more likely to be associated with talocalcaneal coalition.[101]

Although this syndrome has been called peroneal spastic flatfoot, true muscle spasm is rarely found. The peroneal muscles are shortened, and attempts to invert the foot cause pain as the muscles are stretched (Fig. 28-14).[82,86] Electromyography shows that there is no true muscle spasm and that nerve block does not

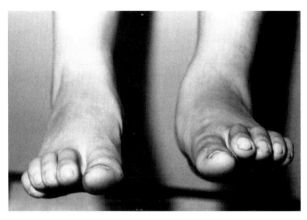

FIGURE 28-14. The patient presented with left foot pain. The left foot was everted, and all attempts at inversion caused pain and reproduced the symptoms.

correct the deformity.[86] Harris and Beath suggested abandoning the term peroneal spastic flatfoot in favor of more descriptive anatomic terms. Stormont and Peterson found muscle spasm in only 2 of 22 patients in their series.[201]

Any condition that injures the subtalar joint can produce the same clinical picture. The most common disorders that must be considered in the differential diagnosis are traumatic, arthritic, and infectious processes. An extensive list is provided in Mosier and Asher's review.[154]

Radiographic Evaluation

The clinical diagnosis should be confirmed by radiographic imaging. Anteroposterior, lateral, and oblique radiographs of the foot should be obtained initially, and they are usually diagnostic in calcaneonavicular

coalition, particularly on the 45 degree oblique view. In some patients, a coalition is plainly visualized. In others in whom the bar has not ossified, the diagnosis is suggested by an elongated process of the calcaneus or prolongation of the navicular bone. Oestreich and colleagues have described the "anteater nose" as a direct sign of calcaneonavicular coalition on the lateral radiograph.[156] A total of 30 feet of 21 children were evaluated for the appearance of the calcaneus and its relation to the navicular bone on films. As with calcaneonavicular bar, in children that were at least 9 years of age, there was a tubular prolongation anteriorly of the superior calcaneus that the researchers thought fancifully resembled the nose of an anteater. This prolongation approaches or overlaps the midportion of the navicular bone and occurred in the 30 feet with calcaneonavicular bar but not in 125 feet of 100 patients reviewed in the second decade who did not have a calcaneonavicular bar.

The subtalar joint surfaces overlap and are oblique, making diagnosis of talocalcaneal coalition by plain radiography difficult. Bony overlap in the anterior and middle facet articulations of the subtalar joint obscures the joint space. Secondary bony changes caused by this tarsal coalition may be revealed on the plain films, indicating the need for additional views or other studies. These changes include talar beaking, broadening or rounding of the lateral process of the talus, narrowing of the subtalar joint, a concave undersurface of the neck of the talus, and failure to see the middle subtalar joint (Fig. 28-15). The ball-and-socket ankle is another secondary sign that appears to develop, probably to compensate for the loss of subtalar motion. Although some have thought this sign was a congenital change, Takakura and colleagues showed by arthrography that the ankle appeared normal in

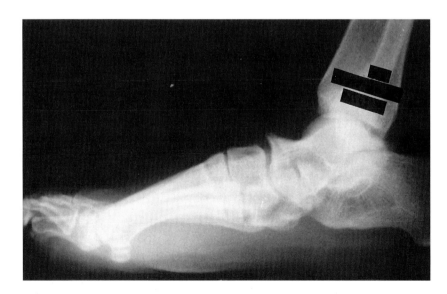

FIGURE 28-15. Lateral radiograph of a foot in a patient with a talocalcaneal coalition, showing a shortened talar neck, talar beaking, loss of definition of the anterior aspect of the subtalar joint, and elongation of the sustentaculum tali.

seven patients younger than 10 months of age but gradually developed the ball-and-socket appearance by 4 or 5 years of age.[126,210]

Harris and Beath developed special axial views taken at different angles in an attempt to demonstrate talocalcaneal coalition, but these views are difficult to take and interpret.[86] Jayakumar and Cowell suggested a technique of taking these views at different angles to increase the chances of demonstrating a coalition.[106] Plain tomography may show narrowing of the joint space and disruption of bone, but this appearance is also difficult to interpret, because these findings are similar to those seen in trauma.[31] Arthrography using 3 to 5 mL of contrast material injected in the dorsum of the talonavicular joint is said to be helpful.[111] Lack of filling of the space between the sustentaculum tali and the talus on Harris views and the lack of contrast material on the lateral view above the sustentaculum are thought to be diagnostic of a coalition. Scintigraphy has also been used but is nonspecific and lacks morphologic detail, which is the key to the diagnosis and management of this condition.[44] Although all of these methods have been used and may provide some information, most coalitions can be diagnosed using the combination of plain radiography and CT.[92,195,202,222]

With CT scanning, patients are positioned in the gantry with the hips and knees flexed and the soles of the feet flat on the table and side by side. Images using 4- or 5-mm slices of both feet are obtained.[195] Several small series have compared plain radiography, scintigraphy, or arthrography with CT. In one series, five patients had talocalcaneal bars and one a calcaneonavicular bar.[202] Routine radiography, including Harris views, was abnormal in four, arthrography abnormal in two, and scintigraphy abnormal in two. CT clearly demonstrated the talocalcaneal coalition in all five. The largest series, by Herzenberg and colleagues, is a combination anatomic and clinical study.[92] Results of plain radiography, plain tomography, and CT were compared with anatomic findings of the three subtalar joints in fresh cadaver feet. CT was superior to the other modalities for clearly identifying the anatomy. In the second part of the study, 22 patients with peroneal spastic flatfoot were evaluated with CT. Coalitions were demonstrated in 14 of the 22 patients, and in the other 8, the diagnosis was clearly ruled out. CT was comparable to the other imaging modalities in cost and radiation exposure.

CT is simple to perform, noninvasive, and accurate (Fig. 28-16). It provides precise delineation of the anatomy if surgery is contemplated. CT also gives some idea of whether the tissue is bony, cartilaginous, or fibrous. Coronal sections are useful for the talocalcaneal bar and longitudinal sections or for the calcaneonavicular bar. The procedure requires the patient to remain still for several minutes. Because the other foot is included in the study, it provides a reference if the anatomy is normal or may demonstrate as asymptomatic coalition in the other foot.

Cowell has admonished that patients may have more than one coalition.[34] The emergence of CT has revealed patients with multiple coalitions.[222] The patient in Figure 28-15 was thought to have only a calcaneonavicular coalition until the CT was obtained. The indications for CT are uncertain. Until more information is available about the frequency of multiple coalitions, it may be indicated for all patients suspected of having a coalition.[230] It may be the best single study to demonstrate coalitions.

MRI has also been used to delineate coalitions. Because it can demonstrate cartilage and fibrous tissues, it may eventually replace CT as the procedure of choice to image all coalitions.[140,162] Pizzutillo and colleagues reviewed their experience with use of MRI in diagnosing tarsal coalition.[95] Sixteen feet of eight patients were evaluated, and nine were surgically explored. Radiographs and CT scans revealed four of five calcaneonavicular coalitions and two of four medial facet talocalcaneal coalitions, but they failed to show two talocalcaneal coalitions and one calcaneonavicular coalition. MRI detected fibrous coalitions in these three patients, which was later confirmed by surgery, and visualized the other coalitions as well. These investigators recommend MRI for patients with suspected tarsal coalition when radiography and CT are both negative.

Pathophysiology

Most of the literature on pathomechanics concerns talocalcaneal coalitions, probably because this condition disturbs the normal subtalar function more than other coalitions. The talus is joined to the calcaneus through the anterior, middle, and posterior facets (Fig. 28-17). The body of the talus articulates with the large posterior facet of the calcaneus in the largest weight-bearing surface of the subtalar joint. This synovial compartment is separated from the anterior compartment by the substantial talocalcaneal interosseous ligament. The anterior compartment contains the anterior and middle facets, which can be separate or joined as one elongated process. The medially located middle facet is a major weight-bearing area and is the facet most often associated with a coalition. The middle and anterior facets are considered a unit because they share a synovial compartment with the head of the talus and the navicular bone. Together with the plantar calcaneonavicular ligament and anterior fibers of the deltoid, they form a modified ball-and-socket joint.

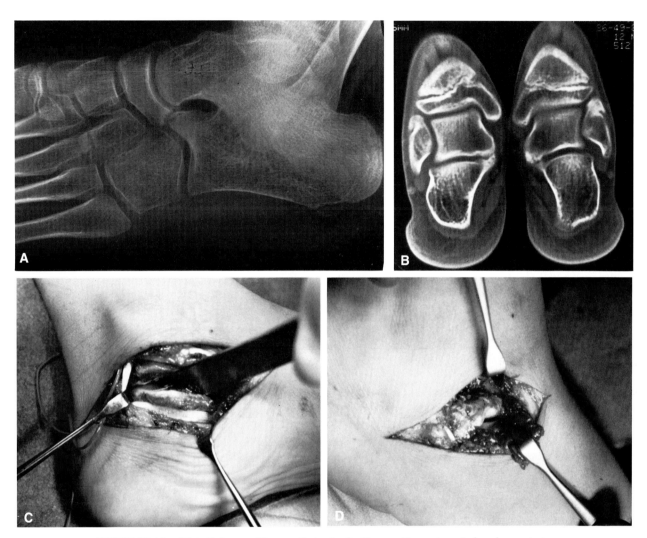

FIGURE 28-16. (A) A 45-degree oblique radiograph of a 12-year-old symptomatic boy demonstrates the calcaneonavicular osteocartilaginous coalition that was present bilaterally. (B) Computed tomography scan of the same patient demonstrates osteocartilaginous talocalcaneal coalition of the middle facet, also present bilaterally. (C) Retraction of the flexor digitorum. An osteotome is inserted in the area of the middle facet coalition. (D) Calcaneonavicular coalition before its removal.

During walking, the subtalar joint has a gliding and a rotary motion. With dorsiflexion, the calcaneus glides forward on the talus. Upward gliding occurs in the calcaneocuboid and talonavicular joints. At the extremes of dorsiflexion, the wide process of the navicular bone moves upward on the talar head but is limited by the talonavicular ligament. Subtalar fusion or a talocalcaneal coalition interferes with this gliding, causing a hinge motion at the midtarsal joints. The navicular bone then impinges on the talus, stretching the talonavicular ligament and resulting in spurring or beaking. Similarly, impingement of the talus on the lateral aspect of the calcaneal sulcus leads to broadening and flattening of the lateral talar process. These effects produce the secondary changes visible on plain radiographs.

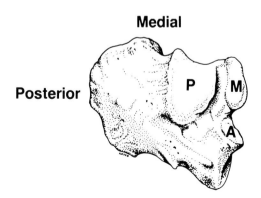

FIGURE 28-17. A right calcaneus viewed from above shows the posterior (P), middle (M), and anterior (A) facets.

Treatment

Most patients who present with a painful foot secondary to tarsal coalition are adolescents. Because we know that many adults with this condition are asymptomatic, the initial treatment should be conservative and should attempt to alleviate the pain.[34,86,130] Injection of the peroneal muscles, nerve blocks, and manipulation under anesthesia are no longer recommended. Scranton reported three adult patients with five involved feet who responded to 3 to 6 weeks of cast immobilization or injection of steroids in the sinus tarsi.[180] Conservative modes that attempt to immobilize the heel are recommended. Because the calcaneus is already relatively immobile, these modes may only relieve or shield the subtalar joint from stress. Empiric methods are usually tried initially, such as Plastizote shoe inserts and modifications that increase the support to the medial side of the foot. Activities that aggravate the pain should be avoided.

Patients not responding to these measures may respond to 3 to 6 weeks of immobilization in a short leg walking cast. This treatment may have to be repeated at intervals during adolescence. Although many series suggest these modalities, very few document their efficacy. Jayakumar and Cowell reported that one third of their patients were successfully managed nonoperatively.[106]

The main indication for surgery (i.e., coalition resection) is persistent pain. Other surgical indications, especially concerning talocalcaneal coalitions, are evolving and are not substantiated by long-term follow-up. The question is whether coalitions should be resected early, before degenerative changes occur. Can we predict which patients will become symptomatic and therefore be justifiable candidates for surgery?

The type of surgery depends on the type of coalition, the age of the patient, and the absence or presence of degenerative changes in the tarsal joints. Although the talar beak has previously been considered a degenerative change, it is actually a periarticular spur and not associated with degenerative changes or with poor postoperative results.[31,34,92,152,207]

For calcaneonavicular bars, resection and interposition of the extensor digitorum brevis is the treatment of choice and is usually associated with good results if there are no degenerative changes.[34,69,150,151,191,202] Cowell has recommended the following guidelines.[34] The patient should be young, and there should be no degenerative changes or other coalitions. Although the presence of other coalitions has not been a frequently documented situation, the use of CT may reveal a higher incidence of associated coalitions than was previously suspected. A rectangle of bone of at least 1 cm long should be resected and

the extensor digitorum brevis sutured in the defect. All cartilaginous portions of the coalition should be removed so the navicular bone and the calcaneus are clearly identified. A short leg walking cast is worn for 7 to 10 days postoperatively, and then subtalar motion is begun. Full weight bearing is not allowed for 4 to 6 weeks.

Of 26 feet treated in this manner at the A.I. DuPont Institute, 23 were symptom free.[106] Of the three feet that did poorly, one had reformation of the bar (8 of 23 had partial reformation of the bar with satisfactory results), one had a talocalcaneal coalition, and one had degenerative changes at the time of resection. The results for 75 feet of 48 patients evaluated 2 to 23 years after this procedure were rated good or excellent for 77% by Gonzalez.[69] The best results were obtained in patients with cartilaginous coalitions and in those who were younger than 16 years of age at the time of surgery.

Stormont and Peterson reported that 20 of 22 patients with this condition were successfully treated with resection and that two required triple arthrodesis.[201] Few patients with this type of coalition require triple arthrodesis.

Swiontkowski and associates reviewed 57 operations in 40 patients with tarsal coalition.[207] Thirty patients with calcaneonavicular coalition had 39 resections of the bar, and five had primary triple arthrodesis. The mean age at diagnosis was 12 years and 2 months, and the symptoms existed for a mean of 25.3 months. At a mean follow-up of 4.6 years, 29 feet were asymptomatic, and 40 (90%) of 44 feet were improved considerably by the surgical procedure. There were no recurrences of the bar.

Talocalcaneal coalitions have been more difficult to diagnose and treat. Calcaneal osteotomy is listed as an option to correct the valgus heel, but review articles, although mentioning it, do not list it as a treatment option in use.[22,154,158] Previous studies have discouraged resection of talocalcaneal bars, stating that resection of the middle facet disturbs the weight-bearing organization of the foot. Until the advent of CT, this coalition was difficult to diagnose, and in some series, the diagnosis was not made until the time of surgery. Although little has been written on this subject, a variety of interpositional materials have been used in talocalcaneal coalitions, and no large series has appeared to document the efficacy of any one procedure or determine whether the interpositional material is necessary.

Morgan and Crawford reported on 12 patients with coalitions, four of whom had talocalcaneal bars not responding to conservative care.[152] No consideration was given at the time of surgery to the presence or absence of degenerative changes on radiographs. Two patients had talocalcaneal coalitions resected, one bilaterally. Both were able to return to sports. Follow-up for the entire group was 31 months on average. Another study claimed successful resection of eight talocalcaneal coalitions in athletes, with improvement in subtalar motion and decreased pain, but no length of follow-up was mentioned.[55]

In Swiontkowski's series, the mean age at diagnosis of the patients with talocalcaneal coalition was 13.8 years, and the mean duration of symptoms was 4 years and 1 month.[207] Among the 10 patients with talocalcaneal coalition, five resections were attempted, four of which were successful. No interposition material was mentioned. At surgery, the coalition was found to involve the middle fact in four cases and the posterior facet in one. The mean follow-up period was 3.1 years. The remaining five patients with talocalcaneal bars required a variety of primary fusion procedures, depending on the anatomy found. The investigators recommended resection of coalitions under certain conditions. There should be no articular degenerative changes. Talar beaking is not considered a degenerative change but rather a talonavicular ligament traction spur. Severe malalignment is a contraindication. Although the bar should not be resected if tomography or CT indicates it is too large, no definition of this size was offered. An arthrodesis is preferable if any of these conditions are present.

Scranton reported 14 patients with 12 symptomatic coalitions reviewed at a mean of 3.9 years.[180] Five feet in three patients were successfully managed in casts, and four feet underwent triple arthrodesis. The indications for resection of the coalition were failure of conservative management and involvement of less than one half of the talocalcaneal joint surface area. Ten resected coalitions were medial, and four were lateral. Bone wax was placed on the raw cancellous bone, and fat was interposed. The patients were immobilized for a total of 6 weeks after surgery. Eight patients who had 13 resected coalitions had good results. Triple arthrodesis also provided a satisfactory result in Scranton's patients with symptomatic talocalcaneal coalitions, but he thought the procedure should be reserved for patients who fail to respond to conservative treatment and who have an unresectable coalition or advanced degenerative changes. The question of how extensive a coalition can be successfully resected is still unanswered. Some of Scranton's patients had approximately one half of the joint surface resected.

Olney and Asher reviewed nine patients with 10 talocalcaneal coalitions of the middle facet treated by excision and autogenous fat graft.[158] At an average follow-up of 42 months, results were excellent in five feet, good in three, fair in one, and poor in one. Function was comparable to that reported in patients after calcaneonavicular resection. There was no correlation between results with age, gender, or type of coalition.

One graft reviewed at 9 months was shown to be necrotic fat replaced by fibrous tissue. McCormick has updated the Olney and Asher series, providing a longer-term follow-up.[142] Ten feet in eight patients were followed for an average of 11 years and 8 months (range, 10–16 years). Symptomatically, the feet were rated as excellent in seven, fair in one, and poor in one. Even the fair results were doing well, with eight of nine satisfactory after 10 years. Radiographically, there were no evidence of degenerative changes in the hindfoot or midfoot. One patient with a poor result developed some talar beaking since the original study. The two patients in the original study who had talar beaking had excellent results, and it did not seem to be a contraindication to resection. The researchers think that resection of middle facet coalitions provides long-term relief of symptoms for most patients at 10 years of follow-up.

The surgical management of tarsal coalition continues to evolve, especially with regard to the resection of coalitions. The preceding review indicates that many adults have asymptomatic tarsal coalitions, which argues for an initial trial of conservative management. Most series now indicate that calcaneonavicular coalitions can be successfully managed by resection with interposition of the extensor digitorum brevis. The surgical indications for and results of talocalcaneal coalition resection are more controversial and await larger series with longer follow-up.

Calcaneal osteotomy to bring the heel out of valgus has been reported by Cain and Hyman to produce pain relief in a series of 13 patients with 14 involved feet.[22] The role of this procedure is uncertain, but the technique may be indicated for selected patients, especially those with advanced degenerative changes or severe malalignment. If the pain in these patients is from a stress reaction or fracture through the coalition, an isolated solid fusion of the subtalar joint may relieve the pain and avoid triple arthrodesis. There is no series of patients reported to support this approach. Triple arthrodesis is indicated for patients who have unresectable coalitions and pain that does not respond to conservative measures. It may also be the procedure of choice if there are degenerative joint changes. Triple arthrodesis is not often indicated until late adolescence or adulthood.

ACCESSORY NAVICULAR

The accessory navicular is the most common accessory bone in the foot. It occurs on the medial, plantar border of the navicular in close association with the posterior tibialis tendon. Shands found that 26% of 214 children studied had an accessory bone in the foot.[186] Of these, the accessory navicular bone was the most common, occurring in 20 (9.3%) of the children with accessory bones.

Clinical Features

The patient presents with a prominence on the medial aspect of the foot at the distal aspect of the talus and in the area of the talonavicular joint, along the insertion of the posterior tibialis tendon. Inversion of the foot against pressure usually demonstrates the posterior tibialis tendon closely associated with this prominence. In a symptomatic patient, other findings include presence of a bursa, redness, and irritation over the prominence from a shoe. Local tenderness to palpation is exhibited, and pain may be elicited by foot inversion against resistance.

Radiographic Evaluation

The best radiographic view for demonstrating an accessory navicular is a standard anteroposterior or a 45-degree eversion oblique view (Fig. 28-18). The navicular is the last tarsal bone to appear, occurring in 1- to 3.5-year-old girls and 3- to 5.5-year-old boys, and may ossify from multiple centers.[224] Difficulty with multiple, irregular centers may be encountered in differentiating this ossification from the intermittent stages of Koehler disease. The diagnosis of Koehler disease should not be made on the basis of a radiograph alone; it depends on clinical symptoms and findings.

The role of the accessory navicular in flatfoot has been a controversy since the original description of

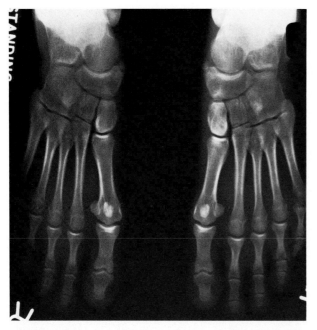

FIGURE 28-18. Anteroposterior standing radiograph demonstrates bilateral accessory naviculars.

Kidner.[113] He wrote that the "prehallux" was a common and previously unrecognized anomaly, which by changes in leverage, interferes with the normal mechanics of the posterior tibialis muscle. The resultant weakness of the longitudinal arch was thought to be highly resistant to the usual conservative methods of treatment. He thought that the loss of the normal insertion transformed the posterior tibialis into an adductor instead of an elevator of the tarsus in the longitudinal arch. Subsequent articles concerning his procedure have not provided a uniform definition of a flatfoot. In a radiographic study of 200 patients presenting with nontraumatic foot complaints who were compared with 19 patients with accessory naviculars, there was no evidence to substantiate the opinion that the longitudinal arches of the patients with accessory naviculars were different from those of normal patients.[204] It is more likely that the accessory navicular, when present in flatfoot, is an incidental findings, and its inclusion among causes of pain for painful symptomatic flatfoot in children is unwarranted.

Accessory naviculars have been classified by their radiographic appearances.[74] Type I is a small ossicle within the substance of the posterior tibialis tendon. This was previously called the os tibiale externum or navicular secondarium. It is posterior and medial to the navicular body. Type II is triangular, larger than type I, and joined to the navicular by a cartilaginous synchondrosis. Repeated fractures through this cartilaginous bridge may account for the pain. Type III is a cornuate navicular resulting from fusion of the accessory navicular with the navicular.

The navicular bone is occasionally bipartite. In this condition, there is a smaller, partially displaced and larger, medially subluxed center.[161] The condition is congenital.

Pathoanatomy

Histologically, accessory naviculars show proliferating vascular mesenchymal tissue, cartilage proliferation, and osteoblastic and osteoclastic activity.[74] Instead of a true joint, there is a synchondrosis in various stages of development. In some patients, it is a separate ossicle; in others, it has more of a cartilaginous connection to the navicular; and in the latter variety, the navicular is successfully prolonged around the medial aspect (cornuate navicular). The histologic findings of Grogan and colleagues were consistent with healing microfractures, substantiating the opinion that the pain is related to chronic, repetitive stress reaction.[74]

Natural History

Most patients are asymptomatic or can be managed conservatively without the need for operative treatment. In the series by Sullivan and Miller, 18 patients who had simple excisions were reviewed to determine the success of the procedure.[204] A second group of 208 patients with nontraumatic foot complaint were reviewed to determine the incidence of accessory navicular. In this second group of patients, 29 cases of previously undetected accessory naviculars were identified, lending credence to the belief that most cases are asymptomatic in adult life.

Treatment

The patient can often be managed symptomatically or by modifying the shoes. The patient can wear softer shoes or have the shoe stretched in the area over the prominence.

Surgical management is indicated for failure to respond to conservative measures. The Kidner procedure was advocated as a means of excising the ossicle within the tendon and reestablishing what he thought was the normal support of the arch by the posterior tibialis tendon.[113] The studies of Basmajian and Smith have indicated that muscular activity is not necessary to maintain the arch of the loaded foot at rest.[8,194] The first line of support is by passive structures. The accessory navicular is seldom symptomatic or detected before adolescence.[186] Simple excision of the prominent ossicle seems to be the surgical procedure of choice when conservative means of management fail.[11,65,204,216] Nothing is done with the tibialis tendon other than place sutures in the area where the ossicle was excised. Patients should be forewarned that there will be a scar in the area of the previous prominence that can become painful with shoe wear.

OSTEOCHONDROSES

Koehler Disease

Koehler disease is a clinical condition associated with pain in the area of the tarsal navicular in combination with density, fragmentation, and eventually narrowing of the tarsal navicular.

Etiology

The cause of Koehler disease is unknown. Waugh studied the vascular pattern of the tarsal navicular.[224] He found that the navicular bone has a network of vessels that often originates from a single artery. Because the navicular is the last tarsal bone to ossify, he suggested that it is subjected to more risk of damage from repeated loading. The result could be fragmentation of the navicular.

Clinical Features

Typically, this condition occurs in a child younger than 6 years of age who presents with midtarsal pain. It is more frequent in boys than girls and may occur bilaterally. Pain is present on weight bearing and relieved by rest. The patient may have palpable tenderness over the navicular.

Radiographic Evaluation

Radiographically, the increased density and fragmentation of the tarsal navicular progresses to flattening (Fig. 28-19). Followed over time, the navicular gradually reconstitutes with new bone formation. The radiographic features may be seen in asymptomatic patients and represent variations in ossification of the navicular.

Pathoanatomy

Pathologic specimens have been rare. In the few cases observed, there have been bone destruction and dead trabeculae, with interference of normal ossification.[231]

Karp concluded that the average age of appearance of the ossific nucleus is between 18 months and 2 years in girls and between 2.5 and 3 years of age in boys.[110] The pattern of development of the navicular varies, and abnormalities of ossification are common. It is a combination of history, physical findings, and radiographic features that leads to the diagnosis.

Natural History

No known cases have been described in adults. The condition is self-limiting, and the navicular gradually reconstitutes.

Treatment

The treatment of this benign, self-limited condition is entirely nonsurgical. Williams and Cowell found a difference in duration of symptoms that depended on treatment.[231] Individuals who were not casted had symptoms that lasted an average of 15.2 months, and those treated with a cast had symptoms lasting only an average of 3.2 months. A walking cast was equally as effective as a nonwalking cast. It is the treatment of choice for those requiring treatment.

Freiberg Infraction

Freiberg infraction is a clinical condition in which there is pain in the second metatarsal head in an adolescent with characteristic radiographic findings.

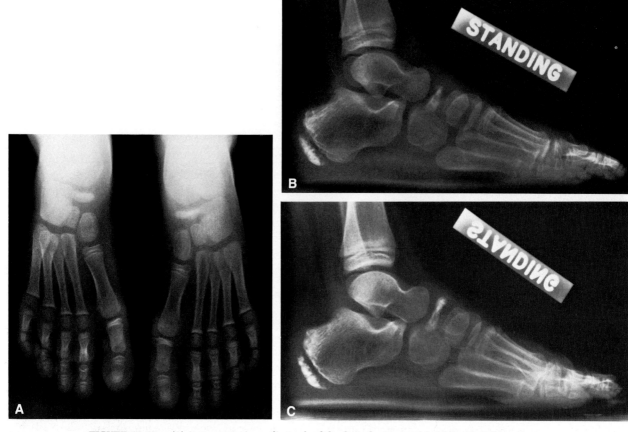

FIGURE 28-19. (**A**) Anteroposterior radiograph of the feet of a 6-year-old child with Kohler disease. (**B**) The right foot showed no symptoms. (**C**) The child had symptoms on the left, emphasizing that the diagnosis is based on radiographic findings.

Etiology

The cause of Freiberg infraction is unknown. As Freiberg said, there is no unanimity of opinion regarding the cause or the essential nature of the condition.[61] This statement made in 1926 remains true today. Smiley suggested that Freiberg infraction was caused by stress fractures secondary to a short first metatarsal.[192] In the Canadian Army study of Harris and Beath of over 7000 feet, 40% had short metatarsals, but there was no increase of foot pain in this group.[83] Braddock performed an experimental study of metatarsals.[17] He used fresh necropsy specimens that were subjected to weights dropped from a height. The experiment showed a relative weakness of the second metatarsal epiphysis at a certain stage of epiphyseal maturation. Even when grossly comminuted, the resultant fractures were not compatible with the radiographic findings of Freiberg infraction.

Clinical Presentations and Radiographic Evaluation

Symptoms occur most often in the second decade. The patients present with a history of pain in the foot.

The findings are pain, decreased range of motion, and tenderness to palpation of the metatarsophalangeal joint.

The anteroposterior radiograph is usually the basis for the diagnosis (Fig. 28-20). If the physis is open, it may show irregularity and collapse. In patients whose physes have closed, the metatarsal head is enlarged, flattened, and irregular on the articular surface. The joint space may be narrowed.

Treatment

Nonoperative treatment should be tried for all patients to allow the condition to heal. Initially, casting may be necessary to relieve the pain. Various orthotic devices have been suggested, including metatarsal bars, shoe inserts to relieve weight-bearing stresses to the metatarsal head, or a change in footwear.

Surgery is rarely necessary in this unusual condition. Operative management is indicated only if conservative care has failed to alleviate symptoms. The metatarsal head may be irregular, and the joint space may show degenerative changes. Margo suggested reshaping and shaving of the metatarsal head with a

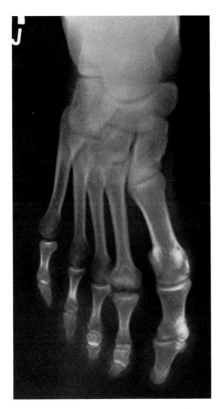

FIGURE 28-20. Typical radiographic findings of a Freiberg infraction in a symptomatic 18-year-old patient.

rasp.[139] He further advised that the base of the adjacent proximal phalanx be excised instead of the metatarsal head to preserve the weight-bearing aspect of the forefoot. Another alternative is excision of the metatarsal head. Complications include a shift in weight bearing, causing metatarsalgia after excision of the metatarsal head or continued pain.

CONGENITAL CLUBFOOT

Congenital clubfoot is a complex foot deformity that consists of hindfoot equinus with varus of the forefoot and heel and an adducted forefoot. It is best thought of as displacement of the navicular, calcaneus, and cuboid bones around the talus. It is also referred to as congenital talipes equinovarus.

Incidence

One study reported the overall incidence in Sweden was 0.93 per 1000 children.[38] Seventy-nine percent of the affected children were boys, and 44% of cases were bilateral. In other studies, congenital clubfoot occurs 1.24 times per 1000 live births in the general population.[36,234–236] Boys are affected twice as often as girls, and 50% of cases are bilateral. First-degree relatives (i.e., siblings and parents) have an occurrence rate

17 times higher than the normal population. Second-degree relatives (i.e., aunts and uncles) have an occurrence rate six times the population rate. Monozygotic twins have approximately a 32.5% rate of concordance (i.e., both twins having the disorder). Wynne-Davies concluded that this supports a pattern of inheritance of a dominant gene with reduced penetrance or multifactorial inheritance system.[236] The conclusions reached by Cowell was that this was multifactorial inheritance modified by intrauterine and environmental factors and possibly affected by a gene acting in a dominant fashion.[36]

Several conclusions have been reached regarding genetic counseling for Caucasians.[36,234–236] If a male baby has the disorder, the chances are 1 in 42 that a subsequent brother will be affected and very low that a sister will be affected. If a female baby has congenital clubfoot the chances are higher that a subsequent sibling will be affected: 1 in 16 for brothers and 1 in 40 for sisters. If a parent and child have the disorder, the chances are about 1 in 4 that a subsequent child will have congenital clubfoot.

Etiology

The cause of congenital talipes equinovarus is unknown. Several extrinsic causes have been related to this disorder in humans. Oligohydramnios with the formation of amniotic bands has a high association with congenital clubfoot.[35] Sodium aminopterin ingestion in an attempt to induce an abortion can induce multiple congenital anomalies, including clubfoot. D-Tubocurarine for treatment of tetanus during the first trimester of pregnancy can result in arthrogryposis and clubfoot in the fetus.[50] Several groups of theories have been suggested for the cause of congenital clubfoot. None has been accepted as the cause in most cases, although the most widely accepted theories are mechanical factors, a germ plasm defect, or a neuromuscular cause.

Some have proposed that congenital clubfoot is a mechanical problem, the result of intrauterine crowding or packing.[20,36] This is not supported by an increased occurrence of clubfoot among high-birth-weight babies, cases of multiparity, or in twins.[27,234,235]

Bohm described five stages of development and concluded that the cause of clubfoot was an embryonic arrest of development in the first stage.[15] Irani and Sherman investigated 11 extremities with equinovarus foot recovered from stillbirths.[100] The head of the talus was deviated medially, with the navicular articulating with the medial side of the head of the talus. They suggested that this was the result of a germ plasm defect.

Others have suggested neuromuscular causes, such as abnormal muscles.[10,135] Clubfoot is associated with underlying conditions such as arthrogryposis, myelomeningocele, and other genetically inherited disorders. Ippolitto and Ponseti thought this was the result of shortening and thickening of ligaments because of retracting fibrosis.[99] Deitz and colleagues thought that a regional growth disturbance on the medial side of the foot was responsible for a local hypoplasia, resulting in clubfoot.[45,46] The cause of clubfoot remains controversial.

Clinical Features

The history should include a family history for other members with congenital clubfoot or any other neurologic problems. The physical examination should confirm that the foot has a fixed deformity in which the hindfoot is in equinus, the heel in varus, and the forefoot is adducted. Cavus may also be evident. Generally, a clubfoot is smaller than a contralateral normal foot. The calf is small, and the involved leg may be shorter.

The term clubfoot refers to a wide spectrum of severity. The degree of rigidity is assessed to determine where any given foot lies within that spectrum. Positional clubfeet are those in which, on the first examination, the hindfoot and forefoot can be brought to neutral varus, adductus, and plantigrade. These usually respond dramatically to a few cast changes. Tachdjian refers to these feet as postural clubfeet and states that they are caused by intrauterine malposture.[208] He makes the point that the skin creases are normal, unlike clubfeet in which there are deep furrows and creases over the heel and the medial sole of the foot. He reserves the term talipes equinovarus for the resistant clubfoot.

The resistant congenital clubfoot cannot be brought to neutral and often has associated creases medially, transversely across the arch, and superior to the heel. Congenital clubfoot must also be separated from those associated with arthrogryposis, myelomeningocele, and other syndromes.

Physical examination should include an examination of the spine, looking for signs of spinal dysraphism or spinal deformity. The neck is examined for torticollis, and the hips and lower extremities for torsional alignment.

Radiographic Evaluation

There is no consensus on the value of radiographs in the routine management of congenital clubfoot. Tachdjian devotes five pages of his chapter on clubfoot to the methods of obtaining and measuring x-ray films.[208] Simons has written extensively on the use of analytical radiography to assess the severity of clubfeet and to monitor their intraoperative correction.[190,211] Beatson used radiography to assess the correction of clubfeet.[9] Wenger and Ponseti wrote that radiography has little role in the decision-making process.[125,226]

If x-ray films are obtained, they should be taken in a standardized manner and must be weight-bearing or forced dorsiflexion views (Fig. 28-21).

The difficulty with all radiographs of congenital clubfeet in the young child is the late appearance of the tarsals and the difficulty in achieving reproducibility. Even when tarsal coalitions and other anomalies are present, they are often not visible during the first year of life. Most agree that the measurement of the anteroposterior and lateral talocalcaneal angles after treatment provides some measure of correction.

I rarely obtain radiographs on the first visit. After 2 or 3 months of casting, a set of radiographs are taken to assess correction and the need for possible surgery. Radiographs are not used to monitor surgical correction, but they are used to verify the position of transfixing pins. Postoperatively, radiographs are obtained at 3- to 6-month intervals for approximately 1 year and then annually or biannually until adolescence.

Other imaging studies are not routinely used. Arthrograms of the ankle or subtalar joint have been used but have not gained wide acceptance. CT scans, occasionally with three-dimensional reconstruction, are used with older children in whom the bones are more fully ossified in contemplating surgery for residual deformity. Ultrasound can be useful in making the prenatal diagnosis of congenital clubfoot.[19,203]

MRI may prove beneficial if it more clearly defines the pathoanatomy. Downey reviewed the MRI findings of 10 infants with congenital clubfoot.[49] The findings were consistent with medial deviation of the talar neck and head. The calcaneus was medially rotated relative to the talar body, with the posterior calcaneus laterally deviated, accounting for the parallelism revealed on plain radiographs.

Pathoanatomy

Howard and associates dissected three clubfeet in stillborns.[96] The soft tissue abnormality demonstrable in their dissection was a dense fibrous knot at the inferomedial aspect of the foot that proved difficult to separate from the tendon and sheath of the tibialis posterior. If the fibrotic mass were contractile, many of the abnormalities of clubfoot could be explained; however, this was not definitely proven.

The most marked deformity Settle found in 16 dissections of infantile clubfeet was in the neck of the talus, which showed marked medial and plantar deviation on the body.[184] The talar articular surface of the navicular was displaced further medially and plantarly on the deviated neck. The articular surfaces were distorted. The calcaneus had a normal contour but was smaller and rotated internally. No abnormalities were found in the biopsies of muscles or nerves.

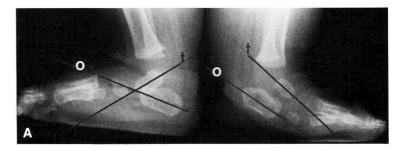

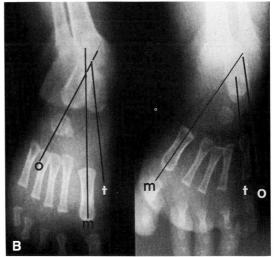

FIGURE 28-21. (A) Lateral radiographs of the feet of a young child. The feet have been positioned so the malleoli are overlapped. The right foot is normal. There is a severe left clubfoot with a rocker-bottom deformity. This figure demonstrates some problems with drawing lines on radiographs. The black lines do not correspond to the lines drawn by the radiologist. (B) Anteroposterior view of the normal right foot and left clubfoot. Notice the parallelism between t and o in the clubfoot and the adductus of the forefoot in the clubfoot. (m, line through the first metatarsal; o, line through the long axis of the os calcis; t, line through the long axis of the talus.)

Irani and Sherman examined 11 extremities with equinovarus deformity of the foot, 14 of which appeared completely normal.[100] They also found that the head of the talus was deviated medially, with the navicular articulating with the medial side. The consistent abnormality was in the anterior part of the talus, which was short, and the angle of the long axis of the forepart of the talus with the long axis was decreased. This angle usually was 150 to 155 degrees, but in clubfeet, it was 115 to 135 degrees. The shape of the forefoot was normal, but it was smaller. The other bones appeared normal. Recent MRI studies have substantiated the changes in the talus and the relation with the calcaneus.[49]

Waisbrod dissected eight fetuses with unilateral clubfoot.[220] The most important abnormality was in the talar angle of declination. Carroll examined 17 normal embryologic and fetal feet and four patients with five clubfeet.[24,26] He found, in addition to tight tendons, capsules, and ligaments, that the lateral malleolus was directed posteriorly and the head of the talus pointed laterally, with the navicular subluxed toward the medial malleolus. The calcaneus compensated by tipping into equinus and rotating into varus. The long axis of the calcaneus and talus become more nearly parallel. He thought that the equinus and varus of the calcaneus could not be corrected until the talus was derotated medially. The foot would assume the

normal position after the navicular was affixed to the head of the talus.

The fact that the talus is displaced is accepted, but there is disagreement about whether it is rotated laterally or medially in the ankle mortise. McKay thought it was a neutral alignment.[145] Goldner thought there was internal rotation.[68] Carroll thought there was external rotation and that the the lateral malleolus was posterior.[24,26]

Hjelmstedt and Sahlstedt paid particular attention to the ankle joint, unlike most other studies of clubfoot anatomy in which the foot was examined as a unit separate from the leg.[90] They found a strong fibrous connection between the medial malleolus and the trochlea, with these fibers occupying space in the trochlea that would ordinarily be articular cartilage.

There is contracture of the short plantar muscles, the plantar fascia, and the spring ligament. The calcaneus and talus are parallel with the calcaneus and the talus in equinus. There is contracture of the triceps, tibialis posterior, flexor hallucis, and flexor digitorum, with contracture of the posterior capsule of the tibiotalar and subtalar joints. There has been disagreement about whether tibial torsion is associated with clubfoot.[99,116,237,233]

Most investigators agree that congenital clubfoot results from an abnormal displacement of the navicular, calcaneus, and cuboid bones about the talus. The major portion of the deformity is centered on the talus, which has a medially and plantarly deviated neck. The configuration of the calcaneus, navicular, and cuboid bones with the talus is best considered as a ball-and-socket joint, similar to the femoral head and acetabulum. In this instance, the talus is analogous to the femoral head, and the other bones with their ligamentous connections form a socket analogous to the acetabulum. In this instance, it is similar to femoral anteversion in which the neck of the femur is abnormally angulated. In addition, the socket formed by the other tarsal is medially and plantarly displaced.

Natural History

Untreated, severe congenital clubfoot develops into a severe deformity (Fig. 28-22). In the severe, untreated foot, a large callus develops on the dorsum of the foot for weight bearing, and painful arthritic changes

develop. Extremely modified shoes are necessary for ambulation with these severely compromised feet.

Treatment

The goal of treatment of congenital clubfoot is a functional, pain-free, plantigrade foot with good mobility and without callus. As near-normal a range of motion as is possible is desirable.

Twenty-nine patients with unilateral clubfoot and 29 controls were reviewed for an average of 10 years after definitive treatment to assess disability.[2] Treatment varied from prolonged casting to early posteromedial release. The most significant findings were a 42% decrease in ankle motion (65% lack of dorsiflexion), 24% decrease in plantar flexion strength (correlated with the number of heel cord lengthenings), and 10% decrease in calf girth, which was unrelated to the time in casts. It should be stressed to parents that a

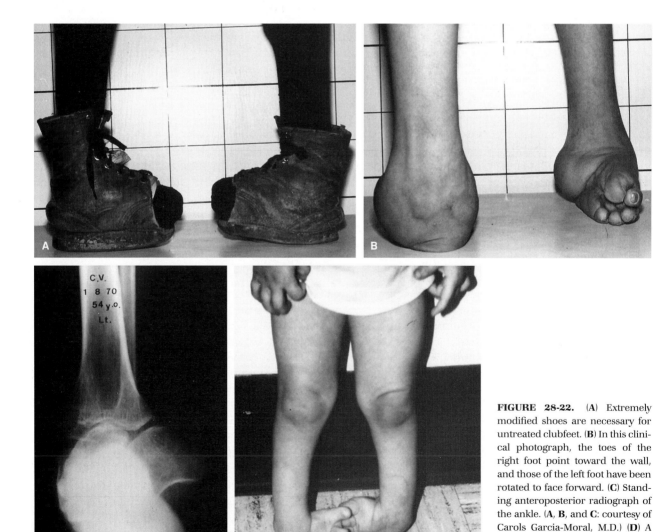

FIGURE 28-22. (**A**) Extremely modified shoes are necessary for untreated clubfeet. (**B**) In this clinical photograph, the toes of the right foot point toward the wall, and those of the left foot have been rotated to face forward. (**C**) Standing anteroposterior radiograph of the ankle. (**A, B,** and **C:** courtesy of Carols Garcia-Moral, M.D.) (**D**) A 3-year-old child who was initially casted but lost to follow-up shows the resultant deformity.

congenital clubfoot will never be an entirely normal foot, regardless of treatment modality, except in the mildest of cases. The foot and calf often are smaller than the opposite side in a unilateral case.

Nonoperative Treatment

Taping has been suggested but is rarely effective except for cases of positional clubfeet. Serial plaster casting at frequent intervals has been the mainstay of treatment for many years. All infant clubfeet should be casted initially to assess the response to casting and the potential for correction. The earlier this is begun, the greater is the likelihood of success. The foot is manipulated at each cast change, taking care not to produce a breach at the ankle or at the midfoot. Although casting has its proponents, it is often difficult to apply on a weekly basis, particularly if patients must travel long distances or have limited incomes.

The technique attempts to correct the deformity about the talus. The forefoot must be brought from its medially displaced position to neutral or beyond to realign the navicular with the talus. The forefoot is everted by pressing on the sole of the first metatarsal (correcting any cavus), attempting to push the cuboid and navicular laterally while abducting the foot by gradually increasing amounts. The medial and plantar ligaments are progressively stretched until the foot is realigned in the horizontal plane about the vertical axis to reduce the talonavicular and calcaneocuboid joints. Only at that point should the surgeon begin to attempt to correct the posteriorly contracted structures by dorsiflexing the foot. Failure to achieve forefoot correction can cause a break at the midfoot and a progressive rocker-bottom appearance. Most orthopaedic specialists advocate at least weekly cast changes with manipulation.

Based on his experiences of manipulation of clubfoot deformity in India, Brand thought that the foot should be serially casted while the child is suckling the breast of the nursing mother. The foot is only corrected to the point that the child loses interest in nursing. Most would find this difficult to achieve in today's population, but it makes the point that manipulation should be gentle.

CAST TECHNIQUE. Several researchers have written excellent descriptions of the closed management of clubfeet.[169,208,226] The reader is urged to read these detailed descriptions of technique.

I prefer to use 5-cm (2-in) cotton padding applied over a slight amount of tincture of benzoin. This extends well out over the toes. Gypsona plaster has the best combination of speed of setting and moldability for these small feet. Although most stress the need to apply a long leg cast, a short leg cast may be used at times.[226] I initially use a long leg cast in most cases. If only the forefoot adductus and heel varus are being corrected, a short leg cast is used. As the foot is brought up to correct the equinus contracture, a long leg cast is used. It may be more difficult to keep a short leg cast from slipping distally on a small, fat, conical leg. For the cast, 5- to 7.5-cm (2–3-in) plaster is best, depending on the size of the child. The application of clubfoot casts requires a team approach, with a parent to hold the child, someone to apply the plaster, and someone to mold the correction.

I prefer to stretch the foot and then hold it while an assistant applies the plaster and I mold the cast. The person rolling the plaster pulls it on snugly and then holds the thigh to immobilize the leg during molding. I prefer to have the parents remove the cast on the evening before coming to the clinic. This allows them time to bathe the baby and provide skin care. Most relate horror stories of having children soak in water for hours. Various additives, such as dishwashing detergent or a small amount of white vinegar, supposedly facilitate the plaster breakdown. By leaving a tag of plaster at the end of the cast, the parents can find a starting point for unrolling it. I have found it more humane to supply a small pair of bandage scissors with a serrated edge to the parents and allow them to cut the cast off after it becomes soggy.

When applying a clubfoot cast, the plaster is applied with some tug to ensure a snug-fitting cast. The right temperature and type of plaster are necessary to achieve a creamy, moldable plaster that will hold in the corrected position without a lot of excessive bulk. During manipulation a clubfoot, I prefer holding the heel. If it is a right foot, the heel is held with the left hand, with the thumb positioned just on the calcaneus behind the calcaneocuboid joint. The right hand grasps the first, second, and third toes, abducting and everting the foot. The thumb of the right hand presses up on the midfoot, pushing the navicular and cuboid laterally. The foot is left in equinus until the forefoot is corrected. Plaster is rolled well out over the toes. The knee is flexed approximately 80 to 90 degrees and the cast applied to the groin in a single unit. Care must be taken to mold an arch to prevent rocker-bottom deformity and mold over the calcaneus with the navicular and cuboid bones being displaced laterally. On the right foot, the left thumb is held on the calcaneus while the finger and thumb of the opposite hand evert and abduct the foot. With care, no trimming is necessary. Adequate circulation to the toes should be evident before the patient leaves the clinic.

RESULTS OF CLOSED TREATMENT. Ponseti described the fine points of the manipulative management of clubfoot.[58,125,169] He attributed poor results to faulty technique and the scant time and space allotted to teaching manipulating techniques. He used six to eight toe-to-groin plaster casts changed weekly and worn for a total of 7 to 10 weeks to obtain the maximum correction possible. For more detail about this technique, the reader is referred to his review.[169]

In Ponseti's experience, 85% to 90% of clubfeet were treated successfully with proper manipulation, casts, splints, and corrective shoes. His group placed more emphasis on the clinical appearance of the foot than on the radiographic appearance. Ponseti also thought that, regardless of the form of treatment, a clubfoot has a tendency to relapse until the child is about 7 years of age. He recommended managing relapses by casting, Dennis Browne splints, and high-top shoes to maintain the correction. Splints were worn full time for 2 to 3 months after casting and thereafter at night for 2 to 4 years. Specific instructions were given about the type of splints and the way they should be crafted. He thought that relapse could be prevented in about 50% of patients with careful supervision and cooperative parents. In addition to casting, he employed percutaneous heel cord tenotomy and, at times, transfer of the anterior tibialis to the third cuneiform. Laaveg and Ponseti reviewed the experience at the University of Iowa Clinics using this approach and found that manipulation and serial casting, supported by limited operative procedures, produced satisfactory functional results in 89% of feet (Table 28-2).[125]

Ruth Wynne-Davies studied 121 feet in 84 patients treated from 1940 to 1951.[233] They were treated initially by manipulation, followed by Hobble splints and then nighttime Browne boots with a crossbar. The average age at final discharge from the clinic was 15 years. One third had closed treatment alone, and two thirds had surgery. At follow-up, few of the patients limited their activities on account of the deformed feet. Few were symptomatic. The average shortening of the limb was 2.5 cm, and each had a thin calf with a smaller than normal foot. Some patients had a false correction, and the foot was broken at the talonavicular level. Clinical assessment correlated with the radiographic appearance, showing the near impossibility of a good foot resulting from false correction.

Ikeda and colleagues studied 25 patients who had received conservative treatment.[98] At 4 to 16 years of age, the outcome was excellent or good by the Laaveg-Ponseti rating system (see Table 28-2). They thought that muscle imbalances that made correction difficult in infancy improved with time.

Complications of closed treatment include increased cavus deformity, rocker-bottom deformity, longitudinal breach, and flattening of the proximal surface of the talus with lateral rotation of the ankle and increased stiffness. Meticulous technique is necessary to prevent skin complications.

Positional clubfeet and some of the less severe resistant congenital clubfeet respond to this treatment. Kite advised that most clubfeet could be successfully corrected by plaster casts and wedging with far better results than with the use of anesthetics, forceful manipulations, or operative procedures.[116] Gradually, others became convinced that more nearly normal results could be obtained with less morbidity by operative treatment. There are no accurate figures for the number of clubfeet considered to be postural or positional and that respond to treatment. According to McKay, only 15% of clubfeet can be treated nonoperatively.[145-147] A majority of pediatric orthopedists think that most clubfeet require surgical treatment.

Surgical Treatment

Surgery is indicated for a failure to achieve satisfactory results by closed methods. Continued forceful manipulations do not reduce the foot and can cause damage to articular surfaces and breakdown of the midfoot, producing a rocker-bottom foot, or the ankle joint.

There is no unanimity about when surgery should be performed or how to evaluate the result. Pous wrote that surgery could be performed in the neonate or child 6 weeks of age, but there has not been wide acceptance of that approach.[172] Turco thought that children should be older than 1 year of age.[213] I think children can be safely operated at 4 months of age. By this time, if closed methods are going to be successful, they should have achieved their goal. This allows a satisfactory period after the operative procedure for casting but does not interfere with the child's normal progression to crawling, standing, and walking.

Just as there is disagreement about the exact pathoanatomy of clubfoot, there is a difference of opinion about surgical goals. In some children with near-normal feet and only residual equinus, a limited procedure, such as heel cord lengthening and perhaps posterior capsulotomy, can achieve a satisfactory result. Multiple limited approaches can be disastrous. In one study of 118 operations that included 57 reoperations, the most frequent cause of relapse was insufficient primary surgery.[219] The second identifiable cause of relapse was surgery on a foot that was originally stiff and not reducible. For most patients, a full, formal release is required.

The type of operative procedure depends on the age of the patient and whether there has been previous treatment. In general, patients younger than 6 years of age are treated by soft tissue procedures. For children between 6 and 12 years of age, a combination of soft tissue releases, occasionally with tendon transfers, and limited bony procedures is indicated. The teenage patient usually has a residual deformity from clubfoot,

TABLE 28-2   *Functional Rating System for Clubfoot*

CATEGORY	POINTS
Satisfaction (20 points)	
I am	
a) very satisfied with the end result	20
b) satisfied with the end result	16
c) neither satisfied nor unsatisfied with the end result	12
d) unsatisfied with the end result	8
e) very unsatisfied with the end result	4
Function (20 points)	
In my daily living, my clubfoot	
a) does not limit my activities	20
b) occasionally limits my strenuous activities	16
c) usually limits me in strenuous activities	12
d) limits me occasionally in routine activities	8
e) limits me in walking	4
Pain (30 points)	
My clubfoot	
a) is never painful	30
b) occasionally causes mild pain during strenuous activities	24
c) usually is painful after strenuous activities only	18
d) is occasionally painful during routine activities	12
e) is painful during walking	6
Position of heel when standing (10 points)	
Heel varus, 0 degrees or some valgus	10
Heel varus, 1–5 degrees	5
Heel varus, 6–10 degrees	3
Heel varus, > 10 degrees	0
Passive motion (10 points)	
Dorsiflexion	1 point per 5 degrees (up to 5 points)
Total varus-valgus motion of heel	1 point per 10 degrees (up to 3 points)
Total anterior inversion-eversion of foot	1 point per 25 degrees (up to 2 points)
Gait (10 points)	
Normal	6
Can toe-walk	2
Can heel-walk	2
Limp	−2
No heel strike	−2
Abnormal toe-off	−2

From Laaveg SJ, Ponseti IV, Long term results of treatment of congenital clubfoot. J Bone Joint Surg [Am] 1980;62:23.

and the surgeon usually must resort to bony procedures.

In the previously untreated infant, complete release of the complex of tarsals about the talus, with lengthening of tight structures and release of capsules, can produce satisfactory reduction of clubfoot. A variety of surgical procedures have been described to achieve this end. The main points of the procedures advocated by Turco, Goldner, Carroll, and McKay are discussed in this chapter, but the original articles should be consulted for greater detail.

In the Turco procedure, a medial incision is made

from the base of the first metatarsal and continued proximally over the heel cord. All medial tendons and neurovascular structures are identified. Posterior, medial, and lateral subtalar releases are performed sequentially. The posterior capsule of the subtalar joint is identified along with the calcaneofibular ligament, which he thinks is an important contributor to clubfoot deformity. A portion of the deltoid on the calcaneus is dissected. Medially, the posterior tibial tendon is cut just above the medial malleolus, and the proximal end is allowed to retract. The talonavicular joint is opened medially. The posterior tibial attachments to the sustentaculum and spring ligament are incised. The talocalcaneal joint is exposed medially, permitting release of the superficial layer of the deltoid from the calcaneus under direct vision. The deep portion of the deltoid must be preserved to prevent, in his opinion, the formation of a flatfoot deformity. The calcaneal interosseous ligament is transected, as is the bifurcate Y-shaped ligament. The navicular is reduced onto the talus and pinned. The other tarsals are carried with it. The subtalar joint is opened like a book, as the calcaneus, which must be released at both ends, everted, and moved laterally at its anterior end while the tuberosity is moved downward and away from the ankle joint. The tendoachilles is repaired. In the older child, Steindler stripping is performed as a part of the operative procedure.

Postoperatively, the patient is immobilized for a total of 4 months. The Kirschner wires remain in place for the first 6 weeks. A walking cast is used after the Kirschner wires are removed in the older child. Turco continues immobilization in a Dennis Browne night splint for 1 year, and a pronator shoe is recommended for 2 years. Turco thought the upper limit for this operative procedure was 6 years of age.

Carroll has described an operative procedure using two separate incisions.[26] His indication for operative management of clubfoot is a foot that cannot be corrected with 3 months of serial manipulation and casting. The steps in the surgical procedure are summarized:

1. A plantar release
2. Release of the Henry knot
3. Identification of the tibialis anterior
4. Protection of the peroneus longus and short plantar ligaments, with the long and short plantar ligaments divided to expose the calcaneocuboid joint
5. Z-plasty of the tendoachilles
6. Z-plasty of the tibialis posterior
7. Posterior capsulotomy, including the posterior calcaneofibular and posterior talofibular ligaments

8. Open reduction of the talonavicular dislocation
9. Placement of Kirschner wire through the back of the talus for correction of the anterior extrusion and external rotation
10. Correction of the forefoot adductus and supination
11. Kirschner wire fixation of the midtarsal joint
12. Repair of tendons, with the foot held in a plantigrade position.

Goldner classified clubfeet in three major categories with eight subgroups.[67,68] The Goldner technique emphasizes correction of the malrotated talus through the tibiotalar joint and release of the deltoid ligament. Tendons lengthened include the flexor hallucis, flexor digitorum, posterior tibialis, and Achilles. The subtalar joint is opened posteriorly, but not circumferentially. The abductor hallucis is released. The calcaneocuboid joint is ordinarily opened through the medial incision, and a plantar dissection is often carried out if there is a cavus component. The talonavicular joint is opened medially. His results for the first 100 cases were reported.[67] Gross is an advocate of the Goldner approach with some modifications to prevent overcorrection and avoid tendon displacement into the ankle joint.[25]

McKay thinks surgery is warranted if closed means fail to achieve reduction within the first 6 weeks or for recurrence despite three attempts at correction with casts.[147] He offered specific indications for surgical correction of clubfoot deformity.[146,147]

1. The child has a rigid foot that causes walking on its lateral border, heel varus, posterior position of the fibula, and an internally rotated gait.
2. On a piece of paper, an angle is drawn that is the relation of the longitudinal plane of the foot to the bimalleolar plane of the ankle. An angle of less than 76 degrees is an indication for surgery.
3. Parallelism between the long axis of the talus and the calcaneus on the anteroposterior and lateral radiographs is an indication for surgery. However, this indication is less reliable than others, because the radiographic findings may be inaccurate and difficult to obtain.

The operative procedure employed by McKay is an extensive medial, posterior, and lateral release performed with the patient supine.[147] The basic tenants are that the posterior tibialis and Achilles tendon are lengthened, and the sheaths of the flexor hallucis and flexor digitorum are dissected free but not opened. The talonavicular and calcaneocuboid joint capsules are released. A talocalcaneal release is performed medially and posteriorly. The lateral talocalcaneal joint is incised from the attachment of the calcaneocuboid joint to the sheath of the flexor hallucis longus posteriorly. The neurovascular bundle is dissected into the arch of the foot, and the plantar structures are released. The deep deltoid is preserved. The interosseous ligament is left intact or partially or completely transected, depending on evaluation at the time of surgery. Guidelines are given in the original article. The talonavicular joint is reduced and held with a pin placed across the joint. The most important aspect of the procedure is correcting the rotation of the calcaneus beneath the talus. The calcaneocuboid joint is pushed anterior to the ankle joint in a lateral direction while pushing the calcaneus posterior to the ankle joint in a medial and plantar direction and secured with a pin.

McKay transfers the flexor hallucis longus tendon to the peroneus longus in patients older than 2 years of age who have had a recurrence despite conservative care. This is done to prevent elevation of the first metatarsal. The distal flexor hallucis longus is sutured to the flexor digitorum.

Postoperatively, the patient is first managed with a compression-type bandage with plaster. A hinged cast with wire cables is applied 7 to 10 days postoperatively to allow motion. This is performed using a U-shaped 14- or 16-gauge stranded electrical wire.

Comparing studies is difficult because of the lack of standard means of evaluating results or the severity of clubfoot preoperatively. A system frequently used is the functional rating system of Laaveg and Ponseti (see Table 28-2).[125,238] One advantage of using this functional rating is that it allows direct comparison of results. A disadvantage is that 50 of the 100 rating points are based on the subjective perceptions of satisfaction and pain. The system uses a questionnaire and clinical examination to grade the feet on a 100-point scale that includes satisfaction (20 points), function (20 points), pain (30 points), heel position (10 points), passive motion (10 points), and gait (10 points). The rating system classifies the results as excellent (90–100), good (80–89), fair (70–79), or poor (<69). It does not include specific references to foot progression angle or inturning.

At follow-up, Turco reviewed 240 resistant congenital clubfeet in 176 patients treated by one-stage posterior medial release with internal fixation.[213] Of the 240, 149 feet reached the endpoint of treatment and were followed for 2 to 15 years. Excellent or good

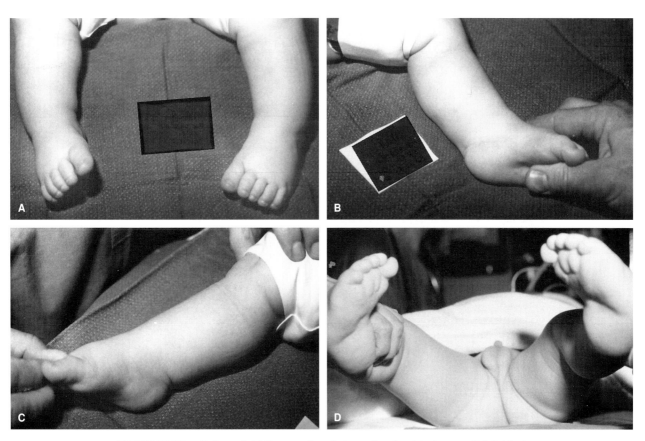

FIGURE 28-23. (A through D) Preoperative photographs of resistant congenital clubfoot.

results were achieved for 83.8%, 10.7% had fair results, and 5.3% were failures. He thought the best age for surgery was between 1 and 2 years.

Yoneda and Carroll reviewed the results of surgical correction of 84 severe cases of clubfeet.[239] The minimum follow-up was 5 years, and 19% required additional surgery in the form of plantar and lateral releases, causing Carroll to advocate a full release as described for severe cases of resistant clubfoot. Porat reviewed 33 feet treated by the Carroll technique after an average of 4 years follow-up.[171] He found 82% had satisfactory results.

Yngve and associates reviewed 52 feet treated by tibiotalar release without wide subtalar release 4.2 to 10.0 years after surgery.[238] Eleven feet (21%) required additional operative procedures at the time of review. The mean talocalcaneal index was 49 degrees (range, 12–76 degrees), indicating that correction of the subtalar joint could occur without wide subtalar release. No pins were used, and casting was continued for 3 to 4 months after surgery. This procedure satisfactorily corrected many feet but undercorrected some. Overcorrection was rare. Subluxation of the navicular bone occurred in 15% of patients and was often associated with recurrence. Because pinning was not a part of the procedure, it may have contributed to the lack of maintenance of correction. The Laaveg and Ponseti

functional rating in Yngve's study was 89 points, compared with 87.5 in Laaveg and Ponseti's series. In a companion study, Yngve used carbon paper to measure the foot progression angle of the treated feet.[237] The most significant cause of inturning was residual metatarsus adductus, but in some, it was caused by internal tibial torsion or internal femoral torsion.

Necessity of additional surgery for loss of correction can also be used as a measure of failure. In comparing the subtalar with the tibiotalar release, several points were observed. Additional surgery was performed in 11 (21%) of 52 feet in the study of Yngve[238] (tibiotalar release) and 9% of those in Thompson's[212] series, in which complete posteromedial releases were carried out. In Carroll's series, 19% required repeat surgery.[239] In the study by DeRosa and Stepro,[43] additional surgery was performed for 5%, and 5% of Turco's series required repeat surgery.[213]

Overcorrection into valgus was found in two of Yngve's patients and was associated with pain.[238] Other researchers have reported valgus for 8% to 20%.[189,213] This is a difficult problem to correct. Turco reported that 70% of his fair results were attributed to overcorrection.[213]

McKay reviewed the results of his technique by evaluating 102 children treated over a 6-year period.[146] Fifty-five previously unoperated feet received the sur-

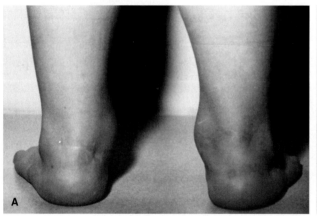

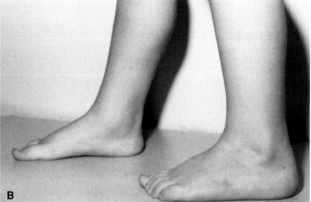

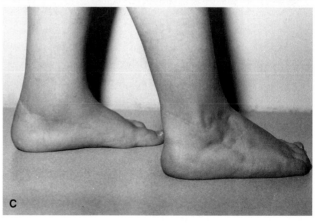

FIGURE 28-24. Postoperative status of the patient in Figure 28-23. (**A** through **D**) Clinical photographs of postoperative result. (**E**, **F**, and **G**) Lateral radiographs of postoperative result.

gical procedure described earlier. The postoperative follow-up period was 2 months to 8.5 years, with an average of 1 year and 3.5 months. The average follow-up was 2 years 3 months. The results for 45 feet were good to excellent, giving an 80% success rate. He concluded that it was best to avoid completely releasing the interosseous ligament unless horizontal rotation of the subtalar joint could not be obtained.

The functional results of a series of patients treated by a modified Turco technique was compared with a series of patients treated by a modified, complete subtalar release.[189] One third of the Turco group required a second procedure for recurrence, but no patient in the second group required further surgery. The investigators related this to the better visualization afforded by the circumferential Cincinnati incision and the more complete subtalar release.

Yngve's review of the patients treated after the recommendations of Goldner revealed a high level of parent satisfaction. Although Yngve stated that over-

correction was rare, I was concerned that some of my patients included in this study did overcorrect (see Fig. 28-26). For the past 12 years, I have used an operative approach that most closely resembles that described by McKay, through a circumferential or Cincinnati incision. The patient is immobilized for 6 weeks in a long leg cast and then in short leg casts after pin removal for a total of 4 months. Although no formal review has compared this approach with my previous series, I have been pleased with the results, and overcorrection has not been a problem (Figs. 28-23 and 28-24).

Additional Operative Procedures

Recurrence of clubfoot or the need for additional surgery occurs in an average of 25% of cases (range, 13%–50%).[4] The surgeon is often faced with a patient who has had one or more operative procedures and an incompletely corrected foot. The deformity must

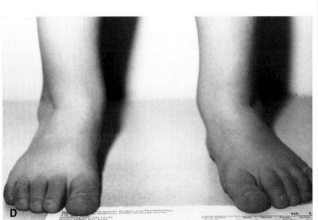
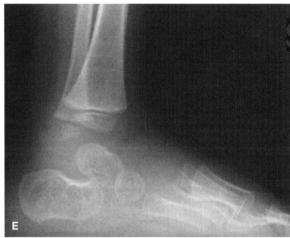
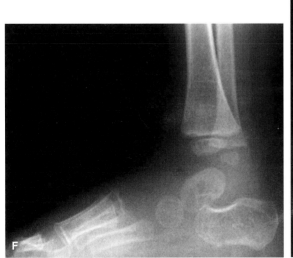
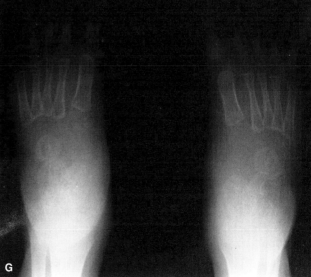

FIGURE 28-24 (*Continued*)

be analyzed for each case. No one operative procedure fits all patients. At the time of surgery, there is often abundant scarring, making the identification of tendons, ligaments, and joint capsules difficult. The structures preventing reduction must be identified and released.

In Ponseti's series of patients treated with casting, 50% had relapses between the ages of 10 months and 7 years.[125,169] Relapses were treated by transfer of the anterior tibialis tendon to the third cuneiform. Further correction of the varus deformity of the heel with manipulation and application of cast could be maintained, and the anteroposterior talocalcaneal angle became normal. Recurrence of cavus deformity was treated with a fasciotomy and transfer of the extensor hallucis tendon to the neck of the first metatarsal. Ponseti thought that operative release of the tarsal joints was seldom needed.[62,63]

In the review by Atar of 24 patients (29 feet), the most common surgical method was soft tissue release alone or combined with calcaneocuboid fusion, plantar release, or additional capsulotomies.[4] One explanation for poor results was the finding of talocalcaneal cartilaginous bars. These have been found on several occasions in my hospital at the time of subtalar release, and they have been resected.

Lichtblau quoted a high recurrence rate for deformity and a considerable amount of foot and ankle stiffness after medial release.[134] He combined medial release with excision of the distal part of the calcaneus to shorten the lateral column and permit good correction without the extensive dissection that he thought was responsible for postoperative stiffness. He also resected the posterior tibialis tendon. In a review of 11 patients, joint mobility was preserved and was clinically demonstrable as long as 6 years after surgery. There was a calcaneocuboid joint space on radiographs. No patients had pain on walking. All had resumed normal activity. Evans had also emphasized the importance of secondary adaptive changes and recommended a wedge resection and fusion of the calcaneocuboid joint.[56]

McHale's treatment of residual clubfoot deformity is by an opening wedge medial cuneiform osteotomy and closing wedge cuboid osteotomy.[144] In a review of 7 feet of 6 patients with residual bean-shaped feet, the procedure produced good correction of the forefoot deformity. It was a simple, direct, and reproducible procedure that addressed residual forefoot adductus and midfoot supination. It can be used in the child who is too old for a soft tissue release by itself or too young for triple arthrodesis. It avoids extensive dissection in previously operated feet.

Dwyer described a lateral closing wedge osteotomy of the calcaneum for pes cavus and later adapted this procedure for the treatment of resistant or elapsed clubfoot by a medial opening wedge osteotomy.[54] The aim of the operation was to correct the varus of the heel and increase its height by an opening medial wedge calcaneal osteotomy, held open by a bone graft from the ipsilateral tibia. Often, this must be combined with soft tissue procedures to achieve satisfactory position of the calcaneus.

Kumar and colleagues reviewed Dwyer's 26 patients after a mean elapsed time of 27 years.[122] For 36 feet, the mean Laaveg and Ponseti grading was 83.7%. In 94%, the heel was in neutral or valgus, and 86% of the feet were plantigrade. A good range of motion was achieved in the ankle or subtalar joint in 83%. All but 2 of the 36 feet could be fitted with normal shoes. Mild adduction of the forefoot persisted in these patients. Problems with wound healing and scar formation in these deformed feet are often quoted as the reasons why this opening wedge osteotomy did not gain great popularity. The weakness of this study is that Dwyer had performed this procedure on 124 patients, but only 26 could be traced by Kumar. Although the results were excellent for these patients, we do not know the results of the remaining 98 patients.

The Ilizarov technique has been suggested as a means of treating relapsed clubfeet, particularly for patients who are 8 to 15 years of age.[3,60,71] It is usually mentioned as an alternative for the patient 6 to 12 years of age when soft tissue procedures are less successful and the patient is too young for triple arthrodesis. Grant and associates described the use of the Ilizarov method to treat complex foot deformities in children, including those with resistant clubfeet. It is a fairly drastic measure that may be required for some complex recurrent clubfeet. Experience has been limited to a few centers, and the follow-up period is short.

Complications of Surgical Management

Surgical procedures, particularly in children in the first year of life, are delicate and require magnification. Wound problems, including dehiscence and infection, occur. With a severe clubfoot, the surgeon sometimes must accept less than complete correction on the first operative day, with additional correction achieved subsequently by casting. The foot usually can be held satisfactorily reduced with pins but not fully corrected in other parameters, taking tension off the skin. The neurovascular bundle must be carefully identified and protected to avoid damage.

Loss of reduction and recurrence is probably the most frequent complication. Overcorrection is a problem that is particularly difficult to remedy. Lateral shift of the calcaneus with a valgus heel can result (Figs. 28-25 and 28-26).

Although cases of flatfoot after posterior tibialis tendon loss in children have not been described, it can occur in adults, and it seems reasonable to pre-

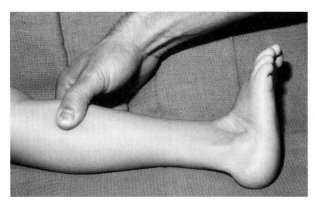

FIGURE 28-25. In this clinical photograph, the patient has had an extensive posteromedial tibiotalar release. The forefoot is dorsiflexed, and the heel is in valgus, with calcaneal impingement against the fibula.

serve the structure in children. Calcaneus deformity can occur from overlengthening of the posterior structures, although it has been unusual in the management of clubfoot.

Dorsal subluxation of the talonavicular joint can occur (Fig. 28-27). Kuo reviewed his personal experience of 168 idiopathic clubfeet in 126 patients.[124] Twelve of 168 feet developed dorsal subluxation of the navicular bone in 11 patients. Factors that appeared to be associated with dorsal subluxation included release of the talonavicular joint, use of a Cincinnati incision, Kirschner wire fixation, flattening of the talar head, and postoperative residual cavovarus deformity. Morphologically, dorsal subluxations were characterized by a wedge-shaped appearance of the navicular bone on the lateral radiograph. Cadaver specimens and subsequent revision surgeries revealed that a counterclockwise rotation of the navicular bone would adequately correct dorsal subluxation. It was postulated that this subluxation is in reality a rotatory deformity of the navicular bone in the coronal plane. The lateral aspect of the navicular bone is tethered to the lateral column. This produces a wedge-shaped navicular bone based dorsally, with the wider medial end of the navicular bone rotating superiorly. This shortens the lateral column and causes plantar flexion, contributing to forefoot adduction, supination, and cavovarus foot. Kuo thought this was preventable if the surgeon pays attention to the position of the navicular bone at the time of fixation and casting after clubfoot releases.

The blood supply of the talus is primarily from the artery of the sinus tarsi and should be protected to prevent aseptic necrosis of the talus. The navicular bone can also lose its vascularity, although this complication is unusual. Persistent forefoot supination and

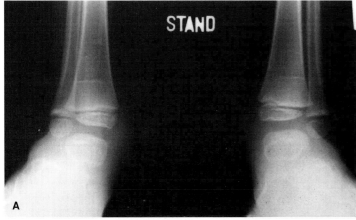

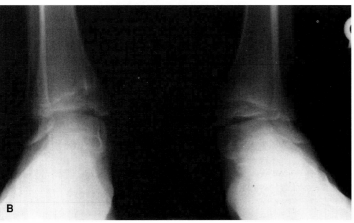

FIGURE 28-26. (A) Standing anteroposterior radiographs of a patient after extensive posteromedial tibiotalar release. Notice the lateral shift of the calcaneus. (B) By 11 years of age, the patient had severe impingement against the fibula and pain. A medial tibial epiphyseodesis was performed.

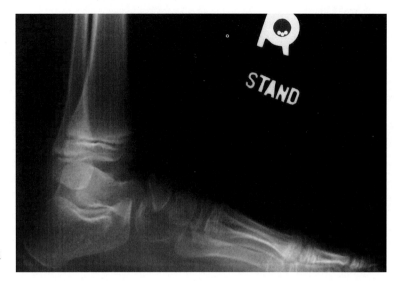

FIGURE 28-27. Lateral radiograph shows dorsal subluxation of the navicular.

a loss of normal motion of the ankle and subtalar joint can occur.

ADOLESCENT BUNION

Adolescent bunion is defined as the medial prominence of the head of the first metatarsal. It is often associated with various degrees of hallux valgus. The term adolescent bunion is sometimes used interchangeably with hallux valgus. Adolescent bunion differs from its adult counterpart in that the range of motion of the joint is usually normal, arthritis is usually not present, and the deformity is less severe. Adolescent bunion usually also implies that the physeal plate of the first metatarsal is still open.

Incidence

Adolescent bunion is more common in girls than boys and has an increased familial incidence. Johnston described one pedigree in which it appeared that hallux valgus was transmitted as an autosomal dominant trait with incomplete penetrance.[107] Although it is thought to be hereditary, the definite mode of inheritance has not been defined. The incidence is also unknown.

Etiology

Various structural changes have been implicated in the genesis of adolescent bunion, but none are proven. These include pronation of the foot, ligamentous laxity, and pes planus. The implication is that, with pronation of the foot, the medial capsule is stretched, causing displacement of the phalanx on the metatarsal head. A long first metatarsal has also been implicated as one of the risk factors for bunion formation.[181]

Kilmartin and Wallace studied the relation of pes planus to hallux valgus.[115] They measured the arch

index on standing radiographs and found that there was no difference in the longitudinal arch of patients with and without hallux valgus. They concluded that pes planus was not the cause of bunion deformity and that arch supports could not be beneficial in preventing the deformity.

Kilmartin, Barrington, and Wallace studied 6000 school children in England and found 36 unilateral and 60 bilateral cases of hallux valgus.[114] They defined this as a metatarsophalangeal angle greater than 14.5 degrees, measured on a standing anteroposterior radiograph. Metatarsus primus varus was found in the early stages of hallux valgus and in the unaffected feet of children with unilateral hallux valgus.

Clinical Features

The typical patient presenting with adolescent bunion is most often a girl between 12 and 15 years of age who presents with a prominent medial first metatarsal head with a mild bursa. The patient complains of pain and difficulty obtaining adequate shoe wear. Patients should be examined for range of motion of the metatarsophalangeal joint and the amount of medial prominence. The passive correctability of the deformity should also be assessed. Examination must include a relaxed sitting and a standing examination. The presence or absence of heel valgus and pronation of the foot should also be assessed. The overall muscle strength and function of the foot should be evaluated. The shoe wear pattern should be inspected.

Radiographic Evaluation

Standard radiographs for evaluating the bunion deformity include standing anteroposterior and lateral weight-bearing views. Although various angles have been used to quantitate the bunion, the most common are the intermetatarsal angle and the metatarsophalangeal angle. The normal angle between the first metatarsal and the first proximal phalanx is 14 to 16 degrees in adolescents.[161] The intermetatarsal angle must be measured on a weight-bearing anteroposterior x-ray film (Fig. 28-28). A line through the center of the articular surface of the first metatarsal head and base is drawn to intersect a similarly drawn line through the second metatarsal. The normal angle is less than 10 degrees (range, 6–9 degrees).[161]

The degree of subluxation of the metatarsophalangeal joint and its congruity are measured. The position of the sesamoids are identified, because they may subluxate laterally. Piggott related the congruency of the joint with the likelihood of progression.[166] He reviewed all the patients seen before 21 years of age at the Royal National Orthopaedic Hospital. In normal patients, he found the mean valgus deviation of the great toe was 14.4 degrees at 14 to 15 years of age and 15.7 degrees in young adults. Valgus of less than 15 degrees was considered normal. He measured this angle and the intermetatarsal angle and then looked at the congruity of the joint. He divided the joints into three groups: congruous, deviated, and subluxated. The congruous joints were most nearly normal, and the subluxated were most displaced. He found that if the joint was congruous in adolescents, progression was unlikely. Subluxation indicated deterioration was likely, and with deviation, it was unpredictable. He thought that metatarsus primus varus was secondary to lateral displacement of the proximal phalanx and lateral deviation of the proximal phalanx was the primary change in hallux valgus.

Some orthopedic specialists place emphasis on the length of the first metatarsal.[181] The status of the growth plate should be determined, because it may affect operative planning.

Mitchell and coworkers found an intermetatarsal angle of 10 to 22 degrees consistently in their bunion patients.[149] Piggott found this to be an uncommon occurrence in adolescent hallux valgus.[166]

Pathophysiology

Subluxation or incongruity of the metatarsophalangeal joint is a bad prognostic sign for progression. Piggott thought that if the joint were congruous and was stable it would not progress to significant hallux valgus.[166] An incongruous joint with a slight deviation was at significant risk for progression of metatarsophalangeal subluxation. Coughlin and Mann examined the orientation of the articular surfaces of the metatarsal in relation to the long axis of the metatarsal and the articular surface of the proximal phalanx.[33] These are evaluated to decide whether the joint is congruous. The metatarsocuneiform joint may also be a factor in the increased intermetatarsal angle.

The most usual anatomic variations associated with adolescent bunion include a widened first intermetatarsal angle associated with cuneiform first metatarsal obliquity. There is a variable degree of hallux valgus. There may be loss of the longitudinal arch and foot pronation. The sesamoids and extensor flexor tendons displace laterally. The anatomic portion called the bunion is the medial prominence of the first metatarsal and is not a true exostosis. Severe incongruity may predispose the joint to arthritic changes.

Treatment

Nonoperative Treatment

As with many orthopaedic conditions, the decisions about treatment involve educating the patient about the realistic outcomes of nonsurgical and operative methods of treatment. The physician must evaluate the severity of the deformity, the degree to which it is interfering with the person's lifestyle, and whether operative means can realistically alter that significantly.

The first line of treatment is to attempt to convince the patient to accept the amount of deformity if it is mild. The nonsurgical means of treatment involves stretching the shoes over the forefoot with bunion stretchers or finding suitable types of shoes. Although athletic shoes and softer shoes may provide relief of the pain, they are not acceptable in all social situations. Dress shoes often come in limited sizes. There are no orthoses that satisfactorily alleviate bunion symptoms.

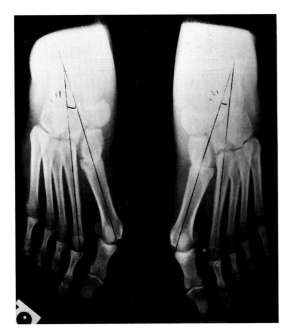

FIGURE 28-28. Standing anteroposterior radiographs of a patient with adolescent bunion. The inner metatarsal angles are 12 degrees on the left and 15 degrees on the right.

Groiso outlined the method of managing juvenile hallux valgus, using a moldable thermoplastic splint at night and incorporating active and passive stretching exercises.[75] In a review of 56 children, 2 to 6 years after the institution of therapy, the metatarsophalangeal joint angle and the intermetatarsal angle were improved in approximately one half of the feet, and no recurrences were detected among the patients who had improved.

Operative Procedures

Kelikian listed more than 130 operations for adolescent hallux valgus.[112] When there are multiple operative procedures available for the treatment of a condition, it is usually true that none is perfect or that virtually anything will work. In the case of adolescent bunion, no single operation can fit each patient, and the selection of the operative procedure depends on the pathoanatomy.

Bunion operations include soft tissue and bony procedures. Soft tissue procedures are intended to release contracted lateral structures or reef medial structures. In most procedures, the medial bony prominence or bunion is excised. If there is widening of the intermetatarsal angle between the first and second rays, an osteotomy is indicated to decrease the angle, along with realignment of the metatarsophalangeal joint. The osteotomy can be accomplished at the base by a closing or opening wedge or achieved by a dome- or crescent-shaped saw blade, which preserves length and allows good correction of the osteotomy.

The Mitchell osteotomy is performed distally.[149] The length of the first metatarsal must be taken into account. If the second metatarsal is longer than the first, it is important not to shorten the first metatarsal unnecessarily by osteotomy, perhaps causing more of a shift of weight bearing to the second metatarsal head.

The Akin procedure is indicated if there is a normal intermetatarsal angle and if only an osteotomy of the proximal phalanx of the great toe is needed to realign the toe.[1] The McBride procedure or a variation is often used to release the conjoint adductor tendon, although it is usually not reinserted into the first metatarsal head but done only as a release.[141]

In the usual patient with adolescent bunion, there is a metatarsus primus varus that is corrected by osteotomy. The hallux valgus is corrected by excision of the bunion, with reefing of the capsule or repair and often a release of the soft tissues on the lateral aspect to realign the toe. For osteotomies of the base of the first metatarsal, internal fixation with a pin or with a single screw is indicated to hold the osteotomy in place and prevent loss of reduction in the cast (Fig. 28-29).

Mann and colleagues reviewed 75 patients (109 feet) treated for hallux valgus with release of the distal soft tissues, excision of the medial prominence with plication of the medial capsule, and a proximal crescentic osteotomy of the first metatarsal.[137] Ninety-three percent of patients were satisfied with the results. There was improvement in the intermetatarsophalangeal angle. Hallux varus occurred in 13 feet (9 patients). There was improvement in 43 of 48 feet that had a symptomatic plantar keratosis beneath the second metatarsal head. Peterson and Newman outlined the procedure of osteotomy with longitudinal pin fixation of the first metatarsal.[165] This was performed on 15 feet. The surgeons thought the procedure was technically easy, provided excellent correction and stability, and

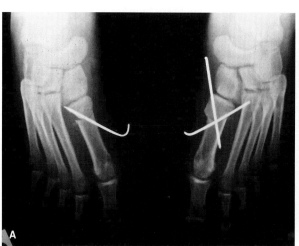
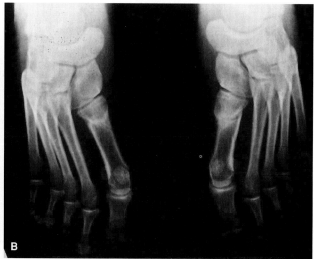

FIGURE 28-29. (A) Postoperative raidograph of the patient in Figure 28-28 with the pins in place. (B) Healed osteotomy.

had a low recurrence rate. The follow-up was 32.5 months.

The chevron osteotomy has been used in adolescents.[177,240] Zimmer reviewed 20 adolescent patients treated with 35 chevron osteotomies for the correction of painful hallux valgus.[240] Eighty-five percent expressed overall satisfaction. The radiographic evaluations did not correlate with the clinical results.

Geissele and Stanton reviewed the surgical management of hallux valgus for 32 feet.[64] There was a 16% (5 feet) recurrence rate, which was attributed to technical errors in all cases. Another 70% of patients were satisfied with the results. In a subgroup of patients treated for metatarsus primus varus, the Mitchell osteotomy provided excellent results for 95% of patients. Correction of the intermetatarsal angle was thought to be the factor that most highly correlated with decreased risk of recurrence and with patient satisfaction.

Complications of Treatment

It has been said that surgery should be delayed until the patient is skeletally mature. Bonney and MacNab found a recurrence rate of 42% in bunion repairs in skeletally immature patients.[16] A 20% recurrence rate was reported by Scranton and Zuckerman for skeletally immature adolescents.[182] Other reasons for failure of osteotomies include inadequate or absent internal fixation or improper immobilization for sufficient time before weight bearing. Recurrence has been attributed to remodeling in the patient with growth remaining. Coughlin and Mann discussed the ages at which skeletal maturity occurs, observing that a 12-year-old girl typically has only 0.8 cm of total foot growth remaining.[33] In 12-year-old boys, there is 2.7 cm of total growth remaining. Coughlin and Mann think that it is unlikely that recurrence can be attributed to remodeling. No one has ever proven conclusively that remodeling is the cause of recurrence. In patients 12 to 14 years of age, surgery should be entertained for the proper indications. The surgeon must be careful not to damage an open physis. Other complications include nonunion at the osteotomy site and avascular necrosis of the metatarsal head after the Mitchell procedure.

A weight-bearing shift from the first metatarsal to the second can occur after bunion operation. This results in a painful second metatarsal head with an overlying callus and occasionally in other affected metatarsals. The incidence has been as high as 32%.[108] The type of osteotomy performed and its internal fixation is probably more important than shortening of the first metatarsal. Allowing the first metatarsal head to ride up or extend shifts the weight to the second metatarsal.

TAILOR BUNIONETTE

Tailor bunion or bunionette is a prominence on the fibular side of the fifth metatarsal head, usually occurring in a wide foot or in a foot with lateral deviation of the fifth metatarsal.[136] A bursa forms over the metatarsal head. This is aggravated by tight shoes. Conservative measures, including stretching of the shoes, should be attempted. If this fails, excision of the prominence is usually sufficient. For an extremely wide intermetatarsal angle of greater than 8 degrees between the fifth and fourth rays, osteotomy of the base of the fifth metatarsal may be indicated.

HEEL PAIN IN CHILDREN

Heel pain is a frequent presenting complaint of children. Although it may alarm patients, parents, and physicians, it usually proves to be the result of overuse. Arriving at that diagnosis and alleviating the pain are not always simple because many causes of pain in the heel have been described.

Clinical Features

The child presenting with heel pain often is involved with athletics and may be participating in more than one sport. Cleated shoes or other types of footwear should be sought as a culprit. A change in training habits, the surface, or the sport can invoke this condition.

Pain may begin after the sport. As symptoms progress, it may interfere with participation. The physical examination usually reveals tenderness, which may be diffuse about the calcaneus or may be localized over the insertion of the tendoachilles. Subtalar motion must be carefully tested and pain in the subtalar joint ruled out. The patient may limp. The x-ray films are often normal. Initially, anteroposterior, lateral, and weight-bearing radiographs of the foot should be done. A bone scan, CT, or MRI may occasionally be done, although the yield from these imaging techniques is quite low, and they therefore are rarely indicated.

The differential diagnosis includes any of the benign tumors that can affect the heel, including unicameral bone cyst, aneurysmal bone cyst, and osteoid osteoma (Table 28-3). Tarsal coalition or any inflammatory process involving the subtalar joint must be considered. Osteomyelitis or septic arthritis, although unusual, must be ruled out. Most often, the classic history and physical findings in addition to the radiograph confirm the diagnosis of an overuse syndrome.

If the Achilles tendon is tight, it should be stretched. Most often, the heel should be rested or

TABLE 28-3 *Differential Diagnosis of Childhood and Adolescent Heel Pain*

Overuse, Overgrowth, or Trauma
Calcaneal apophysitis
Contusion or strain
Stress fracture of calcaneus
Fracture of calcaneus

Developmental Problems
Tarsal coalition

Inflammatory Process
Tendinitis (e.g., Achilles tendon, patellar tendon, flexor hallucis longus)
Plantar fasciitis
Retrocalcaneal bursitis
Periostitis
Os trigonum inflammation

Infections
Soft tissue infection
Abscess
Calcaneal osteomyelitis

Rheumatologic Conditions
Juvenile rheumatoid arthritis
Reiter syndrome
Miscellaneous

Tumors
Benign
  Osteoid osteoma
  Osteochondroma
  Chondroblastoma
  Bone cyst, solitary or aneurysmal
Malignant (rare)
  Leukemia
  Metastatic
Neurologic Problems
  Tarsal tunnel syndrome

Adapted from Micheli LJ, Ireland ML. Prevention and management of calcaneal apophysitis in children: an overuse syndrome. J Pediatr Orthop 1987;7:34.

protected. This can be done with heelcups, with pads, or by elevating the heel to put more weight on the forefoot. Restriction of activities is often the key to successful management but may be difficult to enforce in children. The problem may run its course in several weeks to several months. Oral antiinflammatory medication can be tried. Injection of steroids is not indicated.

Sever Disease

In the infant and young child, the posterior aspect of the calcaneus is not ossified. There is an irregular sawtooth pattern that develops just before the appearance of the calcaneal apophysis, which appears between 4 and 7 years of age in girls and 7 to 10 years in boys.[161] Multiple centers of ossification show up initially, and they gradually coalesce to form one apophyseal center that later unites with the calcaneus at 12 to 15 years of age. An irregular sclerotic apophysis is the rule and is not diagnostic of any clinical condition.

Sever described apophysitis of the os calcis in children who are overweight for their years, physically active, and have strong muscles.[185] His patients presented with heel pain, and the examination showed moderate tenderness over the posterior portion of the calcaneus. He thought the condition resembled "achillobursitis or inflammation of the Achilles tendon." He described the x-ray findings as practically constant, showing irregular ossification in the calcaneal apophysis. He went on to state that the treatment was to elevate the heel or to place a rubber pad in the heel, treatments that we still recommend for many children with heel pain.

Irregularity of the calcaneal apophysis on radiographs is the rule rather than the exception. Ferguson and Gingrich studied the radiographs of 100 children, looking at the calcaneal apophysis.[59] It was usually irregular and less dense than the surrounding bone, and it remained irregular for several years. It also has a tendency to become more dense during development, and deep clefts may divide it into two or three segments. This is the normal sequence of events.

Pump Bump

A pump bump is a calcaneal prominence associated with an overlying bursa. These patients have difficulty with footwear. Some respond to change of shoes. Others eventually require excision of the bony prominence.

CAVUS

Cavus is a complex foot deformity consisting of elevation of the longitudinal arch. It is usually combined with deformity of the hindfoot, forefoot, or both. When there is depression over the first metatarsal (flexion), the condition is called cavovarus. When combined with plantar deviation of the calcaneus, it is called calcaneovalgus.

Etiology

The cause is unknown in all cases. It is said to be idiopathic in a large percentage of cases, but as imaging techniques and diagnostic methods for neuromuscular disease have improved, more causes such

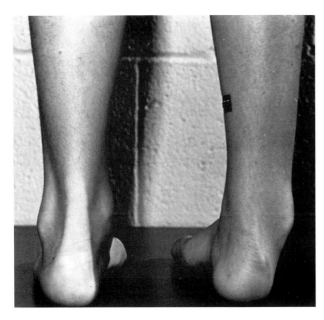

FIGURE 28-30. A 10-year-old patient with a tethered spinal cord and a unilateral cavovarus foot with forefoot adduction, heel varus, and cavus. The affected right leg and foot are smaller than the unaffected left lower extremity.

as tethered cord have been identified for cavus (Fig. 28-30). In the series of Brewerton and associates of 77 patients with cavovarus feet followed with neurologic and electrodiagnostic studies, a definite diagnosis was made for 51 (66%).[18]

Muscle imbalance from neuromuscular diseases can produce this deformity. It is not unusual to see some form of cavus in Charcot-Marie-Tooth syndrome, Friedreich ataxia, cerebral palsy, polio, tethered cord, and myelodysplasia. Sometimes, cavus is seen as a residual sequela of clubfoot.

In cavovarus, the deforming force is anterior tibialis weakness with a tight gastrosoleus. Overpull of the flexors and intrinsic muscles of the foot produces the deformity. In calcaneocavus, it is weakness or paralysis of the calf musculature, allowing muscles to be stretched, combined with the various strengths of the dorsiflexors, plantar flexors, and intrinsic muscles.

Clinical Features

In cavovarus foot, the forefoot is in equinus and pronated. There is plantar flexion of the metatarsals, especially over the first metatarsal. The hindfoot is in varus, and the longitudinal arch is elevated. There are various degrees of flexibility and tightness of the plantar structures. In calcaneocavus, the hindfoot is in calcaneus. Forefoot plantar flexion is combined with a high arch and clawed toes. There are various degrees of fixed contracture.

Other investigators have often made use of the analogy of a tripod or a pyramid to describe cavus

deformity.[29,226] If one limb of the tripod is elevated, it can cause a deviation of the base. In this condition, if the first metatarsal (i.e., one limb of the tripod) is in fixed plantar flexion, it causes deviation of the heel when the foot strikes. If the heel has remained supple, it is inverted into varus. This is the basis of the clinical tests devised by Coleman for flexibility of the longitudinal arch and heel.[29] In the test, the patient's foot is placed on a block approximately 1 inch (2.5 cm) thick (Fig. 28-31). The heel and lateral border of the foot are placed on the block so they can fully bear weight, allowing the first through third or fourth metatarsals to fall into pronation. If after relief of the forefoot equinus the heel is in neutral or valgus, it indicates that the heel is flexible and that correction of the forefoot will simultaneously correct the heel. This is usually a visual test but can be documented to some extent by an anteroposterior or lateral photograph and a standing roentgenogram. Clinical evaluation must include examination of the foot and a meticulous neurologic examination. The spine must be examined for midline skin defects or other signs of spinal dysraphism, which is further evaluated by MRI. Neurologic changes or asymmetric findings warrant further neurologic workup.

Radiographic Evaluation

Standard radiographs are standing anteroposterior and lateral views of the foot (Fig. 28-32). CT or MRI of the nervous system may also be indicated to image the spinal cord or central nervous system. Further workup may include an electromyogram and nerve conduction studies. Muscle biopsy is indicated for some patients with underlying neuromuscular pathology for whom the diagnosis is not definitely known.

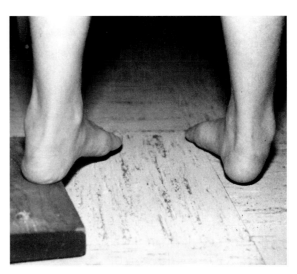

FIGURE 28-31. The Coleman block test. The effect of the first metatarsal plantar flexion is negated by placing the block laterally. If the hindfoot varus is flexible, it corrects as depicted.

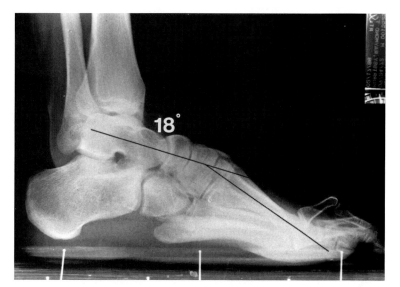

FIGURE 28-32. A 14-year-old patient with a tethered spinal cord. On the lateral view, the Meary angle demonstrates forefoot cavus. Meary angle results from the intersection of the lines drawn along the longitudinal axis of the talus and first metatarsal. The normal angle is 0 degrees. The radiographic appearance of the sinus tarsi results from the varus alignment of the hindfoot.

Natural History

The natural history depends on the neurologic disorder. The surgeon must decide whether the neurologic disorder is progressive or static, and the status also depends on the age at which the foot deformity is detected. Prediction of future function is based on the underlying condition and its known natural history. An untreated cavus foot can result in calluses, arthritis, pain, and difficulty in wearing shoes.

Pathoanatomy

The first metatarsal is in plantar flexion and pronation, which results in forefoot supination. If the heel is flexible, it shifts into varus as the patient stands because of the rigid forefoot. Initially, the deformity is flexible and can be passively corrected. With time and further contractures of the plantar structures, this becomes fixed, as shown by the Coleman block test, and cannot be corrected clinically.

Treatment

Conservative treatment of a very young child with a flexible foot can consist of casting, bracing, shoe inserts, and orthotics to position the foot. These usually do not prevent progression. They should not be used to the extent that the deformity becomes noncorrectable or rigid. They may be used temporarily to alleviate pain.

Operative treatment is indicated for most patients. Soft tissue procedures are indicated to balance the deforming forces or relieve contractures. The surgeon must know the natural history of the underlying disease when selecting the muscle groups to transfer. Transfer of a muscle such as the anterior tibialis that may later be nonfunctional serves no purpose. The operating surgeon must do an accurate manual motor test and be familiar with the muscles available for transfer. It is usual to lose one grade of strength with the transfer. The tendon transfers should be placed in as near a straight line as possible.

A plantar release is done through a medial incision in a location that allows dissection to the dorsum of the foot and well into the plantar surface (Fig. 28-33). The abductor hallucis muscle is traced back to its origin, taking care to protect the neurovascular bundle and the medial and lateral plantar nerves. The abductor hallucis, the short toe flexors, and the plantar fascia are all released from the calcaneus extraperiosteally. The flexor digitorum and flexor hallucis are identified, and the dissection is carried across the calcaneus to the calcaneocuboid joint, releasing all of the soft tissues from the calcaneus. Capsulotomies are performed, as necessary, of the calcaneocuboid and midtarsal joints. The flexor hallucis longus and flexor digitorum sheaths are opened, the tendons are identified, and they are retracted. Fixation is not used unless the first metatarsal is osteotomized.

Claw toes are a common deformity of this condition and should be treated by resection of the proximal interphalangeal joints, transfer of the extensor tendons to the metatarsal necks, or both. Soft tissue procedures used for feet that have hindfoot flexibility are usually plantar fasciotomy and tendon transfers, such as the tibialis posterior or the anterior tibialis if they are providing deforming forces.

Bony procedures include calcaneal osteotomy to shift the calcaneus laterally, sliding osteotomy, and closing wedge osteotomy.[41,53] Occasionally, metatarsal osteotomy is performed; usually the first is performed to bring the first metatarsal out of flexion. Wedge osteotomy of the tarsals have been tried, but their results are variable and frequently unsatisfactory.[105]

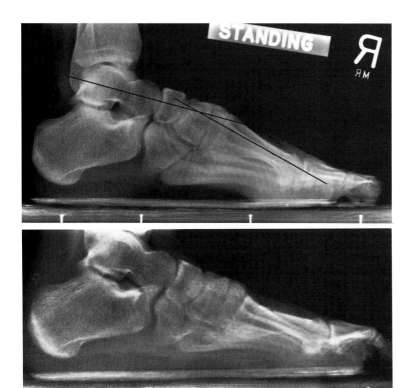

FIGURE 28-33. Preoperative and postoperative radiographs after soft tissue release and a dorsal closing wedge osteotomy of the first metatarsal.

Dwyer described removing a wedge with a base 8 to 12 mm wide from the calcaneus, just below the peroneus longus tendon.[53] The wedge tapered down the medial cortex, which was broken but left intact, with the periosteum left intact to provide some stability. He reviewed 63 cases in 41 children who were between 3 and 16 years of age at the time of surgery. All patients had improvements in gait and their ability to wear normal shoes. Dropping of the foot and clawing of the toes had been less striking. He did not include release of the plantar fascia with his operation.

Dekel and Weissman reviewed 38 osteotomies of the calcaneus with concomitant plantar stripping in 33 children with neuromuscular disease.[41] The operation was prophylactic in slightly more than one half of the cases, done in young children before fixed deformity had occurred. Among 26 patients older than 11 years of age at the time of review, 14 patients (18 feet) did not need further treatment. For three other patients, the deformities recurred, requiring further surgery. In the remaining nine patients, the marked recurrences necessitated tarsal reconstructions.

For the severely deformed foot that is not correctable by soft tissue or individual bony procedures, triple arthrodesis is necessary. This usually requires a very large amount of bone to be removed, as in the method described by Hoke.[94]

Complications of treatment include failure to balance the foot, progression of the deformity, lack of full correction, and neurovascular complications.

CALCANEOCAVUS

Calcaneocavus is a difficult condition to treat because of the weakness of the gastrocnemius muscle group. Poliomyelitis is the most common cause of this deformity worldwide.[227] In the United States, it is more common in children with myelomeningocele.[87,132,133,214]

With weakness of the triceps, the calcaneus assumes a position of dorsiflexion or comes to look like a pistol grip (Fig. 28-34). The calcaneus is dorsiflexed, and the forefoot plantar flexes because of the effect of gravity, the long toe flexors, the anterior tibialis, and the peroneal and intrinsic muscles. The toes are hyperextended at the metatarsophalangeal joint, and the metatarsal heads further plantar flex on weight bearing.

These patients are recognized clinically by the extreme elevation of the longitudinal arch and weakness of the gastrosoleus muscle group. There may be marked callus formation over the metatarsal heads and over the calcaneus. The toes are clawed. Patients often have trouble with footwear and ambulation because of pain and callus formation. The treatment depends on the muscle groups still functioning. Manual muscle testing must be carefully performed.

Nonoperative treatment is futile. In some young children, transfer of the tendon of the triceps surae into the fibula is advised in an to attempt to prevent the development of progressive calcaneus deformity and valgus deformity of the distal tibial plafond.[199] Pa-

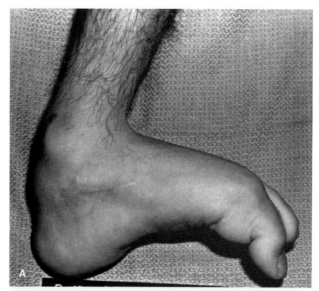

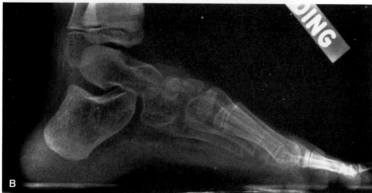

FIGURE 28-34. (A) Typical appearance of a calcaneocavus foot, demonstrating the prominent calcaneus or pistol-grip deformity. (B) The lateral radiograph shows dorsiflexion of the calcaneus, which has resulted in paralysis of the triceps surae secondary to poliomyelitis.

tients 5 to 12 years of age should have extraarticular subtalar joint stabilization at the same time. The plantar soft tissues should be released. If the anterior tibialis is functioning, it should be transferred through the interosseous membrane to the calcaneus in an attempt to improve plantar flexion. Soft tissue releases are performed to allow the foot to correct.

Patients older than 12 years of age usually have fixed bony deformity and ankle deformity. Soft tissue release and triple arthrodesis with tendon transfers may be required. The triple arthrodesis is difficult to perform, because the calcaneus must be brought out of dorsiflexion.

MISCELLANEOUS FOOT PROBLEMS

Congenital Hallux Varus

Congenital hallux varus consists of congenital medial deviation of the great toe and, in some instances, a short first metatarsal (Fig. 28-35). The condition may interfere with the ability to wear shoes, and it can be a difficult problem to manage. The metatarsal can be

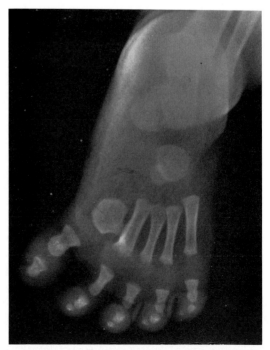

FIGURE 28-35. Anteroposterior radiograph of congenital hallux varus. The short, broad first metatarsal indicates a partial duplication of the great toe.

short or an incompletely duplicated Y-shaped metatarsal. Adequate bone and soft tissue must be removed early in life.

If there is a duplicated Y metatarsal, it is shaved to form a single shaft. It may be bowed, but will remodel to form a normal or almost normal bone. The wide metatarsal head associated with a duplicated phalanx should be narrowed surgically to avoid the development of a painful bunion. Short, block-like metatarsals remain normal.

Polydactyly associated with a short first metatarsal and congenital hallux varus carries a poor prognosis and may require continued treatment. Postoperative casting and taping should be used to prevent angular deformity and encourage normal foot contour.

Mills reviewed the surgical management of 17 feet in 12 patients treated by a variety of soft tissue procedures for congenital hallux varus and short first metatarsal.[148] Arthrodesis of the first metatarsophalangeal joint was necessary in three patients. Twelve of 17 feet achieved satisfactory results. The unsatisfactory results were due to appearance rather than function.

In a series by Steidmann and Peterson, the first metatarsal of six feet in four patients was surgically lengthened by distraction and fibular grafting. The average increased length was 36%, with the fibular graft healing in all patients.

Mubarek and colleagues described a longitudinal epiphyseal bracket that is rare ossification anomaly in which the epiphysis brackets the diaphysis of a phalanx, metacarpal, or metatarsal.[155] This tethers longitudinal growth, resulting in a shortened, oval bone. They reviewed four patients treated by central physeal lysis and followed for a mean of 6 years. All patients had significant hallux varus deformity. Three had duplication of the great toes, and two had tibial hemimelia. Resection of the bar of the longitudinal epiphyseal bracket allowed the proximal and distal epiphyses to resume untethered growth. The interpositional material used was Silastic or methylmethacrylate to prevent bony rebridging. The hallux varus deformity

was treated concomitantly by capsulorrhaphy and Kirschner wire fixation. Correction of the deformity was maintained at follow-up. It has also been called the C-shaped epiphysis. This condition is often associated with numerous other congenital anomalies, such as syndactyly, polydactyly, cleft hand, Apert hand, and ulnar clubhand.

Curly Toes

This is a condition that is present at birth in which the toes are flexed and deviated medially or laterally, most often medially. Commonly, it is the distal phalanx that is deviated, and the most frequently involved are the fourth and fifth toes, with the third less commonly involved (Fig. 28-36).[168]

Etiology and Natural History

The deformity is caused by contractures of the long toe flexors, but the cause of contracture is unknown.

The curly toes are asymptomatic in children. They may become symptomatic in adult life, resulting from callus, blister formation, and irritation of the adjacent toe by pressure from footwear or from the nail of the adjacent toe. Patients presenting to the pediatric orthopaedist are usually young children who are asymptomatic and have flexion contractures.

Clinical Features

Clinical examination reveals medial deviation, with one toe overriding the other. There is usually a flexion contracture at the level of the interphalangeal joints. Most often, the toe can be passively extended if the metatarsophalangeal joint is flexed, indicating that this is a contracture of the long toe flexor tendon. It is more pronounced with weight bearing, as the long toe flexor contracts.

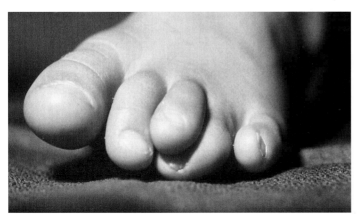

FIGURE 28-36. Clinical appearance of congenital curly toe, with the third toe overriding the fourth.

Treatment

Most affected children do not require treatment. Sweetnam found that, at the average age of 13 years, none of his patients was symptomatic.[206] Twenty-five percent of the patients he studied had improved spontaneously, and he saw no response to the nonoperative methods of treatment. Although taping and stretching can be used, they probably are more for the treatment of the family and the physician than for the patient. Ross and Menelaus advocated open flexor tenotomy in patients requiring treatment.[175] They reviewed 62 children between 3 and 14 years of age (average age, 9.8 years) after flexor tenotomy. No patient was aware of any loss of power in the toes, and for only 5% of the 188 toes were the operations unsuccessful. Browning and McKinnon reported 32 patients with 173 curly toes.[21] These were treated with a very simple operation consisting of tenotomy of the long flexor tendon through a short transverse incision over the middle phalanx.

The other operation that has been advocated is transfer of the long flexor to the extensor. Hamer and colleagues performed a double blind, randomized, and prospective study of the management of curly toe deformity.[78] Nineteen children were randomized into a group with a flexor to extensor tendon transfer, and others had a simple flexor tenotomy. If the patient had the deformity bilaterally, they were allocated at random to receive a flexor tenotomy or flexor extensor transfer, and the corresponding toe of the other foot received the other operation. The operations were tenotomy of the long flexor through a dorsal incision or the toe flexor to extensor transfer described by Taylor and credited to Girdlestone. Of the 19, 13 were reviewed (23 pairs of toes). These were 23 third toes, 22 fourth toes, and 2 fifth toes. The deformities were much improved 4 years later, and the choice of procedure made no difference. The conclusion is that, for patients requiring treatment, tenotomy of the long flexor is the important part of the operation, and transfer of the divided tendon is unnecessary.

Overriding of the Fifth Toe

Overriding of the fifth toe can also be seen at birth and is similar to curly toes, except that the toe, rather than being under the adjacent toe, is superior to the fourth toe. This is a familial problem of unknown cause. Conservative methods such as taping and strapping have proven to be ineffective.[131] Symptoms of pain, callus formation, and problems with footwear are the indications for surgical correction. The procedures include capsular release, plication, and tendon rerouting. Janecki and Wilde reported their results using the Ruiz-Mora procedure.[104] In the procedure, an elliptic segment of skin is removed from the plantar aspect of the fifth toe with flexor tenotomy. The proximal phalanx is removed by subperiosteal dissection. In 22 patients with 31 procedures followed for an average of 3.5 years, there was relief of those symptoms, but 23% had a painful prominent fifth metatarsal head or bunionette. An additional 32% developed a hammertoe deformity of the adjacent fourth toe and a painful corn. They related these problems to excessive shortening of the fifth toe because of excessive bone removal.

Cockin reported the results of a procedure that had been related to him by Butler.[28] A dorsal racquet-shaped incision is made. The extensor to the toe and the dorsal capsule of the metatarsophalangeal joint are cut for correction of the toe. The adherent capsule is freed, allowing the toe to lie in a fully corrected position without any tension (Fig. 28-37). He suggested that the McFarland syndactyly of the fourth and fifth toes and the Ruiz-Mora procedure replaced one deformity with another. This operation seemed to address the primary pathology of the dorsal contracture. De-

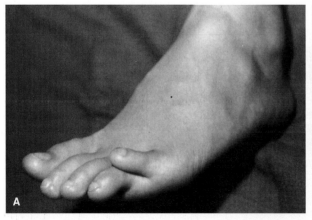
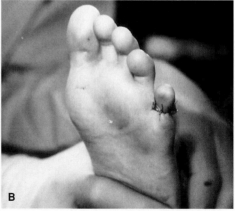

FIGURE 28-37. (A) Clinical appearance of an overriding fifth toe. (B) Postoperative release through a dorsal bracket-shaped incision of the extensor and dorsal capsules of the metatarsophalangeal joint.

spite the extensive incision, there was no circulatory damage to the toes in his series. Of his 55 patients, 45 were younger than 15 years of age. A good result was obtained in 91% of patients. De Boeck reported satisfactory results for 16 of 17 patients.[39]

Idiopathic Toe Walking

A child may walk with a toe-heel pattern without evidence of an underlying neurologic disorder. It has been described as habitual toe walking or congenital short Achilles tendon, but it is usually called idiopathic toe walking. This is a normal occurrence during the early stages of walking. The cause and natural history are unknown. Kalen found a positive family history for 71% of patients, and 20% of these patients had evidence of learning disabilities.[109]

The clinical presentation is that of a child, usually younger than 7 years of age, who does not have a normal heel strike. The differential diagnosis should include cerebral palsy, muscular dystrophy, spinal dysraphism, and acute myopathies. The final diagnosis is determined by exclusion.

Clinical Features

The patient presents with a history of toe walking. Heel wear on the shoes is absent or minimal. The foot is supple, but the heel cord may be contracted. A careful neurologic examination must be done to rule out underlying neurologic disease. Spasticity must be carefully sought. The spine is examined for midline skin defects or signs of underlying spinal dysraphism. If there is evidence of any type of spinal dysraphism or abnormal reflexes, plain radiographs of the spine should be obtained. Radiographs of the foot are not beneficial.

Treatment

NONOPERATIVE. If the foot can be dorsiflexed above neutral, the child should be placed in ankle-foot orthoses in an attempt to break the pattern. Children younger than 5 years of age with heel cord contracture and equinus should be treated with stretching casts until the foot dorsiflexes above neutral and then placed in ankle-foot orthoses. The child can be weaned gradually from the ankle-foot orthoses, but if the toe-walking pattern recurs, the patient must be returned immediately to the ankle-foot orthoses.

OPERATIVE. Surgery is indicated if conservative treatment fails or for a child older than 5 or 6 years of age with definite heel cord contracture. In Hall's series, patients were observed, and if no improvement of the contracture was seen over a 6-month period, surgery was carried out.[76] Twenty patients treated in this manner and followed for 1.5 to 7 years were doing well and walking normally with normal shoes and no recurrences. No sign suggested the development of other conditions.

Griffin and associates reviewed children who were habitual toe walkers electromyographically.[73] There was no electromyographic muscle activity at rest in any of the six normal walkers or six habitual toe walkers. They concluded that habitual toe walking is a diagnosis of exclusion for patients with otherwise normal orthopaedic and neurologic examination results. The muscles appeared normal by electromyography. The pattern remained normal after treatment with serial casts for 6 more weeks to stretch the Achilles tendon.

Kalen, Adler, and Bleck studied 18 idiopathic toe-walking patients, 14 controls, and 13 patients with mild cerebral palsy.[109] The findings on electromyography were that idiopathic toe walkers behaved similar to patients with cerebral palsy with equinus deformities and different from the control group. They suggested this might indicate an unknown central nervous system deficit. Because all other studies show that these patients are normal into adult life, with no recurrence, a central nervous system defect would seem unlikely.

Cleft Feet

Cleft feet are rare, congenital anomalies. Clefts can occur bilaterally in the hands and feet. One or several rays are absent, with normal rays bordering the cleft, resulting in a pincher-like deformity (Fig. 28-38).

Previously referred to as "lobster claw" or "crab claw," these feet should be referred to as cleft feet. The inheritance pattern is autosomal dominant with incomplete penetrance. Associated anomalies include cleft lip and palette, deafness, and urinary tract abnormalities. Children should have a renal ultrasound to determine if they have functioning kidneys. The goal of treatment must be to accommodate the foot to normal shoes. For some children, this only requires counseling for the family and assurance that nothing else need be done.

Sumiya and Monizukia described their experience with an operative procedure.[205] A double-pedicle flap from the cleft is raised and turned down to make a wide third toe. The second and fourth metatarsals are approximated by a strip of fascia lata, and a free skin graft is placed on the dorsal defect. The third toe and the old lateral toe are each divided to make two new toes by using a free graft from the skin defects. They encountered a failure of the newly formed toes to grow. Although the new toes did not appear to inter-

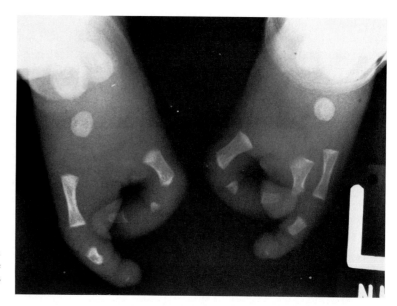

FIGURE 28-38. The forefoot in this patient with congenital cleft foot can accommodate a normal shoe and therefore does not require treatment. The toes deviate toward the midline.

fere with function, they did not improve in function. It would be expected that they would be insensate. Osteotomy can also be performed with closure of the defect to pull the foot together.

Macrodactyly

Macrodactyly is an uncommon, congenital malformation characterized by an increase in size of all of the elements of a digit or foot (Fig. 28-39). All structures are enlarged, and no underlying pathologic condition can be discovered. Data for the natural history and long-term results are lacking. Neurofibromatosis must be ruled out. Similar conditions occur in lymphangioma, multiple hemangiomatosis, and in Sturge-Weber syndrome. Although the growth may be slow or even static, in most patients, because of the overgrowth of fibrous, fatty, and bony tissues, the condition causes unacceptable deformity with time. The eventual treatment usually is surgical, and many procedures have been employed. Amputation of toes, defatting, and even amputations of rays are indicated. Treatment for each patient must be individualized.

Dedrick and colleagues recommended that a ray resection be performed in macrodactyly when the child's foot is two standard deviations larger than normal or than its mate.[40] They reviewed eight boys and 6 girls (10 left and 5 right feet). The initial therapy consisted of soft tissue excision in 13, amputation of phalanges in nine, epiphyseodesis of phalanges in two, and ray resection with complete metatarsal excision and serial cast treatment in one patient each. In 7 feet, a second procedure to reduce foot size was performed at an average of 5 years after the initial procedure. Five patients underwent three or more procedures to

reduce foot size because of continued growth. The patients followed to skeletal maturity had five or more procedures. Problems were encountered with width and height of the forefoot. It was this group of patients with metatarsal and midfoot hypertrophy that seemed to benefit most from ray resection. Usually, the second ray is removed. This seemed to provide the most consistent correction of abnormal height and width and reduced the total number of operations. The removal of the entire metatarsal, including its most proximal portion, is important in achieving the desired reduction in foot size. A threaded Steinmann pin is placed across the remaining metatarsals until full healing has occurred. Standing radiographs and measurements of both feet should be made preoperatively.

Radiographs of the parents' feet are used to predict a proper length for epiphyseodesis. In a limited experience with patients with this condition, one of the complications is devascularization of the flaps at the time of defatting. Plantar incisions are necessary and have not been a problem. Split-thickness skin grafts have also been used on the plantar surface of my patients to manage skin slough and have hypertrophied and fared well.

Polydactyly

Polydactyly is a common congenital abnormality in which one or more toes are duplicated (Fig. 28-40). Polydactyly has an increased familial incidence, and it can be associated with other syndromes. Venn-Watson wrote an excellent review of the topic.[217] Fibular side duplication is more frequent than duplication on the great toe side. The patient is initially seen and counseled that the toes will have to be removed, most often

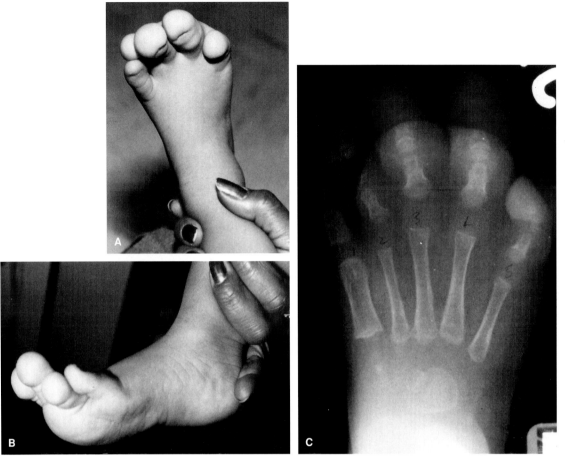

FIGURE 28-39.   (**A** and **B**) Clinical photographs of a foot with macrodactyly. There is extreme involvement of the middle three metatarsals and the greater involvement of the forefoot than the hindfoot. (**C**) Anteroposterior radiograph.

because of difficulty wearing shoes. It is preferable to defer the surgery until near walking time to allow as much ossification as is possible in the extra digit and to plan the operative procedure. Hasty excision may leave behind a cartilaginous anlage that will later require excision. A decision must be made about which toe will be ablated and which will be preserved. Usually, this requires an examination of potential tendon function and the location of the extra toe. An incision should be planned to avoid scars on areas that will be in contact with the shoes. Reconstruction or creation of tissues to substitute for joint capsules ablated by the amputation may be indicated as well.

Venn-Watson reviewed the records of all patients treated at the Carrie Tingley hospital from 1938 to 1972.[217] A total of 72 patients were reviewed. In most cases, the toe amputated was the medial-most toe when the first toe is involved and the lateral-most toe when the fifth is involved. This approach gave the best results. If it is necessary to cut across an epiphysis, he recommends making the cut perpendicular to the

physis, because this is least likely to cause growth arrest.

Ingrown Toenails

Ingrown toenails rarely occur in infants and in children.[6] They begin making their appearance during the adolescent years. In most cases, it is the great toe that is involved. The condition is caused by pressure from shoes or socks, repeated trauma to the nail, or improper trimming of the nail. The nails should be trimmed square. When they are trimmed curved and repeatedly traumatized, the nail edge becomes thickened and rounded. It presses into the surrounding soft tissues. The tissue overgrows, and the medial and lateral nail grooves become covered and obliterated. Infection forms in the skin fold and may spread to the nail and the nail matrix.

Conservative treatment consists of educating the patient about the proper means of trimming the nail square and straight across and keeping them cleaned.

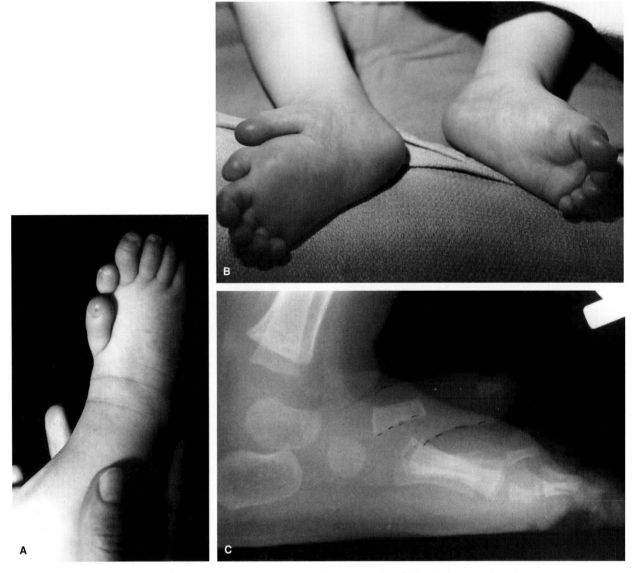

FIGURE 28-40. (**A** and **B**) Clinical photographs of a patient with polydactyly. (**C**) Lateral radiograph of a patient with polydactyly. This patient had entire duplication of an extra ray, and the first ray, which was left after amputation, was also shortened and abnormal.

Elevation of the ingrown nail by conservative means takes time because it requires the nail to grow out. The foot should be soaked and cleaned several times per day, and then some type of nail care device should be used to elevate gently the lateral and medial margins of the nail plate. The first time this is done, it is best done by the physician, who simultaneously instructs the patient. It is a slow process, and if extremely painful, it may require a digital block or sedation. After the nail is properly elevated, a small wisp of cotton or gauze should be packed under the nail, and the patient should be instructed to replace this at least daily, gradually elevating the nail and pushing back the adjacent cuticle. If the toe has overt infection,

antibiotics are prescribed. Additional education includes information about the proper type of shoes to wear. Particularly during the acute phase of management, a shoe with a very broad toe or with the toe cut out is required.

If the nail fails to respond to this treatment, operative procedures are indicated. For treating children, it is unusual to require a bony procedure. The first type of treatment is soft tissue excision of the granulation tissue along the margin of the nail. A portion of the medial nail groove must also be removed and then should be sutured to adjacent healthy skin, obliterating the dead space. Proper trimming and placement of pledgets under the nail are continued until healing is complete. Nail avulsion can be used for recurrent deformity. This works well in only about one third of cases and only for the first time.[47] In long-standing cases or those for which all conservative and other operative means have been exhausted, permanent nail plate avulsion by excision of the nail bed matrix is indicated. Even this must be meticulously and thoroughly carried out, or there can be recurrence of the ingrown nail, and patients may form nail spurs that also may require surgical excision.[47]

Subungual Exostosis

Subungual exostosis is a benign bone tumor found on the distal phalanx of a digit. It is rare. Most occur in the second and third decades of life. The presenting complaint is deformity of the nail or pain. There may be ulcerations and secondary infection. Radiographs are typical. The lesions vary from 5 mm to 2 cm and have a cartilaginous cap. They are histologically benign and are not related to osteochondromas.

The treatment consists of excision with preservation of the nail. If nail ablation is necessary for exposure, it should be replaced to prevent adhesions and to form a splint. Recurrence is possible if the nail is not completely excised. Landon reviewed 44 patients with subungual exostosis on the great toe seen at the Mayo Clinic.[128] Forty-three were treated by local excision, and five had local recurrences.

ACKNOWLEDGMENT

Grateful appreciation is extended to Ms. Linda Fannin for the preparation and assistance in writing this chapter.

References

1. Akin OF. The treatment of hallux valgus—a new operative procedure and its results. Med Sentinel 1925;33:678.
2. Aronson J, Puskarich CL. Deformity and disability from treated clubfoot. J Pediatr Orthop 1990;10:109.
3. Atar D, Lehman WB, Grant AD. Complications in clubfoot surgery. Orthop Rev 1991;20:233.
4. Atar D, Lehman WB, Grant AD, Strongwater AM. Revision surgery in clubfeet. Clin Orthop 1992;223.
5. Badgley CE. Coalition of the calcaneus and the navicular. Arch Surg 1927;15:75.
6. Baile FB, Evans DM. Ingrowing toenails in infancy. Br Med J 1978;2:737.
7. Barlow TG. Early diagnosis and treatment of congenital dislocation of the hip. J Bone Joint Surg [Br] 1962;44:292.
8. Basmajian JV, Stecko G. The role of muscles in arch support of the foot: an electromyographic study. J Bone Joint Surg [Am] 1963;45:1184.
9. Beatson TR, Pearson JR. A method of assessing correction in clubfeet. J Bone Joint Surg [Br] 1966;48B:40.
10. Bechtol CO, Mossman HW. Clubfoot: an embryological study of associated muscle abnormalities. J Bone Joint Surg [Am] 1950;32A:827.
11. Bennett GL, Weiner DS, Leighley B. Surgical treatment of symptomatic accessory tarsal navicular. J Pediatr Orthop 1990;10:445.
12. Berg EE. Reappraisal of metatarsus adductus in skew-foot. J Bone Joint Surg [Am] 1986;68:1185.
13. Bleck EE. Metatarsus adductus: classification and relationship to outcomes of treatment. J Pediatr Orthop 1983;3:2.
14. Bleck EE, Berzinz UJ. Conservative management of pes valgus with plantar flexed talus, flexible. Clin Orthop 1977;122:85.
15. Bohm M. The embryologic origin of clubfoot. J Bone Joint Surg 1929;11:229.
16. Bonney G, Macnab I. Hallux valgus and hallux Rigidus. J Bone Joint Surg [Br] 1952;34:366.
17. Braddock GTF. Experimental physeal injury in Freiberg's disease. J Bone Joint Surg [Br] 1951;41:154.
18. Brewerton DA, Sandifer PH, Sweetnam DR. Idiopathic pes cavus and Investigation into its etiology. Br Med J 1963;2:659.
19. Bronshtein M, Zimmer EZ. Transvaginal ultrasound diagnosis of fetal clubfeet at 13 weeks, menstrual age. J Clin Ultrasound 1989;17:518.
20. Browne D. Congenital deformities of mechanical origin. Arch Dis Child 1955;30:37.
21. Browning WH, McKinnon B. Camptodactyly of the toes (curly toes): a simple surgical treatment of children. Orthop Trans 1986;10:504.
22. Cain TJ, Hyman S. Peroneal spastic flatfoot. J Bone Joint Surg [Br] 1978;60:527.
23. Caldwell GD. Surgical correction of relaxed flat foot by the Durham flatfoot plasty. Clin Orthop 1953;2:221.
24. Carroll NC. Pathoanatomy and surgical treatment of the resistant clubfoot. Instr Course Lect 1988;37:93.
25. Carroll NC, Gross RH. Point/counterpoint: operative management of clubfoot. Orthopedics 1990;13:1285.
26. Carroll NC, McMurtry R, Leete SF. The pathoanatomy of congenital clubfoot. Orthop Clin North Am 1978;9:225.
27. Ching GHS, Chung CS, Nemechek RW. Genetic and epidemiological studies of clubfoot in Hawaii: ascertainment and incidence. Am J Hum Genet 1969;21:566.
28. Cockin J. Butler's operation for an overriding fifth toe. J Bone Joint Surg [Br] 1968;50:78.
29. Coleman SS, Chesnut WJ. A simple test for hindfoot flexibility in the cavovarus foot. Clin Orthop 1977;123:60.
30. Coleman SS, Stelling FH III, Jarrett JJ. Congenital vertical talus: pathomechanics and treatment. Clin Orthop 1970;70:62.
31. Conway HR, Cowell HR. Tarsal coalition: clinical significance and roentgenographic demonstration. Radiology 1969;92:799.
32. Cook DA, Breed AL, Cook T, et al. Observer variability in the radiographic measurement and classification of metatarsus adductus. J Pediatr Orthop 1992;12:86.
33. Coughlin MJ, Mann RA. The pathophysiology of the juvenile bunion. Instr Course Lect 1987;36:123.
34. Cowell HR. Diagnosis and management of peroneal spastic flatfoot. Instr Course Lect 1975;24:94.
35. Cowell HR, Hensinger RN. Relationship of clubfoot congenital annular bands. In: Bateman JE, ed. Foot science. Philadelphia: WB Saunders, 1976:41.
36. Cowell HR, Wein BK. Current concepts review—genetic aspects of club foot. J Bone Joint Surg [Am] 1980;62:1381.
37. Crego CH, Ford LT. An end-result study of various operative procedures for correcting flat feet in children. J Bone Joint Surg [Am] 1952;34:183.
38. Danielsson LG. Incidence of congenital clubfoot in Sweden: 128 cases in 138,000 infants, 1946–1990, in Malmo. Acta Orthop Scand 1992;63:424.
39. De Boeck H. Butler's operation for congenital overriding of the fifth toe. Retrospective 17 year study of 23 cases. Acta Orthop Scand 1993;64:343.

40. Dedrick DK, Kling TJ Jr, Smith WS. Macrodactyly of the foot reduced with ray resection. Proceedings of the American Association of Orthopaedic Surgeons, New Orleans, February 1986.

41. Dekel S, Weissman SL. Osteotomy of the calcaneus and concomitant plantar stripping in children with talipes cavo-varus. J Bone Joint Surg [Br] 1973;55:802.

42. DelSel JM, Grand NE. Cubonavicular synostosis. A rare tarsal anomaly. J Bone Joint Surg [Br] 1959;41:149.

43. Derosa GP, Stepro D. Results of posteromedial release of the resistant clubfoot. J Pediatr Orthop 1986;6:590.

44. Deutsch AL, Resnick D, Campbell G. Computed tomography and bone scintigraphy in the evaluation of tarsal coalition. Radiology 1982;144:137.

45. Dietz FR, Ponseti IV, Buckwalter JA. Morphologic study of clubfoot tendon sheaths. J Pediatr Orthop 1983;3:311.

46. Dietz RF. On the pathogenesis of clubfoot. Lancet 1985;1:388.

47. Dixon GL. Treatment of ingrown toenail. Foot Ankle 1983;3:254.

48. Dodge LD, Ashley RK, Gilbert RJ. Treatment of the congenital vertical talus: a retrospective review of 36 feet with long-term follow-up. Foot Ankle 1987;7:326.

49. Downey DJ, Drennan JC, Garcia JF. Magnetic resonance image findings in congenital talipes equinovarus. J Pediatr Orthop 1992;12:224.

50. Drachman DB, Coulombre AJ. Experimental clubfoot in arthrogryposis multiplex congenita. Lancet 1962;2:523.

51. Drennan JC, Sharrard WJ. The pathological anatomy of convex pes valgus. J Bone Joint Surg [Br] 1971;53:455.

52. Duchenne GB. Physiology of motion. Philadelphia: WB Saunders, 1959:337.

53. Dwyer FC. Osteotomy of the calcaneum for pes cavus. J Bone Joint Surg [Br] 1959;41:80.

54. Dwyer FC. The treatment of relapsed club foot by the insertion of a wedge into the calcaneum. J Bone Joint Surg [Br] 1963;45:67.

55. Elkus RA. Tarsal coalition in the young athlete. Am J Sports Med 1986;14:447.

56. Evans D. Relapsed clubfoot. J Bone Joint Surg [Br] 1961;43:722.

57. Eyre-Brook A. Congenital vertical talus. J Bone Joint Surg [Br] 1967;49:618.

58. Farsetti P, Weinstein SL, Ponseti IV. The long-term functional and radiographic outcome of untreated and nonoperatively treated metatarsus adductus. J Bone Joint Surg [Am] 1994;76:257.

59. Ferguson AB, Gingrich RM. The normal and the abnormal calcaneal Apophysis and tarsal navicular. Clin Orthop 1957;10:87.

60. Franke J, Grill F, Hein G, Simon M. Correction of clubfoot relapse using Ilizarov's apparatus in children 8–15 years old. Arch Orthop Trauma Surg 1990;110:33.

61. Freiberg AH. The so-called infraction of the second metatarsal Bone. J Bone Joint Surg 1926;8:257.

62. Fried A. Recurrent congenital club-foot. The role of the tibialis posterior in etiology and treatment. J Bone Joint Surg [Am] 1959;41:243.

63. Gartland JJ. Posterior tibial transplant in the surgical treatment of recurrent clubfoot. J Bone Joint Surg [Am] 1964;46:1217.

64. Geissele AE, Stanton RP. Surgical treatment of adolescent hallux valgus. J Pediatr Orthop 1990;10:642.

65. Geist E. The accessory scaphoid bone. J Bone Joint Surg 1925;7:570.

66. Glessner JR Jr, Davis GL. Bilateral calcaneonavicular coalition occurring in twin boys. A case report. Clin Orthop 1966;47:173.

67. Goldner JL. Congenital talipes equinovarus—15 years of surgical treatment. Curr Pract Orthop Surg 1969;4:61.

68. Goldner JL. Extensive subtalar arthrotomy is unnecessary in the surgical treatment of congenital clubfoot. J Bone Joint Surg [Br] 1988;70:506.

69. Gonzalez P, Kumar SJ. Calcaneonavicular coalition treated by resection and interposition of the extensor digitorum brevis muscle. J Bone Joint Surg 1990;72:71.

70. Gould N, Moreland M, Alvarez R, et al. Development of the child's Arch. Foot Ankle 1989;9:241.

71. Grant AD, Lehman WB. Clubfoot correction using the Ilizarov technique. Bull Hosp Joint Dis 1991;51:84.

72. Gregersen HN. Naviculocuneiform coalition. J Bone Joint Surg [Am] 1977;59:128.

73. Griffin PP, Wheelhouse WW, Shiavi R, Bass W. Habitual toe walkers. Clinical and electromyographic gait analysis. J Bone Joint Surg [Am] 1977;59:97.

74. Grogan DP, Gasser SI, Ogden JA. The painful accessory navicular: a clinical and histopathological study. Foot Ankle 1989;10:164.

75. Groiso JA. Juvenile hallux valgus. A conservative approach to treatment. J Bone Joint Surg [Am] 1992;74:1367.

76. Hall JE, Salter RB, Bhalla SK. Congenital short tendo calcaneus. J Bone Joint Surg [Br] 1967;49:695.

77. Hamanishi C. Congenital vertical talus: classification with 69 cases and new measurement system. J Pediatr Orthop 1984;4:318.

78. Hammer AJ, Stanley D, Smith TWD. Surgery for curly toe deformity: a double blind, randomized, prospective trial. J Bone Joint Surg [Br] 1993;75:662.

79. Hardy RH, Clapham JCR. Hallux valgus: predisposing anatomical causes. Lancet 1952;1:1180.

80. Hark FW. Rocker-foot due to congenital subluxation of the talus. J Bone Joint Surg [Am] 1950;32:344.

81. Harris BJ. Anomalous structures in the developing human foot. [Abstract] Anat Rec 1955;121:399.

82. Harris RI. Follow-up notes on articles previously published in the journal: retrospect—peroneal spastic flat foot (rigid valgus foot). J Bone Joint Surg [Am] 1965;47:1657.

83. Harris RI, Beath R. The short first metatarsal. J Bone Joint Surg [Am] 1949;31:553.

84. Harris RI, Beath T. Army foot survey: an investigation of the foot ailments of Canadian soldiers. Ottawa: Ottawa National Research Council 1947;1:52.

85. Harris RI, Beath T. Hypermobile flat-foot with short tendo Achilles. J Bone Joint Surg [Am] 1948;30:116.

86. Harris RI, Beath T. Etiology of peroneal spastic flat foot. J Bone Joint Surg [Br] 1948;30:624.

87. Hayes JT, Gross IP, Dow S. Surgery for paralytic defects secondary to myelomeningocele and myelodysplasia. J Bone Joint Surg [Am] 1964;46:1577.

88. Heiple KG, Lovejoy CO. The antiquity of tarsal coalition. Bilateral deformity in a pre-Columbian Indian skeleton. J Bone Joint Surg [Am] 1969;51:979.

89. Helfet AJ. A new way of treating flat feet in children. Lancet 1956;1:262.

90. Helmstedt A, Sahlstedt B. Talocalcaneal osteotomy and soft tissue procedures in the treatment of clubfeet. Acta Orthop Scand 1980;51:349.

91. Herndon CH, Heyman DH. Problems in the recognition and treatment of congenital convex pes planus. J Bone Joint Surg [Am] 1963;45:413.

92. Herzenberg JE, Goldner JL, Martinez S, Silverman PM. Computerized tomography of talocalcaneal tarsal coalition: a clinical and anatomical study. Foot Ankle 1986;6:273.

93. Heyman CH, Herndon CH, Strong JM. Mobilization of the

tarsometatarsal and intermetatarsal Joints for the correction of resistant adduction of the fore part of the foot in congenital clubfoot or congenital metatarsus varus. J Bone Joint Surg [Am] 1958;40:299.

94. Hoke M. An operation for stabilizing paralytic feet. J Orthop Surg 1921;3:494.

95. Horn DB, Pizzutillo PD, Wechsler RJ, et al. Magnetic resonance imaging in the diagnosis of tarsal coalition. Proceedings of the American Orthopaedic Association, Sun Valley, ID 1994.

96. Howard CB, Benson MKD. Clubfoot: its pathological anatomy. J Pediatr Orthop 1993;13:654.

97. Hughes JR. Pathologic anatomy and pathogenesis of congenital vertical talus and its practical significance. J Bone Joint Surg [Br] 1970;52:777.

98. Ikeda K. Conservative treatment of idiopathic clubfoot. J Pediatr Orthop 1992;12:217.

99. Ippolito E, Ponseti IV. Congenital clubfoot of the human fetus: a histologic study. J Bone Joint Surg [Am] 1980;62:8.

100. Irani RN, Sherman MS. The pathological anatomy of club foot. J Bone Joint Surg [Am] 1963;45:45.

101. Jack EA. Bone abnormalities of the tarsus in relation to peroneal spastic flat foot. J Bone Joint Surg [Br] 1954;36:530.

102. Jacobs JE. Metatarsus varus and hip dysplasia. Clin Orthop 1960;16:203.

103. Jacobsen ST, Crawford AH. Congenital vertical talus. J Pediatr Orthop 1983;3:306.

104. Janecki CJ, Wilde AH. Results of phalangectomy of the fifth toe for hammertoe. J Bone Joint Surg [Am] 1976;58:1005.

105. Japas LM. Surgical treatment of pes cavus by tarsal V-osteotomy. J Bone Joint Surg [Am] 1968;50:927.

106. Jayakumar S, Cowell HR. Rigid flatfoot. Clin Orthop 1977; 122:77.

107. Johnston O. Further studies of the Inheritance of hand and foot Anomalies. Clin Orthop 1956;8:146.

108. Joplin RJ. Sling procedure for correction of splay-foot, metatarsus primus varus, and hallux valgus. J Bone Joint Surg [Am] 1950;32:779.

109. Kalen V, Adler N, Bleck EE. Electromyography of idiopathic toe walking. J Pediatr Orthop 1986;6:31.

110. Karp MG. Koehler's disease of the tarsal scaphoid an end result study. J Bone Joint Surg 1937;19:84.

111. Kaye JJ, Ghelman B, Schneider R. Talocalcaneal-navicular joint arthrography for sustentactular-talar tarsal coalitions. Radiology 1975;115:730.

112. Kelickin H. Allied deformities of the forefoot and metatarsalgia. Philadelphia: WB Saunders, 1965;241.

113. Kidner FC. The prehallux in relation to flatfoot. JAMA 1933;101:1539.

114. Kilmartin TE, Barrington RL, Wallace WA. Metatarsus primus varus. A statistical study. J Bone Joint Surg [Br] 1991;73:937.

115. Kilmartin TE, Wallace WA. The significance of pes planus in juvenile hallux valgus. Foot Ankle 1992;13:53.

116. Kite JH. Principles involved in the treatment of congenital club-foot. J Bone Joint Surg 1939;21:595.

117. Kite JH. Flat feet and lateral rotation of legs in young children. J Int Col Surg 1956;25:77.

118. Kite JH. Congenital metatarsus varus. J Bone Joint Surg [Am] 1967;49:388.

119. Kling TF, Kollias SL. Calcaneal lengthening for painful pes planus in children. In: Proceedings of the Pediatric Orthopaedic Society of North America. Memphis: Pediatric Orthopaedic Society of North America, 1994.

120. Kodros SA, Dias LS. Long-term follow-up of single-stage surgical correction of congenital vertical talus. In: Proceedings of the American Academy of Orthopaedic Surgeons annual meeting. New Orleans: American Academy of Orthopaedic Surgeons, 1994.

121. Koutsogiannis E. Treatment of mobile flatfoot by displacement osteotomy of the calcaneus. J Bone Joint Surg [Br] 1971;53:96.

122. Kumar PNH, Laing PW, Klenerman L. Medial calcaneal osteotomy for relapsed equinovarus deformity: long-term study of the results of Frederick Dwyer. J Bone Joint Surg [Br] 1993;75:967.

123. Kumar SJ, MacEwen GD. The incidence of hip dysplasia with metatarsus adductus. Clin Orthop 1982;164:234.

124. Kuo KN, Jansen LD. Rotary dorsal subluxation of the navicular: a Late Complication of clubfoot surgery. In: The proceedings of the Pediatric Orthopaedic Society of North America. Memphis: Pediatric Orthopaedic Society of North America, 1994.

125. Laaveg SJ, Ponseti IV. Long term results of treatment of congenital clubfoot. J Bone Joint Surg [Am] 1980;62:23.

126. Lamb D. The ball and socket ankle joint—a congenital abnormality. J Bone Joint Surg [Br] 1958;40:240.

127. Lamy L, Weissman L. Congenital convex pes valgus. J Bone Joint Surg 1939;21:79.

128. Landon GC, Johnson KA, Dahlin DC. Subungual exostoses. J Bone Joint Surg [Am] 1979;61:256.

129. Larsen B, Reimann I, Becker-Andersen H. Congenital calcaneal valgus. Acta Orthop Scand 1974;45:145.

130. Leonard MA. The inheritance of tarsal coalition and its relationship to spastic flat foot. J Bone Joint Surg [Br] 1974;56:520.

131. Leonard MH, Rising EE. Syndactylization to maintain correction of overlapping fifth toe. Clin Orthop 1965;43:241.

132. Levitt RL, Canale ST, Cooke AJ Jr, Gartland JJ. The role of foot surgery in progressive neuromuscular disorders in children. J Bone Joint Surg [Am] 1973;55:1396.

133. Levitt RL, Canale ST, Gartland JJ. Surgical correction of foot deformity in the older patient with myelomeningocele. Orthop Clin North Am 1974;5:19.

134. Lichtblau S. A medial and lateral release operation for club foot. J Bone Joint Surg [Am] 1973;55:1377.

135. Maffulli N, Capasso G, Testa V, Borrelli L. Histochemistry of the triceps surae muscle in idiopathic congenital clubfoot. Foot Ankle 1992;13:80.

136. Mann RA. Surgery of the foot. St. Louis: CV Mosby, 1986:194.

137. Mann RA, Rudicel S, Graves SC. Repair of hallux valgus with a distal soft-tissue procedure and proximal metatarsal osteotomy. A long-term follow-up. J Bone Joint Surg [Am] 1992;74:124.

138. Mann RA, Thompson FM. A rupture of the posterior tibial tendon causing flatfoot: surgical treatment. J Bone Joint Surg [Am] 1985;67:556.

139. Margo MK. Surgical treatment of conditions of the fore part of the foot. Instr Course Lect 1967;49A:1665.

140. Masciocchi C, D'Archivio C, Barile A, et al. Talocalcaneal coalition: computed tomography and magnetic resonance imaging diagnosis. Eur J Radiol 1992;15:22.

141. McBride ED. A conservative operation for bunions. J Bone Joint Surg [Am] 1928;10:735.

142. McCormack T, Olney B, Asher M. Long-term follow-up of middle facet talocalcaneal coalition resections. In: The proceedings of the Pediatric Orthopaedic Society of North America. Memphis: Pediatric Orthopaedic Society of North America, 1994.

143. McCormick DW, Blount WP. Metatarsus adductovarus: "skewfoot." JAMA 1949;141:449.

144. McHale KA, Lenhart MK. Treatment of residual clubfoot deformity—the "bean-shaped" foot—by opening wedge medial cuneiform osteotomy and closing wedge cuboid osteotomy.

Clinical review and cadaver correlations. J Pediatr Orthop 1991;11:374.

145. McKay. New concept and approach to congenital clubfoot—morbid anatomy. J Pediatr Orthop 1982;2:347.

146. McKay DW. New concept of an approach to clubfoot treatment: section III. Evaluation and results. J Pediatr Orthop 1983;3:141.

147. McKay DW. New concepts of an approach to clubfoot treatment: section II. Correction of the clubfoot. J Pediatr Orthop 1983;3:10.

148. Mills JA, Menelaus MB. Hallux varus. J Bone Joint Surg [Br] 1989;71:437.

149. Mitchell CL, Fleming JL, Allen R, et al. Osteotomy-bunionectomy for hallux valgus. J Bone Joint Surg [Am] 1958;40:41.

150. Mitchell G. Spasmodic flatfoot. Clin Orthop 1970;70:73.

151. Mitchell GP, Gibson JMC. Excision of calcaneonavicular bar for painful spasmodic flatfoot. J Bone Joint Surg [Br] 1967;49:281.

152. Morgan RC, Crawford AH. Surgical management of tarsal coalition in adolescent athletes. Foot Ankle 1986;7:183.

153. Mosca V. Skewfoot deformity in children: correction by calcaneal lengthening and medial cuneiform opening wedge osteotomies. Personal communication.

154. Mosier KM, Asher M. Tarsal coalition and peroneal spastic flat foot. J Bone Joint Surg [Am] 1984;66:976.

155. Mubarak SJ, O'Brien TJ, Davids JR. Metatarsal epiphyseal treatment by central epiphyseolysis. J Pediatr Orthop 1993;13:5.

156. Oestreich AE, Mize WA, Crawford AH, Morgan RC. The "ant-eater nose": direct sign of calcaneonavicular coalition on the lateral radiograph. J Pediatr Orthop 1987;7:709.

157. Ogata K, Schoenecker PL. Congenital vertical talus and its familial occurrence: an analysis of 36 patients. Clin Orthop 1979;139:128.

158. Olney BW, Asher MA. Excision of symptomatic coalition of the middle facet of the talocalcaneal joint. J Bone Joint Surg [Am] 1987;69:539.

159. Oppenheim W, Smith C, Christie W. Congenital vertical talus. Foot Ankle 1985;5:198.

160. Osmond-Clark H. Congenital vertical talus. J Bone Joint Surg [Br] 1956;38:334.

161. Ozonoff MB. Pediatric orthopaedic radiology. 2nd ed. Philadelphia: WB Saunders, 1992.

162. Pachuda NM, Lasday SD, Jay RM. Tarsal coalition: etiology, diagnosis, and treatment. J Foot Surg 1990;29:474.

163. Penneau K, Lutter LD, Winter RD. Pes planus: radiographic changes with foot orthoses and shoes. Foot Ankle 1982;5:299.

164. Peterson HA. Skewfoot (forefoot adduction and heel valgus). J Pediatr Orthop 1986;6:24.

165. Peterson HA, Newman SR. Adolescent bunion deformity treated with double osteotomy and longitudinal pin fixation of the first ray. J Pediatr Orthop 1993;13:80.

166. Piggott H. The natural history of hallux valgus in adolescent and early adult life. J Bone Joint Surg [Br] 1960;42:749.

167. Pineda C, Resnick D, Greenway G. Diagnosis of tarsal coalition with computed tomography. Clin Orthop 1986;208:282.

168. Pollard JP, Morrison PJM. Flexor tenotomy in the treatment of curly toes. Proc R Soc Med 1975;68:480.

169. Ponseti IV. Current concepts review: treatment of congenital club foot. J Bone Joint Surg [Am] 1992;74:448.

170. Ponseti IV, Becker JR. Congenital metatarsus adductus: the results of treatment. J Bone Joint Surg [Am] 1966;48:702.

171. Porat S, Kaplan L. Critical analysis of results in clubfeet treated surgically along the Norris Carroll approach: seven years of experience. J Pediatr Orthop 1989;9:137.

172. Pous JG, Dimeglio A. Neonatal surgery on clubfoot. Orthop Clin North Am 1978;9:233.

173. Rao UB, Joseph B. The influence of footwear on the prevalence of flat foot. A survey of 2300 children. J Bone Joint Surg 1992;74:525.

174. Reinmann I, Werner HH. Congenital metatarsus varus: a suggestion for possible mechanism in relation to other foot deformities. Clin Orthop 1975;110:223.

175. Ross ERS, Menelaus MB. Open flexor tenotomy for hammertoes and curly toes in children. J Bone Joint Surg [Br] 1984;66:770.

176. Rushforth GF. The natural history of hooked foot. J Bone Joint Surg [Br] 1978;60:530.

177. Sammarco GJ, Brainard BJ, Sammarco VJ. Bunion correction using proximal chevron osteotomy. Foot Ankle 1993;14:8.

178. Sato K, Sugiura S. Naviculo-cuneiform coalition—report of three cases. Nippon Seikeigeka Gakkai Zasshi 1990;64:1.

179. Schwartze DJ, Denton JR. Normal values of neonatal lower limbs: evaluation of 1000 neonates. J Pediatr Orthop 1993;13:758.

180. Scranton PE. Treatment of symptomatic talocalcaneal coalition. J Bone Joint Surg [Am] 1987;69:533.

181. Scranton PE, Rutkowski R. Anatomic variations in the first ray: part I. Anatomic Aspects related to bunion surgery. Clin Orthop 1980;151:244.

182. Scranton PE, Zuckerman JD. Bunion surgery in adolescence: results of surgical treatment. J Pediatr Orthop 1984;4:39.

183. Seimon LP. Surgical correction of congenital vertical talus under the age of 2 years. J Pediatr Orthop 1987;7:405.

184. Settle GW. The anatomy of congenital talipes equinovarus: sixteen dissected specimens. J Bone Joint Surg [Am] 1963;45:1341.

185. Sever JW. Apophysitis of the os calcis. NY Med J 1912;95:1025.

186. Shands AR. Congenital anomalies, accessory bones, and osteochondritis in the feet of 850 children. Surg Clin North Am 1953;33:1643.

187. Shephard E. Tarsal movements. J Bone Joint Surg [Br] 1951;33:258.

188. Sim-Fook L, Hodgson AR. A comparison of foot forms among the nonshoe and shoe wearing Chinese population. J Bone Joint Surg [Am] 1958;40:1058.

189. Simons EW. Complete subtalar release in clubfeet: part II—comparison with less extensive procedures. J Bone Joint Surg [Am] 1985;67:1056.

190. Simons GW. A standardized method for the radiographic evaluation of clubfeet. Clin Orthop 1978;135:107.

191. Slomann HD. On coalition calcaneonavicularis. J Orthop Surg 1921;3:586.

192. Smilie IS. Freiberg's infarction (Koehler's second disease). J Bone Joint Surg [Br] 1955;39:580.

193. Smith JT, Bleck EE, Gamble JG, et al. Simple method of documenting metatarsus adductus. J Pediatr Orthop 1991;11:679.

194. Smith JW. Muscular control of the arches of the foot in standing: an electromyographic assessment. J Anat 1951;88:152.

195. Smith RW, Staple TW. Computerized tomography (CT) scanning technique for the hindfoot. Clin Orthop 1983;177:34.

196. Staheli LT, Chew DE, Corbett M. The longitudinal arch: a survey of eight hundred and eighty-two feet in normal children and adults. J Bone Joint Surg [Am] 1987;69:426.

197. Stark JG, Johanson JE, Winter RB. The Heyman-Herndon tarsometatarsal capsulotomy for metatarsus adductus: results in 48 feet. J Pediatr Orthop 1987;7:305.

198. Stern HJ, Clark RD, Stroberg AJ, Shohat M. Autosomal dominant transmission of isolated congenital vertical talus. Clin Genet 1989;36:427.

199. Stevens PM, Toomey E. Fibular-Achilles tenodesis for paralytic ankle valgus. J Pediatr Orthop 1988;8:169.

200. Storen H. On the closed and open correction of congenital

convex pes valgus with a vertical astragalus. Acta Orthop Scand 1965;36:352.

201. Stormont DM, Peterson HA. The relative incidence of tarsal coalition. Clin Orthop 1983;181:28.

202. Stoskopf CA, Hernandez RJ, Kelikian A. Evaluation of tarsal coalition by computerized tomography. J Pediatr Orthop 1984;4:365.

203. Stygar AM, Demidov VN. Prenatal ultrasonographic diagnosis of congenital isolated developmental defects of fetal extremities. [Translated from Russian] Akush Ginekol (Mosk) 1991;22.

204. Sullivan JA, Miller WA. The relationship of the accessory navicular to the development of the flatfoot. Clin Orthop 1979;44:233.

205. Sumiya N, Onizuka T. Seven years' survey of our new cleft foot Repair. Plast Reconstr Surg 1980;65:447.

206. Sweetnam R. Congenital curly toes, and investigation into the value of treatment. Lancet 1958;2:398.

207. Swiontkowski MF, Scranton PE, Hansen S. Tarsal coalitions: long-term results of surgical treatment. J Pediatr Orthop 1983;3:287.

208. Tachdjian MD. The child's foot. Philadelphia: WB Saunders, 1985:556.

209. Tachdjian MO. Congenital convex pes valgus. Orthop Clin North Am 1972;3:131.

210. Takakura Y, Tamai S, Masuhara K. Genesis of the ball-and-socket ankle. J Bone Joint Surg [Br] 1986;68:834.

211. Thometz JG, Simons GW. Deformity of the calcaneocuboid joint in patients who have talipes equinovarus. J Bone Joint Surg [Am] 1993;75:190.

212. Thompson GH, Richardson AB, Westin GW. Surgical management of resistant talipes equinovarus deformity. J Bone Joint Surg [Am] 1982;64:652.

213. Turco VJ. Resistant congenital clubfoot—one stage posteromedial release with internal fixation. J Bone Joint Surg [Am] 1979;61:805.

214. Turner JW, Cooper RR. Posterior transposition of tibialis anterior through the interosseous membrane. Clin Orthop 1971;79:71.

215. VanderWilde R, Staheli LT, Chew DE, Malagon V. Measurements on radiographs of the foot in normal infants and children. J Bone Joint Surg [Am] 1988;70:4077.

216. Veitch JM. Evaluation of the Kidner operation and treatment of symptomatic accessory tarsal scaphoid. Clin Orthop 1978;131:210.

217. Venn-Watson EA. Problems in polydactyly of the foot. Orthop Clin North Am 1976;7:909.

218. Viladot A. Surgical treatment of the child's flatfoot. Clin Orthop 1992;34.

219. Vizkelety T, Szepesi K. Reoperation in treatment of clubfoot. J Pediatr Orthop 1989;9:144.

220. Waisbrod H. Congenital clubfoot: an anatomical study. J Bone Joint Surg [Br] 1973;55:796.

221. Walker AP, Ghali NN, Silk FF. Congenital vertical talus. The results of staged operative reduction. J Bone Joint Surg [Br] 1985;67:117.

222. Warren MJ, Jeffree MA, Wilson DJ, MacLarnon JC. Computed tomography in suspected tarsal coalition. Examination of 26 cases. Acta Orthop Scand 1990;61:554.

223. Waugh W. Partial cubo-navicular coalition as a cause of peroneal spastic flat foot. J Bone Joint Surg [Br] 1957;68:834.

224. Waugh W. The ossification and vascularisation of the tarsal navicular and their relation to Köhler's disease. J Bone Joint Surg [Br] 1958;40:765.

225. Wenger DR, Mauldin D, Speck G, et al. Corrective shoes and inserts as treatment for flexible flatfoot in infants and children. J Bone Joint Surg 1989;71:800.

226. Wenger DR, Rang M. The art and practice of children's orthopaedics. New York: Raven Press, 1993.

227. Westin GW. Tendon transfers about the foot, ankle, and hip in the paralyzed lower extremity. J Bone Joint Surg [Am] 1965;47:1430.

228. Wetzenstein H. The significance of congenital pes calcaneovalgus in the origin of pes plano-velgus in childhood. Acta Orthop Scand 1960;30:64.

229. Wickstrom J, William RA. Shoe correction and orthopaedic foot support. Clin Orthop 1970;70:30.

230. Wiles S, Palladino SJ, Stavosky JW. Concurrent calcaneonavicular and talocalcaneal coalitions. J Foot Surg 1989;28:449.

231. Williams GA, Cowell HR. Koehler's disease of the tarsal navicular. Clin Orthop 1981;158:53.

232. Wray JB, Herndon CN. Hereditary transmission of congenital coalition of the calcaneus to the navicular. J Bone Joint Surg [Am] 1963;45:365.

233. Wynne-Davies R. Talipes equinovarus a review of eighty-four cases after completion of treatment. J Bone Joint Surg [Br] 1964;46:464.

234. Wynne-Davies R. Family studies and aetiology of clubfoot. J Med Genet 1965;2:227.

235. Wynne-Davies R. Genetic and environmental factors in the etiology of talipes equinovarus. Clin Orthop 1972;84:9.

236. Wynne-Davis R. Family studies and the cause of congenital clubfoot–talipes equinovarus, talipes calcaneal valgus and metatarsus varus. J Bone Joint Surg [Br] 1964;46:445.

237. Yngve DA. Foot progression angle in clubfeet. J Pediatr Orthop 1990;10:467.

238. Yngve DA, Gross RH, Sullivan JA. Clubfoot release without wide subtalar release. J Pediatr Orthop 1990;10:473.

239. Yoneda B, Carroll NC. One stage surgical management of resistant clubfoot. J Bone Joint Surg [Br] 1984;66:302.

240. Zimmer TJ, Johnson KA, Klassen RA. Treatment of hallux valgus in adolescents by the chevron osteotomy. Foot Ankle 1989;9:190.

Lovell & Winter's Pediatric Orthopaedics, fourth edition,
edited by Raymond T. Morrissy and Stuart L. Weinstein.
Lippincott–Raven Publishers, Philadelphia © 1996.

Chapter

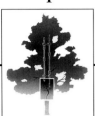

29

The Limb-Deficient Child

John A. Herring
Donald R. Cummings

CLASSIFICATION OF LIMB DEFICIENCIES

The system proposed by Franz and O'Rahilly is widely used to classify extremity anomalies (Fig. 29-1).[35,47] Disorders are first separated into terminal and intercalary deficiencies. Terminal deficiencies are those in which there are no unaffected parts distal to and in line with the missing segment. Intercalary deficiencies are those with a middle portion of the limb missing while portions proximal and distal are unaffected. These major divisions may be subdivided into transverse and paraxial deficiencies based on the nature of the deficit. Transverse deficiencies affect the entire width of the limb, and paraxial deficits affect only the preaxial or postaxial portion of the limb.

Each specific deficiency is named for the part that is missing; fibular absence is fibular hemimelia. If the rays of the foot are deficient, the abnormality is a terminal deficit, but if the foot is normal, the defect is intercalary. Because only the fibular portion of the

extremity is involved, the defect is paraxial rather than transverse. In another example, a congenital below-elbow absence is a terminal, transverse defect. Several general terms for deficiencies should also be defined. Hemimelia is a nonspecific term meaning half a limb, and it is used when one of the paired bones of the forearm or leg is missing. Complete and incomplete are added as modifiers to specify whether part or all of the named bone is missing. Amelia is the complete absence of an extremity. Acheiria means absent hand, and apodia is absence of the foot. Adactylia is absence of the fingers, and aphalangia is absence of phalanges.

CONGENITAL ABNORMALITIES

There are important differences between congenital and acquired absences of a limb. When the team working with the child and family appreciate these differences, they are able to work together much more effectively and avoid many problems. The child with

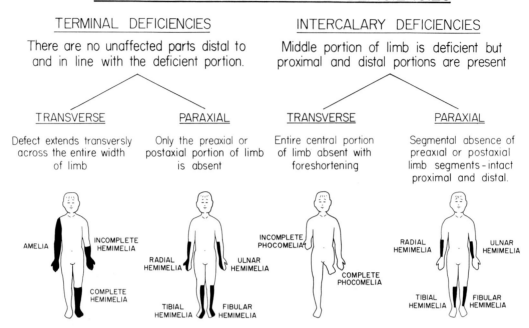

FIGURE 29-1. Franz and O'Rahilly classification of congenital limb anomalies.

a congenital anomaly has no sense of loss and consequently needs no adjustment period. He or she can make remarkable adaptations to meet milestones and attempts to do all activities. Most very young children who have undergone amputations for injury or disease often respond in the same way. However, older children with acquired amputations have a sense of loss and must work through a grieving process. Their desire to be like they were before the amputation may get in the way of productive adaptations.[32]

What to Tell Parents

Etiology

The a parent often asks, "Why did this happen?" The exact cause of limb anomalies is known in only a small number of cases. There are a few hereditable limb anomalies, and most such abnormalities occur sporadically with no known environmental agent, no familial occurrences, and no known injuries. A review of birth defects in Norway showed that mothers of children with limb anomalies have a significantly higher chance of having a second child with a similar defect. Of 957 mothers with a child with a limb anomaly, 25 second infants had a similar defect, compared with an expected rate of only 2.2. They also found that the risk of a birth defect was much lower when the mother moved to another city after the first child was born, suggesting environmental factors.[73] Although many drugs are known teratogens, the only drug

firmly associated with a large number of anomalies is thalidomide.[36,38,54,79,85]

Most parents must be told at the outset that the cause of their child's abnormality is unknown. It is best to give them as much information as is available about the problem, which often helps resolve some of their fears. For example, it is known that most single anomalies have a very small chance of recurring in subsequent children or in the children of the affected individual. This information alone may relieve much parental anxiety. Many mothers are convinced that they did something wrong during their pregnancy that caused this problem. Reassuring them when that is not the case also helps to free them of considerable guilt. Appropriate genetic counseling should be initiated when there is a positive family history of a disorder, when the abnormality resembles those with a known genetic cause, and when necessary to resolve parental anxiety.

In some cases, the mother may have used drugs or may have been exposed to potential teratogens. In those instances, a thorough history should be taken to determine the developmental stage of the fetus at the time of the exposure, as well as dosages and exposure to other agents. It is important to initiate appropriate counseling and child welfare intervention to protect future offspring.

Another known cause of prenatal amputations are amniotic bands (Streeter syndrome; Fig. 29-2). These bands of tissue form constriction rings around different areas of the extremities. In some cases, the bands

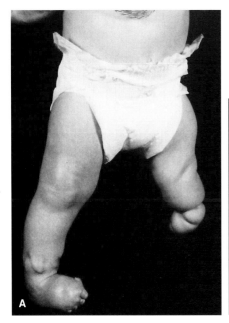
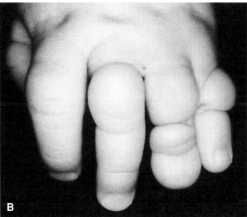

FIGURE 29-2. (A) Lower extremities of a child with amniotic band syndrome. The bands produce deep soft tissue clefts, resulting in deformities and amputations distal to the clefts. The foot deformity distal to a band is often difficult to manage, and the recurrence rate after surgical correction is high. (B) The fingers of a child with amniotic band syndrome. There are soft tissue accumulations proximal to the bands and absence of the nail on the fourth finger.

completely amputate the parts of the extremity distal to the band. In some, the bands constrict venous drainage, resulting in edema, and in others, the bands persist as deep clefts in the soft tissues. Although some late intrauterine amputations in which the amputated extremity is delivered with the baby have been reported, in most cases, there is early disturbance of the limb bud, with failure of the extremity to further develop.[44] Kino reproduced the syndrome in rat fetuses by amniocentesis and concluded that the malformations were caused by "excessive contraction of the uterine muscle during pregnancy with resulting hemorrhages from the marginal blood sinuses of the digital rays." He estimated that the malformation usually occurs at 6 weeks of development.[62]

Timing

Parents need to know when the defect in question occurred. All of the components of the upper and lower extremities are essentially fully formed by 7 weeks of fetal development. Major malformations such as a deficiency of a long bone occur by 7 weeks of embryonic life. Fuller and Duthie pointed out that major upper limb deficiencies occur on the 28th day, major lower limb abnormalities on the 31st day, and distal upper anomalies at 35 days, and distal lower limb anomalies at 37 days.[39] Henkel and Willer demonstrated that anomalies occur in orderly patterns, depending on the timing and severity of the insult.[53] The

knowledge that most anomalies happen in the first 7 weeks may reassure parents that some traumatic event that occurred late in the pregnancy could not have caused the limb anomaly. Many mothers do not remember what agents they used nor which medications they took during the first 6 weeks as they were just becoming aware of their pregnancy. This is often a problem in confirming or eliminating a potential etiologic agent. Deformations, which are changes in already formed structures from some outside influence, may occur at any time during fetal maturation. An example is the deformation distal to a constricting amniotic band.

Chance of an Anomaly in Subsequent Offspring

A burning question for most parents concerns the likelihood of the abnormality occurring in subsequent children. Although there are a few limb anomalies with genetic bases, most are sporadic occurrences that do not affect subsequent children of the same parents or children of the affected child. The incidence of recurrence of the same deformity is just slightly higher than that of the general population, in the range of 1% to 3%. It is important to encourage parents to have more children if they so desire. Tibial hemimelia is one of the few abnormalities that often has an inheritance pattern.[68,98] The combination of femoral deficiency with anomalies of the ulna, known as the ulnar femoral syndrome, may be inherited.

Whose Fault Is It?

Parents often have an unspoken question regarding which parent is at fault for the problem. Unfortunately, when a child is born with an abnormality, the parents and grandparents often begin a process of assigning guilt. This is especially true if there is some preexisting discord in the family. This factor must be recognized, because it often results in anger and hostility that is directed at the medical personnel involved with the child. A direct discussion of guilt may help resolve the issue. For nongenetic problems, no line of responsibility exists. For genetic abnormalities, one side of the family may carry the dominant gene, and the job of the medical team is to see that that information is used constructively. The situation is more difficult if the presence of a genetic abnormality has been kept a secret from the other spouse. Even in this situation, the family must be encouraged to focus on positive issues regarding the child. If drugs or alcohol are implicated, the family may require formal psychological counseling.

The Grieving Process

The birth of a child with a significant abnormality represents a considerable loss to the family, and after any loss, a period of grief is necessary. The family should be dealt with sympathetically and encouraged to work through their feelings of disappointment.[45,97] The positive attitude of medical personnel toward the infant may help the family move forward. A well-organized team, including a prosthetist with a major interest in children, physical and occupational therapists, a social worker, a nurse, and others as needed, provides an excellent resource for managing these children. Many clinics have a program in which "veteran" parents are asked to be available to meet with new parents of children with similar anomalies. These people who have coped with the same feelings and problems often become an ongoing resource for the new family.[108]

Often the best agent for healing these early wounds is the individual child with the abnormality. The passage of early milestones helps the family to focus on positive aspects of the child's future. These children are just as responsive and interactive as others, and that uniquely human interaction communicates much about the true potential of the child. Generally, the first few weeks are the hardest for the family, and accurate information and counseling should be available at the outset.

The Next Steps

Parents need help to move beyond their initial questions, and the first step in helping the family see the child's future in a positive light is to give them a realistic view of what is ahead. Most children with limb abnormalities have normal intellects. Even children who lack several extremities may achieve virtually normal function. The best way to bring this message home is to introduce the family to another child with similar abnormalities. The interaction with the older child answers questions the new parents are not even aware they should ask. Deep down, the parent is asking, "Will he or she be a freak?" Meeting another such child usually puts this to rest. Much as a picture is worth a thousand words, a visit with a child with similar problems answers a thousand questions.

Another important early intervention is to explain clearly what can and cannot be done to improve the child's situation. It is important to realize that parental concerns are often ranked in the reverse order of the medical team's concerns. For example, the parent of a child with a congenital absence of the forearm is most concerned about the child's appearance. The medical team knows that function will be excellent and may overlook the parent's questions, which are focused on the issue of how the abnormality appears to others. If the physician tells the parent that no prosthesis can improve the child's function, the parents will seek help elsewhere. Some families need to try a cosmetic prosthesis to discover that a true cosmetic replacement is impossible.

The physician should tell the parents that they are in for an experience that will be far more positive than they can imagine. The things they will learn from the adaptability of their child will amaze and encourage them. They must be willing to go the distance in supporting and loving the child, and in the long run, nothing will be more gratifying or rewarding than the time spent with their child.

The Future

The probability of future medical advancements is a difficult area to discuss with parents. Many of the "amazing" results performed with external fixation devices were impossible 10 years ago, and the future undoubtedly holds many other unexpected advances. Compounding this scientific uncertainty is the wishful thinking of the parents, who are hoping for nothing short of a miracle.

The physician should deal with these issues in a way that helps the parents differentiate impossible hopes from likely medical advancements. Techniques undoubtedly will improve dramatically over the child's lifetime, but basic biologic principles probably will change little. If a Syme amputation is appropriate, how does the surgeon deal with the parental questions about future methods of treatment that may allow the foot to be saved? To answer this, the long-term interests of the child must be weighed. When there is an absent tibia with the usual unstable knee and ankle, saving the foot causes so much delay in the child's development that, even if it may someday be possible to insert a tibial allograft, the penalty to the waiting child is too great. However, if there is a moderate abnormality, such as a partial fibular hemimelia, that, although challenging, should be correctable at an older age, the foot should be saved.

Guide to Decision Making

Interventions should be planned to complement the normal developmental milestones of the child. We know that most children can sit at 6 months of age. This corresponds with the use of both hands together in the midline. When the child is sitting well and attempting two-handed activities, an upper extremity prosthesis can be fitted, and the child can begin to use it in apposition with the other hand. Most children begin to walk at about 12 months of age. It is best to plan early surgical interventions so they can be completed by that age if possible. For example, the ideal time to perform a Syme amputation for fibular hemimelia is when the child is starting to stand, usually around 10 months of age, so the wounds are healed and the prosthesis is ready by walking age. Because young children have immature balance, there is no need for a knee in a toddler's first above-knee prosthesis. By 3 years of age, articulated knees can be used skillfully.

The developing anatomy is an important consideration in the timing of interventions. Correction of certain deformities is better maintained if the child is weight bearing, and these procedures should be done after the child reaches walking age. A fusion of the upper tibia to the fibula in a case of partial tibial hemimelia may be performed more easily after the tibial anlage is well ossified than when the structure is mostly cartilaginous. A knee fusion for proximal femoral focal deficiency (PFFD) is also easier to perform at 4 or 5 years of age, when the femoral condyles and upper tibia are well ossified, than at 10 months of age, when the ossific nuclei are surrounded by a large amount of cartilage, even though an amputation may be planned for a young age. An alternative plan may be to allow the child to ambulate in an equinus prosthesis with an amputation and knee fusion planned for 3 or 4 years of age.

There are many important social matters to consider. The start of elementary school is often a time when parents and children wish to try an upper extremity prosthesis, after having rejected one earlier. However, the start of the year in a new school is a poor time for a child to go to school on crutches after a surgical procedure. Adolescence is a time of great emphasis on appearance, and any steps designed to avoid embarrassing the child should be taken. Putting a prosthetic foot and shoe on a cast after stump revision surgery may allow the patient to continue to "fool" his comrades into believing he has a foot. Children who were rough users of lower extremity prostheses may desire more fragile, endoskeletal prostheses with cosmetic covers when they reach adolescence. An interesting teenage prosthetic variation is the "Captain Hook" approach. This often occurs with kids involved in sports such as skiing, for whom a colorful prosthesis or a wooden "peg-leg" is the "in" thing to wear. This frank, take it or leave it approach is often a very healthy adaptation.

The physician and the parent working with a team of people including prosthetists, therapists, and others have some exacting decisions to make concerning the long-term plan for the child. A difficult choice often arises between a course of multiple corrective procedures and a less-complicated early solution such as amputation, a common dilemma when the patient has fibular hemimelia. A Syme amputation performed just before walking age will be a successful, single intervention. The child will probably have no future hospitalizations and will function at an almost normal level in sports, but he or she must adjust to having a prosthesis instead of a foot. As an alternative, it is feasible to lengthen the limb and correct much of the deformity using modern limb-lengthening technology. Choosing this path obligates the child to two or three future periods of management in a lengthening device, each of which may last 6 months or longer. The procedures are best performed in late childhood or early adolescence, which leaves a problem of management in the meantime.

The anatomic results of these interventions are well publicized, but functional assessments of such patients are unavailable. For example, there are no studies of the function of the deformed ankle of a fibular hemimelia patient, especially after the pressures of lengthening may have resulted in damage to the articular cartilage and stiffness. These procedures are often difficult and painful, and a successful outcome depends on the patient following through with the second and third stages of the plan. The psychological costs of these interventions have also not been well analyzed, but they must be significant. Whenever possible, the parents and children should meet other children who have had similar procedures and decide which avenue to take with guidance from the medical team. The role of the physician is to be sure the patient and the parents understand fully the risks and benefits of each approach and ensure that choices are not made out of ignorance or wishful thinking.[21]

SPECIFIC LOWER EXTREMITY DEFICIENCIES

Proximal Focal Femoral Deficiency

PFFD is one of several terms applied to a condition in which the femur is short, and there is an apparent absence of continuity between neck and the shaft of the femur. In many instances, the radiographically delineated defect in the upper femur of the infant ossifies as the child matures. A congenitally short femur without an ossification defect is probably a milder form of the same condition and is often considered in discussions of management of femoral deficiency.[49]

Femoral deficiency is one of the anomalies associated with the use of thalidomide in the first trimester of pregnancy. Otherwise, the remainder of cases are of unknown cause, and the disorder is not usually heritable. The combination of femoral deficiency with abnormal facies is known as the femoral hypoplasia–unusual facies syndrome and is thought to be an autosomal dominant disorder.[59]

Classification

There are many classifications of femoral deficiency. The Aitken classification is the most commonly used, and it has some clinical relevance. In Aitken's scheme there are types A through D (Fig. 29-3). Type A has a radiographic defect in the upper femur in the young child that later ossifies (Fig. 29-4). There is a femoral head present and a well-formed acetabulum, and a pseudarthrosis in the subtrochanteric area usually heals by skeletal maturity. There is usually a varus deformity of the proximal femur, and the femoral shaft may lie above the femoral head. In the Aitken type B defect, the femoral segment is shorter than in type A, there is often a tuft at the proximal end of the femur, and the acetabulum is well formed (Fig. 29-5). The femoral head may not be ossified at birth, but it appears as the child gets older. The upper portion of the femur usually lies proximal to the acetabulum, and at maturity, there is no ossific connection of the shaft to the head segment of the femur. In type C, the femoral shaft is short with a proximal tuft, the femoral head is absent, and the acetabulum is poorly formed with a flat lateral wall of the pelvis in the place of the acetabulum (Fig. 29-6). In type D, as in type C, the femoral head is absent and the acetabulum poorly formed; in addition, the femoral shaft is extremely short or even absent (Fig. 29-7).

A more comprehensive classification proposed by Hamanishi has 10 gradations of femoral maldevelopment, ranging from a shortened femur without a ra-

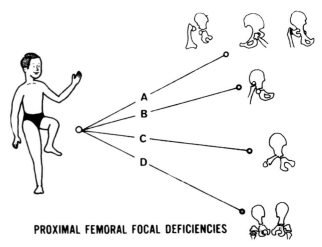

FIGURE 29-3. The Aitken classification of proximal femoral deficiencies.

diographic defect to complete absence of the femur. This classification supports the concept that the disorder is a continuous spectrum of response to an insult rather than a group of different clinical entities (Fig. 29-8).[49] The differences in pathology represent different degrees of inhibition of growth and development, and there is a category for almost any deformity. Hemanishi also observes that isolated congenital coxa vara is a different entity that is not related to PFFD.

Gillespie proposed a clinical classification that places patients into two categories. In group I, the femur is 40% to 60% shorter than the normal femur, and the hip and knee can be made functional. Group II includes those with more severely short femurs and with "useless" hip and knee joints.[42] Group I patients are candidates for lengthening procedures, and group II patients require amputation or rotationplasty and prosthetic management.

Fixsen and Lloyd-Roberts described three radiographic categories based on the appearance of the upper femoral shaft. In type I, there is a bulbous proximal femur, always followed by continuity of the head, neck, and greater trochanter. A pseudarthrosis may develop below the greater trochanter. In type II, there is a tuft or cap of ossification separated from a blunt proximal shaft by an area of lucency. The hip is usually unstable, and even if the pseudarthrosis heals, the neck is in varus. In type III, there is no tuft, and the femur is not bulbous, but it is blunt or pointed, and all these developed unstable pseudarthroses. He recommends operative stabilization of those that may be unstable (types II and III).[33]

Clinical Features

The clinical appearance of a PFFD is distinctive. The thigh is very short; the hip is flexed, abducted, and externally rotated; and there is usually a flexion

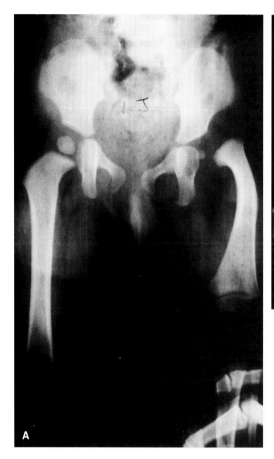

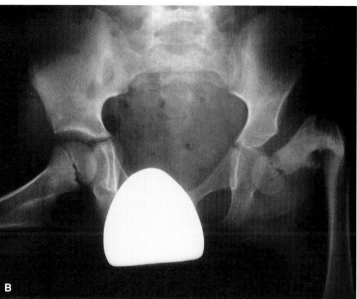

FIGURE 29-4. (A) An Aitken type A proximal focal femoral deficiency. This example has a widened lucent area between the head and neck of the femur, without a true defect. The femur is short and anterolaterally bowed. (B) An Aitken type A hip in a 4-year-old boy. There is a severe varus deformity, or a "shepherd's crook," of the upper femur; the acetabulum is well formed.

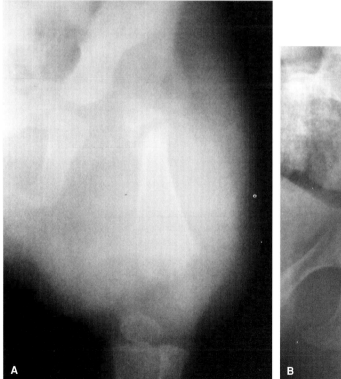

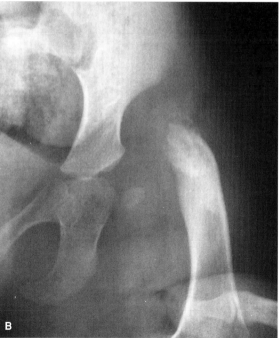

FIGURE 29-5. (A) Aitken B type of proximal focal femoral deformity. There is a tuft at the proximal end of the femur, and at this age, the proximal segment is unossified. (B) At 8 years of age, the femoral head has formed in the acetabulum, and there is no continuity between the head and shaft of the femur, a defining characteristic of Aitken type B deformity.

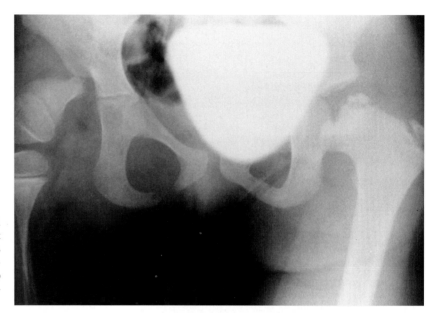

FIGURE 29-6. Aitken C type of proximal focal femoral deformity of the patient's right lower extremity. The femoral segment is short, and there is no ossification of the proximal segment. The pelvic wall is flat, with no acetabular formation. The left hip is also abnormal, with a shortened left femur.

contracture of the knee. The foot usually lies at the level of the contralateral knee (Figs. 29-9 and 29-10). Flexion contractures of the hip and knee add to the apparent shortening, and the true discrepancy can be more accurately appreciated by comparing the length of the two extremities in a sitting position. The hip abductors and extensors are present but are foreshortened and cannot function normally because of the altered anatomy of the upper femur. The knee joint lies in the groin and functions as an unstable intercalary segment.[7] In about 45% of cases, there is an associated ipsilateral fibular hemimelia, resulting in shortening of the tibia and an equinovalgus deformity of the foot.[63] There may also be deficient lateral rays of the foot.

In the related disorder known as congenital shortening of the femur, the appearance is less dramatic. The extremity is shortened, and there is an anterolateral femoral bow with a valgus deformity of the knee. The thigh and the leg may be shortened, and the knee is externally rotated. There is usually anteroposterior laxity of the knee, often with absence of the cruciate ligaments. In some cases, there is limited straight leg raising due to shortened hamstrings.[57] These children also frequently have an associated ipsilateral fibular hemimelia.

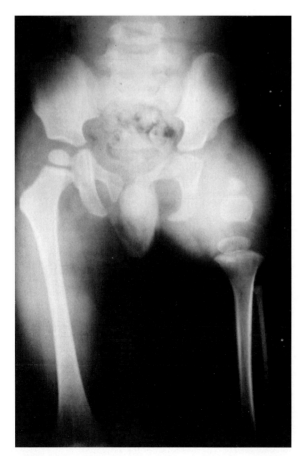

FIGURE 29-7. Aitken D type of proximal focal femoral deformity, with an extremely short femoral segment. As in the Aitken C type deformity, there is no acetabular formation.

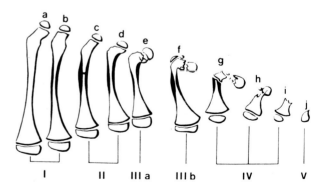

FIGURE 29-8. THe Hamanishi classification of proximal focal femoral deformities. Virtually every variation of upper femoral abnormality can be placed in one of these categories.

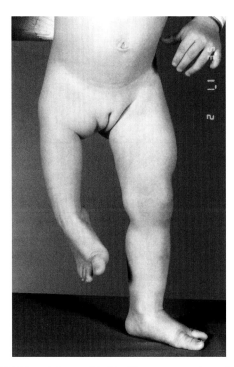

FIGURE 29-9. A 1-year-old girl with an untreated proximal focal femoral deficiency. The foreshortened thigh has a funnel shape, the extremity is externally rotated, and the foot is at the level of the contralateral knee.

Developmental milestones are usually not delayed in children with femoral deficiency. Children with marked shortening of one lower extremity walk by bearing weight on the knee of the normal extremity and the foot of the deficient side, and they begin ambulating at the usual walking age (see Fig. 29-10). Children with a congenitally short femur walk with hip and knee flexion on the normal side and with equinus on the affected side to equalize the limb length.

Treatment Considerations

The first step in the decision-making process is to determine the existing leg length discrepancy and estimate the final discrepancy at maturity. The percentage of limb length discrepancy is determined from measured radiographs. The relative shortening of the extremity remains constant throughout growth,[10] and the probable final discrepancy is determined by multiplying the average adult femoral length by the percentage of discrepancy. The eventual limb length discrepancy may also be predicted by using the standard methods of Green and Anderson and Moseley with longitudinal radiographic measurements. If the final discrepancy of the lower extremity is more than 20 cm, some form of prosthetic management is necessary. If a final discrepancy of less than 20 cm is predicted, as is common with congenital shortening of the femur, a lengthening procedure may be considered. Stability

of the hip and femoral segment must be established to lengthen the femur successfully.

If shortening will exceed 20 cm at maturity and prosthetic management is planned, several options must be weighed. The first decision is choosing among performing an ankle disarticulation, performing a rotationplasty using the foot to control the prosthetic knee, or maintaining the foot to fit the child with an equinus prosthesis. If amputation or rotationplasty is chosen, the next decision is between fusion of the knee to provide a stable proximal limb and fusion of the proximal femur to the pelvis to provide a more stable gait. Rarely, surgical intervention to fuse the proximal femoral pseudarthrosis must be considered

PROSTHETIC MANAGEMENT

Patients with shortening of greater than 50% of the contralateral femoral length, usually with a final discrepancy of greater than 20 cm, require prosthetic management. These fit into Gillespie's group II.[42] The upper femoral deformity varies and may fit any of Aitken's groups. In these patients, the discrepancy is too great to be overcome with lengthening procedures, and some form of prosthetic management is necessary. Young children are able to function well in an equinus prosthesis or an extension orthosis. As the child gets older, however, the prosthetic management becomes more difficult, and amputation of the foot or rotationplasty should be considered.

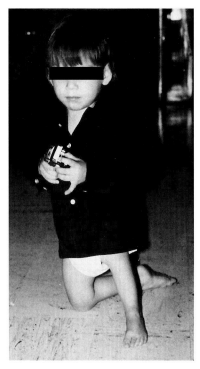

FIGURE 29-10. A boy with proximal focal femoral deformity, who has begun knee walking on the affected side to equalize his limb length discrepancy. He was managed with a Syme amputation and a knee arthrodesis.

Amputation of the foot with prosthetic management is a well-established method of managing these major femoral deficiencies, and it is commonly combined with a knee arthrodesis (Fig. 29-11). An alternative of fusion of the femur to the pelvis to provide hip stability should be considered before fusing the knee. A modified Syme or Boyd amputation maintaining the malleoli provides a residual limb that is well adapted to prosthetic wear and end weight bearing.[7,61,83,116] Heel pad migration is usually not a problem after the Syme disarticulation, and the more complicated Boyd procedure is rarely indicated. In the modified Syme procedure, the ankle is disarticulated and the malleoli are left intact. Reduction of the size of the malleoli is unnecessary and would probably cause a growth disturbance if done. After the amputation, the child can walk at an early age using an above-knee prosthesis and can also walk without a prosthesis by bearing weight on the end of the affected limb and the knee of the contralateral limb.

In the older child, the short femoral segment with the knee at the upper brim of the prosthesis usually does not provide enough stability for a satisfactory gait. The prosthesis tends to displace proximally and anteriorly as the knee and hip flex during stance phase of gait. This problem can be corrected by performing an arthrodesis of the knee to create a straight residual limb with the prosthesis directly under the acetabulum. The timing of the procedures varies. Some prefer to perform the amputation just before walking age and defer the knee arthrodesis until the child is 3 or 4 years of age. Others perform both procedures together at 2 or 3 years of age and use a nonstandard prosthesis in the interim.

A common problem after Syme amputation and knee arthrodesis is that the end of the residual limb lies at or below the contralateral knee at skeletal maturity. When this is the case, the tibial segment of the prosthesis must be shortened to accommodate the prosthetic knee mechanism, resulting in a discrepancy of knee heights (see Fig. 29-11). The length discrepancy can be reduced by performing an epiphysiodesis of

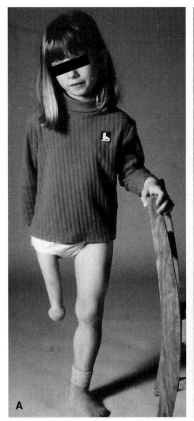 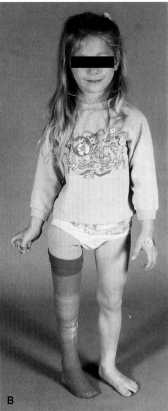 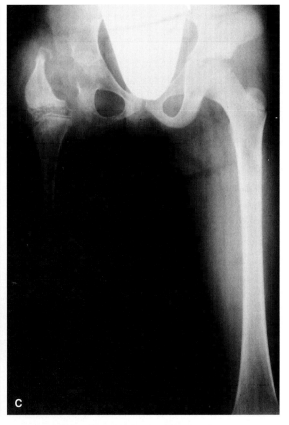

FIGURE 29-11.   (**A**) A girl who has had a Syme amputation and a knee arthrodesis for proximal focal femoral deficiency. The end of her residual limb is at the level of the contralateral knee. Ideally, the end of the limb should lie at least 5 cm (2 in) above the knee to have room for the prosthetic knee. (**B**) The same girl with her prosthesis, which is an ischial weight-bearing prosthesis with a cosmetic cover. A neoprene band provides suspension. (**C**) Radiographs of an Aitken type D deformity. The knee arthrodesis was performed with excision of the distal femoral epiphysis, followed by fusion of the femoral metaphysis to the proximal tibial epiphysis. The epiphyseal excision allows the extremity to gradually shorten to a more desirable length.

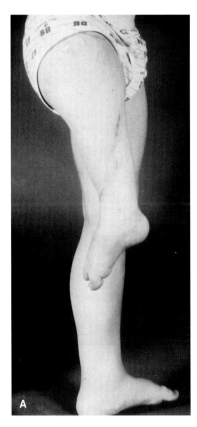
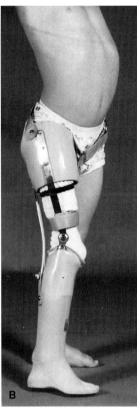

FIGURE 29-12. A child after a Van Nes rotationplasty for proximal focal femoral deformity. In this case, the rotation was performed through the tibial segment. The disadvantage to this technique is that the foot gradually derotates as the limb grows. (**B**) The same child wearing his prosthesis. The ankle provides motor and sensory control of the prosthetic knee.

the distal femur or the proximal tibia at the time of knee arthrodesis. A simple way to do this is to excise either epiphysis, usually the femoral, at the time of the arthrodesis, and the tibial epiphysis is fused to the distal femoral metaphysis. When this is done at 3 or 4 years of age, the ultimate length is usually satisfactory. The final discrepancy may be calculated from growth charts, but the flexion of the hip and knee before fusion often makes these measurements inaccurate.

Van Nes described a rotationplasty of the tibia in which the foot is rotated 180 degrees, and the toes face posteriorly to enable the ankle and foot to control a prosthetic knee (Fig. 29-12). The motor control of the ankle is primarily through the gastrocsoleus muscle, which becomes a "knee" extensor in the new configuration. In addition to motor control, the sensory feedback from the ankle allows better proprioceptive control of the knee.[48,64,67,113] Gillespie reported good initial function after the Van Nes procedures, but the feet gradually derotated as the children grew, with 10 of 21 cases requiring repeated rotationplasty procedures.[42] Similarly, 12 of the 20 cases reported by Kostuik had to be rerotated, with 6 having a second rerotation surgery.[64] Other techniques have evolved in which the rotation is performed partially through an arthrodesis of the knee, with additional rotation gained through a tibial osteotomy. Torode and Gillespie reported the results of a procedure in which the most of the rotation

(about 120 degrees) is obtained by rotating the tibia on the femur at the time of knee arthrodesis, with additional rotation through a tibial osteotomy.[111] They reported good functional results, but a report with longer follow-up is needed to evaluate long-term rotational stability. When there is rotational malalignment, the function of the Van Nes rotationplasty deteriorates, and prosthetic fitting is especially difficult.

Controversy exists about the need for stabilization of the upper femoral defect. Kruger recommends performing osteosynthesis between 3 and 6 years of age.[70] Others report that the defect usually may be left alone unless progressive deformity or instability occurs. We have found that most upper femoral defects are stable and require no intervention. The indication for osteosynthesis of the femoral defect is documentation of progressive deformity.

Patients with PFFD who are treated with the previously described procedures are able to lead active lives and have good functional outcomes. They walk without aids and usually hop twice on the sound leg when attempting to run. The main problem in gait is related to hip instability.[29] Deformities of the upper femur—usually a short, varus femoral neck, coupled with acetabular abnormalities—are such that the abductor muscles cannot support body weight in stance, and an abductor lurch is inevitable. This is often barely evident in the young child but becomes a major cosmetic and functional problem in the adolescent and

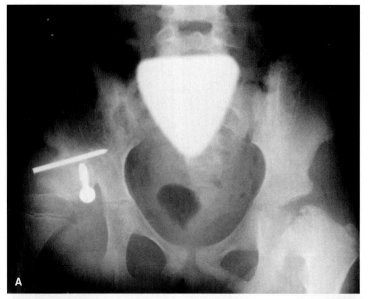

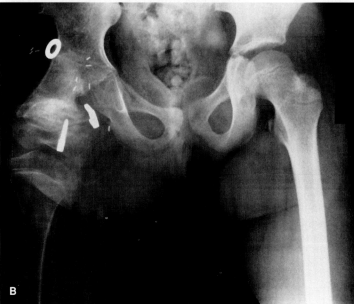

FIGURE 29-13. (**A**) A patient with proximal focal femoral deformity after fusion of the femoral segment to the pelvis as described by Steel.[105] (**B**) An example of fusion of the femoral segment to the pelvis in a reversed, extended position as described by Brown. The reversed knee joint acts as a hinged hip joint, with the gastrocnemius functioning as a hip flexor. (Courtesy of Kenneth Brown, M.D., Vancouver.)

adult. In an attempt to eliminate the abductor lurch, several operative procedures have been developed. Steel described an approach in which the femur is fused to the pelvis in a flexed position, with the knee functioning as a hip joint.[105] This may be combined with a Van Nes rotationplasty or Syme amputation (Fig. 29-13). To keep the limb in line with the body mass, the femur should be shortened and the femoral epiphysis fused. In Steel's series, revisions were always necessary for overgrowth of the femoral segment. To avoid this problem, we have fused the femoral condyles to the pelvis after excising the remaining femoral metaphysis and physis. In the short term, the gait is improved and the abductor lurch minimized. There is usually little active hip flexion power, but this is not a major functional deficit. The follow-up period in

Steel's series was 5 years, and longer follow-up is not available to establish the efficacy of the procedure.

Brown adapted a limb-salvage approach to the management of PFFD. He recommends rotating the femur 180 degrees before fusing it to the pelvis, with excision of excess soft tissue. The femur remains in an extended position, and the knee functions as a hip joint, with the gastrocnemius soleus as a hip flexor (see Fig. 29-13). The retained foot and ankle function as a knee joint, as in the Van Nes procedure. He reports that the abductor lurch is eliminated, and derotation cannot occur. Long-term follow-up is not available for this procedure.

The pertinent decisions to be made in management of the patient with severe shortening and PFFD may be summarized in questions of saving, rotating,

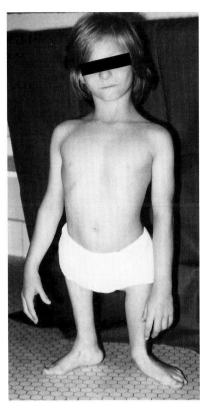

FIGURE 29-14. A patient with bilateral proximal focal femoral deformity. Equinus prostheses may be useful, but surgical treatment is not indicated. The main functional problems of a child like this are the shortness of stature and waddling gait.

or amputating the foot and a decision to fuse the knee or to fuse the femur to the pelvis. A knee fusion with Syme amputation provides good function but allows a Trendelenburg gait, and a rotationplasty with femoropelvic fusion may provide better prosthetic knee control and less of an abductor lurch. The significant functional advantages of the rotationplasty must be weighed against the cosmetic concerns of a "backward" foot. The advantages include the ability to control the knee with the foot, and the proprioceptive feedback from the ankle.[43] Parents and children should meet other families with similar problems to fully understand the implications of their decision. Psychological counseling may also be helpful.

Bilateral PFFD is fortunately rare (Fig. 29-14). Treatment is usually limited to improving the patient's height by using extension prostheses, and amputations are contraindicated.

LIMB LENGTHENING

When a discrepancy of less than 20 cm is projected, as in most cases of congenital short femur and in some cases of PFFD, lengthening of the extremity is often the ideal management. These patients fit into group I of the classification of Gillespie and Torode[42] and have a femur that is at least 40% to 60% of the

length of the normal femur. The foot of the affected side usually reaches the midtibial level of the normal leg. The anatomy of the proximal femur and hip must be such that hip stability can be achieved.

In this condition, the goal of treatment is equalization of the limb lengths. In some cases, a single femoral lengthening combined with contralateral epiphysiodesis can correct the leg length discrepancy,[42] but in other cases, two femoral lengthenings are necessary. Sometimes, the tibia must also be lengthened.

Lengthening procedures for congenital femoral shortening are arduous and prone to many complications, and they should not be undertaken lightly.[63,83,87,114,116]

There are unique aspects of the PFFD that should be considered before undertaking a lengthening procedure. The hip and proximal femur may require procedures to correct preexisting deformity (Fig. 29-15). Mild acetabular dysplasia is common, and muscle forces created by femoral lengthening causes the dysplastic hip to dislocate if the dysplasia is not corrected. A pelvic osteotomy may be done to prevent this complication, and the nature of the acetabular deficiency should be determined preoperatively. If there is anterolateral acetabular insufficiency, a Salter procedure is appropriate, and if the deficiency is posterior, a Dega osteotomy is preferred. Deformity of the upper femur that is often retroverted should also be corrected before lengthening. The neck-shaft angle should be corrected to normal (about 135 degrees), but the femur should not be placed in valgus, because this favors hip dislocation.[21,74] The patient should be fully recovered from such procedures before beginning a femoral lengthening. The iliotibial band is often contracted and should be released before femoral lengthening.

Femoral lengthening is usually not undertaken in early childhood, making it necessary to manage the shorter limb in ways that allow normal childhood activities. Simple extension prostheses or sometimes large shoe lifts are useful for very young children, but they are unsightly for the older child. In the school-age child, an equinus prosthesis effectively equalizes leg length and allows full function, and shoe lifts are used for milder discrepancies (Figs. 29-16 and 29-17).

Fibular Deficiency

Congenital absence of the fibula, also called fibular hemimelia, has several manifestations. These range from complete absence of the fibula with missing lateral rays of the foot (i.e., terminal longitudinal deficiency) to absence of only a portion of the fibula without foot involvement (i.e., intercalary longitudinal deficiency).

Congenital fibular deficiency usually occurs spo-

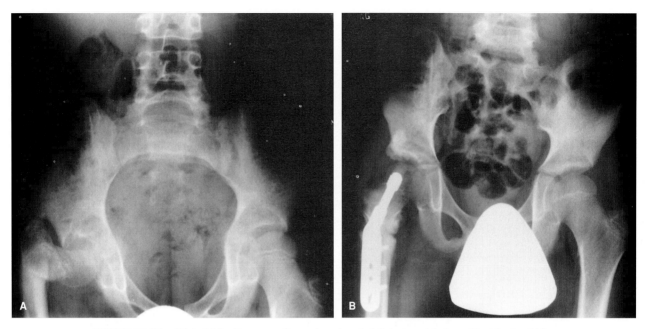

FIGURE 29-15. (A) A child with a varus femoral neck and deficient acetabulum. The hip should be stabilized in preparation for femoral lengthening. (B) The same patient after femoral valgus osteotomy and Dega acetabuloplasty to improve hip stability.

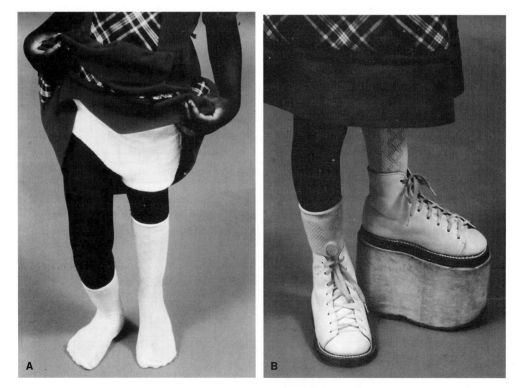

FIGURE 29-16. (A) A girl with an Aitken type A deformity with mild shortening. (B) Early treatment of this girl was accomplished with a shoe lift.

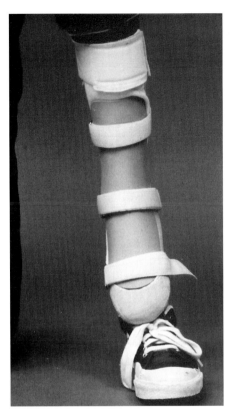

FIGURE 29-17. An equinus prosthesis is useful for correcting leg length discrepancy in a patient with proximal femoral deficiency. This device is more cosmetic than a large shoe lift.

radically, without a known cause. Fifteen percent of patients have associated femoral deficiencies.[9] Kruger found that patients with five-rayed feet always had femoral shortening, and one half of those with fewer rays had femoral shortening.[68]

Classification

In the Franz and O'Rahilly classification, the fibular deficiency may be a terminal deficiency with absent rays of the foot or an intercalary deficiency with a normal foot. It is always a paraxial (longitudinal) deficiency.

Coventry and Johnston classified fibular hemimelia into three types: type I with partial absence of the fibula, type II with complete fibular absence, and type III that includes bilateral cases and unilateral cases with other skeletal anomalies.[24] Achterman and Kalamachi have classified the entity based on the degree of fibular deficiency (Fig. 29-18), and their classification is more clinically useful.[1] Type I includes all cases with a portion of the fibula present. In their type IA, the proximal fibular epiphysis is distal to the level of the tibial growth plate, and the distal fibular physis is proximal to the dome of the talus. In type IB, there is 30% to 50% decrease in the length of the proximal

fibula, and distally, the fibula did does not support the ankle. In type II, the fibula is completely absent. They report eventual total limb length discrepancy at maturity of 12% in type IA, 18% in type IB, and 19% in type II. The tibial discrepancy was 6% in IA, 17% in IB, and 25% in type II.[1]

The child with complete absence of the fibula presents clinically with an anterolateral bow of the tibia, an equinovalgus deformity of the foot, and a tarsal coalition. The talotibial joint is usually malformed; with the fused talocalcaneus having a flat upper surface that articulates with the tibia in a valgus and equinus position. The foot may be missing one or two lateral rays. There is always significant shortening of the leg and frequently additional shortening of the ipsilateral femur (Figs. 29-19 through 29-21).[9,68,117]

The clinical syndrome of partial fibular hemimelia is distinctive, and the abnormalities affect the entire lower extremity. There is a variable degree of femoral shortening, valgus of the knee, deficiency of the anterior cruciate ligament with absence of the tibial spine, and a tarsal coalition (Fig. 29-22). The lateral malleolus is proximal in the ankle mortise, and there is mild ankle valgus. The ultimate leg length discrepancy is made up of femoral and tibial shortening and ranges from 12% to 18% of the length of the extremity.[1]

Treatment

There is a reasonable consensus that complete fibular hemimelia is best treated by performing an ankle disarticulation in early childhood and fitting a Syme-type prosthesis.[7,9,30,68,117] In the past, many other procedures were performed to attempt centralization of the foot and lengthening of the extremity. Badgley, in the early 1940s, pioneered ankle disarticulation as

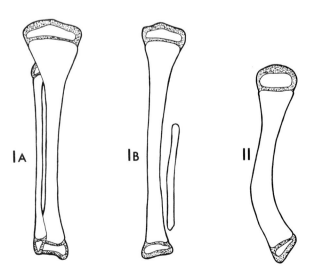

FIGURE 29-18. The Achterman and Kalamachi classification of fibular hemimelia.

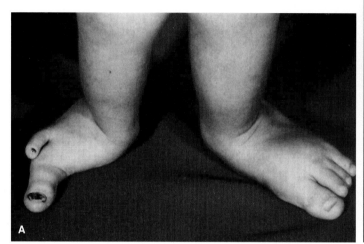
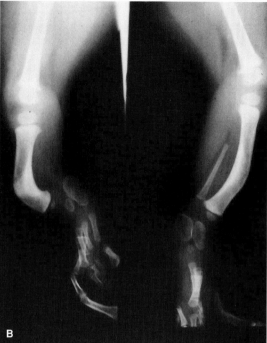

FIGURE 29-19.   (A) Clinical appearance of a child with partial fibular hemimelia on the left and complete hemimelia on the right. On the right, there is only one fully formed ray, and the left foot is missing the fifth ray. (B) The bowing of the tibia, which is usually present with complete fibular hemimelia, is evident on the right in this radiograph.

definitive treatment for fibular hemimelia.[68] The report of Kruger and Talbot of 48 cases was the first large series to document the advantages of amputation.[68] Although most series report good results from modified Syme amputation, some physicians prefer the Boyd amputation, using the retained calcaneus for heel pad stability. Kruger recommends this for older boys.[70] Eilert found good results with the Boyd and Syme amputations and found that the best results correlated with central placement of the heel pad by either method.[28] In our experience, migration of the

heel pad after Syme amputation was fairly common and produced little difficulty for the prosthetist or the patient, and we have found little need to perform the more complicated Boyd procedure (Fig. 29-23).[55]

The amputation is best done at the time when the child is pulling to stand, usually at 9 or 10 months of age, so the child will be able to ambulate in a prosthesis at 1 year of age. Children so treated function almost normally and are able to run and play all sports (Fig. 29-24).[55] If the tibial bowing produces too great an anterior prominence, a tibial osteotomy may be done at the time of amputation. Mild bowing of the tibia is well tolerated and does not require corrective osteotomy. Subsequent prosthetic management is relatively simple as the leg assumes a cylindrical shape, with only slight enlargement distally. Soft liners and foam shell designs have eliminated the need for a window in the prosthesis (Figs. 29-25 and 29-26).

Newer limb-lengthening techniques have resulted in renewed interest in correcting deformity and limb length discrepancy in patients with complete fibular hemimelia.[20,34] We agree with Kruger that children with large discrepancies (>5 cm at birth) and those with major foot deformities are better managed with amputation.[70] Those with lesser discrepancies may be candidates for lengthening procedures, but the exact indications and results of these procedures have not been well defined. These children usually need several lengthenings and may be left with significant func-

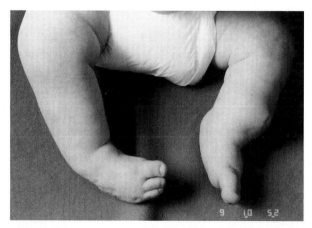

FIGURE 29-20.   A child with a left fibular hemimelia. Notice the marked anterior bow of the tibia, the diminutive foot, and shortening of the leg.

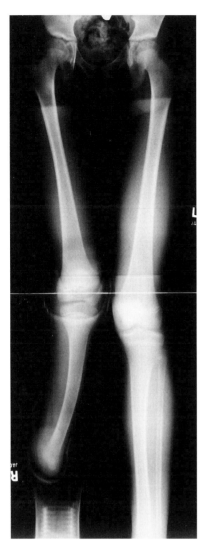

FIGURE 29-21. Radiographs of a child with a complete fibular hemimelia after a Syme amputation. The shortening of the femur, valgus of the knee, and absence of the tibial spine are often seen with fibular hemimelia. The valgus was subsequently corrected in this child with a medial hemiepiphyseodesis of the proximal tibia.

tional deficits due to abnormalities of the foot and ankle. The advantages of maintaining the foot should be weighed against the disadvantages of repeated surgical procedures, time spent with the external fixator in place, and the significant social and psychological costs, which are hard to measure.

Treatment decisions are also difficult for patients with partial fibular hemimelia. Single or staged leg lengthenings with repositioning of the foot may be successful, and the short fibula may be differentially lengthened relative to the tibia to restore a more normal tibial-fibular relation. Almost all patients with fibular hemimelia have a tarsal coalition and an abnormal talotibial articulation, and the long-term function of the foot and ankle are difficult to predict. The degree of discrepancy is proportional to the likelihood of complications of lengthening procedures. The child with

6 cm of shortening predicted at maturity and a functional foot and ankle is an ideal candidate for lengthening. The child with 18 cm of discrepancy, severe valgus of the ankle, and a diminutive foot is better off with a Syme amputation. Children with intermediate abnormalities require individualized decisions, but long-term results are not available to assist with decision making.

Some of these children develop progressive valgus of the knee, regardless of the type of initial treatment. This is best left alone until 1 or 2 years before skeletal maturity, when a partial growth arrest procedure may be performed. With more than 15 degrees of valgus and at least 2 cm of growth remaining, a medial proximal tibial or distal femoral growth arrest (depending on the site of the valgus) can bring about gradual correction of the deformity. Staples should not be used, because they are poorly tolerated beneath the prosthesis. The patient should be carefully observed in the first 6 to 9 months after the epiphysiodesis, because the deformity may overcorrect into varus. If the limb reaches neutral alignment after the arrest and the lateral portion of the proximal tibial physis is still open, a lateral epiphysiodesis should be performed to prevent overcorrection.

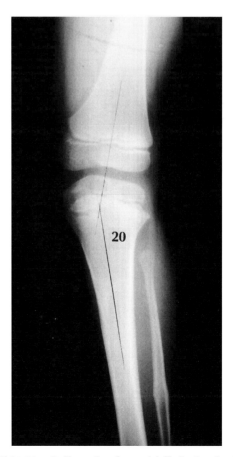

FIGURE 29-22. Radiographs of a partial fibular hemimelia. Notice the distal position of the fibular head, the absence of the tibial spine, and the valgus of the knee.

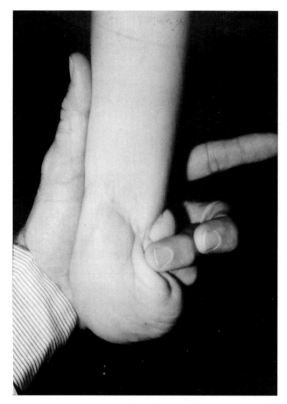

FIGURE 29-23. A well-formed residual limb after a Syme amputation. The child can grip the prosthesis by contracting his gastrocnemiussoleus muscle, which can enhance suspension while running.

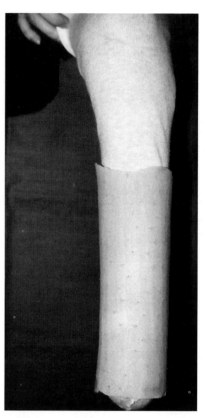

FIGURE 29-25. A removable socket liner may be worn between socks to give a snug fit to a Syme amputation. This liner is molded at the time of prosthetic fitting and allows the residual limb to fit into a cylindric socket despite a bulbous distal end.

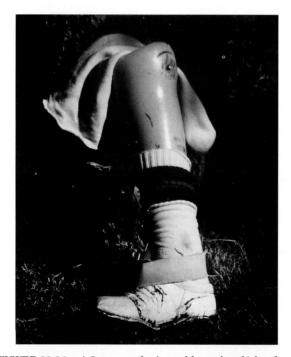

FIGURE 29-24. A Syme prosthesis used by a place kicker for a major college football team. He kicked with the prosthetic foot, which was squared off at the toe for a perfect kicking surface. Children with Syme amputations are capable of high levels of athletic competition and should not be given any arbitrary limitations.

The treatment of a child with bilateral fibular hemimelia involves other considerations (Fig. 29-27). These children usually have minimal discrepancy between the length of the two limbs, but a significant discrepancy between the lengths of the legs relative to the rest of the body. This discrepancy is not objectionable in the young child, but at an older age, the disproportion between femoral and tibial lengths produces an unsightly "dwarfism" due to the short tibias. If the tibial shortening is not too great and if the foot is well aligned, the feet should be preserved, and lengthening of the tibias may be considered. However, if there is major shortening of the tibias and if the feet are malpositioned, the patient is better treated with ankle disarticulations. A study by Kruger estimated that 50% of the patients with bilateral fibular hemimelia in his clinic should have been treated with amputation rather than limb-saving procedures.[68] This study was done before the advent of modern limb-lengthening techniques.

Tibial Deficiency

Etiology

There is no known cause for most patients with tibial hemimelia. There are several forms of the disor-

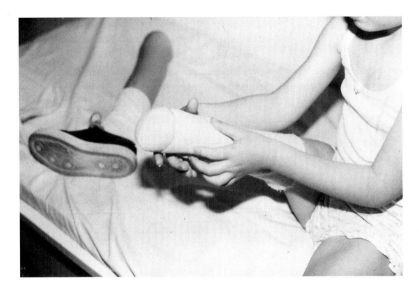

FIGURE 29-26. A child applying her prosthesis with the liner in place. This results in an intimate fit of the prosthesis, and no other suspension is necessary.

der that are hereditable in an autosomal dominant pattern.[23,72,98] In the hereditable type, the deformity is usually bilateral, there is duplication of the toes, and there may be hand anomalies. Geneticists have recognized at least four autosomal dominant tibial hemimelia syndromes: tibial hemimelia–foot polydactyly–

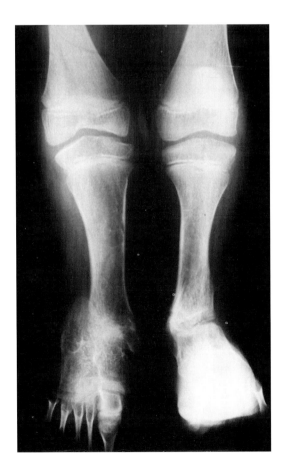

FIGURE 29-27. Radiographs of a bilateral fibular hemimelia. Although controversial, Syme amputation is often the best method of managing these patients because of difficulties with foot and ankle function.

triphalangeal thumbs syndrome (Warner syndrome), tibial hemimelia diplopodia syndrome, tibial hemimelia–split hand and foot syndrome, and tibial hemimelia–micromelia-trigonobrachycephaly syndrome. There are also cases that suggest autosomal recessive inheritance.[96] The multitude of associated anomalies includes split hand and foot, syndactyly, polydactyly, foot oligodactyly, five-fingered hand, anonychia, bifid femurs, ulnar reduplication, fibular reduplication, radial ray agenesis, radioulnar synostosis, micromelia, diplopodia, joint hyperextensibility, trigonomacrocephaly, and deafness.[96]

Classification

Jones has classified tibial hemimelia into four categories (Fig. 29-28). In type I, the tibia is not seen radiographically at birth. In subtype IA, there is an upper tibia, and in IB, the upper tibia is late to ossify (Fig. 29-29). If there is no ossification of the distal femoral epiphysis or it is small, it is likely that no upper tibia is present. In type II, the proximal tibia is ossified, and the distal tibia is absent (Fig. 29-30). In type III, the distal tibia is ossified, and the proximal tibia is absent, an exceedingly rare variation. Type IV consists of the entity formerly called congenital diastasis of the ankle (Fig. 29-31). In these cases, the tibia and fibula diverge at the ankle, the tibia is short, the talus is proximally displaced, and the distal tibial articular surface is absent.[58]

Clinical Examination

When the tibia is completely absent (Jones type IA), there is a knee flexion contracture, with the lying proximal and lateral to the femoral condyles (Figs. 29-32 and 29-33). The upper portion of the leg should be carefully examined, because there may be a palpable tibial segment present that has not ossified and is

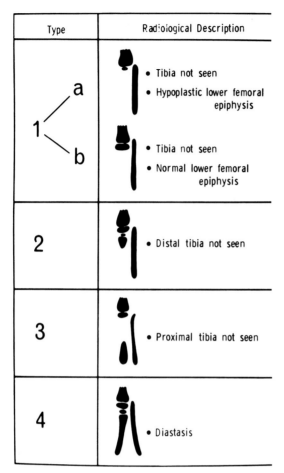

Type	Radiological Description
1 (a)	• Tibia not seen • Hypoplastic lower femoral epiphysis
1 (b)	• Tibia not seen • Normal lower femoral epiphysis
2	• Distal tibia not seen
3	• Proximal tibia not seen
4	• Diastasis

FIGURE 29-28.   The Jones classification of tibial hemimelia.

not visible radiographically. An ultrasound scan or magnetic resonance image may better demonstrate this finding.[46] Children with complete tibial absence usually have hamstring function but rarely have quadriceps function, and the patella is usually absent. The foot is in a severe varus position relative to the distal fibula and has little functional movement.

When the distal tibia is absent and the proximal tibia present (Jones type II), the knee moves normally, and quadriceps and hamstring functions are intact. The head of the fibula is proximally and laterally displaced, and the leg is in varus, with marked varus instability. At the ankle, the foot is displaced medially relative to the fibula and is in a varus position.

When there is a diastasis of the distal tibia and fibula (Jones type IV), the leg is moderately shortened, and the foot is wedged between the tibia and fibula with a rigid varus deformity.

Treatment

Treatment of complete tibial hemimelia usually requires a knee disarticulation. Brown described centralization of the fibula combined with Syme amputation for this condition (Fig. 29-34).[18,19] The Brown procedure has frequently been performed for these patients, but most have subsequently required knee disarticulation.[76,90] Failure most often results from progressive flexion contracture of the knee caused by unopposed hamstring pull. The marked knee instability makes prosthetic management difficult and contributes to the ultimate failure of the procedure. The absence of the patella and the lack of femoral condylar notch precludes anterior transfer of the hamstrings to provide active knee extension. In the rare cases in which the child presents with good quadriceps function, the Brown procedure has been reported to be effective.[22] In our experience, there has been a gradual deterioration of knee function over a number of years, and most cases have resulted in eventual amputation. We have concluded that the procedure is rarely indicated for complete tibial hemimelia.

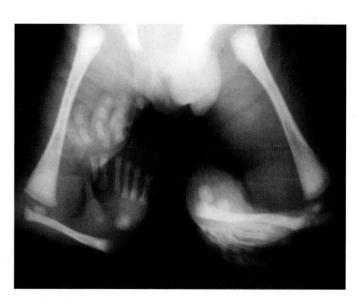

FIGURE 29-29.   A case of bilateral complete tibial hemimelia with polydactyly (Jones type Ia). Complete instability of the fibula at the knee and severe flexion contractures are evident.

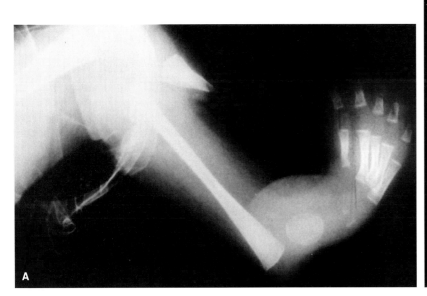
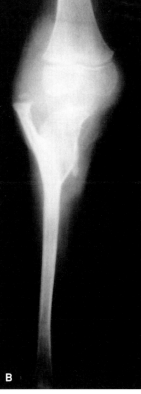

FIGURE 29-30. (A) A patient with Jones type II partial tibial hemimelia. The short proximal tibial segment often lies in a soft tissue envelope that protrudes from the anterior surface of the leg. (B) The same patient after synostosis of the fibula to the upper tibia and Syme amputation. This limb functions as well as a fibular hemimelia after a Syme amputation.

When knee disarticulation is necessary, the surgeon can anticipate a good functional result. Loder reported six patients with nine knee disarticulations and found that the physiologic cost index, which is a measure of energy consumption in gait, was within the normal range in these patients. The children were able to run, but their 50-yard dash times were below the fifth percentile.[75]

For partial tibial hemimelias, the outlook is much better, comparable to that for fibular hemimelia. When the proximal portion of the tibia is present (Jones type II deformity), fusion of the proximal fibula to the upper tibia provides an excellent functional result (see Fig. 29-30).[6,51,58] In infancy, the upper tibia may be largely cartilaginous, and fusion should be done after there is enough bone in the proximal tibia to achieve a synostosis with the fibula. The fibula may be fused to the tibia in a side-to-side position with screw fixation or an end-to-end position using an intramedullary pin. Because of the extreme instability of the foot and ankle, the best treatment of the distal segment is a Syme amputation followed by prosthetic management. These children function as well as other Syme-level amputees, and normal sports activities are the rule.

The distal diastasis abnormality (Jones type IV) is best managed with a modified Syme ankle disarticulation. The procedure should be done as the child reaches walking age, and the expected functional result is excellent. With other options, which include tibial lengthening and foot repositioning procedures, it is sometimes possible to achieve a plantigrade foot, but the abnormalities of the talus and calcaneus, as well as the absence of a distal tibial articular surface, make functional reconstruction difficult.[58] Although current limb-lengthening techniques may offer other treatment options for the diastasis abnormality, there are few published reports, and these procedures should be considered investigational.

Foot Deficiencies

Etiology and Classification

Congenital absence of the foot is an uncommon anomaly, and the most common cause is constriction band formation (Streeter bands). Traumatic partial foot amputations are common after injuries with power mowers and other equipment.

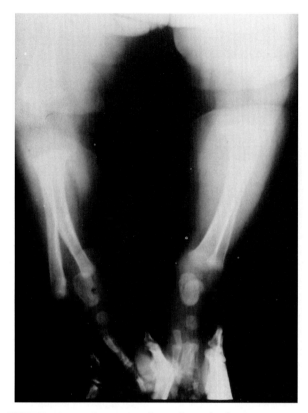

FIGURE 29-31.   Anteroposterior radiograph of a Jones type IV distal tibial fibular diastasis. This patient was treated with a Syme amputation. Functional reconstruction of the foot and ankle is extremely difficult in this condition because of the absence of a distal tibial articular surface.

These amputations are transverse and are classified by level as transmetatarsal, tarsometatarsal (Lisfranc), and midtarsal (Chopart).

Treatment

The prosthetic management of these amputations is usually simple. The transmetatarsal amputation may require only a toe-filler device to prevent shoe distortion. Periosteal overgrowth may occur and require revision surgery to remove the sharp ends of the metatarsals. Tarsometatarsal and midtarsal amputations function well with a slipper-type prosthesis that is a modified plastic shoe insert (Figs. 29-35 and 29-36). When the residual foot is too short to suspend a prosthesis, a modified ankle-foot orthosis with a partial prosthetic foot may be used. Children with congenital partial foot amputations rarely have problems with equinus deformity. The foot also remains in a neutral position after a traumatic tarsometatarsal amputation provided the tibialis anterior and toe extensor tendons are sutured to the talus at the time of amputation to balance the pull of the tendo Achillis.

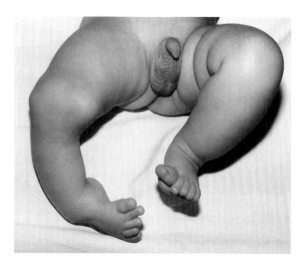

FIGURE 29-32.   A child with right tibial hemimelia. The knee flexion contracture is 45 degrees, and the foot is fixed in varus.

ACQUIRED AMPUTATIONS

Etiology

Malignant tumors result in more amputations in children than any other disease and are only exceeded by trauma as a cause of acquired amputation. The management of these children and adolescents often differs significantly from the management of traumatic amputees. The child with a malignancy often needs to be fitted with a prosthesis while recovering from

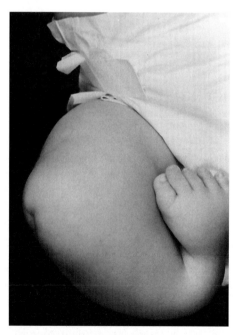

FIGURE 29-33.   A child with a severe deformity due to complete tibial hemimelia. There is a 90-degree knee flexion contracture, and the varus of the foot places it in the perineum. A through-knee amputation is the only treatment option in this situation.

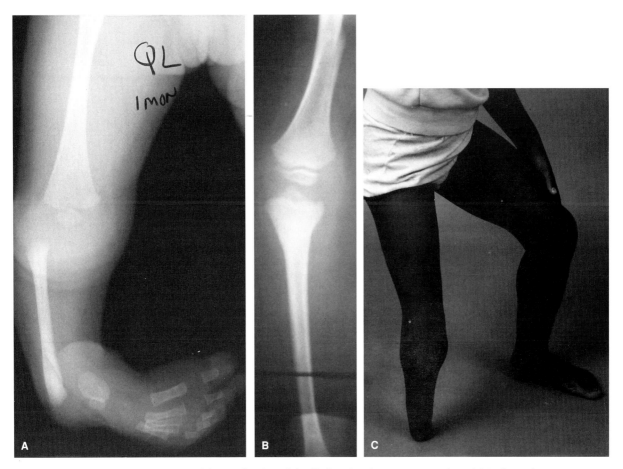

FIGURE 29-34. Successful centralization of the fibula using the Brown procedure. (**A**) Radiographs taken in an infant with a complete tibial hemimelia. (**B**) Radiographs of the lower extremity 8 years after the centralization procedure. The fibula has remodeled and enlarged to resemble a tibia. (**C**) At 9 years of age, the patient has a good gait and is able to ambulate on her limb without a prosthesis. The range of motion of the knee has gradually decreased to a 60-degree arc. Most such procedures fail because of knee instability and the development of knee flexion contractures. Results of this type are the exception, and the procedure is recommended only if quadriceps function is present preoperatively.

events that are physically and emotionally traumatic. The amputation may have been preceded by chemotherapy, and the child may be undergoing chemotherapy or irradiation at the time of beginning prosthesis use. In addition to these physical insults, the emotional impact of dealing with a life-threatening illness is almost impossible to imagine. We are continually amazed at the courage and perseverance of these children and their families.

The prosthetic team must deal with many issues. The child receiving chemotherapy has intermittent periods of weight loss that alter the fit of a prosthesis. Sockets that can be adapted to volumetric changes should be used in these instances (Fig. 29-37). The child should be mobilized as quickly as possible. His or her life span may be shortened, and the periods of medical intervention should be minimized. Early prosthetic fitting is important for the child's body im-

age, but it is done with the knowledge that the residual limb will change size and shape rapidly. It may be helpful to begin with a temporary prosthesis or socket that can easily be replaced as the residual limb matures. Children with more than one site of tumor present even more complex problems. For example, a secondary lesion in the upper extremity may preclude the effective use of crutches.

Another cause of multiple extremity amputations is purpura fulminans (Fig. 29-38). This devastating disease is usually caused by meningococcal septicemia that results in gangrene of extremities. Some children sustain four extremity amputations from this life-threatening disease, and others lose one or two limbs. Septicemia from other organisms such as *Haemophilus influenzae* may result in a similar clinical picture. These children often have an apparent level of demarcation of gangrene at the middle of the extremities. The

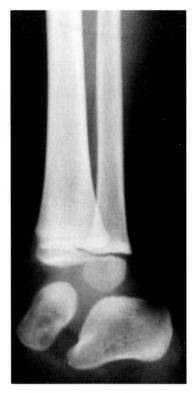

FIGURE 29-35. Radiograph of a child with congenital absence of the foot at the Chopart level. This is a very functional level of amputation that allows full weight bearing.

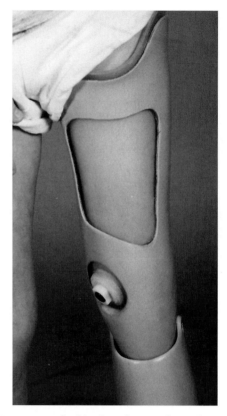

FIGURE 29-37. A flexible above-knee socket with a windowed outer frame. If limb volume fluctuation is anticipated, as in a child receiving chemotherapy, this design simplifies prosthetic modifications. Because the inner socket is pliable and removable, the prosthetist can modify the frame, add material between the frame and the socket, or replace the entire socket.

surgeon may find vascularized, viable tissue extending well distal to the proximal margin of the gangrenous skin and subcutaneous tissue eschar. The amputation should be done at the level of deep gangrene, not at the margin of the eschar, and this often allows saving the knee and sometimes saving the elbow. The wound may then be covered with skin grafts, which usually function surprisingly well, even in weight-bearing areas.

The most frequent cause of traumatic extremity amputations in children is power tools, especially power lawn mowers. We hope that better public education about the danger of these machines will reduce the incidence of these mutilating injuries. Other causes of traumatic amputation, in order of frequency, are motor vehicle accidents, gunshot wounds, explo-

sions, and railroad injuries.[110] Certain surgical principles apply to the treatment of children who have sustained such injuries, and the first is to preserve length whenever possible. It is especially important to maintain a cartilaginous surface at the end of the residual limb to avoid the problems of periosteal overgrowth. When the femoral condyles or the distal tibial articular surfaces are preserved, the child is usually able to bear full weight, even on hard surfaces. At the ankle, the medial and lateral malleoli are not usually prominent and should only be removed in patients who are approaching skeletal maturity at the time of amputation.[8,37] Epiphyses should be preserved so that the limb

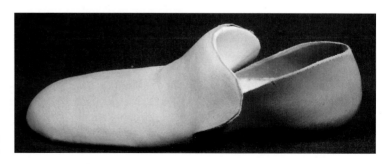

FIGURE 29-36. A slipper-type prosthesis aids in shoe wear for the patient with a partial absence of the foot.

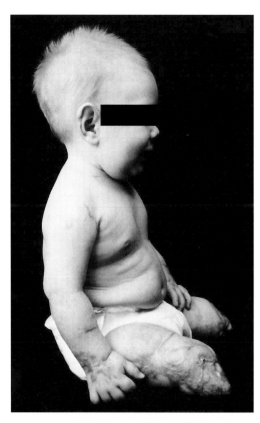

FIGURE 29-38. A child who has had bilateral below-knee amputations after purpura fulminans. Despite the severe skin loss, prosthetic wear has been satisfactory.

can continue to grow. It is especially important to remember that the distal femoral epiphysis is responsible for 80% of the growth of the femur, and early loss of that growth center ultimately leaves the femur very short.

Complications

Amputations through long bones, although often necessary, do not fare well and tend to have overgrowth of bony spicules at the ends of the bone. This is the result of periosteal bone formation, not epiphyseal growth, and frequently requires a surgical revision to remove the bone (Fig. 29-39). When the condition is untreated, a painful bursa forms, and the bone eventually grows through the skin. The humerus, fibula, tibia, and femur are the most common sites of overgrowth, in that order.[4,104] Efforts to avoid overgrowth have been tried, such as placing silicone sleeves over the end of the bone, but these have usually failed.[82,106] Marquardt described a procedure in which the transected bone end is capped with autogenous cartilage-bone graft to prevent overgrowth.[80] Despite these efforts, repeated revisions as the child grows are often necessary.

Phantom pain is unusual in younger children who have an amputation, and it does not occur with con-

genital absences. Older children may have phantom sensations, but these are rarely disabling. Painful phantom sensations may be managed by various techniques, including tactile stimulation, physical therapy, and medical management with tricyclic antidepressants such as amitriptyline. The symptoms of phantom pain usually wane over time. Neuromas may form, and to prevent this, nerves should be tensioned, cut sharply, and allowed to retract away from the end of the limb at the time of amputation. Persistent neuromas may require excision and replacement of the severed nerve into healthy tissue.

After burns or purpura fulminans, residual limbs are often covered with split-thickness skin grafts. These are quite resilient to weight bearing in a prosthesis despite their appearance (see Fig. 29-38).[5] Occasionally, they must be replaced with a free tissue transfer. Although providing excellent coverage, free tissue transfers take some time to develop protective sensation and may break down if weight bearing is begun while they are insensate.

Immediate prosthetic fitting is hazardous in younger children and may result in wound dehiscence if the child assumes early full weight bearing. Postoperative casts often fall off as the residual limb rapidly

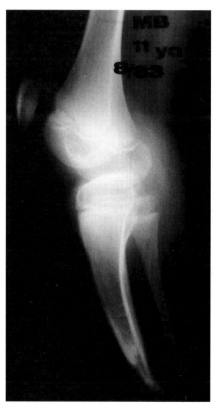

FIGURE 29-39. A radiograph shows periosteal bone overgrowth at the distal tibia and fibula. Amputations through the long bones frequently require revision for distal overgrowth, sometimes as often as every 2 or 3 years.

shrinks, and we prefer soft elastic bandages for shaping the residual limb.

Above-Knee Amputation

Some aspects of above-knee amputation in children differ from adult management. A longer femur is better, provided there is adequate soft tissue coverage distally. In the stance phase of gait, the abductor muscles must support the rest of the body, and the base of support for the abductors is the femur and its contact with the prosthesis. The patient with a short femoral segment and a fleshy thigh is obliged to walk with an abductor lurch, because there is no way for the femur to counter the abduction force of the abductor muscles. However, a long femoral segment provides a broad surface of contact with the prosthesis, resulting in a stable base for abductor function. The patient with a long femur should have little or no abductor limp.

In performing a transfemoral amputation, the femur should be shortened enough to allow closure of a muscle flap over the end. It may be helpful to attach the muscles to the bone. Even extremely short femoral segments should be preserved, because it may be feasible to lengthen them in the future. Periosteal bony overgrowth is common after above-knee amputation,

especially in younger children, and several revisions may be necessary as the child grows.

Knee Disarticulation

A knee disarticulation is a very functional amputation level in children (Fig. 29-40).[75] Full weight bearing at the knee is usual in a prosthesis or when knee walking in the child with bilateral disarticulations. At the time of amputation, the hamstrings may be sutured to the stump of the cruciate ligaments to provide better hip extension power.[93] The femur grows at an almost normal rate and becomes almost as long as the contralateral femur, which presents a minor prosthetic problem. When the knee mechanism is added below the residual limb, the tibial segment of the prosthesis is shorter than the contralateral tibia. This disproportion may be prevented by performing a distal femoral epiphysiodesis several years before skeletal maturity to shorten the residual limb 4 or 5 cm to allow room for a prosthetic knee.

Below-Knee Amputation

At the time of amputation, any viable portion of the proximal tibia should be retained if the knee joint is intact and soft tissue coverage can be obtained. Split-thickness skin over the proximal tibia may perform

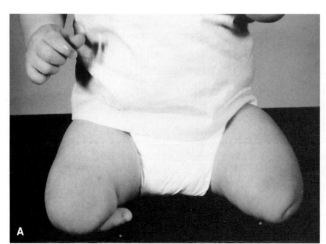
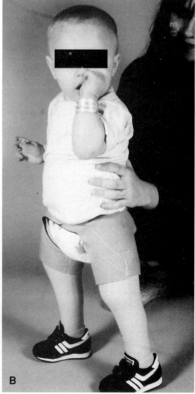

FIGURE 29-40.   (A) A child with bilateral through-knee congenital absences. He will be able to ambulate without prostheses, fully bearing weight on his distal femurs. (B) Bilateral knee disarticulation prostheses. He is 12 months of age, and these first prostheses do not have knee joints. The prostheses are suspended with a neoprene total elastic suspension belt.

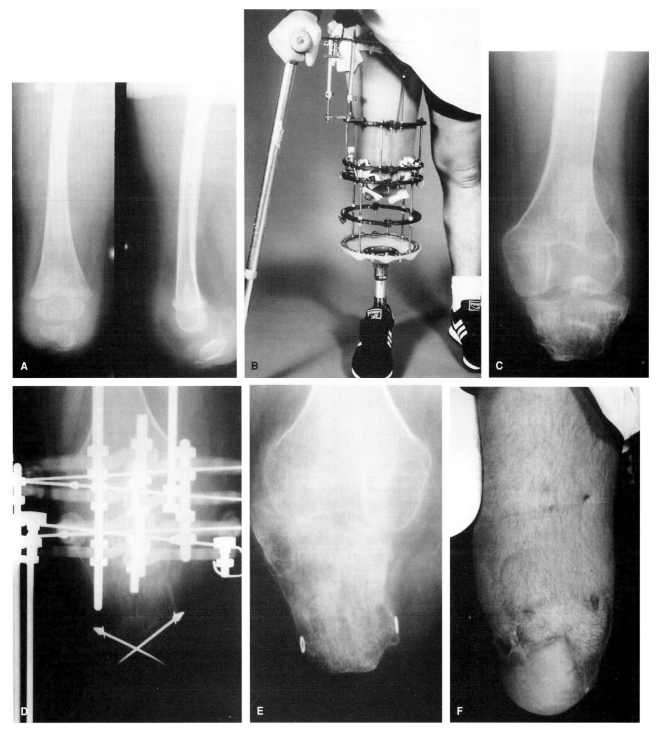

FIGURE 29-41.   (**A**) Radiographs of a child with an amputation at the level of the upper tibial physis. (**B**) The patient is placed in an Ilizarov apparatus to lengthen the residual limb. (**C**) Radiographs after the first of two lengthenings with the Ilizarov device. (**D**) Radiographs during the second stage of lengthening. (**E**) Radiographs after the final lengthening. (**F**) Appearance of the residual limb after lengthening. A free flap was applied before the second lengthening procedure. (Courtesy of John Birch, M.D., Dallas.)

well and can be replaced later with free tissue if necessary.[70] Newer materials and methods for managing sheer forces and pressure within the socket also reduce the problems of skin breakdown.

Very short below-knee stumps have been length-ened with Ilizarov and other techniques.[118] Although these procedures may be arduous, the functional gain accomplished when the patient advances from a knee disarticulation level to a below-knee level is worth the effort (Fig. 29-41). The advantages of the below-knee amputation include control of the knee, propriocep-tion of knee position, reduced energy expenditure with gait, and simpler prosthetic construction. A residual limb below the knee of at least 6 cm in a mature individual is necessary for adequate prosthetic fitting.

As children with below-knee amputations get older, several unique problems may develop. The knee may gradually develop a valgus deformity, which can usually be managed with prosthetic modifications. Some patients develop recurrent patellar dislocation that may in part be related to the valgus deformity. They also develop patella alta, which contributes to patellar instability.[86] Occasionally, the prosthesis be-comes twisted during sports activities, and the medial prosthetic brim may force the patella to dislocate. Bony overgrowth of the distal tibia and fibula is a common problem, often requiring revision.[3] To treat recurrent fibular overgrowth, a synostosis can be cre-ated surgically between the distal fibula and the tibia.

Upper Extremity Amputations

The same principles described for lower extremity amputations apply to upper extremity ablations. Transhumeral amputations are especially prone to periosteal overgrowth and frequently require revi-sions. Length should be preserved whenever possible. Small residual carpals and metacarpals have been suc-cessfully lengthened, providing the ability to pinch that had been lost. Because weight bearing is not usually required of the upper extremity, split-thickness skin grafts provide excellent coverage.

MULTIPLE CONGENITAL AMPUTATIONS

Children with multiple congenital limb deficiencies make remarkable functional adaptations by using whatever limb components they have to substitute for those that are missing (Figs. 29-42 through 29-44). Cer-tain functional patterns are common to all children with the same deficit. Children with bilateral upper extremity absences do not use prostheses for their functional activities. They can learn prosthetic wear and may use prostheses at times, but they inevitably perform almost all functional activities better with the sensory surfaces available to them: their feet. Children with bilateral wrist disarticulations have prehensile elbows and often movable carpals, which have pre-

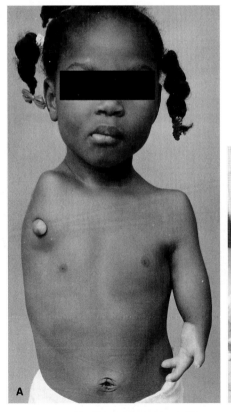

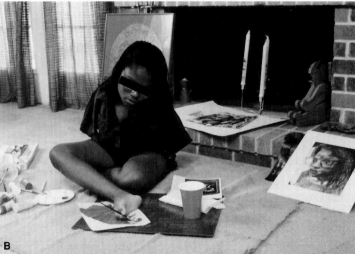

FIGURE 29-42. (A) A child born with absence of the right arm and a short left arm with a stiff elbow and three-rayed hand. (B) The same child in adolescence, using her feet for functional activities. She is an accomplished artist and independent individual. Children with bilateral upper extremity absence rarely use prostheses functionally.

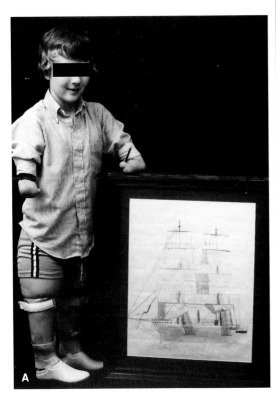

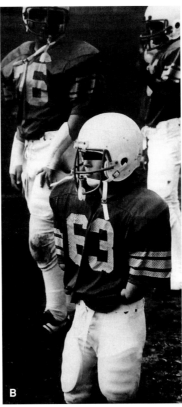

FIGURE 29-43. (**A**) A boy with quadrimelic congenital absences. As a young child, he ambulated with stubby prostheses. In adolescence, he mastered prostheses with articulated knees. (**B**) The same boy playing junior high school football.

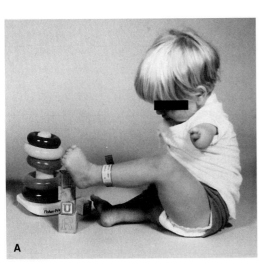

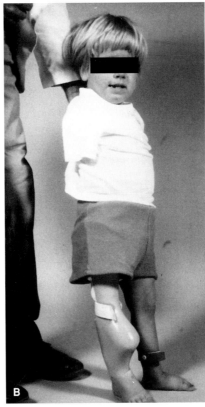

FIGURE 29-44. (**A**) A boy with bilateral upper extremity absences and a right proximal focal femoral deformity. He uses his feet for all manual activities. (**B**) This extension prosthesis is designed for ease of entry and exit, so the child can quickly remove it to use his feet as hands.

hensile function. Individuals with bilateral below-elbow levels function well using the elbows for prehension and by using both arms for holding larger objects. Children with bilateral above-elbow absences use the arms together in the midline if the limbs are long enough and, with shorter limbs, use the arm against the cheek. Children with very short humeri use their feet for most manual activities and are able to perform any task they can reach. They usually can reach just above their heads. Older individuals can drive an unaltered car with automatic shift. Toileting is a challenge, but bathroom adaptations solve most of the problems.

Bilateral lower extremity amputees have unique problems at the knee disarticulation level and above. A bilateral knee disarticulation requires a forceful knee extension at heel strike to maintain knee stability. Going up hill is difficult, and uneven ground is challenging. Bilateral above-knee amputations increase the need for the same compensations, and the short bilateral above-knee levels may need external support, such as canes or crutches for ambulation. As they age, the bilateral higher-level patients may choose wheelchair ambulation, especially for sports. When bilateral lower extremity absences are combined with bilateral upper extremity deficits, the problems are compounded (see Figs. 29-43 and 29-44). With above-knee levels, the absence of arms makes rising from a chair difficult and the use of crutches impossible. Prosthetic sockets attached to crutches or a walker may be used by the quadrimelic person with below-elbow amputations. The shorter the upper extremities, the more difficult is ambulation. For these persons, very short lower extremity prostheses (i.e., stubbies) may be the only prostheses they can ambulate with (see Fig. 29-43).[71]

PROSTHETICS

Parents usually are anxious to know when their child will be able to receive a first prosthesis. For children with congenital deficiencies requiring prosthetic fitting, the decision is usually based on the child's developmental readiness for the prosthesis. Usually, children with lower limb deficiencies are ready to be fit with a prosthesis when they first begin attempting to stand (9–16 months).[14,69] Children with upper limb deficiencies are generally considered ready for fitting with a passive prosthesis when they begin gaining independent sitting balance.[91] In either case, the clinic team's focus on matching the child's developmental readiness can extend to surgical intervention, training, and prosthetic design. For example, a toddler's first above-knee prosthesis may be nonarticulated or include a lockable knee. With training, by 3 or 4 years

of age, the child may be able to adapt to a prosthesis with an articulated knee.

During the child's growing years, the prosthesis may require replacement every 12 to 24 months. A follow-up examination for growth adjustments to the prosthesis is usually scheduled every 3 to 6 months.

Parents also need information about the fabrication of the prosthesis. Although the sequence can be compressed into a shorter period if necessary, most lower limb prostheses require three or four appointments separated by a week or two. The process begins when the prosthetist evaluates and measures the patient and makes a cast of the residual limb. This negative cast is then filled with plaster, and the prosthetist sculpts or "modifies" the model so the pressures are applied where tolerated and relieved where necessary. A clear plastic "test" socket is then fabricated over the model and removed for initial evaluation of socket fit.

In many orthopaedic practices, prosthetists design sockets by using computer-aided design and manufacture (CAD-CAM). Computerization is a means of enhancing, not substituting for, the abilities and skills of the prosthetist. After the mold of the patient's limb has been digitized, this relatively new technology enables the prosthetist to modify a three-dimensional computer graphic of the residual limb. Any changes made to the model can then be recorded and reproduced precisely. A computer-driven milling machine carves the model, after which the prosthetist fabricates a test socket.[84]

During the second appointment, the prosthetist evaluates the prototype socket to ensure the socket fits well and can be adjusted as the child grows. Because the success or failure of the prosthesis depends largely on a comfortable, total-contact fit between the socket and the residual limb, the prosthetist may make several test sockets and design changes before moving on to the next stage.

After an appropriate socket and suspension system have been designed, the third appointment usually involves dynamic alignment of the prosthesis. In most cases, the prosthetist temporarily attaches the socket to an adjustable leg or uses components that allow alignment changes as the patient ambulates with the prosthesis. Pediatric patients or recent amputees often begin gait training at this time, and the prosthetist may make alignment changes over a period of several days as the child gains independence with the temporary prosthesis. For older, more experienced patients, dynamic alignment may only require a single office visit of several hours.

After an appropriate alignment and overall prosthetic design have been determined, final fabrication may require from several hours to several days before the finished prosthesis can be delivered. Additional physical therapy may be required after delivery of the prosthesis. Upper limb prostheses follow a similar sequence of casting, test socket fitting, prototype fitting, and delivery.

Lower Extremity Prosthetics

Most children who use lower extremity prostheses are active and healthy, and they consequently place unique demands on their prostheses (Fig. 29-45). They can be expected to wear out or destroy their prostheses through play and sports activities. Soft, cosmetic covers over modular, endoskeletal components may wear out in weeks in young children and are only appropriate when weight-saving or adjustable components are more important than durability or for older, less active adolescents. Children often outgrow their socket in a year and may require lengthening every 3 to 6 months. As they grow, they lose the intimate fit of the socket, and frequent prosthetic adaptations are necessary to keep them functioning. The prosthetist must be able to make a prosthesis that is lightweight but strong. It needs to be durable enough to take much abuse and remain reasonably cosmetic. It must fit intimately and yet be easy to modify to accommodate

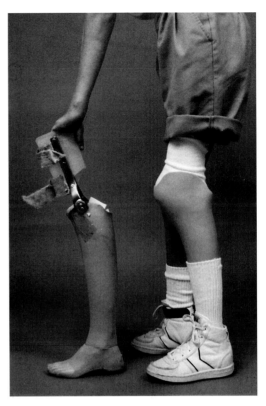

FIGURE 29-46. A child holding his old hinged prosthesis and wearing his new patellar tendon–bearing supracondylar type of below knee prosthesis. The high walls of the prosthesis are necessary because the boy has an unstable knee.

growth. These are difficult demands that often challenge knowledgeable and experienced professionals.

The term "nonstandard prosthesis" is usually applied to a device used with an extremity anomaly that has not undergone an amputation (Fig. 29-46; see Fig. 29-18). These are often hybrids between an orthosis and a prosthesis, and they require considerable expertise to fabricate. McCollough proposed four reasons for their use: when surgical conversion of the anomaly has been refused, when surgical conversion is delayed, during early periods of observation of longitudinal deficiencies, and when lower extremity anomalies that would usually be treated with amputation are combined with upper limb absences that require the use of the feet for hand function.[81] So many variables of anatomy must be managed by the children's prosthetist that most of the prostheses are "nonstandard."

Cummings and Kapp reviewed common methods to deal with changing size and length of residual limbs due to growth.[25] Easily altered socket liners allow modifications for changes in shape and size of the residual limb. An alternative method is to fit a prosthesis over extra socks, which can be reduced as growth occurs. Another technique is the use of "triple-wall" sockets, which enable the prosthetist to remove a thin inner socket when necessary to accommodate growth.[40] The

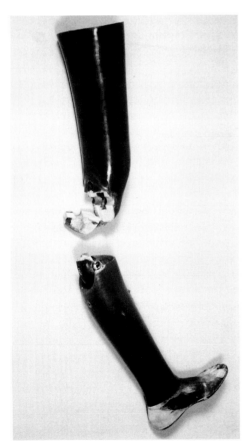

FIGURE 29-45. An above-knee prosthesis that suffered a major injury on the football field. This may be hard on the prosthesis, but the enormous benefits of participation outweigh any disadvantages.

best technique to accommodate growth in length of transtibial amputations is the use of distal end pads that can be replaced with smaller "pour pads" as the limb grows. If distal bone overgrowth occurs, this technique also enables the prosthetist to repour pads to relieve pressure. Flexible sockets with open frame designs are also useful, especially for oncology patients whose limbs change size rapidly.[25] These sockets are easier to modify as the residual limb changes than standard sockets (see Fig. 29-37).

Some children have never been seen without their prostheses, and they may need spares to wear in case extensive repairs to their primary prostheses are necessary. Children also need to play, swim, ride bicycles, play football, and ride horses, and a refurbished old prosthesis is useful.

Above-Knee Prosthesis

Among the most common topics of discussion in a prosthetic clinic where children with transfemoral amputations are being treated are socket design, suspension, prosthetic knees, and gait deviations. The most frequently used sockets are the quadrilateral socket and the ischial containment socket. A key feature of the quadrilateral design is a vertical weight-bearing "shelf" beneath the ischial tuberosity and gluteal musculature. To accomplish this, the prosthetist reduces and socket dimension from front to back to position the ischium on the shelf.[94] In contrast, the ischial containment socket includes the ischium within the socket. This is achieved, in part, through a reduced medial to lateral socket dimension.[77,99]

Because ischial containment is a relatively recent evolution, both designs are generating much debate and investigation (Fig. 29-47).[92] A panel of experts concluded that, although there were no clear contraindications for either design, some generalities may aid the clinic team in recommending one over the other. For example, the panel felt it may be unwise to convert a satisfied wearer of a quadrilateral socket to any new design. Quadrilateral sockets are more successful on longer residual limbs with good muscle tone, and shorter, fleshier residual limbs do better in ischial containment sockets. The panel also thought that, more often than not, active individuals prefer ischial containment over quadrilateral sockets.[101]

For pediatric patients, advantages and disadvantages of the two designs are even less defined. Because ischial containment theory dictates that the socket "locks" the tuberosity within the socket brim through a carefully controlled dimension between the ischium and the lateral femur, the design may require a less aggressive approach in the pediatric population. For example, a gradually sloping brim of flexible plastic may enable some enclosure of the ischium without

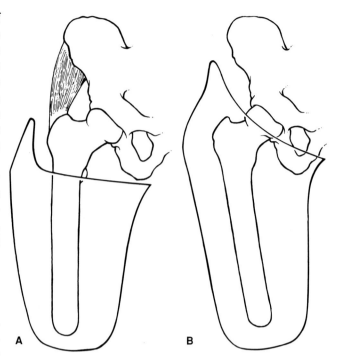

FIGURE 29-47. **(A)** A quadrilateral socket positions the ischium on a shelf using a tight anteroposterior dimension. **(B)** An ischial containment socket includes the ischium within the socket through a narrow mediolateral dimension.

generating uncomfortable pressure as the child grows (see Fig. 29-37).

Suspension of a transfemoral prosthesis for a child is complicated by growth and development. Suction suspension, the method of choice for most adults with stable limb volume, is generally not recommended for young children. The suction socket requires a distal one-way valve for air release, and the prosthesis is suspended by a combination of negative air pressure, surface tension between the skin and socket, and muscular contraction against the socket walls (see Fig. 29-37). Because the socket must be donned precisely, the child should possess the cognitive ability and maturity necessary to take a little extra time getting into the prosthesis. If there is lack of distal contact in a suction socket, the high negative pressures created in the air space may result in local circulatory congestion and edema.[16] To avoid this, frequent socket modifications or replacements may be necessary as the limb grows in length and circumference. Although it is technically possible to fit young children with suction suspension, it may be more trouble than it is worth until the child is at least 6 or 7 years of age.[109] Thereafter, suction should still be prescribed judiciously, but by adolescence, most children with transfemoral amputations should do well with suction sockets. If suction suspension is prescribed for a growing child, the design should also include a flexible socket and frame or some other appropriate means of accommodating growth changes (see Fig. 29-37). Contraindications to suction include deep fissured scars, volumetric fluctuation (e.g., patients undergoing chemotherapy or dialysis), extremely short residual limbs, or upper limb involvement that would make getting into the prosthesis more difficult. Some modern adaptations of suction suspension such as flexible sockets and silicon suction allow easier growth adjustments and may be useful in the future for younger children.[102]

The most common method of suspending a transfemoral prosthesis for young children is a Silesian belt. The belt attaches to the socket laterally near the trochanter, passes around the child's back and opposite iliac crest, and then fastens with Velcro or a buckle at a single or double attachment point on the proximal anterior socket. A popular variation of this is the total elastic suspension belt (TES). Made of elastic neoprene lined with nylon and using a Velcro closure, it is quite comfortable, growth adjustable, and prefabricated in children's sizes (see Fig. 29-40*B*).[102] Some children find these belts constricting and hot to wear. The also need to be removed for regular cleaning. Silesian belts and their variations may be used as auxiliary suspension for suction sockets or as the sole form of suspension. As children grow, this form of suspension allows them to adjust the fit of their prosthesis for as much as a year by reducing the "ply" or thickness of their prosthetic sock. The belt allows simple donning and doffing of the prosthesis and is growth adjustable.

In cases of an extremely short residual limb, weak hip abductors, obesity, or an unstable or painful hip, suspension of the prosthesis by a hip joint with a pelvic band and belt may be indicated. For children, this should be considered a last resort for problems such as rotational control of the prosthesis or for mediolateral stability of the pelvis.

Until the mid-1980s, while adults and adolescents had many choices, relatively few prosthetic knees were available for young children. However, more knee components engineered for children have been made available. Michael has simplified the large array of knee components by classifying them according to their function. Within each class, the knees may differ greatly by appearance, material, size, weight, or structural design, but their functional characteristics are similar.[84]

MANUAL-LOCKING KNEES. Although some of the other knee classes have locking options, the traditional manual locking knee is a single-axis knee with a lock. The young child generally walks with the knee locked, and the parents, therapist, or child can unlock it for sitting by pushing a button or pulling a cable-activated lever. A manual lock or a nonarticulated knee is appropriate for children just learning to walk. By 3

or 4 years of age, most unilateral amputees can make the transition to an articulated knee. Children with bilateral amputations may keep one or both knees locked until age 6 or later before using unlocked knees.

CONSTANT-FRICTION KNEES. These have a single axis of rotation and a mechanism for creating constant friction to control the knee during swing phase. This constant-friction feature provides a smooth, controlled gait at only one speed, and adolescents who frequently vary their cadence may prefer a hydraulic knee. Stability is not inherent and must be provided by muscular control or by the alignment of the knee axis. Because of a lack of alternatives, these knees were frequently prescribed for children up to 5 or 6 years of age who had less need for changing cadence. There are no appropriate fluid-controlled knees available for children younger than 9 or 10 years of age.

STANCE-CONTROL OR WEIGHT-ACTIVATED FRICTION KNEES. These are single-axis constant-friction knees with an adjustable braking mechanism activated by the patient's weight during the first 20 degrees of knee flexion. This braking mechanism is designed to provide an "antistumble" feature in addition to the stability provided by muscle action and alignment. Recent amputees or those with short residual limbs may benefit from this feature, particularly during early gait training. There are no true pediatric knees in this class, and their use is generally limited to adolescents with recent amputations.

POLYCENTRIC OR FOUR-BAR KNEES. Instead of a single axis of rotation, prosthetic knees in this class simulate the rocking and gliding motion of the anatomic knee by curved bearing surfaces or by means of linkages. The most common polycentric knee is the four-bar linkage knee. The moving center of rotation in a four-bar knee gives the wearer greater control against buckling and is therefore more stable. Several variations that allow the prosthetist to more closely match knee centers are designed specifically for knee disarticulations or long amputations. Unfortunately, only a few polycentric knees are available for children younger than 10 years of age. Four-bar knees are appropriate for children and adolescents with knee disarticulations, transfemoral amputations, or for those who would benefit from some extra knee stability.

FLUID-CONTROLLED KNEES. These are generally single-axis knees with hydraulic or pneumatic control of the swing phase. The hydraulic fluid and, to a lesser degree, the air respond to changes in cadence and therefore provide a smooth gait pattern for velocities from slow walking to running. Some units also provide stance-phase control and optional locks for certain activities. Hydraulic knees add weight and maintenance to the prosthesis, and they are generally indicated for healthy, active adolescents. They are ideally suited to the active lifestyle of children, but until recently, none have been available for children younger than 8 or 10 years of age. One exception that may be used for some children as young as 7 or 8 years of age and for adolescents is the Total Knee. This polycentric knee combines a unique hydraulic swing-phase control with a stance-phase braking mechanism.[112]

Feet Prostheses

Prosthetic feet also come in a wide variety. The SACH foot (solid ankle cushion heel) is used by younger children with almost all prostheses. In older children and adolescents, dynamic response feet, which have a flexible keel, improve running skills and athletic performance. Multiple-axis ankles are available but are not often used in children because of complexity and lack of durability.

Knee Disarticulation

Knee disarticulation offers many functional advantages and a few cosmetic disadvantages compared with more proximal transfemoral levels (see Figs. 29-40 and 29-43). It is the preferred transfemoral level for children because it preserves both femoral epiphyses, eliminates osseous overgrowth, and enables end weight bearing. Many prosthetic socket variations and knee mechanisms have been designed to take advantage of the supracondylar suspension capacity, long lever arm, and end weight-bearing tolerance of the level.[56]

Socket design for the knee disarticulation is often dictated by the degree to which distal weight bearing is tolerated and the size of the femoral condyles relative to the thigh. To facilitate comfortable end weight bearing, a thin distal pad is usually built into the socket. Whenever possible, the flaring of the femoral condyles should be used to suspend the prosthesis. This may be accomplished much in the manner of Syme prosthesis, through expandable inner socket liners, or pads. Particularly among pediatric amputees who have the knee disarticulation for a congenital deficiency, the distal femur may be underdeveloped and unable to provide adequate suspension of the prosthesis. In such cases, conventional suspension methods such as suction or a Silesian or TES belt may be indicated.

Virtually any knee mechanism could conceivably be used with a knee disarticulation prosthesis. This is particularly true among children in whom growth disturbances or surgical epiphysiodesis may cause femoral length to be significantly shorter and the condyles less bulky than the contralateral sound side. In such cases, the patient often benefits from all of the advantages of knee disarticulation, but none of the traditional cosmetic disadvantages associated with bulkiness and nonmatching knee centers. In this group, almost any knee unit may be appropriate, depending on the individual goals and needs of the patient.

In most cases, however, knee disarticulation results in femoral length virtually equal to the contralateral side. Because conventional knees add 5 cm (2 in) or more of additional length to the prosthetic thigh, such mechanisms are not appropriate in most cases for knee disarticulations, and a polycentric knee should be used. Because of the proximal hinges and attachment hardware, even a polycentric knee linkage lengthens the thigh by 2 to 3 cm, but this discrepancy appears to be acceptable to most patients.[88] If epiphysiodesis is planned to provide room for a prosthetic knee, 3 cm should be sufficient to accommodate a polycentric knee, and 6 cm permits the use of virtually any knee.

Hip Disarticulation

The socket for a hip disarticulation encapsulates the remaining pelvis on the amputated side and extends around the contralateral pelvis for suspension. Modern, flexible materials and socket designs make for a more comfortable prosthesis (Fig. 29-48). An anteriorly located hip joint allows flexion and extension to a neutral position. The hip must be anterior and the knee posterior to the midline of the body for the joints to be stable in a standing position. Endoskeletal components are used to reduce the weight of the prosthesis.

The young child with a hip disarticulation usually starts with a prosthesis with an articulated hip to facilitate walking and sitting, but without a knee joint. The prosthesis should be prescribed when the child is actively pulling to stand and seems developmentally ready to begin walking. By 4 or 5 years of age, the child can usually learn to walk with a prosthetic knee joint.[25]

Proximal Focal Femoral Deficiency

There are four methods of managing PFFD that require prosthetic fittings. In the usual case, the child's weak, unstable hip and extreme proximal knee and foot provide the prosthetist with cosmetic and functional challenges. Nevertheless, these children can be fitted with prostheses to compensate for their major leg length discrepancies, and when not wearing the

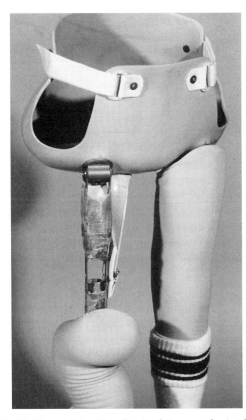

FIGURE 29-48.   A bilateral hip disarticulation prosthesis. The side openings in the socket accommodate phocomelic feet. The hinge joint and endoskeletal components are concealed beneath a cosmetic cover.

prostheses, most are able to tolerate full weight bearing on the affected side. To counteract the piston action of the unstable hip, the prosthetic socket generally provides ischial or gluteal weight bearing. The patient's knee is usually included in the socket, and the foot is positioned in equinus, primarily for cosmetic reasons. The prosthesis may be suspended by a heel strap or waist belt. As the child approaches adolescence, the leg length discrepancy may be large enough to allow the prosthetist to include a prosthetic knee joint below the child's foot. For less severe discrepancies, the prosthesis may simply provide an extension with a prosthetic foot below the patient's plantar-flexed foot (see Fig. 29-17). As with all prostheses for children, components should be as light as possible to maximize function. As a general rule, children with bilateral PFFD should not have amputations, but they may benefit from a pair of extension prostheses for certain activities at school or work.[66]

The second management option is a Syme amputation alone, followed by conventional fitting of a Syme prosthesis. In most cases, the child is able to bear weight distally in the prosthesis, and the device can be self-suspended over the prominent malleoli. The gait is quite good, although the abnormal hip and shorter, weaker hip abductors may cause a Trendelenburg lurch. One notable disadvantage of this approach is that the affected femur is noticeably shorter than the sound side, and the knee joint is more proximal. The relatively long prosthesis and high knee joint are most noticeable when the child sits. Despite this cosmetic drawback, there are major functional benefits from keeping the functional knee.

Syme amputation with knee fusion, the third management option, usually applies only when the short femur is less than 50% of the length of the sound side. Knee fusion is performed to create a single, straight lever arm for prosthetic fitting in an "above-knee" prosthesis and generally eliminates the child's hip flexion contracture (see Fig. 29-11).[60,61] Syme amputation with knee fusion converts the limb to a functional above-knee amputation, usually with the added benefit of distal loading tolerance. Prosthetic fitting can begin when the incisions are well healed and the child is developmentally ready. The prosthetic socket generally provides ischial or gluteal weight bearing to diminish any pistoning of the unstable hip. The prosthesis is usually suspended by a waist belt, but in some cases, the malleoli and heel pad may be sufficiently bulbous to "self-suspend" the prosthesis. Self-suspension may also be accomplished by an expandable inner "bladder" that grips above the malleoli but allows the flared distal limb to pass in or out of the prosthesis.[107] Another method uses a compressible suspension pad placed directly over the residual limb distally. When the child is ready for a prosthetic knee joint, the inherent stability and cosmetic advantages of a polycentric four-bar knee are ideal for this level.

The fourth surgical option that requires a prosthesis is the Van Nes rotationplasty. In this procedure, the goal is to convert the extremity to a functional "below-knee amputation" in which the rotated foot acts as a knee joint (see Fig. 29-23).[61] For optimum prosthetic function, it is critical that the ankle joint of the involved extremity is normal and capable of at least a 60-degree arc of motion after the procedure.[109] The ankle should be at the same level as the opposite knee, and the ankle joint should be rotated by a full 180 degrees.[65]

The typical Van Nes prosthesis encloses the foot in a position of comfortable equinus within the socket and provides weight bearing through the plantar, now anterior, aspect of the foot and calcaneus (see Fig. 29-12).[15] Room for growth of the toes is provided distally, and a forgiving socket liner is used. To provide medio-lateral stability for the ankle, single-axis joints extend from the socket and up to a rigid, bivalved shell or corset around the thigh. If the hip is unstable, the thigh section should extend proximally to provide ischial-gluteal weight bearing. If the hip has been stabilized, ischial weight bearing may be unnecessary, and weight may be borne by the foot. Suspension is often through a heel strap or a waist belt. Components and alignment depend on the case. Gait usually is not normal, because the deficient hip joint and musculature produce a Trendelenburg lurch. Strength and range of motion of an appropriately rotated ankle determine the degree of functional "knee" control.

Fibular Deficiency

Prosthetic management is relatively simple, because the leg assumes a cylindrical shape with only slight enlargement distally. Despite the fact that the lateral malleolus is usually absent, children with an ankle disarticulation are able to fully bear weight on the heel pad. In the prosthesis, a protective but firm distal pad combined with a total-contact patellar tendon-bearing (PTB) socket design are used. If anterior bowing of the tibia exists, special padding or relief in the socket may be necessary (see Fig. 29-26). The length discrepancy associated with fibular hemimelia can actually be an asset after amputation, because the prosthetist has more space in the prosthesis distal to the residual limb in which to place a foot. Instead of being able to use only a few prosthetic feet designed specifically for the Syme amputee, the prosthetist may use any type of foot. Prosthetic suspension for a child who is just learning to walk usually requires a cuff above the femoral condyles, a waist belt, or neoprene sleeve. By their second or third prosthesis, many children may be able to hold the device on by actively contracting their heel pad against the contoured inner wall of the socket or may self-suspend through the use of pads or an expandable inner socket (see Figs. 29-24 through 29-26).[25]

To provide rotational control and some mediolateral stability, the proximal brim of the socket should extend high on either side of the knee. Genu valgum, commonly associated with fibular hemimelia, can be accommodated in the prosthesis by medial displacement of the prosthetic foot. If the valgus progresses to create a functional or cosmetic problem, medial growth-plate arrest (i.e., hemiepiphysiodesis), or a tibial osteotomy may be justified.[41]

Tibial Deficiency

Prosthetic requirements depend on surgical management. In the case of complete absence of the tibia, if the fibula has been centralized, the child is fitted with a below-knee prosthesis with knee joints and a thigh corset to provide mediolateral knee stability (see Fig. 29-46). An unstable knee, often lacking quadriceps function, combined with a tendency toward knee flexion contracture makes this a difficult level to man-

age prosthetically, and recurrent deformity often requires repeated surgical revisions.[70]

After a knee disarticulation has been performed, the child can be fitted when developmentally ready with an end-bearing above-knee prosthesis. The knee of the first prosthesis usually includes a manual lock or is nonarticulated. By 3 years of age, the child should be able to manage well with an articulated knee and should eventually be capable of a high activity level including running.[75]

If the proximal tibia is present and the fibula has been centralized along with an ankle disarticulation, the child may use a conventional Syme prosthesis. If the knee is stable and the hamstrings and the quadriceps are functioning well, joints and a thigh corset are not needed.

Below-Knee Prosthesis

Several socket designs are commonly used with below-knee prostheses (see Fig. 29-46). All use some degree of patellar tendon weight bearing with additional support through the medial flare of the tibia in the area of the pes anserinus and through total contact. The fibular head and anterior distal tibia are relieved. The socket may extend with pads over the femoral condyles for suspension, as does the patellar tendon-bearing supracondylar (PTS) design. The supracondylar design is also used when additional mediolateral stability of the knee is indicated, but in the presence of damaged or absent collateral ligaments, the greater stability provided by joints and a thigh corset may be required. Soft sockets and gel liners may solve problems caused by poor skin coverage.[78] Suspension straps are used by younger children to keep the prosthesis on while crawling but are later replaced by the PTS socket or by neoprene sleeves. Silicone has been used as a forgiving, shear-reducing socket interface and a means of suspension. Silicone suspension methods include the 3S design (silicone suction socket) and ICEROSS (Icelandic roll-on silicone socket).

The most common silicone below-knee system consists of a pliable silicone sleeve with a ribbed stainless steel pin protruding distally from the sleeve. To apply the prosthesis, the patient rolls the sleeve directly over his or her residual limb. If necessary, a prosthetic sock with a small distal hole may be worn over the sleeve to accommodate changes in limb volume. When silicone suction is used with children, socks are recommended to enable growth adjustments. When the limb is slipped into the socket, the distal retaining pin slides into and locks firmly within a clutch lock located inside the prosthesis. A push-button release is used to remove the prosthesis. Suction, combined with the viscoelastic nature of the silicone, provides excellent suspension and minimizes shear and up and down pistoning of the prosthesis.

Such systems are not without a few disadvantages. The silicone is heavy, adds bulk, is expensive, and tears easily. Relative contraindications to silicone suction among children include frequent kneeling or crawling, fluctuating limb volume, bony overgrowth, neuromas, considerable adhesive scar tissue, long residual limbs such as with Syme amputation, and physical or mental inability to operate the lock mechanism.[31] Soft distal pads are used to allow longitudinal growth and possible terminal bone overgrowth. When the child begins to experience distal discomfort, a new pad of silicone with a foaming agent can be fabricated to relieve pressure.[25] The same feet are used as with above-knee prostheses.

Partial Foot Prostheses

In the early postoperative period after an acquired partial foot amputation, it may be necessary to use a modified ankle-foot orthosis to prevent an equinus contracture. A padded cosmetic toe filler is added to a polypropylene ankle-foot orthosis. This system provides maximum ankle stability, good rotational control, and an extended toe "lever arm." Less restrictive slipper-style flexible prostheses may be fit a year or so later if no predisposition to contracture is present (see Fig. 29-36).

Children with congenital partial foot absences usually need no surgical intervention, do not develop contractures, and have minimal if any functional limitations.[13] For this group, plastic, leather, or silicone slipper-style prostheses with padded toe fillers are used. These systems are less restrictive than the ankle-foot orthosis–type of prosthesis and provide excellent cosmesis. With congenital partial foot deficiencies rudimentary toes or "nubbins" are common and rarely problematic. Adequate padding in the prosthesis combined with frequent modifications for growth should prevent pressure problems over rudimentary toes.

Bilateral Lower Limb Prostheses

The child with bilateral lower limb deficiencies generally attempts to stand on the remaining limbs when developmentally ready. For levels below the knee, prosthetic fitting is the same as it is in unilateral cases, although at the outset, it may be advantageous to keep the first pair of prostheses an inch or two short to assist the child in balancing. The child with bilateral through-knee or higher amputations is managed much differently, with particular attention paid to a gradual progression in prosthetic height and complexity.

The child with bilateral transfemoral amputations

is first fitted with short "stubby" prostheses (see Fig. 29-43). These include feet or blocks positioned directly beneath the prosthetic sockets. This design gives the young child an extremely low center of gravity to ensure initial success during standing and enables the prosthetist to evaluate the prosthetic socket fit with the child in a secure, comfortable weight-bearing position.

As the child begins gait training, the stubbies may be gradually lengthened as needed.[50] In some cases, the child may progress quickly, allowing transition to taller prostheses with knees in a matter of weeks or months (see Fig. 29-42). When the limbs are very short or in the presence of upper limb involvement, ambulation with full-length legs and articulated knees may be difficult or impossible. Other devices or approaches that may enable children to use longer prostheses include manually locking knees, knees with stance-phase braking, polycentric knees, knee spring-extension assists; assistive devices such as a walker, crutches, and canes; and physical therapy.

Gait Evaluation

Gait deviations for lower limb prostheses, their causes, and possible solutions have been well described.[11,17,95,100] There are some specific gait problems in children that have unique causes and solutions, including "whips," lateral trunk bending, excessive adduction of the prosthesis, circumduction, and vaulting.

A whip is a swing-phase gait deviation seen with above-knee prostheses, and the cause is usually malorientation of the artificial knee axis relative to the line of forward progression. Usually, the prosthetic knee axis is rotated externally relative to the line of progression by 5 degrees. When the knee axis is not optimally aligned, swing-phase whips may be observed. These are best viewed from behind the patient at the very beginning of swing phase on the prosthetic side. If the prosthesis shank and foot whip laterally, the prosthetic knee is too internally rotated, and a medial whip is caused by excessive lateral rotation of the knee axis. To avoid confusion, it should be remembered that the direction of the malrotation of the prosthetic knee is always opposite to the direction of the whip.[26]

Whips may also be a result of poor socket fit. For example, a loose-fitting or poorly suspended socket may rotate on the limb during stance and swing phases, producing a similar malrotation of the prosthetic knee. An excessively tight socket may tend to rotate as muscles contract during ambulation. A whip may also develop as the residual limb grows too large for the socket. This may occur because the child the child applies the prosthesis in a different orientation than when the prosthesis was new. In such cases, the prosthetist may modify the socket or instruct the child to wear fewer prosthetic socks. Sometimes whips cannot be corrected through prosthetic adjustment or gait training. Examples include whips as a result of hip joint pathology, congenital deficiencies, or muscular abnormalities.

Lateral bending of the trunk to the prosthetic side during stance phase (Trendelenburg lurch) may occur with above-knee or below-knee prostheses. This usually occurs when the prosthesis is too short because of the child's growth and is easily corrected by lengthening the prosthesis. Lateral trunk bending is seen in the above-knee amputee when the socket does not provide an adequate surface for the femur to stabilize against. It also occurs when there is excessive pressure on the distal end of the femur causing the child to widen the base of support and lean over the prosthesis. The pressure on the femur is often noticed distally and laterally as the child begins to outgrow the socket and no longer completely enters the prosthesis. Trunk bending is also caused by excess tissue bulging uncomfortably over the proximal medial brim of the socket. Leaning the trunk laterally tends to allow the child to balance over the prosthesis. By shifting weight over the prosthesis, the hip abductors are required to do much less work, and any lateral forces against the residual femur are minimized. In addition to socket fit and alignment, other factors may be involved. For example, when an abduction contracture of the hip must be accommodated in the alignment of the prosthesis, the patient has a lateral trunk lean during midstance.

Even when alignment and socket fit are optimal, patients with weak hip abductors or a very short residual limb (consequently, a very short lever arm for lateral stabilization) may need to lean laterally over the prosthesis. Children with PFFD often exhibit this deviation with their above-knee prostheses because the hip is unstable and the hip abductors usually are quite weak. A short residual limb also provides less surface area over which pressure may be spread. When patients present with short residual limbs and weak abductor strength, the prosthetist must provide auxiliary support and additional stability by adding a pelvic band and hip joint. Patients with long residual limbs, however, tend to have a mechanical advantage over those with sorter limbs, because less muscle is sacrificed, and the longer femoral lever arm provides greater surface area for dispersion of forces.

Another prosthetic gait abnormality seen in young children is the adducted or laterally leaning prosthesis. This may be incorrectly assumed to be caused by poor alignment, although it is actually caused by developmental changes.[50] Fitting goals for a child just pulling to stand may be only the facilitation of standing and cruising, and prosthetic alignment in the tradi-tional sense may not occur until the child is ready for his next prosthesis. If the child initially received a prosthesis between 12 and 24 months of age, he or she probably began walking as most children do, using a wide-based gait with hips and knees flexed. As children mature, they tend to walk with a narrower base that causes the prosthesis to appear incorrectly aligned. For this reason and because young children grow rapidly, the first prosthesis should not be expected to last as long as subsequent ones.

Other deviations such as vaulting on the sound side or circumduction of the prosthesis may be the result of habits developed when the child first began walking. Particularly among children wearing above-knee prostheses, such deviations may be related to compensations they develop as they learn to use a prosthetic knee joint or new prosthesis. Children who wear prostheses are masterful at quickly adapting their gait patterns and are not generally concerned about the cosmetic appearance of their gait. At times, they may benefit from physical therapy to correct undesirable gait patterns.

Upper Extremity Prosthetics

The management of a child with congenital upper limb deficiency is very different from managing an adult or an adolescent who has an acquired amputation. In a challenging paradox, the more the child is missing, the less likely is that child to use a prosthetic device. For example, children with bilateral upper amelia use their feet for all functional activities (see Figs. 29-42 and 29-44). They can learn to operate upper extremity prostheses and will do so if coerced, but the child will always revert to foot use when allowed to do so. The prosthetic team should first nurture the relation with the family so they understand and accept this fact of their child's future. Although prostheses of the future may have full sensory feedback and rapid voluntary control, currently available devices are insensate and inefficient to operate. Adult amelics have expressed their anger at being forced as children to comply with devices that hampered rather than enhanced their function.

The child born with an absent portion of an upper extremity functions by adapting the structures they are born with, no matter how unusual or malformed, to their needs. These adaptations are always efficient and energy conserving. Unless the prosthetic team understands this reality, the prosthetic prescription will be inappropriate. In the best of circumstances, the child may perceive a prosthesis for the upper extremity as more of an imposition from the parents and the doctors than it is functional necessity. When appropriately used, the upper extremity prosthesis is a helpful tool and an imperfect, but sometimes useful

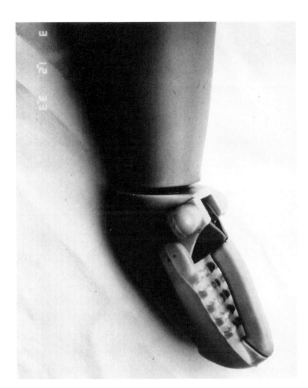

FIGURE 29-49. The CAPP terminal device was designed to enable children to view and grasp objects easily. The soft, serrated cover makes it safe for young children and prevents objects from slipping out of its grasp. Some parents object to its claw-like appearance, but it is a low-cost, functional alternative for younger children.

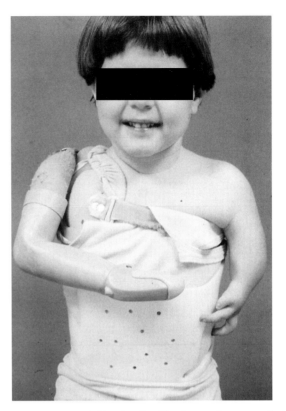

FIGURE 29-50. A child with a shoulder disarticulation prosthesis suspended from a scoliosis orthosis. The shoulder and elbow are passive, and the CAPP terminal device is activated. The prosthesis was never functionally useful for this patient, who used her feet for manual activities.

cosmetic substitute. This is the antithesis of a lower extremity prosthesis, which a child will quickly incorporate into his or her body image and insist on wearing. The physician cannot overestimate the cosmetic significance of a missing or abnormal hand, and the desire to appear ''normal'' is often the underlying motivation for seeking a prosthesis. There are great variations in the reported use rates of upper extremity prostheses, and true functional evaluations in children are not available. Rates of rejection of myoelectric prostheses have been reported from none to 50%.[27,52,89,103,115]

How then should the team manage a child with a missing upper extremity? First, it is important to plan intervention around normal developmental milestones. Most centers fit upper prosthesis at the time of independent sitting, which is also the time when two-handed activities develop. A passive prosthesis usually is tried at around 6 months of age. At some time between 1 and 2 years of age, a new prosthesis with an active terminal device is used. The choices include the CAPP terminal device, body-powered hooks and hands, and myoelectric hands (Figs. 29-49 through 29-53). Parents and their understanding of prosthetic options are key determinants of a child's experience with a prosthesis. Before a decision is made, they should see and understand the function of various devices, and ideally, they should be given the opportunity to talk with other parents of children with similar diagnoses.

Absence of the forearm below the elbow is a common congenital anomaly and an occasional traumatic level. These children learn to use the elbow for prehensile activities and have little functional need for a prosthesis. Many such children wear prostheses at times and use them for certain specific activities. Myoelectric hands are popular because of their appearance and the fact the prosthesis requires no harness above the elbow (see Fig. 29-51). The socket requires an intimate fit with the electrodes in contact with a muscle mass. The child uses a lubricant or a donning sock to enter the prosthesis. Grasping and hooking functions are easily mastered. A trend in fitting children from 1 to 3 years old has been to use a myoelectric prosthesis that requires only one electrode located over one muscle site. When the child contracts the muscle, preferably an extensor group in the forearm, the hand opens. As long as the child continues contracting the muscle, the hand stays open, but the hand closes as soon as the child relaxes. Often referred to as a ''cookie crusher circuit,'' this system enables the

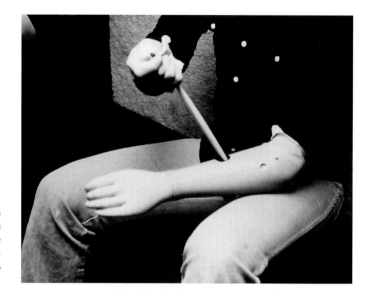

FIGURE 29-51. A young man uses a thin cotton stockinette to break the surface tension between his skin and the plastic socket and to "pull" his arm into a self-suspending myoelectric arm. The socket is contoured to grip above the humeral epicondyles and fits directly against the skin to allow the electrodes to respond to the electrical impulses from the muscles.

young child to quickly gain control over the myoelectric hand. Later, usually within 1 or 2 years, it is advisable to switch the system so that the child uses two electrodes and two muscle sites, controlling opening and closing of the hand independently. Children as young as 3 years of age can be taught to control a hand with a two-site electrode system.[12]

A variety of body-powered terminal devices are available. The CAPP device is especially adapted for younger children. The open design allows easy visual control, and the soft cover is nice to chew on (see Figs. 29-49 and 29-50). Children are often first fitted with a passive prosthesis when they have learned to sit independently, at approximately 9 months of age. At about 18 to 24 months of age, an active terminal body-powered or myoelectric device is used. With voluntary opening hooks, the pinch strength is determined by the number of rubber bands around the base of the

device (see Fig. 29-52). Voluntary closing hooks have a light elastic cord that keeps the hook open, and the child uses the harness to close it. This hook provides some sensory feedback through the harness, and allows the child to vary the amount of grip force. Myoelectric hands many be fit after 18 months, the only limits being the expense, weight, and size of the components.

Other devices also have occasional uses. The sport mitt is popular and helps the child do tumbling and volleyball. The baseball glove adaptation is useful for some children, although most play baseball without a prosthesis at all. Some desire a prosthesis for specific activities such as bike riding, horseback riding, and gymnastics, and many ask for prostheses to improve cosmesis. Unfortunately, the prosthetic hand rarely appears "real" enough to solve this problem. Peak times for desiring a prosthesis are the start of

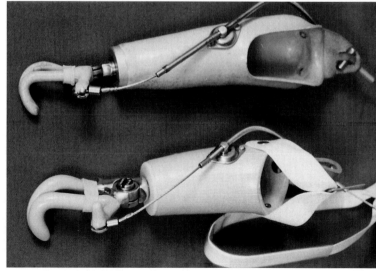

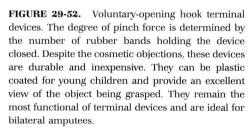

FIGURE 29-52. Voluntary-opening hook terminal devices. The degree of pinch force is determined by the number of rubber bands holding the device closed. Despite the cosmetic objections, these devices are durable and inexpensive. They can be plastic coated for young children and provide an excellent view of the object being grasped. They remain the most functional of terminal devices and are ideal for bilateral amputees.

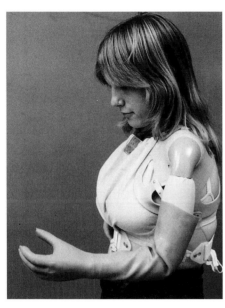

FIGURE 29-53. A shoulder disarticulation prosthesis with a switch-operated electric hand. This patient learned to use the prosthesis but never found it to be functional for her. Like most bilateral upper extremity amputees, she uses her feet for all manual activities. In our clinic, we no longer recommend prostheses for children with bilateral congenital amputations of the upper extremities.

school, going to a new school, and reaching adolescence.

A variety of above-elbow devices are used by children. At first, a passive, friction elbow that may be positioned with the other hand is used with a body-powered or myoelectric terminal device. Later, a body-powered or myoelectric elbow may be added, but these complex devices are not often used by the child with a congenital absence.

Shoulder disarticulation prostheses are even more difficult for children to wear and use (see Figs. 29-50 and 29-53). The shoulder joint is usually passive, and the elbow may also be passive, because the patient with a shoulder disarticulation lacks the excursion necessary for a body-powered elbow. Myoelectric elbows and terminal devices may also be used but are rarely successful for use by the congenital amputee.

Indications for Replacement

One of the biggest challenges in a pediatric prosthetic clinic is to determine when a child has outgrown a prosthesis. Often, there is little doubt about the need for replacement because the child has been so active with the prosthesis that it is essentially demolished. At other times, however, the indications are more subtle.

One indication that the prosthesis needs replacement occurs when continued prosthetic adjustments cannot restore a comfortable socket fit. This usually occurs when no further length or growth adjustments can be made without significant compromises in safety, comfort, or cosmesis. This is often a judgment call by the prosthetist who has already make numerous repairs to the limb.

When weight-bearing surfaces or relief areas in the socket no longer correspond to the patient's anatomy, the prosthesis should be replaced. For example, a transtibial PTB socket probably needs replacement when the tibial tubercle can be palpated above the patellar "bar" in the socket, and the head of the fibula as well as the anterior distal tibia are receiving excess pressure. A transfemoral socket may need replacement when the patient's ischial tuberosity is completely out of the socket and further modifications to the socket cannot restore the ischium to its correct location within the socket or on the "ischial seat." A self-suspending below-elbow prosthesis should be replaced when it can no longer be donned or the olecranon and humeral epicondyles are no longer within the socket.

If the patient's weight or activity level nears or exceeds the maximum values specified by the manufacturer of the prosthetic components, the limb or at least the component should be replaced. For example, many prosthetic pediatric knees and endoskeletal systems have weight limits between 80 and 100 lb. If a child has been wearing the prosthesis for more than 1 year, the weight limit may have been exceeded. Components such as the Seattle Child's Play Foot and the Flex Foot are selected according to a patient's weight and activity level and may need replacement after 1 or 2 years if the patient has significantly changed in weight or activity level.

The prosthesis should be replaced when developmental changes in gait or posture can no longer be accommodated for in the prosthesis. For example, a child with a transfemoral prosthesis first fit at 12 to 15 months of age tends to ambulate with a wide base, hips abducted, knees flexed, and ankles dorsiflexed. During the course of a year, this pattern may change considerably, and a new prosthesis will be needed.

If angular changes cannot be accommodated within the prosthesis, it should be replaced. For example, a patient with a longitudinal deficiency of the fibula and a Syme amputation may exhibit progressive genu valgum. This may spontaneously resolve or may require corrective hemiepiphysiodesis. During the interim, the resulting angular changes require multiple alignment changes or even replacement of the prosthesis.

References

1. Achterman C, Kalamchi A. Congenital deficiency of the fibula. J Bone Joint Surg [Br] 1979;61:133.
2. Aitken G. Amputation as a treatment for certain lower-extremity congenital abnormalities. J Bone Joint Surg [Am] 1959;41:1267.

3. Aitken G. Osseous overgrowth in amputations in children. In: Swinyard C, ed. Limb development and deformity: problems of evaluation and rehabilitation. Springfield, Ill: Charles C. Thomas, 1969.

4. Aitken G. Overgrowth of the amputation stump. J Assoc Child Prosthet Orthot Clin 1962;1:1.

5. Aitken G. Surgical amputation in children. J Bone Joint Surg [Am] 1963;45:1735.

6. Aitken G. Tibial hemimelia. In: A symposium on selected lower limb anomalies: surgical and prosthetic management. Washington, DC: National Academy of Sciences, 1971:1.

7. Aitken GT, ed. Proximal femoral focal deficiency: a congenital anomaly. Washington, DC: National Academy of Sciences, 1969:1.

8. Aitken GT, Frantz CH. Management of the child amputee. Instr Course Lect 1960;17:246.

9. Amstutz H. The natural history and treatment of congenital absence of the fibula. J Bone Joint Surg [Am] 1972;54:1349.

10. Amstutz HC. The morphology, natural history, and treatment of proximal femoral focal deficiency. Washington, DC: National Academy of Sciences, 1969:50.

11. Anderson M, Bray J, Hennessy C. Prosthetic principles: above knee amputations. Springfield, IL: Charles C Thomas, 1960.

12. Baron E, Clarke S, Solomon C. The two stage myoelectric hand for children and young adults. Orthot Prosthet 1983;37:11.

13. Blanco J, Herring J. Congenital chopart amputation: a functional assessment. J Assoc Child Prosthet Orthot Clin 1989;24:27.

14. Bochmann D. Prostheses for the limb-deficient child. In: Kostuik J, Gillespie R, eds. Amputation surgery and rehabilitation. The Toronto experience. New York: Churchill Livingstone, 1981:293.

15. Bochmann D. Prosthetic devices for the management of proximal femoral focal deficiency. Orthot Prosthet 1980;12:4.

16. Bowker J, Keagy R, Poonekar P. Musculoskeletal complications in amputees: their prevention and management. In: Bowker J, Michael J, eds. Atlas of limb prosthetics. St. Louis: Mosby Year Book, 1992:665.

17. Bowker J, Michael J. Atlas of limb prosthetics: surgical, prosthetic, and rehabilitation principles. 2nd ed. St. Louis: Mosby Year Book, 1992.

18. Brown F, Pohnert W. Construction of a knee joint in meromelia tibia (congenital absence of the tibia): a 15-year follow-up study. J Bone Joint Surg [Am] 1972;54:1333.

19. Brown F. Construction of a knee joint in congenital total absence of the tibia (paraxial hemimelia tibia). J Bone Joint Surg [Am] 1965;47:695.

20. Catagni M. Management of fibular hemimelia using the Ilizarov method. Instr Course Lect 1992;61:431.

21. Choi IH, Kumar SJ, Bowen JR. Amputation or limb-lengthening for partial or total absence of the fibula. J Bone Joint Surg [Am] 1990;72:1391.

22. Christini D, Kumar SJ. Fibular transfer in tibial hemimelia: a follow-up study. J Assoc Child Prosthet Orthot Clin 1991;26:8.

23. Clark M. Autosomal dominant inheritance of tibial meromelia. J Bone Joint Surg [Am] 1975;57:262.

24. Coventry M, Johnston E. Congenital absence of the fibula. J Bone Joint Surg [Am] 1952;34:941.

25. Cummings D, Kapp S. Lower-limb pediatric prosthetics: general considerations and philosophy. J Prosthet Orthot 1992;4:196.

26. Cummings D, Knapp S. Manual of transfemoral prosthetics. (In press).

27. Dalsey R, Gomez W, Seitz W Jr, et al. Myoelectric prosthetic replacement in the upper extremity amputee. Orthop Rev 1989;18:697.

28. Eilert R, Jayakumar S. Boyd and Syme ankle amputations in children. J Bone Joint Surg [Am] 1976;58:1138.

29. Epps C. Current concepts review: proximal femoral focal deficiency. J Bone Joint Surg [Am] 1983;65:867.

30. Farmer A, Laurin C. Congenital absence of the fibula. J Bone Joint Surg [Am] 1960;42:1.

31. Fillauer C, Pritham C, Fillauer K. Evolution and development of the silicone suction socket (3S) for below-knee prostheses. J Pediatr Orthop 1989;1:92.

32. Fisk J. Introduction to the child amputee. In: Bowker J, Michael J, eds. Atlas of limb prosthetics: surgical, prosthetic, and rehabilitation principles. St. Louis: Mosby Year Book, 1992:731.

33. Fixsen J, Lloyd-Roberts G. The natural history and early treatment of proximal femoral dysplasia. J Bone Joint Surg [Br] 1974;56:86.

34. Frankel V, Gold S, Golyakhovsky V. The Ilizarov technique. Bull Hosp Joint Dis Orthop Inst 1988;48:17.

35. Frantz C, O'Rahilly R. Congenital skeletal limb deficiencies. J Bone Joint Surg [Am] 1961;43:1202.

36. Frantz C. The upsurge in phocomelic congenital anomalies. J Assoc Child Prosthet Orthot Clin 1994;28:38.

37. Franz C, Aitken G. Management of the juvenile amputee. Clin Orthop 1959;9:30.

38. Franz C. The increase in the incidence of malformed babies in the German Federal Republic during the years 1959–1962. J Assoc Child Prosthet Orthot Clin 1994;28:62.

39. Fuller D, Duthie R. The timed appearance of some congenital malformation and orthopaedic abnormalities. Instr Course Lect 1974;23:53.

40. Gazely W, Ey M, Sampson W. Use of triple wall sockets for juvenile amputees. Interclin Inform Bull 1964;4:1.

41. Gibson D. Child and juvenile amputees. In: Banjerjee S, Khan N, eds. Rehabilitation management of amputees. Baltimore: Williams & Wilkins, 1982.

42. Gillespie R, Torode IP. Classification and management of congenital abnormalities of the femur. J Bone Joint Surg [Br] 1983;65:557.

43. Gillespie R. Principles of amputation surgery in children with longitudinal deficiencies of the femur. Clin Orthop 1990;256:29.

44. Glessner J. Spontaneous intra-uterine amputation. J Bone Joint Surg [Am] 1963;45:351.

45. Gonin-Decarie T. The mental and emotional development of the thaliomide children and the psychological reactions of the mothers. J Assoc Child Prosthet Orthot Clin 1994;28:79.

46. Grissom L, Harcke H, Kumar S. Sonography in the management of tibial hemimelia. Clin Orthop 1990;251:266.

47. Hall C, Brooks M, Dennis J. Congenital skeletal deficiencies of the extremities: classification and fundamentals of treatment. JAMA 1962;181:590.

48. Hall JE. Rotation of congenitally hypoplastic lower limbs to use the ankle joint as a knee. J Assoc Child Prosthet Orthot Clin 1966;6:3.

49. Hamanishi C. Congenital short femur. J Bone Joint Surg [Br] 1980;62:307.

50. Hamilton E. Gait training, part 2: children. In: Kostuik J, ed. Amputation surgery and rehabilitation, the Toronto experience. New York: Churchill Livingstone, 1981:331.

51. Hancock CI, King RE. The one-bone leg. J Assoc Child Prosthet Orthot Clin 1967;7:11.

52. Heger H, Millstein S, Hunter G. Electrically powered prostheses for the adult with an upper limb amputation. J Bone Joint Surg [Br] 1985;67:278.

53. Henkel L, Willert H-G. Dysmelia: a classification and a pattern of malformation in a group of congenital defects of the limbs. J Bone Joint Surg [Br] 1969;51:399.

54. Hepp O. Frequency of congenital defect–anomalies of the extremities in the Federal Republic of Germany. J Assoc Child Prosthet Orthot Clin 1994;28:40.

55. Herring J, Barnhill B, Gaffney C. Syme amputation: an evaluation of the physical and psychological function in young patients. J Bone Joint Surg [Am] 1986;68:573.

56. Hughes J. Biomechanics of the through-knee prosthesis. Prosthet Orthot Int 1983;7:96.

57. Johansson E, Aparisi T. Missing cruciate ligament in congenital short femur. J Bone Joint Surg [Am] 1983;65:1109.

58. Jones D, Barnes J, Lloyd-Roberts G. Congenital aplasia and dysplasia of the tibia with intact fibula: classification and management. J Bone Joint Surg [Br] 1978;60:31.

59. Jones K. Femoral hypoplasia-unusual facies syndrome. In: Jones K, ed. Smith's recognizable patterns of human malformation. Philadelphia: WB Saunders, 1988:268.

60. King R, Marks T. Follow-up findings on the skeletal lever in the surgical management of proximal femoral focal deficiency. Interclin Inform Bull 1971;11:1.

61. King R. Providing a single lever in proximal femoral focal deficiency. A preliminary case report. J Assoc Child Prosthet Orthot Clin 1966;6:23.

62. Kino Y. Clinical and experimental studies of the congenital constriction band syndrome with and emphasis on its etiology. J Bone Joint Surg [Am] 1969;57:636.

63. Koman L, Meyer L, Warren F. Proximal femoral focal deficiency: a 50-year experience. Dev Med Child Neurol 1982; 24:344.

64. Kostuik J, Gillespie R, Hall J, Hubbard S. Van Nes rotational osteotomy for treatment of proximal femoral focal deficiency and congenital short femur. J Bone Joint Surg [Am] 1975; 57:1039.

65. Krajbich I, Bochmann D. Van Nes rotation-plasty in tumor surgery. In: Bowker J, Michael J, eds. Atlas of Limb Prosthetics. Surgical Prosthetic and Rehabilitation Principles. St. Louis: Mobsy Year Book, 1992:885.

66. Krajbich I. Proximal femoral focal deficiency. In: Kalamchi A, ed. Congenital lower limb deficiencies. New York: Springer-Verlag, 1989:108.

67. Kritter A. Tibial rotation-plast for proximal femoral focal deficiency. J Bone Joint Surg [Am] 1977;59:927.

68. Kruger L, Talbott R. Amputation and prosthesis as definitive treatment in congenital absence of the fibula. J Bone Joint Surg [Am] 1961;43:625.

69. Kruger L. Congenital limb deficiencies. Part II: Lower limb deficiencies. In: Bowker J, Michael J, eds. Atlas of limb prosthetics, surgical and prosthetic principles. St. Louis: CV Mosby, 1981:522.

70. Kruger L. Lower limb deficiencies. In: Bowker J, Michael J, eds. Atlas of limb prosthetics: surgical, prosthetic, and rehabilitation principles. St. Louis: Mosby Year Book, 1992:802.

71. Kruger L. The use of stubbies for the child with bilateral lower-limb deficiencies. J Assoc Child Prosthet Orthot Clin 1973;12:7.

72. Kruger LM, Abdo RB, Schwartz AM. Tibial deficiency—a genetic problem. J Assoc Child Prosthet Orthot Clin 1985;20:41.

73. Lie R, Wilcox A, Skjaevren R. A population based study of the risk of recurrence of birth defects. N Engl J Med 1994;331:1.

74. Lloyd-Roberts GC, Stone KH. Congenital hypoplasia of the upper femur. J Bone Joint Surg [Br] 1963;45:557.

75. Loder R, Herring J. Disarticulation of the knee in children. A functional assessment. J Bone Joint Surg [Am] 1987;69:1155.

76. Loder R, Herring J. Fibular transfer for congenital absence of the tibia: a reassessment. J Pediatr Ortho 1987;7:8.

77. Long I. Normal shape–normal alignment (NSNA) above-knee prosthesis. Clin Prosthet Orthot 1985;9:9.

78. Madigan RR, Fillauer KD. 3-S prosthesis: a preliminary report. J Pediatr Orthop 1991;11:112.

79. Marquardt E, Fisk JR. Thalidomide children; thirty years later. J Assoc Child Prost Orthot Clin 1992;27:3.

80. Marquardt E. The multiple limb-deficient child. In: Atlas of limb prosthetics. St. Louis: CV Mosby, Committee on Prosthetics and Orthotics, eds. 1982:595.

81. McCullough N, Trout A, Caldwell J. Non-standard prosthetic applications for juvenile amputatees. J Assoc Child Prosthet Orthot Clin 1963;2:7.

82. Meyer L, Sauer B. The use of porous high-density polyethylene caps in the prevention of appositional bone growth in the juvenile amputee: a preliminary report. J Assoc Child Prosthet Orthot Clin 1975;14:1.

83. Meyer LC, Sauer BW. Problems of treating and fitting the patient with proximal femoral focal deficiency. J Assoc Child Prosthet Orthot Clin 1971;10:1.

84. Michael J. Reflections on CAD/CAM in prosthetics and orthotics. J Pediatr Orthop 1989;1:116.

85. Minnes PM, Stack DM. Research and practice with congenital amputees: making the whole greater than the sum of its parts. Int J Rehabil Res 1990;13:151.

86. Mowery C, Herring J, Jackson D. Dislocated patella associated with below-knee amputation. J Pediatr Orthop 1986;6:299.

87. Murray D, Kambouroglou G, Kenwright J. One-stage lengthening for femoral shortening with associated deformity. J Bone Joint Surg [Br] 1993;75:566.

88. Oberg K. Knee mechanisms for through-knee prostheses. Prosthet Orthot Int 1983;7:107.

89. Patterson DB, McMillan PM, Rodriquez RP. Acceptance rate of myoelectric prosthesis. J Assoc Child Prosthet Orthot Clin 1990;25:73.

90. Pattinson RC, Fixsen JA. Management and outcome in tibial dysplasia. J Bone Joint Surg Br 1992;74:893.

91. Patton J. Developmental approach to pediatric prosthetic evaluation and training. In: Atkins D, Meier R, eds. Comprehensive management of the upper-limb amputee. New York: Springer-Verlag, 1989:137.

92. Pritham C. Biomechanics and shape of the above-knee socket considered in light of the ischial containment concept. Prosthet Orthot Int 1990;14:9.

93. Rab G. Principles of amputation in children. In: Chapman M, ed. Operative orthopaedics. Philadelphia: JB Lippincott, 1993:2469.

94. Radcliffe C. Functional considerations in the fitting of above knee prostheses. Orthot Prosthet 1955;2:35.

95. Radcliffe C. Prosthetics. In: Rose J, Gamble J, eds. Human walking. 2nd ed. Baltimore: Williams & Wilkins, 1994:165.

96. Richieri-Costa A, Ferrareto I, Masiero D, da Silva CRM. Tibial hemimelia: report on 37 new cases, clinical and genetic considerations. Am J Med Genet 1987;27:867.

97. Roskies E. Abnormality and normality: the mothering of thalidomide children. Ithaca, NY: Cornell University Press, 1972:347.

98. Russell JE. Tibial hemimelia: limb deficiency in siblings. Interclin Inform Bull 1965;14:15.

99. Sabolich J. Contoured adducted trochanteric-controlled alignment method. Clin Prosthet Orthot 1985;9:15.

100. Sanders G. Static and dynamic analysis. In: Sanders G, ed. Lower limb amputations: a guide to rehabilitation. Philadelphia: FA Davis, 1986:415.

101. Schuch C. Modern above-knee fitting practice. Prosthet Orthot Int 1988;12:77.

102. Schuch M. Transfemoral amputation: prosthetic management. In: Bowker J, Michael J, eds. Atlas of limb prosthetics. St. Louis: Mosby Year Book, 1992:509.

103. Silcox D, Rooks M, Vogel R, Fleming L. Myoelectric prostheses. J Bone Joint Surg [Am] 1993;75:1781.

104. Speer D. The pathogenesis of amputation stump overgrowth. Clin Orthop 1981;159:34.

105. Steel HH, Lin P, Betz R, et al. Iliofemoral fusion for proximal femoral focal deficiency. J Bone Joint Surg [Am] 1987;69:837.

106. Swanson A. Bone overgrowth in the juvenile amputee and its control by the use of silicone rubber implants. J Assoc Child Prosthet Orthot Clin 1969;8:9.

107. Tablada C. A technique for fitting converted proximal femoral focal deficiencies. Artif Limbs 1971;15:27.

108. Talbot D, Solomon D. The function of a parent group in the adaptation to the birth of a limb-deficient child. Interclin Inform Bull 1979;17:9.

109. Thompson G, Leimkuller J. Prosthetic management. In: Kalamchi A, ed. Congenital lower limb deficiencies. New York: Springer-Verlag, 1989:210.

110. Tooms R. Acquired amputations in children. In: Bowker J, Michael J, eds. Atlas of limb prosthetics: surgical, prosthetic, and rehabilitation principles. St. Louis: Mosby Year Book, 1992:735.

111. Torode I, RG. Rotationplasty of the lower limb for congenital defects of the femur. J Bone Joint Surg [Br] 1983;65:569.

112. Total Knee Geometric Knee System (brochure). Century XXII Innovations, 1993.

113. Van Nes CP. Rotation-plasty for congenital defects of the femur: making use of the ankle of the shortened limb to control the knee joint of a prosthesis. J Bone Joint Surg [Br] 1950;32:12.

114. Velasquez R, Bell D, Armstrong P, et al. Complications of the use of the Ilizarov technique in the correction of limb deformities in children. J Bone Joint Surg [Am] 1993;75:1148.

115. Weaver S. Comparison of myoelectric and conventional prostheses for adolescent amputees. Am J Occup Ther 1988;42:78.

116. Westin GW, Gunderson GO. Proximal femoral focal deficiency: a review of treatment experiences. In: A symposium on proximal femoral focal deficiency: a congenital anomaly. Washington DC: National Academy of Sciences, 1969:100.

117. Wood WL, Zlotsky N, Westin G. Congenital absence of the fibula. Treatment by Syme amputation: indications and technique. J Bone Joint Surg [Am] 1965;47:1159.

118. Younge D, Dafniotis O. A composite bone flap to lengthen a below-knee amputation stump. J Bone Joint Surg [Br] 1993;75:330.

Lovell & Winter's Pediatric Orthopaedics, fourth edition,
edited by Raymond T. Morrissy and Stuart L. Weinstein.
Lippincott–Raven Publishers, Philadelphia © 1996.

Chapter

30

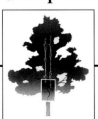

Sports Medicine

Michael T. Busch

CARE OF THE YOUNG ATHLETE

Young athletes sustain musculoskeletal injuries that are different from those of their adult counterparts. Although many of these are the torus fractures, greenstick fractures, and physeal injuries that are common to children, the proliferation of youth athletics has increased the incidence of overuse syndromes and other injuries.[402] The role of rehabilitation in the treatment of sports-related injuries is recognized, and there is a growing emphasis on prevention of these injuries.[137]

The volume of organized sports activities and levels of intensity for youth training and competition have grown tremendously during the past decade. The United States Consumer Product Safety Commission reported that approximately 2 million medically attended sporting injuries occur annually to youths between the ages of 5 and 14 years.[343] In response to this problem, preparticipation physical examinations, heat illness education, safety reviews, school athletic train-

ers, team physicians, and health education programs for grade school and high school sports participants have evolved.[136]

Sports have important effects on strength, speed, and stamina. If appropriately organized, sports can be a positive social experience, with opportunity for character growth and development. Competition is often emphasized, but the lifelong values of health, exercise, and recreation should not be overlooked. Particularly during the elementary school years, programs should be available that emphasize the participation by all children, not just the physically advantaged.[348] Involving younger children in elite-level sports training and competition should be done with caution, because there is a risk of exploiting the child and producing long-term emotional consequences.[342] However, many of the critical behavioral needs of adolescents can be satisfied by athletic participation and competition.[363]

Approximately 2% of children suffer from chronic medical problems that restrict their activity.[135] Besides having to live with the inherent aspects of these conditions, these children are often excessively restricted form physical activities. Most children with asthma, cystic fibrosis, congenital heart disease, or juvenile rheumatoid arthritis can benefit from an appropriately structured exercise and sports recreation program.[22,137] Recommendations are available from the American Academy of Pediatrics for sports participation by youths with special health conditions, although a physician's assessment of the individual situation should always be considered.[77,218]

Programs such as the Special Olympics have grown from the recognition that children with physical impediments can benefit from the personal, social, and physical aspects of sports participation. Children with a variety of chronic illnesses, including asthma, can benefit from exercise conditioning.[303] This should be done with the advice and direction of their physicians.

Nutrition

Everyone seriously involved with youth sports should be familiar with the facts and myths concerning nutrition. This area has received much attention in the medical and lay literature. Inaccurate nutritional information leaves the impressionable and naive young athlete easy prey for food faddists and nutritional charlatans.

Vigorous training increases the consumption of calories but does not significantly alter the athlete's need for essential nutrients.[361] Minerals and electrolytes are replaced by a normal diet unless the athlete is experiencing daily fluid losses of 4% to 6% of body weight because of excessive sweating. Nutritional supplements, such as vitamins and protein powder, are unnecessary if the youth eats a basic mixed daily diet consisting of four fruit or vegetable servings, four grain servings, two diary products, and two high-protein foods.[268,361] As many as 15% to 20% of menstruating female athletes may require an iron supplement. Children from low socioeconomic backgrounds may also lack adequate iron in their diet.[74]

Young athletes have increased energy requirements related to rapid growth and exercise expenditure. The increased need for food energy is best met through complex carbohydrates. A high-carbohydrate diet provides the needed calories while increasing muscle and liver glycogen stores, which are important for athletic performance.[26] Simple sugars provide a readily available source of carbohydrate calories. They may be a needed component of an active athlete's diet to meet total caloric requirements. The disadvantage of simple sugars is that they are absorbed quickly. This induces an insulin response that can lower serum glucose and result in fatigue.

The recommended caloric intake is 50% to 60% carbohydrate, 10% to 15% protein, and 30% to 35% lipids.[210] The ratio of complex carbohydrates to these other components can be achieved with fruits, leafy vegetables, and starches such as potatoes, rice, pasta, and breads. Greasy and salty foods should be discouraged.

Carbohydrate loading during the days before competition can enhance glycogen stores to optimize energy availability for prolonged muscle performance.[78,202] The pregame meal should consist primarily of light carbohydrate foods consumed about 3 hours before the activity.[78] Foods high in fats and salt slow gastric emptying and increase water retention in the gut.[361]

Fats are a rich source of energy, but they are poorly mobilized for a short-term energy expenditure. A diet high in fat fails to enhance the body's glycogen stores, which are important for athletic performance. Excessive consumption of fats also carries the associated risks of elevating serum cholesterol and triglycerides.[210]

Proteins are complex amino acids. They are necessary components for building new muscle tissue. Proteins should account for approximately 15% of total caloric intake, and any surplus is metabolized for energy or excreted in urine.[210] Most protein supplement preparations are solely expensive sources of calories. Gains in muscle strength and mass are made by training and have not been proven to result only from providing a high-protein diet.[202]

A variety of minerals and vitamins are important. Because potassium is primarily an intracellular ion, losses associated with sports are slow and gradual. Potassium does not need to be replenished acutely, but it is needed over the prolonged course of serial competition and training.[210] Magnesium is a key component in the ATP cycle. Bananas are an excellent source of magnesium and potassium. Iron deficiency is still a problem in teens, especially females, vegetarians, and individuals from lower socioeconomic groups.[268] Adolescents should be encouraged to eat iron-fortified foods, such as whole grain breads and lean red meats. When combined with citrus fruits, the bioavailability of iron increases. Athletic activity theoretically depends on all vitamins, but emphasis has been placed on vitamin C and B complex vitamins because of their roles in the metabolism of proteins, fats, and carbohydrates for energy.[210] However, there is no evidence to suggest that an intake in excess of normal requirements improves performance.[206,210]

Heat Illness and Fluids

Between 70% and 80% of the energy consumed in muscle contraction is transformed to heat.[362] Heat loss is promoted by increased blood flow to the skin and by increased sweating. Cooling is provided by thermal conduction, convection, radiation, and evaporation. Extrinsic factors affecting heat exchange include ambient temperature, humidity, clothing, sunlight, and wind.

The spectrum of heat illness can be divided into four clinical entities: heat cramps, heat syncope, heat exhaustion, and heat stroke.[285] Heat cramps are painful muscle spasms that typically occur in the gastrocnemius and soleus, hamstrings, quadriceps, and spine extensors. Because the spasms are primarily caused by fluid depletion, the key elements of treatment are fluid replacement, stretching, and cooling. Heat syncope usually involves a feeling of fatigue and resolves with cooling, fluids and rest. Heat exhaustion is characterized by extreme weakness, exhaustion, headache, altered consciousness, and profuse sweating. This is a much more advanced stage of the heat illness continuum and should be treated aggressively with fluid replacement, cooling, and restriction of further participation in sports for the day. Occasionally, intravenous fluids and hospitalization are necessary.

Heat stroke is a true medical emergency resulting from dehydration with severe hyperthermia. There can be severe abnormalities affecting the brain, heart, clotting system, kidneys, and liver. Edema of the brain and meninges as well as petechial hemorrhage can lead to loss of consciousness, dysphoria, headache, dizziness, weakness, confusion, euphoria, coma, and seizures. Myocardial injury and increased pulmonary vascular resistance can lead to tachycardia, hypotension, and shock. Systemic petechial, gross tissue hemorrhage and consumptive coagulopathy is thought to be triggered by thermal injury to the vascular endothelium. Renal tubular dysfunction and acute tubular necrosis can result in severe dehydration and marked hypokalemia and hyponatremia. Occasionally, there is liver damage, including centrilobular necrosis and cholestasis resulting in hyperbilirubinemia and jaundice.[73] Maximal cooling efforts should be made at the site, and the victim should be rapidly transported for emergency medical care.[285]

Children are less efficient thermal regulators than adults and acclimatize more slowly than adults. They have a lower sweating capacity, especially before puberty. Children also produce more metabolic heat per mass and have a decreased ability to conduct heat to the skin.[74] They have a greater ratio of surface area to mass, which increases heat transfer from the environment on hot days. Additional risk factors for children can include obesity, fever, recent gastroenteritis with dehydration, and cystic fibrosis.[16]

Sweat is hypotonic to body fluids, containing 40

to 80 mEq/L of sodium and less than 5 mEq/L of potassium. Sweating increases serum electrolyte concentrations. Electrolyte solutions for replacement are recommended only after 1 or 2 hours of rigorous activity.[75] Initially, plain water adequately replaces these losses. The water should be cooled to stimulate thirst. Cool liquids do not significantly slow gastrointestinal emptying, but delayed motility can be a side effect of electrolyte solutions with high osmolalities. Salt tablets, once popular, are dangerous because they can produce intracellular dehydration by their osmotic effect in the serum.[362]

Heat illness is almost entirely preventable (Table 30-1).[211] Through awareness and education, changes have come about in workout and competition precautions. The National Collegiate Athletic Association reported 39 heat stroke fatalities in football from 1964 to 1973. Through awareness, education, and precautions, the number dropped to 15 during the next 10 years.[286] The body primarily gains heat from basic metabolism, as a byproduct of muscle work, and from the absorption of the radiant energy of sunlight. The primary means of cooling are the evaporation of sweat and convection to the air. Situations that increase heat gain include rigorous exercise, bright direct sunlight, and dark clothing. Cooling is inhibited by dehydration, high humidity, high air temperature, a lack of wind, and equipment or clothing that acts as insulation. Acclimatization is also important, because it reflects the body's capacity to transfer heat to the skin for convection and the body's ability to produce sweat for evaporation. With this as background, the guidelines in Table 30-1 outline most of the key components for avoiding heat illness.

TABLE 30-1   *Guidelines for Preventing Heat Illness*

Proper acclimatization at the beginning of the workout season
Evaluate weather conditions for temperature, humidity, and sunlight
Schedule rest in the shade
Identify participants at particular risk
Hydrate before practice and competition
Have chilled fluids readily available at the practice site
Enforce periodic drinking
Never use water restriction as discipline
Discourage deliberate dehydration for weight loss
Make appropriate clothing adjustments
Schedule events to avoid peak hours of heat and sun
Educate the players and parents
Record daily weights to ensure adequate rehydration between practices

Strength Training

Weight lifting should be differentiated from weight training. Olympic lifting and power lifting are the two categories of weight lifting. The Olympic lifts consist of snatch and clean-and-jerk lifts. The dead lift, squat lift, and bench press are the three power lifts. In both categories of weight lifting, the object is to perform a one-repetition maximum lift. Weight training refers to the use of free weights and machines to enhance strength and endurance. Submaximal weights are lifted repeatedly with a large variety of exercises typically intended to enhance performance for other sports rather than for a specific contest.[47]

Children can increase strength by 20% to 40% in a well-supervised program with a relatively low risk of injury.[353,399] Females and prepubescent males do not produce significant hypertrophy of their muscles in response to weight training because of insufficient circulating androgens. The strength gains that do occur result from enhanced recruitment of motor units and synchronization rather than significant muscular hypertrophy.

Common injuries associated with weight lifting include patellofemoral pain, meniscal tears, pelvic apophyseal avulsion fractures, and clavicular osteolysis.[38,347] Lumbosacral injuries, including disc herniation and spondylolisthesis, are the most common problems in adolescent weight lifters.[48] The most common injuries from weight lifting are muscle pulls, tendinitis, sprains, and other minor injuries.[48] Stress fractures and a variety of acute physeal, metaphyseal, and diaphyseal fractures have been reported in weight lifters.[47,147,150,344] Despite concerns, there does not seem to be any substantial evidence that weight training using submaximal loads harms the physeal plates. However, power lifting or Olympic weight lifting are not recommended for skeletally immature youths.[76]

Many high schools run successful and safe weight-training programs. A proper strength-conditioning program should be a prerequisite to participation in contact sports. For safe participation, there should be a structured program supervised by an educated and attentive staff. Proper technique should be emphasized, using repetition without maximal weight lifts. Equipment must be in good repair. An attentive partner (i.e., spotter) is important when free weights are used. A conscientious, concurrent stretching program is also important.[147,353] Although the scientific documentation is just evolving for warm-up and stretching, they appear to be important for preventing injuries.[354,381] Stretching and warm-up exercises apparently enhance muscle, tendon, and ligament elasticity and may improve performance by nervous system recruitment and psychologic effects.[354,381]

Drug Abuse

Drug abuse by athletes has become common.[102] Frequently involved substances include amphetamines, analgesics, tranquilizers, diuretics, and anabolic steroids. The evidence for actual performance enhancement is questionable, but the potential complications are well known. Most widely abused are the anabolic steroids used in conjunction with weight training and weight lifting. A 1988 survey of 3400 senior high school students across the United States reported that 6.6% of them had used anabolic steroids. Two thirds of the users had started before 16 years of age.[49,404]

Anabolic steroid use appears to be spreading despite the known side effects, which include premature epiphyseal closure, fluid retention, hematoma, hepatocellular carcinoma, testicular atrophy, and female hirsutism.[56,195,374,383,400] Physicians dealing with adolescent athletes should be aware and suspicious of these problems. Unfortunately, physicians are occasionally the source for these drugs.[49,383,404] The health aspects of drug abuse must be addressed frankly. Rather than concentrating solely on competition or achievement, sports programs should stress the overall importance of health and activity.

Antiinflammatory Drugs

Nonsteroidal Antiinflammatory Drugs

The principles for using nonsteroidal antiinflammatory drugs (NSAIDs) in sports-produced inflammation include decreasing the pain of inflammation to allow compliance of rehabilitation and to avoid pain-induced atrophy, reducing inflammation in freshly healed and relatively vascular tissues during retraining, and limiting the zone of edema-induced tissue necrosis after acute injury. Although their effects, efficacy, and roles are still being clarified, it is important to be familiar with these medications, because they are commonly used by young athletes.

The exact mechanism of action of NSAIDs is not clear, although presumably it is related to the inhibition of prostaglandin synthesis and probably to other effects.[1] Prostaglandin inhibition is the common feature of all of these agents. The three main clinical features are analgesic, antipyretic, and antiinflammatory effects. In inflammatory conditions, the response may take time. In rheumatoid arthritis, only one half of the patients have an adequate response to the NSAID within 2 weeks, and an additional 30% respond by 10 weeks.[44] Fifty percent of patients who experience no relief from the first type of NSAID improve after another is tried, and a trial of several drugs may be needed before a satisfactory response is achieved. In cases of prolonged use, a drug may become ineffective with time, requiring substitution of another NSAID.[44]

The principal metabolic pathway of NSAIDs is hepatic, with renal excretion of the conjugated metabolites. All NSAIDs are extensively bound to proteins, giving them the potential to displace other drugs, but this seldom produces significant potentiation of other drug effects. The potentiation of anticoagulants is therapeutically significant, but these agents are seldom used in children and adolescents. Occasionally, two NSAIDs are used concomitantly, but this should be done under careful scrutiny for toxic side effects.

Aspirin, ibuprofen, naproxen, and tolmetin sodium are the only NSAIDs approved by the U.S. Food and Drug Administration for children younger than 13 years of age. Among the NSAIDs, aspirin is the least expensive but has the highest rate of minor side effects. Most parents are reluctant to administer aspirin because of the well-publicized association with Reye syndrome. Liquid preparations of aspirin derivatives are available, effective, and have reasonably few side effects. Tolmetin sodium and naproxen have the advantage of twice-daily dosing and are available in liquid suspension form. Ibuprofen is used widely because it is relatively inexpensive and available without prescription.

Most of the information available about the use of these agents in younger patients derives from experience in treating juvenile rheumatoid arthritis. Their use in musculoskeletal inflammation secondary to trauma and overuse syndromes is less well documented, particularly in youths. Although these drugs are widely used, their efficacy in sports-related disorders is largely empiric and not well documented in placebo-controlled studies.[1]

Occurring in as many as 10% of patients, the most common side effects of NSAIDs are gastrointestinal: abdominal pain, nausea, diarrhea, and occasionally constipation. Hematuria, proteinuria, and marrow suppression also can occur. Rarely, tinnitus, blurred vision, mood changes, drowsiness, and mouth ulcers are seen. These side effects usually resolve after discontinuance of the medication. Patients on prolonged NSAID therapy should have a hemogram, urinalysis, and liver function profile at 2 weeks, 6 weeks, and then every 2 or 3 months after therapy is begun. Rarely, NSAIDs can cause peptic ulcer, severe liver or renal toxicity, or severe allergic reactions.[44] The use of NSAIDs in young children or for prolonged periods in older children and teens is probably best supervised by a rheumatologist or an experienced pediatrician.

Corticosteroids

Oral and parenterally administered steroids appear to enter the inflammatory cycle earlier than the effect of NSAIDs. This action apparently results in their more potent effect, but it may produce harmful side effects, including the retardation of healing.[226]

There are concerns that intraarticular injection of steroids can damage articular cartilage, possibly by inhibiting the synthesis of chondral matrix.[238] In adults, there are several reports of adults undergoing rapid radiographically evident degeneration after intraarticular injections, but these are probably anecdotal. The risk of adult tendon rupture after steroid injection appears to be substantially more founded.[226] Intraarticular triamcinolone hexacetonide in the management on children with juvenile rheumatoid arthritis has been effective with relatively few side effects.[5] Because there is no definitive evidence regarding the safety and efficacy of oral or parenteral steroids for sports-related maladies in children, these treatment options should probably be avoided or used sparingly.[23]

OVERUSE SYNDROMES

The term "overuse syndrome" categorizes several musculoskeletal maladies that are characterized by connective tissue failure in response to repetitive submaximal loading. In the course of normal activities, a small amount of tissue breakdown usually occurs. With repetition, musculoskeletal tissue hypertrophy occurs, which is the essence of athletic training. If the rate of tissue fatigue exceeds the reparative response, failure occurs. Inflammation ensues and leads to clinical symptoms (Fig. 30-1).[208]

Classic Stress Fractures

Stress fractures are partial or complete disruptions of the bone secondary to an inability to withstand repetitive, nonviolent loads. Normally, the bone remodels itself in response to microtrauma. However, with excessive use, the mechanical fatigue and bone resorption can outpace the osteoblastic response. Although the classic example of stress fractures are the "march fractures" of young adult military recruits,[198,275] stress fractures do occur in adolescent athletes and children.[93,107,302,333]

Adolescents with stress fractures closely parallel their adult counterparts, with a few exceptions.[302,333] In a series of 200 stress fractures occurring in all ages, 36.5% occurred in 16- to 19-year-old adolescents, and 6% occurred in youths 15 years of age or younger.[302] The proximal third of the tibia is the most commonly affected site; metatarsal fractures are rare in youngsters.[302] There is equal distribution among male and female patients. Although most stress fractures in adolescents are associated with endurance running, the average training distance is typically not excessive.[302]

Engh reported stress fractures of the proximal tibia in a series of nine children younger than 12 years

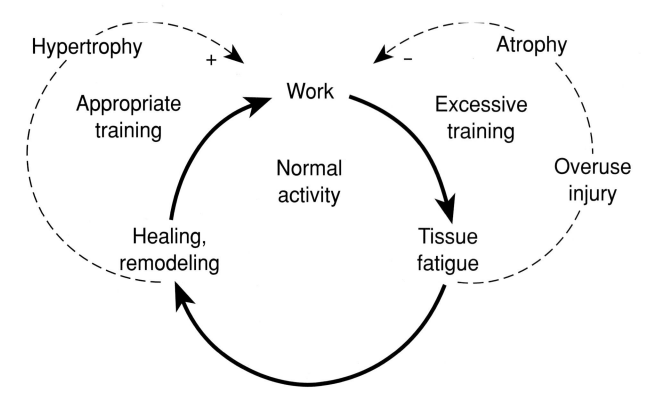

FIGURE 30-1. Cyclic loading of all tissues leads to tissue fatigue. Normally, these tissues heal and remodel, permitting continued activities. Athletic training involves increasing activity and converting the healing and remodeling process into hypertrophy of the tissues. This strengthens tissue, allowing increased tissue loading and greater performance. Excessive training leads to tissue fatigue by exceeding the rate of healing or remodeling.

of age, with the youngest diagnosed at 21 months of age.[107] In many of these cases, there was no clear history of athletic overuse, and these cases seem to represent an entity distinct from sports-related stress fractures.

Stress fractures about the knee can involve the distal femoral physis, the proximal tibial physis, and the patella.[53,96,386,398] Although the lower extremities are most commonly affected, cases of adolescent athletes with stress fractures of the metacarpal, radius, ulna, humerus, and olecranon have been reported.[284,322,325,326] Spondylolysis is often the result of a stress fracture of the pars interarticularis and is most commonly seen in young gymnasts and football linemen (see Chap. 19).[109,187]

The typical history is one of insidious onset of pain in the area of fracture that is initially relieved by rest. The pain eventually increases. It persists after activity and affects normal walking. On examination, the tenderness can be localized to the site of fracture in about two thirds of cases, and swelling occurs in about one fourth.[249]

About 10% of initial radiographs are abnormal.[249] With time, the osteoclastic process may lead to cortical disruption and even to a displaced fracture. Bone scintigraphy is helpful for establishing the diagnosis, espe-

cially during early stages. As many as 50% of adolescents with stress fractures show multiple asymptomatic areas of stress response on bone scan.[333] If clinically asymptomatic, these other areas of bone scan uptake do not warrant treatment.

Osteoid osteoma, malignancies, and infection can have presentations and radiographic appearances similar to stress fractures. The differential diagnosis of tibial stress fracture includes all of the causes of shin splints. Occasionally, a biopsy is indicated, but this should be avoided if possible because the surgical defect may delay healing or precipitate a complete fracture. If a biopsy is performed, an adequate sample must be obtained and the interpretation reviewed carefully. A healing fracture can have many features similar to a malignancy.

Stress fractures of the proximal femur can have serious complications, including avascular necrosis if displacement occurs. These occur in young adults, with a few cases reported as young as 16 years of age.[127,198] Only rarely has stress fracture of the femoral neck been reported in skeletally immature children.[149,406] Other diagnoses, particularly slipped capital femoral epiphysis, should be considered in the young athlete complaining of vague hip, thigh, or groin pain related to activity.

The treatment of most stress fractures involves breaking the cycle of repetitive trauma. This usually can be done by eliminating running while permitting normal walking. Crutches or a cast can be used for fractures that seem to be at particular risk for displacement or for the uncooperative adolescent.[249] Alternative training, such as swimming, cycling, or pool jogging, can be used for maintaining aerobic conditioning in the serious athlete. Compliance is critical in ensuring that a complete fracture does not occur.[97] Healing takes 2 weeks to 3 months.[302] Recommending when to return to sports is a difficult judgment. An appropriate response with radiographic evidence of healing should be documented, especially if there is any question about the diagnosis.

Distal fibular stress fractures have little risk of residual complications. For these, the use of a pneumatic leg brace is useful for the early return to sports.[97] Tibial stress fractures deserve special attention, because nonunion occasionally occurs, even after 4 to 6 months of conservative care.[142] Femoral neck stress fractures should be treated aggressively and may require internal stabilization.

Repetitive Physeal Injuries

Epiphysiolysis of the Proximal Humerus

Adolescents may develop widening of the proximal humeral physeal plate associated with shoulder pain during rigorous upper extremity activities, such as baseball pitching. Coined by Dotter, the descriptive term "Little League shoulder" is not precise because other overhead sports may be involved.[99] The pathol-

ogy has not been delineated because biopsy is not indicated for this self-limiting disorder. The pathomechanics are presumed to be repetitive traction or torsional forces at the physis. This overuse syndrome is clearly different from the acute humeral shaft fracture associated with throwing.[392] The exact incidence of Little League shoulder is unknown.[151]

The typical patient with epiphysiolysis of the proximal humerus is a male baseball player between the ages of 12 and 15 years. There seems to be an association with quantity and intensity of pitching, the age at which pitching was started, and the use of the curve ball pitch. Typically, the pain begins during pitching without an inciting event. Initially, the youth may continue to play despite the pain, with the discomfort resolving between games. Playing ability diminishes as the pain becomes more constant.

Tenderness is primarily in the proximal humerus or shoulder. Pain is elicited with active internal rotation against resistance.[151] The shoulder has a full range of motion.

Plain radiographs demonstrate widening and irregularity of the physeal plate (Fig. 30-2A), and a comparison view of the unaffected shoulder is helpful (Fig. 30-2B).[19] Bone scans do not demonstrate greater than normal activity.[151] The primary differential diagnoses include rotator cuff tendinitis, acromioclavicular joint injury, shoulder instability, and bony lesions of the proximal humerus, such as a solitary bone cyst.

Initially, a sling may be indicated if the shoulder is extremely sore, although treatment primarily involves modification of activity. Gradual return to activity can begin within 1 or 2 months, but radiographic resolution may take up to 6 months.[151] Follow-up radiographs

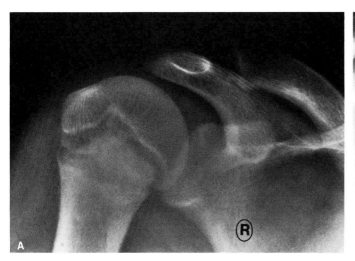
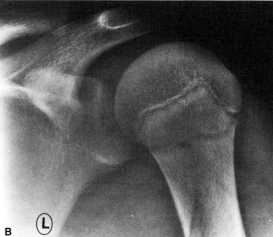

FIGURE 30-2. Radiographs of the proximal humerus in a 14-year-old, right-handed baseball pitcher with shoulder pain that progressed over the final few weeks of the season. (**A**) Widening and irregularity of the physeal plate are present in the right shoulder. (**B**) Radiograph of the left shoulder is provided for comparison.

demonstrate gradual narrowing of the physeal plate. Callus or periosteal new bone may develop.[53] Initially, the athlete should avoid or minimize the precipitating activity, and symptoms should be monitored as sports are resumed. Baseball players can be started in non-pitching positions. Complete elimination of pitching until skeletal maturity is reached probably is not warranted because there are no known sequelae to this condition.[19,53]

Epiphysiolysis of the Distal Radius

Physeal abnormalities of the distal radius have been reported in young female gymnasts.[340] These are most likely stress fractures of the physis. Radiographs demonstrate widening of the growth plate, and there are lucent defects of the adjacent metaphysis and irregularities of the metaphyseal margin (Fig. 30-3).[340,412] Bone scans may be normal.[412] This process resolves with rest, although it may take 3 months or longer for resolution of the radiographic abnormality (Fig. 30-4).[340] Mild cases become asymptomatic in as little as 4 weeks, and there is apparently no growth inhibition or residual deformity.[340,412] However, more severe cases can lead to premature physeal closure of the distal radius.[3] Although the treatment implications of this are not yet clear, prevention and recognition of epiphysiolysis of the distal radius are important.[54]

Apophyseal Conditions

Osgood-Schlatter Disease

In 1903, Osgood and Schlatter separately described the tibial tuberosity disturbance that com-

monly affects active adolescents. Through membranous ossification, the apophysis of the tibial tubercle is formed anterior to the tibial metaphysis. In Osgood-Schlatter disease, there appears to be a partial avulsion of the developing ossification center and overlying hyaline cartilage from the anterior surface of the apophysis.[297]

Patients are usually 10 to 15 years of age at the onset of the disorder, with boys more commonly affected than girls. The lesions typically occur in girls about 2 years earlier than boys.[80,215] Approximately 15% of teenage boys and 10% of teenage girls develop pain in their tibial tubercles.[215] The incidence of bilaterality is 35% to 55% in boys and as low as 18% in girls.[213, 215] The incidence may be as high as 20% in athletic youngsters, compared with 5% in nonathletes.[215] There may be a familial component as well, with an incidence of 20% to 30% among youngsters whose siblings had Osgood-Schlatter disease.[215] Biomechanical malalignment of the lower extremity, including increased quadriceps angle, genu valgum, femoral anteversion, and forefoot pronation, may be a contributing factor.[403] Youths with one of the osteochondroses are likely to develop others; as many as two thirds of athletes with Sever disease later develop symptoms of Osgood-Schlatter disease.[215]

The pain usually is localized to the tibial tubercle, which is often prominent and may have some local swelling. Abnormal findings about the joint itself are absent. Resisted extension of the knee is painful.

The radiographic findings include prominence and irregular ossification of the tibial tubercle (Fig. 30-5A). One or more ossicles may exist. The diagnosis should not rely solely on the x-ray film, because fragmentation of the tibial tubercle may be an asymptom-

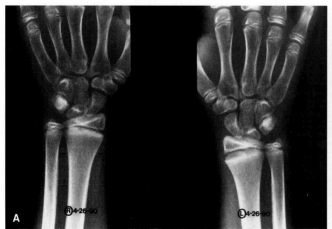
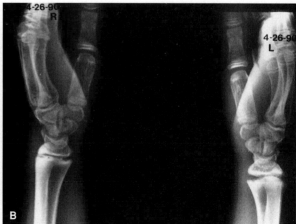

FIGURE 30-3. Bilateral epiphysiolysis of the distal radii in a highly competitive, 11-year-old gymnast. The left is more symptomatic than the right. (**A**) The anteroposterior view shows widening of the left distal radial physis compared with the right. The metaphyseal margins are irregular. (**B**) The lateral view of the wrists shows definite cupping of the distal metaphyses, which is greater on the left than the right.

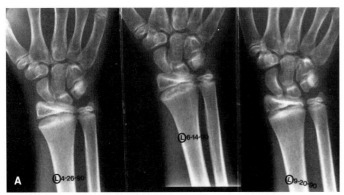

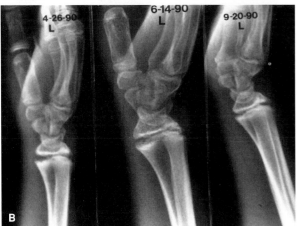

FIGURE 30-4. Sequential radiographs of the patient shown in Figure 30-3. She was asymptomatic 6 weeks after the initial presentation and gradually returned to activities. She remained asymptomatic. The radiographs demonstrate progressive, but incomplete resolution. (**A**) Anteroposterior radiographs were taken at the time of presentation, 6 weeks later, and 5 months after initial presentation. (**B**) Lateral radiographs show gradual resolution of the physeal widening and metaphyseal cupping.

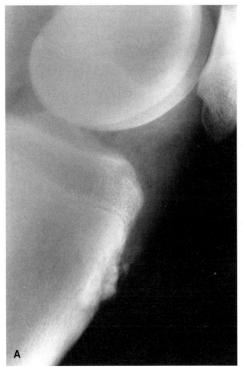

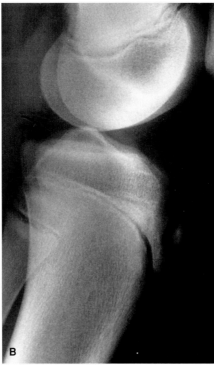

FIGURE 30-5. Osgood-Schlatter disease. (**A**) Typical radiographic findings include a prominence of the tibial tubercle with irregularity of the bone at the insertion of the patellar tendon. (**B**) In some cases, a separate ossicle may form and not unite. If persistently symptomatic, this ossicle may require excision.

atic normal variant. Radiographic blurring of the infra-patellar fat pad has been described and probably results from the associated inflammatory response.[80] Tumor and infection involving the tibial tubercle are rare occurrences but should be considered in the unilateral case. In unilateral cases, radiographs are indicated unless the history is typical of Osgood-Schlatter disease and the findings are directly localized to the tubercle. Radiographs are not usually necessary in bilateral cases. If there is a history of an acute injury, a tibial tubercle fracture may have occurred, and there is the potential of this becoming displaced.[35] Unless the tubercle is elevated or displaced on the radiograph, this diagnosis is made clinically, based on the history and degree of tenderness.

Most symptoms spontaneously resolve with closure of the physeal plate, although as many as 20% of patients have some residual tenderness with kneeling.[213] The treatment is primarily reassurance, symptomatic treatment, and occasional activity modifications. After being assured of the benign nature and self-limited course of this problem, most parents and youngsters are satisfied with tolerating some discomfort during certain activities. Restriction from sports may be necessary to control symptoms. Avulsion of the tibial tubercle associated with Osgood-Schlatter disease has been described in a young athlete.[35] This appears to be a rare complication and probably does not dictate that all young athletes must be curtailed from sports in an attempt to eliminate this risk.

Additional measures that may be helpful for young athletes trying to remain active in sports include ice massage of the tibial tubercle, intermittent NSAIDs, and hamstring stretching. Pads or braces may reduce local trauma, and commercially available straps and knee sleeves appear to help. In view of the risks and unsubstantiated efficacy, steroid injection is not recommended. If a significant biomechanical abnormality such as excessive foot pronation exists, foot orthoses may be helpful.[403] Casts are seldom used because immobilization weakens ligament insertions.[292]

Occasionally, an ossicle and painful bursa forms deep in the tendon, and this remains symptomatic (Fig. 30-5B). If symptoms persist after physeal closure, excision of the ossicle offers simple and successful treatment.[278]

Sinding-Larsen–Johansson Disease

Sinding-Larsen and Johansson independently described a condition in adolescents consisting of painful fragmentation of the patella's inferior pole (Fig. 30-6). Although commonly associated with conditions involving spasticity of the lower extremities, this is commonly seen in healthy, active, and athletic youngsters.[205,335,263] Many analogies are made between this

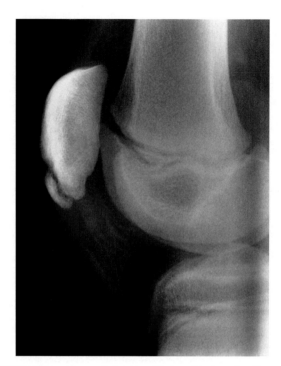

FIGURE 30-6. Larsen-Johannson disease. The lateral radiograph best demonstrates the irregularity at the inferior pole of the patella.

entity and the Osgood-Schlatter lesion, and both processes may occur in the same patient.[263] In the early stages, there may not be radiographically detectable changes in the inferior pole of the patella, and some youngsters with similar clinical findings never develop abnormal calcification. This latter group is often diagnosed with "jumper's knee" or patellar tendinitis, and Sinding-Larsen–Johansson disease may represent a specific variant of this disorder. The cause is presumed to be calcification and ossification at the inferior pole of the patella in response to persistent traction in a growing individual.

The presenting complaints are typically pain in the knee associated with rigorous activities, especially running, climbing stairs, and kneeling. Tenderness is confined to the inferior pole of the patella, with no other significant knee findings. Other conditions that cause inflammation of the fat pad or anterior knee synovium can produce similar findings when the patient is examined with the knee in extension. With 90 degrees of knee flexion, the finding of tenderness at the inferior pole of the patella is more precisely indicative of Sinding-Larsen–Johansson disease or patellar tendinitis. A lateral radiograph of the knee should be able to confirm the presence of a calcified area separated from the patella.

This entity is self-limited. Typically lasting 3 to 12 months, it is shorter in duration than the Osgood-Schlatter condition. Management focuses on reassurance, and for discussion with parents, the term "condition'' may be more appropriate than ''disease.'' Activity modification, ice, and NSAIDs may be helpful. Immobilization is seldom needed, and surgery is not indicated.[263] Restriction from athletics is not absolutely indicated, but activity modifications may reduce symptoms.

Calcaneal Apophysitis

Heel pain in the area of the calcaneal apophysis is a common complaint in young athletes. The age of onset is typically 9 to 14 years of age.[259] The condition is bilateral in 60% to 80% of cases.[274]

This was first described by James Sever in 1912 and is often referred to as ''Sever disease.'' Although histologic analysis is lacking, the clinical condition is an inflammation of the apophyseal growth plate of the calcaneus. It is a self-limited disorder, without documented complications or residual problems. The symptoms resolve after fusion of the apophysis, and treatment is therefore symptomatic. As for the other apophyseal overuse conditions, ice, oral NSAIDs, and activity modification can be helpful. Heal pads or lifts seem to improve symptoms. Cast immobilization may be indicated for the unusual case with severe, unremitting symptoms.[274] For athletes such as gymnasts for whom shoe wear modifications are not practical, taping the heel and arches may provide symptomatic relief.[259]

Apophysitis of the Fifth Metatarsal

Often referred to as Islen disease, apophysitis at the base of the fifth metatarsal is much less common than an apophysitis of the tibial tubercle or calcaneus. Symptoms typically occur in adolescents, who have tenderness of the prominence of the proximal fifth metatarsal without acute trauma. Typically, there is a prominence of the tubercle, soft tissue swelling, and pain with resisted eversion. Oblique radiographic views may show enlargement and irregular ossification of the apophysis.[55,227]

The natural history is apparently benign. Like the unresolved Osgood-Schlatter lesion, a persistently symptomatic ossicle has been described.[55] Treatment is primarily symptomatic, consisting of ice, oral NSAIDs, and reassurance. Arch supports or foot taping may have a role.[227] A cast may be indicated if the symptoms are severe.[55]

Olecranon Apophysitis

Pain at the tip of the olecranon can occur in young athletes and may be associated with ossification irregularity.[84] This is thought to result from repetitive trac-

tion forces[182] or may result from hyperextension impingement, particularly in young gymnasts. Olecranon apophysitis is relatively uncommon.[84] It appears to have a benign natural history and should respond to conservative measures.

Iliac Apophysitis

The iliac crest is one of the less common sites for apophysitis, but it can be troublesome, particularly for young runners.[66,117] Tenderness is localized to the iliac apophysis, and it is often bilateral.[197] Resisted trunk rotation produces pull by the abdominal oblique muscles and reproduces the athlete's pain. This is different from an iliac contusion or hip pointer, because there is no history of direct injury. Osteomyelitis of the ilium typically has symptoms and signs of infection such as fever, malaise, swelling, and warmth, but infection should be considered in the differential diagnosis. Avulsion of the anterior superior iliac spine or anterior inferior iliac spine, Perthes disease, and slipped capital femoral epiphysis should also be considered. Radiographs are negative in iliac apophysitis. It is a self-limited disorder that improves with rest and training modifications.[66,117,197]

Tendinoses

Overuse injuries of tendons and their surrounding sheaths have been classified into three groups by Puddu.[317] Group I tenosynovitis or tenovaginitis is an inflammation of only the paratenon, whether lined by synovium or not. Tendinitis and tenosynovitis often occur together, and it is difficult to differentiate the two clinically. Group II tendinitis is an injury or symptomatic degeneration of the tendon from a resulting inflammatory reaction of the surrounding paratenon. Group III tendinosis involves degeneration of the tendon due to aging, accumulated microtrauma, or both. Although tendinitis is much more common in adults, it is seen in younger athletes. Typically, young athletes have tinosynovitis and occasionally have tendinitis; tendinosis degeneration and tendon rupture is rare.

Achilles Tendinitis

Inflammation of the Achilles tendon is typically localized 2 to 6 cm above the insertion of the tendon into the calcaneus.[225] Contributing factors include overtraining, sudden changes in training, extreme forefoot pronation, poor gastrocnemius-soleus flexibility, and inappropriate training surfaces or shoes.[72,286] Tenderness should be localized to the tendon itself.

The differential diagnosis includes calcaneal apophysitis, retrocalcaneal bursitis, symptomatic pump bumps, and symptomatic os trigonum. Radiographs are usually unnecessary, but they may show minor soft tissue changes.

Treatment in young athletes is almost exclusively nonoperative. Training modification, heel lifts, custom foot orthotics, ice, stretching, and oral NSAIDs are used in combination, depending on the individual circumstances. If an underlying training error is identified, educating the patient and parent about the principles of overuse syndromes is helpful for treatment and prevention of recurrence. Immobilization and surgery are rarely indicated in young individuals.

Popliteus Tendinitis

The popliteus muscle and tendon resist internal rotation of the tibia during gait.[20] Excessive internal rotation and repetitive popliteus function are associated with excessive forefoot pronation during running.[300] This is exacerbated by running on banked surfaces and down hills.[253] As the popliteus tendon courses beneath the fibular collateral ligament, there may be additional irritation of the tendon caused by friction.

Young athletes are particularly prone to tendinitis at the beginning of a sport season, when they are often out of shape, inexperienced and impatient with proper stretching and warm-up exercises. The lateral joint line pain of popliteus tendinitis is typically brought on by activity. Pain may subside during the workout, only to return after practice.

On physical examination, the course of the popliteus tendon along the lateral femoral condyle and beneath the fibular collateral ligament is tender (Fig. 30-7). Sitting cross-legged exacerbates the pain. Joint effusion or ligamentous instability usually is not present.[253] Popliteus tendinitis is occasionally associated with clicking and may simulate a discoid meniscus or iliotibial band friction syndrome. Although typically negative, radiographs should be obtained to exclude any osseous pathology. Occasionally, a small site of ossification is adjacent to the origin of the tendon.[253]

Treatment of popliteus tendinitis consists of "relative rest." This involves diminishing the running component of training and, for the serious athlete, substituting other activities, such as swimming, cycling, pool running, and weight training.[253] NSAIDs and ice massage are helpful. The runner's shoes should be checked for any obvious imbalance related to uneven wear. A foot orthosis may be helpful to control excessive pronation.[239] A graduated, progressive running program with proper warm-up and stretching exercises is begun as symptoms resolve. Steroid injection usually is ineffective for this condition and not recommended in young athletes; steroids are never injected into the tendon itself. Arthroscopy may have a role in excluding other sources of symptoms.

Shin Pain

Shin pain is a common problem in young athletes, accounting for as many as 10% of all athletic complaints.[154,318] These problems can significantly interfere with training and performance, but most forms of shin pain have no long-term sequelae. The term shin splints has been applied to a variety of symptom complexes characterized by exercise-induced pain in the middle part of the leg.[358] Although there may be multi-

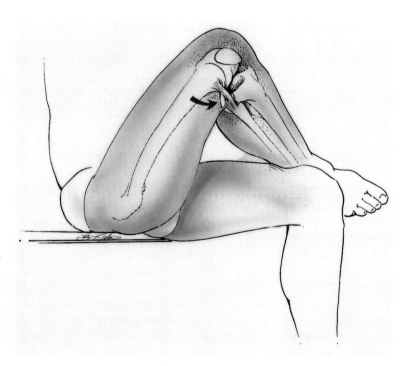

FIGURE 30-7. Popliteus tendinitis is most easily detected with the leg in a figure-four position. The popliteus tendon courses from the proximal tibia to the distal femur, passing beneath the fibular collateral ligament. In this position, the lateral collateral ligament is prominent, and tenderness is elicited along its anterior and posterior margins, where the tendon passes.

ple factors involved in the biology of this problem, periostitis seems to be the most common source of the pain. For the purpose of this discussion, these problems are grouped as periostitis, chronic compartment syndrome, and other causes of shin pain.

Periostitis

Medial tibial stress syndrome, also called the soleus syndrome, is the most common form of periostitis in athletes and is characterized by localized tenderness over the posterior medial edge of the distal third of the tibia.[273,281] About 75% of running athletes with shin pain have posteromedial tenderness.[9] The pain probably results from periostitis, which has been documented histologically and by bone scan.[170,273,281] The soleus muscle and its investing fascia originate in this area and are also implicated in causing the syndrome.[273] These patients do not have elevated posterior compartment pressures, eliminating chronic compartment syndrome as the cause of their pain.[82,281,318]

The pain is bilateral in as many as one half of the cases.[377] Both sexes are equally affected.[281] Predisposing factors include muscle weakness, running shoes with a lack of heel cushion, inadequate arch support, and hard running surfaces. Training errors such as sudden increases in intensity or mileage are common factors.[235] Contributing biomechanical abnormalities include varus hindfoot alignment, excessive forefoot pronation, genu valgum, excessive femoral anteversion, and external tibial torsion.[192]

Initially, the pain is related to activity; later, it persists after the activity is stopped. There is no associated numbness. The history should include the intensity of sports participation, training and competition schedule, any recent change in regimen or shoes, and surface training conditions. The localization of pain, intensity, onset, duration, and any associated numbness are important in the differential diagnosis.

The physical examination should include evaluation of gait, leg lengths, sagittal-plane alignment, rotational abnormalities, muscle laxity or tightness, joint motion, and muscle strength.[234,239] An attempt should be made to localize the painful site. The only significant physical finding is tenderness localized to the margin of the bone. The discovery of a fascial defect, for example, may indicate that the pain is secondary to muscle herniation. A positive Tinel sign indicates sensory nerve compression. Tenderness along the subcutaneous margin of the bone may indicate stress fracture, whereas tenderness over the muscle compartments is suggestive of chronic compartment syndrome.

The differential diagnosis of shin pain should also include stress fractures, sciatica, deep venous thrombosis, popliteal artery entrapment, varicose veins, muscle strain, tumor, and infection.[358] Shin pain in youths should be evaluated for a specific diagnosis, because shin splints are uncommon in patients younger than 15 years of age.[377] Radiographs are likely to be positive if the nonacute symptoms are caused by a tumor or infection. If the radiographs are negative, a bone scan may be needed to rule out more subtle pathology or stress fractures.[170]

Radiographs occasionally show periosteal new bone. When positive, bone scans demonstrate a diffuse longitudinal area of uptake along the bone rather than the transverse pattern characteristic of a stress fracture.[273] Radiographs and bone scans are indicated when there is a clinical suspicion that symptoms and findings are not typical of periostitis.

Regardless of the cause of pain, patients with shin splints and most of those with more specific diagnoses for shin pain often respond to the same fundamental empiric treatment. The first stage of treatment is to diminish inflammation by relative rest, NSAIDs, and the application of ice after activity.[71] An isometric strengthening program can be started early, and the athlete advances to progressive resistance exercises as pain permits. Therapeutic modalities such as ultrasound may help. Crutches may be indicated. Casts are seldom used, but a foot orthosis may be appropriate for the patient with an obvious biomechanical abnormality.[234] The issues of good shoe wear, training surface, and exercise program should be addressed before running is resumed. Rest and shoe modifications may be the most effective components of this program.[9] After the patient is pain free during walking and strengthening exercises, a graduated running program is begun and monitored closely.

If the patient is unresponsive to the usual treatments for shin splints, release of the periosteum localized to the area of pain may provide relief.[273,318] Surgery should be undertaken only after a substantial attempt at nonoperative treatment has failed.[281]

Chronic Compartment Syndromes

In contrast to the acute compartment syndrome that results from trauma or arterial insufficiency, chronic compartment syndromes are induced by exertion, relieved by rest, and seldom result in tissue necrosis or residual disability.[319] The elevated interstitial pressure of chronic compartment syndromes is secondary to inadequacy of the osseofascial compartments to accommodate exercise-induced volume and pressure changes. When compartment pressures exceed capillary filling pressure, the muscle becomes ischemic and produces pain. The anterior compartment is the most commonly involved, although any of the four compartments in the lower leg may be affected.[92]

Typically, the patient complains of aching pain, tightness, or a squeezing sensation brought on by and interfering with athletics.[92] A history of bilateral symptoms should be specifically sought. After unilateral surgical release, patients frequently increase their activity levels, only to develop pain on the side that had been asymptomatic.[92] The pain usually lasts only a short time after exercise. The athlete may experience transient footdrop. Typically, there are paresthesias across the dorsum of the foot with an anterior compartment involvement or plantar paresthesias with chronic posterior compartment syndrome. Fascial defects with muscle herniation may be discernible over the anterior and lateral compartments.[323]

Mubarak pointed out that the symptoms attributed to a chronic deep compartment syndrome frequently are clinically indistinguishable from periostitis.[281] Because the physical findings are nonspecific, the diagnosis is made by measuring compartment pressures.[282] In chronic compartment syndrome, resting pressures typically are not elevated. With exercise, the pressures rise to 70 to 100 mm Hg, while normal compartments rise to less than 30 mm Hg.[319] The degree of compartment pressure elevation correlates with the level of symptoms.[319] All compartments should be assessed because symptoms may not be adequate to identify all involved compartments.

As in any other form of shin pain, initial treatment includes activity modification, orthoses, physical therapy, and time. About one third of patients find these efforts to be helpful.[92] Definitive treatment involves fasciotomy, which can be performed by a variety of techniques. All involved compartments should be released. This can be done through limited skin incisions rather than through the extensive releases suggested for adequate management of the acute compartment syndrome.[92,250,280,332] Care must be taken to protect the saphenous vein, saphenous nerve, and the superficial branch of the peroneal nerve.[332]

A success rate of at least 90% can be expected with surgery. Failure can result from not recognizing preoperatively that multiple compartments can be involved; from inadequate decompression, especially of the deep posterior compartments; and from excessive scar tissue response.[92,332] Few patients require repeat compartment releases.[92,332] Recurrence secondary to excessive scarring is best treated by fasciectomy, although this is not recommended as the primary procedure because it may reduce strength.[92]

Muscle Herniation and Superficial Peroneal Nerve Compression

Styf's series of 90 patients with exercise-induced anterior leg pain included 13 patients with documented compression of the superficial peroneal nerve.[379] Compression of this nerve can be caused by increased muscle pressure within the compartment during exercise. Muscle herniation through a fascial defect, entrapping the nerve, may also produce these symptoms. Patients typically experience diminished sensation over the dorsum of the foot with exertion, and they have point tenderness where the nerve exits the compartment. Nerve conduction velocities can help confirm the diagnosis, but one half are normal at rest and require exercise testing for documentation of this problem.[377]

Ischemia of the entrapped tissue in cases of muscle herniation has been theorized to cause shin pain during activity. This may occur in as many as 60% of chronic compartment syndromes.[323]

Limited fasciotomy is performed for persistently symptomatic peroneal nerve compression or muscle herniation. Specific attention should be directed to the exit point of the superficial peroneal nerve to ensure it is free.[279]

Iliotibial Band Friction Syndrome

Iliotibial band friction syndrome is an overuse phenomenon caused by the iliotibial tract rubbing over the lateral epicondylar prominence during repetitive knee motion.[200,324] Although most commonly seen in adult distance runners, adolescents involved in recreational and team sports also can be affected.[379] Iliotibial band friction syndrome is more common in males and often is associated with physical findings of genu varum, external tibial torsion, pes planovalgus, and pes cavus.[171,288,377,379]

Symptoms typically commence at the beginning of a sports training season. Two thirds of cases are associated with a recent increase in running intensity or distance.[288] The athlete complains of pain over the lateral aspect of the knee, especially during running or cycling, and the pain occurs with every knee flexion.[171] Usually, there is no history of injury or mechanical symptoms such as locking or catching. Slight swelling may occur if a bursitis develops, but there usually is no joint effusion. Tenderness extends from the lateral epicondyle to the joint line from the anterior to posterior margins of the condyle. Frequently, there is a contraction of the iliotibial band that can be detected by the Ober test (Fig. 30-8). This maneuver reproduces pain and demonstrates restricted motion.[289] Radiographs are normal.

The differential diagnosis includes lateral meniscus tear, discoid lateral meniscus, stress fracture, popliteus tendinitis, biceps femoris tendinitis, and patellofemoral pain syndrome.[246] These usually can be differentiated by careful history and physical examination.

Initial treatment involves relative rest or a change in training habits, ice massage, NSAIDs, and a rigorous iliotibial band stretching program.[171,246,301] This condi-

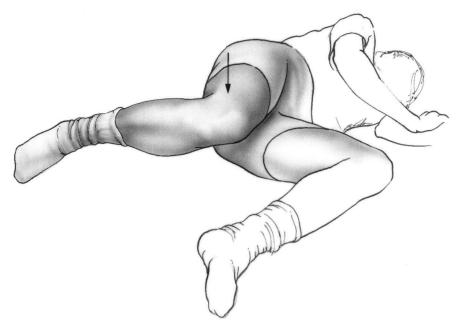

FIGURE 30-8. The Ober test is used to detect tightness of the iliotibial band. With a patient lying on his or her side, the hip is first abducted and extended with the knee held flexed. The test is then performed by attempting to adduct the knee to the midline. Palpation along the lateral femoral epicondyle typically elicits tenderness at this site if iliotibial band friction exists.

tion may take 6 weeks or more to resolve.[324,379] Foot orthoses are often helpful, particularly if an alignment abnormality exists. Extraarticular steroid injection may help recalcitrant cases.[288] In young athletes, surgical release of the distal iliotibial band and excision of the bursa rarely are required.[171,246]

Breaststroker's Knee

Competitive breaststroke swimmers are prone to develop medial knee pain along the course of medial collateral ligament, medial facet of the patella, and the plica.[376,395] The whip kick technique, which is a more powerful modification of the frog kick, has certain variations that are strongly implicated in the cause.[376] This condition may begin in the first few years of competitive swimming and may occur in swimmers as young as 6 years of age,[376] although the frequency is related to increasing age of the swimmer, increasing years of competitive swimming, increasing breaststroke training distance, and decreasing warm-up time.[339] Other than medial knee tenderness, there are no other consistently associated physical or radiographic findings.

Initially, the symptoms are reversible with rest or training alterations, although with time, chondromalacia and medial facet patellar arthritis may occur.[339,376,395] Measures to quiet inflammation of the medial plica, such as ice, NSAIDs, and phonophoresis, may help.[339] Most important is altering the swimmer's whip kick technique, particularly by keeping the legs together during the recovery and rapid extension phase of kicking.[376] Because arthroscopy usually shows medial synovitis without other significant derangements, it is only occasionally indicated.[207]

Valgus Overload Injuries of the Elbow

For elbow injuries, the most commonly involved athletes are baseball players (particularly pitchers), gymnasts, American football quarterbacks, and potentially other throwing athletes.[357,386] These activities can lead to a variety of abnormalities of the capitellum, radial head, and medial epicondyle.[45] These result from excessive and repetitive compression forces through the radiocapitellar joint and tension across the medial epicondyle and collateral ligaments, which are collectively referred to as *Little League elbow*. During the throwing motion, these stresses are induced by the significant valgus moment generated at the elbow (Fig. 30-9).

Osteochondral Lesions of the Capitellum

Lesions of the capitellum can be divided into three groups: Panner disease, osteochondrosis of the capitellum, and acute traumatic osteochondral fractures.

Panner described a lesion of a young boy's capitellum that he compared with Legg-Calvé-Perthes disease.[306] In children younger than 10 years of age who have Panner disease, the course is usually benign.[360,408] The entire ossific nucleus of the capitellum may demonstrate irregular ossification, but an osteochondral loose body does not form. The lesion completely resolves with reconstitution of the capitellum.

Adolescent baseball pitchers and gymnasts can develop fragmentation of the capitellum's subchondral bone and dislodgment of the articular surface. Based on the belief that a low-grade inflammatory process was responsible, Franz Konig called this condition osteochondritis dissecans. Histologically, there

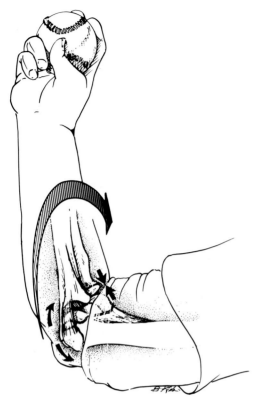

FIGURE 30-9. Pitching produces a valgus moment (*large curved arrow*) at the elbow. There are compressive forces (*straight arrows*) across the radiocapitellar joint and tension (*curved arrows*) across the medial epicondyle and medial collateral ligament.

are no inflammatory cells present, and the term osteochondrosis seems more appropriate.[261,357]

Osteochondral fractures of the elbow can occur from a direct blow or a forceful movement. The onset is acute, and the treatment principles are those of any intraarticular fracture.[6]

The causes of Panner disease and osteochondrosis of the capitellum are unknown. The two entities may represent the same process in persons of different ages, but the course and prognosis contrast sufficiently to consider the disorders separately. Heredity may be a factor.[357,386] Repetitive microtrauma frequently occurs in throwing athletes, and disturbance of the blood supply has also been implicated. By 8 years of age, the capitellum's vascularity is solely from a group of end vessels.[152] These vessels traverse the chondroepiphysis from posteriorly, with no significant collateral contribution. On closure of the physis, the blood supply of the epiphysis and metaphysis becomes interconnected.[357]

Patients with Panner disease and osteochondrosis of the capitellum typically complain of pain with throwing. Tenderness is maximal over the radiocapitellar joint, and there may be crepitus. The elbow typically lacks 10 to 20 degrees of full extension, and flexion is mildly limited.[261,408]

Initial assessment should include bone detail radiographs with anteroposterior, lateral, and oblique views. There is irregular ossification of the capitellum and rarefaction within a crater (Fig. 30-10A).[392,408] Tomograms or computed tomography (CT) scans are occasionally helpful to better define bony pathology (Fig. 30-10B). Loose bodies may be present. Arthrograms are unreliable for cartilaginous loose bodies, because filling defects related to synovial convolutions can lead to false-positive studies. False-negative results can occur if the loose bodies are completely enveloped by synovium or hidden in joint space recesses.[261]

Initial treatment should include restriction of forceful upper extremity activities, application of ice, and NSAIDs. A sling or splint is occasionally needed.[386] It may take 6 or more weeks for the pain to subside,

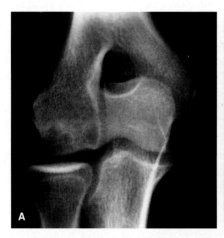
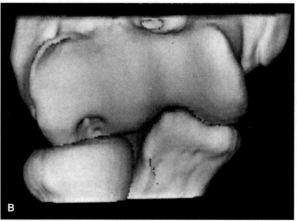

FIGURE 30-10. Osteochondral lesion of the capitellum in a 15-year-old baseball player with a painful elbow. (**A**) The subchondral plate of the capitellum appears intact. Subchondral cysts are present. (**B**) The computed tomography scan with three-dimensional reconstruction demonstrates the bony defect of the capitellum, including loss of the subchondral plate in that area.

at which time range of motion and strengthening exercises are begun.

After almost full and pain-free range of motion with good strength is achieved, a graduated and well-supervised program for returning to upper extremity activity is initiated. Throwing technique should be reviewed to minimize unnecessary valgus load to the elbow. Particularly stressful moves or "tricks" are modified from a gymnast's workout. The prognosis for return to competitive pitching, however, is guarded.[386,408] Baseball players should be switched to a position, such as the infield, that requires less throwing.

The athlete is monitored for recurrent symptoms. Radiographs may remain abnormal, and symptoms are followed closely. Activities are gradually advanced and readjusted if pain recurs.[357] Persistent difficulty should prompt further investigation for a loose body or a chondral flap in the articular cartilage. In this situation, given the indeterminate reliability of CT and magnetic resonance imaging (MRI), arthroscopy may be the most prudent next diagnostic step and offers the advantage of being potentially therapeutic.

Indications for surgery include a locked elbow, a symptomatic intraarticular loose body, or failure of nonoperative program to adequately diminish pain and restore motion.[261,386] Whether open or arthroscopic surgery is performed, loose bodies should be searched for carefully.[146] Flaps of articular cartilage from the surface are debrided, because loose chondral fragments produce synovial inflammation.[64] Bone grafting and internal fixation of the fragment are rarely indicated, because most procedures other than simple excision have been unfavorable in the elbow.[386,408] Drilling of the base of the defects may stimulate a fibrocartilaginous response, but the advantage of this over simple debridement of the lesion is not well documented.[386]

The prognosis for the more advanced lesions is less favorable. After surgery, many athletes are unable to resume their prior levels of competitive throwing.[261,386] The most important lesson about this condition is the opportunity for prevention. Junior baseball programs should all have rules limiting the duration that a youngster pitches. Typically, this is a maximum of 3 innings per game and up to 6 innings per week. Training and practice are difficult to regulate, making it essential to educate parents, coaches, and physicians.

Osteochondral Lesions of the Radial Head

Osteochondral lesions of the radial head are much less common than those of the capitellum.[2,390] Most patients are boys between 8 and 15 years of age.[390] Because repetitive valgus loading occurs, the mechanical stress of throwing is implicated as the cause. Because osteochondrosis of the radial head is an uncommon problem, it may be part of a more generalized disorder.[390] Radiographs should be obtained of the other elbow, and if abnormal, a radiographic survey should be done of the other major joints. The treatment principles are similar to those for symptomatic lesions of the capitellum.

Injuries of the Medial Epicondyle

Traction on the medial elbow structures is the counterpart to radiocapitellar compression during valgus stress. With excessive throwing, the medial epicondyle may become prominent and intermittently painful. Active adolescent baseball players frequently develop accelerated growth, and widening of the medial epicondylar apophysis with fragmentation of the medial apophysis sometimes occurs.[2] The prognosis is excellent, with the pain usually resolving after rest.[360]

Avulsion of the medial epicondyle can occur with forceful throwing. This results from the tension forces exerted by the ulnar collateral ligament and the pull of the forearm flexor muscles. If the elbow is stable and the fragment is minimally displaced, the elbow is immobilized for 3 weeks, after which range of motion is begun, and the athlete is gradually returned to activity.

Displaced fractures should be repaired. Elbow instability can be disabling to throwing athletes, wrestlers, and gymnasts.[407] If there is question of valgus instability, a stress radiograph should be obtained.[401] A positive study should prompt surgical repair of the medial epicondyle fracture in athletes who depend on upper extremity activity. Other standard indications for internal fixation include intraarticular incarceration of the fragment and ulnar nerve dysfunction.[401]

SPORTS TRAUMA

Epidemiology

The number of youth sports participants, the amount of coaching, the intensity of training, and the level of competition are increasing. In 1981, there were approximately 35 million nonschool sports participants in the United States between 6 and 18 years of age, with 5 million involved in high school sports.[247] Injuries are inevitable, and parents often seek advice regarding the risk of injury from sports participation, particularly contact sports. Most trauma in children occurs from activities such as running, tree climbing, and skate boarding.[63] Organized sports account for only about one third of sports injuries, with the remainder occurring in physical education classes and nonorganized sports.[217,414]

In youths 5 to 14 years of age, the sports related to the most total injuries, in order of frequency, are football, baseball, basketball, gymnastics, other ball sports, soccer, wrestling, volleyball, and ice hockey.[139,343] When injury data are adjusted for the number of participant hours, the general trend is for American football to be the highest-risk sport, followed by basketball, gymnastics, soccer, and baseball.[63] Injuries occur most frequently in contact sports. Each year, as many as 20% to 40% of high school football players are injured; however, about 75% of these injuries are minor, resulting in a loss of fewer than 7 days of participation.[315,316,385] The risk of injury in sports must also be weighed against the risk in normal activities. As many as one third of junior sports participants are sidelined by injuries they sustained outside of their sports program.[333]

Although it may seem that the younger child is at greater risk in contact sports, the converse is true, with fewer injuries occurring among younger athletes. Soccer, for instance, results in injuries to about 3% of players in elementary school, 7% in junior high school, and 11% in high school.[365,378] In junior American football programs (9–15 years of age), the incidence of injury is only 2%. Of an estimated 463,000 football-related injuries treated in 1980, 37% occurred in 5- to 14-year-old children, and 63% occurred in athletes 15 years of age and older.[343]

Contusions, sprains, and simple fractures of the upper extremity account for most injuries in younger athletes.[217,260] Teenagers have more lower extremity trauma, with the knee injuries being common and the knee reinjury rate being as high as 25% to 60%.[88,312,315,316] Most injuries are mild, with about 10% resulting in hospitalization, 15% requiring minor procedures, and 2% needing reconstructive surgery.[217,260]

Tragic injuries do occur occasionally in youth sports. The U.S. Consumer Product Safety Commission reported that almost 1.8 million sports-related, medically attended injuries occurred in 5- to 14-year-old children from 1973 through 1980. Of these, 93 were fatalities. Baseball accounted for 40 deaths, with most related to bat or ball blows to the chest or head. Football resulted in 19 fatalities, almost all secondary to head and neck injuries. Surprisingly, golf was related to 13 deaths, with 11 children being struck by clubs and 2 with balls. Many of these children were not actually participating in golf at the time; they were struck by an adult who was playing or by a playmate. Eight children were killed by equipment falling on them, including four soccer goals, two football goal posts, one baseball backstop, and one trampoline.[343]

Prevention

Although the prevention of all injuries related to sports participation is not realistic, the rate and severity of injuries can be reduced. Many sports injuries can be avoided or ameliorated with conscientious supervision, appropriate rules, safe equipment, and adequate rehabilitation of injuries.[137,414] Stretching and warm-up exercises are key components of injury prevention,[354,394] although the scientific basis of these standard training techniques are just starting to be understood.[369,381] Because there is significant individual variation in body types, accurate and specific advice is still evolving.[141,283,394] A preseason conditioning program consisting of warm-up, stretching, running, weight training, and skill development appears to have a positive impact on preventing injuries, especially in collision and contact sports.[52]

Medical evaluations are commonly required before young athletes are allowed to participate in sporting programs, particularly on the interscholastic level. This is often done through a preparticipation screening evaluation. The principle is to identify young athletes at high risk for sports-related injuries or illness. Unfortunately, there is no consensus of opinion regarding the components of an optimal screening program.[341] The yield of identifying disqualifying conditions is low on initial sports screening examinations and becomes even lower on repeated examination.[136,229] Although the cost of doing such screening may appear minimal at first look, unnecessary exclusions and referrals can result in a significant health care cost.[327]

To produce a favorable cost-benefit ratio, the screening process must focus on the relevant history and physical components. Medical history is the most sensitive and specific component. The history should include prior musculoskeletal injury, neurologic injury, infectious disease, and cardiopulmonary problems. Questions related to general health, immunization status, hospitalizations, and limitations of function are helpful. Athletes should be specifically asked about prior history of concussion, unconsciousness, paryesthesias, and prior musculoskeletal treatment or rehabilitation.[341] Syncope can be an important clue to undetected heart disease, specifically idiopathic hypertrophic subaortic stenosis, which is one of the most common causes of sudden death in young athletes.[242] Despite conscientious screening, this uncommon but tragic event is not completely preventable. Athletes and parents should always be informed that screening cannot ensure detection and prevention of all injuries.

The general medical examination should include blood pressure measurement, cardiopulmonary examination, and review for any contagious skin lesions.[31] Ideally, a dynamic evaluation of recovery after exercise should be performed, but this is usually impractical.[375]

The musculoskeletal examination should focus on prior injuries and any residual problems from them.

Inadequate rehabilitation probably accounts for almost one fourth of sports-related injuries in children.[137] A screening examination of the ankles, knees, and neck range of motion should be included for all athletes, and other areas of the musculoskeletal system examined based on the individual's prior history.

Evaluation of athletic performance, joint laxity, and visual acuity are optional components. Otoscopy, ophthalmoscopy. and hernia evaluations are probably unnecessary. Routine laboratory testing does not appear to be cost effective.[136,229,341]

Athletic Trainers

Athletic trainers have been caring for sports injuries since ancient times. The education, ability, and role of athletic trainers have evolved considerably since the founding of the National Athletic Trainers' Association in 1950. These allied health professional have rigorous credentialing requirements. They can provide valuable help in recognition, initial management, triage, prevention, and rehabilitation of athletic injuries. Used effectively, athletic trainers are liaisons between physicians and athletes and provide important educational information for athletes, partners, and coaches.

Although they are widely used for college and professional sports programs, it is estimated that only about 10% of the United States high schools have certified athletic trainers.[315] An estimated 636,000 injuries occur annually among American high school football players. Half of these occur during practice, when physician medical coverage is seldom available.[315] Many injuries can be prevented through safe equipment, proper supervision, appropriate instruction, training, and injury rehabilitation.[137,343,414] To take advantage of this opportunity, the involvement of certified athletic trainers in high school and other youth sports programs should be strongly encouraged.

Types of Injuries and Treatment

Ankle Sprains

Ankle sprains are among the most common injuries in sports. They occur in approximately 6% of all high school sports participants and as many as 70% of all high school basketball players annually.[131,188,364] Most ankle sprains involve the lateral ligaments. Approximately 3% of sprains are medial, with wrestling being the only sport that is associated with a significant number of these.[40,131] Inversion and supination injuries sequentially tear the anterior ankle capsule, the anterior talofibular ligament, and the calcaneofibular ligament.[79,94] Although most ankle sprains are minor, one third of these injuries lead to more than 2 weeks of disability.[364] For severe ankle sprains, a minimal intervention approach is not universally favorable, and treatment can have a positive impact.[370]

For the purpose of this discussion, the following classification is used:

Grade I: mild sprains involve stretching and minimal interstitial tearing of the ligament, with little swelling, limp, and disability.

Grade II: moderate sprains involve partial disruption of the ligaments, with modest swelling, diffuse tenderness, and difficulty with weight bearing.

Grade III: severe sprains result in complete ligament disruption, often with extensive bleeding swelling, instability, and disability.

Knowing the mechanism of injury can be helpful. Anterior tibiofibular sprains typically result from a dorsiflexion injuries, but the more common lateral ligament complex sprain usually results from an inversion injury. Recollection of a popping sensation varies, but a history of prior ankle injuries is important for the assessment of acute or chronic instability.

If the patient is first seen after considerable swelling has developed, it may be difficult to localize the tenderness. Examination of the acute injury should be directed toward pinpointing the maximally tender structures. The entire length of the tibia and fibula should be inspected, with specific attention to the area of the physeal plates. Gentle percussion of the physis and epiphysis by the examiner's fingertip is a useful technique for differentiating physeal fractures from ankle sprains. A more reliable assessment of tenderness and stability can often be achieved after several days of rest, ice, elevation, and compression.

The anterior drawer maneuver primarily tests the stability of the anterior talofibular ligament complex. This can be performed by securing the distal leg with one hand and applying an anterior pull on the heel with the foot held in gentle plantar flexion (Fig. 30-11A). Alternatively, with the patient supine on a table and with the knees flexed about 90 degrees, a posterior force is applied to the lower leg while the foot is held flat on the table top (Fig. 30-11B).

Routine views of the ankle should include anteroposterior, lateral, and "mortise" views. Clinical judgment ultimately dictates the decision to obtain radiographs. For adults, tenderness along the posterior edge of malleoli or inability to bear weight are reliable indicators to prompt ankle radiography. Tenderness over the navicular, cuboid, and base of the fifth metatarsal should prompt additional views of the foot.[373] Although not as well studied in youths, similar criteria probably apply.

The indication for other studies depends on the index of suspicion for injury and treatment philosophy. Anteroposterior or lateral view stress radiographs can be obtained.[346] Unfortunately, the reliability is affected by individual variation, timing, muscle spasm, the patient's pain tolerance, foot position, and variabil-

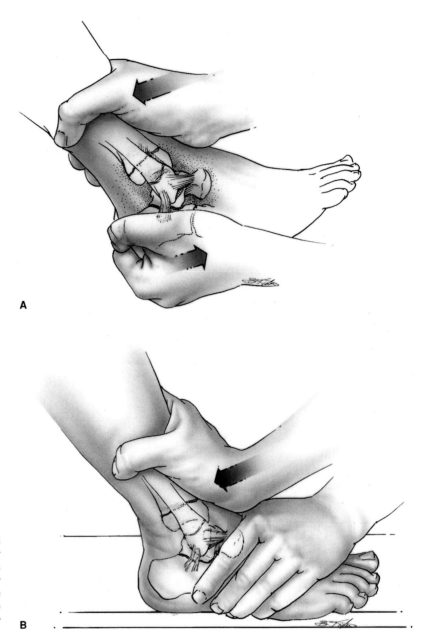

A

FIGURE 30-11. The ankle drawer test is used to evaluate stability of the anterior talofibular ligament. (**A**) The heel is pulled anteriorly with the foot held in gentle plantar flexion. Counter force is applied at the tibia. (**B**) Alternatively, the foot is held firmly on a table top, with the hip and knee flexed at 90 degrees, and posterior force is applied to the lower leg.

B

ity of manual technique.[116] Even with an apparatus and local anesthesia, the overlap between normal and abnormal is considerable.[148] Ankle arthrography can reliably detect anterior talofibular and calcaneal fibular injuries, although the clinical relevance is unproven.[320]

Because tarsal coalitions are associated with ankle sprains, oblique views of the foot may be indicated. The presence of tarsal coalition increases the athlete's risk for recurrence, but it is probably not an indication for resection of the bar.[365]

The primary differential diagnoses include physeal fracture of the distal fibula, triplane fracture, osteochondral fracture of the talus, subluxation of the peroneal tendons, fracture of the base of the fifth metatarsal, sprains of the midfoot ligaments, and Maison-

neuve fracture.[79] Accessory ossification centers at the tip of the medial and lateral malleoli in youths should not be confused with avulsion fractures.[296] Localization of maximal tenderness and radiographs can differentiate most of these. Nondisplaced Salter-Harris type I physeal fractures of the distal fibula is the most commonly occurring problem that closely imitates an ankle sprain. Fingertip percussion over the physeal plate usually differentiates the two by being distinctly positive for a fracture. If doubt remains, immobilizing the ankle in a cast for 3 weeks can adequately treat the fracture, and it is usually not significant overtreatment of a sprain.

Although treatment of ankle sprains varies considerably, a few sound principles have evolved.[204] Sprains are initially treated with ice, compression, immobilization, and elevation. The goal of the initial treatment is to limit bleeding, edema, and any further soft tissue injury. Ideally, these occur at the time and site of injury. After the degree of injury is determined, an appropriate course is planned. Each progressive step of the rehabilitation is based on functional goals rather than an arbitrary calendar.[130]

A grade I sprain is a minor injury. The pain usually resolves and motion returns in 1 week.[188] Satisfactory strength of all muscle groups, particularly the peroneals, must be restored to ensure dynamic protection from a repeat injury. Proprioceptive training may be helpful as well.[391] The athlete must have minimal pain and be able to run, cut, and perform specific tasks relevant to the activity to which he or she is about to return. In some cases, the athlete may be able to return immediately to competition.

Supporting the ankle by taping, a laced stabilizer, or a semirigid orthosis facilitates early return and diminishes the risk of recurrent injury.[144,338] Taping restricts extremes of ankle motion and shortens reaction time of the peroneal muscles, probably by affecting the proprioceptive function of the ankle.[201] The lace stabilizers and semirigid orthotics may offer an advantage over tape, which loosens after a short period of exercise.[221,321,338]

Grade II sprains involve more extensive tissue injury and result in an average of 2 weeks of disability.[188] Crutches are often helpful for several days as weight bearing is progressively increased. For the athlete concerned about an early return to sports, early phases of a supervised rehabilitation program should be directed toward diminishing the swelling and regaining motion. Initially, ice pack and intermittent compression boots are useful modalities.[168] Isometric exercises are started immediately, and progressive resistance exercises are subsequently introduced.

For the serious athlete, aerobic conditioning is continued during rehabilitation by swimming, using an upper body ergometer, running in a pool, or cycling. With minor adjustments, upper body weight conditioning can be continued. The use of ankle supports in grade II sprains is the same as that for a grade I sprain.

Treatment of grade III sprains remains the most controversial.[36] Options include taping, casting, and surgical repair. Tape and immediate motion theoretically minimize stiffness. Treatment with a dorsiflexion cast reduces the talus in the mortise and theoretically reapproximates the torn ligament fibers to their premorbid location.[364] Advocates of surgical treatment feel that other soft tissues may prevent anatomic reduction of the torn ligament fibers, especially if there is an associated bony fragment. Most series reporting surgical outcomes report no difference[108] or fail to provide an adequate control group[370] to demonstrate a clear superiority of surgery over immobilization and ther-

apy protocols.[39] Few reports provide an adequate control group to demonstrate a clear superiority of one treatment approach over another.

I prefer to treat grade III sprains initially with a posterior plaster mold and compression dressing. This controls the initial hemorrhage and swelling. In 7 to 10 days, as swelling starts to resolve, the patient is placed in an articulated ankle orthosis.[163] This permits plantar flexion and dorsiflexion but protects against inversion and eversion. An intermittent compression boot device is used to reduce residual swelling. Weight bearing is progressed as tolerated. The rehabilitation program is advanced as outlined for grades I and II sprains. The orthosis is used continuously for 8 weeks. The athlete may return to competition wearing the device if pain-free motion and adequate strength have been regained. This typically occurs 4 weeks after injury.[163]

Recurrent severe sprains occasionally lead to chronic ligamentous laxity. A variety of reconstructive procedures are available but are uncommonly needed in youths.[65,368] Results of delayed reconstruction are comparable to primary surgical repair, further supporting the approach of nonoperative treatment of most ankle sprains, particularly in young athletes.[59]

Anterolateral Ankle Impingement

After ankle sprains, chronic anterolateral ankle pain occasionally develops because of impingement of the anterior inferior tibiofibular ligament or the synovium in that area.[21,265] Tenderness is localized along the anterolateral corner of the joint. Some patients experience popping with dorsiflexion of the ankle. Radiographs are normal, and the efficacy of MRI is yet unproven. Rest, immobilization, NSAIDs, and physical therapy modalities can be tried to reduce the symptoms.[255] If pain persists, arthroscopic debridement of the reactive synovium and resection of the inferior fibers of the tibiofibular ligament should resolve the problem.[21,265]

Distal Tibiofibular Sprains

Isolated injuries of the distal tibiofibular syndesmosis are uncommon but need to be recognized.[120] These may be associated with injury of the deltoid ligament. Pain and tenderness are located principally at the anterior aspect of the syndesmosis and interosseous membrane. Tenderness is elicited by squeezing the tibia and fibula together and by dorsiflexing and dorsally rotating the foot at the ankle.[173,372] Radiographs occasionally demonstrate an osseous avulsion. The CT scan and bone scan are occasionally helpful in demonstrating occult degrees of injury to the tibiofibular ligament complex.[248]

Sprains of the distal tibiofibular ligament and syndesmosis are usually treated nonoperatively with rehabilitation principles similar to those for lateral complex sprains.[106] The athlete should be aware that the recovery process is typically twice as long as for a severe ankle sprain.[173] Impingement of the ankle joint created by disrupted fibers can cause chronic pain.[21] In rare circumstances, immediate surgical repair or reconstruction of the syndesmosis becomes necessary. If there is significant diastasis, surgical correction may be necessary.[106]

Collateral Ligament Injuries of the Knee

The collateral ligaments of the knee originate from the distal femoral epiphysis and insert into the proximal tibial epiphysis, with the exception of the superficial portion of the medial collateral ligament, which inserts into the proximal tibial metaphysis distal to the physeal plate (Fig. 30-12).[89] Because the ligaments are generally stronger than the physeal plates, significant bending injuries usually produce physeal fractures. Pure ligament disruption can occur in children, and complete rupture of the medial collateral ligament has been reported in children as young as 4 years of age.[37,68,196] The results after these injuries are apparently the same in children and adults.

The grading of collateral ligament sprains requires comparison of the injured with the uninjured knee, because the normal degree of laxity varies. A mild sprain (grade I) has little or no disruption of the ligament's mechanical integrity and no increased laxity. Moderate sprains (grade II) result in plastic deformation of the ligament without complete disruption; the examination demonstrates increased laxity, but there is a distinct endpoint. Severe sprains (grade III) are complete ligament disruptions resulting in significant laxity and having no distinct endpoint.[25]

Because the history of injury obtained from youngsters is often poor, the examination must be relied on heavily. Often tenderness can be localized to the physeal plate or to the path of the collateral ligaments themselves. The collateral ligaments are tested with the knee flexed 20 to 30 degrees to relax the posterior capsule and posterior cruciate ligament.[177] The joint line should be palpated while varus and then valgus stresses are applied. If there is instability, a stress radiograph must be obtained to differentiate opening of the joint space due to severe sprain from motion through the bone due to an unstable physeal fracture. Standard radiographs are obtained to look for physeal fractures or bony avulsions. If an effusion is present in the knee, it can be aspirated, and the area can be

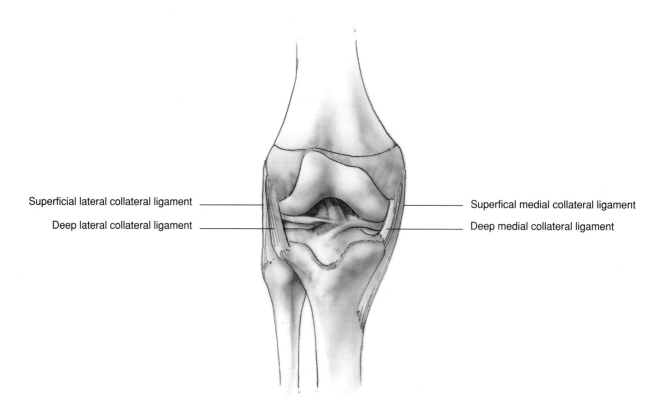

Superficial lateral collateral ligament

Deep lateral collateral ligament

Superfical medial collateral ligament

Deep medial collateral ligament

FIGURE 30-12.   The collateral ligaments of the knee insert into the epiphyses, with the important exception of the distal insertion of the superficial medial collateral ligament. Bending injuries of the immature knee typically disrupt the physeal plates, which are usually the "weak link in the chain."

infused with a local anesthetic to facilitate the examination. Rarely, examination under anesthesia becomes necessary, especially for the uncooperative child.

If hemarthrosis is detected, a cruciate ligament injury should be suspected. Unstable physeal fractures can mimic a severe-grade collateral ligament sprain. Stable physeal fractures may imitate lesser sprains, and the stress radiograph may be normal or show only subtle changes. When in doubt, the knee should be splinted for 1 week and then reevaluated. If there is persistent tenderness at the physeal plate, the problem is assumed to be a physeal fracture, and the extremity is immobilized for 3 to 4 weeks. If there is significant doubt about the clinical findings, a bone scan may help by showing increased uptake of radionuclide in the injured physis.

Isolated collateral ligament sprains in the knee are treated according to the degree of injury and by the same principles that are established for adults. Definitive studies of collateral ligament sprains in children are not available. All partial tears are treated nonoperatively. Most sprains are immobilized only until pain subsides.[292] Sports are resumed when there is full motion, good muscle strength, and ability to run, cut, and perform necessary sport-specific activities.[25,293,371] The use of these functional criteria is particularly helpful for the adolescent athlete who is anxious to return to sports. Grade I sprains result in an average of 10 days lost from activities, and grade II sprains average 20 days.[91] Advising the adolescent athlete to refrain from sports for a sustained period after one of these injuries can be a problem if the recovery is underestimated, because they often tolerate disappointment poorly.

Although a few studies have suggested operative treatment for grade III collateral ligament sprains of the knee, isolated injuries in adults appear to have good clinical results without surgery.[111,119,183] Successful nonoperative treatment is predicated on establishing that the grade III sprain is isolated. If concomitant meniscal tears or an anterior cruciate disruption is present, surgical repair is recommended.

Because of the opportunity for anatomic restoration and bone-to-bone healing, displaced bony avulsions of the collateral ligaments are best managed operatively.[68] Double upright hinged functional braces provide medial stability and therefore have a logical role in the protection of healing medial collateral ligament sprains.[13]

Anterior Cruciate Ligament Injuries

Anterior cruciate ligament (ACL) injuries occur far less commonly in children than in adults. Throughout adolescence and young adulthood, these injuries be-come more frequent. The principles of evaluation and treatment are very similar to those used for adults although the specifics must take into account the open physes and high activity level of youngsters.

In children, the collagen fibers of the ACL blend from ligament to perichondrium to epiphyseal cartilage. Adult ligaments insert directly into bone by means of the Sharpey fibers.[251] This difference probably accounts for the childhood tibial eminence avulsion fracture, which usually spares the ligament itself, although interstitial tears of the ligament can occur in children. Midsubstance disruption has been reported in a 3-year-old child.[396] Avulsion of a bony fragment from the femoral attachments occurs less often and rarely from both ends of the ligament.[104,330] Avulsion from the distal insertion through the chondral-bony interface also can occur.

An ACL injury can easily be overlooked in the treatment of a physeal fracture about the knee. The presence of a physeal fracture does not preclude ligament damage. Fractures of the distal femoral and proximal tibial physes have a significant incidence of associated ligament injuries.[28]

Meniscal tears are commonly associated with ACL sprains.[85,291] Evaluation of the menisci by arthrography or MRI can be useful, particularly if nonoperative treatment is being considered.[295]

The history of injury in the adolescent is usually one of hyperextension, direct blow, or sudden twisting in the open field or court. Occasionally, a pop is heard, and the early onset of swelling due to hemarthrosis is common.[291] The younger child is typically a poor historian of the event. As in tibial eminence fractures, bicycle accidents commonly cause ACL injuries in children.[287,329] The amount of initial pain is variable, with discomfort lasting over the ensuing days. Instability may be noticed if the youngster attempts to return to play.

The physical examination typically reveals effusion, diffuse tenderness, and limited motion. Although the anterior drawer test has been the classic test of anterior cruciate stability, the Lachman test and pivot-shift signs are felt to be more sensitive and specific.[112,128,177,243] Instrumented knee laxity testing is useful if the physical examination is equivocal.[299] The degree of inherent or congenital laxity must be considered in grading these tests, particularly for children. The other knee can usually provide a control against which the injured extremity is compared.

Routine anteroposterior and lateral radiographs of the knee are obtained to look for osteochondral fractures and physeal fractures. A tunnel view may show bony fragments avulsed from the femoral origins of the cruciate ligament. A hypoplastic intercondylar notch with a diminished tibial spine is a sign of congenital absence of the cruciate ligaments.[193,384]

MRI is fairly reliable for identifying injuries of the ligaments, menisci, and cancellous bone. Because most clinically significant ACL injuries are adequately diagnosed by history and manual examination, the indications for MRI must be weighed against its cost.[32,189,314] Imaging studies should only be ordered if management decisions will be influenced by the results. MRI is particularly useful if the presence of an associated injury, such as a meniscal tear, is going to influence the decision to operate. If a reconstruction is already decided on, the menisci can be evaluated at the time of arthroscopy.

The natural history of ACL tears in adults depends on patient age, activity level, expectations, degree of instability, ability to rehabilitate muscle strength, and the patient's resolve to modify activities as needed.[67,113,158,257] Similarly, the decision to stabilize a young person's knee must be individualized, and the risk of reinjury leading to subsequent damage of the menisci should be given strong consideration.[169]

Left unstabilized, complete ACL disruption and instability generally have unfavorable results. Of McCarroll's 16 patients treated without reconstruction, 9 gave up their sport because of instability. Each of the remaining seven had episodes of instability; four of them had multiple reinjuries, recurrent effusions, and pain.[254]

Young athletes with partial tears (grade II, using the system previously defined for collateral ligament sprains of the knee) of the ACL can be treated without surgery if there is no significant meniscal pathology. This usually is successful if the knee does not demonstrate significant instability on examination. The examination is most accurately done under anesthesia with arthroscopy to document the instability, degree of ACL disruption, and associated meniscal tears. The knee should be soundly rehabilitated before returning to sports. Bracing may have a role. If instability with episodes of subluxation and pain develop, or if there is a subsequent injury, the activities must be substantially modified or the knee surgically stabilized. This is done to prevent further injury, especially to the menisci.

For complete ACL tears, nonoperative treatment is an option, particularly if the physeal plates are open and the patient is relatively inactive. However, children and adolescents tend to be active, rambunctious, and poorly attentive to rehabilitation. Despite the guarded prognosis, nonoperative treatment is occasionally selected, and it is preferable in very young patients with substantial growth ahead. Healing of complete midsubstance ACL disruptions is apparently no more favorable in youths than in adults, and primary suturing as an isolated procedure is minimally effective.[10,37,89,244]

Numerous braces have been developed with the intent of protecting the ligaments of the knee. The first were functional braces that had double upright knee hinges. Although the hinges, strapping, brace fitting, and materials have evolved considerably, the stabilizing characteristics of most of these braces appears comparable. Braces may prevent hyperextension injury, but rotational control is questionable and therefore raises doubt about the overall efficacy. A simple upright "prophylactic" brace was developed as a less cumbersome measure to protect uninjured athletes. Most well-designed studies have failed to demonstrate any statistically significant effect of the lateral stabilizing knee braces.[166,382]

For the skeletally mature adolescent, the indications for reconstructive techniques standardly used for adults apply. Reconstruction using the autologous central third of the patellar tendon is the most common choice.

The remaining growth is best evaluated in adolescents by bone age.[7,143] Because little growth occurs during the last year that the physes are open, the risk of growth arrest complications are minimal. The affected and open tibial tubercle on the integrity of an autologous patellar tendon graft is not well documented.

Several techniques for reconstruction of the ACL can be considered in patients with open physes. Extraarticular procedures avoid the physeal plates.[8,254,366] They are probably not adequate to prevent a significant pivot shift and thereby protect the menisci.[57] Intraarticular procedures more accurately reproduce the anatomic and biomechanical properties of the ACL. Anatomic placement of the graft is critical to prevent subsequent loosening.[310] Most intraarticular ACL reconstructions involve crossing the physeal plates. The potential complications of shortening or angular deformity are particularly worrisome in the knee region, because approximately 65% of the leg's growth occurs from the combined distal femoral and proximal tibial physeal plates.[98] Complications were uncommon in two reported series of intraarticular reconstructions in patients with open physeal plates.[230,254] However, caution must be used in extrapolating these data to significantly younger patients.

For the active adolescent with open physeal plates and more than 1 year of growth remaining, I think a semitendinosus and gracilis graft makes the most sense. Drilling a hole across the physis and filling it with a soft tissue graft is analogous to resecting a physeal bar. If a central bridge does occur in the proximal tibia of an adolescent, it is unlikely to produce an angular deformity or functionally significant shortening. The primary concern rests with the femoral tunnel because the distal femoral physis has the most rapid growth in the lower limb, and the eccentric location of the resulting physeal bar could lead to a significant angular (valgus) deformity. This is still a controversial area.

Posterior Cruciate Ligament Injuries

Posterior cruciate ligament (PCL) sprains are much less common in children than ACL injuries.[252,345] They are significant because of the serious potential morbidity. The mechanism of injury can be hyperextension or a fall onto a flexed knee. The patient typically has popliteal fossa tenderness, and recurvatum may be present if the injury was caused by hypertension. The results of the posterior drawer and reverse pivot-shift tests are usually positive, although examination under anesthesia may be necessary to demonstrate this resultant laxity. Although midsubstance injuries may occur, avulsion of the femoral origin of the ligament should be suspected, even if a bony fragment is not seen on radiographs.

Primary repair of osteochondral avulsions appears superior to nonoperative treatment. Repair of a femoral end avulsion can be done through an anterior approach, with sutures passed through the epiphysis without crossing the physeal plate.[252,345] Tibial end avulsions are better handled through a posterior approach. If a midsubstance PCL tear is encountered in an adolescent, the principles of adult PCL injury treatment should be applied.[67,83,178,272]

Meniscal Tears

The menisci serve several important functions in the knee and are no longer considered expendable. The menisci provide stability for the joint and apparently nourish the articular cartilage by distributing synovial fluid.[304] They transmit and distribute load between the articular surfaces.[397] Decreases of joint contact surface between 10% and 75% result in decreased contact forces of 65% to 235%.

The exact incidence of meniscal tears in youths is unknown. Large series of meniscectomy cases typically include about 5% of cases involving youths younger than 15 years of age. Fewer than one third of these cases are acute traumatic tears. Most meniscal tears in children are related to discoid menisci or occur with concomitant injury to the cruciate ligaments.[162,328] Both menisci seem to be equally vulnerable to injury.[328] Most meniscal disorders in children younger than 10 years of age are related to discoid menisci, and this accounts for a slightly higher overall incidence of lateral meniscus tears in youths. Most tears in young individuals are sports related, with some injuries resulting from falls and automobile accidents.[240]

Adolescent meniscal tears usually result from a significant injury and typically involve a twisting mechanism. A pop often is heard or felt. After injury, complaints of popping, intermittent swelling, limping, and giving way are common.[264,328,393] Concomitant ligament injuries are common. The diagnosis may be delayed

as long as 12 months.[240] Younger children typically have a more vague history of injury.[209] Rarely, the onset is atraumatic, as is so often the case in the middle-aged patient.[328]

Joint line tenderness and effusion are the most common signs.[264] The McMurray test, Apley grind test, and quadriceps atrophy may be helpful in the diagnosis of a chronic lesion, but typically, the acutely injured knee is too painful for these maneuvers to be performed effectively.[174] Ligamentous laxity common in children results in hypermobility that can produce a false-positive McMurray test.[209] With a bucket-handle tear, the knee may become locked.

Routine radiographs of the knee should be obtained. Further investigation must be tailored to the degree of suspicion for a tear and the perceived urgency for definitive diagnosis and treatment. A high index of suspicion or persistent discomfort after 10 to 14 days of rest and gradual mobilization may prompt definitive investigation. Imaging is particularly useful in diagnosing the patient with a known medial collateral ligament sprain for whom joint line pain from the sprain cannot be separated from that potentially caused by a concomitant meniscal tear.[25] Imaging can help determine whether early arthroscopy or trial rehabilitation should be recommended.[186]

Although arthrography is minimally invasive and relatively inexpensive, it is rarely used for the diagnosis of meniscal injuries since the advent of arthroscopy and MRI. MRI can identify the soft tissue elements of the knee, including the menisci. MRI scanning for meniscal tears has a reported accuracy of 45% to 98%.[189,314,355]

The differential diagnosis includes collateral ligament sprain, synovial contusion, acute plica syndrome, osteochondritis dissecans, chondral fracture, patellar subluxation, discoid meniscus, and popliteus tendinitis.[50]

Several series of total meniscectomy in youths have shown that well over one half of the patients are symptomatic within 5 to 8 years of surgery. Most of these have significant degenerative changes revealed on radiography.[240,264,393,413] Long-term studies and evaluation of arthroscopic partial meniscectomy lie ahead. Meniscal injuries in youths should not be neglected because of the predictable consequences.

The key issue to meniscal healing appears to be vascularity. Although the embryonic human meniscus has vessels throughout its substance, with age and development, the inner portion becomes completely avascular.[69,199] Microangiographic studies have shown that about 30% of the capsular margin of the adult meniscus receives its blood supply from a plexus of circumferential vessels arising from the medial, lateral, and middle geniculate arteries (Fig. 30-13).[11] A proliferation from the interstitial vessels and the adja-

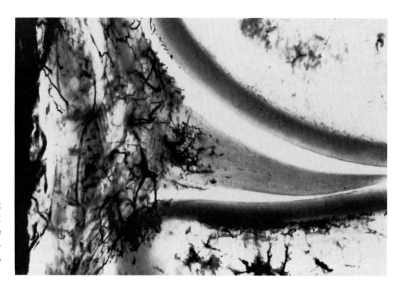

FIGURE 30-13. Vascularity of the human meniscus, as seen in a frontal section of the medial compartment of the knee. Branching vessels from the perimeniscal capillary plexus penetrate the capsular third of the adult meniscus. (From Arnoczky SP, Warren RF. Microvasculature of the human meniscus. Am J Sports Med 1982;10:91.)

cent synovium had been experimentally shown in dogs in response to injury. Mesenchymal cells fill the gap with a cellular fibrovascular scar tissue. With time, the lesion remodels to reflect the contours of the normal meniscus.[10,132]

Children and adolescents seem to have a high percentage of peripheral detachments and longitudinal tears near the capsular margin, which are good candidates for repair.[61,209] Repair yields an 80% to 90% success rate and minor deterioration over time.[245,367] Several open and arthroscopic techniques for meniscal repair have been developed, and each has its merits. There are several key principles. The meniscus should be reduced anatomically and secured by multiple closely placed sutures.[352] Because healing is slow, the sutures should be a nonabsorbable or a slowly resorbable material. They must be passed carefully to avoid neurovascular structures and should be tied down directly on the knee capsule.[61,352] Rasping the synovium to stimulate a vascularized tissue response, much like a pannus formation, seems to augment healing.[61,352] Puncturing the capsular margin of the meniscus may create channels for vascular ingrowth, and the addition of fibrin clot into the repair may augment healing.[12]

Because of the slow healing of the meniscus, the aim of rehabilitation after surgery is to shield the repair from the mechanical stresses of extreme motion and weight bearing. The knee is placed in a brace to limit motion for 6 weeks, and weight bearing is restricted. Rigorous strengthening is started after 6 weeks. Cycling is started at 3 months postoperatively. Straight-ahead jogging is started at 4 months, with full-speed running and sports at 6 months.[86]

If a discoid meniscus is an asymptomatic, incidental finding, excision of the discoid meniscus is not recommended. A study of total meniscectomy for discoid lateral meniscus showed a 75% rate of degenerative articular changes, although 70% of cases were clinically acceptable 20 years after surgery.[216] The results of partial discoid meniscectomy to contour or sculpt the remaining meniscal tissue are hopeful but await long-term follow-up data.[121] Minor tears of the discoid meniscus may heal or become asymptomatic with nonoperative treatment. Some lesions are amenable to partial meniscectomy, and others can be sutured.[95] A symptomatic Wrisberg ligament–type discoid lateral meniscus has been reattached successfully, but long-term success depends on adequate vascularity and collagen healing.[334]

Quadriceps Contusion

Although simple contusions may be an almost daily event, significant quadriceps hematomas can result in marked disability. Because continued participation despite injury can significantly worsen the prognosis, players and coaches should be educated to recognize the injury.[336]

Blunt trauma to the anterior thigh musculature is a common sports injury, occurring most often in football, lacrosse, and rugby.[190] Bleeding typically occurs in the fascial compartment, and a variable amount of thigh swelling results. Swelling and muscle spasm then limit knee flexion.

The differential diagnosis should include fracture of the femoral shaft, physeal fracture, myositis ossificans, and sarcomas of the soft tissues. The keys to the correct diagnosis are a careful history, detailed review of the radiographs, and timely follow-up. The radiographs must be of good quality and checked for subtle evidence of bone resorption and periosteal new bone that may indicate the problem to be an infection, tumor, or stress fracture that has come to attention because of incidental trauma.

Initial treatment consists of rest, ice, compression, elevation, immobilization, and crutches. After pain and spasm subside, gentle active range of motion exercise is begun. After good motion is achieved, progressive strengthening and conditioning are pursued. Athletes with greater than 90 degrees of knee flexion within 48 hours of injury have an average of 1 week of disability. Severe contusions of the quadriceps may take several months to resolve.[190]

Premature return to activity can result in recurrent hemorrhage. The athlete is returned to sports based on the functional parameters of pain, motion, strength, and agility. A padded guard should be fashioned to protect the area from reinjury. Aspiration of the hematoma and injection of proteolytic enzymes or steroids have not been proved efficacious. These may create complications and are not recommended.

Ossification may be an incidental finding after minor trauma. Myositis ossificans traumatica can occur after severe contusions, particularly if reinjury occurs during the healing phase.[231] Ossification of the soft tissue typically appears on radiographs 2 to 4 weeks after injury.[231,336] After localized trauma, the course of myositis ossificans is much more benign than after head trauma. Ossification in the midportion of the muscle belly rarely produces significant limitation of motion.[190] The patient is cautiously rehabilitated until normal function is regained. Excision of the lesion is rarely indicated.[231,336]

Avulsion Fractures of the Pelvis

Avulsion fractures of the apophysis about the hip and pelvis are most commonly related to athletic injuries during adolescence.[110,175,271] The usual mechanism is a sudden forceful concentric or eccentric muscle contraction. This occurs with rapid acceleration or deceleration. Excessive passive lengthening or stretch, such as a cheerleading split, and a variety of gymnastic maneuvers may also be responsible. Rarely does a direct blow produce these injuries.

The amount of displacement is related to the degree of injury and the associated soft tissue attachments (Fig. 30-14). The anterior inferior iliac spine is avulsed by the direct head of the rectus femoris, but migration is limited by the reflected head. The iliac crest apophysis is avulsed by the abdominal muscles and tethered by the attachment of the gluteus medius, iliacus, and tensor fascia lata muscles. The pull of the iliopsoas on the lesser trochanter, the sartorius on the anterior superior iliac spine, and the hamstrings on

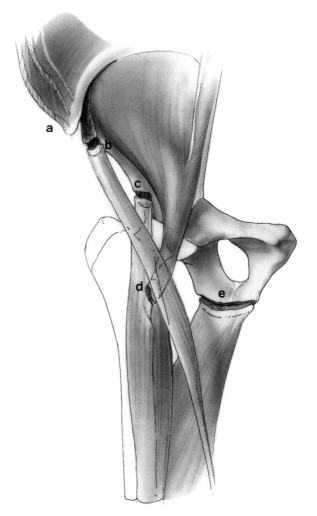

FIGURE 30-14. Avulsion fractures of the growing pelvis result from traction injuries where major muscle groups insert into or originate from apophyses about the pelvis. (**A**) The abdominal and trunk muscles inset into the iliac apophysis. (**B**) The sartorius originates from the anterior superior iliac apophysis. (**C**) The direct head of the rectus femoris originates from the anterior inferior iliac apophysis. (**D**) The iliopsoas inserts into the lesser trochanteric apophysis. (**E**) The hamstrings originate from the ischial apophysis.

the ischium are relatively unopposed, resulting in greater potential for displacement.

Typically, the athlete experiences an acute onset of pain that may be accompanied by a popping sensation. Tenderness is usually confined to the area of avulsion. The patient is most comfortable in a posture with the offending muscle-tendon unit relaxed. Pain is reproduced by active or passive stretch. Anteroinferior iliac spine avulsions may be particularly hard to localize because of their location, and the inciting event may not be recalled.[110] The avulsed fragment usually is seen on routine radiographs. Occasionally, special views are needed, but for most cases, tomography and radionuclide scans are unnecessary.[110]

Neoplasm and infection should be considered, especially if the history is atypical.[159,167] The differential diagnosis should also include muscle strain and a "hip pointer," which is a contusion of the iliac crest.[133,271] Persistent tenderness of the anterior iliac crest can result from an apophysitis, which may be associated with radiographic discontinuity of the apophysis.[232]

Initially, the patient rests with the injured region in a relaxed position. Most physicians recommend the use of crutches for the first 2 weeks, with a phased rehabilitation program guided by functional improvement. The goal should be to restore motion, strength, and sports-specific functioning. Premature return to play may delay recovery or further displace the apophysis. The decision for early or safe return to competition is not easily made and must weigh the clinical findings and radiographic evidence of healing. Complete healing may take 6 weeks to several months.

With time, bone is laid down in response to the injury. Relative shortening of the muscle, prominence of the bony mass, and potential interference of the sciatic nerve have been sighted as causes of residual disability. Limitation of athletic ability rarely occurs and is apparently only related to severely displaced ischial avulsions.[349] In rare cases, troublesome bony fragments should be resected.[405] Surgical reduction and fixation is seldom indicated.[175,271]

Spinal Injuries

Serious injuries to the head and neck are infrequent but often devastating. Football, trampoline, ice hockey, rugby, and diving are the most common activities associated with these injuries to younger athletes.[256,388] Between 1979 and 1984, American high school students sustained 285 serious cervical spine injuries, with 48 permanent quadriplegics.[389]

American football remains a serious risk to the young athlete despite improved equipment and changes in tackling techniques; 72% of high school athletes suffering quadriplegia were attempting to make tackles. Defensive backs are the most commonly injured players. Ironically, the improved protective capabilities of the helmet and face mask during the 1960s and 1970s resulted in the use of the head as a primary point of contact in blocking and tackling.[389] Fifty-two percent of quadriplegics between 1971 and 1975 were injured by "spearing," which is the use of the head to ram an opponent. In 1975, the National Collegiate Athletic Association and the National Federation of State High School Associations adopted football rule changes that prohibit spearing. Since then, there has been a downward turn in the incidence of serious cervical spine injuries and a dramatic decline in quadriplegia.[389] Although the incidence of spine injuries is approximately 5 per 100,000 players (1 quadriplegic per 100,000), this remains a serious problem because of the tragic nature of the injury.

In the United States, trampolines and gymnastics are second to football in causing sports-related spinal cord injuries.[70] At least 114 cervical spine injuries resulting in quadriplegia are known to have resulted from the trampoline and minitrampoline.[387] In 1977, the American Academy of Pediatrics issued a policy statement that prompted most schools to eliminate trampolines. Since then, the estimated frequency of head and neck injuries associated with trampolines has declined by almost two thirds. The trampoline is a dangerous apparatus, and spine injuries can occur even in experienced athletes taking reasonable precautions.[387]

Cineradiography has shown that most cervical spine injuries from sports are caused by axial loading with the neck in a slightly flexed position.[380,387] Improper tackling (American football), checking into the boards (ice hockey), diving into shallow water, and trampolines are clearly causes of spine fractures and paralysis.

Recognizing that these injuries are not just freak accidents provides the opportunity to diminish their occurrence by research, education, rule changes, technique modifications, and equipment improvements. Players should be informed of the hazards, and programs for strengthening neck muscle are essential.[380] Management of these injuries is beyond the scope of this text, but prevention should be a primary interest of everyone dealing with young athletes.

PATELLOFEMORAL DISORDERS

Disorders of the patellofemoral joint include a variety of overuse syndromes, congenital and developmental abnormalities, and instabilities. In adolescents, patellofemoral problems account for almost 10% of all sports "injuries."[88]

Anatomy and Biomechanics

Evolving in upper-level primates, the patella is a sesamoid bone of the quadriceps mechanism.[165] The patella furnishes a site of convergence for the four components of the quadriceps muscle to provide an extension moment arm through the entire knee range of motion.[180,203] Phylogenically, the vastus medialis was the last of the quadriceps group to develop.[118] The hyaline cartilage of the patella is the thickest in the body. It provides a low-friction surface that is able to bear high compressive loads, and the patella protects the distal femoral surface from direct blows during a fall.[180] The trochlear shape of the distal femur stabilizes the patella's tracking.

The inferior pole of the patella first contacts the trochlea at 20 degrees of flexion with a relatively low-contact surface area.[138] With further flexion, the contact site moves more superiorly, and the surface area increases. The most medial facet or "odd facet" only comes into contact with the trochlea between 90 and 130 degrees of knee flexion.

The patellofemoral articulation is subject to extremely high compressive loads, particularly with progressive knee flexion.[241] With the knee flexed 9 degrees during walking, the patellofemoral joint reactive force is approximately one half of the body weight. This increases to 3.3 times body weight at 60 degrees of flexion during activities such as stair climbing. The contact forces reach 7.8 times body weight with full knee flexion during a deep knee bend.[180]

The alignment of the quadriceps relative to the patellar tendon has a valgus relation, much like that of the tibia and femur. This angle is influenced by the patient's height and pelvis width. The quadriceps vector is approximated by a line from the anterosuperior iliac spine to the center of the patella. The line of pull through the patellar tendon runs from the center of the patella to the tibial tubercle. The relation between these two lines is referred to as the quadriceps angle or Q angle. As this angle increases, the vector created by the extensor mechanism tends to translate the patella laterally (Fig. 30-15A). As the Q angle increases, so does the degree of that laterally directed force.[309] The Q angle increases even further with external rotation of the tibia, which occurs dynamically as the tibia externally rotates during terminal extension. There may be a developmental degree of outward rotation of the upward tibia as well. The lateral retinaculum, including the lateral patellofemoral and lateral meniscopatellar ligaments, add to the laterally directed moment of the extensor mechanism.[123] The sum of these forces is resisted by the medial parapatellar stabilizing soft tissues, and the pull of the vastus medialis (Fig. 30-15B). The lateral patellotrochlear articulation is the other key component balancing these forces, and any deficiency of any of these components can exacerbate lateral maltracking or instability of the patellofemoral joint (Fig. 30-15C).[118,241,309]

Anterior Knee Pain

Mechanics and Diagnosis

Patellofemoral pain syndrome is a descriptive term applied to patients with nonspecific anterior knee pain. Malalignment or maltracking appears to be a significant predisposing factor. Lateral tracking or subluxation of the patella demonstrated arthroscopically is highly correlated with the patellofemoral pain syndrome. In some people, lateral tracking is associated with pain and instability. Other patients complain primarily of instability and have relatively little pain. For the purpose of this discussion, patellofemoral pain syndrome is separated from patellofemoral instability, although some patients have components of both.

Several hypotheses have been proposed for the mechanism of pain production. Ficat and associates have proposed that excessive pressure from the lateral facet is transmitted to the sensate subchondral bone, leading to the perception of pain.[114] Hejgaard and Diemer found increased interosseous pressure of the patella in many patients with patellofemoral pain.[160] James proposes that the cause in many patients is an underlying overuse syndrome, resulting in excessive rotational forces in the peripatellar soft tissues.[191] True chondromalacia is not typically found in these younger patients.

Factors predisposing to patellofemoral pain syndrome include habitual overloading related to overuse, a variety of lower extremity malalignments, poorly developed quadriceps muscles, and various dysplastic changes about the patellofemoral articulation. One particularly common aggregate of these abnormalities is commonly seen in adolescent girls and has been called the "miserable malalignment syndrome." These patients have increased femoral anteversion, external tibial torsion, genu valgum, excessive Q angles, heel cord contracture, and pronated feet.[34,191]

The pain in most patellofemoral disorders is generalized to the anterior part of the knee. The pain is typically related to activity, and patients feel more comfortable at rest. Climbing stairs is particularly troublesome because of the excessive patellofemoral loads. Prolonged sitting may produce discomfort and the need to move the knees. Patients may complain of stiffness after prolonged sitting. Erythema and effusion are uncommon. The patient may experience catching or giving way, but true locking is unusual. Training errors—usually related to the change in intensity, duration, or training surface—are common factors in patellofemoral disorders.[191] The complaints are frequently bilateral, although not necessarily concurrent.

The physical findings include diffuse medial and lateral peripatellar tenderness. The combination of increased femoral anteversion and external tibial torsion causes the patellas to face toward each other to some degree when the feet are directed forward; this has been called "squinting patellae." Frequently, the lateral retinaculum is contracted; this can be demonstrated by the inability to elevate the lateral margin of the patella during the tilt test. Crepitus may signal significant articular irregularity, although this must be tested in at least 20 degrees of flexion to ensure that the patella is articulating with the trochlea rather

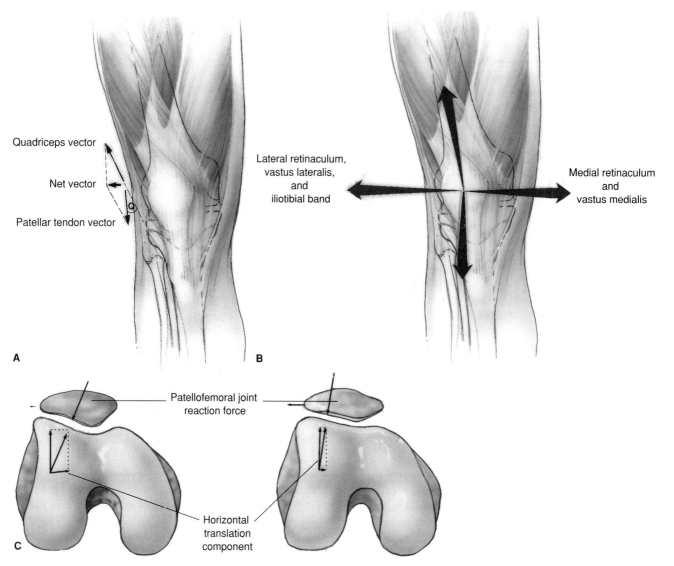

FIGURE 30-15.   Patellofemoral biomechanics. (**A**) The Q angle relates the direction of pull of the quadriceps mechanism to that of the patellar tendon. These are the two most powerful forces exerted on the patella. Their vector sum is directed laterally. (**B**) There are additional soft tissue forces applied to the patella. (**C**) The laterally directed net vector is opposed by the patellofemoral articulation. If the groove is shallow, there is less potential resistance to horizontal translation than for knees with a deeper femoral groove. The dysplastic patellofemoral articulation results in less resistance to lateral translation and therefore greater articular surface sheer forces.

than with the femoral metaphysis. Perhaps the most important finding is the lack of other specific abnormalities, because patellofemoral pain syndrome is primarily a diagnosis of exclusion. For instance, localization of tenderness to the superolateral quadrant or inferior pole of the patella would suggest that the correct diagnosis might instead be bipartite patella (see Chap. 27), Sinding-Larsen–Johansson disease, or patellar tendinitis.

Because underlying biomechanical abnormalities are common, the evaluation must include a thorough inspection of the entire lower extremities and the ath-

lete's shoes, which may demonstrate asymmetrical wear patterns, a finding that can be particularly helpful if the problem is unilateral.[191,234,239] Even if wear is symmetrical, breakdown of the medial counter of the shoe indicates excessive pronation. A wedged pattern of heel wear suggests a valgus heel strike, which is typical of runners with excessive pronation. As the foot rolls during pronation, the tibia rotates inward, and the extensor mechanism experiences greater stresses to resist this.[239] If the shoes demonstrate wear on the lateral edge of the heel, this suggests a hindfoot varus strike, possibly due to a cavus foot. The more rigid cavus foot pattern can result in less shock absorption at the foot and relatively greater ground reaction forces being translated to the knee.[233]

The Q angle, patellar tilt, and lateral glide should be considered.[308] Medial and lateral peripatellar tenderness most often is related to inflammation of the soft tissues rather than a painful articular surface. Thigh circumference and vastus medialis atrophy are signs of long-standing dysfunction and may even be contributing factors.[309] Tightness of the hamstrings and iliotibial band should be checked, because they can lead to increased patellofemoral contact forces.[155,411] Anterolateral or anteromedial joint line tenderness may overlap the symptoms and findings associated with meniscal problems.[140,269]

Radiographic evaluation should include anteroposterior, lateral, and tangential views of the patella. The anteroposterior and lateral views may identify bipartite patella, Larsen-Johansson disease, osteochondritis dissecans, and dorsal defects of the patella. The lateral view can be used to identify patients with patella alta or patella infera. Insall and Salvati described a ratio of the maximal patella length to the patellar tendon length; normal was defined as a ratio of 1 : 1 ± 20%.[185] Lancourt and Cristini have correlated patellar instability and chondromalacia to a decrease in this ratio.[219]

Various tangential views have been developed to evaluate the patella's anatomic relation to the trochlear groove and to the femur.[114,176,267] Merchant's technique is performed with the knee minimally flexed over the edge of the table and supported by an apparatus (Fig. 30-16).[267] Supine positioning relaxes the quadriceps and avoids direct pressure to the patella. This allows a maltracking patella to rest in a subluxated position, probably making the Merchant's view the most sensitive plain radiographic technique. Patellar views done with the knee simply flexed, often called "sunrise views," pull the patella into the distal femoral sulcus and can lead to a false impression that the patella is tracking centrally. CT and MRI can also demonstrate patellar subluxation but are probably not indicated for the routine case.[125,351] A variety of lines, angles, and ratios have been developed to quantitate static patellar tilt and subluxation as an indicator of tracking.[125,224,267] However, the usefulness of this information in determining treatment has not been demonstrated.[140,222]

Bone scans may demonstrate increased radionuclide activity in the patella, suggesting increased metabolic activity of the bone, but for patellofemoral pain, the sensitivity, specificity, and predictive values of bone scans in younger patients have not been proved.[101,115,160,212]

Many patients only need reassurance that the problem is not more serious. The intermittent use of NSAIDs, a knee sleeve, and other isolated modalities may be adequate to control the symptoms. If the symptoms are persistent and troublesome, a more formalized program is helpful. The importance of genuine and concerted efforts at nonoperative management of the patellofemoral pain syndrome should be emphasized. At least 80% of patients can be successfully managed without surgery.[87,100,164,294,411]

Treatment

The treatment program can be divided into four phases, which blend together rather than being separate steps.[87,309,333]

Phase 1 concentrates on symptom reduction. The initial management of symptoms includes modifica-

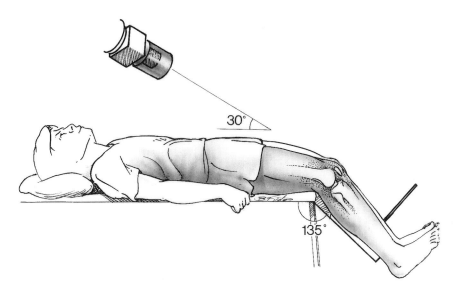

FIGURE 30-16. Tangential x-ray view for evaluating the patellofemoral joint. Merchant's view allows the quadriceps mechanism to relax. The patella is not artifically held reduced in the distal femoral groove.

tion of activities, ranging from elimination of activities such as stair climbing or hill running to complete cessation of sports. For the serious athlete, modification of training or substitution of an alternative such as swimming is critical. NSAIDs may be helpful. Many patients find that use of a knee sleeve with a patella cutout reduces pain, especially when they have pain with daily activities.[305] Isometric quadriceps strengthening exercises and hamstring stretching should be started in this initial phase (Fig. 30-17). Ice is used in conjunction with exercise. Occasionally, the knee may require a brief period of splinting. Crutches are rarely needed. Several bracing and strapping techniques have been advocated to improve patellar tracking. The McConnell taping technique appears to be the most successful of these. An experienced therapist can work with this technique and, if successful, teach it to the patient.

Phase 2 concentrates on reconditioning. When the patient is able to tolerate isometrics comfortably, a quadriceps strengthening program is advanced. Straight leg raising and terminal extension quad arc strengthening exercises are begun. Weights are later added. Isometrically loading the quadriceps or the use of terminal range of motion strengthening exercises

minimizes the excessive patellofemoral contact forces generated in flexion past 20 degrees.[180] DeHaven achieved excellent results with the use of a simple knee extension exercise apparatus or the use of a weight boot.[87] Specific instructions are necessary, and most adolescents require some supervision to ensure compliance. When using the exercise machine, the knee is placed in full extension before the weight is applied. After 5 to 10 seconds, the load is relieved and the quadriceps relaxed (Fig. 30-18).

Isokinetic exercise has been shown to be an excellent method of strengthening muscles; however, there can be disadvantages to its use in the early phases of rehabilitation. Isokinetics may result in excessive patellofemoral contact forces being generated by a rigorous contraction. With appropriate precautions, eccentric strengthening can be used effectively, although this is usually unnecessary until the advanced stages of reconditioning.[24]

A general lower extremity strengthening program, including hamstring stretching and strengthening, is included in phase II. Physical therapy modalities such as high-voltage galvanic stimulation (i.e., Highvolt) or transcutaneous electrical nerve stimulation may be helpful, particularly for the athlete who has limited

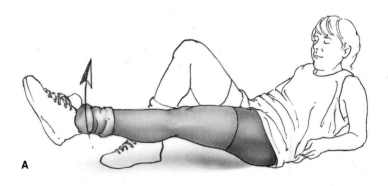

A

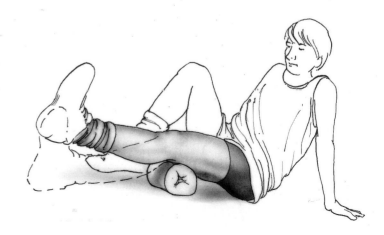

FIGURE 30-17. Patellofemoral rehabilitation. (**A**) Straight leg raising exercises and (**B**) terminal knee extension exercises are used in the initial phases of rehabilitation. Avoiding significant degrees of knee flexion minimizes the patellofemoral contact forces.

B

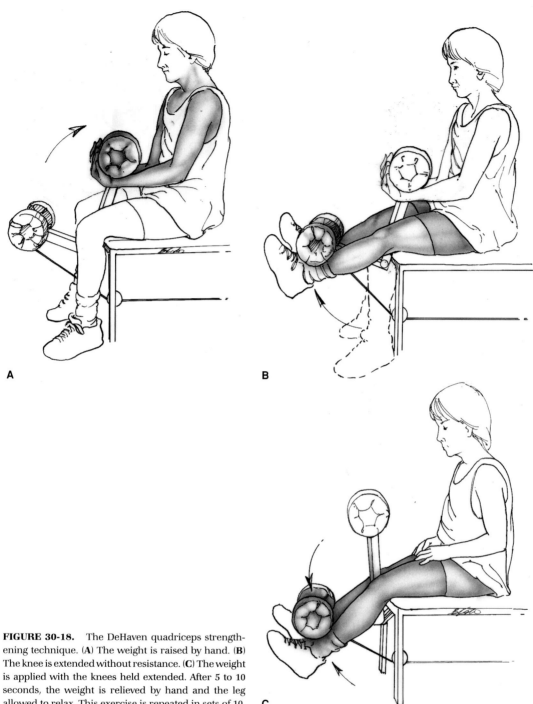

A

B

FIGURE 30-18. The DeHaven quadriceps strengthening technique. (**A**) The weight is raised by hand. (**B**) The knee is extended without resistance. (**C**) The weight is applied with the knees held extended. After 5 to 10 seconds, the weight is relieved by hand and the leg allowed to relax. This exercise is repeated in sets of 10. **C**

exercise capacity because of pain. A patellar "stabilizing" sleeve may also be helpful in controlling pain and facilitating weight lifting.[235]

In phase 3, activities are gradually resumed. After a patient demonstrates consistent progress in quadriceps strengthening, a graduated running program is instituted. This can commence when the patient is performing quadriceps strengthening at about one

half of projected goal. DeHaven outlined recommendations for this in terms of a young adult male eventually progressing to 60 pounds, using a weight-added isometric technique.[87] If using a weight boot or ankle weights, the goal should be 10 pounds for straight leg raises and terminal extensions before initiating a running program.

The running program is based on prior training

experience and ability, but it should include a period of stretching and warm-up exercises, gradually increased duration and speed, initial avoidance of hills, ice after running, good shoe wear, and a foot orthoses if there appears to be a significant biomechanical anomaly. Running should initially be done every other day, with the phase II weight program on the alternate days.

In phase 4, a maintenance level is reached. Stretching and warm-up exercises before all activities are continued. In addition to the athlete's usual training program, weight training is continued two or three times each week. The athlete is advised that minor setbacks can be expected; the program is backed up to the prior comfortable step and progressed more gradually as symptoms permit.

Although the results of surgical treatment for patellofemoral pain are generally good, failure can result in significant disability. This emphasizes the importance of a sincere effort to have patients persevere with a conservative rehabilitation program until all reasonable attempts have been made. Patellofemoral pain syndrome typically does not resolve until adequate strength gains are made. Often, the stumbling block is that adequate strength gains cannot be made because of the pain encountered with each attempt to progress the exercise program. Surgery is not a substitute for exercise therapy; instead, it should be viewed as an aid to improve the patellar tracking and thereby facilitate strengthening.[30]

LATERAL RETINACULAR RELEASE. Contracture of the lateral retinaculum is a common finding in patellofemoral pain syndrome. The contracture may be the underlying cause of the problem or a manifestation of it. A tight lateral tether contributes to maltracking.[228] The principle is to release the tight structures, which improves tracking.

The indications for lateral release include intractable patellofemoral pain, findings such as tenderness over the lateral retinaculum with a tight lateral retinaculum, and no other explanation for the problem.[124] The prerequisites include failure of conservative measures, a tight lateral retinaculum with evidence of lateral tracking, and peripatellar pain.[126,266] Evidence of lateral tracking or subluxation should be confirmed arthroscopically.[58,60,269] The relative contraindications include reflex sympathetic dystrophy, poor cooperation with rehabilitative exercises, psychosomatic illness, and ulterior motives such as a desire to establish a compensation-related disability.[43,51,313] Arthroscopy should be performed at the time of lateral release to thoroughly assess the knee, identifying concurrent pathologic processes or other problems with symptoms that could lead to misdiagnosis.[269] The incidental

finding of lateral tracking in an otherwise asymptomatic knee should not be an indication for lateral retinacular release.[30,269]

Lateral retinacular release can be performed through an open incision or percutaneously.[29,62,103,140,155,214,220,223,258,266,269,356] The release should transect the lateral meniscopatellar fibers inferiorly and extend just above the superior pole of the patella. Adequacy of the release should be demonstrated by an intraoperative manual tilt test.[366] The vastus lateralis should not be detached from the superolateral pole of the patella, because this can be associated with significant atrophy of the vastus lateralis and postoperative medial subluxation of the patella.[179]

Hemarthrosis is a relatively common complication and can be associated with delayed rehabilitation, persistent synovitis, and poor overall results.[366] Specific attention is paid to the superolateral branch of the geniculate artery, which is typically transected.[103] Although cautery is theoretically an advantage of the open technique, the arthroscopic use of electric cautery has also been proven effective.[27,276]

Postoperatively, the use of a sleeve that fills with ice water, such as the Cryocuff (Aircast Corporation, Summit, NJ), seems to greatly reduce pain, swelling, and hemarthrosis. Therapy is begun a few days later to restore the range of motion and prevent adhesions from forming. Within a short time, strengthening should be better tolerated than before surgery.[30]

The overall results of most studies of lateral retinacular release are 75% to 85% favorable.[30,140,214,258,266,269,298,356] Complications include persistent pain, painful hemarthrosis, synovitis, reflex sympathetic dystrophy, recurrent medial subluxation, patellofemoral osteoarthritis, saphenous neuritis, and thrombophlebitis. Factors associated with poor results include reflex sympathetic dystrophy, ligamentous instability, and high-grade chondromalacia.[43,51,176,298,356]

CHONDRAL SHAVING. Cartilaginous debris in a joint produces synovitis. This is the rationale for debriding or shaving articular cartilage in the treatment of patellofemoral pain with advanced grades of chondromalacia patella.[64] Ogilvie-Harris and Jackson demonstrated reasonable results from chondral debridement in cases of trauma where there is no underlying maltracking.[298] In these cases, a lateral retinacular release is only indicated if there is demonstrated concurrent maltracking. In cases of patellofemoral pain with concurrent grade II or III chondromalacia, cartilage debridement should be viewed as an adjuvant procedure only.

OTHER PROCEDURES. Advancement of the vastus medialis and distal realignment procedures may be indicated for specific cases with medial soft tissue defects or excessive Q angles.[124] For patellofemoral pain without overt symptoms of instability, lateral retinacular release is usually the first line of treatment. If the lateral retinacular release fails, secondary procedures should be approached cautiously, first confirming that there is no other diagnosis to explain the symptoms.

Chondromalacia

The term chondromalacia refers to softening and degeneration of the articular cartilage.[138] Adults with maltracking frequently have these cartilage changes, but it is probably incidental in many cases. Significant cartilage fibrillation or fissuring is not typically present in younger patients with signs of patellofemoral pain syndrome. Occasionally, these cartilage changes are seen in larger adolescents and sometimes results from direct trauma to the patella or occurs after patellar dislocations. Symptomatic chondromalacia is much less responsive to rehabilitation efforts than patellofemoral pain. These patients occasionally respond to arthroscopy and chondral shaving, but the physician must beware of other concurrent or underlying processes that have led to the chondromalacia.

Saphenous Nerve Entrapment

Anterior thigh pain extending to the superomedial pole of the patella can be produced by an entrapment syndrome of the saphenous nerve. This branch of the femoral nerve enters the adductor canal alongside the superficial femoral artery. It then penetrates anteriorly through the dense fascia connecting the adductor magnus to the vastus medialis 10 cm proximal to the medial femoral condyle.

Although most reported cases have involved patients past their teens, this condition can be seen in adolescents.[409] Medial thigh and knee pain is typically produced with walking or running. It is often aggravated by quadriceps exercises. The most reliable finding is point tenderness where the nerve exits Hunter canal. Saphenous nerve entrapment should be considered in the differential diagnosis of anterior knee pain and not mistaken for patellofemoral maltracking or plica syndrome.

Injection of a local anesthetic into the affected site relieves the pain and produces an area of numbness in the distribution of the saphenous nerve. If the condition is unresponsive to rest and NSAIDs, a steroid can be injected. This may need to be repeated, and the pain may not completely resolve.[331]

The results of surgical release and neurolysis are mixed, with failures apparently secondary to scar tissue entrapping the nerve. Neurectomy may be necessary, but the patient must be warned of the resultant numbness.[409]

Dorsal Defects of the Patella

Haswell and associates first described a lesion, now called dorsal defect of the patella, that was round and radiolucent, surrounded by a zone of sclerosis typically located in the superolateral aspect of the patella (Fig. 30-19).[156] This defect has been estimated to occur in nearly 1% of the population.[194] It occurs in persons as young as 10 years of age and rarely persists past 30 years.[134,156,172] Histologically, it is composed of a vascular fibrous connective tissue surrounded by sclerotic bone without inflammation.[181] Some necrotic bone may be present.[90,172] The cause is unknown, but the evidence suggests that dorsal defects of the patella result from irregular ossification. This may result from stress exerted by the vastus lateralis insertion, and bipartite patella may have a similar cause.[172]

Although a rare occurrence, almost any benign or malignant tumor can appear as a radiolucent lesion in the patella.[4] Osteomyelitis, Brodie abscess, and osteochondritis dissecans of the patella should be considered in the differential diagnosis.[105,277]

A dorsal defect of the patella usually is an asymptomatic, incidental radiographic finding. It undergoes

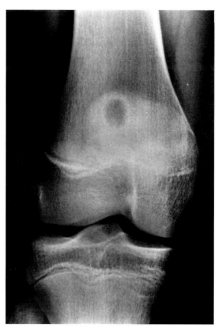

FIGURE 30-19. Dorsal defect of the patella. The typical lesion is a round, radiolucent area in the superolateral pole of the patella. The margins of the lesion are well circumscribed. This is best seen on the anteroposterior radiograph. Typically, the lateral radiograph is normal.

spontaneous regression in most cases and requires no medical treatment.[90,156] In the adolescent, however, it may become symptomatic and can be associated with an underlying articular cartilage defect.[90,129,181] Most patients with this lesion respond to rest, but surgical excision and grafting occasionally may be necessary.[90,129,181]

Fat Pad Impingement

Impingement of the anterior fat pad and its associated synovium is not a well-documented disorder. Described in 1904 by Hoffa, this condition appears to be a distinct entity and should be considered in the differential diagnosis of anterior knee pain.[271] The fat pad may be hypertrophic. The characteristic histopathologic findings include the presence of mononuclear inflammatory cells and some degree of fibrosis. In chronic cases, the adipose tissue becomes replaced by fibrocartilage.[270]

Most patients are females in their teens and early twenties.[270,359] The cause is unknown, although it is postulated that hypertrophy or trauma initiates repetitive impingement, inflammation, and fibrosis.

Typically, the pain is related to activity and localized to the anterior knee joint. There may be a history of trauma. Prominence of the fat pad on each side of the patellar tendon is by no means diagnostic. Hoffa described a test performed by applying fingertip pressure to the fat pad while the knee is passively extended.[271] If pain is elicited near terminal extension, the test result is considered positive. This test is not specific, because several other problems, including patellofemoral pain and chondromalacia, can inflame the fat pads.

Radiographs typically are negative, and the value of other imaging studies has not been proven. The diagnosis is presumptive until confirmed at arthroscopy. The differential diagnosis includes meniscal cyst, meniscal tear, soft tissue trauma, patellofemoral pain, patellar tendinitis, and patellar instability.[359]

Nonoperative treatment includes rest, ice, NSAIDs, and a sequential exercise program. Because terminal quadriceps extension often produces impingement, the exercise range of motion is modified to avoid terminal extension. Physical therapy modalities including high-voltage galvanic stimulation and phonophoresis with hydrocortisone may be helpful.

Nonoperative therapy is usually effective, but if the condition persists, arthroscopy may be indicated. A knowledge of the anatomy, including the normal basal prominences of fat the variability of fat pad size, is essential.[270] The difficulty in differentiating pathologic changes from normal anatomy fuels the controversy in diagnosing this entity. A normal fat pad should not be resected. Generally, the texture and contour of the fibrotic fat pad differs appreciably from the soft texture and yellow color of normal fat. This can be used as a guide during arthroscopic resection, but unfortunately, no proven guidelines are available.[359]

Postoperatively, range of motion exercise is resumed early to minimize scarring. A standard patellofemoral rehabilitation protocol is used, and the patient should demonstrate full return of function before participating in sports activities.

Plica Syndrome

The symptomatic medial patellar plica can be considered the great imitator of knee disorders. The challenge is to recognize this disorder without diagnosing plica syndrome for every case of knee pain having a tender synovial fold.

Embryologically, the synovial cavity of the knee begins as three separate compartments that fuse during the fourth fetal month. The remaining membranes give rise to the three commonly encountered plicae (Fig. 30-20). The infrapatellar plica is also called the

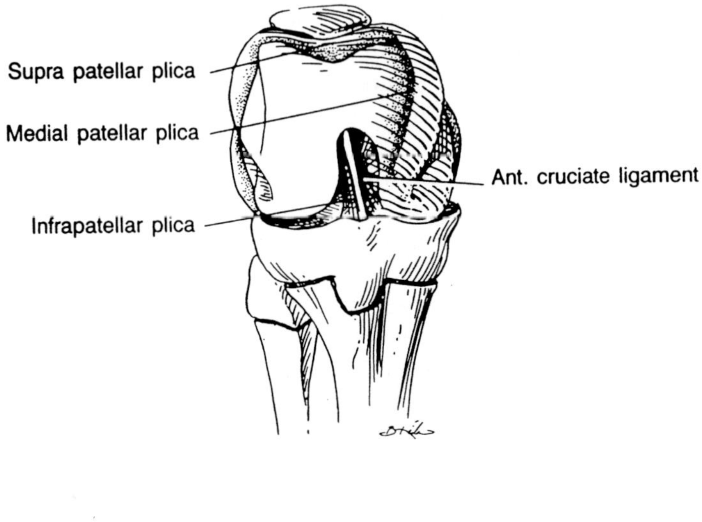

Supra patellar plica

Medial patellar plica

Infrapatellar plica

Ant. cruciate ligament

FIGURE 30-20. Plicas of the knee. (**A**) Superior plica. (**B**) Medial plica, the one most commonly symptomatic. (**C**) Inferior plica (ligamentum mucosum) overlying the anterior cruciate ligament.

ligamentum mucosum. It runs parallel to the ACL. Occasionally, the infrapatellar plica persists as a complete septum, although it is rarely symptomatic.

The suprapatellar plica may result in complete separation of the suprapatellar bursa from the knee. There may be a small opening in the suprapatellar plica called the porta. The suprapatellar plica usually is a crescent-shaped fold originating beneath the quadriceps tendon. It extends to the medial or lateral walls of the joint.[153] The suprapatellar plica is rarely symptomatic.[311]

The medial parapatellar plica is implicated most often as a cause of symptoms.[290,307,337] It lies along the medial wall of the joint, originating near the suprapatellar plica and coursing obliquely downward to attach near the infrapatellar fat pad.[307]

The incidence of plica varies from 5% to 50%, depending on the examiner's criteria for how large of a fold must be to constitute a plica. The lesions range from a small cord to a large shelf. The plica may completely cover the surface of the medial femoral condyle, and it may be fenestrated.[18]

Inflammation can produce thickening and fibrosis of the plica. This leads to further impingement of the plica in the patellofemoral joint, which is a self-propagating problem. Pain may be secondary to mechanical compression of the plica or to the plica applying traction to the fat pad.[290] In advanced cases, the articular surface may erode.[153]

The presenting symptoms of plica syndrome include anteromedial knee pain, popping, snapping, and giving way. The pain may be referred to the medial or lateral joint line. Symptoms often begin after repetitive activities such as running, jumping, and climbing stairs.[153,290] Occasionally, the plica becomes acutely inflamed after a twisting injury or direct blow, and the patient may present with pseudolocking of the knee.[290,307]

The plica can usually be palpated along the medial surface of the femoral condyle in symptomatic and asymptomatic patients. Tenderness is invariably present, but it is not a pathognomonic finding. Many abnormalities produce localized or generalized synovitis that secondarily affects the plica. To further confuse the examiner, the patient with an inflamed plica may also have a false-positive Apley test, McMurray test, or a patellar compression test. The lateral joint line may be tender anteriorly, and an effusion may be present.[290]

Radiographs usually should be normal, and other studies have not proven to be efficacious.[153] The diagnosis is based on compilation of all available data and the exclusion of other lesions. Even at arthroscopy, the determination of a pathologic plica from an incidental finding is not always clear, thus the potential for underdiagnosis and overdiagnosis.[190]

It is imperative to search for other pathologic processes of the knees, such as a meniscus tear, loose body, chondromalacia, significant patellofemoral maltracking, or instability.[153] Initial treatment should include rest, ice, NSAIDs, and a gradual patellofemoral exercise program. Because terminal extension may impinge the plica, exercises are modified to avoid that range. McConnell taping may be helpful. Intraplical steroid injection has been used, although the ability to inject the plica specifically without placing steroids into the knee is questionable.[337] If persistently symptomatic, the synovial band is easily resected arthroscopically, and the rest of the joint is carefully inspected. Good and excellent results of more than 90% have been achieved with appropriate patient selection.[153,290,307] Because scarring may occur from simple division of the plica, complete resection is recommended. The surgeon must keep in mind that the symptomatic plica may be the early signs of patellofemoral maltracking, and this is a common cause of surgical failure.

Acute Patellar Dislocation

Dislocation of the patella is usually related to an underlying dysplasia or a malalignment of the patellofemoral articulation.[41] In as many as 75% of patients with patellofemoral instability, at least one element of deficiency can be identified.[58] The depth of the patellofemoral articular groove, patella alta, excessive Q angle, and ligamentous laxity have been cited as predisposing factors.[222] There is a positive family history for one fourth of these patients.[41] A direct blow to the medial aspect of the patella accounts for only 10% of cases.[222] Most patellofemoral dislocations are lateral, although medial dislocations are a recognized complication of overzealous lateral retinacular release.[176]

Most patellar dislocations occur or begin in patients from 14 to 20 years of age.[41,58,164,222] Although football, baseball, and basketball commonly are involved, significant numbers of patellar dislocations occur from simple falls, gymnastics, dancing, cheerleading, and a wide variety of other activities.[236] Although significantly affecting more girls than boys, patellar dislocations must be considered in the differential diagnosis of acute knee injuries in young male athletes.[14,58,64,176,236]

A patient with an unreduced patellar dislocation presents with the knee flexed and the hamstrings in spasm. With the patellar displaced laterally, the femoral condyles become prominent medially, often leading the patient or lay observer to report that the dislocation was medial rather than lateral. Most patellar dislocations reduce spontaneously or shortly after they occur, especially if the episodes are recurrent. A wide array of activities can precipitate the episode, but the mechanism usually involves a twisting event. A history of prior episodes of subluxation, anterior knee pain, and a family history may help to support the diagnosis.

After reduction, the residual findings include diffuse parapatellar tenderness and a positive apprehension test. Medially, there may be a palpable defect from avulsion of the vastus medialis insertion into the patella. The medial capsule and retinaculum may have been stretched or torn, and tenderness may extend to the medial femoral epicondyle.

Hemarthrosis may result from a capsular tear or a concurrent osteochondral fracture. The ligaments should be examined carefully, because the mechanism of injury and findings with patellar dislocation are similar to those of a cruciate sprain.

Postreduction radiographs should be inspected for evidence of osteochondral fragments. Bony fragments seen along the medial patellar margin may not be free in the joint, but rather result from avulsion of the vastus medialis insertion. A Merchant view of both patellas may demonstrate significant residual maltracking.

The natural history of acute patellar dislocation in children is such that approximately 1 of 6 will develop recurrent dislocations, 2 of 6 will have some minor residual symptoms, and 3 of 6 will remain asymptomatic.[262] The incidence of redislocation after nonoperative treatment diminishes considerably with advancing age. Cash and Hughston found a 60% incidence among patients between 11 and 14 years of age, 30% incidence among patients between 19 and 28 years of age, and only 1 affected patient older than 28 years of age.[58]

Acutely, the extensor mechanism holds the patella trapped over the margin of the distal femoral condyles. With the patella posterior to the axis of the knee and the hamstrings contracted in response to pain, the knee is firmly held in flexion. The reduction is performed without forceful manipulation. The knee is gradually and steadily extended. Reduction is facilitated by turning the patient into a prone position so the hip is extended and the hamstrings become relaxed. After reduction, the joint can be aspirated if a tense hemarthrosis develops. The surface of the bloody fluid should be inspected for fat droplets that would suggest an osteochondral fracture.

Rehabilitation begins as soon as practical, particularly after a repeat dislocation from which there may be little acute damage to the medial stabilizers. The knee is placed in an immobilizer for comfort, but it is unnecessary to continue immobilization arbitrarily for 6 weeks as some have suggested.[222,262]

Straight leg raising exercises are begun immediately to minimize quadriceps atrophy. The knee is periodically reexamined (for up to 6 weeks), and when comfortable, a formal patellar rehabilitation program is begun. The immobilization is discontinued, and a flexible knee sleeve with the patellar cutout is used once the extensor mechanism is working adequately to support the knee. Criteria such as full range of motion and the ability to do straight leg raises with 5 lb (2.25 kg) of ankle weights can be used as the objective measure for this.[305] As strength is gained, activities are progressed, starting with biking and straight-ahead running. Cutting and twisting activities are then reintroduced. The patient is encouraged to continue with quadriceps exercises, particularly emphasizing the vastus medialis.

After an acute patellar dislocation treated with an adequate rehabilitation program, most patients do not require surgical stabilization.[58] If there is an associated osteochondral fracture from the lateral femoral condyle or patellar surface, removal of the fragment or internal fixation is required, depending on the size and location of the injury. Small pieces avulsed from the medial edge of the patella usually are attached and may not require removal. Small loose bodies can be removed arthroscopically. There are preliminary reports of successful arthroscopic repair of a torn medial retinaculum and capsule.[58,410]

Early repair or advancement of the vastus medialis and distal realignment procedures are sometimes indicated. If there is an underlying malalignment or dysplasia accompanying a significant osteochondral fracture, both problems should be addressed. Occasionally, there is significant avulsion of the vastus medialis that requires primary repair.[237] Cash and Hughston had acceptable results after nonoperative care for 75% of appropriately selected patients. Rather than surgically stabilizing all patients, a group at high risk can be identified.[58]

One risk factor for recurrent dislocation is a young age, with those less than 14 years of age having the highest incidence of recurrent dislocation (Table 31-2).[58] Highly active and competitive athletes may also benefit from immediate stabilization.[33] Those with congenital dysplasia may be at higher risk for recurrence. The signs of this dysplasia include hypermobility of the patella, radiographic evidence of a shallow intercondylar groove, contralateral subluxation, a positive family history, patella alta, and a mechanism of injury other than a direct blow.[41,42,58,185]

Recurrent Patellar Dislocations

Although the risk of ongoing patellofemoral instability increases with each subsequent dislocation, many patients are successfully managed without surgery. In most cases, even young, active youths with other risk factors deserve a thorough trial of rehabilitation after

TABLE 30-2 *Risk Factors for Recurrent Patellar Dislocation*

Osteochondral fracture
Child younger than 14 years of age
Highly active or competitive youth
Mechanism other than direct blow
Palpable medial defect
Contralateral evidence of dysplasia
Hypermobility of the patella
Multiple prior dislocations
Positive family history
Patella alta

a first patellar dislocation. Knee sleeves and foot orthoses for those with severe pronation and tibial torsion may be helpful. Activity modifications are another option.

The decision to treat recurrent patellar instability surgically must be individualized. The degree of instability and disability should be weighed against the risks and benefits. Age is a factor to be considered, because tibial tubercle transfers are generally contraindicated if the physes are open.

Most aspects of the lateral retinacular release procedure are discussed in the patellofemoral pain section of this chapter. Many studies of lateral retinacular release mix patients with patellofemoral pain among those with patellofemoral instability. Metcalf analyzed the 14 cases of recurrent patellar dislocation in his series of 79 patients and found that none dislocated subsequent to a lateral retinacular release.[269] Nine were rated good and three rated excellent, with no instances of medial instability. Although it appears the lateral retinacular release has a role in the treatment of patellofemoral instability, the degree of instability that responds to this as an isolated procedure is yet to be defined.[350] A lateral retinacular release is routinely combined with medial advancements and distal realignments.

Patients with an obvious defect of the vastus medialis insertion are probably best served with advancement of the medial retinaculum and muscle. A variety of techniques have been described, but the fundamental elements include lateral release and plication of the vastus medialis.[15,184,237] The vastus medialis is advanced one third to one half of the width of the patella. The

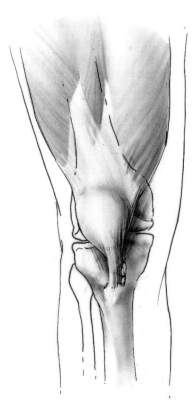

FIGURE 30-21. The Roux-Goldthwait procedure splits the patellar tendon. The lateral half is transferred beneath the medial side and sutured to the periosteum along the metaphysis. This redirects the patellar tendon vector more medially.

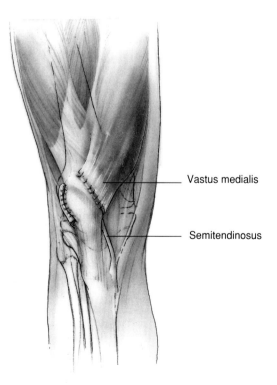

Vastus medialis

Semitendinosus

FIGURE 30-22. The Galeazzi procedure transfers the semitendinosus to the inferior pole of the patella. From there, it courses through a drill hole placed obliquely through the patella, exiting the superior lateral aspect. The tendon is then sutured to the soft tissues. This provides a medial tether and effectively alters the net vector of the patellar tendon toward the medial side. Typically, the vastus medialis is advanced approximately one third the width of the patella.

suture repair needs to be protected for at least 4 weeks after surgery.

Patients with an excessive Q angle can benefit from a distal realignment to medialize the pull of the patellar tendon. This can be accomplished by moving part of the patellar tendon itself, by transferring another tendon to the patella, and by moving the tibial tubercle. If there is significant growth remaining for the patient, the Roux-Goldthwait procedure should be considered. Tibial tubercle transfers can lead to distal migration of the tubercle or genu recurvatum secondary to growth arrest.[161,236] The Roux-Goldthwait operation involves splitting the patellar tendon and transferring the lateral half beneath the medial side (Fig. 30-21). For recurrent patellar dislocations, Chrisman reported 93% acceptable results with this procedure when combined with lateral retinacular release and medial reefing.[64] How much of the effect is the result of the distal transfer is unknown.

The Galleazzi procedure transfers the proximal end of the semitendinosus to the inferomedial pole of the patella, leaving the distal end of the semitendinosus attached to the tibia (Fig. 30-22). This effectively redirects the vector of force of the extensor mecha-

nism. Baker and colleagues had 81% successful results with this procedure.[14] Patients with excessive ligamentous laxity have the highest risk of persistent instability. Because the next most common complication is necrosis of the skin flap, undermining should be minimized.

For adolescents with closed physeal plates, the tibial tubercle can be transferred medially. This must be done in a manner that does not move the insertion of the tibial tubercle posteriorly along the face of the upper tibia, as did the Hauser procedure.[81,157]

The Elmslie-Trillat technique avoids this problem by shifting a long segment of bone, including the tubercle (Fig. 30-23A). For patellofemoral instability, good results can be expected in 80% of cases.[46] Tibial tubercle transfers are routinely combined with a lateral retinacular release. A vastus medialis obliquus advancement should be added if the patella drifts laterally when the knee reaches full extension and the quadriceps relaxes.[145,185]

If there is a significant component of patellofemoral pain or marked chondral injury of the patella, the Fulkerson modification of the Elmslie-Trillat procedure can reduce patellofemoral contact forces.[122,241]

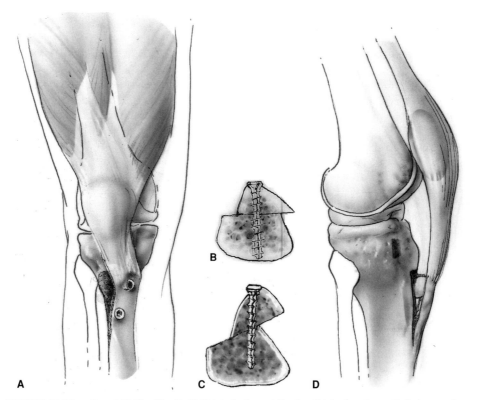

FIGURE 30-23. (**A** and **B**) The Elmslie-Trillat technique shifts the tibial tubercle medially by rotating a segment of bone. (**C**) The Fulkerson modification involves an oblique cut that results in anterior translation as the tubercle is moved medially. This reduces the patellofemoral contact forces while shifting the pull of the patella medially. (**D**) The Maquet procedure moves the tibial tubercle anteriorly by inserting a block of bone. This diminishes the patellofemoral contact forces but does not medialize the pull of the patellar tendon.

Instead of the osteotomy being in the coronal plane, it is tilted toward the sagittal plane such that the tubercle migrates anteriorly as it shifts medially (Fig. 30-23B).

The Maquet procedure reduces the patellofemoral contact forces by elevating the tubercle through the use of a bone block (Fig. 30-23C). This does not medialize the pull of the tendon, but it may be useful in cases of isolated patellofemoral chondromalacia.

All of these procedures require adequate rehabilitation to restore knee motion and maximize dynamic stability from the quadriceps.

The care of young athletes presents many challenges. Many of the principles of adult sports medicine and sports orthopaedics apply to youths, but there are many unique problems related to the growing musculoskeletal system. The evolving biology and psychology of young athletes makes working with them a pleasure and challenge.

References

1. Abramson SB. Nonsteroidal anti-inflammatory drugs: mechanism of action and therapeutic considerations. In: Leadbetter WB, Buckwalter JA, Gordon SL, eds. Sports-induced inflammation. Park Ridge, IL: American Academy of Orthopaedic Surgeons, 1990:421.
2. Adams JE. Injury to the throwing arm. Calif Med 1964;102:127.
3. Albanese S, Palmer A, Kerr D. Wrist pain and distal growth plate closure of the radius in gymnasts. J Pediatr Orthop 1989;9:23.
4. Alexander JE, Seibert JJ, Aronson J. Dorsal defect of the patella and infection. Pediatric Radiology 1987;30:325.
5. Allen RC, Gross KR, Laxer RM, et al. Intraarticular triamcinolone hexacetonide in the management of chronic arthritis in children. Arthritis Rheum 1986;29:997.
6. Alvarez E, Patel MR, Nimberg G, Pearlman HS. Fracture of the capitulum humeri. J Bone Joint Surg [Am] 1975;57:1093.
7. Anderson M, Green WT, Messner MB. Growth and predictions of growth in the lower extremities. J Bone Joint Surg 1963;45:1.
8. Andrews JR, Sanders R. A "mini reconstruction" technique in treating anterior lateral rotatory instability. Clin Orthop 1983;172:93.
9. Andrish JT, Bergfeld JA, Walheim J. A prospective study on the management of shin splints. J Bone Joint Surg [Am] 1974;56:1697.
10. Arnoczky SP, Rubin RM, Marshall JL. Microvasculatures of the cruciate ligament and its response to injury. J Bone Joint Surg 1979;61:1221.
11. Arnoczky SP, Warren RF. Microvasculature of the human meniscus. Am J Sports Med 1982;10:90.
12. Arnoczky SP, Warren RF. The microvasculature of the meniscus and its response to injury. Am J Sports Med 1983;11:131.
13. Baker BE, VanHanswyk E, Bogosian S, et al. A biomechanical study of the static stabilizing effect of knee braces on medical stability. Am J Sports Med 1987;15:566.
14. Baker RH, Carroll N, Dewar FP, Hall JE. The semitendinosus tenodesis for recurrent dislocation of the patella. J Bone Joint Surg [Br] 1972;54:103.
15. Baksi DP. Restoration of dynamic stability of the patella by pes anserinus transposition. J Bone Joint Surg [Br] 1981;63:399.
16. Bar-Or O. Climate and the exercising child—a review. Int J Sports Med 1980;1:53.
17. Baratz ME, Fu FH, Mengato R. Meniscal tears: the effect of meniscectomy and of repair on intraarticular contact areas and stress in the human knee. Am J Sports Med 1986;14:270.
18. Barber FA. Fenestrated medial patella plica. J Arthosc Rel Surg 1987;3:253.
19. Barnett LS. Little League shoulder syndrome: proximal humeral epiphyseolysis in adolescent baseball pitchers. J Bone Joint Surg [Am] 1985;67:495.
20. Basmajian JV, Lovejoy JF. Functions of the popliteus muscle in man. J Bone Joint Surg [Am] 1971;53:557.
21. Bassett FH, Gaits HS, Billys JB, et al. Talar impingement by the anteroinferior tibiofibular ligament: a cause of chronic pain in the ankle after inversion sprain. J Bone Joint Surg [Am] 1990;72:55.
22. Beekman RH. Exercise recommendations for adolescents after surgery for congenital heart disease. Pediatrician 1986;13:210.
23. Behrens TW, Goodwin TW. Oral corticosteroids. In: Leadbetter WB, Buckwalter JA, Gordon SL, eds. Sports-induced inflammation. Park Ridge, IL: American Academy of Orthopaedic Surgeons, 1990:405.
24. Bennett JG, Stauber WT. Evaluation and treatment of anterior knee pain using eccentric exercise. Med Sci Sports Exerc 1986;18:526.
25. Bergfield J. First-, second-, and third-degree sprains. Am J Sports Med 1979;7:207.
26. Bergstrom J, Hultman E. Nutrition for maximal sports performance. JAMA 1972;221:999.
27. Bert JM. The use of 1.5% glycine as a non-conductive fluid medium for arthroscopic electrosurgery. Arthroscopy 1987;3:248.
28. Bertin KC, Goble EM. Ligament injuries associated with physeal fractures about the knee. Clin Orthop Rel Res 1983;177:188.
29. Betz RR, Lonergan R, Patterson R. The percutaneous lateral retinacular release. Orthopedics 1982;5:57.
30. Bigos SJ, McBridge GG. The isolated lateral retinacular release in the treatment of patellofemoral disorders. Clin Orthop 1984;186:75.
31. Blum RW. Preparticipation evaluation of the adolescent athlete. Adolesc Athlete 1985;78:52.
32. Boger DC, Kingston S. Magnetic resonance imaging of the normal knee. Am J Knee Surg 1988;1:99.
33. Boring TH, O'Donoghue DH. Acute patellar dislocation: results of immediate surgical repair. Clin Orthop 1978;136:182.
34. Boucher JP. Am J Sports Med 1992.
35. Bowers KD Jr. Patellar tendon avulsion as a complication of Osgood-Schlatter's disease. Am J Sports Med 1981;9:356.
36. Bowker JH, Thompson EB. Surgical treatment of recurrent dislocation of the patella. J Bone Joint Surg [Am] 1964;46:1451.
37. Bradley GW, Shives TC, Samuelson KM. Ligament injuries in the knees of children. J Bone Joint Surg [Am] 1979;61:588.
38. Brady TA, Cahill BR, Bodnar LM. Weight training-related injuries in the high school athlete. Am J Sports Med 1982;10:1.
39. Brand RL, Collins MDF, Templeton T. Surgical repair of ruptured lateral ankle ligaments. Am J Sports Med 1981;9:40.
40. Brastrum. Sprained ankles anatomic lesions in recent sprains. Acta Orthop Scand 1964;188:483.
41. Brattstrom H. Shape of the intercondylar groove normally and in recurrent dislocation of patella. Acta Orthop Scand 1964;68:1.
42. Brattstrom H. Patella alta in non-dislocating knee joints. Acta Orthop Scand 1970;41:578.
43. Bray RC, Roth JH, Jacobsen RP. Arthroscopic lateral release for anterior knee pain. Arthroscopy 1987;3:237.
44. Brewer EJ, Arroyo I. Use of nonsteroidal anti-inflammatory drugs in children. Pediatr Ann 1986;15:575.

45. Brogdon BG, Crow NE. Little Leaguer's elbow. AJR 1960;83:671.

46. Brown DE, Alexander AH, Lichtman DM. The Elmslie-Trillat procedure: evaluation in patellar dislocation and subluxation. Am J Sports Med 1984;12:104.

47. Brown EW, Abani K. Kinematics and kinetics of the dead lift in adolescent power lifters. Med Sci Sports Exerc 1985;17:554.

48. Brown EW, Kimball RG. Medical history associated with adolescent power lifting. Pediatrics 1983;72:636.

49. Buckley WE, Yesalis CE, Friedl K, et al. Estimated prevalence of anabolic steroid use among male high school seniors. JAMA 1988;260:3441.

50. Busch MT. Meniscal injuries in children and adolescents. Clin Sports Med 1990;9:661.

51. Busch MT, DeHaven KE, Panni AS. Two- to ten-year results of lateral retinacular release for patellofemoral pain. Las Vegas, American Academy of Orthopaedic Surgeons Meeting, 1989.

52. Cahill BR, Griffith EH. Effect of preseason conditioning on the incidence and severity of high school football knee injuries. Am J Sports Med 1978;6:180.

53. Cahill BR, Tullos HS, Fain RH. Little League shoulder. Am J Sports Med 1974;2:150.

54. Caine D, Roy S, Singer KM, Broekhoff J. Stress changes of the distal radial growth plate. Am J Sports Med 1992;20:290.

55. Canale ST, Williams KD. Iselin's disease. J Pediatr Orthop 1992;12:90.

56. Carrasco D, Prieto M, Pallardo L, et al. Multiple hepatic adenomas after long-Term therapy with testosterone enanthate. J Hepatol 1985;1:573.

57. Carson Jr. WG. Extra-articular reconstruction of the anterior cruciate ligament: lateral procedures. Orthop Clin North Am 1985;16:191.

58. Cash JD, Hughston JC. Treatment of acute patellar dislocation. Am J Sports Med 1988;16:244.

59. Cass JR, Morrey BF, Katoh Y, Chao EYS. Ankle instability: comparison of primary repair and delayed reconstruction after long-term follow-up study. Clin Orthop Rel Res 1985;198:110.

60. Cassells SW. Clin Orthop.

61. Cassidy RE, Shaffer AJ. Repair of peripheral meniscus tear: a preliminary report. Am J Sports Med 1981;9:209.

62. Ceder LC, Larson RL. Z-plasty lateral retinacular release for the treatment of patellar compression syndrome. Clin Orthop 1979;144:110.

63. Chambers RB. Orthopaedic injuries in athletes (ages 6 to 17). Am J Sports Med 1979;7:195.

64. Chrisman OD, Fessel JM, Southwock WO. Experimental production of synovitis and marginal articular exostoses in the knee joints of dogs. Yale J Biol Med 1965;37:409.

65. Chrisman OD, Snook GA. Reconstruction of lateral ligament tears of the ankle. J Bone Joint Surg [Am] 1969;51:904.

66. Clancy WG, Folotz AS. Iliac apophysitis and stress fractures in adolescent runners. Am J Sports Med 1976;4:214.

67. Clancy WG, Shelbourne KD, Zoellner GB, et al. Treatment of knee joint instability secondary to rupture of the posterior cruciate ligament. J Bone Joint Surg [Am] 1983;65:310.

68. Clanton TO, DeLee JC, Sanders B, Neidre A. Knee ligament injuries in children. J Bone Joint Surg [Am] 1979;61:1195.

69. Clark CR, Ogden JA. Development of the menisci of the human knee joint. J Bone Joint Surg [Am] 1983;65:538.

70. Clarke KS. A survey of sports-Related spinal cord injuries in schools and colleges. J Safety Res 1977;9:140.

71. Clement DB. Tibial stress syndrome in athletes. J Sports Med 1975;2:81.

72. Clement DB, Tauton JE, Smart GW. Achilles tendinitis and peritendinitis: etiology and treatment. Am J Sports Med 1984;12:179.

73. Clowes GH, O'Donnell TF. Heat stroke. N Engl J Med 1974;291:564.

74. Committee on Sports Medicine, American Academy of Pediatrics. Climactic heat stress and the exercising child. Pediatrics 1982;69:808.

75. Committee on Sports Medicine, American Academy of Pediatrics. Nutrition and sports performance. In: Smith N, ed. Sports medicine health care for young athletes. Evanston, IL: American Academy of Pediatrics, 1983:161.

76. Committee on Sports Medicine, American Academy of Pediatrics. Thermoregulation and fluid and electrolyte needs. In: Smith N, ed. Sports medicine health care for young athletes. Evanston, IL: American Academy of Pediatrics, 1983:142.

77. Committee on Sports Medicine, American Academy of Pediatrics. Weight training and weight lifting: information for the pediatrician. Physician Sports Med 1983;11:157.

78. Committee on Sports Medicine, American Academy of Pediatrics. Recommendations for participation in competitive sports. Pediatrics 1988;81:737.

79. Costill DL, Hargreaves M. Carbohydrate nutrition and fatigue. Sports Med 1992;13:86.

80. Cox JS. Surgical and nonsurgical treatment of acute ankle sprains. Clin Orthop 1985;198:118.

81. Crigler NW, Riddervole HO. Soft tissue changes in x-ray diagnosis of the Osgood-Schlatter lesion. Virginia Med 1982;109:176.

82. Crosby EB, Insall J. Recurrent dislocation of the patella. J Bone Joint Surg [Am] 1976;58:9.

83. D'Ambrosia RD, Zelis RF, Chuinard RG, Wilmore J. Interstitial pressure measurements in the anterior and posterior compartments in athletes with shin splints. Am J Sports Med 1977;5:127.

84. Dandy DJ, Pusey RJ. The long-term results of unrepaired tears of the posterior cruciate ligament. J Bone Joint Surg [Br] 1982;64:92.

85. Danielsson LG, Hedlund ST, Henricson AS. Apophysitis of the olecranon. A report of four cases. Acta Orthop Scand 1983;54:777.

86. DeHaven KE. Diagnosis of acute knee injuries with hemarthrosis. Am J Sports Med 1980;8:9.

87. DeHaven KE. Meniscus repair in the athlete. Clin Orthop 1985;198:31.

88. Dehaven KE, Dolan WA, Mayer PJ. Chondromalacia patellae in athletes. Am J Sports Med 1979;7:5.

89. DeHaven KE, Lintner DM. Athletic injuries: comparison by age, sport, and gender. Am J Sports Med 1986;14:218.

90. DeLee JC, Curtis R. Anterior cruciate ligament insufficiency in children. Clin Orthop Rel Res 1983;172:112.

91. Denham RH. Dorsal defect of the patella. J Bone Joint Surg [Am] 1984;66:116.

92. Derscheid GL, Garrick JG. Medial collateral ligament injuries in football. Am J Sports Med 1981;9:365.

93. Detmer DE, Sharpe K, Sufit RL, Girdley FM. Chronic compartment syndrome: diagnosis, management, and outcomes. Am J Sports Med 1985;13:162.

94. Devas MB. Stress fractures in children. J Bone Joint Surg [Br] 1963;45:528.

95. Dias LS. Lateral ankle sprain: an experimental study. Journal of Trauma 1979;4:266.

96. Dickhaut SC, DeLee JC. The discoid lateral meniscus syndrome. J Bone Joint Surg [Am] 1982;64:1068.

97. Dickson JM, Fox JM. Fracture of the patella due to overuse syndrome in a child: a case report. Am J Sports Med 1982;10:248.

98. Dickson JM, Kichline PD. Functional management of stress fractures in female athletes using a pneumatic leg brace. Am J Sports Med 1987;15:86.

99. Digby KH. The measurement of diaphyseal growth in proximal and distal directions. J Am Physiol 1915;50:187.

100. Dotter WE. Little Leaguer's shoulder. 1953.

101. Doucette SA, Goble EM. The effect of exercise on patellar tracking in lateral patellar compression syndrome. Am J Sports Med 1992;20:434.

102. Dye SF, Boll DA. Radionuclide imaging of the patellofemoral joint in young athletes. Orthop Clin North Am 1986;17:249.

103. Dyment PG. The adolescent athlete and ergogenic aids. J Adolesc Health Care 1987;8:68.

104. Dzioba RB, Strokon A, Mulbry L. Diagnostic arthroscopy and longitudinal open lateral release: a safe and affective treatment for "chondromalacia patella." Arthroscopy 1985;1:131.

105. Eady JL, Cardenas CD, Sopa D. Avulsion of the femoral attachment of the anterior cruciate ligament in a seven-year-old child. J Bone Joint Surg [Am] 1982;64:1376.

106. Edwards DH, Bentley G. Osteochondritis dissecans patellae. J Bone Joint Surg 1977;59:58.

107. Edwards GSJ, DeLee JC. Ankle diastasis without fracture. Foot Ankle 1984;4:306.

108. Engh CA, Robinson RA, Milgram J. Stress fractures in children. J Trauma 1970;10:532.

109. Evans GA, Hardcastle P, Frenyo AD. Acute rupture of the lateral ligament of the ankle. J Bone Joint Surg [Br] 1984;66:209.

110. Ferguson RJ, McMasters MC, Stanitski CL. Low back pain in college football lineman. J Bone Joint Surg [Am] 1974;58:1300.

111. Fernbach SK, Wilkinson RH. Avulsion injuries of the pelvis and proximal femur. AJR 1981;137:581.

112. Fetto JF, Marshall JL. Medial collateral ligament injuries of the knee: a rationale for treatment. Clin Orthop 1978;147:29.

113. Fetto JF, Marshall JL. Injury to the anterior cruciate ligament producing the pivot-shift sign. J Bone Joint Surg [Am] 1979;61:710.

114. Fetto JF, Marshall JL. The natural history and diagnosis of anterior cruciate ligament insufficiency. Clin Orthop Rel Res 1980;147:29.

115. Ficat RP, Philippe J, Hungerford DS. Chondromalacia of the patella: a system of classification. Clin Orthop 1979;144:55.

116. Fogelman I, McKillop JH, Gray HW. The "hot patella" sign: is it of any clinical significance? J Nucl Med 1983;24:312.

117. Fordyce AJW, Horn CV. Arthrography in recent injuries in the ligaments of the ankle. J Bone Joint Surg [Br] 1972;54:116.

118. Fox IM. Iliac apophysitis in teenage distance runners. J Am Podiatr Med Assoc 1986;76:294.

119. Fox TA. Dysplasia of the quadriceps mechanism. Surg Clin North Am 1975.

120. Frank C, Woo SL, Amiel D. Medial collateral ligament healing: a multidisciplinary assessment in rabbits. Am J Sports Med 1983;11:379.

121. Fritschy D. An unusual ankle injury in top skiers. Am J Sports Med 1989;17:282.

122. Fujikawa K, Iseki F, Mikura Y. Partial resection of the discoid meniscus in the child's knee. J Bone Joint Surg [Br] 1981;63:391.

123. Fulkerson JP. Anteromedialization of the tibial tuberosity for patellofemoral malalignment. Clin Orthop 1983;177:176.

124. Fulkerson JP, Gossling HR. Anatomy of the knee joint lateral retinaculum. Clin Orthop 1980;153:183.

125. Fulkerson JP, Schutzer SF. After failure of conservative treatment for painful patellofemoral malalignment: lateral release or realignment? Orthop Clin North Am 1986;17:283.

126. Fulkerson JP, Schutzer SF, Ramsby GR, Bernstein RA. Computerized tomography of the patellofemoral joint before and after lateral release or realignment. J Arthosc Rel Surg 1987;3:19.

127. Fulkerson Jp, Shea Kp. Disorders of patellofemoral alignment. J Bone Joint Surg [Am] 1990;72:1424.

128. Fullerton LR, Snowdy HA. Femoral neck stress fractures. Am J Sports Med 1988;16:365.

129. Galway HR, MacIntosh DL. The lateral pivot shift: a symptom and sign of anterior cruciate ligament insufficiency. Clin Orthop Rel Res 1980;147:45.

130. Gamble JG. Symptomatic dorsal defect of the patella in a runner. Am J Sports Med 1986;14:425.

131. Garrick JG. "When can I. . .?" Am J Sports Med 1981;9:67.

132. Garrick JG, Requa RK. Injuries in high school sports. Pediatrics 1978;61:465.

133. Ghadially FN, Wedge JH, LaLonde J. Experimental methods of repairing injured menisci. J Bone Joint Surg [Br] 1986;68:106.

134. Godshall RW, Hansen CA. Incomplete avulsion of a portion of the iliac epiphysis. J Bone Joint Surg [Am] 1973;55:1301.

135. Goergen TG, Resnick D, Greenway G. Dorsal defect of the patella (DDP). Radiology 1979;130:333.

136. Goldberg B. Children, sports, and chronic disease. Physician Sports Med 1990;18:45.

137. Goldberg B, Saraniti A, Witman P, et al. Pre-participation sports assessment—an objective evaluation. Pediatrics 1980;66:736.

138. Goldberg B, Witman PA, Gleim GW, Nicholas JA. Children's sports injuries: are they avoidable? Physician Sports Med 1979;7:93.

139. Goodfellow J, Hungerford DS, Woods C. Patello-femoral joint mechanics and pathology. J Bone Joint Surg [Br] 1976;58:291.

140. Grana WA. Summary of 1978–79 Injury Registry for Oklahoma secondary schools. Okla State Med Assoc J 1979;72:369.

141. Grana WA, Hinkley B, Hollingsworth S. Arthroscopic evaluation and treatment of patellar malalignment. Clin Orthop 1984;186:122.

142. Grana WA, Moretz JA. Ligamentous laxity in secondary school athletes. JAMA 1978;240:1975.

143. Green NE, Rogers RA, Lipscomb AB. Nonunions of stress fractures of the tibia. Am J Sports Med 1985;13:171.

144. Green WT, Anderson M. Skeletal age and the control of bone growth. Instr Course Lect 1960;17:199.

145. Gross MT, Bradshaw MK, Ventry LC, Weller KH. Comparison of support provided by ankle taping and semi-rigid orthosis. J Orthop Sports Phys Ther 1987;9:33.

146. Gruber MA. The conservative treatment of chondromalacia patellae. Orthop Clin North Am 1979;10:105.

147. Guhl JF. Arthroscopy and arthroscopic surgery of the elbow. Orthopedics 1985;8:1290.

148. Gumbs VL, Segal D, Halligan JB, Lower G. Bilateral distal radius and ulnar fractures in adolescent weight lifters. Am J Sports Med 1982;10:375.

149. Hackenbruch W, Noesberger B, Debrunner HU. Differential diagnosis of ruptures of the lateral ligaments of the ankle joint. Arch Orthop Traum Surg 1979;93:293.

150. Hajek MR, Noble HB. Stress fractures of the femoral neck in joggers. Am J Sports Med 1982;10:112.

151. Hamilton H. Stress fracture of the diaphysis of the ulna in a body builder. Am J Sports Med 1984;12:405.

152. Hansen NM. Epiphyseal changes in the proximal humerus of an adolescent baseball pitcher. Am J Sports Med 1982;10:380.

153. Haraldsson S. On osteochondrosis deformans juveniles capituli humeri including investigation of intra-osseous vasculature in distal humerus. Acta Orthop Scand 1959;38:1.

154. Hardaker WT, Whipple TL, Bassett FH. Diagnosis and treatment of the plica syndrome of the knee. J Bone Joint Surg [Am] 1980;62:221.

155. Harvey JS. Overuse syndromes in young athletes. Pediatr Clin North Am 1982;29:1369.

156. Harwin SF, Stern RE. Subcutaneous lateral retinacular release for chondromalacia patellae: a preliminary report. Clin Orthop 1981;156:207.

157. Haswell DM, Berne AS, Graham CB. The dorsal defect of the patella. Pediatr Radiol 1976;4:238.

158. Hauser ED. Total tendon transplant for slipping patella. Surg Gynecol Obstet 1938;66:199.

159. Hawkins RJ, Misamore GW, Merritt TR. Follow-up of the acute nonoperated isolated anterior cruciate ligament tear. Am J Sports Med 1986;14:205.

160. Hedstrom SA, Lidgren L. Acute hematogenous pelvic osteomyelitis in athletes. Am J Sports Med 1982;10:44.

161. Hejgaard N, Diemer H. Bone scan in the patellofemoral pain syndrome. Int Orthop 1987;11:29.

162. Hejgaard N, Skive L, Perrild C. Recurrent dislocation of the patella. Acta Orthop Scand 1980;51:673.

163. Helfet AJ. Mechanisms of derangements of the medial semilunar cartilage and their management. J Bone Joint Surg [Br] 1956;41:319.

164. Henning CE, Egge LN. Cast brace treatment of acute unstable lateral ankle sprain. Am J Sports Med 1977;5:252.

165. Henry JH, Craven PR. Surgical treatment of patellar instability: indications and results. Am J Sports Med 1981;9:82.

166. Herzmark MH. The evolution of the knee joint. J Bone Joint Surg 1938;20:77.

167. Hewson GF Jr, Mendini RA, Wang JB. Prophylactic knee bracing in college football. Am J Sports Med 1986;14:262.

168. Highland TR, Lamont RL. Osteomyelitis of the pelvis in children. J Bone Joint Surg 1983;65:230.

169. Hocutt JE, Jaffe R, Rylander R, Beebe JK. Cryotherapy in ankle sprains. Am J Sports Med 1982;10:316.

170. Holden DL, Jackson DW. Treatment selection in acute anterior cruciate ligament tears. Orthop Clin North Am 1985;16:99.

171. Holder LE, Michael RH. The specific scintigraphic pattern of "shin splints in the lower leg." J Nucl Med 1984;25:869.

172. Holmes JC, Pruitt AL, Whalen NJ. Iliotibial band syndrome in cyclists. Am J Sports Med 1993;21:419.

173. Holsbeeck MV, Vandamme B, Marchal G, et al. Dorsal defect of the patella: concept of its origin and relationship with bipartite and multipartite patella. Skeletal Radiol 1987;16:304.

174. Hopkinson WJ, St. Pierre P, Ryan JB, Wheeler JH. Syndesmosis sprains of the ankle. Foot Ankle 1990;10:325.

175. Hoppenfeld S. Physical examination of the spine and extremities. New York: Appleton-Century-Croft, 1976.

176. Howard FM, Piha RJ. Fractures of the apophysis in adolescent athletes. JAMA 1965;192:150.

177. Hughston JC. Subluxation of the patella. J Bone Joint Surg [Am] 1968;50:1003.

178. Hughston JC, Andrews JR, Cross MJ. Classification of knee ligament instabilities. Part I. The medial compartment and cruciate ligaments. J Bone Joint Surg [Am] 1976;58:159.

179. Hughston JC, Bowden JA, Andrews JR, Norwood LA. Acute tears of the posterior cruciate ligament. J Bone Joint Surg [Am] 1980;62:438.

180. Hughston JC, Deese M. Medial subluxation of the patella as a complication of lateral retinacular release. Am J Sports Med 1988;16:383.

181. Hungerford DS, Barry M. Biomechanics of the patellofemoral joint. Clin Orthop 1979;144:9.

182. Hunter LY, Hensinger RN. Dorsal defect of the patella with cartilaginous involvement. Clin Orthop 1979;143:131.

183. Hunter LY, O'Connor GA. Traction apophysitis of the olecranon. A case report. Am J Sports Med 1980;8:51.

184. Indelicato PA. Non-operative treatment of complete tears of the medial collateral ligament of the knee. J Bone Joint Surg [Am] 1983;65:323.

185. Insall J, Falvo KA, Wise DW. Chondromalacia patellae. J Bone Joint Surg [Am] 1976;58:1.

186. Insall J, Goldberg V, Salvati E. Recurrent dislocation and the high-riding patella. Clin Orthop Rel Res 1972;88:67.

187. Ireland J, Trickey EL, Stoker DJ. Arthroscopy and arthrography of the knee. J Bone Joint Surg 1980;62:3.

188. Jackson D, Wiltse L, Cirincone R. Spondylolysis in the female gymnast. Clin Orthop 1976;117:68.

189. Jackson DW, Ashley RL, Powell JW. Ankle sprains in young athletes. Clin Orthop Rel Res 1974;101:201.

190. Jackson DW, Jennings LD, Maywood RM. Magnetic resonance imaging of the knee. Am J Sports Med 1988;16:29.

191. Jackson MDW, Feagin LCJA. Quadriceps contusions in young athletes. J Bone Joint Surg [Am] 1973;55:95.

192. James SL. Chondromalacia of the patella in the adolescent. 1979; 205.

193. James SL, Bates BT, Osternig LR. Injuries to runners. Am J Sports Med 1978;6:41.

194. Johansson E, Aparisi T. Congenital absence of cruciate ligaments. Clin Orthop;182:108.

195. Johnson JF, Brogdon BG. Dorsal defect of the patella: incidence and distribution. AJR 1982;139:339.

196. Johnson MD, Jay MS, Shoup B, Rickert VI. Anabolic steroid use by male adolescents. Pediatrics 1989;83:921.

197. Joseph KN, Pogrund H. Traumatic rupture of the medial ligament of the knee in a four-year-old Boy. J Bone Joint Surg [Am] 1978;60:402.

198. Julsrud ME. Iliac apophysitis and a review of the osteochondroses. J Am Podiatr Med Assoc 1985;75:586.

199. Kaltsas D-S. Stress fractures of the femoral neck in young adults. J Bone Joint Surg [Br] 1981;63:33.

200. Kaplan EB. Discoid lateral meniscus of the knee joint. J Bone Joint Surg [Am] 1957;39:77.

201. Kaplan EB. The iliotibial tract—clinical and morphological significance. J Bone Joint Surg [Am] 1958;40:817.

202. Karlsson J, Andreasson GO. The effect of external ankle support in chronic lateral ankle joint instability. Am J Sports Med 1992;20:257.

203. Karlsson J, Saltin B. Diet, muscle glycogen, and endurance performance. J Appl Physiol 1971;31:203.

204. Kaufer H. Mechanical function of the patella. J Bone Joint Surg [Am] 1971;53:1551.

205. Kay DB. The sprained ankle: current therapy. J Foot Ankle 1985;6:22.

206. Kay JJ, Freiberger RH. Fragmentation of the lower pole of the patella in spastic lower extremities. Radiology 1991;101:97.

207. Keren G, Epstein Y. The effect of high-dosage vitamin C intake on aerobic and anaerobic capacity. J Sports Med 1980;20:145.

208. Keskinen K, Eriksson E, Komi P. Breaststroke swimmer's knee: a biomechanical and arthroscopic study. Am J Sports Med 1980;8:228.

209. Kibler WB. Concepts in exercise rehabilitation of athletic injury. In: Leadbetter WB, Buckwalter JA, Gordon SL, eds. Sports-induced inflammation. Park Ridge, IL: American Academy of Orthopaedic Surgeons, 1990;759.

210. King AC. Meniscal lesions in children and adolescent: a review of the pathology and clinical presentation. Injury 1984;15:105.

211. Klepping J, Boggio V, Guilland JC, et al. The nutritional requirements of young athletes. Ann Nestle 1986;44:1.

212. Knochel JP. Dog days and siriasis. JAMA 1975;233:513.

213. Kohn HS, Newton GN, Collier BD. Chondromalacia of the patella: bone imaging correlated with arthroscopic findings. Clin Nucl Med 1988;13:96.

214. Krause BL, Williams JPR, Catterall A. Natural history of Osgood-Schlatter's disease. J Pediatr Orthop 1990;10:65.

215. Krompinger WJ, Fulkerson JP. Lateral retinacular release for intractable lateral retinacular pain. Clin Orthop 1983;179:191.

216. Kujala UM, Kvist M, Heinonen O. Osgood-Schlatter's disease in adolescent athletes. Am J Sports Med 1985;13:236.

217. Kurosaka M, Yoshiya S, Ohno O. Lateral discoid meniscectomy: a 20-year follow-up. San Francisco, American Academy of Orthopaedic Surgeons Meeting, 1987.

218. Kvist M, Kujala UM, Heinonen OJ, et al. Sports-related injuries in children. Int J Sports Med 1989;10:81.

219. Lambert GP. Children and sports medicine in the 1990's. N J Med 1991;88:635.

220. Lancourt JE, Cristini JA. Patella alta and patella infera: their etiological role in patellar dislocation, chondromalacia and apophysitis of the tibial tubercle. J Bone Joint Surg 1975; 57:1112.

221. Lankenner PA, Micheli LJ, Clancy R, Gerbino PG. Arthroscopic percutaneous lateral patellar retinacular release. Am J Sports Med 1986;14:267.

222. Larsen E. Taping the ankle for chronic instability. Acta Orthop Scand 1984;55:551.

223. Larsen E, Lauridsen F. Conservative treatment of patellar dislocations. Clin Orthop 1982;171:131.

224. Larson RL, Cabaud HE, Slocum DB. The patellar compression syndrome: surgical treatment by lateral retinacular release. Clin Orthop 1978;134:158.

225. Laurin CA, Dussault R, Levesque HP. The tangential x-ray investigation of the patellofemoral joint. Clin Orthop 1979; 144:16.

226. Leach RE, James S, Wasilewski S. Achilles tendinitis. Am J Sports Med 1981;9:93.

227. Leadbetter WB. Corticosteroid injection therapy in sports injuries. In: Leadbetter WB, Buckwalter JA, Gordon SL, eds. Sports-induced inflammation. Park Ridge, IL: American Academy of Orthopaedic Surgeons, 1990:527.

228. Lehman RC, Gregg JR, Torg E. Iselin's disease. Am J Sports Med 1986;14:494.

229. Lindberg U, Lysholm J, Gillquist J. The correlation between arthroscopic findings and the patellofemoral pain syndrome. J Arthosc Rel Surg 1986;2:103.

230. Linder CW, DuRant RH, Seklecki RM, Strong WB. Preparticipation health screening of young athletes. Am J Sports Med 1981;9:187.

231. Lipscomb AB, Anderson AF. Tears of the anterior cruciate ligament in adolescents. J Bone Joint Surg [Am] 1986; 68:19.

232. Lipscomb AB, Thomas ED, Johnston RK. Treatment of myositis ossificans traumatica in athletes. Am J Sports Med 1976; 4:111.

233. Lombardo SJ, Retting AC, Kerlan RK. Radiographic abnormalities of the iliac apophysis in adolescent athletes. J Bone Joint Surg [Am] 1983;65:444.

234. Lutter LD. Cavus foot in runners. Foot Ankle 1981;1:225.

235. Lutter LD. Runner's knee injuries. Instr Course Lect 1984; 33:258.

236. Lysholm J, Nordin M, Ekstrand J. The effect of a patella brace on performance in a knee extension strength test in patients with patellar pain. Am J Sports Med 1984;12:110.

237. MacNab I. Recurrent dislocation of the patella. J Bone Joint Surg [Am] 1952;34:957.

238. Madigan R, Wissinger HA, Donaldson WF. Preliminary experience with a method of quadricepsplasty in recurrent subluxation of the patella. J Bone Joint Surg [Am] 1975;57: 600.

239. Mankin HJ, Conger KA. The acute affects of intraarticular hydrocortisone on articular cartilage in rabbits. J Bone Joint Surg [Am] 1966;48:1383.

240. Mann RA, Baxter DE, Lutter LD. Running symposium. Foot Ankle 1981;1:190.

241. Manzione M, Pizzutillo PD, Peoples AB, Schweizer PA. Menis-

cectomy in children: a long-term follow-up study. Am J Sports Med 1983;11:111.

242. Maquet P. Mechanics and osteoarthritis of the patellofemoral joint. Clin Orthop 1979;144:70.

243. Maron BJ, Roberts WC, McAllister HA, et al. Sudden death in young athletes. Circulation 1980;62:218.

244. Marshall JL, Wang JB, Furman W, et al. The anterior drawer sign: what is it? Am J Sports Med 1975;3:152.

245. Marshall JL, Warren RF, Wickiewicz L. The anterior cruciate ligament: a technique of repair and reconstruction. Clin Orthop 1979;143:97.

246. Marshall SC. Combined arthroscopic/open repair of meniscal injuries. Contemp Orthop 1987;14:15.

247. Martens M, Libbrecht P, Burssens A. Surgical treatment of the iliotibial band friction syndrome. Am J Sports Med 1989;17:651.

248. Martens R. Sports for children and youths. Champaign, IL: Human Kinetics Publishers, 1986.

249. Marymont JV, Lynch MA, Henning CE. Acute ligamentous diastasis of the ankle without fracture: evaluation by radionuclide imaging. Am J Sports Med 1986;14:407.

250. Matheson GO, Clement DB, McKenzie DC, et al. Stress fractures in athletes. Am J Sports Med 1987;15:46.

251. Matsen FA, Winquist RA, Krugmire RB. Diagnosis and management of compartment syndromes. J Bone Joint Surg [Am] 1980;62:286.

252. Matz SO, Jackson DW. Anterior cruciate ligament injury in children. Am J Knee Surg 1988;1:59.

253. Mayer PJ, Micheli LJ. Avulsion of the femoral attachment of the posterior cruciate ligament in an eleven year old boy. J Bone Joint Surg [Am] 1979;61:431.

254. Mayfield GW. Popliteus tendon tenosynovitis. Am J Sports Med 1977;5:31.

255. McCarroll JR, Rettig AC, Shelbourne KD. Anterior cruciate ligament injuries in the young athlete with open physes. Am J Sports Med 1988;16:44.

256. McCarroll JR, Schrader JW, Shelbourne KD, et al. Meniscoid lesions of the ankle in soccer players. Am J Sports Med 1987;15:255.

257. McCoy GF, Piggott J, MacAfee AL, Adair IV. Injuries of the cervical spine in schoolboy rugby football. J Bone Joint Surg [Br] 1984;66:500.

258. McDaniel Jr. WJ, Dameron TJ Jr. Untreated ruptures of the anterior cruciate ligament. J Bone Joint Surg [Am] 1980;62:696.

259. McGinty JB, McCarthy JC. Endoscopic lateral retinacular release. Clin Orthop 1981;158:120.

260. McKenzie DC, Taunton JE, Clement DB, et al. Calcaneal epiphysis in adolescent athletes. Can J Appl Sports Sci 1981;6:123.

261. McLain LG, Reynolds S. Sports injuries in a high school. Pediatrics 1989;84:446.

262. McManama GB Jr, Micheli LJ, Berry MV, Sohn RS. The surgical treatment of osteochondritis of the capitellum. Am J Sports Med 1985;13:11.

263. McManus F, Rang M, Heslin DJ. Acute dislocation of the patella in children. Clin Orthop 1979;139:88.

264. Medlar RC, Lyne ED. Sinding–Larsen–Johansson disease. J Bone Joint Surg [Am] 1978;60:1113.

265. Medlar RC, Mandiberg JJ, Lyne ED. Meniscectomies in children. Am J Sports Med 1980;8:87.

266. Meislin RJ, Rose DJ, Parisien JS, Springer S. Arthroscopic treatment of synovial impingement of the ankle. Am J Sports Med 1993;21:186.

267. Merchant AC, Mercer RL. Lateral release of the patella: a preliminary report. Clin Orthop 1974;103:40.

268. Merchant AC, Mercer RL, Jacobsen RH, Cool CR. Roentgenographic analysis of patellofemoral congruence. J Bone Joint Surg [Am] 1974;56:1391.

269. Meredith CN, Dwyer JT. Nutrition and exercise: effects on adolescent health. Annu Rev Public Health 1991;12:309.

270. Metcalf RW. An arthroscopic method for lateral release of the subluxating or dislocating patella. Clin Orthop 1982;167:9.

271. Metheny JA, Mayor MB. Hoffa disease: chronic impingement of the infrapatellar fat pad. Am J Knee Surg 1988;1:134.

272. Metzmaker JN, Pappas AM. Avulsion fractures of the pelvis. Am J Sports Med 1985;13:349.

273. Meyers MH. Isolated avulsion of the tibial attachment of the posterior cruciate ligament of the knee. J Bone Joint Surg [Am] 1975;57:669.

274. Michael RH, Holder LE. The soleus syndrome. Am J Sports Med 1985;13:87.

275. Micheli LJ, Ireland ML. Prevention and management of calcaneal apophysitis in children: an overuse syndrome. J Pediatr Orthop 1987;7:34.

276. Milgrom C, Giladi M, Stein M. Stress fractures in military recruits. J Bone Joint Surg [Am] 1985;67:732.

277. Miller GK, Dickason JM, Fox JM. The use of electrosurgery for arthroscopic subcutaneous lateral retinacular release. Orthopedics 1982;5:309.

278. Miller WB, Murphy WA, Gilula LA, Kantor OS. Brodie's abscess of the patella. JAMA 1977;238:1179.

279. Mital MA, Matza RA, Cohen J. The so-called unresolved Osgood-Schlatter lesion. J Bone Joint Surg [Am] 1980;62:732.

280. Mubarak S, Hargens A. Symposium on the foot and legs in running sports. St. Louis: CV Mosby, 1982:141.

281. Mubarak SJ, Owen CA. Double incision fasciotomy of the leg for decompression in compartment syndromes. J Bone Joint Surg [Am] 1977;59:184.

282. Mubarak SJ, Gould RN, Lee YF, et al. The medial tibial stress syndrome. Am J Sports Med 1982;10:201.

283. Mubarak SJ, Hargens AR, Owen CA, et al. The wick catheter technique for measurement of intramuscular pressure. J Bone Joint Surg [Am] 1976;58:1016.

284. Munnings F. Does stretching really help performance and prevent injuries? Your Patient Fitness 1990;3:10.

285. Murakami Y. Stress fracture of the metacarpal in an adolescent tennis player. Am J Sports Med 1988;6:419.

286. Murphy RJ. Heat illness in the athlete. Am J Sports Med 1984;12:258.

287. Nelen G, Martens M, Burssens A. Am J Sports Med 1989;17:754.

288. Nichols JN, Tehranzadeh J. A review of the tibial spine fractures in bicycle injury. Am J Sports Med 1987;15:172.

289. Noble CA. Iliotibial band friction syndrome in runners. Am J Sports Med 1980;8:232.

290. Noble HB, Hajek MR, Porter M. Diagnosis and treatment of iliotibial band tightness in runners. Physician Sports Med 1982;10:67.

291. Nottage WM, Sprauge NF, Auerbach BJ, Shahriaree H. The medial patellar plica syndrome. Am J Sports Med 1983;11:211.

292. Noyes FR. Functional properties of knee ligaments and alterations induced by immobilization. Clin Orthop 1977;123:210.

293. Noyes FR, Bassett RW, Grood ES, Butler DL. Arthroscopy in acute traumatic hemarthrosis of the knee. J Bone Joint Surg [Am] 1980;62:687.

294. Noyes FR, Butler DL, Grood ES, et al. Biomechanical analysis of human ligament grafts used in knee-ligament repairs and reconstructions. J Bone Joint Surg [Am] 1984;66:344.

295. O'Connor GA. Collateral ligament injuries of the joint. Am J Sports Med 1979;7:209.

296. O'Neill DB, Micheli LJ, Warner JP. Patellofemoral stress: a prospective analysis of exercise treatment in adolescents and adults. Am J Sports Med 1992;20:151.

297. Odensten M, Lysholm J, Gillquist J. The course of partial anterior cruciate ligament ruptures. Am J Sports Med 1985; 13:183.

298. Ogden JA, Lee J. Accessory ossification patterns in injuries of the malleoli. J Pediatr Orthop 1990;10:306.

299. Ogden JA, Southwick WO. Osgood-Schlatter's disease and tibial tuberosity development. Clin Orthop 1976;116:180.

300. Ogilvie-Harris DJ, Jackson RW. The arthroscopic treatment of chondromalacia patellae. J Bone Joint Surg [Br] 1984;66:660.

301. Oliver JH, Coughlin LP. Objective knee evaluation using the Genucom knee analysis system. Am J Sports Med 1987;15:571.

302. Olson WR, Rechkemmer L. Popliteus tendinitis. J Am Podiatr Med Assoc 1993;83:537.

303. Orava S. Iliotibial tract friction syndrome in athletes. Br J Sports Med 1978;12:69.

304. Orava S, Jormakka E, Hulkko A. Stress fractures in young athletes. Arch Orthop Traum Surg 1981;98:271.

305. Orenstein DM, Reed ME, Grogan FTJ, Crawford LV. Exercise conditioning in children with asthma. J Pediatr 1985;106:556.

306. Orethorp N, Anders A, Ekstrom H. Immediate effects of meniscectomy in the knee joint: the effect of tensile load on knee joint ligaments in dogs. Acta Orthop Scand 1978;49:407.

307. Palumbo RM. Dynamic patellar brace: a new orthosis in the management of patellofemoral disorders. Am J Sports Med 1981;9:45.

308. Panner HJ. An affection of the capitellum humeri resembling Calvé-Perthes disease of the hip. Acta Radiol 1927;10:234.

309. Patel D. Arthroscopy of the plicae—synovial folds and their significance. Am J Sports Med 1978;6:217.

310. Paulos L, Drawbert JP, Rosenberg TD. Knee and leg: soft tissue trauma. Orthop Knowledge Upade 1986–87;2:418..

311. Paulos L, Rusche K, Johnson C, Noyes FR. Patellar malalignment. Phys Ther 1980;60:1624.

312. Penner DA, Daniel DM, Wood PFL. An in vitro study of anterior cruciate ligament graft placement and isometry. Am J Sports Med 1988;16:238.

313. Pipkin G. Lesions of the suprapatellar plica. J Bone Joint Surg 1950;32:363.

314. Pitman MI. Sports injuries in children. Resident Staff Physician 1986;32:47.

315. Poehling GG, Pollock FE, Koman LA. Reflex sympathetic dystrophy of the knee after sensory nerve injury. Arthroscopy 1988;4:31.

316. Polly DW, Callaghan JJ, Sikes RA. The accuracy of selective magnetic resonance imaging compared to the findings of arthroscopy of the knee. J Bone Joint Surg [Am] 1988;70:192.

317. Powell J. 636,000 Injuries annually in high school football. Athlet Train 1987;22:19.

318. Pritchett JW. A statistical study of knee injuries due to football in high-school athletes. J Bone Joint Surg [Am] 1982;64:240.

319. Puddu G, Ippolito E, Postacchini F. A classification of Achilles' tendon disease. Am J Sports Med 1976;4:145.

320. Puranen J. The medial tibial syndrome. J Bone Joint Surg [Br] 1974;56:712.

321. Puranen J, Alavaikko A. Intracompartmental pressure increase on exertion in patients with chronic compartment syndrome in the leg. J Bone Joint Surg [Am] 1981;63:1304.

322. Raatikainen T, Putkonen M, Puranen J. Arthrography, clinical examination, and stress radiograph in the diagnosis of acute injury to the lateral ligaments of the ankle. Am J Sports Med 1992;20:2.

323. Rarick GL, Bigley G, Karst R, Malina RM. The measurable support of the ankle joint by conventional methods of taping. J Bone Joint Surg [Am] 1962;44:1183.

324. Read MT. Stress fractures of the distal radius in adolescent gymnasts. Br J Sports Med 1981;15:252.

325. Reneman RS. The anterior and lateral compartment syndrome of the leg due to intensive use of muscles. Clin Orthop 1975;113:69.

326. Renne JW. The iliotibial band friction syndrome. J Bone Joint Surg [Am] 1975;57:110.

327. Rettig AC. Stress fracture of the ulna in an adolescent tournament tennis player. Am J Sports Med 1983;11:103.

328. Rettig AC, Beltz HF. Stress fracture in the humerus in an adolescent tennis tournament player. Am J Sports Med 1985;13:55.

329. Risser WL, Hoffman HM, Bellah GG Jr, Green LW. A cost-benefit analysis of preparticipation sports examinations of adolescent athletes. J School Health 1985;55:270.

330. Ritchie DM. Meniscectomy in children. Aust N Z J Surg 1965;35:239.

331. Roberts JM, Lovell WW. Fractures of the intercondylar eminence of the tibia. J Bone Joint Surg [Am] 1970;52:827.

332. Robinson SC, Driscoll SE. Simultaneous osteochondral avulsion of the femoral and tibial insertions of the anterior cruciate ligament. J Bone Joint Surg [Am] 1981;63:1342.

333. Romanoff M, Cory T, Kalenak A. Saphenous nerve entrapment at the adductor canal. Atlanta, American Academy of Orthopaedic Surgeons Meeting, 1988.

334. Rorabeck CH, Bourne RB, Fowler PJ. The surgical treatment of exertional compartment syndrome in athletes. J Bone Joint Surg [Am] 1983;65:1245.

335. Rosen CPR, Micheli LJ, Treves S. Early scintigraphic diagnosis of bone stress and fractures in athletic adolescents. Pediatrics 1982;70:11.

336. Rosenberg TD, Paulos LE, Parker RD. Discoid lateral meniscus: case report of arthroscopic attachment of a symptomatic Wrisberg ligament type. Arthroscopy 1987;3:277.

337. Rosenthal RK, Levine DB. Fragmentation of the distal pole of the patella in spastic cerebral palsy. J Bone Joint Surg [Am] 1979;59:934.

338. Rothwell AG. Quadriceps hematoma. Clin Orthop Rel Res 1982;171:97.

339. Rovere GD, Adair DM. Medial synovial shelf plica syndrome. Am J Sports Med 1985;13:382.

340. Rovere GD, Clarke TJ, Yates CS, Burley K. Retrospective comparison of taping and ankle stabilizers in preventing ankle injuries. Am J Sports Med 1988;16:228.

341. Rovere GD, Nichols AW. Frequency, associated factors, and treatment of breaststroker's knee in competitive swimmers. Am J Sports Med 1985;13:99.

342. Roy S, Caine D, Singer KM. Stress changes of the distal radial epiphysis in young gymnasts. Am J Sports Med 1985;13:301.

343. Runyan DK. The pre-participation examination of the young athlete. Clin Pediatr 1983;22:674.

344. Rutenfranz J. Ethical considerations: the participation of children in elite sports. Pediatrician 1986;13:14.

345. Rutherford GW, Miles R. Overview of sports related injuries to persons 5 to 14 years of age. Washington, DC, U.S. Consumer Product Safety Commission, 1981.

346. Ryan JR, Salciccioli GG. Fractures of the distal radial epiphysis in adolescent weight lifters. Am J Sports Med 1976;4:26.

347. Sanders WE, Wilkins KE, Neidre A. Acute insufficiency of the posterior cruciate ligament in children. J Bone Joint Surg [Am] 1980;62:129.

348. Sauser DD, Nelson RC, Lavine MH, Wu CW. Acute injuries of the lateral ligaments of the ankle: comparison of stress radiography and arthrography. Radiology 1983;148:653.

349. Scavenius M, Iversen BF. Nontraumatic clavicular osteolysis in weight lifters. Am J Sports Med 1992;20:463.

350. Schaffer. Competitive sports for children of elementary school age. Phys Sports Med 1981;9:140.

351. Schlonsky J, Olix ML. Functional disability following avulsion fracture of the ischial epiphysis. J Bone Joint Surg [Am] 1972;54:641.

352. Schonholtz GJ, Zahn MG, Magee CM. Lateral retinacular release of the patella. J Arthosc Rel Surg 1987;3:269.

353. Schutzer SF. Orthop Clin North Am.

354. Scott GA, Jolly BL, Henning CE. Combined posterior incision and arthroscopic intra-articular repair of the meniscus. J Bone Joint Surg [Am] 1986;68:847.

355. Sewall L, Micheli LJ. Strength training for children. J Pediatr Orthop 1986;6:143.

356. Shellock FG, Prentice WE. Warming-up and stretching for improved physical performance and prevention of sports-related injuries. Sports Med 1985;2:267.

357. Silva I, Silver DM. Tears of the meniscus as revealed by magnetic resonance imaging. J Bone Joint Surg 1988;70:199.

358. Simpson LA, Barrett JP Jr. Factors associated with poor results following arthroscopic subcutaneous lateral retinacular release. Clin Orthop Rel Res 1984;186:165.

359. Singer KM, Roy SP. Osteochondrosis of the humeral capitellum. Am J Sports Med 1984;12:351.

360. Slocum DB. The shin splint syndrome. Am J Surg 1967;114:875.

361. Smillie IS. Diseases of the knee joint. New York: Churchill Livingston, 1974.

362. Smith MG. Osteochondritis of the humeral capitellum. J Bone Joint Surg [Br] 1964;46:50.

363. Smith NJ. Nutrition and the athlete. Orthop Clin North Am 1983;14:387.

364. Smith NJ. The prevention of heat disorders in sports. Am J Dis Child 1984;138:786.

365. Smith NJ. Is that child ready for competitive sports? Contemp Pediatr 1986;3:30.

366. Smith RW, Reischl SF. Treatment of ankle sprains in young athletes. Am J Sports Med 1986;14:465.

367. Snyder RB, Lipscomb AB, Johnston RK. The relationship of tarsal coalitions to ankle sprains in athletes. Am J Sports Med 1981;9:313.

368. Snyder RW, Andrews JR. Combined arthroscopy and "mini-reconstruction" techniques in the acutely torn anterior cruciate ligament. Orthop Clin North Am 1958;16:171.

369. Sommerlath K. Meniscus repair: 6- to 10-year follow-up. Am J Knee Surg 1988;1:169.

370. St. Pierre R, Allman JF, Bassett I, et al. A review of lateral ankle ligamentous reconstructions. Foot Ankle 1982;3:114.

371. Stanish WD, Curwin SL, Bryson G. The use of flexibility exercises in preventing and treating sports injuries. In: Leadbetter WB, Buckwalter JA, Gordon SL, eds. Sports-induced inflammation. Park Ridge, IL: American Academy of Orthopaedic Surgeons, 1990:731.

372. Staples OS. Result study of ruptures of lateral ligaments of the ankle. Clin Orthop Rel Res 1972;85:50.

373. Steadman JR. Rehabilitation of first and second degree sprains of the medial collateral ligament. Am J Sports Med 1979;7:300.

374. Steihl JB. Complex ankle fracture dislocations with syndesmotic diastasis. Orthop Rev 1990;14:499.

375. Stiell IG, Greenberg GH, McKnight RD, et al. Decision rules for the use of radiography in acute ankle injuries. JAMA 1993;269:1127.

376. Strauss RH, Wright JE, Finerman GAM, Catlin DH. Side effects of antibiotic steroids in weight trained men. Physician Sports Med 1983;11:87.

377. Strong WB, Steed D. Cardiovascular evaluation of young athletes. Pediatr Clin North Am 1982;29:1325.

378. Stulberg SD, Shulman K, Stuart S, Culp P. Breaststroker's knee: pathology, etiology, and treatment. Am J Sports Med 1980;8:164.

379. Styf J. Diagnosis of exercise-induced pain in the anterior aspect of the lower leg. Am J Sports Med 1988;16:165.

380. Sullivan JA. Evaluation of injuries in youth soccer. Am J Sports Med 1980;8:325.

381. Sutker AN, Jackson DW, Pagliano JW. Iliotibial band syndrome in distance runners. Physician Sports Med 1981;9:69.

382. Tator CH, Edmonds VE. National survey of spinal injuries in hockey players. Can J Neurol Sci 1984;130:875.

383. Taylor DC, Dalton JD, Seaber AV, Garrett WE. Viscoelastic properties of muscle-tendon units. Am J Sports Med 1990; 18:300.

384. Teitz CC, Hermanson BK, Kronmal RA, Diehr PH. Evaluation of the use of braces to prevent injury to the knee in collegiate football players. J Bone Joint Surg [Am] 1987;69:2.

385. Terney R, McLain LG. The use of anabolic steroids in high school students. Am J Dis Child 1990;144:99.

386. Thomas NP, Jackson AM, Aichroth PM. Congenital absence of the anterior cruciate ligament. J Bone Joint Surg [Br] 1985;67:572.

387. Thompson N, Halpern B, Curl WW. High school football injuries: evaluation. Am J Sports Med 1987;15:117.

388. Tivnon MC, Anzel SH, Waugh TR. Surgical management of osteochondritis dissecans of the capitellum. Am J Sports Med 1976;4:121.

389. Torg JS. Epidemiology, pathomechanics, and prevention of athletic injuries to the cervical spine. Med Sci Sports Exerc 1985;17:295.

390. Torg JS, Das M. Trampoline-related quadriplegia: review of the literature and reflections on the American Academy of Pediatrics' position statement. Pediatrics 1984;74:804.

391. Torg JS, Truex JR, Quedenfeld TC, et al. The national football head and neck injury registry. JAMA 1979;241:1477.

392. Trias A, Ray RD. Juvenile osteochondritis of the radial head. J Bone Joint Surg [Am] 1963;45:576.

393. Tropp H, Askling C, Gillquist J. Prevention of ankle sprains. Am J Sports Med 1985;13:259.

394. Tullos HS, King JW. Lesions of the pitching arm in adolescents. JAMA 1972;220:264.

395. Vahvanen V, Aalto K. Meniscectomy in children. Acta Orthop Scand 1979;50:791.

396. Van Mechelen W, Hlobil H, Kemper HCG, et al. Prevention of running injuries by warm-up, cool-down, and stretching exercises. Am J Sports Med 1993;21:711.

397. Vizsolyi P, Taunton J, Robertson G, et al. Breaststroker's knee: an analysis of epidemiological and biomechanical factors. Am J Sports Med 1987;15:63.

398. Waldrop JI, Broussard TS. Disruption of the anterior cruciate ligament in a three-year-old child. J Bone Joint Surg [Am] 1984;66:1113.

399. Walker PS, Erkman MJ. The role of the menisci in force transmission across the knee. Clin Orthop 1975;109:184.

400. Weber PC. Salter-Harris type II stress fracture in a young athlete. Orthopedics 1988;11:309.

401. Weltman A, Janney C, Rians C. The effect of hydraulic resistant strength training in pre-pubertal males. Med Sci Sports Exerc 1986;18:629.

402. Whitehead R, Chillag S, Elliott D. Anabolic steroid use among adolescents in a rural state. J Fam Pract 1992;35:401.

403. Wilkins DE. Fractures and dislocations of the elbow region in fractures in children. Philadelphia: JB Lippincott, 1984.

404. Wilkins KE. The uniqueness of the young athlete: musculo-skeletal injuries. Am J Sports Med 1980;8:377.

405. Willner P. Osgood-Schlatter's disease: etiology and treatment. Clin Orthop 1969;62:178.

406. Windsor R, Dumitru D. Prevalence of anabolic steroid use by male and female adolescents. Med Sci Sports Exerc 1989; 21:494.

407. Winkler H, Rapp IH. Ununited epiphysis of the ischium: report of a case. J Bone Joint Surg 1947;29:234.

408. Wolfgang GL. Stress fracture of the femoral neck in a patient with open capital femoral epiphyses. J Bone Joint Surg [Am] 1977;59:680.

409. Woods GM, Tullos HG. Elbow instability and medial epicondyle fracture. Am J Sports Med 1977;5:23.

410. Woodward AH, Bianco Jr. AJ. Osteochondritis dissecans of the elbow. Clin Orthop Rel Res 1975;110:35.

411. Worth RM, Kettelkamp DB, Defalque RJ, Duane KU. Saphenous nerve entrapment. Am J Sports Med 1984;12:80.

412. Yamamoto RK. Arthroscopic repair of the medial retinaculum and capsule in acute patellar dislocations. J Arthosc Rel Surg 1986;2:125.

413. Yates C, Grana WA. Patellofemoral pain: a prospective study. Orthopedics 1986;9:663.

414. Yong-Hing K, Wedge JH, Bowen CV. Chronic injury to the distal ulna and radial growth plate in an adolescent gymnast. J Bone Joint Surg 1988;70:1087.

415. Zaman M, Leonard MA. Meniscectomy in children: results in 59 knees. Br J Accident Surg 1981;12:425.

416. Zaricznyj B, Shattuck LJM, Mast TA, et al. Sports-related injuries in school-aged children. Am J Sports Med 1980;8:318.

Lovell & Winter's Pediatric Orthopaedics, fourth edition,
edited by Raymond T. Morrissy and Stuart L. Weinstein.
Lippincott–Raven Publishers, Philadelphia © 1996.

Chapter

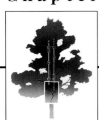

31

Management of Fractures and Their Complications

Dennis P. Devito

Musculoskeletal trauma accounts for approximately 15% of all childhood injuries. The fracture rate increases as children grow, with the incidence peaking for young adolescent boys. Children who are the victims of high-energy trauma usually sustain extremity fractures as part of the injury complex, and almost 50% of all deaths of children 14 years of age and younger result from trauma.[60] Fortunately, most fractures injure a single extremity and are minor, sustained from low-energy impact, such as a fall on the outstretched hand. Although many trauma management principles can be applied equally to children and adults, there are definite anatomic, biomechanical, and physiologic differences between the two groups. The pediatric skeleton is dynamic, constantly changing as the child grows and matures, and the purpose of this chapter is to highlight the features that are unique to the skeletally immature. The mechanisms of injury, healing principles, and age-appropriate treatment guidelines are delineated in this chapter.

GENERAL FEATURES OF FRACTURES IN CHILDREN

Anatomic Differences

Pediatric bone is less dense and more porous than adult bone because of more vascular channels and less mineral content. The surrounding periosteum is thicker and stronger, although it is loosely attached and more easily elevated with trauma, especially from the diaphysis. The periosteum attaches most firmly in the metaphyseal-epiphyseal region and helps to stabilize the physis. The periosteum usually is not cirumferentially torn, even with displaced fractures, and often is found intact on the compression side of the injured bone. Consequently, the fracture site is partially stabilized by the periosteum, and subsequent fragment reduction is facilitated by this intact structure. Other anatomic differences include the presence of a growth plate (i.e., physis) and the secondary ossification center (i.e., epiphysis). These chondrosseous structures are radiolucent, making the diagnosis of injury a greater challenge. Physeal fractures account for approximately 20% to 30% of all children's fractures, creating the possibility of additional problems that require special attention.

Biomechanical Differences

Because of the different composition of bone in children, which is more porous and has less mineral content, the modulus of elasticity and bending strength is lower than adult bone. As a result, there is a greater capacity for plastic deformation, and less energy is required to cause the fracture.[35] Pediatric bone can fail in tension and compression, producing unique fracture patterns. The torus or buckle fracture is an example of compression failure of bone. This usually occurs at the diaphyseal-metaphyseal junction, where the more rigid diaphyseal cortex is driven into the trabecular metaphysis (i.e., thinner cortex).

Plastic deformation of bone can occur, in which case the bone does not return to its original shape. Microscopic mechanical failure, not evident on routine radiographs, has transpired on the compression side of the bone. As a result, there is no fracture hematoma and minimal periosteal reaction.

Greenstick or incomplete fractures occur only in the immature skeleton. In this instance, the bone demonstrates failure on the tension side, and plastic deformation on the compression side. Complete fractures display transverse, oblique, or spiral configurations, depending on how the injury force was applied. Comminuted fracture patterns are less commonly seen, partly because the cortical porosity thwarts fracture line propagation and because less force usually is required to bend the bone.

The largely cartilaginous epiphysis in young children is less frequently injured, transmitting injury forces to the metaphysis. With growth, the ossification center enlarges, imparting more rigidity to the otherwise resilient cartilage, and epiphyseal fractures are thus more common in older children. Intraarticular fractures, joint dislocations, and ligamentous disruptions are less common in children, approaching adult incidence only in the maturing adolescent. It is more common to see fractures that involve physeal separation or the metaphyseal region, because these areas are relatively weaker than the surrounding ligaments. With maturation, there is an increase of bone in the epiphysis, and there is decreased porosity of all regions. The increase in the amount of dense cortical bone, with a more compact lamellar structure, changes the mechanical characteristics of the bone to a more rigid and brittle structure.

Physiologic Differences

Children experience considerably more rapid healing of fractures than adults because of increased blood flow and increased cellular activity. This local vascular response to a fracture can result in growth acceleration of the involved bone, allowing some fractures to heal in an overlapped position.

The periosteum is responsible for the rapid healing of children's fractures, largely because of its osteogenic activity (Fig. 31-1). When the periosteum is stripped from the bone, it carries the osteogenic cells with it. The fracture hematoma is soon stabilized by the formation of a rim of periosteal new bone formation, further aiding the healing process. If the periosteal tube is intact after a displaced fracture, the entire bone segment can sometimes regenerate, even if there has been bone loss. Significant damage to the periosteum, as may occur in open fractures, delays fracture healing in children and adults.

Healing rates are also affected by the age of the child; younger children have more rapid bone union than older patients. Healing time also is influenced by the area of the bone injured. Physeal fractures unite more rapidly than metaphyseal fractures, which heal

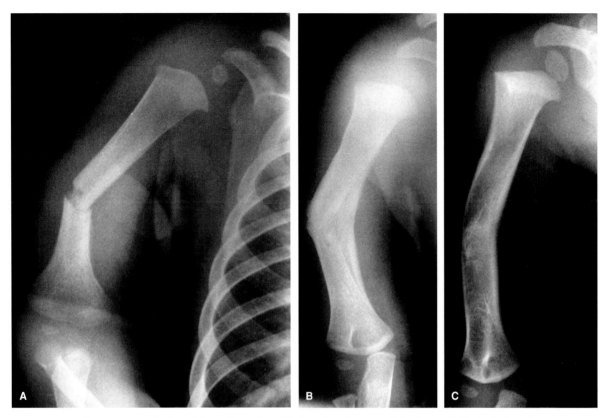

FIGURE 31-1.   Periosteal bone formation. (**A**) Complete fracture of the humeral diaphysis in a 6-month-old child. The periosteum is presumed to be intact on the compression (concave) side. (**B**) Four weeks later, the periosteum has formed a complete column of new bone. (**C**) Six months after injury, there has been significant remodeling, with a 50% correction of the angular deformity.

faster than the diaphyseal region. Nonunion usually is not a feature of children's fractures under normal conditions.

Although accurate anatomic reduction should be the goal in treating any displaced fracture, perfect alignment is unnecessary for a good result in non-intraarticular fractures because of the often dramatic bone remodeling capabilities of children; acceptable fragment alignment depends on the anticipated final shape. Remodeling depends on several factors. The more growth remaining (i.e., younger patient), the more time there is for remodeling, and the more active is the process. Fractures close to the physis demonstrate a greater capacity to remodel, especially if the residual angulation is in the plane of joint motion. Immature bone is very responsive to the normal stress of body weight, muscle forces, and joint motion, which provide further stimuli for remodeling. The metaphyseal area demonstrates more remodeling than the diaphyseal region, where reshaping is largely the result of deposition of periosteal new bone along the concave (compression) side of the fractured bone.

To a much smaller degree, resorption of mechanically unnecessary bone can also occur. The physis also responds with eccentric growth as a result of asymmetric pressures, reorienting itself perpendicular to the major reaction forces.

Remodeling is most pronounced closer to the end of the bone that contributes the most to longitudinal growth. The proximal humerus (80% growth), the distal femur (70% growth), and the distal radius (75% growth) are areas where significant remodeling is expected to occur in each of these bones. Conversely, fractures about the elbow display less remodeling ability, and alignment must be kept within a narrower threshold. Because fracture malrotation has relatively little capacity to change over time, it should be accurately obtained from the outset. There is great individual variation variability with regard to the amount of remodeling and growth stimulation that is displayed in response to a fracture. The expectation of remodeling is not a substitute for attention to detail and quality fracture management.

INJURY TO THE PHYSIS

Physeal Anatomy

The physis contains the cells responsible for bone growth and is located at the ends of all long bones, oriented perpendicular to the long axis. Longitudinal growth is the primary function of the physis and is accomplished through the process of endochondral bone formation. The peripheral portion of the physis also produces latitudinal growth. Most physes are extraarticular, although the femoral, proximal radial, and a portion of the proximal humeral physes are intraarticular. Distal physes have a greater propensity for injury than those located proximally.[125] The peak age for injury to the growth plate is early adolescence (11–12 years), and physeal fracture is uncommon in children younger than 5 years of age. Boys are affected twice as often as girls.[125] Despite the fact that the physis is the weakest area of the immature skeleton, only about 20% of all children's fractures occur in this region.

The ultrastructure of the physis reveals four distinct zones and is organized in longitudinal columns. The first two zones have an abundant cartilage matrix and are relatively strong. They consist of the germinal or growth cells and the maturation layer. In the third zone, the chondrocytes enlarge as they begin their transformation from cartilage to bone matrix, and they have a decreased ability to resist shear forces. The final zone is strengthened by the mineralization process, but it is still weaker than the first two zones. Fractures tend to occur through the zone of hypertrophic cartilage (zone 3), especially in younger children.[148] In the maturing physis, there is thinning of the cartilage zones, and consequently, the fracture plane is likely to course through all portions of the growth plate. Typically, the germinal part of the plate stays attached to the epiphyseal side of the fracture fragment.

The physis is stabilized externally by the firmly attached perichondrium and internally by undulations known as mammillary processes. Rotational forces are most likely to produce a physeal fracture. The physis has a rich blood supply from the epiphyseal and metaphyseal side and from the perichondrium. This contributes to the rapid healing rate of physeal fractures, combined with the high cellular activity that typifies this region.

Physeal Fractures

The most widely used classification system of physeal fractures is that detailed by Salter and Harris.[148] This classification scheme is based on the radiographic identification of five types of fracture, although a sixth fracture pattern was subsequently added by Rang (Fig. 31-2).[139]

The type I injury involves a transverse fracture through the entire physis, without evidence of a metaphyseal fragment. This type of fracture is most commonly seen in infants or young children. The epiphyseal fragment is usually minimally displaced if the periosteum is not torn, and the diagnosis of a recent fracture is confirmed by localized swelling and point tenderness. Delayed fracture diagnosis may be confirmed by the radiographic presence of periosteal new bone formation around the physis.

Type II fractures represent 75% of physeal frac-

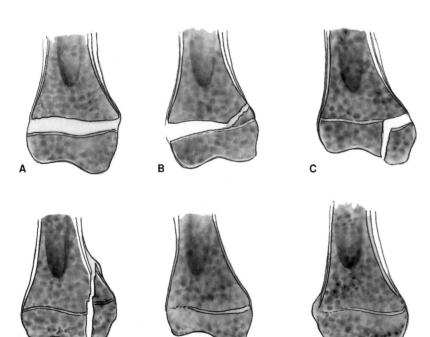

FIGURE 31-2. Salter-Harris classification. (**A**) Type I transepiphyseal separation without evidence of a metaphyseal fragment. (**B**) In type II, the fracture line is through the physis, exiting into the metaphysis, leaving a small triangular portion attached to the physeal plate (i.e., Thurston-Holland fragment). (**C**) The type III fracture is an intraarticular fracture, with the fracture traversing the physis and exiting through the epiphysis. (**D**) Type IV describes a vertical fracture line that is intraarticular. It passes through the epiphysis, physis, and metaphysis. (**E**) Type V fracture describes a crush injury to the physis that usually is not apparent on initial injury films. (**F**) Type VI fracture is a localized injury to a portion of the perichondral ring. Subsequent healing produces bone formation across the perimeter of the physis, connecting the metaphysis to the epiphysis.

tures and entail a fracture line that passes through a variable portion of the physis before exiting across the metaphysis. The metaphyseal fragment (i.e., Thurston-Holland sign) is on the compression side of the fracture, where the periosteum often is intact. The prognosis is good in most instances, but growth disturbance occurs in 10% to 30% of the patients, depending on the location of the fracture.

The type III injury is caused when the fracture splits a portion of the epiphyseal ossification center in addition to the physeal separation. This is an intraarticular fracture, and the prognosis is directly related to the ability to restore anatomic alignment.

Type IV lesions describe a vertical splitting of all zones of the physis. The fracture is intraarticular and traverses the epiphysis, physis, and metaphysis. There is a propensity for fragment displacement, which results in partial growth arrest.

When a significant crushing force is applied to the growth plate, a type V injury can occur. Unfortunately, this may not be apparent on radiographs obtained immediately after the injury, because it does not always involve fracture fragment displacement. Crush injury to the germinal physeal cells can occur in combination with other Salter-Harris fracture patterns.

The type VI physeal injury is a peripheral bruise, burn, or avulsion of the perichondrial ring, and it does not technically damage the main portion of the physis. Problems with growth occur as a result of the healing process as new bone forms across the physis, connecting the epiphysis to the metaphysis.

The significance of properly identifying a physeal fracture is that a growth disturbance may result, and parents need to be appraised of the relative risk of this problem occurring. Certain fracture patterns require operative realignment and stabilization to reduce the likelihood of growth disturbance. Closed manipulation of displaced physeal fractures should be performed gently to avoid additional physeal cell damage. Distraction of the distal fragment should be a component of the reduction maneuver to reduce shearing across the fracture. Repeated reduction attempts may increase the chance for iatrogenic growth plate disturbance. Surgical principles involve minimal soft tissue exposure, especially around the periosteum in the region of the physis (identified by a change in the resistance to periosteal elevation). Internal fixation should not cross the physis whenever possible; if necessary, smooth pins should be used and then removed as soon as early healing is evident. The placement of compression screws across epiphyseal fragments, parallel to the physis, is an effective means of restoring stable articular congruity. This fixation is facilitated by the use of cannulated screws that are placed over smooth provisional fixation pins.

Physeal Arrest

Trauma is the most common cause of physeal damage that results in growth arrest. This complication ensues when a bridge of bone forms across the metaphysis to the epiphysis, tethering any further longitudinal growth. This bridge is also referred to as a bony bar, whose size and location determine what kind of deformity eventually develops.

The magnitude of the deformity depends on how much growth remains in the child. Although complete growth cessation is possible, typically, a partial physeal arrest occurs and may present in three different patterns (Fig. 31-3). The first is a peripheral bar, which produces an angular deformity. This is the most common pattern. The second is a central bar, which results in tenting of the physis and epiphysis with eventual articular surface distortion. The perichondrial ring is circumferentially intact, but a longitudinal growth deficiency usually ensues because of the central growth tether. The third pattern of bar formation involves portions of the peripheral and central physis (i.e., combined arrest) and is referred to as a linear bar. This is often the result of a Salter-Harris type IV fracture that has healed in a displaced position. The result is intraarticular incongruity and a progressive angular growth disturbance (Fig. 31-4). Complete physeal arrest may be seen after a crush injury to the growth plate, producing a significant limb length discrepancy in young children.

Partial growth arrest is first recognized 3 to 6 months after physeal injury but may also manifest as long as 2 years later. It may appear as a blurring and narrowing of the physis, or as an area of reactive bone condensation. Adjacent metaphyseal bone growth may be distorted. Another early sign of growth disturbance is the development of asymmetric Harris lines. This sclerotic line often appears in the metaphysis 6 to 12 months after a fracture.[56] If the line remains parallel to the physis across the entire width of the metaphysis during subsequent growth, the entire physis is probably healthy (Fig. 31-5). However, partial growth arrest is likely if the Harris line is oblique (i.e., tilted) to the physis in the coronal or sagittal plane.[82] The most common areas for growth arrest are the distal femur, the distal tibia, the proximal tibia, and the distal radius.

Once suspected, the extent of physeal bar formation should be accurately delineated. This involves obtaining plain radiographs with the beam centered and in line with the inclination of the physis. Traditionally, hypocycloidal tomography has been used to detail the bony bar, but computed tomography (CT) scanning is more readily available. Thin CT sections are required, and reformations in the sagittal and coronal planes are necessary. Axial reconstruction is not help-

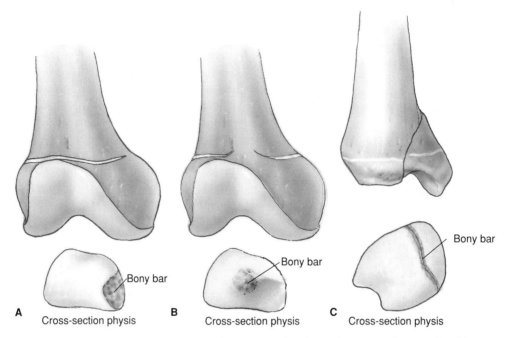

FIGURE 31-3. Growth arrest patterns. (**A**) Type I peripheral growth arrest, with a peripheral bony bar. (**B**) Type II central growth arrest, with central physeal tethering. The peripheral physis and perichondral ring are intact. (**C**) Type III combined growth arrest, demonstrating a linear bar involving the peripheral and central portions of the physeal plate. This type of growth arrest is more typical after a Salter-Harris type III or IV fracture.

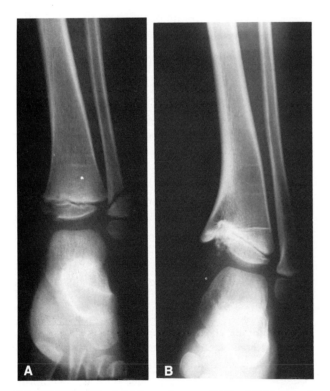

FIGURE 31-4. Distal tibial growth arrest. (**A**) Distal tibial physeal Salter-Harris type IV injury treated by cast immobilization without reduction. (**B**) Two years later, there is varus angulation to the distal tibia from a medial physeal bar. The Harris growth arrest line is not parallel to the distal physis and does not extend across the entire width of the metaphysis.

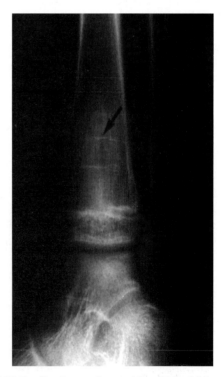

FIGURE 31-5. Harris growth arrest line. This child sustained a fracture of the distal tibial physis approximately 16 months earlier. Two sclerotic lines in the distal tibial metaphysis represent Harris growth arrest lines; they extend parallel to the growth plate across the entire width of the tibial metaphysis. This indicates continued symmetrical physeal growth since the healing of the fracture.

ful, because the sections are taken in the same plane as the physis. The drawbacks of CT scanning include the problem of proper orientation of the x-ray beam to the irregular contour of the physis and the inability to easily differentiate normal physeal undulations from the abnormal bone bridge. Magnetic resonance imaging (MRI) provides another means for imaging the physis, but it has yet to be proven as the preferred technique. The size and location of the physeal bar should then be mapped to determine what kind of surgical approach can be taken.[26] Physeal bar resection is a treatment possibility only if at least 50% of the cross-sectional area of the growth plate remains undamaged. The exception to this may be the very young child with a central growth arrest.

There are many treatment options for partial growth plate damage, depending on the location of the bone bridge, the size of the bar, and the age of the patient. Once identified, a partial arrest can be surgically converted to a complete arrest to prevent further angulation. Contralateral limb epiphysiodesis is required if there is enough growth remaining to produce a significant length discrepancy. An alternate plan entails later lengthening of the shorter ipsilateral limb (i.e., side with the growth arrest), especially if the length discrepancy will exceed 5 cm. If there is more than 2 years of growth remaining and less than 50% of the physis is damaged, bar resection can be considered.

Peripheral bone bridges are approached directly with excision of the overlying periosteum and removal of the abnormal bone until normal physeal cartilage is uncovered. Interposition material is inserted to prevent bone from respanning the physis. Fat and Cranioplast are the two most widely used materials for interposition, and the material must remain in contact with the physis during further growth. This is accomplished by securing the interposed substance to the epiphysis. Radioapparent markers usually are inserted in the bone to facilitate the measurement of subsequent growth (Fig. 31-6). Growth acceleration may occur after bar excision, spontaneously correcting smaller degrees of angulation. However, corrective osteotomy to realign the limb may be necessary if the angular deformity exceeds 15 to 20 degrees.[101]

Central bars are approached through a metaphyseal window, carefully protecting the peripheral margins of the physis. Because of this indirect approach, the abnormal portions of the physis are more difficult to see, especially in the region closest to the metaphyseal window. If an angular deformity is to be corrected simultaneously, the bone bar can sometimes be more easily resected through the osteotomy site. A linear bar is approached directly where it contacts the periphery, and then the physeal scar is resected from one side to the other, creating a tunnel that follows the original fracture line. The best results of physeal bar resection are obtained with central bridges because of the ability of the peripheral physis to maintain longitudinal growth. Unfortunately, injured physeal plates tend to close prematurely, before the contralateral side, despite successful restoration of growth.

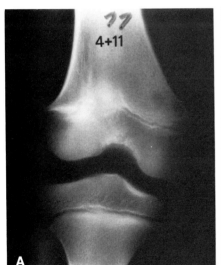
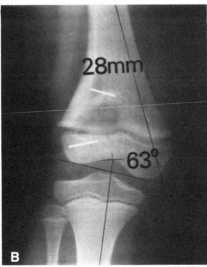
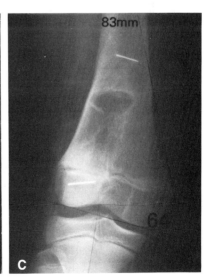

FIGURE 31-6. Physeal bar resection. (**A**) A distal femoral physeal bar is depicted on this anteroposterior hypocycloidal tomogram. (**B**) This condition was treated by bar excision and insertion of cranioplast. Five months later, the physis remains open, and the two metal markers inserted at the time of surgery are 28 mm apart. There is residual femoral tibial valgus deformity. (**C**) Four years later, there has been some improvement in the femoral tibial alignment, and growth of the distal femur has resumed. The markers are 83 mm apart.

FRACTURES OF THE SHOULDER REGION

Clavicle Fractures

The clavicle is a curved bone that is flat laterally and triangular medially. It connects the shoulder girdle to the axial skeleton at the sternoclavicular joint. It is attached to the scapula at the acromioclavicular joint and held in place by the coracoclavicular ligaments. The sternoclavicular joint is more mobile than the scapular end. Beneath the clavicle lies the subclavian vessels, the brachial plexus, and the apex of the lung.

The clavicle is frequently fractured in children, and the most common portion injured is the shaft. The mechanism of injury is usually a fall on the shoulder or any excessive lateral compression of the shoulder girdle. Clavicle fractures are also seen as a result of a

difficult birth delivery, and the newborn's lack of arm movement may be confused with brachial plexopathy or proximal humeral fracture (i.e., pseudoparalysis).

Clavicle Diaphysis

Shaft fractures usually are managed closed, and uneventful, rapid healing is the rule. Treatment is designed to provide comfort for the child and consists of a sling for small children and a figure-eight harness for the older child or adolescent. These external supports are often discontinued after 2 to 3 weeks.

Operative indications include open fractures, severe displacement with the bone end impaled through the trapezius, or irreducible tenting of the skin by the bone fragments. Flail chest with other associated shoulder girdle fractures (e.g., scapula) may also be

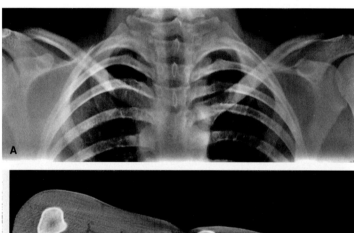

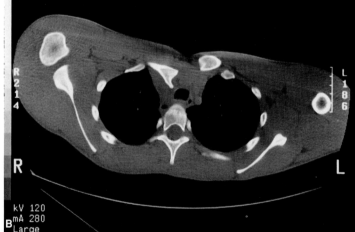

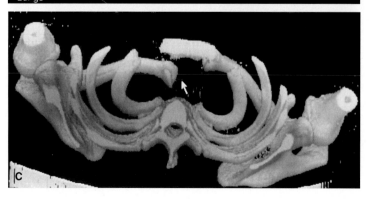

FIGURE 31-7. Sternoclavicular separation. This 14-year-old boy sustained an injury to the right clavicle during a wrestling match as his shoulder was compressed against his chest wall. He complained of shortness of breath, especially when he extended his neck. (**A**) The anteroposterior radiograph demonstrates asymmetry of the sternal position of the clavicle. (**B**) The computed tomographic scan demonstrates posterior displacement of the medial end of the right clavicle, which is in close proximity to the trachea. (**C**) A three-dimensional reconstruction with a cephalic projection demonstrates the posterior and midline displacement of the clavicle.

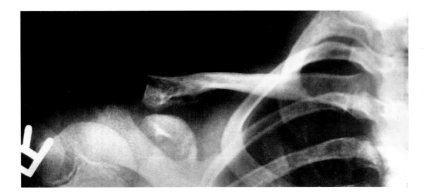

FIGURE 31-8. Lateral clavicle fracture. The swelling and dorsal prominence of the clavicle may suggest an acromioclavicular (AC) separation; however, the distal end of the clavicle and the AC joint remain reduced. Periosteal bone beneath the clavicle indicates that the coracoclavicular ligaments have held the periosteum in a reduced position despite the elevation of the clavicle. This defect will fill in with new bone and subsequently remodel.

another relative indication for open reduction and internal fixation of the clavicle.

Techniques for stabilization are intramedullary pinning or anterior plating with a 2.7-mm reconstruction plate and compression screws. Intramedullary pins are to be used with caution because of their tendency to migrate. Nonunion generally occurs only in fractures that have had open periosteal stripping, as in open fractures or reductions.[114]

Medial Clavicle

Fractures of the medial end of the clavicle consist of physeal separations, mimicking a true sternoclavicular dislocation. These are Salter-Harris type I or II injuries, although the epiphyseal fragment is not well visualized on radiographs. The medial clavicular physis does not close until the person is 20 to 25 years of age.[41]

Injury results from a lateral force applied to the shoulder, compressing the shoulder toward the midline, and the direction of pseudodislocation can be anterior or posterior. Posterior displacement can cause dysphagia or respiratory compromise, especially when the child's head and neck are extended. Apical lordotic radiographs are helpful, but the deformity is best visualized by CT scan (Fig. 31-7). Reduction by closed technique is possible, usually requiring a general anesthetic. The reduction maneuver entails percutaneous forceps' capture of the medial clavicle, followed by lateral and upward pulling combined with longitudinal arm traction. Posteriorly displaced fractures are usually stable after reduction, and a shoulder immobilizer or figure-eight harness is sufficient immobilization. Anteriorly displaced epiphyseal separations are less stable, and partial redisplacement may occur. However, remanipulation or operative treatment is unnecessary, because fracture remodeling will occur.

Lateral Clavicle

Fractures of the distal (lateral) end of the clavicle involve an epiphyseal separation. The acromioclavicular and coracoclavicular ligaments are firmly attached to the thick periosteum of the clavicle (Fig. 31-8). Typically, the lateral metaphysis displaces through the injured dorsal periosteum, leaving the epiphyseal end of the clavicle reduced in the acromioclavicular joint.[36] Rockwood classified these distal fractures as types I through VI, according to the magnitude of vertical displacement or the direction of displacement of the clavicle. Although there is residual displacement, the strong coracoclavicular ligaments have remained attached to the periosteal sleeve; consequently, there is considerable remodeling. Reduction is unnecessary, except for the rare instance in which the clavicle is posteroinferiorly displaced (i.e., type IV or VI). Most distal clavicle fractures are treated with a sling or shoulder immobilizer for 3 weeks.

Acromioclavicular Separation

True acromioclavicular separation can occur in adolescents and is caused by a blow to the point of the shoulder. Sports injuries are the most common mechanism. Three degrees of separation are described, with increasing severity of sprain of the acromioclavicular ligament from type I to type III.[3] Mild joint subluxation occurs with type II separations, and type III injuries demonstrate upward displacement of the clavicle because of a complete tear of the coracoclavicular ligament. The distance between the coracoid process and the clavicle is increased compared with the contralateral side, and the acromioclavicular joint is dislocated.

Treatment of acromioclavicular separations is usually conservative, even in competitive athletes, because shoulder strength and range of motion are not impaired after rehabilitation.[164,169,177] In complete separations (type III), the clavicle remains prominent, but usually asymptomatic. Type II separations can produce late symptoms of pain because the joint is incongruous, and this may require resection of the distal clavicle.[164]

Scapular Fracture

Scapular fracture is a rare injury in children; older adolescents are more commonly affected. Fractures can involve the body, glenoid, or acromial region of the scapula. A significant blunt force directly applied to the scapula is required to cause the injury, as may occur in a motor vehicle accident. Initial evaluation should also determine the presence of other blunt injuries to the chest wall, such as rib fractures, pulmonary or cardiac contusion, and injury to the thoracic vascular system.

Scapulothoracic dissociation is the result of high-energy thoracic trauma and is diagnosed by identifying lateral displacement of the scapula on the anteroposterior chest radiograph. This injury essentially is a subcutaneous avulsion of the midline scapular muscles, and a clavicle fracture may also be present. Significant associated injuries include avulsion of the brachial plexus nerve roots (proximal and distal), subclavian arterial rupture, and cervical spine fracture or dislocation. Depending on the degree of neurovascular damage, later reconstruction is possible, but it usually entails a shoulder disarticulation or forequarter amputation.

Most scapular body fractures are nondisplaced, and the thick mantle of surrounding muscle prevents fragment displacement. CT scans are essential for delineating scapular fracture anatomy. Treatment of most scapular fractures is achieved with a sling and early shoulder motion after the pain has subsided. However, displaced lateral border fractures occasionally need internal fixation. Glenoid rim fractures, often seen in conjunction with shoulder dislocation, may need to be repaired to confer shoulder joint stability. Intraarticular fractures with more than 3 mm of displacement should be restored to anatomic positions. An anterior surgical approach is recommended for glenoid fractures, and a posterior approach is used for scapular neck and glenoid fossa fractures.[72]

Shoulder Dislocation

Glenohumeral dislocation is rarely seen in children younger than 10 years of age; it is a problem usually encountered in young adults. Approximately 20% of all shoulder dislocations occur in persons between the ages of 10 and 20 years. Most displace anteriorly and produce a detachment of the anteroinferior capsule from the glenoid neck (i.e., Bankart lesion). There is a 10% incidence of nerve injury associated with this injury, involving the axillary nerve or the brachial plexus. Rarely does the physician see associated greater tuberosity fracture or rotator cuff tear in children. Reduction is accomplished by providing adequate pain relief, muscle relaxation, and longitudinal traction that is gravity assisted or using the modified Hippocratic method. Treatment is achieved with a shoulder immobilizer or sling for 2 to 3 weeks before initiating shoulder muscle strengthening, especially for the internal rotators. The most frequent complication is recurrent dislocation, which has an incidence between 60% to 85%, usually within 2 years of the primary dislocation.[78,81]

Humeral Fractures

Proximal Humerus

In children, shoulder trauma usually results in a proximal humeral fracture instead of joint dislocation. The proximal physis is an undulating structure and forms a peak in the posteromedial quadrant of the middle of the humeral head. A portion of the metaphysis is intracapsular. Proximal humeral fractures consist of metaphyseal fractures and physeal separations. Generally, three fracture patterns are displayed, each common to a specific age group.

Salter-Harris I fractures are seen in the neonate and in children younger than 5 years of age. Only clavicle fractures are more common in the neonate. Neonatal fractures are usually the result of obstetric trauma in which the arm is excessively rotated and hyperextended, and the affected newborn demonstrates decreased use of the upper extremity (i.e., pseudoparalysis).[37] Because physeal separation in the infant may also be the result of physical abuse, a thorough history should be obtained. Closed reduction is not indicated because remodeling is pronounced and because the proximal growth plate provides 80% of the longitudinal growth of the humerus. Healing is rapid, especially in the younger child. Immobilization is achieved with a sling and swathe for 2 to 3 weeks (Fig. 31-9).

Metaphyseal fractures occur in children between 5 and 10 years of age, presumably because of the rapid growth during this period that results in thinning of the metaphyseal cortex, making it more susceptible to fracture. Most fractures are transverse or short oblique (80%). These fractures generally do not require a reduction; bayonet apposition is acceptable in patients up to 10 to 12 years of age (Fig. 31-10). Rarely, the distal fragment is impaled through the deltoid muscle, or the fracture angulation exceeds 50 degrees; both require closed manipulation to improve alignment. In children older than 12 years of age, bayonet

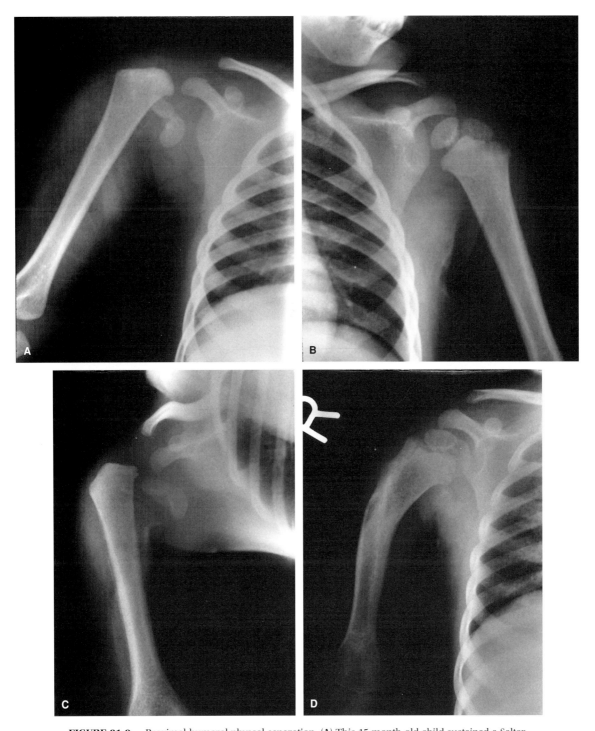

FIGURE 31-9.   Proximal humeral physeal separation. (**A**) This 15-month-old child sustained a Salter-Harris type I complete physeal separation of the proximal humerus. (**B**) The contralateral, uninjured shoulder. (**C**) Twelve days after injury, the fracture is stable, and periosteal new bone formation is seen along the humeral head and shaft. Abduction of the arm was limited to 70 degrees. (**D**) The appearance of the shoulder only 6 months after injury demonstrates extensive remodeling.

healing may limit abduction and forward flexion of the shoulder, and the fracture should be reduced.

Salter-Harris II fractures are seen in the adolescent, generally after 11 years of age. Seventy-five percent of fractures in this age group are of this variety, and the remainder are type I fractures. Fracture dis-

placement is in an anterior direction because the periosteum is thinner and weaker in this region than it is posteriorly, where the periosteal sleeve remains intact. The proximal fragment is flexed and externally rotated because of the pull of the rotator cuff, while the deltoid muscle tends to elevate the distal fragment, producing

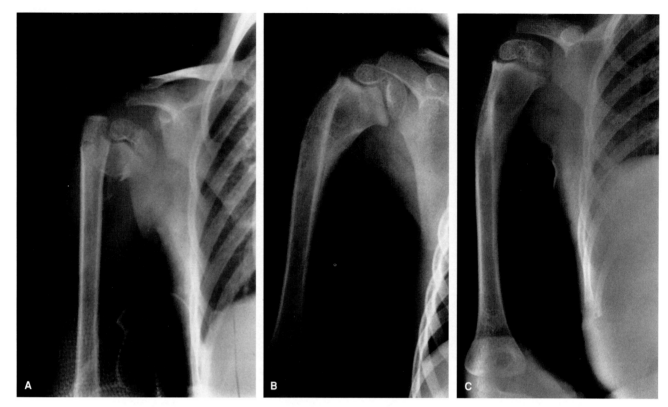

FIGURE 31-10. Proximal humeral metaphyseal fracture in a 5-year-old child. **(A)** The metaphyseal portion of the distal fragment was palpable in the deltoid muscle, and alignment was not improved despite the use of a hanging arm cast. **(B)** As early as 3 months after healing, extensive remodeling occurred, but limited abduction persisted. **(C)** Nine months after injury, there is a full range of motion, and further remodeling has occurred. The original fracture site is farther away from the proximal growth plate.

shortening of the arm. Adduction of the distal fragment is caused by the pectoralis major muscle. Fractures with less than 20 to 30 degrees of angulation and less than 50% displacement can be managed in a shoulder immobilizer, without a reduction, especially if the fracture is impacted (i.e., stable). Greater degrees of displacement adequately remodel in children younger than 11 years of age, precluding the need for fracture reduction.[96,128] The adolescent approaching physeal closure can remodel bone to a lesser extent and consequently tolerates less deformity. In this instance, displaced fractures heal shortened by 1 to 3 cm and in varus, although shoulder function is not significantly compromised.[128,155]

In adolescents, fractures with excessive angulation (>35 degrees) or with more than 50% displacement, should be managed with closed reduction.[155] The arm is externally rotated, abducted, and forward flexed to align the fragments. Percutaneous pin fixation is implemented to secure the reduction (Fig. 31-11), because closed reduction without fixation usually results in recurrence of the original deformity.[10] Pins are left in place for approximately 3 weeks, allowing early fracture healing, and then the use of a sling is sufficient. Hanging arm casts and skeletal traction are not effective techniques for producing fracture align-

ment.[10,96] Shoulder spica casts with the arm in the salute position may control proper fragment position, but they are cumbersome and can produce brachial plexus neuropathy.

Humeral Shaft

Humeral shaft fractures are less common in children than adults and are typically seen in the teenager as a result of blunt trauma. Spiral fractures are caused by a twisting force, and in young children and infants, these fractures may represent nonaccidental trauma. Physical abuse is the most common cause of humeral shaft fractures in children younger than 3 years of age. However, no particular fracture pattern is diagnostic of child abuse; transverse diaphyseal fractures are also consistent with this mechanism of injury.[92]

Treatment of humeral shaft fractures consists of closed management using a coaptation splint to maintain alignment of the arm. Adjustments in fragment position can be performed for as long as 3 weeks after injury, when early healing has occurred, and may be facilitated by the use of an abduction orthosis. Occasionally, a cast can be placed high enough above the fracture site to effectively control fragment position, and it can be converted to a functional humeral splint

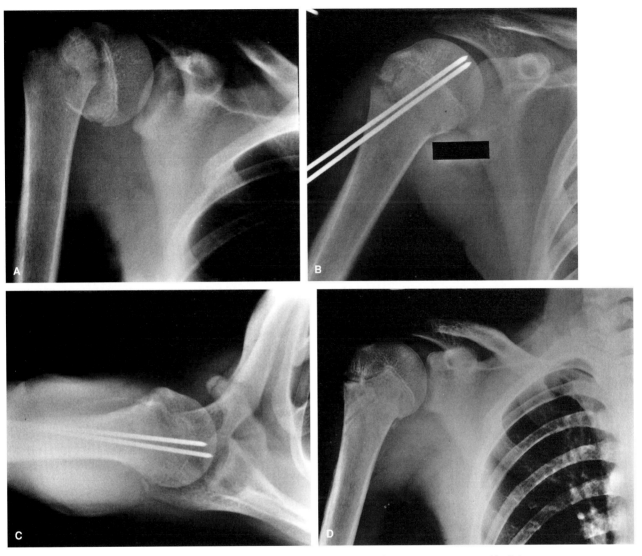

FIGURE 31-11.   Salter-Harris type II fracture of the proximal humerus in a 15-year-old adolescent. (**A**) Displaced fracture with 70 degrees of angulation. The proximal fragment is abducted and externally rotated because of the rotator cuff attachments. The shaft is displaced proximally by the pull of the deltoid muscle and is generally adducted by the action of the pectoralis muscle. The distal fragment is also internally rotated if the arm is placed in a sling. (**B** and **C**) Anteroposterior and lateral radiographs after closed reduction and percutaneous pinning. The arm is externally rotated and abducted with longitudinal traction to achieve this position. (**D**) Final alignment after removal of the pins in 4 weeks.

or brace after early bone union has commenced. The functional humeral orthosis is especially effective when healing is delayed, allowing the recovery of shoulder and elbow joint motion while providing adequate fracture stability. Fractures located at the junction of the middle and distal third of the humerus may be associated with a radial nerve palsy because of the proximity of the nerve to the bone at this point. Most radial nerve palsies resolve spontaneously in 2 to 4 months.

Operative indications include open fractures, polytrauma victims, and ipsilateral forearm fractures in adolescents (i.e., "floating elbow"). Fixation techniques include flexible intramedullary nails, antegrade insertion of a Rush rod, or compression plate and screws. Severe open fractures can also be stabilized with an external fixator, converting to a functional brace after wound healing is complete and there is some fracture stability resulting from periosteal bone formation.

FRACTURES AND DISLOCATIONS ABOUT THE ELBOW

The elbow region is injured frequently in growing children, especially those between 5 and 10 years of age. Supracondylar fracture of the distal humerus is the most common, representing 75% of all elbow fractures, followed by lateral condylar (17%) and medial epicondylar injuries. T-condylar, medial condyle, and lateral epicondyle fractures are rare and have a combined incidence of less than 1%. Delineating exact fracture patterns is a challenge in young children because of the large cartilage composition of the distal humerus; at birth, the distal epiphysis of the humerus is still completely cartilaginous. There are also multiple ossification centers, appearing at different ages (Fig. 31-12). The capitellum is the first to appear at 6 months of age, followed by the radial head and the medial epicondyle at 5 years of age. The trochlea ossifies at 7 years, and the lateral epicondyle and olecranon appear at 9 and 11 years of age, respectively. The lateral epicondyle, trochlea, and the capitellum coalesce to form a single epiphysis by 12 years of age.

The elbow is a complex joint and has three major articulations: radiohumeral, ulnar-humeral, and radioulnar joints. Except for the medial and lateral epicondyles, the other ossification centers are intraarticular. Other intraarticular structures include the olecranon fossa and the coronoid fossa and process. There are two fat pads: one in the olecranon fossa posteriorly and the other in the coronoid fossa anteriorly. Displacement of the posterior fat pad is a reliable indication of intraarticular effusion, as may occur with an occult fracture. The anterior fat pad is sometimes seen under normal conditions. The distal humerus has a good collateral circulation, with most of the interosseous blood supply entering posteriorly.

The clinical carrying angle of the normal elbow is a slight valgus alignment, averaging approximately 7 degrees. There are several helpful radiographic lines and angles that can be measured to decide if there is adequate postinjury alignment; a comparison view of the other elbow often is needed as a reference. All measurements are subject to the inaccuracies of how the extremity is positioned, and this should be kept in mind when making clinical decisions. The Baumann angle is used to assess the varus attitude of the distal humerus, usually after a supracondylar elbow fracture. It is the angle formed between the capitellar physeal line and a line perpendicular to the long axis of the humerus (Fig. 31-13). This measurement should be within 5 to 8 degrees of the contralateral elbow. An anteroposterior view of the distal humerus, positioned parallel to the radiographic plate, is necessary to reduce the variation of the Baumann angle that occurs by rotating the arm; 10 degrees of rotation produces a 6-degree change in the angle.[23] The lateral capitellar angle indicates the normal forward-flexed position of the capitellum and averages 30 to 40 degrees. The anterior humeral line is a similar way to assess the position of the capitellum and is measured on a true lateral radiographic projection. A line along the anterior humeral cortex should pass through the center of the capitellum (see Fig. 31-13).

The medial epicondylar epiphyseal angle is measured from the long axis of the humerus and a line through the medial epicondylar physis.[15] It has the advantage of being reliably measured while the elbow is held in flexion (i.e., Jones view), as during the reduction process. The mean angle is 38 degrees, and less than 34 degrees implies cubitus varus. It is not a good measurement for children younger than 3 years or older than 10 years of age.

Supracondylar Fracture

This is the most common elbow fracture, and the mechanism of injury is an acute hyperextension load

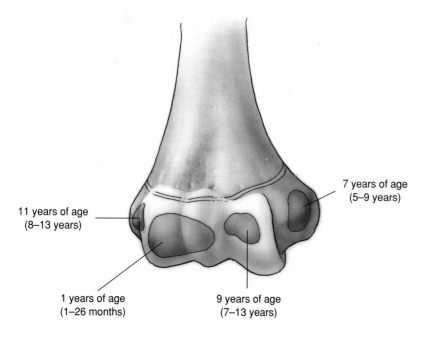

11 years of age
(8–13 years)

1 years of age
(1–26 months)

9 years of age
(7–13 years)

7 years of age
(5–9 years)

FIGURE 31-12.   Ossification of the secondary centers of the distal humerus. The average ages are specified, and the age ranges are indicated. The ossification ranges are earlier for girls than boys. The lateral epicondyle, capitellum, and trochlea coalesce between 10 and 12 years of age, subsequently fusing to the distal humerus between 13 and 16 years of age. This is about the time that the medial epicondyle fuses to the proximal humerus.

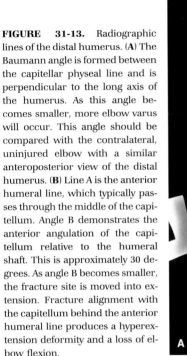
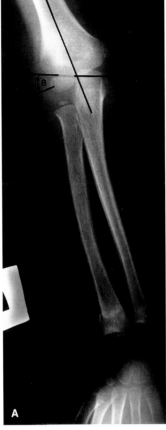
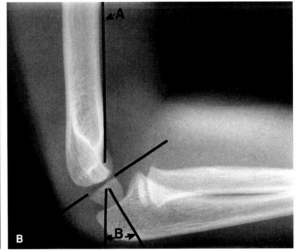

FIGURE 31-13. Radiographic lines of the distal humerus. (A) The Baumann angle is formed between the capitellar physeal line and is perpendicular to the long axis of the humerus. As this angle becomes smaller, more elbow varus will occur. This angle should be compared with the contralateral, uninjured elbow with a similar anteroposterior view of the distal humerus. (B) Line A is the anterior humeral line, which typically passes through the middle of the capitellum. Angle B demonstrates the anterior angulation of the capitellum relative to the humeral shaft. This is approximately 30 degrees. As angle B becomes smaller, the fracture site is moved into extension. Fracture alignment with the capitellum behind the anterior humeral line produces a hyperextension deformity and a loss of elbow flexion.

on the elbow from falling on the outstretched arm. The distal fragment displaces posteriorly (i.e., extension) in more than 95% of fractures. The medial and lateral columns of the distal humerus are connected by a very thin area of bone between the olecranon fossa posteriorly and the coronoid fossa anteriorly. The central thinning and the surrounding narrow columns predispose this area to fracture. As the elbow is forced into hyperextension, the olecranon impinges in the fossa, serving as the fulcrum for the fracture. The collateral ligaments and the anterior joint capsule also resist hyperextension, transmitting the stress to the distal humerus and initiating the fracture.[1]

After complete fracture, a small amount of rotational malalignment allows tilting of the fragments, heralding instability (Fig. 31-14). If the fracture heals with excessive tilting, cubitus varus or, less commonly, cubitus valgus results. The classification system, modified from Gartland's system,[57] describes three major types of fracture patterns:

Type IA: nondisplaced or minimally displaced
Type IB: minimally displaced, medial impaction
Type II: intact posterior cortex, posterior angulation
Type III: completely displaced, usually in the posteromedial direction

Associated injuries include nerve, vascular, and other ipsilateral upper extremity fractures. The incidence of nerve injury is approximately 15% and most often is a neurapraxia that resolves spontaneously within 4 months. The nerve injured is related to the position of the displaced fragment, and the anterior interosseous nerve is the most common deficit.[33] However, radial and ulnar nerve palsies are also encountered. Median nerve palsy associated with vascular insufficiency suggests that these neurovascular structures are entrapped in the fracture site.[33] Forearm fractures can coexist with supracondylar elbow injuries and are typically distal both-bone forearm fractures. The general approach is closed reduction and pinning of the elbow followed by closed reduction and cast application of the distal fracture.

Type IA injuries are treated with an above-elbow cast for 3 weeks, with the elbow flexed 90 to 100 degrees. Type IB fractures may need closed manipulation if the varus alignment is significantly different from the contralateral elbow; otherwise, casting without reduction is adequate. Unrecognized medial or lateral column impaction or comminution allows fragment migration, producing a varus or valgus deformity that cannot remodel. If the elbow has required realignment, it is prudent to pin the fracture to maintain the desired position.

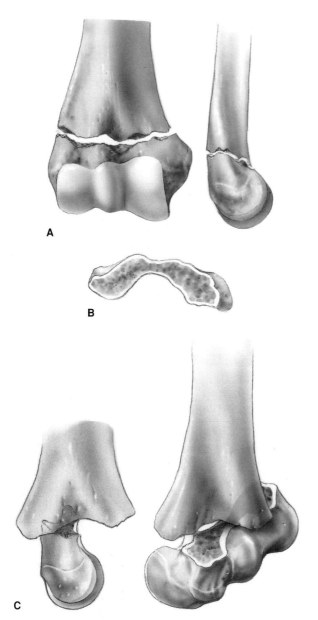

FIGURE 31-14. (**A**) The typical orientation of the fracture line in the supracondylar fracture. Sagittal rotation of the distal fragment generally results in posterior angulation, although less commonly, it can be flexed. (**B**) The cross-sectional area through the fracture demonstrates the thin cross-sectional area of the supracondylar region. (**C**) Any horizontal rotation tilts the distal fragment. Typically, medial tilting occurs, producing cubitus varus. The lateral projection readily demonstrates this horizontal rotation, producing a fish-tail deformity. In this instance, the distal portion of the proximal fragment is obliquely profiled, although there is a true lateral view of the distal humeral fragment.

Occasionally, type II fractures can be treated with closed reduction and casting alone, especially if the fracture is not rotated (extended only). However, the elbow should be flexed to 120 degrees to hold the reduction, because displacement occurs in 80% of cases if the elbow is more extended.[123] Excessive swell-

ing and a reduction in radial arterial inflow may prevent this extreme positioning. Follow-up radiographs are made at weekly intervals until there is sufficient healing, usually 3 to 4 weeks. Type II fractures in which the capitellum is posterior to the anterior humeral line signify too much extension of the distal fragment and should be closed reduced (Fig. 31-15). Percutaneous pinning is also recommended.

Primary closed reduction and percutaneous pinning is the preferred treatment regimen for type III injuries. Multiple series have demonstrated the best results with this type of fracture management.[65,136] Type III fractures treated with closed reduction and casting, without fixation, have the highest incidence of residual deformity, usually cubitus varus.[99] No cases of forearm compartment syndrome (i.e., ischemic contracture) have been identified in the cases treated with early pinning, compared with those treated with only closed reduction and casting.[136] This is probably because the elbow does not have to be positioned above 90 degrees of flexion to hold the reduction if the fracture has been pinned.

The rare irreducible fracture can be managed with open reduction through a medial approach, adding a lateral incision if necessary. An anterior surgical interval (i.e., S-curved incision over the antecubital fossa) can also be used and is recommended if the neurovascular structures need to be exposed. A posterior approach is not preferred, because it disrupts any remaining intact soft tissue and is the location of the primary vascular supply to the distal humeral fragment.

Skin or skeletal traction has been used in the management of supracondylar fractures, but this technique requires longer hospitalizations and does not provide any advantage over immediate reduction.[133] The idea that the arm is too swollen for a reduction is not valid, because the appropriate bony landmarks are usually palpable. After closed reduction and pinning, the edema lessens.

The technique for closed reduction involves extension of the elbow, followed by correction of the medial and lateral translation. Traction is applied, and the elbow is flexed, using digital pressure over the olecranon to bring the distal fragment forward. The elbow is then held in hyperflexion to lock in the position of the distal fragment. If the fracture is medially displaced, the lateral periosteum is torn. For this condition, the forearm is pronated, tightening the reduction against the intact medial periosteum while helping to maintain closure of the lateral column.[5,64] Pronating the forearm is ineffective in holding some type III fractures if the periosteal sleeve is completely disrupted. Occasionally, the proximal fragment is in a subcutaneous position, producing the ''pucker'' sign, and this fracture is unreducible unless the muscles

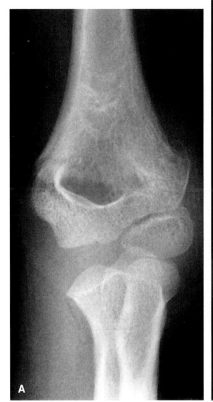
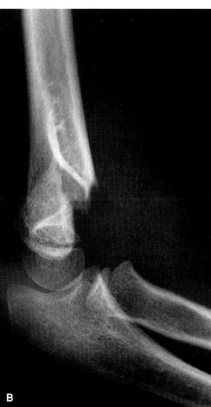

FIGURE 31-15. Impacted type II supracondylar fracture. (**A**) Anteroposterior projection, showing some lateral impaction with valgus angulation. (**B**) Lateral projection, showing hyperextension of the fracture. The capitellum is posterior to the anterior humeral line. This will produce a hyperextension and valgus deformity of the elbow if left unreduced.

can be manipulated back over the end of the bone. The elbow must be flexed while this is attempted.

After reduction and with the elbow in maximal flexion, anteroposterior radiographic images are obtained with the arm slightly internally and externally rotated to evaluate the quality of the reduction. The shoulder can be gently externally rotated to yield a true lateral view of the elbow. The most stable pinning configuration is with single medial and lateral column pins, crossing above the fracture line (Fig. 31-16).[187] If the medial landmarks are difficult to palpate, the lateral pin can be inserted first, and then the elbow is taken out of hyperflexion to a neutral position. This makes palpation of the ulnar groove easier. An alternative is to make a small medial incision to identify the ulnar groove or to use two lateral pins (less stable pinning, especially for type III fracture). Confirmation of satisfactory alignment after pinning is documented with anteroposterior and lateral radiographs of the distal humerus. Immobilization is maintained for 3 to 4 weeks, after which the pins are removed and active range of motion exercises are instituted.

In the event of a pulseless extremity, prompt reduction of the supracondylar fracture usually restores palpable arterial inflow.[153] Complete vascular injury is uncommon because the thick local muscle envelope protects the artery. Vascular evaluation requires differentiation of a pulseless but viable extremity from one

with true vascular insufficiency. The collateral circulation is vast and often provides enough distal perfusion despite brachial artery disruption. A Doppler-detected pulse at the wrist does not signify that the brachial artery is functioning. Brachial artery disruption can be reliably determined by obtaining differential Doppler pulse pressures in the hand. However, the collateral circulation can produce a warm, normal-colored hand, with brisk capillary refill and 100% oxygen saturation, that is viable. There is no clear evidence of a clinical problem with cold intolerance or exercise-induced muscle fatigue for the hand surviving on collateral vascularity, but long-term studies addressing this problem are lacking.

For persistent true vascular insufficiency (e.g., avascular hand), especially if there is nerve palsy or inadequate reduction, an anterior open reduction is recommended. Frequently, the neurovascular bundle is found kinked at the fracture site, and liberation of the artery restores the pulse. There may also be evidence of brachial artery injury. The decision to perform vascular reconstruction if the vessel does not respond to local measures (e.g., adventitia stripping, lidocaine, papaverine) is less clear. Reconstruction is unnecessary if the distal extremity is well perfused, in which case the grafted vessel may not even remain patent. The pulse sometimes spontaneously returns within 48 hours, indicating resolution of arterial

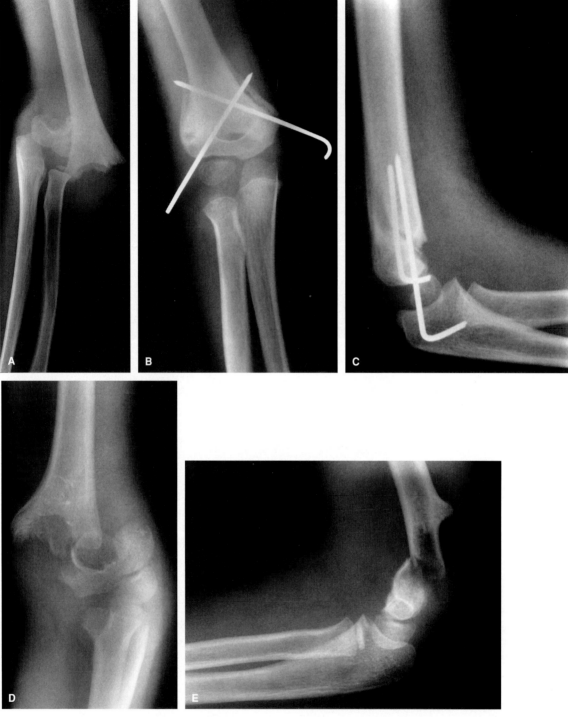

FIGURE 31-16.   Type III supracondylar elbow fracture. **(A)** Complete displacement in the typical posteromedial direction. The distal fragment is in extension. **(B)** Anteroposterior (AP) projection, showing treatment with crossed medial and lateral Kirschner wires. **(C)** The lateral projection, showing that the normal forward tilt of the capitellum has been restored. **(D)** This type III fracture demonstrates lateral displacement. **(E)** The lateral projection also shows flexion of the distal fragment. The treatment for this less common position is the same as for extension fractures. The posterior periosteum is torn, and hyperflexion of the elbow will forward flex the distal fragment excessively. The elbow is best pinned at slightly less than 90 degrees of flexion, because it is technically difficult to pin the elbow in extension. **(F** and **G)** Show AP and lateral postreduction and pinning films.

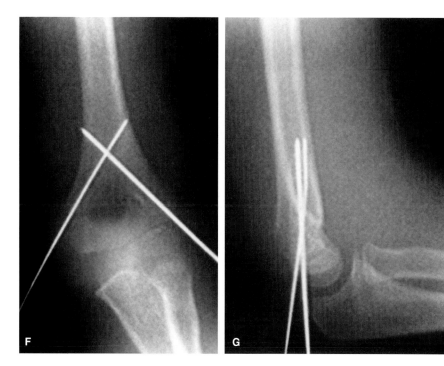

FIGURE 31-16 (*Continued*)

spasm. If vascular repair is performed, the elbow fracture should be stabilized first. Fortunately, open reduction does not adversely affect long-term functional results, which are comparable to closed reduction and percutaneous pinning.[32]

T-Condylar Fracture

The T-condylar fracture is a variation of the supracondylar fracture. The mechanism of injury is axial impaction, with resultant intraarticular fracture. This injury occurs predominantly in adolescents, around physiologic physeal closure, but it can also occur in younger children. The capitellum and trochlea usually are separated from each other, and the two from the proximal humerus. The fracture line transects the epiphyseal plate. In young children, a closed reduction and percutaneous pinning may be sufficient treatment, provided adequate reduction of the condylar fragments is obtained. In adolescents, management usually requires an open reduction with the primary goal of anatomic alignment of the articular surface. Transverse fixation of the trochlea to the capitellum is performed first, and this unit is secured to the distal humerus with crossed Kirschner wires or cancellous screws (Fig. 31-17). Alternatively, 2.5-mm reconstruction plates are applied to the medial and lateral columns of the distal humerus. Internal fixation should be stable to allow early motion, which may be difficult to completely restore.[85]

Lateral Condyle and Epicondyle Fracture

Fracture of the lateral condylar physis is the second most common elbow fracture in children and has two proposed mechanisms of injury. The first is a result of a varus force on the supinated forearm, in which the extensor longus and brevis muscles avulse the condylar fragment.[84] The second mechanism involves a compression force from the radial head, which pushes off the lateral condyle. Although the peak age range for this injury is between 5 and 10 years, younger children may also sustain this fracture.

This is a complex fracture because it involves the physis and the articular surface. A significant portion of the fragment is unossified, especially in children younger than 5 years of age. Usually, a thin lateral metaphyseal rim of bone is identified, indicating the injury, and the remaining fracture line extends through the cartilage of the lateral third of the trochlear epiphysis into the elbow joint.

Milch classified this injury into two fracture patterns (Fig. 31-18). Type I is a fracture lateral to the trochlear groove, coursing through the ossification center of capitellum. This represents a Salter-Harris type IV physeal fracture. The type II fracture line passes into the trochlear region between ossification centers. This fracture is more unstable and may be associated with an apparent elbow dislocation. This injury more closely resembles a Salter-Harris type II fracture, because the fracture line starts in the metaphysis and then courses along the physeal cartilage; there is no contact between the ossification center of the epiphysis and the exposed bone in the metaphysis.

Minimally displaced fractures may not be recognized on standard anteroposterior and lateral radiographs, but they can be visualized by obtaining an oblique view with the arm internally rotated. Displace-

(*text continues on p. 1250*)

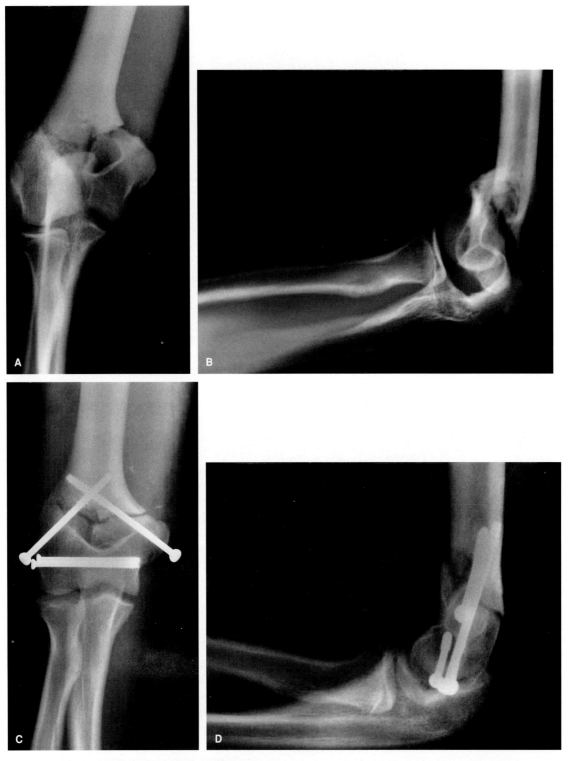

FIGURE 31-17. T-condylar elbow fracture in a 13-year-old adolescent. (**A**) Anteroposterior projection, demonstrating separation of the medial and lateral condyles, with disruption of the normal alignment of the articular surface. (**B**) Lateral projection, showing some anterior comminution. (**C**) Postoperative treatment with restoration of the articular surface using transcondylar compression screws and crossed medial and lateral column cancellous screws. (**D**) Lateral projection, demonstrating restoration of the normal forward-flexed position of the capitellum. Range of motion exercises were begun 2 weeks after open reduction and internal fixation.

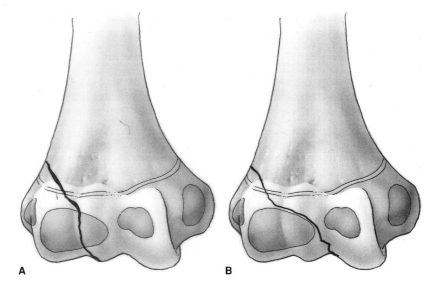

FIGURE 31-18. Milch classification of lateral condyle fractures. (**A**) Type I fracture, traversing the ossification center of the capitellum. (**B**) More common type II pattern, in which the fracture line courses between ossification centers. In type II fractures, if there is wide displacement of the lateral condylar fragment, the ulna may translocate laterally, with the condylar fragment appearing clinically as an elbow dislocation.

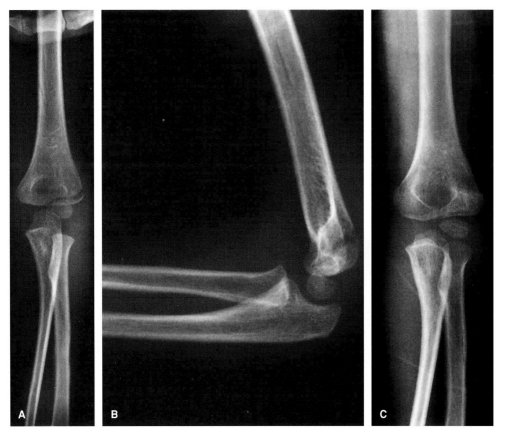

FIGURE 31-19. Lateral condylar fracture. (**A**) The anteroposterior projection shows a 3-mm gap. The fracture is wider radially than it is medially, probably representing a stage II fracture, although the articular cartilage could be intact. Stability of this fragment is not easily determined radiographically and must be closely followed for displacement. (**B**) Lateral projection demonstrates minimal sagittal rotation of the lateral condylar fragment. (**C**) Six weeks later, there was complete fracture healing after closed treatment in an above-elbow cast.

ment has been described as occurring in three stages, depending on whether a cartilage bridge remains intact at the joint line.[84] The bridge anchors the fragment to the remainder of the distal humeral epiphysis, preventing further displacement. In stage I, the articular surface is intact, and there is minimal fragment displacement. Stage II describes a fracture into the elbow joint, but there is no significant fragment rotation. The condylar piece may or may not be further displaced. In stage III, the fracture is displaced and rotated and therefore completely unstable. If the fracture gap is seen only on lateral views and cannot be followed to the trochlear epiphysis, it is probably an intact cartilage bridge (Fig. 31-19). However, if the metaphyseal fracture gap is as wide medially as it is laterally, the cartilage bridge must be severed, suggesting a complete fracture, and the subsequent stability of the fragment is less predictable. The significance of determining the stability of the fracture is that closed management of most stage I and II fractures has a high success rate with a low rate of later displacement (approximately 2%). Fractures with complete fragment separation have a higher rate of unacceptable later displacement if managed closed, and consequently, they must be closely monitored.[168]

Treatment depends on the degree of initial displacement and the assessment of fragment stability.

Fractures displaced 3 mm or less can be treated with cast immobilization. A follow-up radiograph out of the cast must be reviewed 7 to 10 days later to screen for significant additional displacement of the fragment. Immobilization can be discontinued when bridging callus is identified, usually by the fourth week. Healing for these minimally displaced fractures, treated in this fashion, is the expected outcome.[172] When fracture gaps as large as 4 mm are included, successful treatment with cast immobilization alone is still likely, with healing in more than 85% of cases.[51] However, the time to complete healing may be extended, sometimes taking as long as 12 weeks. Minor displaced fractures sometimes fail to heal and are diagnosed later as a nonunion. These probably represent fractures that were unrecognized and untreated, rather than those that failed closed management.[50,86]

The overall incidence of late displacement is 10% to 15%, but the rate depends on the magnitude of the initial fracture gap. It has been reported that those with 3 mm or more of initial separation are likely to displace.[51] Those that do are presumably stage II separations and demonstrate movement within the first 2 weeks from injury. The displacement may not be significant; the original closed treatment plan is altered for only one half of the cases in which fragment movement occurred.[168] Percutaneous pinning of frac-

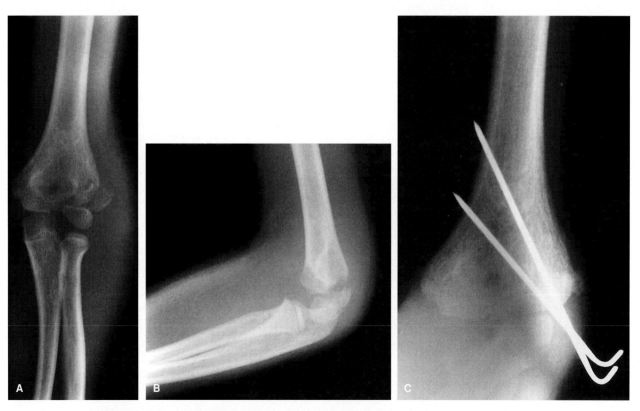

FIGURE 31-20. Lateral condylar fracture. (**A**) The anteroposterior projection shows stage III separation with significant rotation of the condylar fragment. (**B**) The lateral projection shows some sagittal rotation of the fragments. (**C**) Treatment consisted of open reduction and fixation with Kirschner wires crossing in the condylar fragment for greater stability.

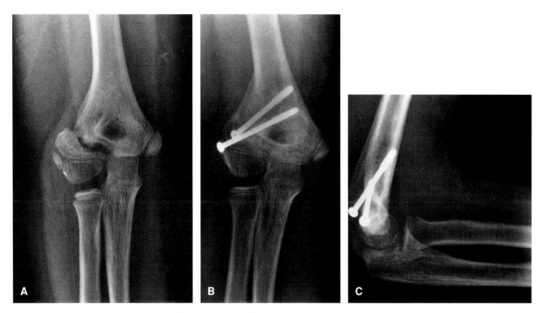

FIGURE 31-21.   Nonunion of the lateral condyle. (**A**) Anteroposterior (AP) view of a child who sustained this fracture 4 months earlier. Symptoms consisted of pain and decreased range of motion. (**B**) AP projection after stabilization of the condylar fragment with bone screws and bone grafting of the nonunion. (**C**) Lateral projection.

tures separated between 3 and 4 mm can be performed, provided joint surface congruity is documented with an arthrogram.[116,124] Although this procedure ensures that there is no further fragment displacement, it is unnecessary in most cases.

Fractures displaced 4 mm or more usually display rotation of the condylar fragment (stage III), denoting significant instability and joint incongruity (Fig. 31-20). In this situation, primary open reduction should be performed, with restoration of articular congruity. Pin stabilization is best achieved with two divergent lateral pins crossing before the fracture or with two parallel pins. Pins must engage the far cortex. Excessive soft tissue stripping of the condylar fragment should be avoided, especially posteriorly (i.e., entrance of blood supply) to prevent avascular necrosis of the capitellum.

Controversy exists about the management of the late presenting lateral condyle fracture. Some investigators recommend no treatment until later problems arise, suggesting that early operation may produce worse results.[42,71,84] Fractures probably can be anatomically reduced and pinned with good results for as long as 6 weeks after the injury.[42,146] After this time, the ability to reduce the fragment precisely is lessened because of remodeling of the fracture surfaces and soft tissue contracture. Excessive stripping of the condylar portion results in avascular necrosis. However, establishing union between the lateral condyle and the distal humerus can prevent further fragment migration, ameliorating the development of some of the adverse late sequelae of the untreated nonunion. This includes ulnar neuritis, progressive valgus deformity, and elbow instability with decreased strength.

In established nonunions, the lateral condyle frag-

ment should be pinned in a position that preserves the best functional range of elbow motion, realizing that anatomic restoration is not possible. Bone grafting is necessary to achieve union (Fig. 31-21). Any residual valgus deformity can be corrected with a supracondylar osteotomy.[117] Ulnar nerve transposition may be needed, especially if there are preoperative symptoms.[146]

Lateral epicondyle fracture is a rare elbow injury that does not involve the articular surface. This ossification center does not appear until the second decade. It is often misdiagnosed as an avulsion fracture of the lateral condyle. Treatment is usually immobilization and early motion when comfortable.

Medial Epicondyle and Condyle Fracture

The medial epicondylar apophysis is fractured when a valgus load is applied to the extended elbow. The displacement is encouraged by the pull of the forearm flexor wad, which is attached to this region. The medial collateral ligament also originates from this apophysis and may play a role in the initial fracture displacement, especially when there is an associated elbow dislocation. The typical age of children sustaining this injury is 9 to 14 years, later than the age peak for most other elbow fractures. Almost 50% of these fractures occur concomitantly with a posterolateral elbow dislocation.

Management of this fracture depends on the degree of displacement and understanding that the fragment tends to rotate forward from its posteromedial origin. There are many advocates for the closed treatment of this injury, especially if there is less than 10

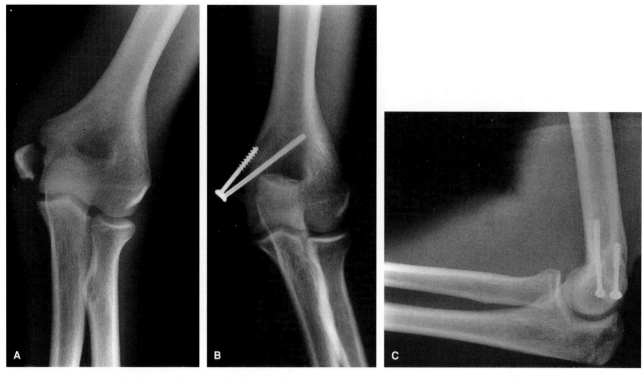

FIGURE 31-22. Displaced medial epicondyle fracture in an adolescent. It is difficult to quantitate the amount of displacement based on the anteroposterior projection, because the fragment has also moved anteriorly. It also may be malrotated. (**B**) Treatment with bone screws and early motion. (**C**) Lateral projection. A single screw is sufficient if it is placed in a posterior to anterior direction, capturing the anterior cortex of the distal humerus.

mm of displacement. Although nonunion is a frequent result of closed management, it does not appear to be a clinical problem.[89] Late symptoms from a nonunion can be treated with excision of the fragment. In cases with valgus instability or greater than 5 to 10 mm of displacement, open reduction and pinning is performed. The goal is to restore the integrity of the medial collateral ligament and to retension the forearm flexors for optimal elbow function.[43,184]

In adolescents, fragment fixation can be accomplished with a cancellous bone screw, directed from a posterior position to capture the anterior humeral cortex (Fig. 31-22). This allows early postoperative elbow range of motion after 2 to 3 weeks of immobilization, which is important because stiffness is the most common complication of this fracture. This is especially the case when there has been an associated elbow dislocation. Preadolescents require Kirschner wire fixation of the fracture and cast immobilization for approximately 4 weeks. In fractures that show significant displacement of the medial epicondyle, especially if the fragment is at the level of the joint, it is imperative to rule out intraarticular entrapment. This problem is another indication for open reduction.

Fracture of the medial condyle, an unusual injury, is caused by a mechanism similar to that for the medial epicondylar fracture: valgus force and ligament avulsion. The fragment usually includes the intact medial epicondyle, and the elbow joint tends to be unstable. If the intraarticular fracture is displaced, it needs open reduction and internal fixation. Because healing may be slow, even in minimally displaced fractures, bone union should be documented radiographically before discontinuing treatment.

Fracture-Separation of the Distal Humeral Physis

Fracture-separation of the distal humeral physis usually is an injury of infants and can even be seen in the newborn. Three age ranges have been described: 0 to 9 months, 7 months to 3 years, and 3 to 7 years.[39] The diagnostic challenge lies in the two younger age categories because of the lack of ossification of the distal humeral epiphysis. In older children, there is usually a Thurston-Holland fragment visible, simplifying the diagnosis. The mechanism of injury involves rotatory shear forces resulting in a Salter-Harris type I or type II fracture pattern. Three clinical settings provide information for the cause of the fracture; birth trauma, accidental trauma (e.g., fall), and child abuse.

Diagnosis of this fracture relies on a good physical examination and an understanding of the relation of the proximal radius and ulna to the distal humerus. There is usually significant soft tissue swelling and soft crepitus with elbow motion. The proximal radius lines up with the capitellum ossification center, and this serves as the main reference point (Fig. 31-23). Typically, the distal fragment is posteromedially displaced.

The differential diagnosis includes elbow dislocation, lateral condyle fracture, and supracondylar fracture. Elbow dislocation is an extremely rare injury in young children and especially in infants. Most dislocations demonstrate posterolateral displacement. The long axis of the radius also is lateral to the capitellum. A lateral condyle fracture in a 2- to 3-year-old child may be confused with transphyseal separation, especially if there is joint subluxation. In this instance, the radius axis line does not pass through the capitellum, which is medial to this ossification center. The entire distal fragment may be displaced laterally, unlike the medial direction consistent with physeal separation. A supracondylar fracture line usually is visible above the epiphyseal plate, although the relation of the radius to the capitellum is preserved.

Arthrography can help confirm the diagnosis of separation of the entire distal humeral physis and is a helpful adjunct at the time of definitive treatment to confirm the quality of fracture reduction. The information obtained at the time of arthrography may alter treatment.[2] Treatment consists of closed reduction and placement of the elbow in a position of flexion and pronation, followed by casting. A single lateral pin can be placed percutaneously to prevent redisplacement (Fig. 31-24). Late-diagnosed fractures should not be manipulated, because there is evidence that normal alignment can occur even in those that have healed in a translated position.[39] Growth disturbance does not seem to occur.

Fractures of the Proximal Radius and Ulna

Fractures of the proximal radius usually involve the radial neck; the radial head is largely cartilaginous and is rarely injured, unlike the skeletally mature elbow. However, if there is evidence of radial head subluxation without bony fracture, the examiner should suspect a partial chondral separation of the radial head or capitellum, and a diagnostic arthrogram or explor-

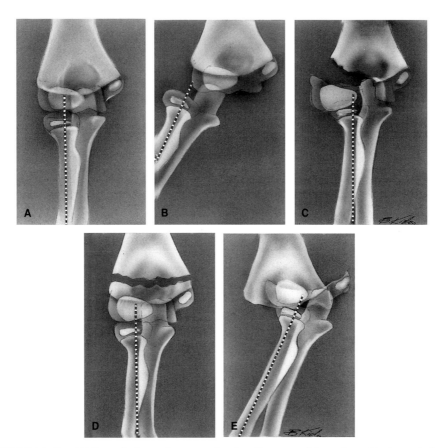

FIGURE 31-23.   (A) Normal elbow, demonstrating the alignment of the radius with the capitellum. (B) In a dislocation of the elbow, there is disruption of the radial capitellar alignment. Most dislocations are posterolateral. (C) In a displaced lateral condyle fracture, there is again disruption of the radial capitellar alignment. (D) Supracondylar elbow fracture, in which the radius and capitellum remain aligned despite displacement of the distal humeral fragment. (E) A fracture-separation of the distal humeral physis. The radiocapitellar relation is preserved, and typically, the distal segment is posteromedially displaced. (Adapted from DeLee J, Wilkins K, Rogers L, et al. Fracture separation of the distal humeral epiphysis. J Bone Joint Surg [Am] 1980;62:46.)

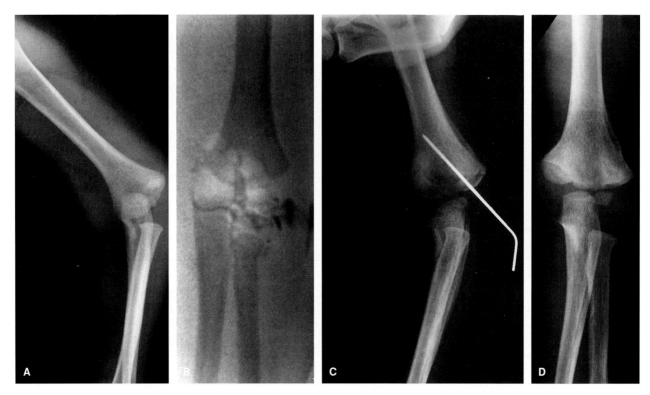

FIGURE 31-24. Fracture-separation of the distal humeral physis in a 2-year-old child. (**A**) On the anteroposterior projection, there is a varus alignment to the elbow with medial displacement of the radial capitellar alignment. (**B**) The intraoperative arthrogram demonstrates the large cartilaginous component of the distal humerus and a partial reduction of the deformity. (**C**) The reduction was stabilized with a single lateral Kirschner wire for 3 weeks. (**D**) Six weeks after injury and pin removal, the radiograph demonstrates good alignment with the elbow. There may be slight residual medial displacement of the distal fragment. The radial capitellar relation has been maintained.

atory arthrotomy is indicated. Proximal radius fractures occur most commonly in 9- to 12-year-old children. The mechanism of injury is most likely a fall on the extended elbow, producing valgus stress. Because most of the radial neck is extraarticular, a fracture may not produce a fat pad sign.

Radial Neck Fracture

Fracture of the radial neck typically produces an angular deformity, and approximately 35 to 45 degrees of angulation is acceptable for successful closed management. Angulation greater than this needs to be reduced, which usually can be accomplished by closed manipulation (Fig. 31-25). Less angulation (approximately 15–20 degrees) is accepted in children older than 10 years of age. The manipulation technique consists of traction and varus stress combined with digital pressure over the radial head.[134] Alternatively, a percutaneous pin can be used to manipulate the proximal fragment and improve alignment.[13]

Three fracture patterns are observed: Salter-Harris type I or II, Salter-Harris type IV, or a metaphyseal fracture distal to the physis. Salter type IV injuries are the least common. The metaphyseal fracture can have a transverse or an oblique fracture line. The displacement can be angulation, translation, both, or complete

separation from the radius. Translation greater than 10% is not acceptable, because the radial head can no longer rotate in a circle, and the congruity of the proximal radioulnar joint is disrupted. Supination and pronation become limited. Radial neck fractures can occur as isolated fractures but are commonly associated with elbow dislocation, or they can be part of the Monteggia-type injury. Well-centered anteroposterior and lateral radiographs of the proximal forearm best delineate the fracture.

Indications for open reduction include complete displacement of the radial head, irreducible angulation greater than 45 degrees, or a displaced Salter-Harris IV fracture. Fixation is best accomplished with a Kirschner wire placed obliquely across the fracture, avoiding the use of a transhumeral (radiocapitellar) pin. If there is a large enough metaphyseal fragment, a minifragment screw can be used instead of the Kirschner wire. Complications of open reduction include injury to the posterior interosseous nerve and significant loss of elbow motion.

Olecranon Fractures

Olecranon fractures are not common in children, but when present in young patients, they are often

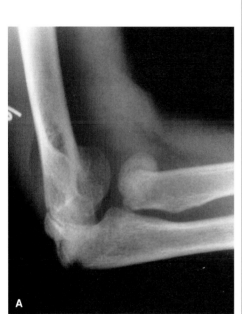

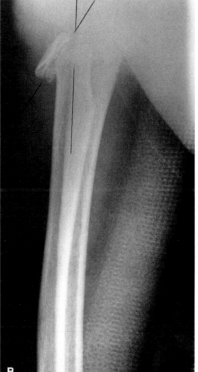

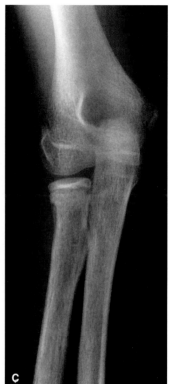

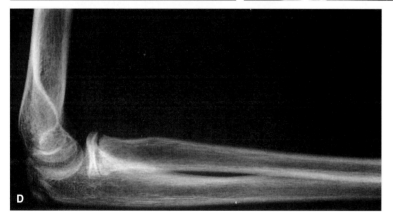

FIGURE 31-25. Radial neck fracture. (**A**) A lateral radiograph demonstrates deformity of the radial head. (**B**) The anteroposterior (AP) view shows a metaphyseal fracture of the radial neck with 50% translation and 60 degrees of angulation. This was treated with a closed reduction and casting. (**C**) The AP radiograph 3 weeks later shows correction of the translation and angulation. (**D**) Lateral projection.

minimally displaced. In adolescents, a displaced fracture is more typically seen. The most common mechanism of injury is an avulsion. In younger children, extension injuries to the elbow can produce angulated metaphyseal fractures of the olecranon, usually in conjunction with proximal radial fracture or medial epicondyle separation.

Displaced transverse fractures are best managed by standard osteosynthesis (AO) tension band technique or its modification, which involves placing the distal wire hole anterior to the axis of the intramedullary Kirschner wires (Fig. 31-26).[145] This provides additional compression forces across the articular surface of the olecranon. Oblique fractures of the olecranon can be treated by lag screw compression, using 3.5- or 4-mm cannulated cancellous screws (Fig. 31-27). Angulated metaphyseal fractures that do not align with closed reduction and that do not involve the articular surface often can be straightened with the insertion of an intramedullary pin.

Elbow Dislocation

Elbow dislocation is a relatively uncommon injury in young children; the peak incidence is in the second decade of life. Often, there is an associated fracture, most commonly the medial epicondyle but occasionally a coronoid process or a proximal radius fracture. Elbow dislocation is predominantly a male injury (70%), involving the nondominant arm (60%), and associated fractures are common (60%).[25]

The most common pattern is displacement of the proximal radius and ulna articulation from the humerus without disruption of the radioulnar articulation. Most are posterolateral, but medially directed dislocations can occur. The injury may tear the ante-

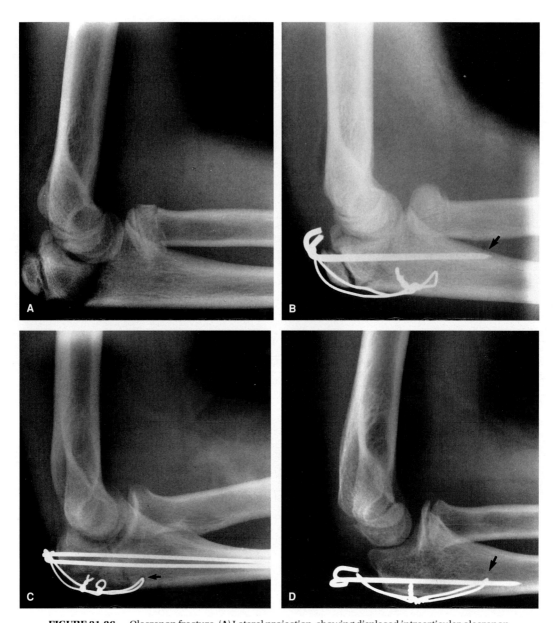

FIGURE 31-26. Olecranon fracture. (**A**) Lateral projection, showing displaced intraarticular olecranon fracture. There is also an impacted radial neck fracture. (**B**) This is treated with standard tension band technique. The slight variation from standard fixation is to capture the anterior cortex of the ulna with the Kirschner (K) wires (*arrow*). (**C**) Standard AO technique used in a similar case with parallel intramedullary K-wires with the tension band transverse hole inferior (*arrow*). (**D**) Modified AO technique performed by placing the transverse hole anterior to the K-wires (*arrow*). The compressive force is anterior to the pin, which prevents the articular surface of the semilunar notch from gapping. Ideal joint compressive forces are obtained with placement of the K-wires down the middle axis of the ulna and the transverse hole anterior to this axis.

rior elbow joint capsule, rupture of the ulnar collateral ligament or the equivalent (e.g., medial epicondyle separation), disrupt the brachialis muscle, and damage the collateral arterial system.

Treatment is accomplished by prompt closed reduction, usually in the emergency department, after establishing pain control. The surgeon should beware of interposed fragments, such as the medial epicondyle, or unsatisfactory postreduction alignment, suggesting soft tissue or cartilaginous interposition. A pos-

terior splint is applied for 2 to 3 weeks; thereafter, elbow range of motion can commence. Approximately 11% of dislocations demonstrate mild neurapraxia involving the median or ulnar nerves. Rarely is there significant arterial disruption.

Radial Head Dislocation

Occasionally, isolated radial head dislocation occurs, usually in an anterior direction (Fig. 31-28). This

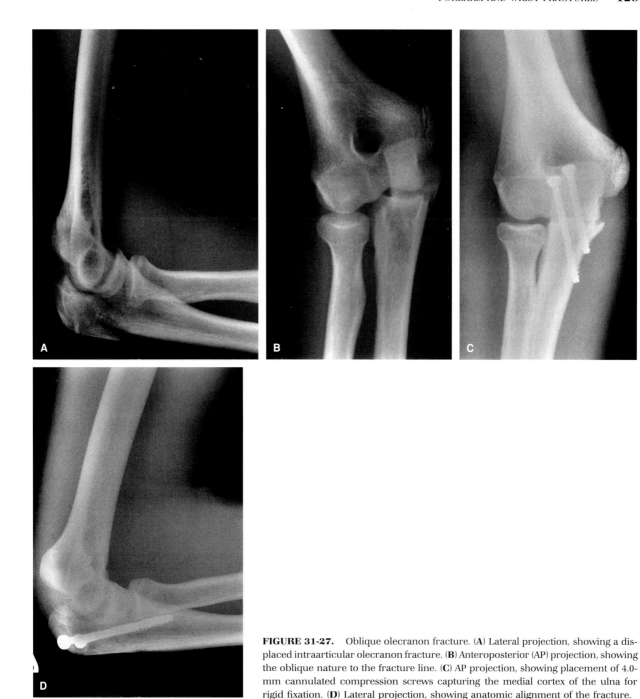

FIGURE 31-27. Oblique olecranon fracture. (**A**) Lateral projection, showing a displaced intraarticular olecranon fracture. (**B**) Anteroposterior (AP) projection, showing the oblique nature to the fracture line. (**C**) AP projection, showing placement of 4.0-mm cannulated compression screws capturing the medial cortex of the ulna for rigid fixation. (**D**) Lateral projection, showing anatomic alignment of the fracture.

is treated with closed reduction, and the elbow is placed in flexion of greater than 90 degrees. Subluxation of the radial head is a common injury and represents a partial tear and displacement of the orbicular ligament over the radial head. The mechanism of injury is traction on the extended, pronated elbow in children younger than 5 years of age. Most often, they are girls with ligamentous laxity. Reduction is obtained with supination and flexion of the elbow, and immobilization is unnecessary, unless the child is still not using the arm normally (pain). In this situation, a posterior splint is applied and removed at home after 3 to 5 days.

FOREARM AND WRIST FRACTURES

Fractures involving the forearm and wrist are common in children, accounting for slightly more than one half of all children's fractures.[112] Most forearm fractures occur in children older than 5 years of age. The location of the fracture advances distally with increasing age of the child, probably because of the anatomic changes in the radial shaft–metaphyseal junction that occur with maturity and place different areas at risk for fracture.[171] Physeal separations are primarily fractures of early adolescence rather than childhood. The distal forearm is the site of 70% to 80%

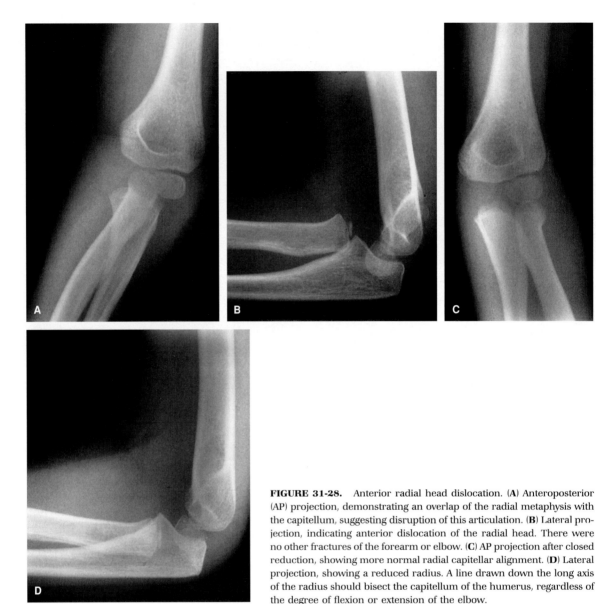

FIGURE 31-28. Anterior radial head dislocation. **(A)** Anteroposterior (AP) projection, demonstrating an overlap of the radial metaphysis with the capitellum, suggesting disruption of this articulation. **(B)** Lateral projection, indicating anterior dislocation of the radial head. There were no other fractures of the forearm or elbow. **(C)** AP projection after closed reduction, showing more normal radial capitellar alignment. **(D)** Lateral projection, showing a reduced radius. A line drawn down the long axis of the radius should bisect the capitellum of the humerus, regardless of the degree of flexion or extension of the elbow.

of fractures. Most of these are nonphyseal injuries. The remainder of the fractures are in the middle of the forearm, and approximately 5% are located in the proximal one third. The usual mechanism of injury is a fall on the outstretched hand. In 13% of patients, elbow fractures occur in conjunction with forearm fractures. This highlights the importance of a thorough clinical and radiographic examination of the injured extremity.

The ulna is triangular but is configured straight, and the radius has a more complex, curved shape, with a cylindrical proximal portion, a triangular middle, and a flattened distal third. The radius rotates around the ulna during forearm supination and pronation. There are three areas of soft tissue interconnection between the radius and the ulna. Proximally, there is the radioulnar articulation, which is stabilized by the annular ligament, and the interosseous mem-

brane connects the two bones over most of the forearm. Distally, the radioulnar articulation is stabilized by the triangular fibrocartilage complex and by the ulnar collateral and the volar and dorsal radiocarpal ligaments. The proximal and distal radioulnar joints are most stable in supination, and the interosseous membrane is widest when the forearm is in a position of neutral to 30 degrees supination. Because of these interconnections, both bones are usually injured at the time of fracture, or one bone is broken in conjunction with damage to the proximal or distal radioulnar articulation.

Displaced forearm fractures demonstrate angular deformity that also involves a component of rotational malalignment. Supination and flexion are coupled motions, as are pronation and extension. This concept is especially evident when considering a dorsally angulated radius fracture that has rotated around an intact ulna. The magnitude of angular deformity that is tolerated for the closed management of forearm fractures is highlighted in the discussion of each regional fracture. An angular deformity is a dynamic problem, because remodeling changes the shape of the injured bones over time, influencing the final range of motion.

Remodeling potential depends on several factors, which should be reviewed when designing a treatment plan for each fracture. Perhaps the most significant factor is the age of the child and therefore how many years of growth remain. The farther the fracture site is away from the distal physis (the most active growth center), the less effect the growth plate has on remodeling. It has been estimated that 10 degrees per year of correction of residual angulation is from distal epiphyseal growth, and the rate of correction is proportional to the severity of the deformity.[53] Rotational deformity cannot be relied on to remodel, although some studies suggest small degrees of malrotation spontaneously correct through reshaping of the bones.[137,165] Clinical, subjective, and functional results are generally excellent after treatment of forearm and wrist fractures, although some permanent loss in rotational range of motion can often be demonstrated.

The most important factor in maintaining fracture alignment after closed reduction is the quality of the applied immobilization, provided there is some fracture site stability. A three-point mold with no space between cast padding, the skin, and the cast material provides good fracture support. The forearm should be immobilized in any position in which the angula-

tion is minimized and the reduction feels stable. The width of the proximal and distal fragments should match, helping to confirm correct rotational alignment. Although muscle forces exert some influence on the ability to maintain bone position in plaster, their importance is perhaps overstated. The position of the forearm in the cast does not affect the ability to maintain the reduction.[28,59,90,174] Significant redisplacement occurs in 7% to 13% of cases within the first 2 weeks of treatment, despite good-quality initial alignment. Fortunately, remanipulation of the fracture does not adversely affect the outcome, except perhaps for physeal injuries.[59,174]

Midshaft Fracture

Fractures of the midshaft of the radius and ulna tend to follow three injury patterns: plastic deformation, greenstick fracture, and complete fracture. Plastic deformation of cortical bone is possible because of the elastic properties of young children's bones. This injury represents a series of microfractures that are not seen on radiographs. If the deformity is pronounced, a prolonged corrective force must be applied to straighten the bone, followed by the placement of a well-molded cast. Treatment by fracture manipulation in children older than 4 years of age is recommended if there is greater than 20 degrees of angulation. For fewer degrees of angulation, sufficient remodeling occurs in the younger child.[111]

Greenstick fractures are characterized by a com-

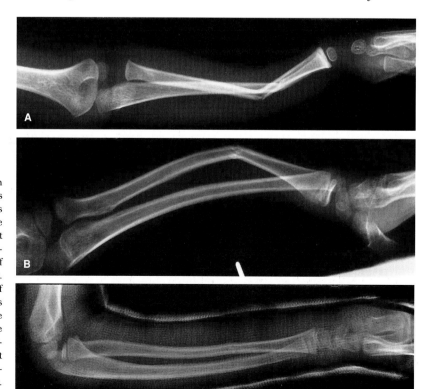

FIGURE 31-29. Coupled relation of rotation and angulation. (**A**) This fracture demonstrates volar angulation. The mechanism of injury was falling on the outstretched hand. When the fracture of the radius and ulna are at different levels, angulation cannot occur without rotation. Notice the anteroposterior appearance of the elbow and the lateral projection of the wrist. This deformity is corrected with pronation of the distal fragment. (**B**) The radiograph shows the opposite deformity with pronation of the distal fragment and dorsal angulation of the radius. The ulna has undergone plastic deformation. When a single bone angulates, it must rotate around the other. (**C**) Alignment is restored with supination of the distal fragment. The lateral projections of the elbow and the wrist are now matched.

plete fracture of one cortical margin and plastic deformation of the opposite side. Most greenstick fractures represent a rotational malalignment in which dorsal angulation (apex volar) suggests a supinating deforming force, and volar angulation is caused by a pronating force (Fig. 31-29). Reduction is accomplished by reversing the injury mechanism with pronation or supination, respectively. Completing the fracture of the opposing cortex is unnecessary in this situation, although this frequently occurs during the reduction maneuver. Occasionally, greenstick fractures involving the radius and the ulna are caused by a direct force, producing mostly an angular deformity without much malrotation. In this situation, it is often necessary to break the opposite cortex to prevent recurrent angulation (this requires adequate analgesia). Although the goal is to complete the cortical fracture, excessive forceful manipulation is avoided because it tears the surrounding intact periosteum, significantly increasing fracture instability.

Complete both-bone fractures usually assume a position dictated by local muscle forces, depending somewhat on the precise level of the fracture. Most proximal fragments are in a position of supination because of the action of the biceps and supinator muscles. The distal fragment is usually pronated, influenced by the pronator quadratus, thumb abductors, and the brachioradialis. The pronator teres has a more neutral effect on rotation, unless the fracture site is proximal to its insertion, in which case it tends to pronate the distal portion. After fracture reduction, the forearm is rotated so the distal segment is aligned to the position of the proximal portion, neutralizing the muscular pull. Alternatively, the fragments can be aligned by observing the bone widths on radiographs and matching their contours by rotating the forearm. The bicipital tuberosity may be a helpful landmark in children, provided it is visible on radiographs. The tuberosity points ulnarward in maximal supination, aligning with the full profile of the ulnar styloid. With neutral forearm rotation, the tuberosity is in midposition, superimposed over the radial shaft.[49] Severely displaced fractures may be held in an abnormal position because of soft tissue interposition, reflecting the force of the injury and subsequent fragment displacement rather than the influence of local muscle pull.

Treatment requires adequate pain relief and muscle relaxation, usually provided through regional (i.e., Bier or axillary block) or general anesthesia. The reduction technique typically involves increasing the angular deformity, applying longitudinal traction, and correcting any malrotation by supinating or pronating the forearm. Postreduction casting entails a flat interosseous mold along the volar forearm, creating an oval shape while keeping a straight lateral border along the ulnar side. An above-elbow cast should be used.

Fracture stability is improved with at least 50% bone apposition. If one bone disengages, shortening occurs, usually followed by an increase in angulation. Shortening of the radius at the level of the wrist (i.e., radioulnar joint) should not exceed 4 mm to ensure a good result.[34] Bayonet apposition is acceptable for patients younger than 8 years of age, with no adverse effect on final alignment or rotational motion if there is no interosseous impingement.

Reduction of the interosseous space by bony angulation reduces the arc of motion the radius takes around the ulna during forearm rotation. In children younger than 8 years of age, 15 to 20 degrees of midshaft angulation is acceptable. For a more proximal radius fracture, less deformity should be the goal, because remodeling is less pronounced.[91] Children older than 8 years of age should not be allowed to develop more than 10 degrees of midshaft angulation and should be held to less than 15 degrees for fractures located at the junction of the middle and distal thirds.[185] A 10-degree angle in the diaphysis of the forearm causes an approximately 20-degree loss of rotation. There is also a 1-degree loss in forearm rotation for each 1 degree of fracture malrotation. Fortunately, 20 to 30 degrees of malrotation is clinically acceptable for a good outcome.[137] The closed treatment of forearm fractures usually produces excellent results (90% of patients) with less than 10 degrees of loss of rotation, especially when the physician is able to stay within these management guidelines.[137]

There are several indications for operative intervention in diaphyseal forearm fractures in children. If closed reduction is not successful or if casting has failed to maintain acceptable position despite repeat manipulation, a different approach is implemented, depending on the problem. For example, if soft tissue interposition is suspected, open treatment of the fracture is required. If the fracture reduction is then stable, a cast alone may be applied. Alternatively, internal fixation to one or both bones can be performed. Unstable fractures may also be treated with primary intramedullary pinning. This usually consists of retrograde insertion (proximal to distal) of an ulnar pin and antegrade insertion of a radius pin (Fig. 31-30). Supplemental casting usually is required, unless three-point intramedullary fixation is obtained with an elastic flexible rod, which allows early unprotected motion.[102] Intramedullary fixation is well suited for young adolescents and children, because healing is rapid and the hardware is easily removed after sufficient bone union is established. Soft tissue disruption is minimal because the pins usually are inserted percutaneously.

Adolescents with displaced both-bone forearm fractures are usually treated with open reduction and compression plating of the bones (Fig. 31-31). This provides anatomic fracture alignment and allows

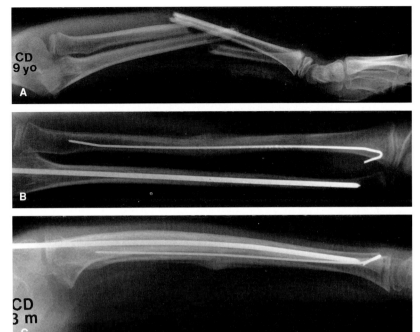

FIGURE 31-30. Both-bone forearm fracture in a 9-year-old child. (**A**) There was a grade I open injury of the radius. After irrigation and debridement, the closed reduction was unstable. (**B**) The anteroposterior projection shows insertion of the intramedullary Steinmann pins. (**C**) Lateral projection shows alignment. Intramedullary fixation was augmented with the use of an above-elbow splint for 2 weeks, followed by a below-elbow cast for an additional 2 weeks.

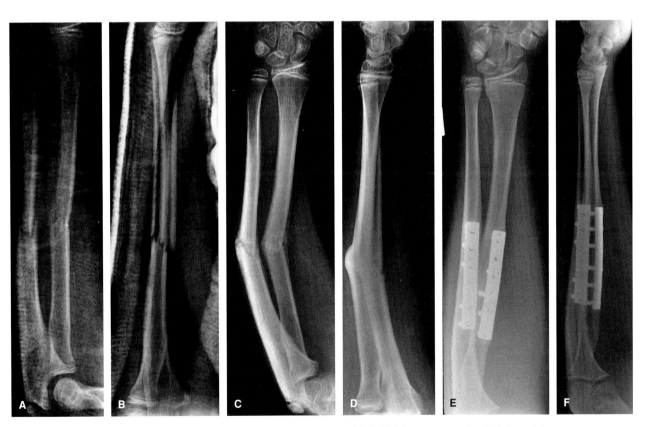

FIGURE 31-31. Malunion of the forearm in a 14-year-old child. (**A**) Anteroposterior (AP) view of the alignment after closed reduction and casting. (**B**) The lateral projection shows acceptable alignment. (**C**) The AP projection 12 weeks after treatment shows malunion of the radius and ulna. (**D**) A lateral projection shows dorsal angulation. Clinical evaluation demonstrated only 15 degrees of rotation of the forearm. (**E**) An AP projection after osteotomy and internal fixation with 3.5-mm compression plates. (**F**) The lateral projection shows restoration of anatomic alignment. The range of motion was significantly improved, with full supination but with a loss of the last 20 degrees of pronation.

early, unprotected range of motion. Plating is rarely used in younger children, but it is indicated for comminuted fractures or when the fracture site is too distal on the ulna or too proximal on the radius for adequate intramedullary pinning. Plating has the disadvantage of possible later hardware removal, which entails the added risk of neurovascular injury and refracture.[12,40]

Except for grade I open fractures, which can usually be managed by closed reduction after appropriate wound care, more significant open injuries are best managed by the addition of internal or external fixation, depending on the severity of soft tissue damage and fracture stability. Children and especially adolescents with ipsilateral humeral fracture may be candidates for primary internal stabilization of their fractures to allow early mobility of the extremity. A relative indication for internal fixation is a refracture in an older child after completing a course of closed management.[137] The goal is to prevent further loss of range of motion through stable fracture fixation and early movement. However, it is important to realize that

operative intervention with anatomic alignment does not guarantee recovery of full motion. The final range of motion is determined by the degree of soft tissue scarring that occurs, especially that which involves the interosseous membrane.[91]

Distal-Third Fracture

Distal-third both-bone forearm fractures are common and are usually caused by a fall onto the wrist with the hand in a pronated position. Unicortical fractures (i.e., torus or "buckle" fractures) of the radius and ulna are frequently encountered and are stable injuries. Treatment aims for patient comfort and protection of the forearm from further injury. Immobilization with a below-elbow cast or splint for 2 to 3 weeks is sufficient. This simple injury should be differentiated from the minimally displaced bicortical fracture that has a propensity for significant later volar angulation (Fig. 31-32). A well-molded above-elbow cast is recommended, especially if there is pain with forearm rotation, and 1-week follow-up radiographs are recommended for bicortical fractures.

In complete fractures, the distal fragment is usually dorsally displaced, but the dorsal periosteum is not torn. Fracture reduction is accomplished by increasing the deformity, which relaxes the intact concave periosteum. Longitudinal traction is then applied with digital pressure at the fracture site until length is restored. The angular deformity then is corrected (Fig. 31-33). The goal should be to obtain at least 50% bone apposition combined with neutral angulation. More reduction force is required if the ulna is not completely broken, and pronating the distal segment during the reduction maneuver assists in fragment realignment. The wrist should be placed in slight palmar flexion and ulnar deviation, and the cast is molded with pressure dorsally over the distal fragment and proximally on the volar forearm.

The cast molding technique is designed to counter the tendency for later radial and dorsal fracture displacement (Fig. 31-34). Most often, an above-elbow cast is used for immobilization, but it has been demonstrated that a well-molded below-elbow cast can also effectively control these fractures, highlighting the importance of casting technique. Chess treated 558 distal forearm fractures with below-elbow casting, reporting that 90% displayed less than a 5-degree change in angular alignment during the course of treatment.[28] Fracture alignment should be monitored for the first few weeks after the injury, when there is the greatest potential for repeat displacement.

Initially, displaced distal forearm fractures are manipulated to start treatment with as near-normal anatomic positioning as possible, especially if there is also a clinical deformity. However, because of the proximity of these fractures to the distal growth plate,

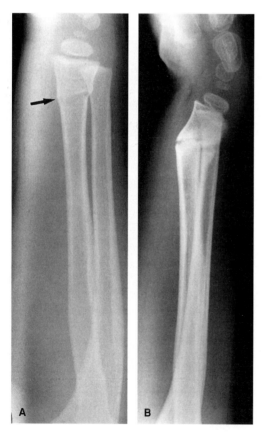

FIGURE 31-32. Bicortical fracture. **(A)** This minimally displaced bicortical fracture (*arrow*) of the distal radius can easily be mistaken for a simple dorsal buckle fracture. **(B)** Three weeks later after cast removal, 35 degrees of dorsal angulation has occurred. Although this probably will remodel over the next year, there is considerable clinical deformity and a loss of rotation until this angulation resolves. This problem can be avoided through the use of a well-molded cast placed above the elbow to control rotation.

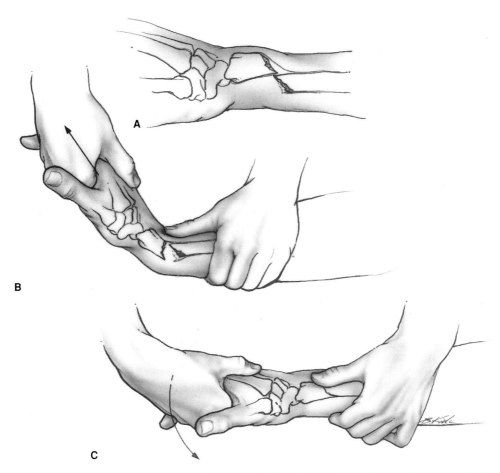

FIGURE 31-33. Reduction technique for a distal both-bone fracture. (**A**) The fracture is 100% translated and shortened. The dorsal periosteum is generally intact. Longitudinal traction alone can tighten the soft tissues, preventing reduction of the fragment. (**B**) The dorsal soft tissues need to be completely relaxed by hyperextending the fracture and then providing longitudinal traction, restoring length to the dorsal cortex. Digital pressure on the distal fragment generally helps with this maneuver. (**C**) The reduction is completed with volar flexion of the distal fragment. The goal is at least 50% apposition of the bony surfaces and no angulation.

the remodeling potential is great. This may allow the correction of rather significant degrees of malalignment during subsequent growth. The guidelines for acceptable residual angulation are age dependent and only serve as a general indicator of expected results. Children younger than 5 years of age who display 25 to 35 degrees of volar angulation can be allowed to complete healing in this position, and children between 5 and 10 years of age should be held in the 20- to 25-degree range. Between 10 and 12 years of age, 15 degrees is a better goal, and those older than 12 years should be controlled at less than 15 degrees to ensure a good outcome. Radial deviation remodels much less than does angulation in the plane of active wrist motion; therefore, this deformity should be kept to less than 15 degrees in children younger than 10 years of age and to less than 10 degrees in older children.

Occasionally, a distal-third fracture is unreducible with closed manipulation because of soft tissue interposition, usually entrapment of the pronator quadra-

tus. In young children, maintaining adequate alignment with closed treatment yields a good result if the radius is not excessively shortened (Fig. 31-35). In older children, a small volar incision allows removal of the soft tissue hindering the reduction, and then closed management can proceed.

The isolated distal-third radius fracture may represent a more difficult fracture to control with casting, especially if there is an oblique fracture configuration.[68] The reported incidence of significant fracture redisplacement varies considerably.[28,59] Most can be successfully managed with closed reduction and application of an above-elbow cast, although Chess treated 45 isolated distal radius fractures in below-elbow casts and reported only 10% with significant redisplacement.[28] Supination of the forearm may also reduce the incidence of delayed dorsal angulation by negating the pull of the brachioradialis.[68] Occasionally, fractures that do not maintain their position by closed treatment can be percutaneously pinned to avoid repeated fracture manipulation.[59] On close inspection,

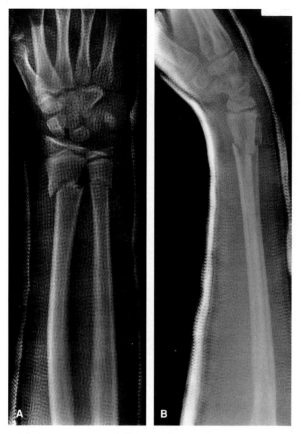

FIGURE 31-34. A distal both-bone forearm fracture with a well-molded cast. (**A**) The anteroposterior projection shows a small amount of translation of the fracture fragments but no significant angulation. The radial border of the cast is well molded, and the wrist is in neutral to slight ulnar deviation. A common error is to have the wrist in radial deviation, which allows fragment displacement in this direction. (**B**) The lateral projection shows some palmar flexion of the wrist with a flat mold over the dorsum of the wrist and a flat volar mold proximal to the fracture site.

many isolated radius fractures also show fracture of the ulnar styloid.

Distal Physis Fracture

Fracture of the distal radial physis is the most common physeal fracture in children, comprising 14% to 18% of all distal forearm fractures. Eighty percent are Salter-Harris type I or II fractures. Closed reduction may be performed under a regional block, including local Xylocaine "hematoma" infiltration or by pharmacologic sedation. Above-elbow casting is recommended for 2 weeks, followed by below-elbow casting for an additional two. The wrist must be palmar flexed and the dorsal portion of the cast well molded for three-point fixation. This fracture is easily reduced, and it also readily redisplaces, usually by the first week of follow-up. However, this is not a problem if the angulation is not excessive (Fig. 31-36).

In type I and II physeal separations, the germinal cells remain with the distal epiphyseal fragment, and an anatomic reduction is unnecessary for continued normal growth. Approximately 50% apposition of the distal fragment is acceptable, but the angulation should not be greater than 25 to 30 degrees in children younger than 10 years of age. In children older than 12 years of age, angulation in excess of 15 degrees is to be avoided. Multiple reduction attempts may lead to growth plate damage; two or more attempts have produced growth arrest in slightly more than 25% of these patients.[103] Repeat manipulation should not be attempted more than 10 days after the injury, because physeal healing has already commenced, and further growth plate trauma will probably occur. Compression injury to the distal physis (i.e., Salter-Harris type V) is uncommon but is associated with the later presentation of growth disturbance.

Forearm Fracture-Dislocations

The combination of forearm fracture with proximal radiohumeral or distal radioulnar joint dislocation is a less common injury than the other types of forearm fracture. The peak incidence occurs between 4 and 10 years of age, and the most common mechanism of injury is a fall on the outstretched hand. The Monteggia lesion occurs at the elbow, and the Galeazzi lesion is located at the wrist. The classic Monteggia complex describes a fracture of the ulna, with a dislocation of the radial head. The radial dislocation is in the direction of the apex of the ulnar deformity—anterior, posterior, or lateral.

Bado devised a classification system of four basic types of injury and several equivalent lesions.[9] Type I describes anterior radial head dislocation (i.e., ulnar apex deformity anterior), and this is the most common childhood pattern (Fig. 31-37). The type II fracture entails posterior or posterolateral radial head dislocation. The second most common Monteggia fracture seen in children is the type III lesion, in which the radial head is displaced laterally. In this instance, the ulna fracture is usually in the proximal metaphyseal region. Type IV fracture-dislocations involve anterior dislocation of the radial head in combination with a proximal-third radius fracture. Because the dislocation is anterior, this may be considered a variant of the type I lesion.

There are numerous Monteggia lesion equivalents that represent the multitude of fracture-dislocation variations. For example, the ulna fracture may be combined with radial neck fracture or a complete radial physeal separation, rather than a simple radial head dislocation. Segmental fracture of the ulna, usually of the diaphysis and the olecranon, or plastic deformation of the ulna with radial head dislocation are other forms. The surgeon must be wary of any apparent isolated proximal-third ulna fracture, recognizing the

(*text continues on p. 1267*)

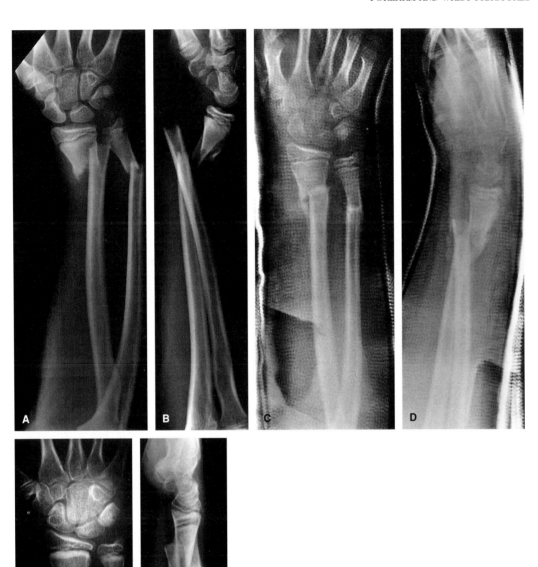

FIGURE 31-35. Distal both-bone forearm fracture with bayonet apposition. (**A**) An anteroposterior (AP) projection of a completely displaced distal radius and ulnar fracture. (**B**) A lateral projection shows significant displacement. (**C**) The AP projection after closed reduction and casting shows there is a slight radial deviation of the distal fragments. (**D**) A lateral projection shows bayonet apposition but no significant angulation. A well-formed cast has held this position. (**E**) The AP projection 3 months after injury shows healing of the fracture and good alignment. (**F**) A lateral projection shows no significant angulation. In this 8-year-old child, complete remodeling is expected, with the return of a normal range of motion.

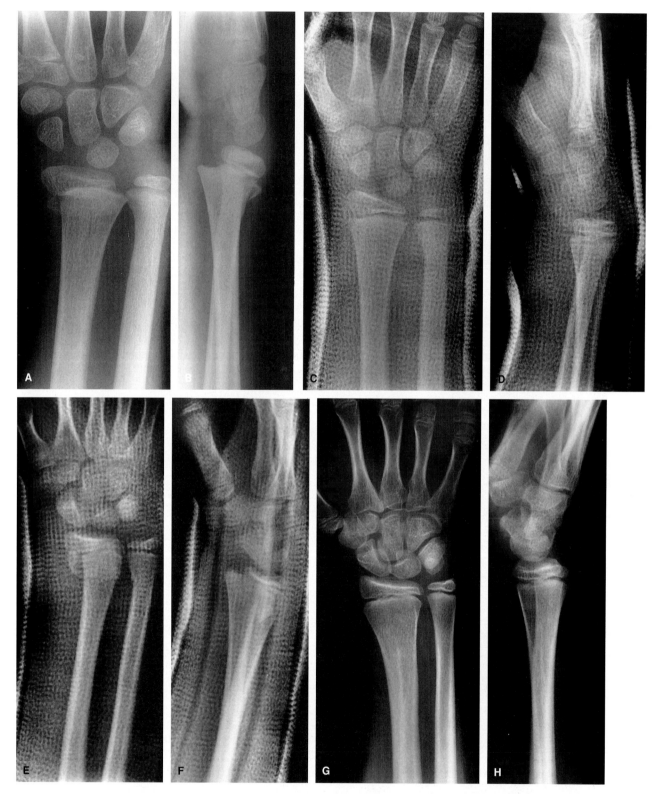

FIGURE 31-36. Salter-Harris distal radius physeal fracture in a 10-year-old child. (**A**) The anteroposterior (AP) projection demonstrates displacement of the distal radial epiphysis. The small metaphyseal fragment classifies this radiographically as a Salter-Harris II fracture. (**B**) The lateral projection shows dorsal displacement. (**C**) The AP projection after closed reduction and casting. (**D**) A lateral projection shows anatomic alignment. (**E** and **F**) Twelve days later, there has been redisplacement on AP and lateral radiographs. (**G** and **H**) AP and lateral projections 1 year later show complete remodeling of the fracture with restoration of normal growth.

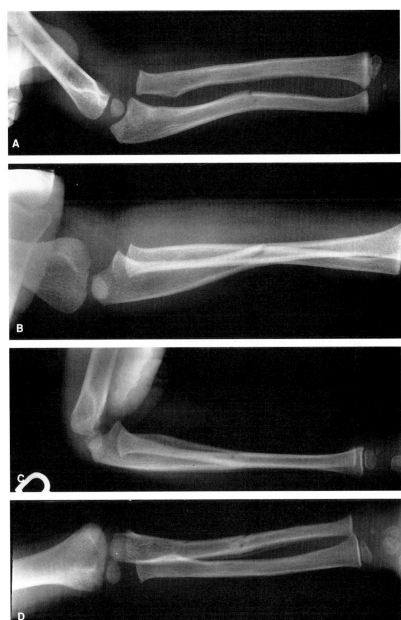

FIGURE 31-37. Type I Monteggia lesion. (**A**) The lateral projection shows an ulnar fracture angulated anteriorly, with dislocation of the radial head in the same direction. (**B**) Anteroposterior projection shows malalignment of the radiocapitellar joint. (**C**) Alignment after closed reduction and correction of the ulnar angulation. A line through the central axis of the radius points to the capitellum. This fracture must be followed closely for recurrent angulation. (**D**) The anteroposterior projection shows early healing of the ulna and normal alignment of the radiocapitellar joint.

high incidence of concomitant radiohumeral joint disruption or its equivalent.

In children, most Monteggia fractures can be successfully managed by closed reduction and above-elbow casting.[105,132,181] Because the ulna fracture often is incomplete, the reduction is stable. It is imperative to review a lateral radiograph that demonstrates anatomic radial head relocation. The key to successful treatment is maintaining ulnar length, which is accomplished by eliminating the angulation, keeping the radial head reduced. The forearm is held in a position of full supination, which provides for maximal radial head stability. Weekly follow-up is suggested for 2 to 3 weeks to detect recurrent radial head subluxation. Nerve palsies associated with Monteggia fractures oc-

cur in approximately 10% of patients, and the posterior interosseous nerve is most frequently injured.[132]

Operative intervention is indicated when the ulnar angulation cannot be controlled, as may be the case with an oblique or segmental ulnar fracture. The percutaneous insertion of an ulnar intramedullary pin is a simple and effective way to manage this problem (Fig. 31-38); alternatively, the ulnar shaft can be plated. If the radial head is not reduced after correction of the ulnar length and alignment, open examination of this joint is necessary. Typically, there is interposition of the annular ligament or, less often, an intraarticular osteochondral fragment. Transcapitellar pinning of the reduced radial head usually is unnecessary and inadvisable. The Monteggia equivalent that consists of

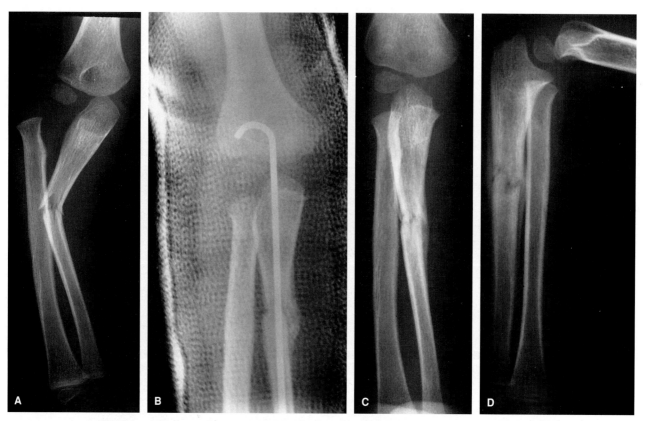

FIGURE 31-38. Type III Monteggia lesion. (**A**) The anteroposterior (AP) projection shows lateral angulation of the ulna and lateral dislocation of the radial head. A satisfactory closed reduction could not be maintained in the ulna. (**B**) An intramedullary Kirschner wire has been inserted to maintain alignment of the ulna, and consequently, it stabilized the radiocapitellar joint. (**C**) The AP view, 4 weeks later, after pin removal. (**D**) The lateral view shows anatomic alignment.

radial neck or head fracture has been identified as an injury that often requires open reduction (Fig. 31-39).[132]

The classic Galeazzi lesion is a fracture of the distal third of the radius without fracture of the ulna and is associated with a dislocation of the distal radioulnar joint. This is an uncommon injury in children, occurring in approximately 5% of all distal radial shaft fractures. The triangular fibrocartilage complex is disrupted, and the distal ulna is dorsally displaced, as viewed on a lateral radiograph. Injury to the distal radioulnar joint is frequently overlooked, and persistent joint subluxation is responsible for poor long-term results.[176] Management consists of closed reduction and above-elbow casting with the forearm in full supination. It is rarely necessary to place a smooth Kirschner wire across this joint to maintain the reduction.

The Galeazzi-equivalent injury is represented by physeal separation of the distal ulna instead of a triangular fibrocartilage tear.[106] The ulna metaphysis is displaced and is reduced with forearm supination. Long-term problems include premature physeal arrest and a loss in supination range of motion.

PELVIC FRACTURES

Fractures of the pelvis in children usually involve significant direct trauma to the child, as occurs in motor vehicle accidents. In children younger than 10 years of age, the most common mechanism of injury is a pedestrian–motor vehicle collision. The immature pelvis is more malleable than that of an adult, largely because a much greater component is cartilage and the corresponding joints are more flexible. Greater energy is absorbed with impact, and the resultant fractures are less displaced and therefore more stable. Single breaks in the pelvic ring can also occur in children. Small degrees of displacement seen on radiographs may be misleading as the elasticity of the bones and soft tissues can allow some recoil.

Because of the high-energy trauma, it is possible that there are other associated injuries local and remote to the pelvic fracture site. The most frequent concurrent injury is to the central nervous system; closed head injury or cervical spine injury occurs in 40% to 75% of cases. Intraabdominal damage is seen in 10% to 20% of the patients, and 20% to 40% of the

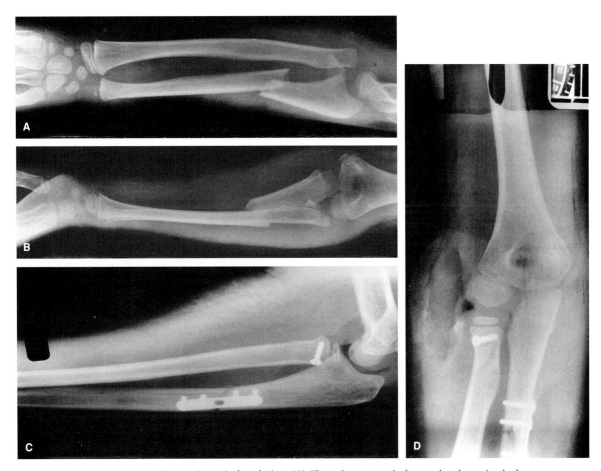

FIGURE 31-39. Monteggia-equivalent lesion. (**A**) There is an anteriorly angulated proximal ulnar fracture with an anterior displaced radial shaft. There also is a fracture of the radial neck, with malalignment of the radiocapitellar joint. (**B**) The anteroposterior (AP) projection. (**C**) This fracture configuration usually requires open reduction. In this instance, a small plate was used on the ulnar shaft. An alternative would have been an intramedullary rod. The radial neck fracture was treated with a minifragment compression screw. (**D**) The AP projection shows restoration of alignment.

children have sustained another skeletal fracture.[141,179] Anterior ring fractures should alert the examiner to the possibility of genitourinary system trauma. Between 5% and 10% of patients have urethral or bladder disruption, especially if there is a double break in the pelvic ring. Injury to the lumbosacral nerve plexus or to the sciatic nerve occurs in 1% of patients and is seen with posterior ring injuries (e.g., sacrum, sacroiliac joint). Mortality rates are about 12%, and death usually is caused by an associated cerebral injury.

Classification

The importance of the classification system is to recognize which injury patterns are associated with pelvic fragment instability. This assessment helps guide the subsequent treatment regimen. Key and Conwells divide the injuries into four categories:

1. Marginal fractures or avulsions that do not involve the pelvic ring (stable)

2. Single breaks of the pelvic ring, involving the rami or symphysis separation (stable)

3. Double breaks of the pelvic ring, including bilateral rami fractures, anterior and posterior ring disruptions, vertical displacement, and multiple fractures (unstable)

4. Any of the above three types associated with an acetabular fracture.

Although these categories are helpful, AO/ASIF classification provides further information about the increasing severity of the fracture pattern and possible management of the injury. This system is based on Tile's modification of Pennal's adult pelvic fracture classification. The AO/ASIF system identifies three modes of injury: anteroposterior compression, lateral compression, and vertical shear.

Type A injuries are stable and include avulsions (e.g., anterosuperior or inferior spine, ischial tuberosity) and isolated fracture of the iliac wing. Also included are minor rami fractures not associated with posterior ring disruption.

Type B injuries are rotationally unstable but vertically stable and include open book injuries (e.g., symphysis pubis diastasis) and lateral compression fractures (e.g., ipsilateral or contralateral sacral alar fracture, sacroiliac joint separation combined with anterior ring disruption). Pubic diastasis of greater than 3 cm is associated with disruption of the anterior sacroiliac joint ligaments.

Type C injuries are rotationally and vertically unstable and may be unilateral or bilateral. Vertical shear or instability occurs when anterior ring disruption, such as symphysis separation or bilateral rami fracture, is combined with a displaced fracture of the posterior iliac crest, sacrum, or sacroiliac joint. Any weight-bearing load increases the amount of vertical migration of the hemipelvis. Type C injuries also include associated acetabular fractures.

Management

The clinical assessment of the child with a presumed pelvic fracture begins with a detailed physical examination. Attention is directed toward any area with significant contusion, and the perineum must be inspected for lacerations signifying an open fracture. Rectal examination is needed to look for evidence of hemorrhage signifying bone penetration into the rectum and to verify intact perineal sensation (i.e., sacral plexus function). Pelvic stability should be tested with anteroposterior and lateral compression of the hemipelvis. The peripheral arterial circulation is also documented.

Initial radiographic evaluation is accomplished by standard anteroposterior projection. Pelvic inlet (40-degree caudal) and outlet (40-degree cephalad) views can be obtained to assess pelvic ring integrity and malrotation of the hemipelvis. If an acetabular fracture is suspected, 45-degree oblique views (Judet) are taken. The obturator view highlights the anterior column, the posterior acetabular wall, and the obturator foramen, and the iliac view defines the posterior column, the anterior acetabular wall, and the iliac wing. CT scanning is the study of choice for complex fractures and for the identification of intraarticular loose fragments. CT imaging also clarifies injuries of the sacrum, sacroiliac joints, and acetabulum.

Treatment options depend on the age of the child, the stability of the fracture pattern, and the general medical condition. Most pediatric pelvic fractures can be managed by bed rest and protected weight bearing, especially if there is a stable fracture pattern (type A). Cast immobilization is used in the unreliable or very young child who may bear weight too early. Type B fractures that are not significantly displaced may also be treated by casting. Skeletal traction is occasionally used to secure a fracture that is vertically unstable, but radiographic follow-up is needed to show that further migration of the fragment does not occur. A cast is applied after early healing has stabilized the fragments. Traction is not very effective for reducing the degree of initial vertical displacement, especially in a child older than 8 years of age, and healing with significant malalignment leads to limb length discrepancy and poor functional results.[179] The child is confined to bed, which is less desirable for the patient who has multiple injuries.

Open reduction and internal fixation is recommended for significantly displaced fractures and for open fractures. Surgical intervention is usually delayed 48 to 72 hours to allow hematoma formation. Symphysis pubis diastasis greater than 3 cm can be stabilized with the application of a two-hole anterior compression plate. Vertically unstable fractures usually are approached by securing the posterior injury by either anterior plating or posterior cancellous compression screws across the sacroiliac joint (Fig. 31-40).[118] The anterior injury can be treated with plating of the symphysis or with the application of an external fixator. Sometimes, the stabilization of one region of the pelvic ring allows the closed reduction and cast stabilization of the other region.

External fixation is useful for the management of open fractures or a fracture in an adolescent that would probably fail closed reduction and casting. Severe injuries of the anterior and posterior pelvic ring may not be sufficiently held with an external fixator alone. Life-threatening hemorrhage from pelvic fracture in children is seen less commonly than in adults. However, bilateral anterior and posterior ring fractures correlate with significant bleeding. This may require that emergent pelvic stability be provided by the application of external fixator. Subsequent angiography with arterial embolization is a useful adjunct.[120]

Acetabular Fractures

Acetabular fractures in young children tend to be nondisplaced and consist largely of linear fractures associated with pelvic disruptions. Fractures of the acetabulum also occur frequently with dislocation of the hip (50% incidence) and are small, avulsed fragments or minimally displaced linear fractures.[73] Rarely do central fracture-dislocations occur. The adolescent may sustain the more typical adult fracture patterns, which are best classified by Letournel.[104] These include fracture of the posterior wall or posterior column, anterior wall or anterior column, transverse acetabular fracture, and combinations of these patterns. Most are easily managed by bed rest and cast immobilization if they are nondisplaced. Confirmation of the extent of injury is best made by obtaining a CT scan. Open reduction and internal fixation are indicated for any

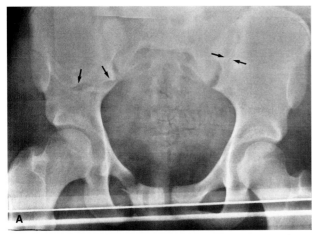

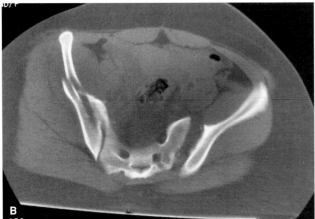

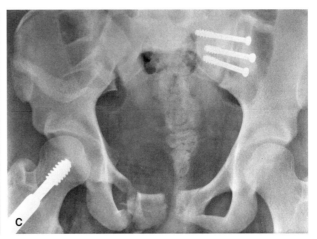

FIGURE 31-40.   Complex pelvic fracture (*arrows*) in a 13-year-old child. (**A**) The anteroposterior (AP) view of the pelvis shows a fracture of the iliac wing and superior inferior pubic rami, with contralateral sacroiliac joint widening. This is classified as a type B-3 injury. (**B**) The computed tomography scan demonstrates complete disruption of the sacroiliac joint and a contralateral iliac wing fracture. (**C**) The sacroiliac joint injury was stabilized with large-fragment cancellous bone crews, performed through a posterior approach with the patient prone on a radiolucent table. A posterior approach is made to the sacroiliac joint, and after reduction, drill holes are made approximately 1.5 cm anterior to the crista glutea and at the midpoint between the iliac crest and the sciatic notch. The angle of drilling is perpendicular to the ilium. The 40-degree caudad, direct AP and 40-degree cephalad projections are viewed with an image intensifier to guide screw positioning. There has been some displacement of the iliac wing fracture, which could have been stabilized by internal fixation.

intraarticular fragments or fracture displacement greater than 2 mm (Fig. 31-41).

Injuries to the acetabular triradiate cartilage are unique to the immature skeleton and may have grave long-term results in young children. This is especially true for children younger than 10 years of age at the time of growth plate damage. The triradiate cartilage is responsible for growth in the height and width of the acetabulum. Disturbance in growth results in the acetabulum becoming more shallow and can lead to some degree of hip subluxation.[151] This is less of a problem for patients who are older than 11 years of age at the time of injury.[20]

Acetabular growth plate injury is estimated to occur in 15% to 20% of children's pelvic fractures. Salter-Harris type I or II is the pattern usually seen, with central displacement of the distal fragment. Crush injury (type V pattern) can also occur and carries a worse prognosis because growth arrest invariably occurs. This injury can often go unrecognized, detected only after acetabular dysplasia has developed. The sacroiliac joint may also suffer growth inhibition after impact injury.[74]

FRACTURES AND DISLOCATIONS OF THE HIP

Proximal Femur Fractures

Proximal femur fractures represent approximately 1% of all pediatric fractures and are usually the result of high-energy trauma, typically a motor vehicle accident or a fall from a substantial height. In 30% of the cases,

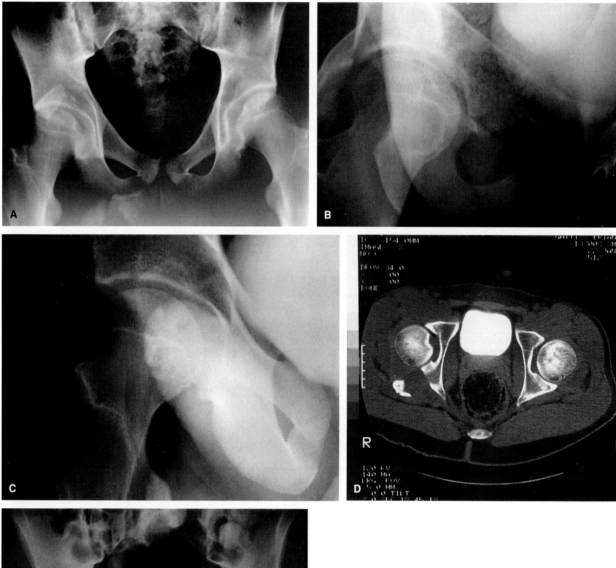

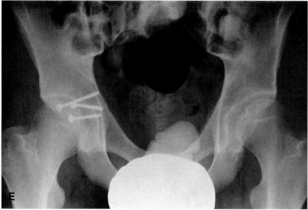

FIGURE 31-41. Posterior acetabular wall fracture. **(A)** The antero-posterior (AP) projection suggests a right acetabular fracture. **(B)** The obturator view shows an intact anterior column and demonstrates the posterior wall fracture. **(C)** The iliac view defines an intact posterior column and an intact anterior acetabular wall. **(D)** A computed tomography scan shows significant displacement of a large posterior wall fragment. This requires internal fixation to confer stability to the hip joint. **(E)** An AP projection after internal fixation with cancellous bone screws.

there is another significant associated injury to the chest, head, or abdomen. The exceptions to this mechanism of injury are children younger than 2 years of age who have been subjected to child abuse or fracture through a pathologic lesion of the femoral neck (e.g., bone cyst). Fortunately, proximal femur fractures are rare. The consequences of this injury are significant, including femoral head avascular necrosis, physeal damage with growth arrest, malunion, and nonunion. Long-term studies indicate an overall 47% avascular

necrosis rate for proximal femur fractures, with a 30% malunion rate.[24,38,140] Most patients who develop avascular necrosis need later reconstructive hip surgery, with almost one half requiring total hip arthroplasty.[38]

Anatomy

In the infant, the proximal femur is composed of a single, large cartilaginous growth plate. The medial portion becomes the epiphyseal center of the femoral head (ossifying around 4 months of age), forming the proximal femoral physis. The lateral portion of the proximal femur forms the greater trochanter physis, and this epiphysis ossifies by 4 years of age. Injury to the proximal femur can affect one or both centers of growth. The proximal femoral physis is responsible for the metaphyseal growth of the femoral neck and provides 13% of the total length of the femur. The greater trochanter helps shape the proximal femur, and damage to this apophysis in children younger than 10 to 12 years of age produces an elongated, valgus femoral neck.[138]

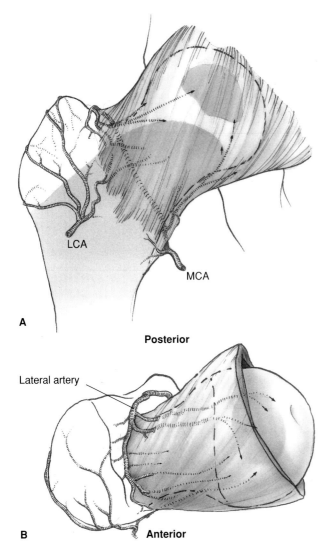

A

Posterior

Lateral artery

B   **Anterior**

FIGURE 31-42. Arterial supply of the developing proximal femur. (**A**) The anterior view demonstrates the lateral circumflex artery (LCA), which supplies the metaphysis and greater trochanter. The medial circumflex femoral artery (MCA) is the dominant vessel to the femoral head. (**B**) The superior view shows the lateral ascending artery, which sends numerous epiphyseal and metaphyseal branches (*arrows*) that supply the greatest volume of the femoral head and neck. These ascending cervical branches traverse the articular capsule as the retinacular arteries. The interval between the greater trochanter and the hip capsule is extremely narrow and is the area where the lateral ascending cervical artery passes. This may be a site of vascular compression or injury.

The vascular supply of the growing child's proximal femur is jeopardized by these fractures, and the extent of damage greatly affects the final outcome. The dominant arterial source for the femoral head is the lateral epiphyseal vessels, which are the terminal extension of the medial femoral circumflex artery. These posterosuperior and posteroinferior vessels are found at the level of the intertrochanteric groove, where they penetrate the capsule and course along the femoral neck toward the head, supported by the retinacular and periosteal tissue in the region (Fig. 31-42).[29,131] The lateral circumflex system can supply a portion of the anterior femoral head until 2 to 3 years of age, after which it primarily supplies the metaphysis. In children older than 14 to 18 months of age, the proximal femoral physeal plate becomes an absolute barrier to the metaphyseal blood supply, preventing direct vascular penetration of the femoral head.[29,131] Subsequently, the metaphyseal and epiphyseal vascular networks remain separate in children until complete physeal closure occurs. This may in part account for the higher incidence of avascular necrosis among children than adults. The vessels of the ligamentum teres do not contribute a significant portion of the blood supply of the femoral head, especially in children younger than 8 years of age.

Management

Provided other associated injuries have been thoroughly evaluated and stabilized, these fractures should be treated as urgent cases, within 12 hours of the injury. Other than the degree of initial fragment displacement, the delay in fracture reduction and stabilization may be the most significant factor affecting the incidence of avascular necrosis. Displaced fractures can leave the vascular leash intact but occluded until realignment is established.[163] All other musculoskeletal injuries should be addressed after the proximal femur fracture. Nondisplaced fractures do not have the same incidence of avascular necrosis as displaced ones, further supporting the concept that the magnitude of initial fragment separation is a major determinant of vascular damage.[100] It has also been suggested that prompt decompression of the intracapsular hematoma contributes to the restoration of normal vascular flow, preventing the continuance of an adverse internal pressure gradient.[163] However, there is no clear evidence that femoral neck fracture hematoma produces physiologically significant intracapsular pressures or that emergent anterior capsulotomy reduces the incidence of femoral head avascular necrosis.[58,167]

Delbet's classification (Fig. 31-43) offers a simple yet useful system for the treatment and prognosis of proximal femur fractures. Type I fractures are transphyseal separations, and in children, severe violence is necessary to produce this injury. Although this physeal

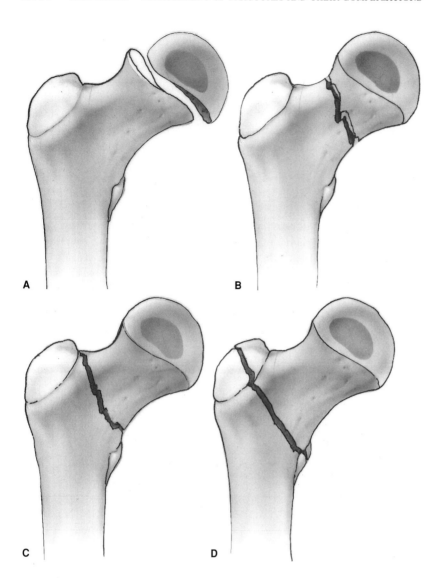

FIGURE 31-43. Delbet's classification for proximal femur fractures. (**A**) Type I is a transepiphyseal fracture. (**B**) Type II is a transcervical fracture. (**C**) Type III is a cervicotrochanteric fracture (basicervical). (**D**) Type IV is an intertrochanteric fracture.

separation is occasionally seen as a birth fracture, it may also be the result of child abuse, unless there is a corroborating history of significant trauma. Transphyseal fracture is associated with dislocation of the epiphyseal fragment from the acetabulum in 50% of cases involving high-energy trauma.[126] This carries an especially poor prognosis, with certain avascular necrosis and probable proximal femoral growth arrest.

Treatment with closed reduction and casting is appropriate for minimally displaced fractures and for children younger than 2 years of age. Obstetric fracture-separations uniformly have excellent clinical results without avascular necrosis, despite frequent delayed diagnosis and no apparent treatment.[166] This young age group has a better prognosis than older children with type I fractures, who experience an 80% avascular necrosis rate. This difference is mainly the result of the mechanism of injury, which involves less force and prevents disruption of the vital vascularity. More rapid healing and the reestablishment of transphyseal vascularity are unique to children younger

than 18 months of age and may help to prevent clinical avascular necrosis. In children older than 2 years of age, stabilization of the reduced fracture should be accomplished with two smooth pins and supplemented with spica casting. Open reduction is necessary if the epiphysis is dislocated.

Type II fractures occur in the neck of the femur between the epiphyseal plate and the base of the neck and are called transcervical fractures. They comprise approximately one half of all fractures of the proximal femur.[38] These fractures can usually be reduced by closed methods and are fixed by the percutaneous insertion of a cancellous bone screw into the metaphyseal portion of the proximal fragment (Fig. 31-44). Preferably, two screws are inserted, depending on the size of the femoral neck, to provide greater fracture stability. If the proximal metaphyseal fragment is too small to hold a screw, smooth pins can be placed across the physis to allow subsequent growth. In the adolescent near the end of growth, threaded screws may be placed across the physis for better fixation.

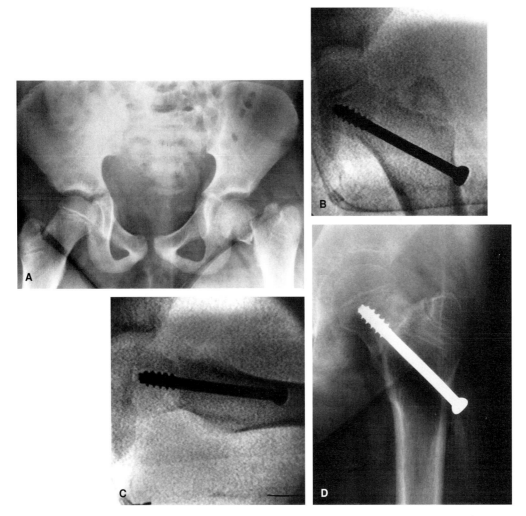

FIGURE 31-44.   Femoral neck fracture in a 6-year-old child. (**A**) The anteroposterior projection shows a displaced type II femoral neck fracture. (**B**) The intraoperative radiograph shows the fracture after closed reduction and stabilization with a single 7.0-mm cancellous bone screw. The metaphyseal portion of the proximal fragment was just large enough to hold all the threads of the screw, enabling compression at the fracture site. The femoral neck is not large enough for an additional screw of this size. Care was taken to avoid the physis. Alignment of the medical calcar is imperative for fracture stability. (**C**) A lateral projection shows the central placement of the screw. This internal fixation was supplemented with a spica cast for 6 weeks. (**D**) Six weeks after injury, there is evidence of fracture healing and bridging callus medially. There has been some displacement and settling of the fracture.

Spica casting is used to augment fixation in children, especially when smooth pins have been used. Nondisplaced fractures in patients younger than 6 years of age can be treated by spica cast alone with good results.[38] Open reduction is occasionally required if suitable alignment is not obtained by closed means. An anterolateral (Watson-Jones) approach is recommended, with opening of the anterior capsule to avoid damaging the posterior vascular network.

Complications are frequent with type II fractures, for which the incidence of avascular necrosis and physeal growth arrest approaches 50% to 60%. The nonunion rate is 15%. The proximal femoral physis is responsible for ⅛ in (0.3 cm) of femoral length per year, and a significant limb length discrepancy is only a problem for the preadolescent with a growth arrest.

Type III fractures occur in the cervicotrochanteric or basal neck region of the femoral neck. This is the second most common location of proximal femoral fractures in children. Nondisplaced fractures in young children can be treated in a spica cast if there is anatomic alignment, especially of the medial cortex. Serial radiographs are necessary to monitor possible fracture migration that would lead to varus malalignment. Displaced fractures are reduced by gently flexing the hip while traction is applied. The limb is then externally rotated and abducted. Biplanar radiographs are obtained to confirm reduction. Two cancellous bone screws provide compression across the fracture site and are sufficient fixation if supplemented with a spica cast. Nondisplaced fractures in the older child or adolescent should be treated with internal fixation to pre-

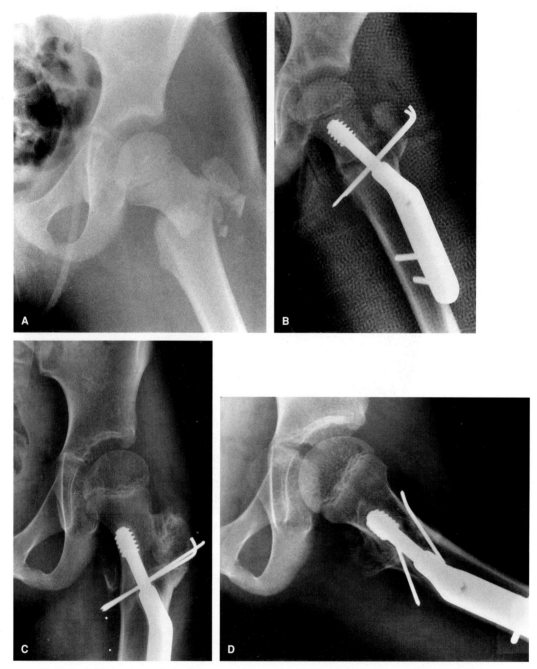

FIGURE 31-45. Comminuted type III femoral neck fracture. (**A**) The anteroposterior projection shows a basicervical neck fracture with an associated fracture of the greater trochanter. (**B**) Open reduction and internal fixation are necessary to provide stability for this fracture and avoid varus malunion. Lag screw fixation was used because of the location of the fracture, and the greater trochanter was stabilized with Kirschner wires. A cast was used. (**C**) Eighteen months later, there is complete healing of the fracture and no evidence of avascular necrosis to the femoral head. However, there may be evidence of growth arrest of the greater trochanter, and this hip should be followed for later development of femoral neck deformity. (**D**) A lateral projection just before implant removal.

vent late displacement. The indication for open reduction is the inability to obtain adequate alignment; the anterolateral approach is used (Fig. 31-45). Avascular necrosis occurs in 30% of displaced cases, and the malunion (i.e., varus) rate is 20%. Because the fracture line is vertically oriented, shear forces can inhibit bone union; nonunion occurs in 10% of these patients. This problem may be lessened by precise fracture reduc-

tion combined with compression across the fracture site through cancellous bone screws (i.e., lag technique).

Type IV fractures occur in the intertrochanteric region, and this fracture carries the least risk to the local vascular supply. The incidence of avascular necrosis is between 0% and 10%. This fracture does not demand the urgency of the type I, II, and III fractures, but in polytrauma, the prompt stabilization of this injury improves general management. Although skeletal traction, followed by casting, can be employed as a treatment option, hospitalization is too lengthy. For small children, early closed reduction and casting, using a percutaneous cancellous screw to provide fixation is preferred if the fracture is unstable. Open reduction is employed if the normal neck shaft angle cannot be established by closed means. In adolescents, a sliding hip screw or angled blade plate is necessary for fixation, avoiding the need for a supplemental body cast. The malunion rate is approximately 30%, and malunion usually is more pronounced in fractures treated by closed methods.[38,126]

Hip Dislocation

Dislocation of the hip in children can be the result of minor trauma, such as tripping or falling; moderate force, as in football or other sports injuries; or high-energy impact, as in a motor vehicle accident. The mechanism of injury somewhat depends on the age of the child. For example, dislocations in children older than 10 years of age are likely as a result of moderate or severe trauma; mild trauma is responsible for producing a dislocation in one half the children younger than 10 years of age.[130] Adequate radiologic assessment of the pelvis and entire femur is necessary to identify other fractures, such as those of the femoral neck, acetabulum, or the femoral shaft. Detailed clinical examination reveals evidence of sciatic nerve injury in approximately 24% of cases.

Dislocation of the hip is uncommon, representing only 5% of all pediatric dislocations. Most hip dislocations are posterior, but anterior displacement has been described.[18] Most dislocations can be reduced by closed methods with muscle relaxation and analgesia, although a general anesthetic sometimes is required. The reduction technique involves longitudinal traction of the lower limb, with the knee flexed and the hip flexed to some degree. In older children, an assistant is needed for countertraction and may also apply direct digital pressure over the palpable displaced proximal femur. After the hip is reduced, stability should be assessed while the hip is put through a full range of motion, especially flexion. A concentric reduction must also be radiographically confirmed, and a CT scan is recommended if there is any suggestion of joint space widening or acetabular fracture on plain radiographs (Fig. 31-46). Associated minimally displaced acetabular rim fractures, subluxation with extremes of hip motion, and young children are indications for spica cast immobilization. Stable closed reductions in older children can be managed with protected ambulation and activity restriction for approximately 6 weeks.

The indications for open reduction include an unstable closed reduction, a nonconcentric reduction, or an acetabular rim fragment with more than 2 mm of displacement. Open reduction is approached in the direction of the dislocation, such as the posterior interval (i.e., Kocher-Langenbeck approach) for posterior dislocations. Children who have required an open reduction should be placed in a spica cast for 3 to 4 weeks and then mobilized.

The rate of avascular necrosis is between 3% and 10% and positively correlates with reductions delayed by more than 12 hours. The preferred timing is within 6 hours of injury.[47] Prognosis is also related to the amount of energy involved in producing the dislocation; avascular necrosis is not typical of minor traumatic dislocations. Damage to the femoral head because of loss of the blood supply is usually apparent 4 to 6 months after injury. Although MRI scanning may identify this condition sooner, its role in the clinical management has not been defined. Long-term radiographic results show that coxa magna develops in the absence of avascular necrosis in almost one half of the patients, but this does not affect the clinical outcome.[130]

FEMORAL SHAFT FRACTURES

Femoral fractures are common childhood fractures, and these patients may present in several clinical settings. Fortunately, there is great variety in the types of treatment available, allowing a specific plan to be designed for each patient and each clinical problem. Fracture patterns are a reflection of the force involved in producing the injury. Direct forces cause transverse fractures, with occasional minor comminution. Torsional forces generate spiral patterns or short, oblique fractures if bending is also a component of the injury. Comminution, segmental breaks, or open wounds imply that greater forces were applied to initiate the fracture. Recognizing the mechanism of trauma and correlating it with the injury history is necessary to determine if the fracture was the result of accidental trauma. This is especially relevant for children younger than 4 years of age, among whom the incidence of child abuse is higher.[67]

Most femur fractures have significant displacement, and the location of the break is in the diaphyseal region in 70% of patients. However, infants and toddlers have an especially thick periosteum that prevents significant fragment separation and shortening. The femur has a rich endosteal and periosteal blood supply supported by a thick, soft tissue envelope. This abundant muscle layer helps promote rapid healing, and restoration of bone mass occurs quickly. Because this muscle cuff protects the neurovascular structures from injury, vascular disruption is rare. However, displaced fractures of the distal-third metaphyseal-diaphyseal junction may damage the femoral artery, and

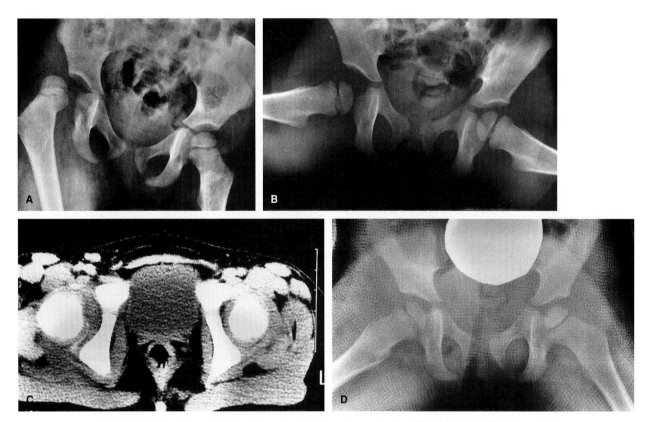

FIGURE 31-46. Traumatic hip dislocation. (**A**) An anteroposterior (AP) projection of a 3.5-year-old child with a low-energy injury producing a posterior hip dislocation. (**B**) An AP view of the pelvis after closed reduction of the hip, taken in the emergency department. Clinically, a stable reduction was obtained, but there is significant joint space widening, suggesting an intraarticular obstruction. (**C**) The computed tomography scan confirms incomplete reduction. There is some radiodense material in the posterior acetabulum. (**D**) A posterior open reduction of the hip was performed and the interposed soft tissue removed. There was no osteochondral fracture. An AP radiograph of the pelvis confirms concentric symmetrical reduction of the hip. A spica cast was applied for 4 weeks.

the peripheral circulation must be carefully evaluated. Soft tissue interposition at the fracture site, blocking bony alignment, is rarely a problem.

Subsequent fracture position is a reflection of the large thigh muscles acting unopposed across the fracture site. The proximal femoral fragment angulates in flexion and external rotation, midshaft fragments tend to flex (i.e., anterior bow), and the distal shaft portion tends to adduct (i.e., varus alignment). Supracondylar femoral fractures displace into recurvatum, especially if the knee is extended, as a result of pull from the gastrocnemius muscle.

Management

Fracture treatment regimens are classically organized according to the age of the child. However, there are often many other issues that can alter these routine treatment plans that are just as significant as chronologic age. It is more logical to list the various available treatment options and match them with the specific clinical situations.

The clinical variables that influence the type of treatment rendered include the age and weight of

the child, isolated femur fracture or component of polytrauma, fracture pattern and stability, and the severity of soft tissue injury (i.e., open or closed fracture). Coexistent neuromuscular, metabolic, or immune disorders and the socioeconomic status can influence treatment. Another factor that affects many of these clinical variables is whether the fracture was the result of high- or low-energy impact. High-energy fractures are more displaced, with greater disruption of the periosteal sleeve and surrounding soft tissues. The likelihood of open injury and femoral shaft comminution is increased, creating a mechanically less stable fracture site. The result is more potential complications and longer times to complete bone healing.

There are many treatment alternatives, most of which can be applied to any injured child, regardless of age. They include closed reduction and early casting, skeletal traction and delayed casting, external fixation, rigid intramedullary fixation with or without intramedullary reaming, flexible intramedullary fixation, and open reduction with compression plating. Selecting a final strategy involves integrating the major clinical variables with the appropriate available treatment options. This choice also depends on the physician's preference and skill with each treatment alternative. The goals are to maintain appropriate limb length and alignment safely and reliably. Remodeling is an active process, especially in preadolescents, and this should be recognized when designing a treatment plan.

The following sections highlight the various types of fracture management, with emphasis on the common indications.

Nonsurgical Treatment

EARLY-FIT SPICA CAST. The typical candidate for early-fit spica cast treatment is a child between 2 and 10 years of age with an isolated femoral shaft fracture.[75,83] The ideal fracture pattern is a spiral fracture, usually because the periosteum is still intact, facilitating the closed reduction. Subsequent fracture healing is also rapid. The alignment of transverse or short oblique fractures is harder to control, relying more on a well-fitted cast, and must subsequently be monitored closely for changes in length and angulation. Preoperatively, the child is confined to bed rest with several pounds of skin traction and pillow support of the lower limb. Closed reduction and casting are performed under general anesthesia, usually within 24 hours of injury. If the delay in treatment exceeds 48 hours, it is better to stabilize the femur in balanced skeletal traction for the patient's comfort.

The cast application technique begins with an assessment of fracture stability by gently manipulating the limb under the image intensifier. After obtaining fracture alignment, a bent-knee cylinder cast is applied, molding the thigh flat anteriorly and laterally, anticipating the tendency for later fragment displacement into flexion and varus. The foot is left free. The popliteal area must be well padded, because traction is maintained on the cylinder cast while the hip is flexed to between 70 and 90 degrees. The limb is abducted and placed in slight external rotation while the torso and contralateral thigh is incorporated into the cast. Anteroposterior and lateral radiographs are obtained to confirm acceptable alignment.

The weight and body habitus of the child are also important determinants of the feasibility of spica cast treatment. Obesity precludes cast treatment; conversely, a thin or small adolescent may be a good cast candidate despite an older age, especially if there is a favorable fracture configuration, such as a spiral fracture. In general, children who weigh more than 80 pounds are too large to manage in an immediate-fit spica cast. Open fractures or other significant soft tissue injuries and unstable fracture patterns (e.g., segmental, comminuted) preclude the use of this technique. There must be a reliable home environment for proper care of the casted child, although this is

seldom a problem. Proximal subtrochanteric, distal supracondylar, and bilateral femur fractures are more difficult fractures to control with an early-fit spica cast.

After casting, patients are able to be discharged to their homes within 24 hours. Two or three weekly follow-up visits are necessary to monitor alignment, because most of the shortening and angulation occurs during this time (Fig. 31-47). There is some evidence that initial severe fragment overlap or shortening greater than 10 mm at the time of spica application is associated with subsequent unacceptable fracture shortening.[115] The amount of residual angulation that is acceptable largely depends on the age of the child. In children younger than 10 years of age, frontal-plane (i.e., varus-valgus) alignment should not surpass 15 to 20 degrees of neutral. Anterior bow should not exceed 35 degrees, and recurvatum is tolerated up to 10 to 15 degrees. Infants can adequately remodel bone with even more deformity. In children older than 10 years of age, frontal-plane angulation should be controlled to within 5 to 7 degrees. Because malrotation deformity remodels poorly, more than a 10-degree difference between limbs should be avoided. Small amounts of angular deformity can be corrected by wedging the cast, and occasionally, the entire cast must be changed. Unacceptable shortening (>20 mm) or poorly controlled angulation requires a different treatment plan. Options include skeletal traction, followed by recasting, or preferably, operative stabilization with an external fixator or intramedullary device.

Growth acceleration after fracture healing is unique to the immature skeletal system, and this phenomenon occurs in patients 2 to 10 years of age. Typically, this amounts to 1 to 2 cm of longitudinal growth, and in this age group, it is acceptable for 10 to 15 mm (not exceeding 20 mm) of fragment overlap to occur, but the amount of overgrowth is unpredictable for each child.

Knee stiffness is not a problem in the closed management of femur fractures, and it occurs only if there has been significant damage to the quadriceps muscle. There may be some residual thigh muscle weakness after cast immobilization, but it does not seem to present as a clinical problem, especially in the preadolescent.[76] It has not been demonstrated that operative stabilization of femur fractures prevents the development of this subclinical muscle weakness. Ligamentous knee injury can occur in conjunction with femoral shaft fracture in children and is identified after the fracture has stabilized. Distal femoral physeal crush injury (i.e., Salter-Harris type V) can occur despite apparent energy dissipation that should have occurred at the fracture site. Because this problem does not manifest itself until later, follow-up radiographs in 6 to 12 months should include an evaluation of the distal femoral physis.

Infants and children younger than 2 years of age

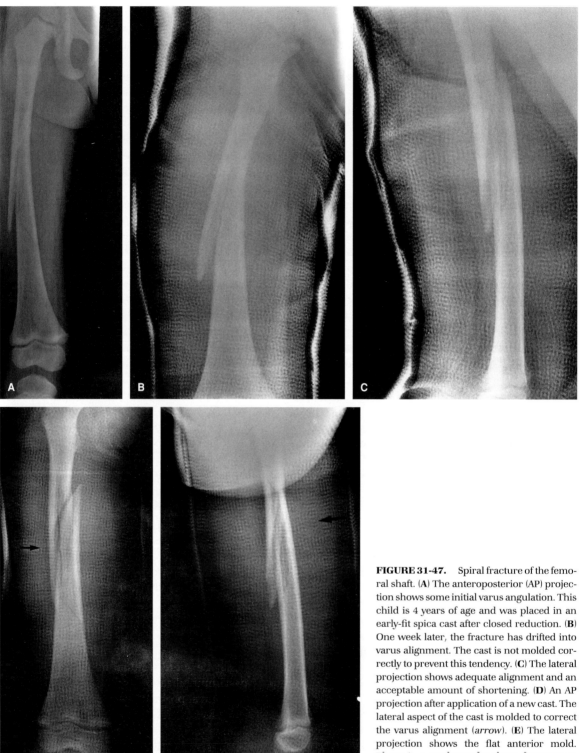

FIGURE 31-47.   Spiral fracture of the femoral shaft. (**A**) The anteroposterior (AP) projection shows some initial varus angulation. This child is 4 years of age and was placed in an early-fit spica cast after closed reduction. (**B**) One week later, the fracture has drifted into varus alignment. The cast is not molded correctly to prevent this tendency. (**C**) The lateral projection shows adequate alignment and an acceptable amount of shortening. (**D**) An AP projection after application of a new cast. The lateral aspect of the cast is molded to correct the varus alignment (*arrow*). (**E**) The lateral projection shows the flat anterior mold. There is a tendency for these fractures to angulate anteriorly, and it is important to have a flat anterior mold proximal to the fracture (*arrow*).

with femoral shaft fractures are readily managed by the immediate application of a spica cast. The thick periosteum usually prevents significant fracture shortening. The cast can be applied in the emergency department with appropriate sedation. The lower limb is placed in 70 to 90 degrees of flexion, 30 to 40 degrees of abduction, and slight external rotation. Healing is usually sufficient for cast removal after 4 weeks.

SKELETAL TRACTION. Skeletal traction is a safe, reliable, and easily instituted form of management for almost any femur fracture in any age group.[83,158] There are several ways balanced traction can be constructed, but the simplest is the 90-90 position (i.e., hip and knee flexed 90 degrees) for preadolescents and for proximal femur fractures. Adolescents are usually placed in balanced traction, with a thigh sling (e.g., Thomas splint) and an adjustable knee support (e.g., Pearson sling) to allow 45 degrees of knee flexion. Skeletal traction can be instituted if there is going to be a significant delay before spica cast application is possible, usually when other medical systems need to be closely monitored, as for a visceral injury.

The typical patient for which skeletal traction is indicated is younger than 12 years of age and has a subtrochanteric, supracondylar, or an unstable fracture pattern that is likely to fail primary cast treatment. In small children, bilateral femur fractures can be managed in traction provided there are not other serious systemic injuries or multiple fractures.

The technique entails the insertion of a small-caliber, threaded pin in a lateral to medial direction into the metaphyseal region of the distal femur of a patient under local anesthesia. Proximal tibial pins usually are avoided. The pin should be 2 cm above the growth plate and must be placed parallel to the knee joint to avoid axial malalignment.[6] A traction bow (e.g., Kirschner) is attached to the threaded pin, and longitudinal traction is applied. A well-padded below-knee cast is used to prevent ankle equinus. Periodic radiographs are obtained to guide the amount of weight and direction of traction vectors needed to restore alignment. Frontal-plane alignment should be maintained within 5 to 7 degrees of neutral, and femoral length must be restored in the child older than 10 years of age. After relative fracture stability has occurred (17–21 days) and callus formation is confirmed on radiographs, a cast is applied after correcting any residual deformity. Casting is necessary for an additional 6 to 9 weeks.

Skeletal traction involves hospitalization for 2 to 3 weeks, followed by an additional lengthy period of immobility in a cast.[77,142] The total expense for in-hospital skeletal traction is three times greater than for early-fit spica casting and of the same magnitude as

major surgery, such as intramedullary rodding.[129] Adolescents require even longer periods of treatment because of slower healing rates, and independent mobility with a return to school is delayed. Cast treatment of femur fractures in adolescents is associated with an increased incidence of complications, including malunion (i.e., limb length discrepancy and angular deformity), compared with operative stabilization.[6,77,93,142] This is especially true in the setting of multiple extremity fractures or an ipsilateral tibial fracture.[17,119] Children with multiple trauma frequently need to be taken out of traction for ongoing diagnostic tests and trips to the operating room. Bilateral femur fractures treated in traction make nursing and skin care more difficult, especially for the older child. Head-injured patients usually are not good candidates for skeletal traction because of their combative movements as they recover.[55]

Surgical Treatment

Surgical management of a femoral shaft fracture is indicated for the larger and usually older child, especially if the fracture is not amenable to casting. Another relative indication is bilateral femoral shaft fractures. The polytrauma victim, with other fractures or systemic injuries (especially closed head injury) is also best treated with prompt operative stabilization of the femur fracture. Grade II or III open fractures or other significant soft tissue injuries should be managed by fracture stabilization at the time of soft tissue repair. These indications are essentially independent of the age of the child.

The degree to which overgrowth can occur in children between the ages of 2 to 10 years is based on studies of closed (i.e., cast) treatment of femur fractures.[159,162] Other modes of fracture treatment in this young age group, such as external or internal fixation, may produce a different standard to which limb lengths should be set.

EXTERNAL FIXATION. The prime indication for external fixation is a fracture with significant associated soft tissue damage, as in open fractures or burns. It may be considered as a form of ambulatory traction, enabling the child to be partially weight bearing and independent several days after sustaining the injury. Hospitalization is subsequently reduced to a few days. This treatment modality may be used as first-line treatment for uncomplicated fractures in the young adolescent too large for a cast and too immature for a conventional intramedullary rod (i.e., 8–12 years of age).

Spiral and oblique fracture patterns are ideally suited for external fixation because fracture healing usually is rapid, with enough new bone formation to allow frame removal approximately 12 weeks after injury. Transverse fractures seem to display less abundant callus formation with slower rates of healing and may be better treated with intramedullary fixation. External fixation is also used as secondary management for failure of early-fit spica casting. Other relative indications include polytrauma, in which the multiple fractures and the child's general medical condition favor rapid and bloodless bony stabilization that is possible with this technique (Fig. 31-48). Malalignment can also be easily adjusted on a delayed basis, if necessary, after the patient's overall condition has stabilized. External fixation of femoral fractures is also helpful if blood loss must be kept to a minimum (e.g., Jehovah witness patient) or if there is an underlying neuromuscular disorder.[94]

The technique involves the sequential insertion of two pins above and below the fracture site, attaching them to a unilateral frame. Pin location should be approximately 2 cm from the fracture site and should avoid penetrating the femoral neck calcar or the distal femoral physis. Under fluoroscopic guidance, final

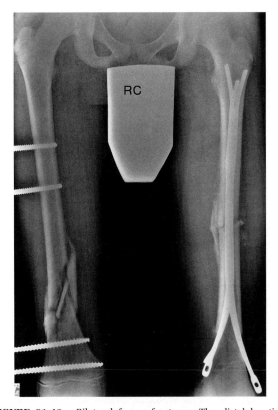

FIGURE 31-48. Bilateral femur fractures. The distal location, proximity to the growth plate and marked comminution of the right femur fracture are best managed through the application of an external fixator. Although this could have been applied to the contralateral fracture, intramedullary fixation was chosen because of the transverse pattern of the fracture.

alignment can be adjusted as the pins are secured to the body of the fixator (Fig. 31-49).

The most frequent problem encountered with the use of external fixators is pin tract infections, occurring in approximately 5% to 10% of patients.[8,62] These are usually superficial and are managed by local skin cleaning and oral antibiotics. Rarely, deep infection ensues, and the pins must be changed or removed. In this instance, fixator removal before complete bone union is managed by the application of a cast, because other forms of internal fixation increase the risk for subsequent osteomyelitis. It is sometimes difficult to assess when complete fracture healing has occurred, especially if only a small amount of external callus has formed. Premature frame removal can then result in refracture. Limb lengths are set anatomically in the older child and adolescent or up to 10 mm of shortening in children younger than 8 years of age, because growth acceleration is not as pronounced with this type of fracture fixation.[8]

INTRAMEDULLARY FIXATION. Two types of intramedullary fixation are rigid nails (reamed or unreamed) and semirigid (flexible) unreamed nails. Rigid nails are ideally suited for children older than 12 years of age, when the intramedullary canal is close to adult proportions. Although rigid femoral nails are available as small as 8 mm in diameter, reaming of the proximal segment is still necessary (to 12 mm), but not at the level of the fracture. The nails can also be interlocked proximally and distally to control shortening and rotation (Fig. 31-50). Interlocking nails are recommended for unstable fracture patterns, especially if there is not at least 50% cortical bone contact.[182] The combination of closed stabilization of the fracture with the biomechanical advantage of a load-sharing device yields an almost 100% healing rate. The use of rigid intramedullary nails in children younger than 12 years of age is associated with a higher risk of proximal femoral growth plate injury, with premature epiphysiodesis of the greater trochanter, resulting in femoral neck deformity (i.e., valgus).[138] Avascular necrosis of the femoral head is also reported.[11] This may be related to direct damage of the vascular supply during the process of opening the proximal femoral canal in the region of the intertrochanteric fossa or to the extent of reaming of the proximal bone segment.

Flexible or elastic intramedullary nails have the advantage of being applicable to the smaller and younger child, without risking damage to the growth plate or to the vascular supply of the femoral head, because the rods are commonly inserted from the distal femoral metaphysis retrograde toward the proximal end of the femur, avoiding the physes.[113] The ideal patients are children, 8 to 12 years of age, who are too large for a spica cast and too immature for a

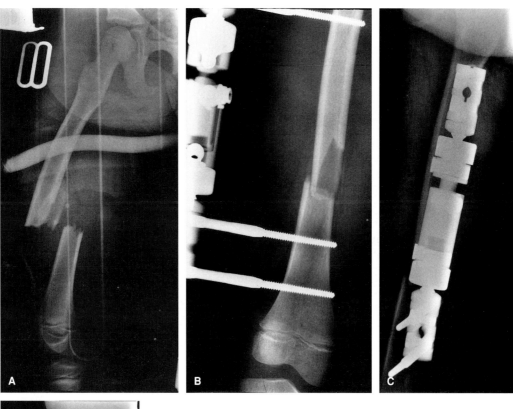

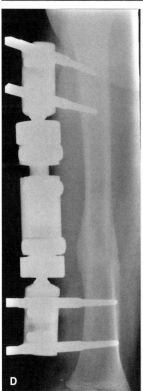

FIGURE 31-49. External fixation for open fracture. (**A**) Injury film of grade III open femur fracture in a 7-year-old child. (**B**) Alignment and stabilization with external fixation after irrigation of the wound and removal of the devitalized segment of femoral shaft. (**C**) The lateral projection shows anatomic alignment. (**D**) Twelve weeks later, there is good callus formation and new bone formation in the area of segmental bone loss. The child was ambulatory with full weight bearing without assistance. The fixator was removed at this time.

standard rigid intramedullary nail. A transverse fracture is the best pattern for this mode of internal fixation. The nails should be "stacked" in the femoral canal to provide the most effective stable immobilization (Fig. 31-51), although two nails, one medial and one lateral, are sufficient if three-point intramedullary contact is obtained.[110] Comminuted, spiral, or segmental fractures are unstable and are not well suited for this kind of fixation. The addition of a cast can supplement provisional unstable internal fixation, but this partially defeats the advantages of operative stabilization.

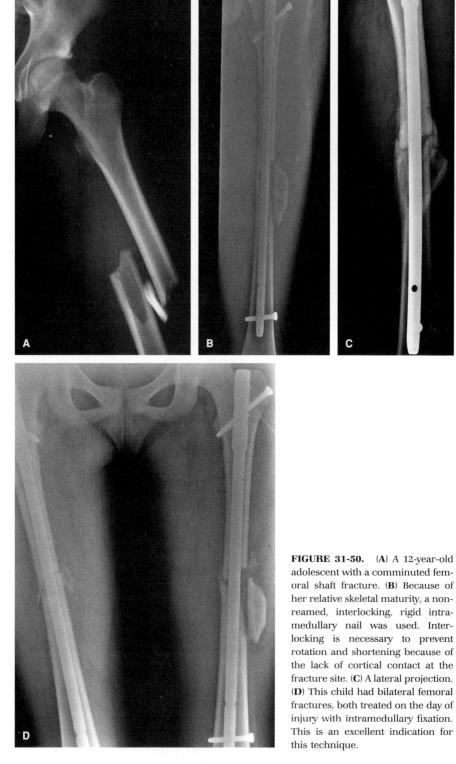

FIGURE 31-50. (A) A 12-year-old adolescent with a comminuted femoral shaft fracture. (B) Because of her relative skeletal maturity, a nonreamed, interlocking, rigid intramedullary nail was used. Interlocking is necessary to prevent rotation and shortening because of the lack of cortical contact at the fracture site. (C) A lateral projection. (D) This child had bilateral femoral fractures, both treated on the day of injury with intramedullary fixation. This is an excellent indication for this technique.

COMPRESSION PLATES AND SCREWS. This technique requires an open reduction of the fracture, with application of a variety of different-sized plates and screws, depending on the size of the femur. There are several clinical settings in which the use of this technique is advantageous. The polytrauma patient who has sustained multiple fractures, especially ipsi-lateral tibial injury, can be approached by anatomic reduction of the femur fracture. The head-injured child also benefits from this treatment regimen, which facilitates nursing care and treatment of the other injuries.[98] A bilevel femur fracture (i.e., femoral neck and shaft) can be approached by plating the shaft fracture after fixation of the proximal lesion. Bilateral

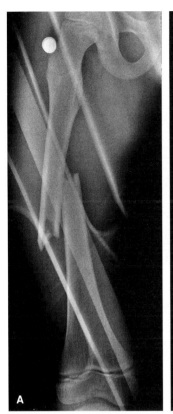
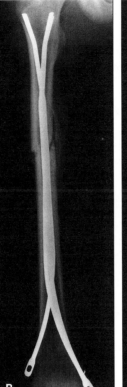
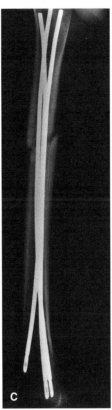

FIGURE 31-51. Flexible intramedullary fixation. (**A**) Short, oblique midshaft femur fracture in a skeletally immature child. (**B**) Flexible nails placed distal to proximal. The starting point is in the metaphyseal flare of the distal femur and three-point fixation is obtained by using curved nails. (**C**) The lateral projection shows that three nails were used to stack the femoral canal. A cast is unnecessary.

femur fractures that are located in an area difficult to secure with an intramedullary nail or an external fixator (e.g., subtrochanteric), if skeletal traction is not selected, can be treated with plate and screw fixation (Fig. 31-52). If medial femoral cortical deficiency exists, it may result in hardware failure and nonunion. In this circumstance, bone grafting should be performed at the time of internal fixation.[178]

One problem associated with internal fixation of this sort is the need for later removal of the stress-shielding implant, especially in a growing child. Extensive surgical exposure is required for spiral fractures, especially if there is comminution, to secure at least six cortices above and below the fracture line. Any less fixation requires cast supplementation. In young children, the plate alone may not be sufficiently strong to preclude the use of a cast for 4 to 6 weeks. Anatomic fracture reduction in the child who is susceptible to overgrowth (2–10 years of age) may produce a later limb length discrepancy, although this has not been reported as a significant problem.[178]

FRACTURES AND DISLOCATIONS ABOUT THE KNEE

Injuries about the knee in children usually result in a fracture, although isolated ligamentous injury can occur in the maturing adolescent.[30] The collateral and cruciate ligaments largely insert on the femoral epiphysis, exposing the physeal plate to bending stresses. Although the young child may sustain a fracture through the thin metaphyseal bone, the adolescent usually sustains a physeal separation at the same degree of force. Physical examination can usually determine the site of injury by noticing point tenderness along the physis and by testing for ligamentous integrity. Plain radiographs usually confirm the diagnosis of a fracture. Stress views can be obtained if there is any remaining question about the nature of the injury. Unfortunately, physeal fracture about the knee does not exclude the possibility of concurrent ligament injury, especially to the anterior cruciate ligament.[14] Follow-up ligamentous examination is recommended after fracture stabilization or healing.

Distal Femoral Physeal Fractures

Distal femoral physeal fractures constitute approximately 5% of all physeal fractures. The direction of displacement reflects the direction of the injuring force. Hyperextension of the knee produces anterior epiphyseal displacement, and valgus or varus stress produces medial or lateral displacement. Impact with the knee flexed causes posterior displacement of the femoral epiphysis.

All of the Salter-Harris fracture patterns are seen, but type I and II are the most common. Salter-Harris

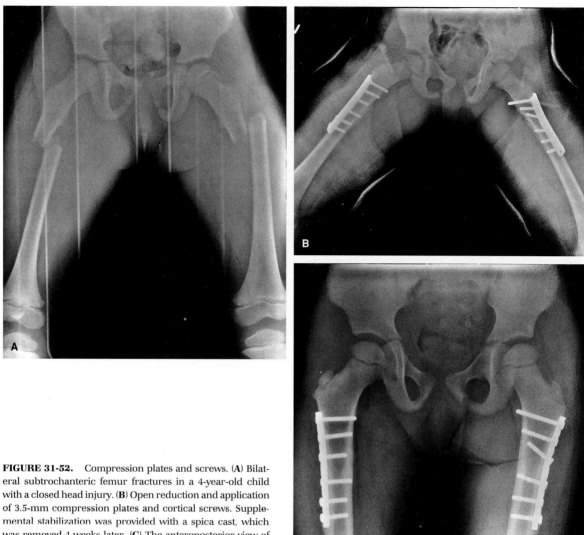

FIGURE 31-52. Compression plates and screws. (A) Bilateral subtrochanteric femur fractures in a 4-year-old child with a closed head injury. (B) Open reduction and application of 3.5-mm compression plates and cortical screws. Supplemental stabilization was provided with a spica cast, which was removed 4 weeks later. (C) The anteroposterior view of the pelvis 3 months after injury shows complete healing.

I fractures can be nondisplaced and stable; they can be treated with cylinder immobilization until the fracture site is nontender, about 3 to 4 weeks. Displaced Salter-Harris I or II fractures are usually easily reduced and can be held with an above-knee cast. Anteriorly displaced fractures require excessive knee flexion to maintain reduction, and these are best treated with crossed percutaneous pins. Casting is then possible with the knee in less than 90 degrees of flexion. Pins should cross well above the growth plate. They are preferably placed from a proximal to distal direction to avoid leaving exposed pins that traverse the synovium of the knee joint (Fig. 31-53). Posteriorly displaced fractures are less common, but the reduction is maintained in extension and is more stable. This fracture can be sufficiently controlled in an above-knee cast.

If the metaphyseal portion of the Salter-Harris II fracture is large enough (2–2.5 cm), fixation can be accomplished with the percutaneous insertion of one or two cancellous bone screws (Fig. 31-54). The surgical approach is usually on the side with the Thurston-Holland fragment, allowing good screw purchase in the larger metaphyseal fragment. The fixation is supplemented with casting. Cannulated screw systems simplify the insertion of this implant, and 6.5-mm screws are recommended. Salter-Harris type III and IV fractures are much less common and require precise open reduction and internal fixation, especially if there is fragment displacement (Fig. 31-55).

Several potential problems are associated with these fractures, especially if there was significant displacement of the fragment. Occasionally, the thick periosteum of the distal metaphysis infolds into the fracture site, preventing anatomic alignment and rendering the reduction unstable. Open reduction is approached on the side opposite the Thurston-Holland fragment, with extraction of the infolded soft tissue, facilitating fracture reduction. At this time, the fracture

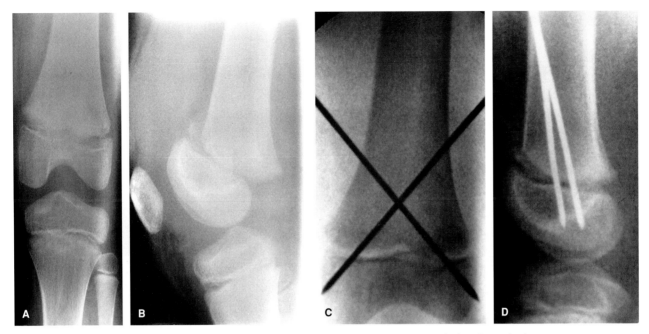

FIGURE 31-53.   Distal femoral physeal fracture. **(A)** An anteroposterior (AP) radiograph shows a widening of the distal femoral physis. **(B)** The lateral view shows an anteriorly displaced Salter-Harris II fracture. **(C)** The intraoperative AP view after closed reduction and crossed Kirschner-wire fixation. The pins are placed from a proximal to distal direction. Smooth pins are used when crossing the physis. **(D)** The lateral projection shows the pins in the midaxis of the femur.

is usually stabilized with internal fixation, placing the threaded portion of the screw into the Thurston-Holland fragment. Varus or valgus residual angulation does not remodel well, and no more than 5 degrees of angulation should be accepted.

Anteriorly displaced fractures are capable of damaging the popliteal neurovascular structures. If pulses are absent, the fracture should be promptly reduced and stabilized. Usually, the pulse returns. Pulse pressures in both extremities should be documented and followed. The child should be admitted to the hospital for observation because delayed vascular insufficiency can occur. Arteriography is suggested if there is a significant difference in pulse pressure between the two extremities. The peroneal nerve can also be injured in cases of displaced fractures.

Unlike most Salter-Harris I and II physeal fractures in other bones, injuries at the distal femoral physis produce a growth disturbance in 40% to 50% of these patients. This is primarily because a significant amount of force causes the shear or crush injury, producing direct damage to the physis during fragment displacement. Various amounts of limb length discrepancy occur, usually because of central physeal growth arrest.[143] Angular deformity is also common. The degree to which growth plate damage causes a clinical problem depends on the skeletal maturity of the child at the time of the injury. Fortunately, birth separations of the distal femoral physis are rarely asso-

ciated with growth arrest. This is probably because of the low-energy aspects of the injury mechanism, unlike the juvenile who sustains this injury from a high-energy impact. There is less interdigitation of the physis with the metaphysis (i.e., mammillary processes) in infants and less resistance to shear forces than in older children. The adolescent most commonly sustains this fracture from a high-energy impact, as in football. Although physeal arrest is prevalent, a clinical problem ensues only if significant longitudinal growth remains. This can be determined by identifying the skeletal age and by monitoring growth with serial radiographs every 6 months.

Knee Dislocation

This is a rare injury in children but can occur in the older adolescent. The most important aspect of management is to be aware that a severe ligamentous disruption of the knee may be the only sign that a dislocation has occurred. This is especially likely if the mechanism of injury was from high-energy impact, as in a motor vehicle accident or from a tackle in football. The vascular status must be carefully evaluated by comparing Doppler pulse pressures to the contralateral limb in all patients suspected of having knee dislocation. If the pulses are reduced or absent, intraoperative arteriography is recommended to prevent any further delay in vascular reconstruction.[52]

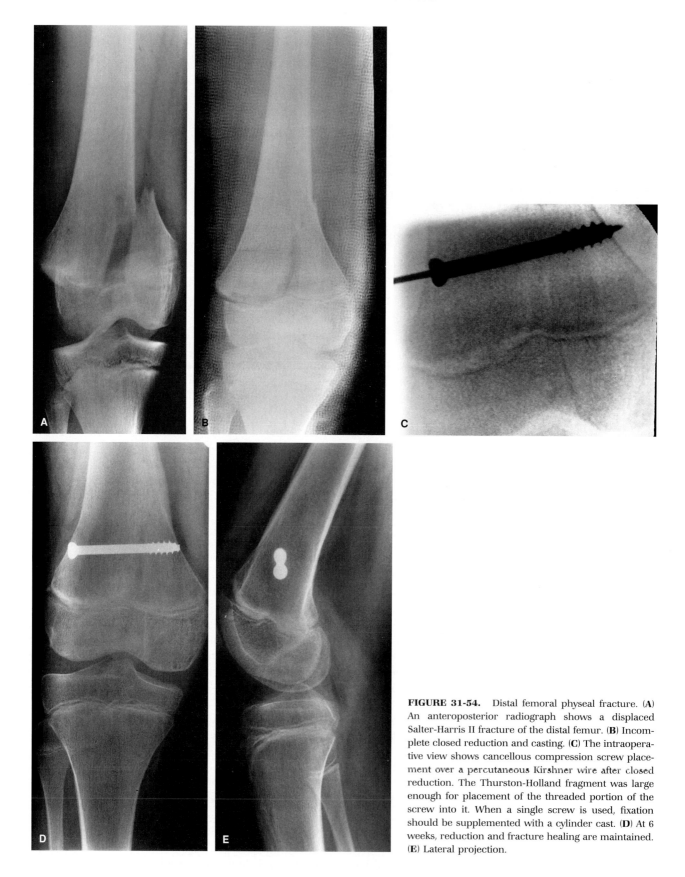

FIGURE 31-54. Distal femoral physeal fracture. (**A**) An anteroposterior radiograph shows a displaced Salter-Harris II fracture of the distal femur. (**B**) Incomplete closed reduction and casting. (**C**) The intraoperative view shows cancellous compression screw placement over a percutaneous Kirshner wire after closed reduction. The Thurston-Holland fragment was large enough for placement of the threaded portion of the screw into it. When a single screw is used, fixation should be supplemented with a cylinder cast. (**D**) At 6 weeks, reduction and fracture healing are maintained. (**E**) Lateral projection.

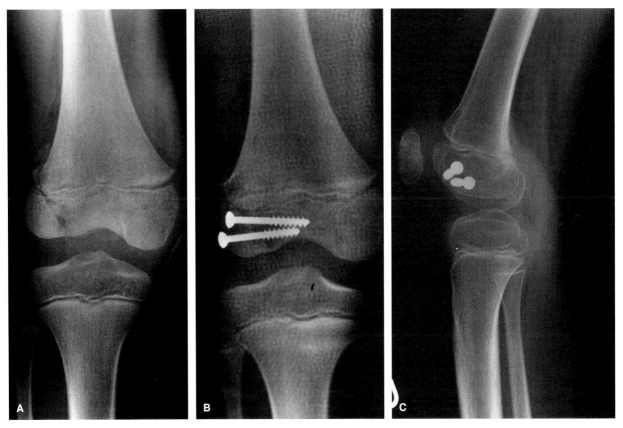

FIGURE 31-55.   Distal femoral physeal fracture. (**A**) Salter-Harris IV fracture involving the lateral condyle of the distal femur. Although the injury film does not show significant displacement, fragment stabilization is recommended to maintain this alignment. (**B**) An anteroposterior projection after placement of cancellous bone screws. (**C**) Lateral projection.

The amputation rate approaches 90% when surgery is not completed within 8 hours of injury.[61] Children tolerate warm ischemia less well (i.e., threshold of only 6 hours) than adults.[160] The patient with knee dislocation and intact pulses needs to be monitored for 48 hours to verify the maintenance of an intact peripheral circulation, ruling out delayed arterial thrombosis. The limb should also be evaluated for impending compartment syndrome. Ligamentous damage can be repaired during the initial surgical procedure, after the vascular status of the extremity has been restored.

Intraarticular Avulsions

Tibial eminence avulsion (i.e., anterior tibial spine fracture) is the most frequent fracture of this type and represents a separation of the anterior cruciate insertion point. The femoral origin of the anterior cruciate ligament is rarely fractured. This tibial avulsion is classified by the degree of apparent displacement of the fragment; type I is minimally displaced, type II is intermediate, and type III completely separated.[122]

Management is by closed reduction and cylinder cast with the knee in full extension, usually requiring general anesthesia for treating type II or III displaced eminence fragments (Fig. 31-56). Although hyperextension of the knee may aid in the reduction maneuver, this position should not be maintained for immobilization. Full knee extension or slight flexion (5–10 degrees) is preferred. Persistent displacement of a type III avulsion implies that the fragment, which is often much larger than it appears on plain radiographs, is blocked from returning to its bony bed, probably by the meniscus. This requires an open reduction, and after the piece is returned to its anatomic position, it can be sutured in place. The sutures can be passed through small drill holes made in the anterior tibial epiphysis, exiting into the center of the eminence fragment. Tilting the fragment when tightening the sutures can be avoided by central to posterior placement of the fixation holes. Although a small cancellous screw can be used, it must remain intraepiphyseal to avoid damage to the proximal tibial growth plate.

Despite anatomic repair, long-term evaluation often demonstrates increased anterior laxity of the knee, suggesting that there is stretch injury to the anterior

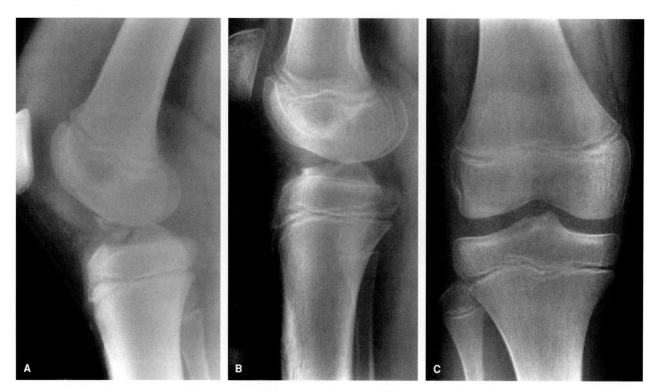

FIGURE 31-56. Tibial eminence fracture. (**A**) Lateral projection of type II avulsion fracture. This fracture is probably in transition between type II and type III displacement. However, when the knee was placed in full extension, the fragments were reduced to an acceptable degree. Treatment was in a cylinder cast. (**B**) Six weeks after injury, reduction has been maintained, and there is evidence of healing. (**C**) The anteroposterior projection shows no significant elevation of the tibial spine.

cruciate ligament.[156] Eminence fragments that are allowed to heal in a displaced position (e.g., incompletely reduced type II or III fracture) provide a mechanical block to full knee extension, and anterior knee laxity is excessive, increasing the chances for late symptoms and instability.[66]

The posterior cruciate ligament may pull off a bony fragment from the posterior tibial epiphysis, and it is usually identified on standard radiographs of the knee. Open reduction and internal fixation are indicated through a posterior approach to the knee to restore ligamentous stability and prevent later symptoms.[121] Internal fixation is achieved with a cancellous screw placed within the epiphysis. The knee is immobilized in 30 degrees of flexion for about 3 to 4 weeks before commencing muscle rehabilitation.

Patellar Disorders

Patellar Fracture

Displaced patellar fractures are usually transverse and are typically the result of direct trauma. This injury is most often seen in the older adolescent. Avulsion injuries also can occur and should be differentiated from bipartite (i.e., secondary ossification center) patella. Treatment of displaced fractures consists of open reduction of the fragments and stabilization with parallel Kirschner wires and tension band compression. The quadriceps extensor mechanism must be repaired.

Patellar sleeve fracture is unique to children, usually between the ages of 8 and 12 years.[80] It is an avulsion of the inferior pole of the patella with a variable amount of articular cartilage attached. The bony portion may not be obvious because most of the fragment is cartilaginous, but the lateral radiograph reveals patella alta (Fig. 31-57). On clinical examination, a gap is palpable between the patellar tendon and its origin. Active knee extension is absent. Repair is necessary to restore normal function, and AO tension band technique is employed.

Patellar Dislocation

Patellar dislocation affects girls more than boys, probably because of the combination of relative greater ligamentous laxity and an increased Q angle in girls. The mechanism of traumatic injury is usually a twisting of the knee with the foot planted, causing a lateral dislocation of the patella. Reduction frequently occurs spontaneously with extension of the knee. Hemarthrosis is present, and the medial retinaculum is

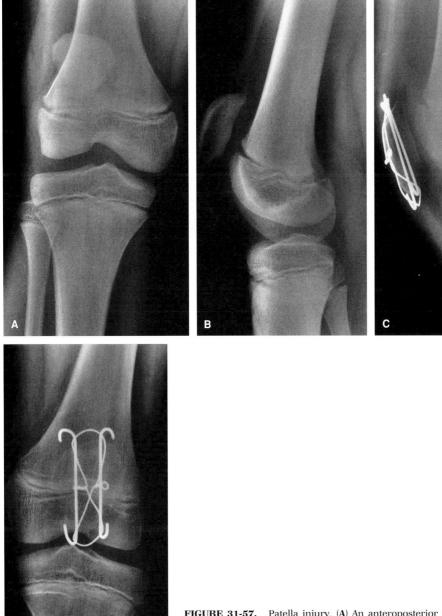

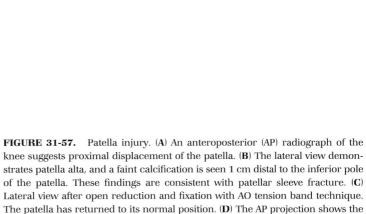

FIGURE 31-57. Patella injury. (**A**) An anteroposterior (AP) radiograph of the knee suggests proximal displacement of the patella. (**B**) The lateral view demonstrates patella alta, and a faint calcification is seen 1 cm distal to the inferior pole of the patella. These findings are consistent with patellar sleeve fracture. (**C**) Lateral view after open reduction and fixation with AO tension band technique. The patella has returned to its normal position. (**D**) The AP projection shows the configuration of the internal fixation.

very tender to palpation. Apprehension is displayed with laterally directed pressure on the patella. Management is immobilization in knee extension for 2 to 3 weeks or until the pain and swelling subside enough to begin a program of extensor strengthening. For patients younger than 14 years of age, the recurrence rate for another dislocation is 60%.

Patellar dislocation is the most common cause of osteochondral fractures about the knee and may involve a portion of the femoral condyle or the patella. These fragments are best visualized on the patella "skyline" view. A hemarthrosis with fat globules in the aspirate suggests an osteochondral fracture. Although only a thin wafer of bone may be identified, the actual size of the fragment can be considerable because of the cartilage component. Arthroscopy can be used to assess if the fragment is large enough to be reattached. A double-threaded "headless" screw allows fixation.

If fixation is not possible, the loose piece can be removed.

Acute Hemarthrosis of the Knee

The clinical setting of a traumatic acute hemarthrosis, without evidence of fracture, suggests internal soft tissue derangement of the knee. This is common in the child older than 12 years of age but can occur in younger children. The anterior cruciate ligament is the structure most frequently torn, followed closely by the medial meniscus. The medial meniscus is injured five times more often than the lateral meniscus. The two injuries can coexist but do so less frequently than is seen in the skeletally mature population. Osteochondral fractures are sometimes the cause of the hemarthrosis, although considerably less often than ligament damage. Diagnostic evaluation is recommended if there is not a return to normal in 3 weeks, although some physicians have suggested early arthroscopy.[161]

Tibial Tubercle Avulsion

The tibial tubercle is the anterior and distal extension of the proximal tibial epiphysis. It develops a secondary ossification center and serves as the insertion site of the patellar tendon. Fracture of the tibial tubercle is an injury of the adolescent knee joint, usually in a boy between 13 and 16 years of age, and occurs during forceful quadriceps contraction (e.g., jumping). The proximal tibial physis is in the process of physiologic closure, beginning centrally and proceeding centrifugally and distally to involve the tubercle; this fracture pattern therefore is seen in adolescents.

The diagnosis is confirmed on a lateral radiograph by identifying the displaced fragment and a high-riding patella. Type I fracture is through the distal ossification center, type II at the junction of the tubercle and the tibial ossification centers, and type III involves the articular surface of the tibia, essentially a Salter-Harris type III fracture (Fig. 31-58). Displaced fractures, typically type II and III, result in the inability to actively extend the knee, and operative correction is necessary. In type III separations, joint congruity must also be restored, and intraarticular exploration is required. Usually, disruption of the proximal tibial periosteum and extensor retinaculae occurs, and significant swelling can ensue. The extensor retinaculum should be repaired. Associated injuries include the knee ligaments and menisci. Internal fixation is accomplished through the insertion of an anteriorly placed cancellous bone screw (Fig. 31-59). Knee immobilization is used for 3 to 4 weeks before establishing active range

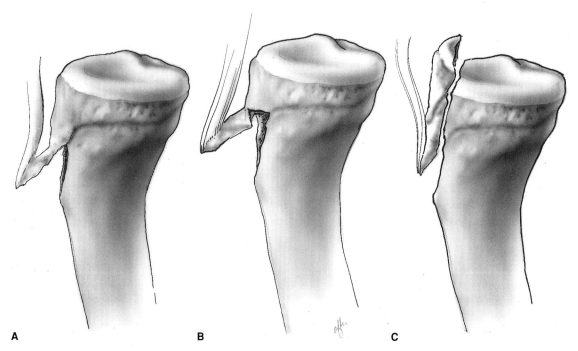

A **B** **C**

FIGURE 31-58. Classification of tibial tuberosity fractures. (**A**) Type I fracture through the secondary ossification center. (**B**) Type II fracture, located at the junction of the primary and secondary ossification centers. Sometimes, this fragment is in two pieces. (**C**) Type III fracture, which is an intraarticular fracture (Salter-Harris Type III). This can also be a two-part fracture.

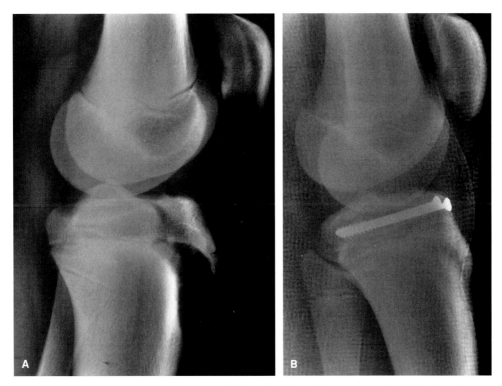

FIGURE 31-59.   Tibial tubercle fracture. (**A**) The lateral radiograh shows type III tibial tubercle avulsion. This is a Salter-Harris III fracture. Open reduction and internal fixation are indicated. (**B**) The postoperative lateral radiograph demonstrates reduction of the fracture with intraepiphyseal cancellous screw placement. This type of fixation was chosen because this is a 13-year-old boy who had significant growth remaining. In the older adolescent with less than 2 years of growth remaining, the screws can cross the physis.

of motion. Progressive recurvatum deformity of the proximal tibia is not usually a clinical problem because of the advanced age of the child at the time of injury. However, young adolescents with this fracture pattern need to be followed longitudinally for growth arrest.

TIBIAL FRACTURES

Tibial fractures are the most common lower limb fracture in children and make up 15% of all pediatric fractures. Proximal epiphyseal and metaphyseal regions are less commonly fractured than the diaphyseal region. The type of tibial fracture depends largely on the age of the child and the mechanism of injury. Most are low-energy fractures occurring from minor falls, twisting injuries, or sports. Treatment is usually by closed means, and healing is rapid and uneventful, especially the younger the child.

Motor vehicle accidents are the most common cause for the significantly displaced tibia-fibula fracture, and the subsequent clinical course is more protracted. Soft tissue injury adds to the complexity of fracture management.

Regions of Tibial Fracture

Proximal Tibial Epiphysis

Despite the frequent exposure of the child's knee to trauma, the proximal tibial epiphysis is rarely fractured. This is probably because of the many musculotendinous units that span the epiphysis without actually inserting into this region. The physis is irregularly shaped, with an anterior downward extension of the tibial tuberosity. Because the lateral collateral ligament inserts on the fibula and the medial collateral inserts on the epiphysis and metaphysis, varus and valgus stresses are not propagated to the tibial epiphysis.

The mechanism of injury is usually direct force to the knee, as can occur in motor vehicle accident. Hyperextension injuries from sports can produce this fracture. The peak age for this fracture is 14 years, close to the time of epiphyseal closure. A second and smaller peak incidence occurs between 2 and 6 years of age, and these fractures usually are sustained by direct injury to the proximal tibia in lawn mower accidents.[22] Most proximal epiphyseal injuries are Salter-Harris type II fractures, demonstrating posterolateral or posteromedial displacement. These are followed in frequency by type I separations, which tend to displace posteriorly, threatening the neurovascular bundle (Fig. 31-60). Any displaced fracture can place the popliteal artery at risk for injury because of its proximity to the bone and the fact that it is tethered to the posterior aspect of the tibia by the anterior tibial artery, which passes into the anterior compartment just distal to the fracture.

Most of these fractures are managed by closed reduction with percutaneous pinning if the fracture is unstable. Cancellous screw fixation is used if the metaphyseal fragment in a type II fracture is large enough. In the adolescent, insufficient growth remains to correct spontaneously any residual deformity after an imprecise reduction. The fractures treated closed must be well aligned and followed closely for any angular displacement. Displaced type III and IV fractures require precise reduction and internal fixation and are secured with transepiphyseal cancellous bone screws. Growth arrest has occurred in 25% to 33% of these patients, regardless of the type of Salter-Harris physeal separation.[22,154]

Vascular compromise from a displaced fracture requires prompt reduction and is an indication for internal fixation. After reduction, Doppler pulse pressures are compared with the contralateral limb, and a significant difference is an indication for arteriography. It is recommended that this be performed in the operating room, in preparation for arterial exploration, to avoid further delay in vascular reconstruction. Symmetrical Doppler pulse pressures allow observation of the extremity or elective arteriography if so desired. If vascular repair is necessary or if warm ischemia has exceeded 4 hours, prophylactic fasciotomy is recommended.[127] This prevents reperfusion compartment syndrome from developing.

Proximal Tibial Metaphysis

Metaphyseal fractures of the proximal tibia occur most commonly in children between the ages of 2 and 8 years, and they are usually incomplete fractures. Typically, the leg is in valgus alignment, although the fracture may also be extended (i.e., recurvatum). Pronounced displacement is uncommon, despite the fact that many fractures are the result of motor vehicle accidents. An associated fibular fracture indicates a greater force was involved in sustaining the injury.

General management consists of closed reduction and above-knee casting, with the knee in almost full extension. This position allows more effective three-point cast molding and makes subsequent radiographic analysis of fragment alignment easier. Healing is usually complete after 6 weeks. Displaced proximal tibial fractures in adolescents sometimes require operative stabilization to control alignment and expedite mobilization. During the 48 hours after closed reduction and casting, the extremity should be monitored for signs of excessive compartment swelling.

Despite initial anatomic alignment and the relative innocuous appearance of the fracture, progressive valgus deformity of the leg frequently develops in young children (Fig. 31-61). The severity of the valgus angulation peaks at 4 to 6 months after injury, and the magnitude of deformity stabilizes after 1 year. The cause of this problem remains somewhat obscure, but it probably results from selective overgrowth of the medial tibial physis in response to asymmetric vascular stimulation.[88] This problem can develop even if the fibula is broken. Torus fractures of the proximal metaphysis generally do not produce this complication. Close review of initial postreduction radiographs occasionally reveals that an imprecise reduction was responsible for at least part of the deformity. Treatment is first by observation, because smaller degrees of angulation resolve, partly because of compensatory remodeling from the distal tibial physis. Surgical correction is delayed until the child is closer to maturity.[144,186] Some physicians think that greater than 15 degrees of valgus angulation is an indication for early

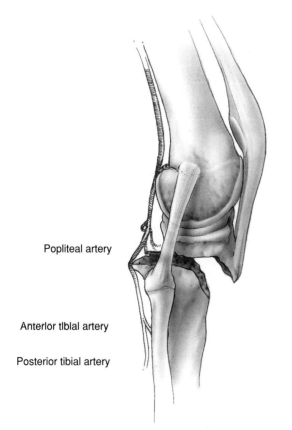

Popliteal artery

Anterior tibial artery

Posterior tibial artery

FIGURE 31-60. Proximal epiphyseal fracture. The distal tibial segment is displaced posteriorly, producing vascular occlusion of the popliteal artery.

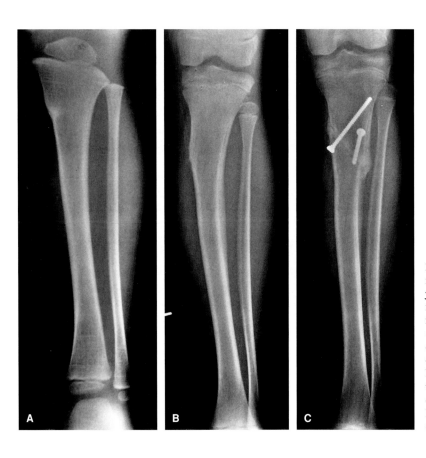

FIGURE 31-61. Traumatic tibial valgus deformity. (**A**) An anteroposterior radiograph of a 3-year-old child 9 months after sustaining a proximal tibial metaphyseal fracture. The clinical deformity was most apparent 6 months after injury. (**B**) Same tibia, 9 years later. The region of valgus deformity has moved distally, but there has been only a minimal reduction in angulation. There has been some adaptive remodeling of the distal tibia. (**C**) Six weeks after corrective oblique osteotomy of the proximal tibia performed at the level of the deformity, there has been restoration of the anatomic axis of the tibia.

corrective osteotomy, but there is significant risk for recurrence of the deformity in the young child.[147]

Tibial Diaphysis

In infants and young children, the tibial shaft is more porous, and it is more likely to bend or buckle than it is to comminute. The surrounding periosteum is strong and imparts stability to the fracture site, limiting displacement. These are low-energy fractures that are usually caused by a torsional force (e.g., indirect trauma), and the fibula is often intact. These uncomplicated fractures usually heal in 8 to 10 weeks. Children with associated closed head injuries or displaced fractures in the older child have longer healing rates, averaging 12 to 16 weeks. Open fractures also display delayed healing rates, averaging 20 weeks.[183] Compared with the young child, the adolescent tibial shaft is composed of more dense cortical bone and a thinner and weaker periosteum, resulting in more fracture displacement, comminution, and slower rates of healing. These fractures are also more often the result of high-energy trauma.

The most useful information about a tibial fracture includes a description of the mechanism of injury, the anatomic location, the fracture pattern, the amount of displacement (including shortening), and the magnitude of soft tissue injury. Mild injuries consist of less than 50% diaphyseal offset, minimal angulation, and no soft tissue damage. Moderate injuries show greater fracture displacement with more angulation and include minor (grade I) open soft tissue wounds. Severe injuries display comminuted or segmental fracture patterns (possible bone loss), marked displacement, and grade II or III soft tissue damage.

Management

Most childhood tibial fractures can be managed by closed techniques. Early assessment of the stability of the fracture pattern helps to predict the success of cast treatment and what problems to anticipate. Stable fracture patterns resist shortening and have the following characteristics:

An intact fibula imparts stability with regard to maintenance of length, but it may contribute to the development of varus angulation.

Spiral fractures have an intact periosteum and large surface area for rapid healing. Fracture alignment is not difficult to maintain. The exception is the distal diaphyseal spiral fracture with greater than 50% shaft-width displacement. This implies that the interosseous membrane is torn, and subsequent angulation is difficult to prevent.

Transverse fractures with displacement less than 50% of the diameter of the shaft usually are stable. The control of angulation is the main challenge, and cast adjustment is frequently needed. Distal one-third fractures may angulate into recurvatum when the ankle is dorsiflexed to neutral. It is necessary to keep an equinus posture until early healing is evident, and then the foot can be gradually dorsiflexed. Complete fractures of the tibia and fibula are more unstable, but axial alignment is easier to control than when the fibula is intact. The tendency is for the fracture to drift into valgus and procurvatum because of the greater muscle bulk posterolaterally in the leg.

When managing a tibial fracture closed, an early weight-bearing cast program helps to promote healing. Above-knee casting should be replaced by a patellar-tendon–bearing cast and then by below-knee immobilization as soon as fracture stability has become evident. If there is delayed healing and persistence of the fracture line, a full-contact removable orthosis can be applied.

Final axial alignment should be within 5 degrees of a varus or valgus position. Although some remodeling occurs at the diaphysis through convex bone resorption, most angular compensation is achieved at the physeal level through asymmetric longitudinal growth. Residual diaphyseal deformity may persist. Infants and young children can correct approximately 50% of the angulation with growth. In children older than 10 years of age, only 25% of the axial malalignment improves. Hansen reported only a 13.5% correction of angular deformity with subsequent growth,[70] but Shannak demonstrated that one third of children with more than 10 degrees of angulation at healing had persistence of the malunion at the final follow-up assessment.[152] In general, varus malalignment seems to remodel more completely than valgus deformity, but compensation at the level of the foot and ankle is poorly tolerated. Recurvatum of more than 10 degrees is also slow to remodel.

The ability to compensate for shortening decreases with age. Children younger than 5 years of age show the greatest capacity, and those older than 10 years of age display the least. Unlike the fractured femur, this increase in tibial growth rate is less dramatic, and predictable growth acceleration greater than 5 to 7 mm is unusual.[63] In a review of 142 tibial fractures, Shannak reported an average of only 4.35 mm of growth acceleration.[152] Comminuted and long spiral fractures displayed the greatest amount of overgrowth, including those that were treated with anatomic reduction and internal or external fixation.

Overgrowth is not routinely seen in girls older than 8 years or in boys older than 10 years of age.

Operative Indications

The indications for operative intervention for tibial fractures in children include failure of closed management, associated soft tissue damage, polytrauma, and compartment syndrome.

FAILURE OF CLOSED MANAGEMENT. Angulation not controlled by repeated cast adjustment and excessive fragment shortening are approached with surgical stabilization. Unstable fracture patterns that are likely to fail cast treatment also qualify for other means of stabilization. In the rare instance of delayed union or nonunion, operative intervention is necessary. This may include internal or external fixation, frequently combined with autologous bone grafting.

SOFT TISSUE DAMAGE. Open fractures, notably grade III, require operative stabilization to facilitate soft tissue healing and wound management. Soft tissue defects combined with unstable fracture patterns are prone to shortening and are difficult to manage in a cast. Associated vascular injury is another indication for primary surgical fixation of the tibial fracture. Compartment syndrome is also a relative indication for operative control of a tibial fracture. Early fracture stability promotes soft tissue recovery and allows easier management of the fasciotomy sites.

POLYTRAUMA. Children who have sustained multiple long bone fractures are candidates for operative stabilization of some or all the fractures. Bilateral tibial fractures or concurrent femoral shaft fracture (ipsilateral or contralateral) are other indications for surgery. Fractures associated with multisystem injuries should be fixed, greatly enhancing patient care. The child with a significant closed head injury exemplifies this approach.

High-energy tibial fractures are also associated with delayed union, especially if there has been segmental bone loss. In this instance, early prophylactic posterolateral bone grafting is advantageous.[16] This is performed approximately 3 to 6 weeks after soft tissue healing, long before there is established delayed union or nonunion (Fig. 31-62).

TODDLER'S FRACTURE. Fracture of the tibia in infancy and early childhood is usually caused by low-energy torsional forces, as when the child twists the leg. The fibula is usually not injured. The child refuses to walk on the affected lower limb or limps. Examination may reveal subtle swelling of the leg, but

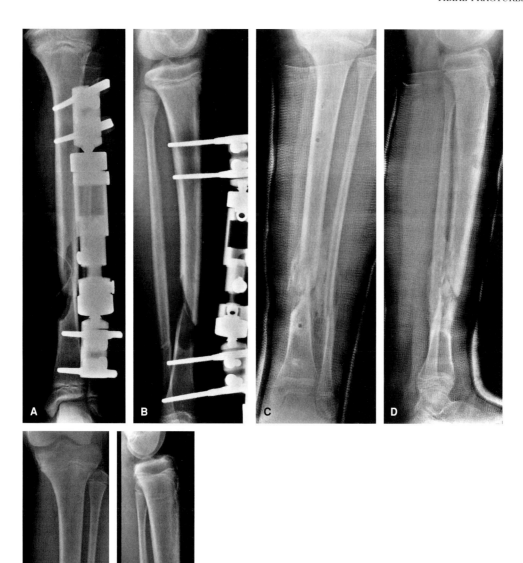

FIGURE 31-62. High-energy tibia fracture. (**A**) Grade III open distal tibial diaphyseal fracture with segmental bone loss in a 10-year-old child. After treatment of the soft tissues, alignment was obtained with an external fixator. (**B**) The lateral radiograph further delineates the bone loss. Approximately 6 weeks after soft tissue healing, posterolateral autologous bone grafting was performed. (**C**) An anteroposterior (AP) radiograph 6 weeks after bone grafting. The external fixator has been removed and a below-knee cast applied. (**D**) A lateral radiograph shows maintenance of the alignment and early bone graft consolidation. (**E**) An AP radiograph 1 year later shows complete healing and maturation of the bone graft. (**F**) A lateral radiograph demonstrates mature bone and synostosis between the fibula and the tibia.

usually an area of point tenderness is located along the distal-third diaphysis of the tibia. Oblique radiographs may show a spiral fracture, but often the fracture line is initially not evident.

Toddler's fracture is differentiated from hip pathology by the child's ability to crawl despite a refusal to bear weight and by a normal range of motion of the hip joint. Acute osteomyelitis of the tibia is typically metaphyseal in location, and laboratory studies for the sedimentation rate, C-reactive protein, leukocyte count, and differential blood counts are abnormally elevated. More chronic conditions of bone usually are well demonstrated on routine radiographs. Occasionally, a triphase bone scan is employed to help with the diagnosis of the acute limping toddler, if the standard workup remains equivocal.[7] The diagnosis of toddler's fracture is radiographically confirmed 10 to 14 days later, when periosteal new bone has formed. Treatment consists of a below-knee walking cast for approximately 3 weeks.

OPEN FRACTURES.   Open fractures constitute 3% to 19% of all tibial fractures and are classified by Gustillo (modified by Mendoza) in Table 31-1.[69] Unfortunately, this grading system does not accurately portray the severity of all open fractures, especially when there is a small external wound combined with severe underlying soft tissue damage (e.g., extensive periosteal stripping) or bone comminution. For greater accuracy, separate grading of the skin, soft tissues, and bone injuries is suggested.

Management of the open fracture requires prompt operative irrigation and debridement of the wound, removing all necrotic or devitalized material. Bone devoid of soft tissue attachments usually is removed, especially if grossly contaminated. Avascular segments of bone that are clean may be preserved if needed to provide fracture stability. In this instance, external fixation pins should not be placed in this segment, because the risk of subsequent osteomyelitis is significant. Bone should be stabilized to create optimal conditions for soft tissue recovery. Cultures are best obtained after complete irrigation of the wound. The occurrence of a positive postirrigation culture is indicative of a high risk for the development of deep infection with that organism.[135] Early soft tissue coverage is advantageous and may require local or free-flap reconstruction. Patients with open wounds are returned to the operating room in 48 hours for repeat irrigation and possible delayed primary closure or flap coverage. Antibiotics are used for 72 hours. Cephalosporins are used for grade I injury, and an aminoglycoside is added for grade II or grade III injuries. Specific antibiotic selection is made after the culture results become available.

Open fractures of the tibia in children share many of the same complications reported in the adult literature, despite their apparent greater healing capacity.[21,79] This includes associated vascular injury in 5%, superficial infection rate of 10% with osteomyelitis in 2%, delayed union in 14%, malunion in 6% to 7%, and compartment syndrome in 5%. The major differences between children's open fractures and those in adults are the occurrence of tibial overgrowth (10 mm in 20%) and the subsequent remodeling of angular deformities.[21] Grade I injuries have the same good prognosis as closed fractures after appropriate initial wound management. Long-term morbidity of open tibial fractures in children may be an understated problem. Some researchers have shown that chronic pain, reduced sporting performance, stiffness, and poor cosmesis are common, especially after grade III fractures.[79]

COMPARTMENT   SYNDROME.   Compartment syndrome can occur after what appears to be a relatively minor, minimally displaced tibial fracture. Although an open fracture often spontaneously decompresses local tissue pressures, it does not preclude the syndrome (5% incidence). The typical fracture associated with compartment syndrome is located in the proximal or middle tibia, but it can develop with

TABLE 31-1.   *Classification of Open Fractures*

WOUND TYPE	*EXTERNAL WOUND SIZE*	*FRACTURE PATTERN*	*SOFT TISSUE DAMAGE*
Type I	<2 cm	Simple	Minimal muscle contusion
Type II	2–10 cm	Simple; minimal comminution	Mild muscle damage; no crush
Type IIIA	Extensive or gunshot wound	Comminuted or segmental fracture	Adequate local soft tissue coverage
Type IIIB	Extensive or crush injury	Extensive periosteal stripping, bone loss	Incomplete coverage, exposed bone
Type IIIC	Same as above	Same as above	Neurovascular injury

distal diaphyseal fractures as well. A constricting dressing or cast may contribute to increased tissue pressures. The clinical findings rely heavily on patient cooperation; unfortunately, this approach is frequently not possible in treating children, and intracompartmental pressures must be measured in all questionable cases. This is especially applicable for the child with a closed head injury who is unable to report any symptoms.

A tense, swollen extremity should alert the examiner, especially if there is pain with passive stretching of the muscles in the involved compartment. Any sensory deficit is an absolute sign, unless there is a more proximal primary nerve injury; nerve injuries are not associated with pain on passive stretch, and measured compartment pressures are normal. Impending syndromes are heralded by complaints of pain out of proportion to that expected from the fracture or that has not been relieved by the usual amount of analgesic. The injured leg should not be excessively elevated, because this maneuver reduces mean arterial pressure, causing a reduction in oxygen perfusion that leads to further muscle ischemia, perpetuating the compartment syndrome. Plantar flexion of the foot may also help reduce compartment pressures.

The diagnosis of acute compartment syndrome is based on signs and symptoms, tempered by the patient's overall medical condition (e.g., hypotension lowers tolerance for increased compartment pressures). Tissue pressure measurements are obtained for all four compartments if there is any suggestion of a compartment syndrome. The pressure threshold for fasciotomy depends somewhat on the technique used. Surgical decompression is performed when pressures rise to within 20 to 30 mm Hg of the diastolic blood pressure, combined with positive clinical findings, or if the absolute value is greater than 35 mm Hg in the unresponsive patient.[19] Muscle and nerve damage commence as soon as 4 to 6 hours after the onset of abnormal pressures. The peroneal nerve is considerably more sensitive than skeletal muscle to changes in tissue pressure. Fibulectomy is not recommended in children because it can lead to a progressive valgus deformity of the ankle.[54]

FLOATING KNEE. The floating knee configuration occurs after fracture of the femur and the ipsilateral tibia. This injury pattern has been classified by Letts.[107] The fracture usually is the result of high-energy trauma, as typically occurs in a pedestrian–motor vehicle collision. This problem is more widespread among children older than 10 years of age.[17] Knee ligament damage occurs in approximately 10% of these patients and is better assessed if juxtaarticular fractures are stabilized. The closed management of float-

ing knee fractures is associated with a higher incidence of complications, especially malunion (30%) and limb length discrepancy, than operative stabilization of at least one of the bones.[107,119]

Techniques of Fixation

EXTERNAL FIXATION. The tibia lies in a subcutaneous position and readily accepts an external fixator. Half-pin, monolateral frames provide sufficient stability and are applied under fluoroscopic guidance. Most are applied to the anteromedial surface of the tibial shaft, with two pins above and two below the fracture. When possible, pins should not be placed any closer than 2 cm from the physis or closer than 2 cm from the fracture site.[4] Transfixing full pins are not indicated, unless a thin-wire circular fixator is used. Pin diameters for treating small children should not exceed 4 mm, but 5- to 6-mm pins can be used in adolescents.

The advantages of external fixation are the ease of application, good access to damaged soft tissues, good fracture stability, and early full weight bearing while maintaining motion of the knee and ankle. The problems with external fixation include a pin infection rate of 50%, increased healing times (probably reflecting more severe injuries), and the possibility of refracture after removal. Some of these complications can be reduced by removing the frame when early fracture stability has been obtained and applying a weight-bearing cast.[21,170]

INTRAMEDULLARY NAIL FIXATION. This technique uses flexible nails and rigid nails to treat tibias in adolescents. Rigid nails can be nonreamed and interlocking, but the child must be near the end of growth, because the proximal tibial physis is likely to be damaged (Fig. 31-63). In the younger child, flexible nails can be stacked into the medullary canal through the metaphyseal region of the proximal tibia, avoiding the physis. The narrow internal diameter of the tibial diaphysis in children may limit the number of intramedullary pins that can be inserted, and cast supplementation may be necessary.

COMPRESSION PLATE AND SCREWS. Open reduction and plating of tibial fractures are rarely indicated, largely because of the more extensive surgical exposure required and because of the thin layer of overlying soft tissue. However, internal fixation can be helpful in fractures of the distal metaphysis, particularly if there is comminution. The use of limited internal fixation (i.e., compression screws alone) in combination with casting or external fixation can be helpful

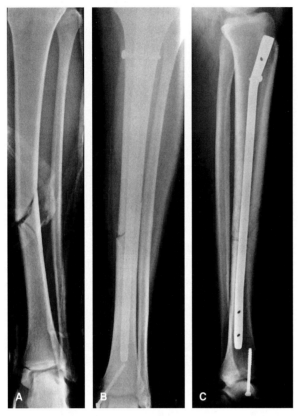

FIGURE 31-63. Mid-diaphyseal tibia fracture. (**A**) Oblique tibia fracture with associated medial malleolus fracture. As an isolated injury, this fracture could be managed by closed reduction and casting. (**B**) A nonreamed interlocking tibial nail was used after internal fixation of the medial malleolus fracture. (**C**) The lateral projection shows anatomic alignment. The proximal tibial physis has already closed, allowing this technique of fixation. This adolescent also sustained an ipsilateral femur fracture, pelvic fracture, and upper extremity injuries. These multiple fractures were the main indication for internal fixation of the tibia, which facilitated the patient's mobility.

in initiating anatomic fracture alignment, but this approach usually fails to provide adequate supplemental fixation, especially over long segments of bone.[157]

Isolated fractures of the fibula are uncommon and are usually the result of direct trauma. Proximal fractures may be associated with peroneal nerve palsy. Closed treatment is combined with casting for 3 to 6 weeks.

ANKLE FRACTURES

Ankle fractures are a relatively common injury in children, and the distal tibial physis is a frequent site of physeal separation, second only to the distal radius. The ankle joint consists of the tibia, fibula, and the talus and is further supported by medial and lateral ligaments. Medial stability is provided by the deep fibers of the deltoid ligament, attaching the tip of the

medial malleolus to the body of the talus. The lateral ligament complex consists of the anterior and posterior talofibular ligaments and the calcaneofibular ligament. Ankle motion is essentially in plantar flexion and dorsiflexion only, rendering this region susceptible to injury with twisting or bending forces. The ligaments attach to the epiphysis, below the level of the physeal plate, on the tibia and fibula. The ligaments display high tensile strength; stress is probably conferred to the surrounding bone during trauma.

Common Patterns of Ankle Fractures

The mechanism of injury is usually indirect violence, with the fixed foot forced into various positions as the leg rotates over the foot. The classification scheme offered by Dias is based on a combination of the adult Lauge-Hansen principles and the Salter-Harris system.[44] The first word is a descriptor of the position of the foot at the time of injury, and the second is the abnormal force applied. The advantage of trying to recreate the injury mechanism is that it is helpful during any attempted reduction maneuver, which is then accomplished by reversing the offending forces.

Supination forces are common about the ankle, comprising 15% to 20% of all injuries. Any mechanism of injury that includes supination also involves an axial load (i.e., crush) to the growth plate. This compression of the physis may contribute to early growth plate closure. External rotation forces about the ankle are also common, causing spiral fractures and transitional fractures in adolescents. Direct trauma to the ankle region may produce comminuted fractures and injury configurations that are not readily classified. The basic classification is discussed in the following sections.

Supination and Inversion

Supination and inversion are adduction injuries in which the talus is driven into the medial malleolus, causing the propagation of a vertical fracture line. This results in a Salter-Harris type III or IV growth plate fracture of the tibia and a type I fracture of the fibula (less commonly a Salter-Harris type II). The injury starts on the lateral side of the ankle with the fibular injury and terminates medially (Fig. 31-64). Avulsion of the tip of the fibular epiphysis by the lateral ligaments is a less commonly seen equivalent to physeal separation. This distal epiphyseal fracture is differentiated from a normal fibular secondary ossification center by the clinical finding of point tenderness.

Pronation or Eversion and External Rotation

Pronation and external rotation fractures are caused by sliding or shear forces, and they usually produce physeal separation. Typically there is a Salter-Harris type II fracture of the distal tibia and a lateral tibial metaphyseal fragment (i.e., lateral Thurston-Holland fragment). The fibula demonstrates a transverse or short oblique fracture above the physis (Fig. 31-65). Displaced fractures result in lateral or posterolateral translation of the distal tibial fragment.

Supination and External Rotation

With the foot supinated, lateral rotation (external) forces produce a Salter-Harris type II fracture of the tibia. The distinguishing anatomic feature of this fracture is a medially based tibial metaphyseal fragment, with a spiral fracture line that starts at the level of the lateral physis. The fibula may have a juxtaphyseal spiral fracture that runs in a posterosuperior direction.

Supination and Plantar Flexion

Plantar-flexion injuries result in Salter-Harris type II physeal fractures with posterior displacement, although a type I separation sometimes occurs. The fracture is best visualized on a lateral radiograph. Typically, the fibula is not injured.

Epiphyseal Injuries

Salter-Harris type I fractures are frequently nondisplaced and are differentiated from ankle sprains by demonstrating point tenderness over the growth plate. This occurs frequently to the fibula and may go unrecognized when combined with tibial injuries because of a lack of displacement. Radiographs may show slight widening of the physis or tilting of the epiphysis. Type I fractures of the fibula can be treated with a below-knee walking cast for 3 to 4 weeks. Follow-up radiographs demonstrating periosteal new bone formation confirm the diagnosis. When significantly displaced, closed reduction is often stable, but occasionally, a smooth Kirschner wire should be placed across the physis to maintain the reduction. Type I fractures of the tibia occur only with external rotation or plantar-flexion forces and are seen in younger children.[31]

Salter-Harris type II fractures are common injuries of the distal tibia and usually are treated by closed reduction and casting. Like most epiphyseal fractures, healing is rapid, and anatomic reduction is not vital for a good result, especially for small degrees of posterior displacement. However, in the adolescent, residual valgus deformity greater than 5 degrees is not acceptable because it cannot sufficiently remodel. This injury occasionally results in premature growth plate closure, although usually only in the adolescent already near the completion of growth. The distal tibia provides approximately ⅛ in (3 mm) of longitudinal growth per year. If significant growth remains, epiphysiodesis of the fibula may be necessary to prevent relative overgrowth.

Salter-Harris type III and IV fractures are most

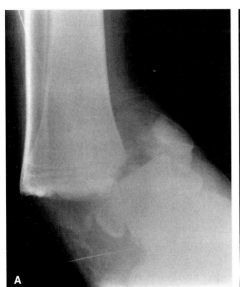
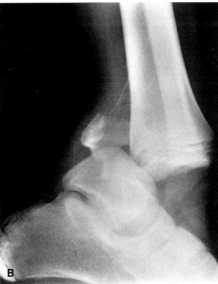
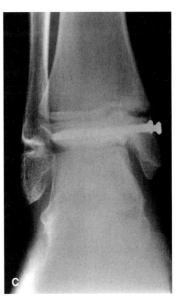

FIGURE 31-64.   Supination-inversion ankle fracture. (**A**) The anteroposterior (AP) radiograph demonstrates a bimalleolar ankle fracture with ankle dislocation. There is a Salter I fracture of the distal fibula and a Salter III fracture of the medial tibial epiphysis. (**B**) Lateral projection. (**C**) An AP radiograph after open reduction and internal fixation. Transepiphyseal screws are used to avoid fixation crossing the growth plate. The joint surface is restored to anatomic alignment. No fixation was required for the fibula fracture. A smooth Kirschner wire can be placed across this physis if needed for ankle stability.

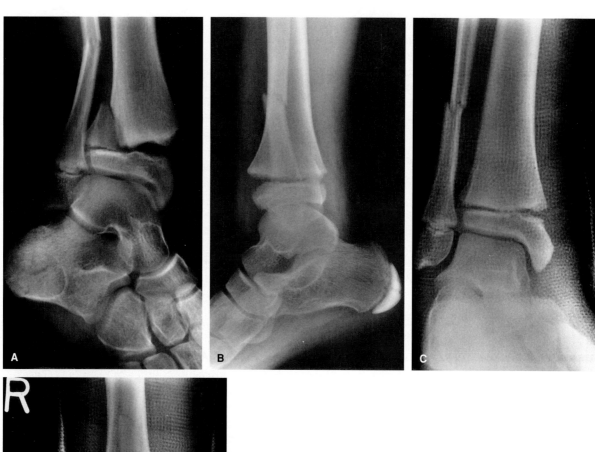

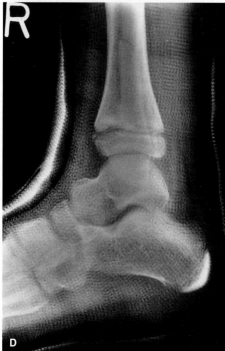

FIGURE 31-65. Pronation and external rotation ankle fracture. (**A**) The antero-posterior radiograph demonstrates a Salter-Harris II fracture of the distal tibia. The Thurston-Holland fragment is lateral. The fibular fracture is transverse and located well above the fibular physis. (**B**) Lateral projection of the same injury. (**C**) This fracture was treated with closed reduction and application of an above-knee cast. (**D**) A lateral radiograph demonstrates acceptable alignment. This fracture was successfully managed by closed reduction.

often caused by inversion (adduction) forces on the ankle, and open reduction and internal fixation are indicated for any residual displacement greater than 2 mm after closed realignment. If there is any vertical displacement, indicating physeal malalignment, anatomic reduction is imperative (Fig. 31-66). These fractures often produce growth disturbance, partly because of the crush component of the injury but most likely because of an imprecise reduction. Restoration of anatomic fragment position has reduced the expected incidence of partial growth arrest reported with these injuries.[95]

Transitional Fractures

Transitional fractures occur in the adolescent as a result of incomplete physeal closure. This physis is completely closed when girls are about 15 years of age

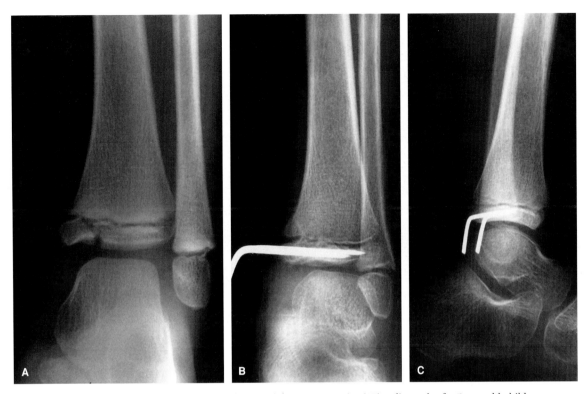

FIGURE 31-66. Distal tibial physeal injury. (**A**) Anteroposterior (AP) radiograph of a 5-year-old child who sustained a Salter-Harris IV fracture of the medial malleolus. This injury has a high risk for growth arrest unless anatomic alignment is restored. There is also a minimally displaced Salter-Harris I fracture of the fibular physis. (**B**) AP radiograph after reduction and stabilization with intraepiphyseal Kirschner wires. (**C**) Lateral radiograph. This fixation was supplemented with a below-knee cast.

and boys are 17 years of age. Closure begins centrally and spreads posteromedially, then anteromedially, and finally laterally. The anterolateral quadrant of the physis is last to close. The entire process requires about 18 months. The mechanism of injury involves external rotation of the foot.

The Tillaux fracture consists of an avulsion of the lateral distal tibial epiphysis by the anterior tibiofibular ligament and is a biplane fracture (Fig. 31-67). This is essentially a Salter-Harris type III fracture. The typical age for this injury is 12 to 14 years, corresponding with early physeal closure. Closed reduction is performed with internal rotation, and the quality of the reduction should be documented. CT scanning is helpful if plain radiographs are inconclusive. If more than minimal displacement remains, open reduction and anatomic internal fixation through an anterolateral approach is recommended. Fixation is accomplished with placement of cancellous screws, crossing the physis if necessary.

Triplane fracture is also caused by external rotation of the foot, and on anteroposterior radiographs, it appears as a Salter-Harris type III injury, but on the lateral projection, it looks like a type II fracture (i.e., posterior metaphyseal fragment). It is most often a two- or three-part fracture (Fig. 31-68).[173] Initial man-

agement of displaced fractures should consist of closed reduction with internal rotation and dorsiflexion of the foot. Confirmation of an acceptable position is recommended with a CT scan, because casting often obscures the fracture line detail. To ensure the best possible long-term outcome, open reduction is performed for fractures with greater than 2 mm of articular surface displacement.[48] The surgical approach entails fixation of the posteromedial fragment to the tibial shaft and securing the lateral epiphyseal fragment to the epiphysis (Fig. 31-69). Inadequate reduction leads to an external rotation deformity of the ankle and articular incongruity that can predispose the area to degenerative arthritis.

FOOT FRACTURES

Talus Fractures

Talus fractures are the result of forced dorsiflexion of the foot. The talus is composed of three parts: head, neck, and body. There is almost no periosteal covering of the talus, because three fifths of the surface is articular cartilage. The neck region is the primary site of vascular entrance to the talus. This is also the site of

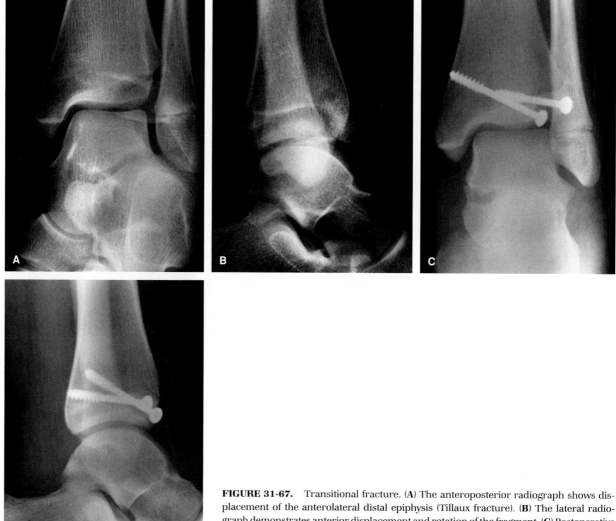

FIGURE 31-67. Transitional fracture. (**A**) The anteroposterior radiograph shows displacement of the anterolateral distal epiphysis (Tillaux fracture). (**B**) The lateral radiograph demonstrates anterior displacement and rotation of the fragment. (**C**) Postoperative x-ray film and open reduction and internal fixation with cancellous bone screws. (**D**) Lateral radiograph. In this instance, the screws can cross the physeal line because this injury occurs in an adolescent after the growth plate has begun physiologic closure.

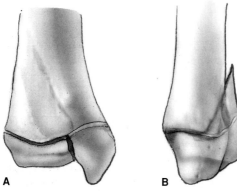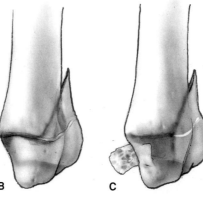

FIGURE 31-68. Triplane fracture. (**A**) On the anteroposterior radiograph, the fracture appears as a Salter-Harris III fracture of the distal tibial epiphysis. (**B**) On the lateral view, the fracture appears as a Salter-Harris II fracture of the distal tibia. (**C**) In the three-part triplane fracture, the anterolateral epiphyseal fragment is displaced as a separate fragment.

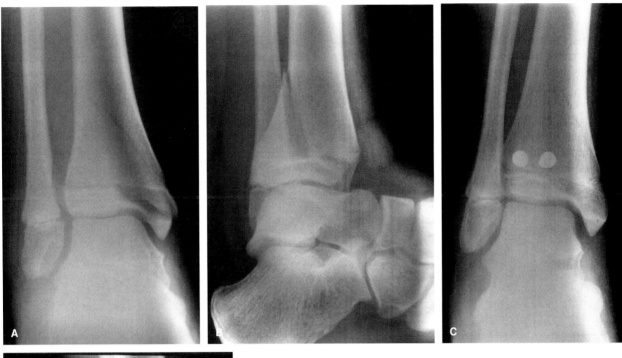

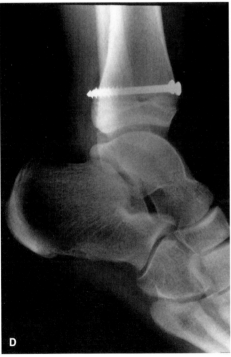

FIGURE 31-69. Two-part triplane fracture. (**A**) The anteroposterior (AP) radiograph shows a Salter-Harris III fracture. In this instance, the fracture line does not come out in the intraarticular portion but exits in the medial distal epiphysis. (**B**) The lateral radiograph shows what appears to be a Salter-Harris II fracture of the distal tibia. Despite closed manipulation, improvement in alignment could not be obtained, and open reduction and internal fixation were performed. (**C**) The AP radiograph shows anatomic alignment and placement of distal metaphyseal screws. (**D**) The lateral view shows reduction of the displaced fracture.

most fractures. Blood is supplied through the tarsal canal artery (i.e., branch of the posterior tibial artery), the dorsalis pedis, and the lateral tarsal artery. They supply the middle one third of the talus, the head and neck, and the lateral one third, respectively. The classification system for talar injuries is helpful in determining the prognosis:

Type I: minimally displaced fracture of the distal talar neck; the incidence of avascular necrosis is low.[108]

Type II: fracture of the proximal neck or body of the talus, also minimally displaced; the avascular necrosis rate is low.[108]

Type III: a displaced talar neck or body fracture; avascular necrosis is a frequent sequela.

Type IV: talar neck fracture combined with dislocation of the body fragment, resulting in avascular necrosis.

Although avascular necrosis of the talus is a dreaded result, it does not prevent healing of the fracture. Favorable outcome is determined more by the restoration of congruence of the ankle and subtalar joints than by the presence of avascular necrosis.

Fractures that are displaced less than 3 mm or angled less than 30 degrees can be managed by closed methods, with the foot casted in slight plantar flexion. This treatment regimen includes most type I and II talus fractures. Until healing is apparent on radiographs, a non–weight-bearing below-knee cast is used, typically for 6 weeks. Then a full–weight-bearing cast can be used. Open reduction is reserved for displaced fractures or if alignment does not improve after

closed manipulation. The anteromedial approach is preferred for fragment reduction, and small cancellous compression screws (3.5 or 4.0 mm) can be placed anterior to posterior or placed retrograde over a cannulated wire, depending on the location of the fracture (Fig. 31-70). Weight bearing is restricted until the fracture has healed.

Forced supination of the foot, as in a sprained ankle, may produce osteochondral fracture of the medial or lateral margin of the talar body. Medial lesions tend to be posteromedial, and lateral lesions tend to be anterolateral. Healing can occur if there is minimal

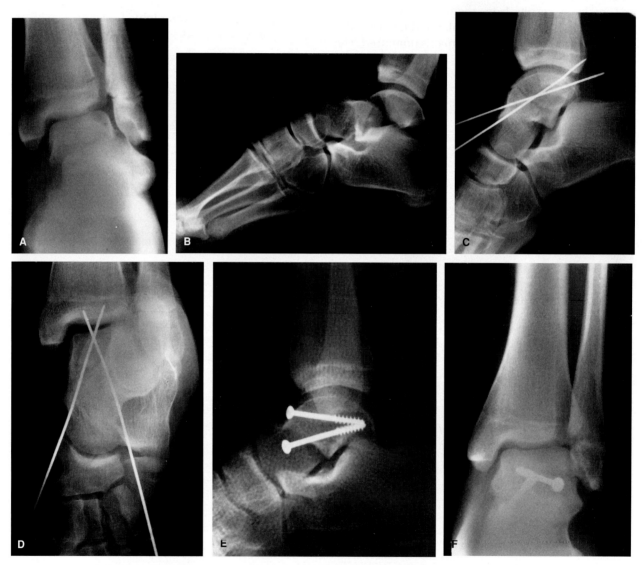

FIGURE 31-70. Talus fracture. **(A)** Anteroposterior (AP) radiograph of the ankle of a 13-year-old gymnast who injured her foot during a dismount. It appears that the head and neck of the talus are displaced laterally toward the fibula. **(B)** The lateral projection shows a type III talus fracture, with subluxation of the talonavicular joint. **(C)** The intraoperative film shows provisional fixation with Kirschner wires. The fracture is reduced with plantar flexion of the foot. **(D)** Another intraoperative AP view shows anatomic alignment of the talar neck with the body. The entry sites for the screws are in the nonarticular portion of the talar neck. **(E)** The postoperative film shows cancellous screw placement. **(F)** An AP radiograph shows restoration of the normal alignment of the ankle. Compared with the injury radiograph, there is no longer a prominence of the talar neck laterally.

displacement; otherwise, pinning of the fragment is suggested. If this is not possible, the loose fragment should be removed. This can usually be accomplished arthroscopically.

Lateral process fractures of the talus may occur with a twisting injury to the foot, and they are easily missed without close inspection of good-quality radiographs. The point of maximal tenderness is medial. Displaced fractures are intraarticular and should be repaired. CT scans may be needed to evaluate the extent of displacement.

Peritalar dislocations are extremely rare in children and are the result of violent twisting of the foot and ankle, as results from motor vehicle accidents. This is a dislocation of the subtalar and talonavicular joints while the tibiotalar joint remains uninjured. The direction is most commonly medial (i.e., clubfoot appearance) but can be lateral (i.e., flatfoot appearance) or even anterior or posterior. This injury is more likely to occur in the older adolescent and occasionally is seen in conjunction with a talar neck fracture.[45]

Calcaneus Fracture

The calcaneus is the most frequently fractured tarsal bone in children. The cortical margin is thin, and high instantaneous loads, as occur in falls from a height, produce fractures. Lawnmower injuries are another common mechanism, resulting in open calcaneal fractures in children.

The calcaneus has four articular surfaces: three subtalar and the calcaneocuboid joint. The posterior facet is the largest and supports the body of the talus. The anterior and middle facets support the head and neck of the talus. Although there are myriad fracture configurations, characteristic primary fracture lines have been described.[27] Shearing forces produce a sagittal split, dividing the calcaneus into medial and lateral fragments. Compression forces split the calcaneus into anterior and posterior pieces. As the anterolateral process of the talus is driven into the calcaneus, the lateral wall collapses (i.e., inverted Y-shaped pattern), and an anterolateral fragment is produced. The byproduct of crush injury is widening of the heel, with later soft tissue problems, such as peroneal tendon impingement.[109] Joint incongruity produces subtalar arthritis.

Most calcaneal fractures in children can be treated in a closed fashion, but accurate images are needed to evaluate joint congruity. The lateral radiograph shows loss of calcaneal height, suggesting intraarticular fracture. The Bohler angle is reduced, and the crucial angle does not reflect the shape of the overlying lateral process of the talus. A Broden view of the foot is taken with the leg internally rotated 30 to 40 degrees and the beam centered over the lateral

malleolus.[97] This projection details the posterior facet and is most helpful during the intraoperative assessment of joint congruity. However, the CT scan has evolved as the best method for imaging calcaneal fractures and is necessary for the complete assessment of displaced fractures. A classification scheme is based on the CT findings.[149]

Type I: nondisplaced intraarticular fractures (<2-mm gap) despite the number of fracture lines

Type II: two-part or split fractures of the posterior facet, with minimal comminution

Type III: three-part fractures that have a centrally depressed portion of the posterior facet

Type IV: highly comminuted fractures, with at least four parts

Extraarticular fractures occur more often in younger children (75% of cases), and in adolescents older than 14 years of age, more than one half of calcaneal fractures are intraarticular.[150] Extraarticular fractures have a good prognosis and are treated with casting and progressive weight bearing. Displaced intraarticular fractures are best managed by open reduction and internal fixation. The recommended approach is lateral through a long L-shaped incision, lifting the peroneal tendons within their sheath and protecting the sural nerve. The lateral wall of the calcaneus is folded down to reveal the medial side, allowing elevation of depressed central fragments. Internal fixation of the posterior facet is accomplished by placing subchondral cancellous screws into the medial sustentaculum, and then buttressing the lateral wall with an H-shaped or Y-shaped plate (Fig. 31-71). Excessive comminution of the sustentaculum precludes this type of surgery.[46] Long-term clinical results show good results after repair of most type II and III injuries but uniformly poor outcomes in type IV fractures. Results deteriorate as the number of articular fragments increase.[149] Open fractures, usually the result of lawn mower accidents, are occasionally seen. Preservation of the heel pad is vital to a good long-term outcome.

Metatarsal Fractures

Metatarsal fractures are common, and the second through fourth metatarsals are the most frequently injured. The base of the fifth metatarsal is also a common site for avulsion fractures and can be mistaken for an ankle sprain. This is also the site of a secondary ossification center. Avulsion fractures must be differentiated from a transverse metaphyseal-diaphyseal fractures (Jones), because they require prolonged casting, and healing must be verified before discharge.

The mechanism of injury is usually direct trauma or crush to the foot, and the associated swelling can be significant. Compartment syndrome can occur in

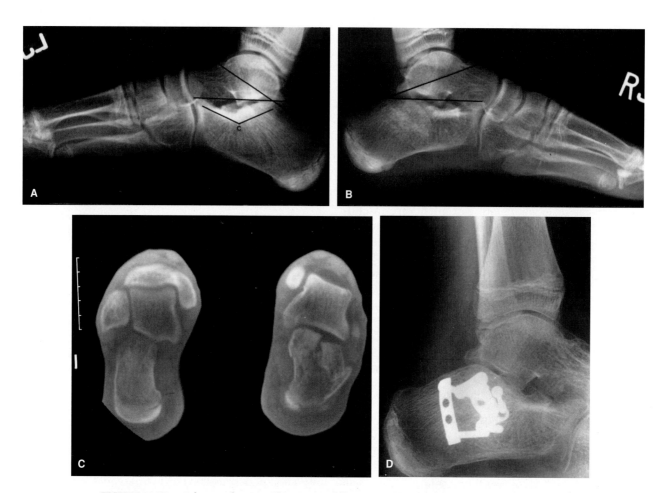

FIGURE 31-71. Calcaneus fracture. This 12-year-old boy injured both feet after jumping off a second-story deck. (**A**) The lateral radiograph of his left foot reveals a minimal fracture of the body of the calcaneus. The Bohler angle is subtended by a line connecting the anterior process of the calcaneus to the highest part of the posterior articular surface, intersecting a line along the most superior point of the calcaneal tuberosity. This angle normally is 25 to 40 degrees and usually is compared with the contralateral side. The crucial angle (c) is directly related to the shape of the overlying lateral process of the talus. In axial compression fractures, the lateral process is driven into the calcaneus, and the crucial angle is distorted. (**B**) The radiograph of the more significantly injured right calcaneus shows flattening of the calcaneus, reduction in the Bohler angle, and flattening of the crucial angle. (**C**) The computed tomography scan demonstrates displacement of the posterior facet of the calcaneus, with impaction of the lateral fragment and widening of the body of the calcaneus. The lateral wall is fractured. This injury should be treated with open reduction and internal fixation. (**D**) After reduction of the posterior facet, a cancellous bone screw is placed through the lateral joint fragment into the sustentacular fragment, securing the subtalar reduction. The lateral wall can be buttressed with a contoured Y-shaped plate or small H-shaped plate. The Bohler angle and the height of the calcaneus are restored.

the foot, involving any of the four zones: medial (i.e., abductor hallucis), central (i.e., flexor brevis, lumbricals, quadratus), lateral, and interosseous. Fasciotomy is indicated to preserve viability of the foot and should be performed as early as the problem is recognized. Fasciotomy is accomplished through a dorsal approach, combined with a second medial incision to release the deep plantar compartments.

The indications for operative treatment include open fractures, significant plantar displacement of the metatarsal head, and displaced intraarticular fractures. Kirschner wire fixation is usually adequate, but the pinning technique requires securing the metatar-

sal-phalangeal joint in a reduced position. If this is not done, extension contracture of the metatarsal-phalangeal joint ensues with the development of a painful, prominent metatarsal head. Kirschner wires are kept in place for 3 to 4 weeks, followed by a weight-bearing below-knee cast. Metatarsal fractures associated with tarsometatarsal dislocation usually are stabilized.

Tarsometatarsal joint injuries usually are seen in the adolescent, although some have described subtle displacements in young children who have jumped from a height (e.g., bunk bed injury).[87] The most common mechanism of injury is forced plantar flexion of the forefoot, usually combined with rotation. Direct

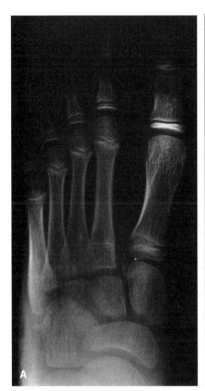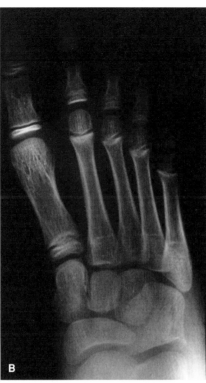

FIGURE 31-72. Tarsal-metatarsal joint injury. This 4-year-old girl had a file cabinet land on the dorsum of her foot. (**A**) There is widening between the first and second metatarsals, and a small fragment of bone is seen in the space. This suggests a partial incongruity, with lateral subluxation of the metatarsals. (**B**) The contralateral foot shows a normal relation of the tarsal-metatarsal joint.

trauma, as in a crushing injury, may also produce this fracture-dislocation (Fig. 31-72). Multiple metatarsal fractures and midtarsal injuries are seen if the injury was the result of high-energy impact (Fig. 31-73). The base of the second metatarsal is almost always fractured (75% of cases), and this is an indication of tarso-metatarsal joint injury.[175,180] This lesion is easily overlooked, and comparison films of the uninjured other foot are sometimes necessary. The dislocation may be in any direction, and soft tissue damage with vascular impairment or compartment syndrome can complicate management. Closed reduction is usually possi-

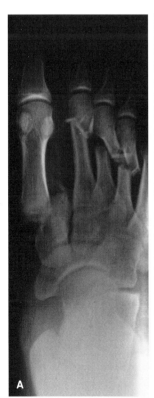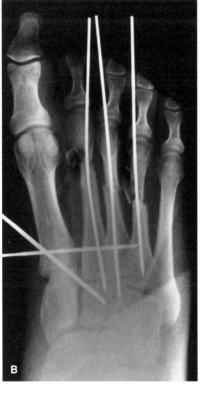

FIGURE 31-73. Tarsal-metatarsal displacement. (**A**) The anteroposterior (AP) projection of the foot in a 14-year-old boy who sustained a plantar flexion injury while involved in a motor vehicle accident. There is complete dislocation of the first metatarsal-cuneiform joint and medial displacement. There are fractures of the second, third, and fourth metatarsal shafts. The ipsilateral tibial fracture was treated with intramedullary fixation. The swelling in the foot was attributed to his tibial shaft injury, and diagnosis of the foot injury was delayed. (**B**) The postoperative AP radiograph demonstrates reduction and pinning of the fracture-dislocation.

ble, and further stability is added by percutaneous pin fixation, especially if there are associated problems. The key to aligning the midfoot is the reduction of the second metatarsal, which should be obtained initially. Open reduction is occasionally required and is approached with a dorsal incision centered between the first and second rays.

References

1. Abraham E, Powers T, Witt P, et al. Experimental hyperextension supracondylar fractures in monkeys. Clin Orthop 1982;171:309.

2. Akbarnia B, Silberstien M, et al. Arthrography in the diagnosis of fractures of the distal end of the humerus in children. J Bone Joint Surg [Am] 1986;68:599.

3. Allman F. Fractures and ligamentous injuries of the clavicle and its articulation. J Bone Joint Surg [Am] 1967;49:774.

4. Alonso J, Horowitz M. Use of the AO/ASIF external fixator in children. J Pediatr Orthop 1987;7:594.

5. Arnold J, Nasca R, Nelson C. Supracondylar fractures of the humerus. J Bone Joint Surg [Am] 1977;59:589.

6. Aronson D, Singer R, Higgins R. Skeletal traction for fractures of the femoral shaft in children. J Bone Joint Surg [Am] 1987;69:1435.

7. Aronson J, Garvin K, Seibert J, et al. Efficiency of the bone scan for occult limping toddlers. J Pediatr Orthop 1992;12:38.

8. Aronson J, Tursky E. External fixation of femur fractures in children. J Pediatr Orthop 1992;12:157.

9. Bado J. The Monteggia lesion. Clin Orthop 1967;50:71.

10. Baxter M, Wiley J. Fractures of the proximal humeral epiphysis. Their influence on humeral growth. J Bone Joint Surg [Br] 1986;68:570.

11. Beaty J, Austin S, Warner W, et al. Interlocking intramedullary nailing of femoral shaft fractures in adolescents: preliminary results and complications. J Pediatr Orthop 1994;14:178.

12. Bednar D, Grandwilewski W. Complications of forearm plate removal. Can J Surg 1992;35:428.

13. Bernstein S, McKeever P, Bernstein L. Percutaneous reduction of displaced radial neck fractures in children. J Pediatr Orthop 1993;13:85.

14. Bertin K, Goble E. Ligament injuries associated with physeal fractures about the knee. Clin Orthop 1983;177:188.

15. Biyani A, Gupta S, Sharma J. Determination of medial epicondylar epiphyseal angle for supracondylar humeral fractures in children. J Pediatr Orthop 1993;13:94.

16. Blick S, Brumback R, et al. Early prophylactic bone grafting of high-energy tibial fractures. Clin Orthop 1989;240:21.

17. Bohn W, Durbin R. Ipsilateral fractures of the femur and tibia in children and adolescents. J Bone Joint Surg [Am] 1991;73:429.

18. Bonnemaison M, Henderson E. Traumatic anterior dislocation of the hip with acute common femoral occlusion in a child. J Bone Joint Surg [Am] 1968;50:753.

19. Bourne R, Rorabeck C. Compartment syndromes of the lower leg. Clin Orthop 1989;240:97.

20. Bucholz R, Ezaki M, Ogden J. Injury to the acetabular triradiate physeal cartilage. J Bone Joint Surg [Am] 1982;64:600.

21. Buckley S, Smith G, et al. Open fractures of the tibia in children. J Bone Joint Surg [Am] 1990;72:1462.

22. Burkhart S, Peterson H. Fractures of the proximal tibial epiphysis. J Bone Joint Surg [Am] 1979;61:996.

23. Camp J, Ishizue K, Gomez M, et al. Alteration of Baumann's angle by humeral position: implication for treatment of supracondylar humerus fractures. J Pediatr Orthop 1993;13:521.

24. Canale S, Bourland W. Fracture of the femoral neck and intertrochanteric region of the femur in children. J Bone Joint Surg [Am] 1977;59:431.

25. Carlioz H, Abols Y. Posterior dislocation of the elbow in children. J Pediatr Orthop 1984;4:8.

26. Carlson W, Wenger D. A mapping method to prepare for surgical excision of a partial physeal arrest. J Pediatr Orthop 1984;4:232.

27. Carr J. Mechanism and pathoanatomy of the intraarticular calcaneal fracture. Clin Orthop 1993;290:36.

28. Chess D, Hyndman J, Leahey J, et al. Short arm plaster cast for distal pediatric forearm fractures. J Pediatr Orthop 1994;14:211.

29. Chung S. The arterial supply of the developing proximal end of the human femur. J Bone Joint Surg [Am] 1976;58:961.

30. Clanton T, DeLee J, Sanders B, et al. Knee ligament injuries in children. J Bone Joint Surg [Am] 1979;61:1195.

31. Cooperman D, Speigel P, Laros G. Epiphyseal fractures of the distal ends of the tibia and fibula. A retrospective review of 237 cases in children. J Bone Joint Surg [Am] 1978;60:1046.

32. Cramer K, Devito D, Green N. Comparison of closed reduction and percutaneous pinning versus open reduction and percutaneous pinning in displaced supracondylar fractures of the humerus in children. J Orthop Trauma 1992;6:407.

33. Cramer K, Green N, Devito D. Incidence of anterior interosseous nerve palsy in supracondylar humerus fractures in children. J Pediatr Orthop 1993;13:502.

34. Creasman C, Zaleske D, Ehrlich M. Analyzing forearm fractures in children: the more subtle signs of impending problems. Clin Orthop 1984;188:40.

35. Currey J, Butler G. The mechanical properties of bone tissue in children. J Bone Joint Surg [Am] 1975;57:810.

36. Curtis R. Operative management of children's fractures of the shoulder region. Orthop Clin North Am 1990;21:315.

37. Dameron T, Reibel D. Fractures involving the proximal humeral epiphyseal plate. J Bone Joint Surg [Am] 1969;51:289.

38. Davison B, Weinstein S. Hip fractures in children: a long term follow-up study. J Pediatr Orthop 1992;12:335.

39. DeLee J, Wilkins K, Rogers L, et al. Fracture separation of the distal humeral epiphysis. J Bone Joint Surg [Am] 1980;62:46.

40. Deluca P, Lindsey R, Ruwe P. Refracture of bones of the forearm after the removal of compression plates. J Bone Joint Surg [Am] 1988;70:1372.

41. Denham R, Dingley A. Epiphyseal separation of the medial end of the clavicle. J Bone Joint Surg [Am] 1967;49:1179.

42. Dhillon K, Sengupta S, Singh B. Delayed management of fracture of the lateral humeral condyle in children. Acta Orthop Scand 1988;59:419.

43. Dias J, Johnson G, et al. Management of severely displaced medial epicondyle fractures. J Orthop Trauma 1987;1:59.

44. Dias L, Tachdjian M. Physeal fractures of the ankle in children. Clin Orthop 1978;136:230.

45. Dimentberg R, Rosman M. Peritalar dislocations in children. J Pediatr Orthop 1993;13:89.

46. Eastwood D, Langkamer V, Atkins R. Intra-articular fractures of the calcaneum. J Bone Joint Surg [Br] 1993;75:189.

47. Epstein H. Traumatic dislocations of the hip. Clin Orthop 1973;92:116.

48. Ertl J, Barrack R, Alexander A, et al. Triplane fracture of the distal tibial epiphysis. J Bone Joint Surg [Am] 1988;70:967.

49. Evans E. Fractures of the radius and ulna. J Bone Joint Surg [Br] 1951;33:548.

50. Flynn J, Richards J. Non-union of minimally displaced fractures of the lateral condyle of the humerus in children. J Bone Joint Surg [Am] 1971;57:1086.

51. Flynn J, Richards J, Salzman R. Prevention and treatment of non-union of slightly displaced fractures of the lateral humeral condyle in children. J Bone Joint Surg [Am] 1975;57:1087.

52. Frassica F, Sim F, Staeheli J, et al. Dislocation of the knee. Clin Orthop 1991;263:200.

53. Friberg K. Remodeling after distal forearm fractures in children. Acta Orthop Scand 1979;50:537.

54. Friedman R, Jupiter J. Vascular injuries and closed extremity fractures in children. Clin Orthop 1984;188:112.

55. Fry K, Hoffer M, Brink J. Femoral shaft fractures in brain injured children. J Trauma 1976;16:371.

56. Garn S, Silverman F, Hertzog K. Lines and bands of increased density: their implication to growth and development. Med Radiogr Photogr 1968;44:58.

57. Gartland J. Management of supracondylar fractures in children. Surg Gynecol Obstet 1959;109:145.

58. Gershuni D, Hargens A, Lee YF, et al. The questionable significance of hip joint tamponade in producing osteonecrosis in Legg-Calve-Perthes syndrome. J Pediatr Orthop 1983;3:230.

59. Gibbons C, Woods D, Pailthorpe C, et al. The management of isolated distal radius fractures in children. J Pediatr Orthop 1994;14:207.

60. Gratz R. Accidental injury in childhood: a literature review on pediatric trauma. J Trauma 1979;19:551.

61. Green N, Allen B. Vascular injuries associated with dislocation of the knee. J Bone Joint Surg [Am] 1977;59:236.

62. Gregory R, Cubison T, Pinder I, et al. External fixation of lower limb fractures in children. J Trauma 1992;33:691.

63. Grieff J, Bergmann F. Growth disturbance following fracture of the tibia in children. Acta Orthop Scand 1980;51:315.

64. Griffin P. Supracondylar fractures of the humerus. Pediatr Clin North Am 1975;22:477.

65. Grimard G, Labelle H, Girard P, et al. Treatment of displaced supracondylar fractures of the humerus in children: a prospective and controlled clinical trial. Orthop Trans 1992: 228.

66. Gronkvist H, Hirsch G, Johansson L. Fracture of the anterior tibial spine in children. J Pediatr Orthop 1984;4:465.

67. Gross R, Stranger M. Causative factors responsible for femoral fractures in infants and young children. J Pediatr Orthop 1983;3:572.

68. Gupta R, Danielson L. Dorsally angulated solitary metaphyseal greenstick fractures in the distal radius. J Pediatr Orthop 1990;10:90.

69. Gustillo R, Mendoza R, Williams D. Problems in the management of type III (severe) open fractures: a new classification. J Trauma 1984;24:742.

70. Hansen B, Grieff J. Fractures of the tibia in children. Acta Orthop Scand 1976;47:448.

71. Hardacre J, Nahigian S, et al. Fractures of the lateral condyle of the humerus in children. J Bone Joint Surg [Am] 1971;53:1083.

72. Hardegger F, Simpson L, Weber B. The operative treatment of scapular fractures. J Bone Joint Surg [Br] 1984;66:725.

73. Heeg M, Klassen H, Visser J. Acetabular fractures in children and adolescents. J Bone Joint Surg [Br] 1989;71:418.

74. Heeg M, Klassen H, Visser J. Injuries of the acetabular triradiate cartilage and sacroiliac joint. J Bone Joint Surg [Br] 1988;70:34.

75. Henderson O, Morrissy R, Gerdes M, et al. Early casting of femoral shaft fractures in children. J Pediatr Orthop 1984;4:16.

76. Hennrikus W, Kasser J, Rand F. The function of the quadriceps muscle after a fracture of the femur in patients who are less than seventeen years old. J Bone Joint Surg [Am] 1993;75:508.

77. Herndon W, Mahnken R, Yngve D, et al. Management of femoral shaft fractures in the adolescent. J Pediatr Orthop 1989;9:29.

78. Hoelen M, Burgers A, Rozing P. Prognosis of primary anterior shoulder dislocation in young adults. Arch Orthop Trauma Surg 1990;110:51.

79. Hope P, Cole W. Open fractures of the tibia in children. J Bone Joint Surg [Br] 1992;74:546.

80. Houghton G, Acroyd C. Sleeve fractures of the patella in children. J Bone Joint Surg [Br] 1979;61:165.

81. Hovelius L. Anterior dislocation of the shoulder in teenagers and young adults. J Bone Joint Surg [Am] 1987;69:393.

82. Hynes D, O'Brien T. Growth disturbance lines after injury of the distal tibial physis: their significance in prognosis. J Bone Joint Surg [Br] 1988;70:231.

83. Irani R, Nicholson J, Chung S. Long-term results in the treatment of femoral shaft fractures in young children by immediate fit spica immobilization. J Bone Joint Surg [Am] 1976;58:945.

84. Jakob R, Fowles J, Rang M, et al. Observations concerning fractures of the lateral humeral condyle in children. J Bone Joint Surg [Br] 1975;57:430.

85. Jarvis J, D'Astous J. The pediatric T-supracondylar fracture. J Pediatr Orthop 1984;4:697.

86. Jeffrey C. Nonunion of the epiphysis of the lateral condyle of the humerus. J Bone Joint Surg [Br] 1958;40:396.

87. Johnson G. Pediatric Lisfranc injury: "bunk bed" fracture. Am J Radiol 1981;137:1041.

88. Jordan S, Alonso J, Cook F. The etiology of valgus angulation after metaphyseal fracture of the tibia in children. J Pediatr Orthop 1987;7:450.

89. Josefsson P, Danielsson J. Epicondylar elbow fracture in children: 35 year follow-up of 56 unreduced cases. Acta Orthop Scand 1986;57:313.

90. Kasser J. Forearm fractures. In: MacEwen G, Kasser J, Heinrich S, eds. Children's fractures: a practical approach to assessment and treatment. Baltimore: Williams & Wilkins, 1993:165.

91. Kay S, Smith C, Oppenheim W. Both-bone midshaft forearm fractures in children. J Pediatr Orthop 1986;6:306.

92. King J, Diefendorf D, et al. Analysis of 429 fractures in 189 battered children. J Pediatr Orthop 1988;8:585.

93. Kirby R, Winquist R, Hansen S. Femoral shaft fractures in adolescents: a comparison between traction plus cast treatment and closed intramedullary nailing. J Pediatr Orthop 1981;1:193.

94. Kirschenbaum D, Albert M, Robertson W, et al. Complex femur fractures in children: treatment with external fixation. J Pediatr Orthop 1990;10:588.

95. Kling T, Bright R, Hensinger R. Distal tibial physeal fractures in children. J Bone Joint Surg [Am] 1984;66:647.

96. Kohler R, Trillaud J. Fracture and fracture separation of the proximal humerus in children. J Pediatr Orthop 1983;3:326.

97. Koval K, Sanders R. The radiologic evaluation of calcaneal fractures. Clin Orthop 1993;290:41.

98. Kregor P, Song K, Routt M, et al. Plate fixation of femoral shaft fractures in multiply injured children. J Bone Joint Surg [Am] 1993;75:1774.

99. Kurer M, Regan M. Completely displaced supracondylar fracture of the humerus in children: a review of 1708 cases. Clin Orthop 1990;256:205.

100. Lam S. Fractures of the neck of the femur in children. J Bone Joint Surg [Am] 1971;53:1165.

101. Langenskiold A. Surgical treatment of partial closure of the growth plate. J Pediatr Orthop 1981;1:3.

102. Lascombes P, Prevot J, Ligier J. Elastic stable intramedullary nailing in forearm shaft fractures in children: 85 cases. J Pediatr Orthop 1990;10:167.

103. Lee B, Esterbai J, Das M. Fracture of the distal radial epiphysis. Clin Orthop 1984;185:90.

104. Letournel E, Judet R. Fractures of the acetabulum. Berlin: Springer-Verlag, 1981.

105. Letts M, Locht R, Wilens J. Monteggia fracture-dislocations in children. J Bone Joint Surg [Br] 1985;67:724.

106. Letts M, Rowhani N. Galeazzi-equivalent injuries of the wrist in children. J Pediatr Orthop 1993;13:561.

107. Letts M, Vincent N, Gouw G. The "floating knee" in children. J Bone Joint Surg [Br] 1986;68:442.

108. Letts R, Gibeault D. Fractures of the neck of the talus in children. Foot Ankle 1980;1:74.

109. Leung K, Yuen K, Chan W. Operative treatment of displaced intra-articular fractures of the calcaneum. J Bone Joint Surg [Br] 1993;75:196.

110. Ligier J, Metaizeau J, et al. Elastic stable intramedullary nailing of femoral shaft fractures in children. J Bone Joint Surg [Br] 1988;70:74.

111. Mabrey J, Fitch R. Plastic deformation in pediatric fractures. J Pediatr Orthop 1989;9:310.

112. Mann D, Rajmaira S. Distribution of physeal and nonphyseal fractures in 2,650 long-bone fractures in children aged 0–16 years. J Pediatr Orthop 1990;10:713.

113. Mann D, Weddington J, Davenport K. Closed Ender nailing of femoral shaft fractures in adolescents. J Pediatr Orthop 1986;6:651.

114. Manske D, Szabo R. The operative treatment of mid-shaft clavicular non-unions. J Bone Joint Surg [Am] 1985;67:1367.

115. Martinez A, Carroll N, Sarwark J, et al. Femoral shaft fractures in children treated with early spica cast. J Pediatr Orthop 1991;11:712.

116. Marzo J, d'Amato C, Strong M, et al. Usefulness and accuracy of arthrography in management of lateral humeral condyle fractures in children. J Pediatr Orthop 1990;10:317.

117. Masada K, Kawai H, Kawabata H, et al. Osteosynthesis for old, established non-union of the lateral condyle of the humerus. J Bone Joint Surg [Am] 1990;72:32.

118. Matta J, Saucedo T. Internal fixation of pelvic ring fractures. Clin Orthop 1989;242:83.

119. McBryde A, Blake R. The floating knee—ipsilateral fractures of the femur and tibia. J Bone Joint Surg [Am] 1974;56:1309.

120. McIntyre R, Bensard D, Moore E, et al. Pelvic fracture geometry predicts risk of life-threatening hemorrhage in children. J Trauma 1993;35:423.

121. Meyers M. Isolated avulsions of the tibial attachment of the posterior cruciate ligament. J Bone Joint Surg [Am] 1975;57:669.

122. Meyers M, McKeever F. Fracture of the intercondylar eminence of the tibia. J Bone Joint Surg [Am] 1959;41:209.

123. Millis M, Singer I, Hall J. Supracondylar fracture of the humerus in children: further experience with a study in orthopedic decision making. Clin Orthop 1984;188:90.

124. Mintzer C, Waters P, Brown D, et al. Percutaneous pinning in the treatment of displaced lateral condyle fractures. J Pediatr Orthop 1994;14:462.

125. Mizuta T, Benson W, Foster B. Statistical analysis of the incidence of physeal injuries. J Pediatr Orthop 1987; 7:518.

126. Morrissy R. Hip fractures in children. Clin Orthop 1980; 152:202.

127. Mubarak S, Carroll N. Volkmann's contracture in children: etiology and prevention. J Bone Joint Surg [Br] 1979;61:285.

128. Neer C, Horwitz B. Fractures of the proximal humeral epiphyseal plate. Clin Orthop 1965;41:24.

129. Newton P, Mubarak S. Financial aspects of femoral shaft fracture treatment in children and adolescents. J Pediatr Orthop 1994;14:508.

130. Offierski C. Traumatic dislocation of the hip in children. J Bone Joint Surg [Br] 1981;63:194.

131. Ogden J. Changing patterns of proximal femoral vascularity. J Bone Joint Surg [Am] 1974;56:941.

132. Olney B, Menelaus M. Monteggia and equivalent lesions in childhood. J Pediatr Orthop 1986;6:58.

133. Palmer E, Niemann K, Vesely D, et al. Supracondylar fracture of the humerus in children. J Bone Joint Surg [Am] 1978;60:653.

134. Patterson R. Treatment of displaced transverse fractures of the neck of the radius in children. J Bone Joint Surg 1934;16:695.

135. Patzakis M, Wilkins J. Factors influencing infection rate in open fracture wounds. Clin Orthop 1989;243:36.

136. Pirone A, Graham H, Krajbich J. Management of displaced extension-type supracondylar fractures of the humerus in children. J Bone Joint Surg [Am] 1988;70:641.

137. Price C, Scott D, et al. Malunited forearm fractures in children. J Pediatr Orthop 1990;10:705.

138. Raney E, Ogden J, Grogan D. Premature greater trochanteric epiphysiodesis secondary to intramedullary femoral rodding. J Pediatr Orthop 1993;13:516.

139. Rang M. The growth plate and its disorders. Baltimore: Williams & Wilkins, 1969.

140. Ratliff A. Fractures of the neck of the femur in children. J Bone Joint Surg [Br] 1962;44:528.

141. Reed M. Pelvic fractures in children. J Can Assoc Radiol 1976;27:255.

142. Reeves R, Ballard R, Hughes J. Internal fixation versus traction and casting of adolescent femoral shaft fractures. J Pediatr Orthop 1990;10:592.

143. Riseborough E, Barrett I, Shapiro F. Growth disturbances following distal femoral physeal fracture-separations. J Bone Joint Surg [Am] 1983;65:885.

144. Robert M, Khouri N, Carlioz H, et al. Fractures of the proximal tibial metaphysis in children. J Pediatr Orthop 1987;7:444.

145. Rowland S, Burkhart S. Tension band wiring of olecranon fractures. Clin Orthop 1992;277:238.

146. Roye D, Bini S, Infosino A. Late surgical treatment of lateral condylar fractures in children. J Pediatr Orthop 1991;11:195.

147. Salter R, Best T. The pathogenesis and prevention of valgus deformity following fractures of the proximal metaphyseal region of the tibia in children. J Bone Joint Surg [Am] 1973;55:1324.

148. Salter R, Harris W. Injuries involving the epiphyseal plate. J Bone Joint Surg [Am] 1963;45:587.

149. Sanders R, Fortin P, DiPasquale T, et al. Operative treatment in 120 displaced intraarticular calcaneal fractures. Clin Orthop 1993;290:87.

150. Schmidt T, Weiner D. Calcaneal fractures in children. Clin Orthop 1982;171:150.

151. Scuderi G, Bronson M. Triradiate cartilage injury. Clin Orthop 1987;217:179.

152. Shannak A. Tibial fractures in children: follow-up study. J Pediatr Orthop 1988;8:306.

153. Shaw B, Kasser J, Emans J, et al. Management of vascular injuries in displaced supracondylar humerus fractures without arteriography. J Orthop Trauma 1990;4:25.

154. Shelton W, Canale S. Fractures of the tibia through the proximal tibial epiphyseal cartilage. J Bone Joint Surg [Am] 1979;61:167.

155. Sherk H, Probst C. Fractures of the proximal humeral epiphysis. Orthop Clin North Am 1975;6:401.

156. Smith J. Knee instability after fractures of the intercondylar eminence of the tibia. J Pediatr Orthop 1984;4:462.

157. Spiegel P, Vander Schilden J. Minimal internal and external fixation in the treatment of open tibial fractures. Clin Orthop 1983;178:96.

158. Staheli L. Fractures of the shaft of the femur. In: Rockwood C, Wilkins K, King R, eds. Fractures in children. Philadelphia: JB Lippincott, 1984:845.

159. Staheli L. Femoral and tibial growth following fracture. Clin Orthop 1967;55:159.

160. Stanford J, Evans W, Morse T. Pediatric arterial injuries. J Vasc Dis 1976;27:1.

161. Stanitski C, Harvell J, Fu F. Observations on acute knee hemar-

throsis in children and adolescents. J Pediatr Orthop 1993;13:506.

162. Stephens M, Hsu L, Leong J. Leg length discrepancy after femoral shaft fractures in children. J Bone Joint Surg [Br] 1989;71:615.

163. Swiontkowski M, Winquist R. Displaced hip fractures in children and adolescents. J Trauma 1986;26:384.

164. Taft T, Wilson F, Oglesby J. Dislocation of the acromioclavicular joint: an end result study. J Bone Joint Surg [Am] 1987;69:1045.

165. Tarr R, Garfinkel A, Sarmiento A. The effects of angular and rotational deformities of both bones of the forearm: an in vitro study. J Bone Joint Surg [Am] 1984;66:65.

166. Theodorou S, Ierodiaconou M, Mitsou A. Obstetrical fracture-separation of the upper femoral epiphysis. Acta Orthop Scand 1982;53:239.

167. Thomas I, Gregg P, Walder D. Intra-osseous phlebography and intramedullary pressure in the rabbit femur. J Bone Joint Surg [Br] 1982;64:239.

168. Thonell S, Mortensson W, Thomasson B. Prediction of the stability of minimally displaced fractures of the lateral humeral condyle. Acta Radiol 1988;29:367.

169. Tibone J, Sellers R, Tonino P. Strength testing after third-degree acromioclavicular dislocations. Am J Sports Med 1992;20:328.

170. Tolo V. External fixation in multiply injured children. Orthop Clin North Am 1990;21:393.

171. Tredwell S, et al. Pattern of forearm fractures in children. J Pediatr Orthop 1984;4:604.

172. Van Vugt A, Severijen R, Festen C. Fractures of the lateral humeral condyle in children: late results. Arch Orthop Trauma Surg 1988;107:206.

173. Von Laer L. Classification, diagnosis, and treatment of transi-tional fractures of the distal part of the tibia. J Bone Joint Surg [Am] 1985;67:687.

174. Voto S, Weiner D, Leighley B. Redisplacement after closed reduction of forearm fractures in children. J Pediatr Orthop 1990;10:79.

175. Vuori J, Aro H. Lisfranc joint injuries: trauma mechanisms and associated injuries. J Trauma 1993;35:40.

176. Walsh H, McLaren C. Galeazzi fractures in children. J Bone Joint Surg [Br] 1987;69:730.

177. Walsh W, Peterson D, et al. Shoulder strength following acromioclavicular injury. Am J Sports Med 1985;13:153.

178. Ward W, Levy J, Kaye A. Compression plating for child and adolescent femur fractures. J Pediatr Orthop 1992;12:626.

179. Watts H. Fractures of the pelvis in children. Orthop Clin North Am 1976;7:615.

180. Wiley J. Tarso-metatarsal joint injuries in children. J Pediatr Orthop 1981;1:255.

181. Wiley J, Galey J. Monteggia injuries in children. J Bone Joint Surg [Br] 1985;67:728.

182. Winquist R, Hansen S, Clawson D. Closed intramedullary nailing of femoral fractures. J Bone Joint Surg [Am] 1984;66:529.

183. Wood D, Hoffer M. Tibial fractures in head injured children. J Trauma 1987;27:65.

184. Woods G, Tullos H. Elbow instability and medial epicondyle fractures. Am J Sports Med 1977;5:23.

185. Younger A, Tredwell S, Mackenzie W. Accurate prediction of outcome after pediatric forearm fracture. J Pediatr Orthop 1994;14:200.

186. Zionts L, MacEwen G. Spontaneous improvement of post-traumatic tibia valga. J Bone Joint Surg [Am] 1986;68:680.

187. Zionts L, McKellop H, Hathaway R. Torsional strength of pin configurations used to fix supracondylar fractures of the humerus in children. J Bone Joint Surg [Am] 1994;76:253.

Lovell & Winter's Pediatric Orthopaedics, fourth edition,
edited by Raymond T. Morrissy and Stuart L. Weinstein.
Lippincott–Raven Publishers, Philadelphia © 1996.

Chapter

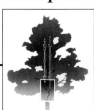

32

The Role of the Orthopaedic Surgeon in Child Abuse

Behrooz A. Akbarnia

Few of us can tolerate with equanimity the concept of small and defenseless children, the weakest members of our species, deliberately and cruelly being harmed by those who care for them. Inflicted trauma is not a new occurrence. Over the centuries, parents have reacted to the stress and frustration of everyday life by striking out at their children, causing soft tissue and bone injuries. As for children, there never has been a golden age. Throughout the history of various societies, children have been killed, abandoned, beaten, and sexually abused. However, it has been only over the past three decades that the attention of the medical community has been focused on child abuse and neglect.

In 1946, Dr. John Caffey,[16] a pediatrician and pediatric radiologist in New York City, reported for the first time in the United States the association of multiple fractures in long bones with chronic subdural hematoma in six infants. None of these children had a his-tory of significant trauma or roentgenographic or clinical evidence of generalized or localized skeletal disease to explain the fractures. He recommended investigation for subdural hematoma in infants with long bone fractures as well as investigation for long bone fractures in patients with subdural hematoma. In 1953, Silverman[52] clearly implicated parents and guardians as the cause of these traumatic lesions and described as part of the syndrome, irregular fragmentation of one or more metaphyses in the tubular bones associated with new bone formation external to the shaft. In 1960, Altman and Smith[4] were the first to report cases of unrecognized trauma in infants and children in the orthopaedic literature.

Although many physicians contributed to the recognition and understanding of child abuse, medicine as a profession did not officially acknowledge child abuse until a paper describing the battered-child syndrome was published by C. Henry Kempe and associates[32] in 1962. The introduction of the term battered-child syndrome was helpful in attracting attention to this still-neglected medical and social problem. Within a few years of the publication of this article, reporting laws were passed in all states mandating that health professionals report suspected cases of abuse. Increased public awareness finally resulted in the passage of the Child Abuse Prevention Act of 1974. The first large series of orthopaedic manifestations of this syndrome was published in 1974.[3] Great strides have been made not only in the passage of child abuse legislation, but also in the diagnosis, management, and understanding of the social, psychological, and epidemiologic aspects of this problem. Unfortunately, the syndrome still remains a major cause of death and of physical and mental disability among our children.

DEFINITION

In 1968, Helfer and Kempe[28] defined child abuse as physical injury inflicted on children by persons caring for them. Since then, the concept of child abuse has been broadened to include physical and emotional neglect, physical abuse, and psychological and sexual abuse. In addition, the list of professionals required to report such abuse has been increased to include virtually all those who are responsible for the care of children. Thus, the definition can vary, depending on the professionals involved. This chapter deals mainly with the diagnosis and management of physical abuse.

PREVALENCE

The prevalence of child abuse is difficult to determine. It has been estimated that 1% to 1.5% of all children are abused each year. The number ranges from 70,000 to 2.6 million.[47,59] In 1991, about 1.7 million reports on an estimated 2.6 million children who were alleged subjects of child abuse and neglect were reviewed by child protective agencies in the United States. Forty-four percent of the substantiated or indicated types of maltreatment were classified as neglect and 24% were classified as physical abuse. The number of childhood deaths due to abuse is difficult to estimate. This is particularly true in infancy, when it is likely that many cases of homicide remain undetected.[32] In 1991, 1081 children were reported to have died of abuse and neglect in 45 states. However, many states have indicated that the actual number may be significantly higher. The number of children subject to a report of alleged maltreatment has more than doubled over the past 10 years.[47] For every case that is reported, many others are not. An estimated 41% of reports

resulted in a substantiated or indicated disposition in 1991. The case reports and statistics are heavily biased toward poor and minority children. Children of the affluent may receive different diagnostic labels for their problems (i.e., "accidents" rather than "abuse"), and practitioners may feel an obligation to protect more affluent families from the stigma of reporting to public agencies. About 30% of fractures in children younger than 3 years of age are nonaccidental.[31,38] In a study of children younger than 1 year of age, 56% of fractures were found to be nonaccidental.[43] If child abuse is overlooked in the emergency department, there is a 35% chance of repeated abuse and a 5% to 10% chance of death.[1] The gender ratio is about equal, but premature babies and stepchildren are at greater risk. Besides parents, boyfriends and stepparents are the most frequent abusers. Although a larger percentage of maltreated children are between 0 and 5 years of age, the number of victims is distributed across most age ranges. However, fatalities from physical abuse are seen most often in children younger than 3 years of age. The highest percentage for any age—7.6% of the total—is for children younger than 1 year of age.[47] Younger children are at greater risk because they are demanding, defenseless, and nonverbal. In a study of 231 abused children, 50% were younger than 1 year of age and 78% were younger than 3 years of age.[3]

DIAGNOSIS

In the spectrum of child abuse and maltreatment, orthopaedic surgeons are involved more often in cases of physical injury and less often in cases of physical and emotional neglect. Because physical abuse as well as chronic neglect of young children tends to be recurrent and often results in permanent sequelae, the orthopaedic surgeon must be satisfied that each injury seen in a child is adequately explained. The role of the orthopaedic surgeon extends beyond simple treatment of the child's fracture.

To differentiate those lesions resulting from inflicted trauma from those caused by accidents, physicians should have a high index of suspicion as well as diagnostic skill. Furthermore, they should be knowledgeable in the patterns of child growth and development as well as common injuries in children.[41,58] The diagnosis of child abuse seldom is made without difficulty. A combination of the history given, the age of the child, the behavior of the parent, and certain clinical manifestations serve as a practical guideline for differentiating nonaccidental injury from that associated with pathologic conditions. Child abuse should be viewed in the same manner as any other medical condition in which facts are gathered and evaluated and a medical judgment based on knowledge and expertise is formulated.[34]

Because all cases of suspected inflicted injuries are possible forensic cases, the diagnosis should include an expression regarding the level of certainty to which the physician is willing to commit. This might be a phrase such as "reasonably medically certain," "more likely than not," or "suspicious." All interventions other than voluntary ones in child abuse cases require that the existence of the abuse be proven at some specific level of certainty.[18]

The given history in a case of child abuse usually is vague and does not explain the objective findings. The history as well as the physician's observation of the behavior of the parent and the child often are more helpful in making the diagnosis than is the physical examination. During the initial visit with the child and the parent, and during the course of the workup, the physician should be able to control his or her attitudes and feelings to create the best possible environment in which the physician, other health professionals, and the family can work together.

The Parents

Parents who are abusive may not readily volunteer information. They may be self-contradictory and display irritation at inquiries regarding their children's symptoms. They may show overreaction with hostility or underreaction with casualness or little evident concern. They may be unavailable or refuse to give information or consent to different tests. Many times, they have inappropriately delayed seeking health care. When they interact with their children, they may seldom touch or look at them, or they may be critical and angry with the children and not mention any positive or good qualities.

No single behavior or combination of behaviors makes a parent abusive by definition. Most cases of child abuse involve parents, and they are not often psychotic. Although the presence of psychological difficulties does not automatically confirm that a parent is abusive, the absence of any apparent psychological disturbance does not rule out the possibility.

Some abusive parents were abused as children and their own needs for nurturing were never met. A history of stress, drug abuse, or family disruption is a cause for suspicion.[54]

The Child

Abused children may be overly compliant and passive or extremely aggressive. They may have developmental delays or show role reversal behavior as a response to the unspoken parental need for nurturing.

CLINICAL MANIFESTATIONS

When confronted with a traumatic lesion, the physician must examine the whole child and look for other possible clues. If there is any question regarding the general medical examination, help should be sought from medical colleagues. Often, it is the nonorthopaedic manifestations of child abuse that lead to the diagnosis.

Failure to thrive or growth retardation secondary to physical and emotional deprivation is common in children who have been subjected to repeated abuse. This should be differentiated from usual causes of growth retardation.

Skin Lesions

A variety of skin lesions, including bruises, burns, welts, lacerations, and scars, are by far the most common finding in cases of child abuse.[48] Typical toddlers have bruises over the shins, knees, elbows, and brow. They may have a few old cuts or scars around the eyes or cheekbones as a result of the usual collisions. However, bruising of the buttocks, perineum, trunk, and back of the legs or back of the head or neck suggests inflicted trauma. These lesions may have the same shapes or configurations as the implements used to create them (Fig. 32-1). Loop marks or scars on the skin are inflicted by a doubled-over cord or rope. Human bite marks are distinctive, paired, crescent-shaped bruises that face each other. The skin lesions may be in various stages of healing (Fig. 32-2). Wilson[60] has suggested some guidelines for estimating the age of a bruise from its color. From 0 to 3 days after injury, a bruise usually is red, blue, or purple. From 3 to 7 days, it is green or green-yellow, and from 8 to 28 days, it is yellow or yellow-brown. These guidelines can be helpful in determining whether bruises are the result of one or more traumatic episodes. When bruises are present, diseases such as leukemia, idiopathic thrombocytopenic purpura, and hemophilia should be ruled out. Other cutaneous manifestations of child abuse include bruises in the shape of a hand print, alopecia or subgaleal hematoma from pulling of the hair, and areas of abraded skin from bindings or restraints. Impetigo in its various forms can be confused with burns or inflicted injuries.

It is essential that photographs of skin lesions be taken for the purpose of documentation and possible future use in the courts. Informed consent should

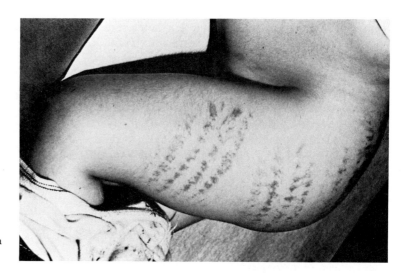

FIGURE 32-1.   Rope marks on an infant who was a victim of repeated physical abuse.

be obtained, and the photographs can be taken by a member of the child abuse team or by a social worker.

Cao-gio, or "scratch the wind" is a Vietnamese folklore medical practice. It consists of using a boiled egg covered with hair, a coin, or a similar object to scratch skin previously massaged with hot oil. This leaves broad bruises or ecchymosis. It is believed that these scratching maneuvers help rid the body of "bad wind." These lesions should not be confused with nonaccidental lesions.[7]

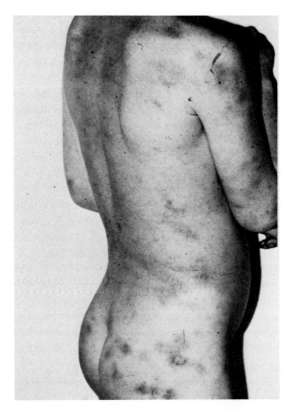

FIGURE 32-2.   Bruising of the back and buttocks, typical of physical abuse. Bruises may be found in different stages of healing.

Burn injuries are common and are seen in 10% of abused children.[1] These lesions can be scalding injuries, cigarette burns, or burns caused by flames. Burns are most common among children between 0 and 5 years of age. The pattern of deliberate immersion burns often is symmetrical, with sharp lines between the burned and unburned skin. Accidental scald burns usually are distributed asymmetrically.[48]

Head Injuries

The head is a convenient and vulnerable target. Because "the face represents the person," it is logical to strike the face to assail the person. The most convenient weapon for striking a child is the human hand. An open palm, the knuckles, or a closed fist is sufficient to produce severe damage to the brain, skull, or scalp when used forcefully. Of 110 physically abused children seen by O'Neill and associates,[51] 32 had evidence of cerebral trauma. Over 50% of all cases of permanent disability occur among children younger than 2 years of age and result, in large part, from inflicted head injuries. The scalp may be swollen. Extension of the swelling and ecchymosis to the eyelids and face is a telltale sign of cranial trauma. Head injuries can be severe and result in immediate death, or less severe and cause various subtle neurologic impairments. Subdural hematoma can occur with or without skull fractures. Many children with brain injuries have no external evidence of trauma. Caffey[15] suggested that violent shaking may cause stretching and tearing of the veins, creating subdural hematoma. If the insult is repeated, causing minor brain injury each time, it may result in additional brain damage manifested by mental retardation, seizure disorders, and other motor and learning disabilities, some of which do not become apparent for months or years after the abusive behavior has ended. Careful neurologic assessment of all suspected cases of abuse or neglect is essential.

Conversely, the unexplained appearance of central nervous system symptoms in an infant should trigger suspicion of abuse. Fractures of the skull are not easy to produce in infants because of the yielding elasticity of the thin cranial bones that are not yet fixed at the sutures. When present, they may be indicative of a forceful nonaccidental impact to the skull. Several cases have been reported of children with inappropriate widening of the cranial sutures, which is believed to result from increased intracranial pressure secondary to cerebral edema or subdural hematoma.[3] Computed tomography (CT) has greatly improved our precision in differentiating accidental and nonaccidental head injuries, and this test should be performed in any child with unexplained acute or chronic neurologic signs. A child with acute and unexplained unconsciousness should undergo head CT immediately after stabilization, often followed by abdominal CT and skeletal survey radiographs.[5] Magnetic resonance imaging (MRI) is not recommended as the primary imaging study because it can fail to reveal subarachnoid hemorrhage in the early stages. After a few days, MRI can be helpful in diagnosing cerebral abnormalities. MRI also is useful in patients with chronic neurologic findings.

Internal Injuries

Child abuse can produce injuries to the internal organs, such as rupture of the pancreas and pseudocyst formation, laceration of the liver and spleen, intramural hematoma of the bowel, hemorrhage behind the peritoneum, laceration or contusion of the kidneys, perforation of the intestine, and rupture of the ureter or bladder.[33] Of the deaths that result from child abuse, many are caused by internal hemorrhage from the rupture of abdominal organs after punches or kicks. Most such deaths occur in children 3 years of age or younger. The high death rate of these injuries is due not only to the severity of the trauma, but also to the delay of the abuser in seeking medical attention. Unfortunately, the lack of a history of trauma and failure of the physician to notice other signs of abuse often result in a delay of diagnosis as well.

ORTHOPAEDIC MANIFESTATIONS

About one third of all physically abused children require orthopaedic treatment.[3] The incidence of fractures in child abuse cases varies from 11% to 55%. Skeletal injuries are significantly more common in the younger age groups. Factors influencing the reported incidence of fractures relate to the age of the patient, the type of abuse, and the type and quality of the imaging techniques used to detect skeletal injuries.

Fractures can occur in almost any bone of the body. However, the long bones, ribs, and skull are common locations. Fractures can be categorized as epiphyseal, metaphyseal, diaphyseal, or miscellaneous.[3]

Physeal Fractures

Physeal fractures, although rare, are seen most often in the femur, tibia, and humerus, and are being recognized in more cases of child abuse.[2,22,25] A fracture through a growth plate, especially when the epiphysis is not visible, can cause difficulty in diagnosis. Metaphyseal lucency or irregularity and soft tissue swelling may be the only findings on radiographic examination. Arthrographic examination of the joint can be helpful in certain cases, such as fractures around the elbow[2] (Fig. 32-3).

Fractures of the proximal femur involving the epiphyseal-metaphyseal region are much less common than those involving the shaft and distal femur. They are identical to those caused by birth trauma. These fractures not only are difficult to diagnose, especially before the ossific nucleus has appeared, but they may result in the most severe deformities of the lower extremities caused by child abuse.

Metaphyseal Fractures

Metaphyseal fractures are classified as corner fractures, impaction injuries, buckle fractures, or irregular metaphyseal deformities. Corner fractures are caused by forceful downward pulling on the extremity and often are bilateral. They may not be visible on the initial roentgenogram, but can result in periosteal separation and subperiosteal hemorrhage, with subsequent new bone formation external to the cortex. The periosteal new bone formation becomes visible in about 7 to 10 days. These patients often have swollen and painful extremities that cannot be moved. If the lesion is already 7 to 10 days old, the swollen and warm extremity with periosteal new bone formation, often associated with fever, can be confused with osteomyelitis.

Metaphyseal injuries, especially corner fractures as opposed to shaft fractures, are highly specific. However, detection of these lesions often requires high-quality radiographic images. Kleinman[35] believes that these lesions are the most diagnostic fractures indicating nonaccidental trauma. He has presented an extensive radiologic histopathologic study and has indicated that the fundamental histologic lesion is a series of microfractures occurring in a planar fashion through the most immature portion of metaphyseal primary spongiosa. The most subtle indication of injury is a transverse lucency within the subepiphyseal region of the metaphysis. These lucent lines occasionally can

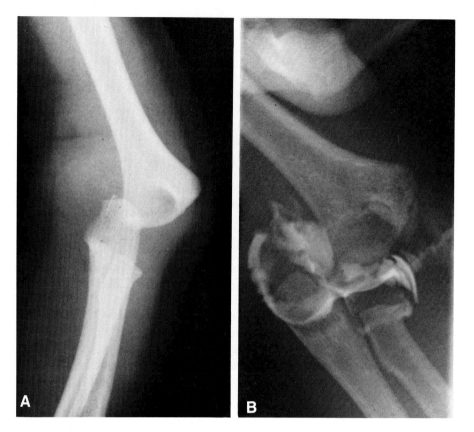

FIGURE 32-3. A 15-month-old infant was seen in the emergency department because she was not able to move her right elbow. (**A**) The exact location and severity of the fracture of the distal humerus cannot be identified. (**B**) An arthrogram of the elbow shows the outline of the distal humeral epiphysis, which is separated.

be indistinguishable from those found in patients with chronic diseases such as leukemia. The fracture fragment is made up of epiphysis, physis, and a thin portion of metaphysis (Fig. 32-4). In the peripheral margin, the disc-like fragment is relatively thick and can show evidence of different degrees of density. It is this peripheral margin that has been called a metaphyseal

corner fracture. A similar fragment often is seen in the lateral and anteroposterior projections, indicating that these apparently separate triangular fragments actually are portions of the same larger disc-like fragment (Figs. 32-5 and 32-6).

In an impaction injury that is severe, the epiphysis is impacted into an expanded metaphysis and exuber-

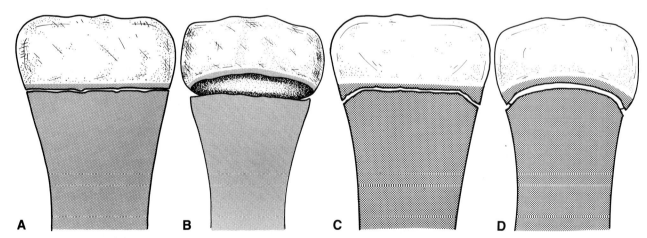

FIGURE 32-4. Metaphyseal lesions. (**A**) A planar fracture through the primary spongiosa produces metaphyseal lucency. (**B**) If the metaphysis is tipped or simply projected at an obliquity to the x-ray beam, the margin of the resultant fragment is projected with a bucket-handle appearance. (**C**) If the peripheral fragment is substantially thicker than the central fragment and the plane of injury is viewed tangentially, a corner fracture appearance will result. (**D**) If the metaphysis is displaced or projected at an obliquity, as in **B**, a thicker bucket handle will be apparent. (From Kleinman PK. Diagnostic imaging of child abuse. Baltimore: Williams & Wilkins, 1987.)

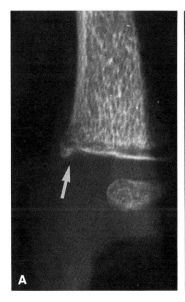
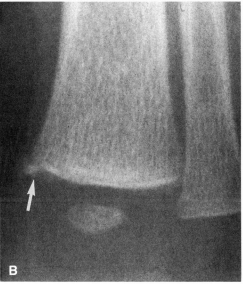

FIGURE 32-5.   Distal tibia of a 3-month-old abused infant. (**A**) Specimen radiograph reveals a corner fracture medially (*arrow*) in addition to a conspicuous metaphyseal radiolucency. (**B**) Ante mortem radiograph tangential to the metaphyseal margin also demonstrates the corner fracture (*arrow*) with the suggestion of a radiolucent band. (From Kleinman PK. Diagnostic imaging of child abuse. Baltimore: Williams & Wilkins, 1987.)

ant periosteal new bone formation subsequently occurs (Fig. 32-7). Simple buckle fractures are common in the metaphysis and often are multiple. Unlike other metaphyseal lesions, they do not produce a significant amount of callus (Fig. 32-8). Gross irregularity of the metaphysis is seen after repeated injuries and frequently is associated with deformity of the joint and limitation of motion.[24]

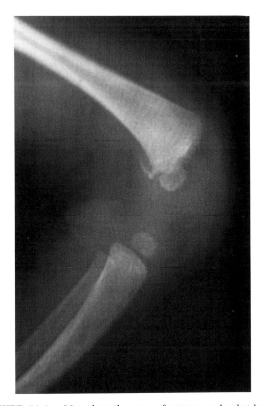

FIGURE 32-6.   Metaphyseal corner fracture or bucket-handle fracture in the lateral view.

Diaphyseal Fractures

Diaphyseal lesions are grouped into three categories:

1. Transverse, spiral, or oblique fractures of the shaft, sometimes associated with exuberant callus because of delay in seeking medical help and lack of proper immobilization
2. Multiple lesions in various stages of healing
3. Gross bony deformities.

The femur and humerus are the two long bones most frequently fractured in abused children. The overall incidence of femoral fractures is 20%.[3,25,51] In a series of 80 femoral fractures in children younger than 4 years of age, 30% were caused by child abuse.[10] Anderson[6] described 117 patients with 122 femoral fractures. Of 24 children younger than 2 years of age, 19 (79%) were abused. Of 18 children younger than 13 months of age, 15 (83%) were abused. In older children, there are more accidental injuries causing femoral fractures.

Some authors have emphasized the frequency of spiral and oblique fractures of the long bones caused by physical abuse.[20] However, it is increasingly evident that usual types of diaphyseal fractures (e.g., transverse fractures) are common in cases of nonaccidental trauma. Therefore, in long bone fractures, especially in the femur, no specific type of fracture (e.g., transverse, oblique) should be considered pathognomonic of child abuse. Other criteria, such as history and patient age, are more helpful in making the diagnosis[21] (Fig. 32-9).

In a review of 429 fractures in 189 abused children, King and associates[33] found the humerus to be the long bone most often affected and transverse fractures to be the most common type. About 50% of their pa-

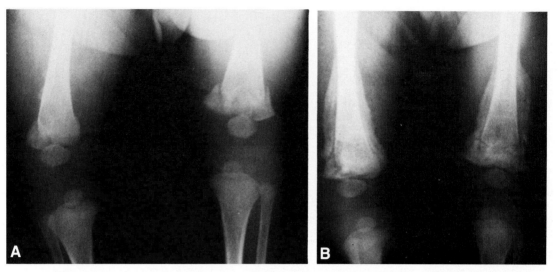

FIGURE 32-7. Bilateral impaction fracture of the distal end of the femur (**A**), with subsequent exuberant periosteal new bone formation (**B**). (From Akbarnia BA, Torg JS, Kirkpatrick J, et al. Manifestations of the battered child syndrome. J Bone Joint Surg 1974;56:1159.)

tients had only a single long bone fracture, 35% in the femur and 29% in the humerus (Fig. 32-10).

Long bone fractures caused by child abuse can be similar to those resulting from accidental trauma. Careful attention to the history and the age of the child could reveal the nonaccidental nature of the injury. Because the risk for accidents begins with mobility, especially walking, when these injuries occur in young nonambulatory infants, they almost always are inflicted in the absence of bone disease.

Miscellaneous Fractures

Rib fractures account for 5% to 27% of all fractures occurring in abused children.[34] Fractures involving the ribs usually are posterior or posterolateral and can be in various stages of healing (Fig. 32-11). They rarely are caused by cardiopulmonary resuscitation. In the absence of radiographic evidence of intrinsic bone disease or obvious major trauma, unexplained rib fractures are specific for abuse. Rib fractures usually are not suspected clinically. Radionuclide bone scanning has been shown to be extremely useful in the detection of rib fractures in abused infants and children.

Other miscellaneous fractures include spinal, clavicular, scapular, and sternal fractures. Spinal and sternal fractures are more specific than are clavicular fractures. Although the clavicle is one of the most common bones to be fractured accidentally in children, it accounts for only 2% to 6% of fractures associated with child abuse.[3,30,45] Therefore, it is not specific for child abuse. Spinal fractures are described separately.

Spinal Injuries

The true incidence of spinal injuries is difficult to determine. The reported incidence has varied from 0% to 3% in large series.[3,6,25] Abused children with spinal injuries occasionally show mild kyphosis, but most do not have significant clinical symptoms referable to the spine. Therefore, many of these injuries go unrecognized. Because spinal injuries are likely to be silent but associated with extremely violent assaults, routine

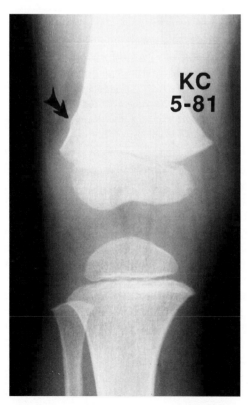

FIGURE 32-8. Metaphyseal buckle fractures involving the distal end of the femur. These fractures often are bilateral.

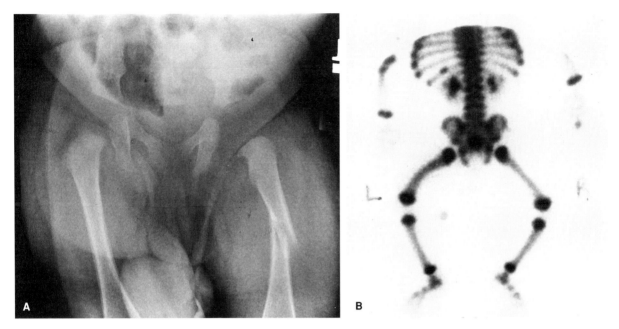

FIGURE 32-9. A 2-month-old boy reportedly fell from a sofa. (A) Femur fracture was not very specific. (B) Because of the patient's age and vague history, a bone scan was obained. The bone scan showed increased uptake in the rib that was not seen in the plain radiographs.

evaluation of the spine is mandatory. Spinal radiographs, especially a lateral projection of the entire spine, should be part of the routine skeletal survey.

In a report of 85 spinal fractures in 41 children, Kleinman[34] found the average patient age to be 22 months. Most of the fractures involved the vertebral bodies. Occasionally, fractures of the posterior arch without involvement of the vertebral bodies are described. Vertebral bodies can show varying degrees of anterior compression. There can be anterior notching, which usually is superior.[56] In cases of disc herniation, intervertebral disc narrowing can be present (Fig. 32-12; see Fig. 32-10). Fracture dislocations with or without neurologic deficits have been reported. Spinal cord injuries or hematomas also can be seen without bony involvement. Significant fracture dislocations, especially those that are not associated with neurologic deficits, may go unrecognized and can result in significant spinal deformity later in life.

The mechanism of injury in most cases is hyperflexion, extension, or both. Therefore, multiple compression fractures in a single patient are common. Occasionally, fractures of the upper extremities are associated with these compression fractures when the child is held above a table or kitchen counter and the buttocks are slammed against the surface. The child uses outstretched arms to break the impact, causing fractures of the upper extremities. Most compression fractures are in the region of the thoracolumbar and lumbar spine. However, fractures and fracture dislocations of the cervical and sacral regions also are seen.

The changes in vertebral bodies and disc spaces

that accompany normal development or infection can cause confusion. The notching of traumatic origin generally involves a large portion of the anterior margin. Disc space narrowing caused by infection usually is more severe than that caused by trauma and disc herniation. The value of a bone scan in detecting spinal injuries is not clear. The standard radiographic studies generally are regarded as the primary method of investigation. In the presence of any neurologic findings, MRI is useful for evaluation of the spinal canal.

DECISION MAKING

Orthopaedic surgeons often are asked to give an opinion regarding the etiology of certain fractures (i.e., accidental versus nonaccidental). The presence of fractures alone may not provide a sufficient basis for making such a determination. However, a major part of the recognition of child abuse still depends on radiologic diagnosis. Certain fractures are more specific than others in these cases. Again, the history and the age of the patient should be considered in making the determination.

In a study of 89 fractures in 36 children, the pattern of fractures was found to be more helpful in making the diagnosis of child abuse than was the presence of multiple fractures in various stages of healing.[25] Suspicious fracture patterns included metaphyseal corner fractures, lower extremity fractures in nonambulatory children, bilateral acute fractures, fractures

(text continues on p. 1326)

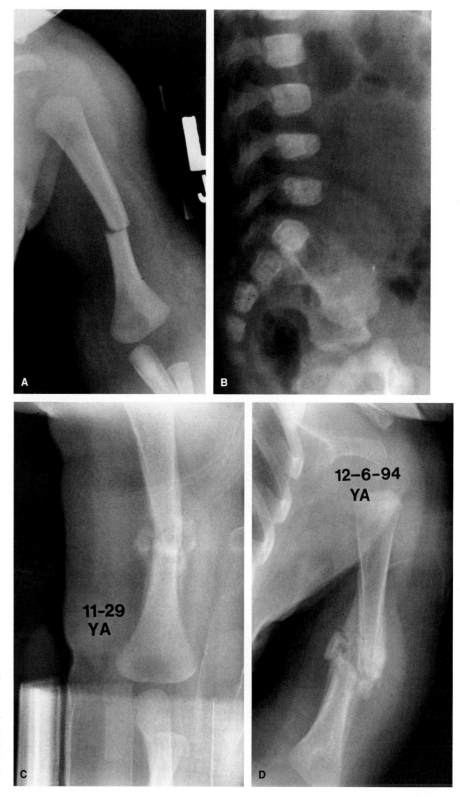

FIGURE 32-10. A 2-month-old infant with a nonaccidental transverse humeral fracture, a spine fracture, and cerebral hemorrhage. (**A**) Transverse humeral fracture. (**B**) L4 compression fracture and anterior wedging. (**C** and **D**) Humeral fracture at 2 and 3 weeks after injury showing progressive healing and new bone formation.

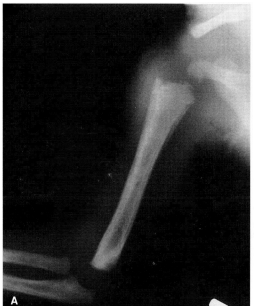
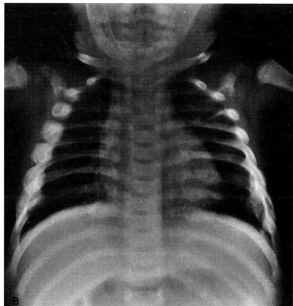
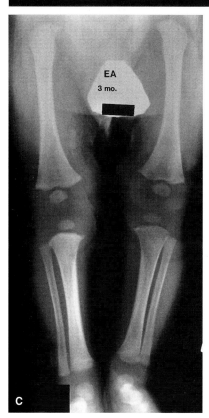

FIGURE 32-11. A 3-month-old infant with a history of a fall. The baby was discharged but returned dead. (**A**) Unusual proximal humerus fracture. (**B**) Lateral and posterior rib fractures. (**C**) Metaphyseal fracture of the proximal right tibia.

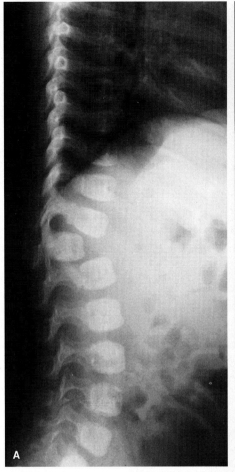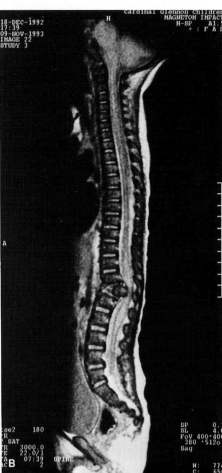

FIGURE 32-12. Fracture-dislocation of the spine in a 10-month-old infant, victim of abuse, who had incomplete paraplegia. (**A**) Lateral radiograph of the spine. (**B**) MRI showing cord compression. (Courtesy of Keith Gabriel, M.D. Cardinal Glennan Children's Hospital, St. Louis, MO.)

in special locations such as the ribs and spine, and physeal fractures in young children.[42] As infants begin walking, they may sustain a classic fracture known as the toddler's fracture,[44,57] which appears as an oblique lucent line in the tibia (Fig. 32-13). Although there can be a good explanation for this fracture, the history and any other available clues should be evaluated carefully before the diagnosis is made. In a patient of the right age without a convincing history, even a fracture of the clavicle should be considered suspicious.

Kleinman[34] suggests that relative specificities can be applied to these fractures based on their nature, location, and chronicity (Table 32-1).

Dating Fractures

The relation between the alleged cause and the timing of an injury is one of the critical elements in the decision-making process. The literature contains little information regarding the dating of fractures based on their radiographic appearance.[36,50] Obliteration of soft tissue planes is the earliest sign of injury. Edema of the soft tissues is associated clinically with pain and swelling that are accentuated with any attempt to move the extremity. When fractures are not displaced, the

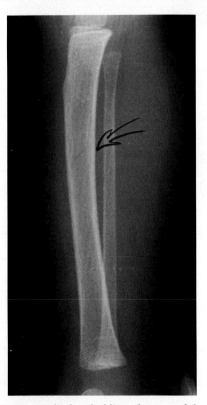

FIGURE 32-13. Undisplaced oblique fracture of the tibia (toddler's fracture).

TABLE 32-1.   Specificity of Radiologic Findings

High Specificity
Metaphyseal lesions
Posterior rib fractures
Scapular fractures
Spinous process fractures
Sternal fractures

Moderate Specificity*
Multiple fractures, especially bilateral
Fractures of different ages
Epiphyseal separations
Vertebral body fractures and subluxations
Digital fractures
Complex skull fractures

Common but Low Specificity*
Clavicular fractures
Long bone shaft fractures
Linear skull fractures

* Moderate- and low-specificity lesions become high-specificity lesions when a history of trauma is absent or inconsistent with injuries.

From Kleinman PK. Diagnostic imaging of child abuse. Baltimore: Williams & Wilkins, 1987:6.

duration of acute inflammation can be only a few days. Infants and children can be free of pain as early as 1 to 2 days after the original injury. Generally, new bone formation occurs between 10 and 14 days after injury. In young infants, this interval is shorter, probably between 7 and 14 days.[50] In addition, solidification and remodeling are more rapid in infants than in older children (Fig. 32-14). The age of the child should be considered in dating a fracture, along with the history, the presence of repetitive injuries, and the degree of immobilization. Although the actual date of a fracture can only be approximated, a few guidelines have been developed. A fracture without periosteal new bone formation usually is less than 7 to 10 days old, and seldom is 20 days old. Slight but definite periosteal new bone formation can be as recent as 4 to 7 days old. A 20-day-old fracture almost always has well-defined periosteal new bone and typically has early (soft) callus. A large amount of callus always indicates a fracture more than 14 days old (see Fig. 32-10). Loss of marginal sharpness of the fracture line can be delayed up to 7 to 14 days. Corner fractures may not cause significant periosteal new bone formation and can be dated only based on their loss of marginal definition. Chronic repetitive trauma and lack of immobilization

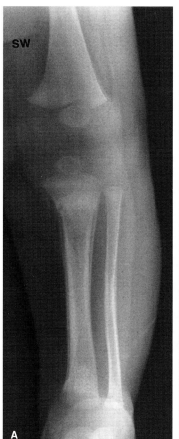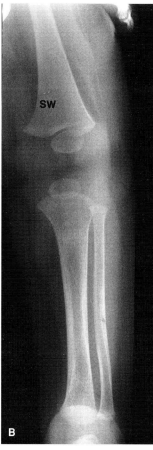

FIGURE 32-14. A 6-month-old baby abused by his babysitter. **(A)** 10-day-old proximal tibial fracture and periosteal new bone formation. **(B)** Significant remodeling has occurred 2 months later.

TABLE 32-2. *Timetable of Radiographic Changes in Children's Fractures**

CATEGORY	EARLY	PEAK	LATE
1. Resolution of soft tissues	2–5 d	4–10 d	10–21 d
2. Periosteal new bone	4–10 d	10–14 d	14–21 d
3. Loss of fracture line definition	10–14 d	14–21 d	
4. Soft callus†	10–14 d	14–21 d	
5. Hard callus	14–21 d	21–42 d	42–90 d
6. Remodeling‡	3 mo	1 y	2 y to epiphyseal closure

* Repetitive injuries may prolong categories 1, 2, 5, and 6.

† The stage of soft callus usually lasts 3 to 4 weeks or until the bony fragments are bridged by lamellar bone and ends clinically when fragments no longer can be easily moved.

‡ In this stage, both periosteal and endosteal bone begin to be converted to lamellar bone and remodeling of the callus begins.

From O'Connor JF, Cohen J. Dating fractures. In: Kleinman PK, ed. Diagnostic imaging of child abuse. Baltimore: Williams & Wilkins, 1987.

can lead to loss of fracture line definition as the earliest finding.

The results of radionuclide bone scans become positive a few hours after injury and remain positive for a long time (1–2 years). They are not helpful in establishing the age of fractures. The role of MRI in the dating of fractures has not been established. O'Connor and Cohen[50] have outlined a timetable of radiographic changes in children's fractures (Table 32-2).

MANAGEMENT

The management of child abuse is divided into two phases: diagnosis and documentation, and treatment. When physical abuse is suspected, documentation is the first step. Skeletal radiographs, bone scans, and CT scans are the usual imaging modalities. However, the indiscriminate use of these tests in all cases of suspected child abuse contributes to unnecessary radiation exposure and rising health care costs. Radiographic skeletal surveys are more helpful in children younger than 5 years of age who have clinical evidence of physical abuse.[40] The yield from skeletal surveys in neglected and sexually abused children is extremely low and does not justify the investigation. The skeletal survey should include anteroposterior and lateral views of the skull and thoracolumbar spine, as well as anteroposterior views of the thoracic cage and extremities. The radiographs of the extremities should include the shoulders, pelvis, hands, and feet. A single film of the entire infant (i.e., babygram) usually is not helpful because it lacks detail and is a single projection. The use of radionuclide bone scanning as a screening procedure for skeletal trauma is controver-

sial. Some authors have suggested that this is a more sensitive screening test in cases of physical abuse and are using it as part of the initial evaluation.[27,55] In a study of 261 cases of suspected child abuse, radiographic skeletal surveys and bone scans were performed, with meticulous attention paid to technique.[55] Abnormalities were found at one or more sites on bone scans in 120 patients and on radiographs in 105 patients. False-negative results were obtained in 32 patients with radiography but in only 2 patients with bone scanning. This report demonstrates the superior sensitivity of bone scanning to radiography under the conditions described by these authors. However, this view is not shared by most pediatric radiologists, who still prefer skeletal surveys as the primary radiologic screening test in cases of suspected child abuse. Bone scans are more sensitive in assessing rib fractures, particularly those involving the costovertebral junction;[37] acute, undisplaced long bone fractures; and subperiosteal hemorrhage.[35] Skeletal surveys are more sensitive in detecting spinal fractures, bilateral metaphyseal injuries, skull fractures, and scapular fractures. Other factors also influence the use of these methods in the initial evaluation. Bone-seeking radionuclides concentrate in areas of increased blood flow and bone formation so that fractures appear as hot spots. However, these findings are not specific for fractures and can be seen in other conditions of rapid bone turnover, such as osteomyelitis or neoplasm. In addition, radionuclide uptake and activity normally are increased near the growth plate, making it more difficult to identify epiphyseal-metaphyseal fractures, especially when they are bilateral. Other disadvantages of bone scanning as the initial skeletal imaging procedure include the limited availability of nuclear medicine services at all hours in many hospitals, the inexperience of many general radiology departments in performing and interpreting pediatric bone scans, and the relatively high radiation dose delivered to the patient's growth plates.[40] In addition, bone scans not only are more costly, but they lack the ability to identify the age and mechanism of the injury, often necessitating additional radiologic examination of suspicious areas for confirmation. Skeletal surveys, on the other hand, are more specific, rarely require patient sedation, and are less subject to interpretive error. Thus, radiographic skeletal surveys should be used first in the evaluation of suspected child abuse cases. If these radiographs do not show any evidence of trauma despite clinical suspicion, a bone scan may prove valuable in identifying subtle or occult injuries to the ribs, the diaphyses, and, occasionally, the epiphysis. Some of these occult fractures are not visible on plain radiographs until 7 to 10 days after injury. In these situations, a second radiograph 1 to 2 weeks later usually is helpful. A bone scan should be done as well if the results of plain radiographs are negative or questionable (see Fig. 32-9). Children older than 5 years of age usually can provide a more reliable history. Radiographic studies in these cases are selected based on the clinical findings and the index of suspicion. CT scans often are helpful when head and abdominal trauma is suspected.

Coagulation disorders, both hereditary and acquired, can produce bruises that can be confused with bruises caused by physical abuse. Hereditary coagulation disorders include hemophilia and von Willebrand disease. Acquired coagulation disorders such as idiopathic thrombocytopenic purpura and leukemia also have been confused with physical abuse.[9] In cases of suspicious or unexplained bruising, blood tests such as a complete blood count, partial thromboplastin time, prothrombin time, platelet count, and bleeding time should be performed. A prolonged partial thromboplastin time is seen in both hemophilia and von Willebrand disease.

Many conditions can cause fractures, periosteal new bone formation, and bone irregularities, and these should be considered in the differential diagnosis of physical abuse. The pitfalls that occasionally lead to errors in diagnosis can result from suboptimal radiographic techniques or errors in interpretation.

The most common difficulty in diagnosis involves the differentiation of accidental from nonaccidental trauma, especially in isolated, nonspecific fractures. An example of this was discussed in the section on diaphyseal femur fractures. Normal variants, such as periosteal new bone formation or the cupping of the metaphysis, can be seen in healthy infants. These findings are observed first at 1 to 3 months of age and usually resolve by 8 months of age.[14]

Conditions to be considered in the differential diagnosis are syphilis, osteogenesis imperfecta, scurvy, Caffey disease, osteomyelitis, septic arthritis, fatigue fractures, osteoid osteoma and other tumors, rickets, hypophosphatasia, leukemia, metastatic neuroblastoma, fractures in neurogenic disorders, congenital indifference to pain, and osteopetrosis. These conditions all have additional signs of the primary disorder and a history of prior disease to distinguish them from nonaccidental trauma. For example, easy bruising is common in osteogenesis imperfecta. A combination of bruises and fractures may lead to the diagnosis of child abuse. The presence of blue sclerae, thin cortices, osteopenia, and a tendency to bowing and angulation distinguishes this condition.[23]

Congenital indifference to pain has an autosomal recessive inheritance. Children have normal intelligence and the only abnormal neurologic finding is insensitivity to painful stimuli. Repeated trauma to the growing skeleton can go unrecognized and result in major changes and deformities of the metaphysis as well as the epiphysis. A careful sensory neurologic examination and history helps in making the diagnosis.

Congenital syphilis involves multiple bones of the body, most commonly the tibia, femur, and humerus. Destructive changes are seen in the metaphysis and diaphysis between the first and sixth months of life. Pathologic fractures of the metaphysis and periosteal new bone formation can mimic the skeletal findings of child abuse. The serologic test for syphilis is most helpful in making the diagnosis.

In most conditions, radiologic features are helpful in differentiating the injuries of child abuse. In other conditions, clinical findings of the disease provide diagnostic clues.

Fractures in the neonatal period often involve the humerus, clavicle, and femur. In these injuries, callus usually appears on radiographs within 2 weeks of life. In this age group, an unusual site or the absence of callus after 2 weeks should alert the physician to the possibility of nonaccidental trauma.[20] Pathologic fractures caused by rickets also are seen in neonates, especially premature babies.

Falling out of bed is a common history frequently related when parents bring the child to the care of a physician. Helfer and associates[29] studied 246 children younger than 5 years of age who fell out of bed. There were only three cranial fractures, three clavicular fractures, and one humeral fracture. None of the children had neurologic impairment from skull fractures. In another prospective study of 436 infants from birth to 1 year of age, 101 (30%) sustained falls.[39] There were no limb fractures and only two skull fractures. Based on these statistics, falling out of bed is rarely the cause of fractures in young infants. A large body of literature exists on the incidence of fractures in children after accidents such as falls.[8,29,39,49,53] The orthopaedic surgeon must be familiar with this literature to interpret properly the history of the accident.

If child abuse is suspected, every effort should be made to protect the child. Although the statistics regarding the incidence of child abuse as well as the resulting mortality are admittedly inaccurate, it is recognized that many children eventually die of these injuries. The home environment in which child abuse occurs is unquestionably pathologic. Returning the child to this home in most cases poses the risk of repeated abuse, additional complications, and possible death. Because child abuse is believed to be a symptom of family distress and a problem with multiple complex origins, it should be managed by an interdisciplinary team that can include a pediatrician, a social worker, a nurse, a psychiatrist, and an attorney. When such a diagnostic unit is not available, the physician must work with a social worker and the protective agencies to which mandated reports are sent in the management of these cases. A social worker should be contacted at the time of the family's presentation to facilitate the social assessment and to form a helping relationship. It is helpful to avoid confrontation and to keep initial conversations to a minimum. The parents should be informed of the physician's responsibility and the fact that other professionals, such as a social worker, will be talking to them. The child should be admitted to the hospital only for medical reasons. In view of the cost of hospitalization, most of the workup and referral should be accomplished in the emergency department or an outpatient facility. If this is not possible, the child should be admitted to the hospital.[26] In most cases, this is acceptable to the parents if the need is clearly explained to them. If the parents refuse admission of the child, the law in most states allows the hospital or the physician to assume custody of the child for a limited period until a court order can be obtained. A report should be made to the local protective services' agency immediately. This usually is an oral report followed by a written report within 24 hours. Under the Child Abuse Prevention and Treatment Act, a central registry of child abuse is required in all states. Laws mandate reporting in all states.

Abuse and neglect must be identified before child protective agencies can deal with it. An increase in public awareness has led to an increase in the number of reported incidents of abuse and neglect. Professionals who work with children are in a unique position to observe child abuse or neglect and are required by law to report suspected cases to the authorities. A reporter does not have to be certain that abuse or neglect has occurred. All that is required is a reasonable suspicion of maltreatment.[46] However, some professionals are hesitant to report suspected cases for a variety of reasons. Among these individuals are nurses, social workers, physicians, day care providers, teachers, and school personnel. Some of the reasons they hesitate to file reports are lack of knowledge of the responsibility to report, lack of knowledge regarding the type of cases to report and to whom to report them, concern about confidentiality conflicts, pressure by others not to report and the threat of lawsuits or other reprisals by parents, reluctance to get involved, and the belief that reporting would not really help and may aggravate the situation.

The amount of time and effort required in these cases also can make orthopaedic surgeons reluctant to get involved. Each case can place a significant demand on a physician's schedule for depositions, testimony, and court appearances. To avoid such involvement, the responsibility can be delegated to a child abuse team in the hospital. In most hospitals, procedures are in place for reporting and subsequent follow-up. All that may be required is that the physician start the process when suspicion of maltreatment exists. When formal teams or other professionals are not available, the orthopaedic surgeon may have no choice but to get involved. However, the legal system is cooperative and understanding. Physicians' schedules usually are accommodated and compensation for their time is provided. Physicians should submit their hourly fees as they do for any other legal work.

Education is the most effective way to overcome the problem of underreporting. Since the creation of a nationwide toll-free telephone hotline for 24-hour reporting, the number of reported cases has risen sharply. A physician or any other reporter has immunity against any civil or criminal liability.[48] This means that a parent or caretaker cannot bring a successful lawsuit against a physician for defamation or for invasion of the family's right to privacy. However, in many states, failure to report subjects the physician to civil or criminal liability.

The most important phase in the management of child abuse cases is the follow-up and rehabilitation of the child and the family. In many cases, failure to provide such follow-up because of lack of funding or personnel has resulted in a higher rate of reinjury or death.

The following seven axioms of child abuse management appear in the literature on child abuse.[11]

1. Once diagnosed, an abused child (especially an infant younger than 1 year of age) is at great risk of reinjury or continued neglect.
2. In the event the child is reinjured, it is likely that the parents will seek care at a different medical facility.
3. There rarely is any need to establish precisely who injured the child and whether the injury

was intentional. The symptoms themselves should open the door to a helping alliance and the development of a comprehensive service plan for the child and the family.

4. If there is evidence that the child is at significant risk, hospitalization may be appropriate to allow time for interdisciplinary assessment. The complex origins of the child's injuries seldom are revealed in the crisis atmosphere at the time of presentation.

5. Protection of the child must be the principal goal of intervention, but protection must go hand-in-hand with the development of a family-oriented service plan.

6. Traditional social casework alone may not adequately protect the abused child in the environment in which the injuries were received. Multidisciplinary follow-up is necessary and frequent contact by all those involved in the service plan may be needed to encourage the child's healthy development.

7. Problems of public social service agencies in both urban and rural areas, especially in the number of adequately trained personnel and the quality of administrative and supervisory functions, mitigate against their effective operation in isolation from other care-providing agencies. Simply reporting a case to the public agency mandated to receive child abuse case reports may not be sufficient to protect an abused child or to help the family.

There is no doubt that prevention is the primary goal. This goal can be achieved by identifying high-risk children and helping families in distress. Orthopaedic surgeons can play an important role in breaking the cycle of child abuse and neglect by remaining aware, facilitating early detection, and helping to initiate therapeutic and rehabilitative measures for both the child and the family.

Medical Neglect

During the usual course of therapy for an orthopaedic condition, parents or caregivers may not follow the instructions provided by their treating physicians and may not adhere to the treatment protocols. For example, the family of a child with developmental dysplasia of the hip who is being treated in a Pavlik harness may fail to bring the child for follow-up appointments, or the family of a child with a positive Ortolani sign who is being treated with a harness may remove the device after returning home and fail to keep follow-up appointments. The family of a child with idiopathic scoliosis may refuse to use a brace when orthotic treatment is likely to be effective. They may allow the curve to progress to 55 to 60 degrees and then refuse surgical intervention. Situations such as these are considered instances of medical neglect.

If the treatment is clearly advantageous and the child is harmed by the lack of treatment, intervention through the proper authorities is indicated. There are situations in which a chronic condition requires more complex treatment and the type and length of the treatment clearly present a hardship for the family. In these cases, help should be provided to the family through appropriate social workers and social service agencies. In some cases, the presence of medical neglect is uncertain. In these instances, the amount of harm caused by the lack of treatment should be compared to the benefits of treatment and an appropriate decision should be made. In more complex cases, it often is helpful for both a physician and a social worker to explain fully the nature of the treatment and the responsibility of the family before treatment is initiated. In this way, any necessary arrangements can be made before treatment is begun to maximize compliance.

THE ORTHOPAEDIC SURGEON, CHILD ABUSE, AND THE LAW

Orthopaedic surgeons should be familiar with the law regarding child abuse. Questions about obtaining informed consent for testing, maintaining medical confidentiality, filing mandated child abuse reports, understanding court actions, and testifying in a courtroom are common. Although the law varies from state to state, the principal issues are the same. Orthopaedic surgeons should obtain appropriate legal counsel whenever necessary. The sensitive management of cases of family violence requires both medical and legal input.[12] In many hospitals, this is facilitated by the use of a team approach and by the maintenance of continuous contact between the department of social services, protective agencies, and the police department.

Legal consent is required for any action taken to treat an abused child. Parents or legal guardians can give this consent. A minor child cannot give consent except in an emergency or other exceptional situation. When there is a conflict with the parent or guardian, it is advisable to consult a hospital lawyer. Consent also is necessary for the release of any information from the medical record and for testifying in court unless a court-ordered subpoena has been issued.

The physician's findings should be recorded as soon as the patient is seen. The record in the chart should be legible and any errors should be corrected by adding follow-up entries rather than removing previous statements. Conclusions should not be made without supporting facts. A conclusion should not be ruled out unless the physician is certain it is medically invalid. For example, a statement such as, "this fracture could not result from child abuse," should not be made.

For the purpose of identifying and protecting abused children, all 50 states have mandatory reporting statutes. The basis of notification is "reasonable suspicion or belief." Legally, it always is better for a mandated reporter to file an abuse or neglect report, even if the allegation later proves erroneous, than to fail to file. All states have an immunity provision protecting mandated reporters. The question of privacy statutes often arises, but abuse reporting requirements override this privilege.[12] After examining the child, the report should be filed by the professional who knows the child best. This usually is the family physician, the pediatrician, or a social worker; however, the orthopaedic surgeon is responsible for reporting if he or she is suspicious and no other report has been filed. Reports should be filed based on the reasonable cause of the injury and not on the characteristics of the family. Many people complain that even if a case is reported, the state does not provide appropriate protection. Again, a report should be filed regardless of whether the state's response is helpful.

Preparation for Court Testimony in Child Abuse Cases

The number of physicians who are being required to testify in court is rising because of the rapid increase in the volume of child abuse reports as well as a continuing trend toward the use of litigation.[17] The orthopaedist should be well prepared before appearing as a witness, and should determine the degree of certainty to which he or she is willing to testify. Although most child abuse reporting laws require reporting at the level of suspicion, actions of any sort require proof at some higher level of certainty. The process of substantiation or verification is always a medical one in cases of physical abuse.

If a physician is not willing to carry out these examinations and to testify in court as an expert witness, no legal action of any kind is possible in most child abuse cases.[17] In court, the burden of proof is on the plaintiff. In the courtroom, for better or worse, it is evidence or proof that matters, not reality or fact. Most judges feel that children should remain with their parents whenever possible. The testimony of the physician as an expert witness is an important part of the process. Many times, court action is the result of a "war between experts." Of greatest concern is what the orthopaedic surgeon does not say on the witness stand or in a deposition that he or she should say,

and most physicians are reluctant to become actively involved in such cases. Brent[13] has called attention to the problem of irresponsible medical experts and has provided guidelines for responsible conduct in court. These have been adopted by the Committee on Medical Liability of the American Academy of Pediatrics in a policy statement[5] (Appendix 32-1).

Preparation is of paramount importance before a deposition or trial.* Physicians should dress appropriately for the courtroom. If they want to show radiographs, they should make sure the necessary equipment is available. Physicians should be objective and act as neutral experts. When a question is asked, they should pause before answering it to consider the form and content of their response and to give their attorneys a chance to object. Physicians should listen carefully to each question and answer only the question asked. They should not expand on the question or open up new issues. It also is a mistake for physicians to assume that they are credible and effective just because they have a medical degree. If they do not know the answer to a question, they should say so. Physicians should not argue with the attorney, but should look to the judge for help. Physicians should be prepared; however, they may review a patient chart to refresh their memory if necessary. In making conclusions, physicians should provide supportive facts and make sure that the link between the facts and the conclusion is clear. Orthopaedists should become accustomed to dating fractures based on the amount of bone repair and the criteria outlined previously. More than anyone else, orthopaedists are in a position to testify when children sustain broken bones. This type of evidence is helpful in cases in which the evidence is cumulative rather than clear-cut. Chadwick† has published an excellent article regarding preparation for court testimony.

Finally, if physicians have any doubt or uncertainty, they should consult with colleagues before testifying to formulate clear and reasonable opinions regarding the degree of certainty to which they are willing to testify. Even when the evidence is almost overwhelming, defense attorneys will attempt to prove that injuries resulted from diseases or accidents rather than abuse, and physicians must be prepared to defend their diagnoses. Although physicians should never present opinions that are not justified by the data, they should not exercise excessive caution when a child has characteristic patterns of abusive injury and abuse is the only reasonable explanation.

---

*Brodeur A, personal communication, July, 1988.

†Chadwick DL, personal communication, October 1994 and March 1995.

ACKNOWLEDGMENT

I wish to thank David L. Chadwick, M.D., for his review and comments on this chapter, and Mel Senac, M.D., for providing selected radiographs.

References

1. Akbarnia BA, Akbarnia NO. The role of orthopaedist in child abuse and neglect. Orthop Clin North Am 1976;7:773.

2. Akbarnia BA, Silberstein MJ, Rende RJ, et al. Arthrography in the diagnosis of fractures of the distal end of the humerus in infants. J Bone Joint Surg [Am] 1986;68:599.

3. Akbarnia BA, Torg JS, Kirkpatrick J, et al. Manifestations of the battered-child syndrome. J Bone Joint Surg [Am] 1974;56:1159.

4. Altman DH, Smith RL. Unrecognized trauma in infants and children. J Bone Joint Surg [Am] 1960;42:407.

5. American Academy of Pediatrics, Committee on Medical Liability. Guidelines for expert witness testimony. Pediatrics 1989; 83:312.

6. Anderson WA. The significance of femoral fractures in children. Ann Emerg Med 1982;11:174.

7. Anh NT. "Pseudo-battered child" syndrome. JAMA 1976; 236:2288.

8. Barlow B, Niemirska M, Gandhi RP, et al. Ten years of experience with falls from a height in children. J Pediatr Surg 1983;18:509.

9. Bays J. Conditions mistaken for child abuse. In: Reece RM, ed. Child abuse: medical diagnosis and management. Malvern, PA: Lea & Febiger, 1994:358.

10. Beals RK, Tufts E. Fractured femur in infancy: the role of child abuse. J Pediatr Orthop 1983;3:583.

11. Bittner S, Newberger EH. Pediatric understanding of child abuse and neglect. Pediatr Rev 1981;2:197.

12. Bourne R. Child abuse and the law. In: Kleinman PK, ed. Diagnostic imaging of child abuse. Baltimore: Williams & Wilkins, 1987.

13. Brent RL. The irresponsible expert witness: a failure of biomedical graduate education and professional accountability. Pediatrics 1982;70:754.

14. Brill PW, Winchester P. Differential diagnosis of child abuse. In: Kleinman PK, ed. Diagnostic imaging of child abuse. Baltimore: Williams & Wilkins, 1987.

15. Caffey J. The whiplash shaken infant syndrome: manual shaking by the extremities with whiplash-induced intracranial and intraocular bleedings, linked with residual permanent brain damage and mental retardation. Pediatrics 1974;54:396.

16. Caffey J. Multiple fractures in the long bones of infants suffering from chronic subdural hematoma. AJR 1946;56:163.

17. Chadwick DL. Preparation for court testimony in child abuse cases. Pediatr Clin North Am 1990;37:955.

18. Chadwick DL. The diagnosis of inflicted injury in infants and young children. (Review) Pediatr Ann 1992;21:477.

19. Cullen JC. Spinal lesions in battered babies. J Bone Joint Surg 1975;57:364.

20. Cumming WA. Neonatal skeletal fractures. Birth trauma or child abuse? J Can Assoc Radiol 1979;30:30.

21. Dalton HJ, Slovis T, Helfer RE, et al. Undiagnosed abuse in children younger than 3 years with femoral fracture. Am J Dis Child 1990;144:875.

22. DeLee JC, Wilkins KE, Rogers LF, Rockwood CA. Fracture separation of the distal humeral epiphysis. J Bone Joint Surg [Am] 1980;62:46.

23. Dent JA, Paterson CR. Fractures in early childhood: osteogenesis imperfecta or child abuse? J Pediatr Orthop 1991; 11:184.

24. Gabriel KR, Akbarnia BA. Complications of child abuse. In: Epps C, Bowen J, eds. Complications in pediatric orthopaedic surgery. Philadelphia: JB Lippincott, 1995.

25. Galleno H, Oppenheim WL. The battered-child syndrome revisited. Clin Orthop 1982;162:11.

26. Gross RH. Child abuse: are you recognizing it when you see it? Contemp Orthop 1980;2:676.

27. Hasse GM, Ortiz VN, Sfakianakis GN, Morse TS. The value of radionuclide bone scanning in the early recognition of deliberate child abuse. Trauma 1980;20:873.

28. Helfer RE, Kempe CH, eds. The battered child. Chicago: University of Chicago Press, 1968.

29. Helfer RE, Slovis TL, Black M. Injuries resulting when small children fall out of bed. Pediatrics 1977;60:533.

30. Herndon WA. Child abuse in a military population. J Pediatr Orthop 1983;3:73.

31. Holter JC, Friedman SB. Child abuse. Early case finding in the emergency department. Pediatrics 1968;42:128.

32. Kempe CH, Silverman FN, Steele BF, et al. The battered child syndrome. JAMA 1962;181:17.

33. King J, Diefendor FD, Apthrop J, et al. Analysis of 429 fractures in 189 battered children. J Pediatr Orthop 1988;8:585.

34. Kleinman PK. Diagnostic imaging of child abuse. Baltimore: Williams & Wilkins, 1987.

35. Kleinman PK, Marks SC, Blackbourne B. The metaphyseal lesion in abused infants: a radiologic-histopathologic study. AJR 1986;146:895.

36. Kleinman PK, Marks SC Jr, Spevak MR, et al. Extension of growth-plate cartilage into the metaphysis: a sign of healing fracture in abused infants. AJR 1991;156:775.

37. Kleinman PK, Marks SC, Spevak MR, Richmond JM. Fractures of the rib head in abused infants. Radiology 1992;185:119.

38. Kowal-Vern A, Paxton TP, Ros SF, et al. Fractures in the under-3-year-old cohort. Clin Pediatr (Phila) 1992;31:653.

39. Kravitz H, Driessen G, Gomberg R, et al. Accidental falls from elevated surfaces in infants from birth to 1 year of age. Pediatrics 1969;44(Suppl):869.

40. Leonidas JC. Skeletal trauma in the child abuse syndrome. Pediatr Ann 1983;12:875.

41. Levinthal JM, Thomas SA, Rosenfield NS, Markowitz RL. Fractures in young children. Distinguishing child abuse from unintentional injuries. Am J Dis Child 1993;147:87.

42. Loder RT, Bookout C. Fracture patterns in battered children. J Orthop Trauma 1991;5:428.

43. McClelland CO, Heiple KG. Fractures in the first year of life. A diagnostic dilemma? Am J Dis Child 1982;136:26.

44. Mellick LB, Reesor K. Spiral tibial fractures of children: a commonly accidental spiral long bone fracture. Am J Emerg Med 1990;8:234.

45. Merten DF, Radkowski MA, Leonidas JC. The abused child, a radiological reappraisal. Radiology 1983;146:377.

46. Myers JEB. Medicolegal aspects of child abuse. In: Kleinman PK, ed. Diagnostic imaging of child abuse. Baltimore: Williams & Wilkins, 1987.

47. National Center on Child Abuse and Neglect: National Child Abuse and Neglect Data System: working paper 2-1991. Summary data component. Washington DC: Government Printing Office, 1993.

48. Newberger EH. Child abuse. Boston: Little, Brown & Company, 1982.

49. Nimityongskul P, Anderson L. The likelihood of injuries when children fall out of bed. J Pediatr Orthop 1987;7:184.

50. O'Connor JF, Cohen J. Dating fractures. In: Kleinman PK, ed. Diagnostic imaging of child abuse. Baltimore: Williams & Wilkins, 1987.

51. O'Neill JA Jr, Meacham WF, Griffin PP, Sawyers JL. Patterns of injury in the battered child syndrome. J Trauma 1973;13:332.

52. Silverman FN. The roentgen manifestations of unrecognized skeletal trauma in infants. AJR 1953;69:413.

53. Smith MD, Burrington JD, Woolf AD. Injuries in children sustained in free falls: an analysis of 66 cases. J Trauma 1975;15:987.

54. Straus MA, Gelles RJ, Steinmetz SK. Behind closed doors: violence in the American family. New York: Anchor Press, 1980:369.

55. Sty JR, Starsha RJ. The role of scintigraphy in the evaluation of the suspected abused child. Radiology 1983;146.

56. Swischuk LE. Spine and spinal cord trauma in the battered-child syndrome. Radiology 1969;92:733.

57. Tenenbein M, Reed MH, Black GB. The toddler's fracture revisited. Am J Emerg Med 1990;8:208.

58. Thomas SA, Rosenfield NS, Leventhal JM, Markowitz RI. Long-bone fractures in young children: distinguishing accidental injuries from child abuse. Pediatrics 1991;88:471.

59. United States Senate. Hearing before the Subcommittee on Children and Youth of the Committee on Labor and Public Welfare. United States Senate, 93rd Congress, First Session, On S.1191, Child Abuse Prevention Act. Washington DC: Government Printing Office, 1973.

60. Wilson EF. Estimation of the age of cutaneous contusions in child abuse. Pediatrics 1977;60:750.

APPENDIX 32-1   *Guidelines for Expert Witnesses*

---

1. The physician should have current experience and on-going knowledge about the areas of clinical medicine in which he or she is testifying and familiarity with practices during the time and place of the episode being considered as well as the circumstances surrounding the occurrence.

2. The physician's review of medical facts should be thorough, fair, and impartial and should not exclude any relevant information to create a view favoring either the plaintiff or the defendant. The ultimate test for accuracy and impartiality is a willingness to prepare testimony that could be presented unchanged for use by either the plaintiff or the defendant.

3. The physician's testimony should reflect an evaluation of performance in light of generally accepted standards, neither condemning performance that clearly falls within generally accepted practice standards nor endorsing or condoning performance that clearly falls outside accepted practice standards.

4. The physician should make a clear distinction between medical malpractice and medical maloccurrence when analyzing any case. The practice of medicine remains a mixture of art and science; the scientific component is a dynamic and changing one based to a large extent on concepts of probability rather than absolute certainty.

5. The physician should make every effort to assess the relationship of the alleged substandard practice to the patient's outcome, because deviation from a practice standard is not always causally related to a less-than-ideal outcome.

6. The physician should be willing to submit transcripts of depositions and/or courtroom testimony for peer review.

7. The physician expert should cooperate with any reasonable efforts undertaken by the courts or by the plaintiffs' or defendants' carriers and attorneys to provide a better understanding of the expert witness issue.

These principles have been adopted as guidelines by the American Academy of Pediatrics for its members who assume the role of expert witness.

From American Academy of Pediatrics, Committee on Medical Liability. Guidelines for expert witness testimony. Pediatrics 1989; 83:312.

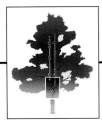

Index

Page numbers followed by f *indicate illustrations; those followed by* t *indicate tabular materials.*